We need your help...

Thank you for your interest in The PDR® Family Guide to Women's Health and Prescription Drugs™. We sincerely hope that this first edition meets your needs; and we want to make sure that future editions are even better. To help us improve the book, your advice is crucial; so please take a moment to tell us what features you'd like to see added or revised. By completing and returning this brief questionnaire, you will be registering to receive product information on a new drug. We will do our best to implement your suggestions.

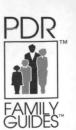

PDR™
FAMILY GUIDES™

1. Why did you purchase this book?
_____
_____
_____
_____

2. What do you LIKE most about this book?
_____
_____
_____
_____

3. What do you DISLIKE most about this book?
_____
_____
_____

4. What would you like added to the book?
_____
_____
_____
_____

5. We are considering publishing other books. What subjects are of most interest to you?
_____
_____
_____

6. Are you interested in an update that will include new drugs? ☐ Yes ☐ No

7. How did you hear about this book?
☐ friend　☐ pharmacist　☐ saw in store
☐ relative　☐ advertising　☐ other
☐ doctor　☐ mailer _____

8. What other healthcare and drug reference books do you own?
_____
_____
_____

And just a few more questions.

9. Please check: ☐ Male ☐ Female

10. How many medications do you take daily?
1　2　3　4　5　6　7　8　9　10 or more

11. In which of these age groups do you fall?

☐ 19 and under　☐ 50-59
☐ 20-29　☐ 60-69
☐ 30-39　☐ 70 and over
☐ 40-49

12. Which of the following best describes your formal education level?

☐ Some high school　☐ Some college
☐ High school　☐ College
　　　　　　　　☐ Graduate school or more

13. Which of the following best describes your family's income?

☐ less than $19,999　☐ $50,000-$59,999
☐ $20,000-$29,999　☐ $60,000-$69,999
☐ $30,000-$39,999　☐ $70,000-$79,999
☐ $40,000-$49,999　☐ over $80,000

Name _____

Address _____

City _____ **State** _____ **Zip** _____

Phone _____

Thank you,

MEDICAL ECONOMICS
Five Paragon Drive
Montvale, New Jersey 07645-1742

WH951

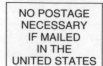
PLEASE FOLD HERE

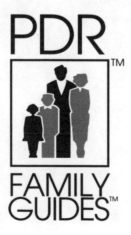

PLEASE TAPE; DO NOT STAPLE

Reaction to
The PDR Family Guide
to Women's Health
and Prescription Drugs

"Factual, yet written in a style that is easily read and understood by those without medical training.... Informative, interesting, and current, the book covers the full range of key issues that concern women today. A must-read for women throughout the country, particularly now that consumers of healthcare want far more information before making an informed choice."

Allan Rosenfield, MD
DeLamar Professor and Dean
Columbia University School of Public Health

"Well-written, concise, and easily understandable....Full of information that is useful on a day-to-day basis."

Charles Kawada, MD
Professor of Obstetrics and Gynecology
Tufts University

"A wonderful table of contents.... The text is clear, to-the-point, and helpful."

Jacob Klein, MD
St. Louis, MO

"This book provides the reader with the tools necessary to preserve her health and become an active participant in her own healthcare. Armed with this information, a woman has the best chance of making the 'right' decisions."

Mace L. Rothenberg, MD, FACP
Assistant Professor of Medicine
The University of Texas Health Science Center at
San Antonio

"An excellent supplement to the education that should occur during every healthcare visit. The Guide allows people to find answers when and where they need them–any time of the day or night in their own home."

Barbara P. Yawn, MD, MS
Associate Professor of Clinical Family Medicine
and Community Health
University of Minnesota

Other Books and Services from Medical Economics

The PDR® Family Guide to Prescription Drugs®

For up-to-the-minute information on the whole family's medications, turn to this first volume in The PDR® Family Guide series. Presents vital facts on all the nation's leading prescription drugs in the same convenient, easy-to-read format. Covers leading pediatric medicines, allergy remedies, pain medications, anticonvulsants, blood pressure medications, heart medicines, skin products, and more. Gives drug interactions, side effects, precautions, and standard doses. Includes hundreds of actual-size, full-color drug photographs, more than 20 chapters on problems ranging from childhood infections to the chronic conditions of later years. Fully illustrated, with over 900 pages. List price: $24.95. To order, call toll-free 1-800-331-0072.

Professional References

Physicians' Desk Reference®
PDR For Nonprescription Drugs®
PDR For Ophthalmology®
PDR Guide to Drug
   Interactions•Side Effects•Indications™
PDR® Drug I.D. System
Pocket PDR™
   (Handheld Electronic Database)
PDR Library on CD-ROM™
PDR Drug Interactions/Side Effects/Indications
   Diskettes™

Medical Device Register™
MDR™ International Edition
Breast Implant Problem Reports™
Directory of Healthcare Group
   Purchasing Organizations™
Directory of Hospital Personnel™
Directory of U.S. Nursing Homes
   and Nursing Home Chains™
HMO/PPO Directory™
Product Development Directory™

Product SOS™ (FDA Problem Reports)
Surgeons' Desk Reference for
   Minimally Invasive Surgery Products™

Red Book®
MicREData
The Red Book® Database

Professional Newsletters

AIDS Alert™
Common Sense About AIDS™
Contraceptive Technology Update™
Emergency Medicine Reports™
Employee Health & Fitness™
Hospital Infection Control™
Hospital Peer Review®
Hospital Risk Management™
Internal Medicine Alert®
Medical Ethics Advisor™
Physician's Managed Care Report™
The Idea Letter for Health Care Managers™
Same-Day Surgery®

THE PDR® FAMILY GUIDE TO

WOMEN'S HEALTH

PDR
FAMILY
GUIDES™

AND PRESCRIPTION DRUGS™

MEDICAL ECONOMICS   **MONTVALE, NEW JERSEY**

1995

Publisher's Note

The drug information contained in this book is based on product labeling published in the 1994 edition of Physicians' Desk Reference®, supplemented with facts from other sources the publisher believes reliable. While diligent efforts have been made to assure the accuracy of this information, the book does not list every possible action, adverse reaction, interaction, and precaution; and all information is presented without guarantees by the authors, consultants, and publisher, who disclaim all liability in connection with its use.

This book is intended only as a reference for use in an ongoing partnership between doctor and patient in the vigilant management of the patient's health. It is not a substitute for a doctor's professional judgment, and serves only as a reminder of concerns that may need discussion. All readers are urged to consult with a physician before beginning or discontinuing use of any prescription drug or undertaking any form of self-treatment.

Brand names listed in this book are intended to represent only the more commonly used products. Inclusion of a brand name does not signify endorsement of the product, absence of a name does not imply a criticism or rejection of the product. The publisher is not advocating the use of any product described in this book, does not warrant or guarantee any of these products, and has not performed any independent analysis in connection with the product information contained herein.

Library of Congress Catalog Card Number: 94-76809

ISBN: 1-56363-086-9 (Medical Economics Data).
Manufactured in the United States of America

10 9 8 7 6 5 4 3

Bulk copy inquiries are invited. Contact the Commercial Sales Department at 1-800-442-6657.

PHYSICIANS' DESK REFERENCE, PDR, PDR For Ophthalmology, PDR For Nonprescription Drugs, and PDR Family Guide to Prescription Drugs are trademarks of Medical Economics Data Production Company, registered in the United States Patent and Trademark Office. PDR Family Guides, PDR Family Guide to Women's Health and Prescription Drugs, PDR Guide to Interactions•Side Effects•Indications, PDR Library on CD-ROM, PDR Drug Interactions/Side Effects/Indications Diskettes, and Pocket PDR are trademarks of Medical Economics Data Production Company.

Officers of Medical Economics: President and Chief Executive Officer: Norman R. Snesil; Executive Vice President and Chief Financial Officer: J. Crispin Ashworth; Senior Vice President, Corporate Operations Group: John R. Ware; Senior Vice President, Corporate Business Development Group: Raymond M. Zoeller; Vice President of Information Services and Chief Information Officer: Edward J. Zecchini.

Contents

Part 1: A Woman's Special Health Concerns

Section I: Common Disorders of the Reproductive System

Section II: General Health Concerns

Section III: Fertility and Family Planning

The PDR® Family Guide to Women's Health and Prescription Drugs™

Editor-in-Chief: David W. Sifton
Pharmaceutical Director: Mukesh Mehta, R Ph
Art Director: Robert Hartman

Part 1: A Woman's Special Health Concerns

Assistant Editors: Lynn H. Buechler; Jayne Jacobson; Eileen McCaffrey; Marcia Ringel; Mildred M. Schumacher; Alice Z. Weiss

Writers: Cynthia Davis, MD; Linda Decker, PA; Nancy J. Groves; Kris Hallam; Ami Havens; Randi Henderson; Jayne Jacobson; Judith K. Ludwig; Jeane M. Malone; Virginia M. Mason; Eileen McCaffrey; Sara Altshul O'Donnell; Marie Powers; Arlene Pressman, RNC, MSN; Marcia Ringel; Heidi Rosvold-Brenholtz; Ronni Sandroff; Deborah J. Shuman; David K. Silver; Hillary M. Wright, M Ed, RD; Ken Zerserson

Illustrations: Christopher Wikoff, MAMS; Cover Photography, Susan Wood

Special Consultant: Jeremy Sugarman, MD, Assistant Professor of Medicine, Duke University, Durham, NC

Part 2: A Woman's Handbook of Medicines

Assistant Editors: Ann Ben Larbi; Beret R. Erway

Writers: Lynn H. Buechler; Jayne Jacobson; Barbara Klink; Theresa Waldron

Pharmaceutical Consultants: Paula R. Ajmera, MS, R Ph; Marion Gray, R Ph; Nancy Jacoby, R Ph

Editorial Production: Marjorie Duffy, Director of Production; Carrie Williams; Assistant Director of Production; Vicki Leal, Production Manager; Gregory Thomas, Product Integration Manager; Beret R. Erway, Production Editor; Lisa Best, Production Assistant; Joanne McCloskey, Electronic Publishing Coordinator; Shawn Cahill, Digital Imaging Coordinator; Kimberly Hiller-Vivas, Electronic Publishing Production Manager; Richard Weinstock, Electronic Publishing Design

Business Staff

Product Manager: Karen B. Sperber

Paul Walsh, Product Support Manager; Robin Bartlett, Commercial Sales Manager; Bill Gaffney, Commercial Sales Account Executive; Michele Barth, Marketing Communications Manager; Laurie Roth, Marketing Communications Coordinator; Roni LaVine, Robert Loeser, Fulfillment Managers; Raul Collado, Database and Systems Development Manager; Martina Murtagh, Administrative Assistant

Foreword

This is a book of solutions—a tool for keeping your health at its peak. It tells you why problems develop, how best to prevent them, and what you and your doctor can do to make them right. Whatever difficulty you face, you'll be amazed at the number of options modern medicine now can offer. Indeed, they are often too numerous, too complex, or too controversial to deal with in a few hurried sessions at the doctor's office. What you need is time to reflect, gain perspective, and sort out the questions you really have to address. This book is designed to help you do that.

It is not a substitute for a physician's advice. After all, only your doctor can judge all the factors that bear on your unique personal situation. But the information you'll find here should give you a good idea of what to expect—how the doctor is most likely to proceed, what information he or she will need from you, the questions you should be asking in turn, and what outcome you can reasonably look forward to.

More often than not, you'll find these facts to be a source of reassurance. However, if they do signal the need for additional discussion with your doctor, that's all for the best. Nobody is going to spend more time thinking about your case than you; and if you find that some factor has been overlooked or feel that some treatment option has been ignored, you need to bring it to the doctor's attention. Good medicine is a partnership: The doctor provides the technical expertise; you provide the knowledge of your body and its reactions. For a treatment to succeed, both you and your doctor must keep the other fully informed.

Unlike most other health guides, this one provides you with complete information on all the medications your doctor is most likely to prescribe, for when it comes to prescription drugs, medicine is an especially collaborative effort. Your doctor can tell you how and when to take a medication, but only you can judge the drug's effects, alerting the doctor to a serious reaction or drug interaction.

The drug profiles in the second part of this book are designed to help you with this effort. They also serve as a reminder of the basic instructions and warnings that all too often are forgotten as soon as you leave the doctor's office. As an extra measure of safety, each profile also highlights the special conditions that might call for a review of your prescription—facts your doctor needs to know in order to assure you the safest, most effective treatment possible.

The information in these drug profiles are drawn from Physicians' Desk Reference® (PDR®), a handbook that has provided doctors with official, FDA-approved prescribing guidelines for almost 50 years. To make these facts—and all the other information in this book—as useful as possible, the editors stripped away the technical shorthand in which medical recommendations are usually cloaked, and attempted to present them in terms any alert consumer can easily understand. To supplement this information,

they've drawn on other sources such as the publisher's Computerized Clinical Information System, used in hospitals throughout the nation. Generally, this additional information describes new uses for an older drug or supplies instructions meant specifically for the patient, such as how to make up a missed dose.

The editors endeavored in this book to include essential information on all the unique physical problems that confront a woman, from fertility and family planning to the disruptive effects of menopause and the many other gynecological problems that trouble women of all ages. Their goal has been to give you all the relevant medical facts. If there's anything they've missed, please let them know about it. You can reach them toll-free at 1-800-331-0072, or write to them at PDR Family Guide, Five Paragon Drive, Montvale, NJ 07645.

The best of health to you.

Penny Wise Budoff, MD
Penny Wise Budoff, MD, Women's Health
  Services, Bethpage, NY
Affiliated with
  North Shore University Hospital

How to Use this Book

Coming to grips with a health problem is always an emotional challenge, filled with uncertainty and dread. To allay unnecessary fears, you need a source you can turn to for immediate answers whenever a problem surfaces. That's what this book is here to do.

In most cases, you'll find the facts surprisingly reassuring. Today medicine offers remedies for all but the gravest of illnesses. And for even the most serious problems, you can at least learn what to expect and how the various treatment options compare. You'll also find out the best ways to prevent a recurrence, and the measures you can take to avoid, delay, or short-circuit development of disorders ranging from osteoporosis to cancer.

This book is not a substitute for a doctor's advice. Only a doctor can weigh all the diverse aspects of your condition and choose the treatment most likely to meet your needs.

What we hope this book can do, however, is help you sort out the facts and questions that deserve further discussion. Your doctor, after all, can respond only to the problems and concerns you mention. And a seemingly unimportant fact could turn out to be a crucial aspect of your particular case.

The book is divided into two major parts. In the first, you'll find an overview of the diseases and disorders that threaten women the most. The second provides you with detailed information on the medicines your doctor is most likely to prescribe.

Part 1: A Woman's Special Health Concerns

Turn to the chapters here whenever you need the basic facts about a health or reproductive problem. Subjects range from infections, chronic disorders, and cancer to the latest in family planning techniques, current guidelines for a trouble-free pregnancy, and the best ways of fighting emotional disorders. Each chapter outlines typical symptoms, your chances of contracting the problem, available tests and treatments, and what to expect in both the short and long terms.

You can read an entire chapter for a thorough background on a problem or, for a quick answer to a specific question, you can turn to the General Index at the end of the book. Each chapter includes a brief description of the medications you'll probably be given. For more detailed information, however, you should turn to the second part of the book.

Part 2: A Woman's Handbook of Medicines

The profiles in this section are designed to give you detailed information on the medicines that women use most. Among them you'll find drugs used only by women—such as oral contraceptives, fertility drugs, vaginal yeast medications, and hormone replacement products—as well as general medications with a major role in gynecology, such as antibiotics for urinary tract infections and drugs for sexually transmitted diseases. Common antidepressants are included, along with tranquilizers, migraine medications, and remedies for PMS; and you'll find a variety of arthritis medications and anticancer agents. Also included are calcium supplements, prenatal vitamins, appetite suppressants, acne treatments, and many other common drugs.

What you will not find here are medicines for the disorders that strike men and women equally. Included in this category are blood pressure medications, heart medicines, asthma drugs, anticonvulsants, diabetes medications, and many specialized antibiotics.

Information on all of these drugs can be found in this book's companion volume, *The PDR® Family Guide to Prescription Drugs®.*

Most prescription products have two names—a generic chemical name and a manufacturer's brand name. Both are listed alphabetically in this book, with a profile of the drug appearing under the more familiar of the two. In most instances, that means the brand name. In a few cases—such as methotrexate, for example—the generic name heads the profile. In either case, the drug's other name gives you a cross-reference to the profile.

If there is more than one brand of a drug, you'll usually find the profile under the name that's most frequently prescribed. For example, information on amoxicillin can be found in the profile of Amoxil, the nation's leading brand. Other brands of amoxicillin, such as Wymox and Polymox, are cross-referenced to the Amoxil entry.

The drug profiles are divided into 10 sections. Here's what you'll find in each.

■ **Why is this drug prescribed?** This section provides an overview of the major diseases and disorders for which the drug is generally given.

■ **Most important fact about this drug.** Highlighted here is one key point—out of the dozens found in a typical profile—that is especially worthwhile to remember. We've placed it here for the sake of emphasis. Never regard this section as a definitive summary of the drug.

■ **How should you take this medication?** Some drugs should never be taken with meals. Others must be. This section details such special instructions including how and when to take the medication, and any dietary restrictions that may apply. Also found here is advice on what to do when you forget a dose, and any special storage requirements that apply.

■ **What side effects may occur?** Shown here are the potential side effects that the manufacturer has listed in the drug's FDA-approved product labeling. Virtually any drug will occasionally cause an unwanted reaction. However, even the most common of these reactions is generally seen in only a small minority of patients. For that reason, presence of a long list of possible side effects does not mean that the drug is unusually dangerous or trouble-prone. Not listed are the few side effects that can be detected only by a physician or analysis in a laboratory.

■ **Why should this drug not be prescribed?** A few drugs are known to be harmful under certain specific conditions, which are detailed here—the most common being hypersensitivity to the drug itself. If you think one of these restrictions applies to you, you should alert your doctor immediately. If you're correct, he or she may decide to use an alternative treatment.

■ **Special warnings about this medication.** This cautionary information is presented as a double check. If it includes any problems or conditions that your doctor may be unaware of, be sure to bring them to his or her attention. Chances are that no change in treatment will be called for, but it's worth making sure.

■ **Possible food and drug interactions when taking this medication.** In this section you'll find a list of specific drugs—and types of drugs—that have been known to interact with the medicine being profiled. Generally, the list includes a few examples of each type. However, it is far from inclusive. If you're not certain whether a medication you're taking falls into one of these categories, be sure to check with your doctor or pharmacist—and don't stop taking either drug without first consulting your doctor.

■ **Special information if you are pregnant or breastfeeding.** Very few medicines have been definitively proved safe for use during pregnancy. On the other hand, only a handful are known to be inevitably harmful. Most drugs fall in between, in a gray area where no harm has been reported, but neither has safety been conclusively proved. If you are pregnant or planning a pregnancy, and one of your medicines falls into this questionable category, the best thing to do is check with your doctor immediately. He or she can tell you whether your need for the medicine outweighs any possible risk.

■ **Recommended dosage.** Shown here are excerpts of the dosage guidelines your doctor uses. They generally present a range of doses recommended for typical cases, and sometimes include a recommended maximum. The information is presented as a convenient double check in case you suspect a misunderstanding or a typographical error on your prescription label. It is not useful for determining an exact dosage yourself.

■ **Overdosage.** As another safety measure, this section lists, when available, the signs of an overdose. Treatment is usually quite complex, and requires specialized medical training, so we have not attempted to summarize it here. If the symptoms listed in this section lead you to suspect an overdose, your best response is to seek emergency medical attention immediately.

Special Features

For easy reference, we've included a number of special sections that focus on specific problems and questions. You'll find most at the end of the book. The first, a color photo section, appears immediately after this overview.

■ **Drug Identification Guide.** It's wise to keep all your prescription medications in their original bottles or vials. However, if they do somehow get mixed up, you may find this section helpful for sorting them out. It includes actual-size photographs of the leading products discussed in the book. Because some of the more common generic alternatives are shown along with the brand-name drugs, the section is arranged by each drug's generic name.

Manufacturers occasionally change the color and shape of a product, so if a prescription does not match the photo shown here, do check with your pharmacist, and don't automatically assume there's been a mistake.

■ **Drug Risks in Pregnancy.** This quick-reference table, which appears immediately following the drug profiles, gives you official FDA use-in-pregnancy guidelines for all leading prescription drugs.

■ **Directory of Support Groups.** This problem-oriented directory lists numbers to call for help, information, referrals, and support when faced with challenges ranging from chronic fatigue syndrome to recovery from rape.

■ **Common Words in Women's Health.** This abbreviated medical dictionary gives plain-English definitions of the words you're most likely to hear in your gynecologist's office.

■ **Safe Medication Use.** Check this brief set of guidelines to make sure that you're telling your doctor and pharmacists all that you should, and that you're using and storing all of your medications as safely and effectively as possible.

■ **Disease and Disorder Index.** To quickly identify drugs available for a particular problem, you can turn to this special index. Arranged alphabetically by ailment, it lists all the alternatives profiled in the book.

■ **General Index.** Turn to this index whenever you need to track down the facts on a specific symptom, syndrome, procedure, or product.

The Doctor-Patient Partnership

Although doctors today can often work miracles with advanced technology and sophisticated medicines, they still need help from you to make most treatments work. No matter how potent the medication, it can still prove worthless if you fail to take it properly. Likewise, if you react badly to a drug, or have a condition that makes it dangerous, there is nothing any doctor can do about it unless you report the problem. Ultimately, it is you who must take charge of your case.

This book is offered as an aid in this cooperative effort with your doctor. We hope its suggests the right questions to ask, while allaying any unwarranted concerns you might have. Most of all, we hope it helps in some small way to make all of your treatments as effective as can be.

Drug Identification Guide

ACETAMINOPHEN/ CODEINE PHOSPHATE

LENOL® W/CODEINE NO.1
MCNEIL PHARMACEUTICAL

300 MG / 7.5 MG

LENOL® W/CODEINE NO.2
MCNEIL PHARMACEUTICAL

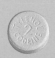

300 MG / 15 MG

LENOL® W/CODEINE NO.3
MCNEIL PHARMACEUTICAL

300 MG / 30 MG

LENOL® W/CODEINE NO.4
MCNEIL PHARMACEUTICAL

300 MG / 60 MG

ACYCLOVIR

ZOVIRAX
BURROUGHS WELLCOME

200 MG

400 MG

800 MG

ALPRAZOLAM

XANAX
UPJOHN COMPANY

0.25 MG   0.5 MG

1 MG

2 MG

AMITRIPTYLINE HCL

ELAVIL
STUART PHARMACEUTICALS

10 MG   25 MG

50 MG   75 MG

100 MG

150 MG

ENDEP
ROCHE LABORATORIES

10 MG   25 MG

50 MG   75 MG

100 MG   150 MG

AMOXAPINE

ASENDIN
LEDERLE LABORATORIES

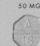

25 MG   50 MG

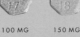

100 MG   150 MG

AMOXICILLIN

AMOXIL
SMITHKLINE BEECHAM

250 MG

500 MG

125 MG CHEWABLE TABLET

250 MG CHEWABLE TABLET

WYMOX
WYETH-AYERST

250 MG

500 MG

TRIMOX
APOTHECON

250 MG

500 MG

AMOXICILLIN/ CLAVULANATE POTASSIUM

AUGMENTIN
SMITHKLINE BEECHAM

125 MG / 31.25 MG CHEWABLE TABLET

250 MG / 62.5 MG CHEWABLE TABLET

250 MG / 125 MG

500 MG / 125 MG

AMPICILLIN

OMNIPEN
WYETH-AYERST

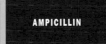

250 MG

500 MG

POLYCILLIN
APOTHECON

250 MG

500 MG

PRINCIPEN
APOTHECON

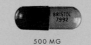

250 MG

500 MG

ASPIRIN

ECOTRIN
SMITHKLINE BEECHAM

325 MG

500 MG

500 MG

EMPIRIN®
BURROUGHS WELLCOME

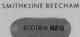

325 MG

ASPIRIN/ CODEINE PHOSPHATE

EMPIRIN® W/ CODEINE NO. 2
BURROUGHS WELLCOME

325 MG / 15 MG

EMPIRIN® /W CODEINE NO.3
BURROUGHS WELLCOME

325 MG / 30 MG

EMPIRIN® /W CODEINE NO.4
BURROUGHS WELLCOME

325 MG / 60 MG

GENERIC
GENEVA

325 MG / 30 MG

GENERIC
GENEVA

325 MG / 60 MG

GENERIC
GOLDLINE

325 MG / 60 MG

GENERIC
UNITED RESEARCH

325 MG / 15 MG

325 MG / 30 MG

325 MG / 60 MG

GENERIC
ZENITH

325 MG / 30 MG

ATROPINE SULFATE/ HYOSCYAMINE/ METHENAMINE/ METHYLENE BLUE

URISED
POLYMEDICA

0.03 MG / 0.03 MG / 40.8 MG / 5.4 MG

AZITHROMYCIN

ZITHROMAX
PFIZER LABS

250 MG

BROMOCRIPTINE MESYLATE

PARLODEL
SANDOZ PHARMACEUTICALS

2.5 MG   5 MG

BUPROPION HCL

WELLBUTRIN
BURROUGHS WELLCOME

75 MG   100 MG

BUSPIRONE HCL

BUSPAR
BRISTOL-MYERS SQUIBB

5 MG   10 MG

BUTALBITAL/ ACETAMINOPHEN/ CAFFEINE

ESGIC
FOREST PHARMACEUTICALS

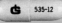

50 MG / 325 MG / 40 MG

50 MG / 325 MG / 40 MG

ESGIC-PLUS
FOREST PHARMACEUTICALS

50 MG / 500 MG / 40 MG

FIORICET
SANDOZ PHARMACEUTICALS

50 MG / 325 MG / 40 MG

BUTALBITAL/ ACETAMINOPHEN/ CAFFEINE/ CODEINE PHOSPHATE

FIORICET® WITH CODEINE
SANDOZ PHARMACEUTICALS

50 MG / 325 MG / 40 MG / 30 MG

BUTALBITAL/ ASPIRIN/ CAFFEINE/

FIORINAL
SANDOZ PHARMACEUTICALS

50 MG / 325 MG / 40 MG

50 MG / 325 MG / 40 MG

ISOLLYL
RUGBY

50 MG / 325 MG / 40 MG

BUTALBITAL/ ASPIRIN/ CAFFEINE/ CODEINE

FIORINAL® W/CODEINE
SANDOZ PHARMACEUTICALS

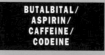

50 MG / 325 MG / 40 MG / 30 MG

CALCIUM

CALTRATE® 600
LEDERLE CONSUMER

600 MG

CALTRATE® 600 + VITAMIN D
LEDERLE CONSUMER

600 MG / 125 IU

CALTRATE® 600 + IRON + VITAMIN D
LEDERLE CONSUMER

600 MG / 18 MG / 125 IU

OS-CAL® 500
SMITHKLINE BEECHAM

500 MG

OS-CAL® 500+D
SMITHKLINE BEECHAM

500 MG / 125 IU

OS-CAL® 500
SMITHKLINE BEECHAM

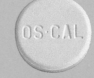

500 MG CHEWABLE TABLET

CEFACLOR

CECLOR
ELI LILLY & COMPANY

250 MG

500 MG

CEFIXIME

SUPRAX
LEDERLE LABORATORIES

200 MG

400 MG

CEFUROXIME AXETIL

CEFTIN
ALLEN & HANBURYS

125 MG

250 MG

500 MG

CEPHALEXIN

KEFLEX
DISTA PRODUCTS

250 MG

KEFLEX
DISTA PRODUCTS

500 MG

CEPHALEXIN HCL

KEFTAB
DISTA PRODUCTS

250 MG

500 MG

CEPHRADINE

VELOSEF
APOTHECON

250 MG

500 MG

CHLORDIAZEPOXIDE

LIBRITABS
ROCHE LABORATORIES

5 MG   10 MG

25 MG

CHLORDIAZEPOXIDE/
AMITRIPTYLINE HCL

LIMBITROL
ROCHE LABORATORIES

5 MG / 12.5 MG

LIMBITROL® DS
ROCHE LABORATORIES

10 MG / 25 MG

CHLORDIAZEPOXIDE
HCL

LIBRIUM
ROCHE LABORATORIES

5 MG

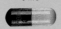

10 MG

25 MG

CHOLINE MAGNESIUM
TRISALICYLATE

TRILISATE
PURDUE FREDERICK

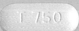

500 MG

750 MG

1000 MG

CIPROFLOXACIN HCL

CIPRO™
MILES INC.

250 MG

500 MG

750 MG

CLOMIPHENE CITRATE

CLOMID
MARION MERRELL DOW

50 MG

CLORAZEPATE
DIPOTASSIUM

TRANXENE® T-TAB®
ABBOTT LABORATORIES

15 MG   3.75 MG

7.5 MG

TRANXENE® · SD™
HALF STRENGTH
ABBOTT LABORATORIES

11.25 MG

TRANXENE® · SD™
ABBOTT LABORATORIES

22.5 MG

CONJUGATED
ESTROGENS

PREMARIN
WYETH-AYERST

0.3 MG   0.625 MG

0.9 MG

1.25 MG

2.5 MG

CONJUGATED
ESTROGENS/
METHYLTESTOSTERONE

PREMARIN® WITH
METHYLTESTOSTERONE
WYETH-AYERST

0.625 MG / 5.0 MG

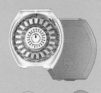

1.25 MG / 10.0 MG

CONTRACEPTIVES/
ORAL

ORTHO-NOVUM 10/11
21 DAY REGIMEN
ORTHO

ORTHO-NOVUM 7/7/7
21 DAY REGIMEN
ORTHO

ORTHO-NOVUM 1/35
21- DAY REGIMEN
ORTHO

ORTHO-NOVUM 1/50
21 DAY REGIMEN
ORTHO

TRIPHASIL®-21
WYETH-AYERST

TRIPHASIL®-28
WYETH-AYERST

CYCLOPHOSPHAMIDE

CYTOXAN
BRISTOL-MYERS ONCOLOGY

25 MG

50 MG

DESIPRAMINE HCL

NORPRAMIN
MARION MERRELL DOW

10 MG   25 MG

50 MG   75 MG

 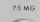

100 MG   150 MG

DIAZEPAM

VALIUM
ROCHE LABORATORIES

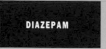

2 MG   5 MG

10 MG

DICLOFENAC SODIUM

VOLTAREN
GEIGY PHARMACEUTICALS

25 MG   50 MG

75 MG

DIETHYLPROPION HCL

TENUATE
MARION MERRELL DOW

25 MG

TENUATE® DOSPAN
MARION MERRELL DOW

75 MG

DIFLUNISAL

DOLOBID
MERCK

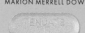

250 MG

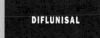

500 MG

DOCUSATE SODIUM

COLACE
ROBERTS

50 MG   100 MG

DOXEPIN HYDROCHLORIDE

SINEQUAN
ROERIG

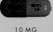

10 MG

25 MG

50 MG

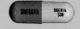

75 MG

100 MG

150 MG

DOXYCYCLINE HYCLATE

DORYX
PARKE-DAVIS

100 MG

VIBRA-TABS
PFIZER LABS

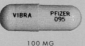

100 MG

VIBRAMYCIN® HYCLATE
PFIZER LABS

100 MG

ERGOLOID MESYLATES

HYDERGINE
SANDOZ

0.5 MG   1 MG

1 MG

HYDERGINE® LC
SANDOZ

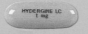

1 MG

ERGOTAMINE TARTRATE/ CAFFEINE

CAFERGOT
SANDOZ

1 MG / 100 MG

ERYTHROMYCIN

ERY-TAB
ABBOTT LABORATORIES

250 MG

333 MG

500 MG

ERYTHROMYCIN
ABBOTT LABORATORIES

250 MG

ERYTHROMYCIN FILMTABS
ABBOTT LABORATORIES

250 MG

500 MG

ERYTHROMYCIN STEARATE

ERYTHROCIN® STEARATE FILMTAB®
ABBOTT LABORATORIES

250 MG

500 MG

ESTRADIOL

ESTRACE
BRISTOL-MYERS SQUIBB

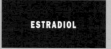

0.5 MG   1 MG

2 MG

ESTROPIPATE

OGEN
ABBOTT LABORATORIES

0.625 MG

1.25 MG

2.5 MG

ORTHO-EST® 1.25
ORTHO

1.5 MG

ETODOLAC

LODINE
WYETH-AYERST

200 MG

300 MG

400 MG

FENOPROFEN CALCIUM

NALFON
DISTA PRODUCTS

600 MG

FLAVOXATE HCL

URISPAS
SMITHKLINE BEECHAM

100 MG

FLUCONAZOLE

DIFLUCAN
ROERIG

50 MG   100 MG

200 MG

FLUOXETINE HCL

PROZAC®
DISTA PRODUCTS

10 MG

20 MG

FLUOXYMESTERONE

HALOTESTIN
UPJOHN COMPANY

2 MG   5 MG

10 MG

FLURBIPROFEN

ANSAID
UPJOHN COMPANY

50 MG

100 MG

FOLIC ACID/ MULTIVITAMINS/ MULTIMINERALS

STUARTNATAL® 1+1
WYETH-AYERST

1 MG

FUROSEMIDE

LASIX
HOECHST-ROUSSEL

20 MG   40 MG

80 MG

HYDROCHLORATHIAZIDE

ESIDRIX
CIBA

25 MG   50 MG

100 MG

HYDRODIURIL
MERCK

25 MG   50 MG

100 MG

IBUPROFEN

BAYER® SELECT™ PAIN RELIEF FORMULA
STERLING HEALTH

200 MG

MIDOL IB
STERLING HEALTH

200 MG

MOTRIN
UPJOHN COMPANY

300 MG

400 MG

600 MG

800 MG

IMIPRAMINE HYDROCHLORIDE

TOFRANIL
GEIGY PHARMACEUTICALS

10 MG   25 MG

50 MG

IMIPRAMINE PAMOATE

TOFRANIL-PM
GEIGY PHARMACEUTICALS

75 MG

100 MG

125 MG

150 MG

INDOMETHACIN

INDOCIN
MERCK

25 MG

50 MG

INDOCIN®-SR
MERCK

75 MG

ISOMETHEPTENE MUCATE/ DICHLORALPHENAZONE/ ACETAMINOPHEN

MIDRIN
CARNRICK

65 MG / 100 MG / 325 MG

ISOSORBIDE DINITRATE

ISORDIL
WYETH-AYERST

5 MG   10 MG

20 MG   30 MG

40 MG

ISOTRETINOIN

ACCUTANE
ROCHE LABORATORIES

10 MG   20 MG

40 MG

KETOCONAZOLE

NIZORAL
JANSSEN PHARMACEUTICA

200 MG

KETOPROFEN

ORUDIS
WYETH-AYERST

25 MG

50 MG

75 MG

ORUVAIL
WYETH-AYERST

200 MG

LEVOTHYROXINE SODIUM

LEVOTHROID
FOREST PHARMACEUTICALS

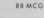

25 MCG   50 MCG

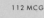

75 MCG   88 MCG

100 MCG   112 MCG

125 MCG   137 MCG

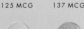

150 MCG   175 MCG

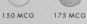 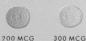

200 MCG   300 MCG

LEVOXINE
DANIELS

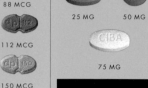 25 MCG	50 MCG
75 MCG	88 MCG
100 MCG	112 MCG
125 MCG	150 MCG
175 MCG	200 MCG
	300 MCG

SYNTHROID
BOOTS

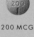 25 MCG	50 MCG
75 MCG	88 MCG
100 MCG	112 MCG
125 MCG	150 MCG
175 MCG	200 MCG
	300 MCG

LORAZEPAM

ATIVAN
WYETH-AYERST

0.5 MG	1 MG
	2 MG

MAPROTILINE HYDROCHLORIDE

LUDIOMIL
CIBA

25 MG	50 MG
	 75 MG

MECLOFENAMATE SODIUM

MECLOMEN
PARKE-DAVIS

50 MG

100 MG

MEDROXY-PROGESTERONE ACETATE

PROVERA
UPJOHN COMPANY

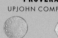 2.5 MG	5 MG
	 10 MG

MEFENAMIC ACID

PONSTEL® KAPSEALS®
PARKE-DAVIS

250 MG

MEGESTROL ACETATE

MEGACE
BRISTOL-MYERS ONCOLOGY

20 MG	40 MG

MENSTRUAL RELIEF

MIDOL
STERLING HEALTH

MIDOL TEEN

Midol PMS

MIDOL MAXIMUM

METHOTREXATE

METHOTREXATE
LEDERLE LABORATORIES

2.5 MG

METHYLERGONOVINE MALEATE

METHERGINE
SANDOZ PHARMACEUTICALS

0.2 MG

METHYLTESTOSTERONE

ANDROID-10
ICN PHARMACEUTICALS

BP 958
10 MG

TESTRED
ICN PHARMACEUTICALS

10 MG

METHYSERGIDE MALEATE

SANSERT
SANDOZ PHARMACEUTICALS

78 58
2 MG

METRONIDAZOLE

FLAGYL
G. D. SEARLE & CO.

250 MG

FLAGYL
500 MG

PROTOSTAT
ORTHO

ORTHO 1570
250 MG

ORTHO 1571
500 MG

MINOCYCLINE HCL

MINOCIN
LEDERLE LABORATORIES

50 MG

100 MG

MULTIVITAMINS/ FLUORIDE

POLY-VI-FLOR
MEAD JOHNSON

487
0.25 MG

POLY-VI-FLOR
MEAD JOHNSON

487
0.25 MG

468
0.50 MG

474
1.0 MG

NABUMETONE

RELAFEN
SMITHKLINE BEECHAM

500
500 MG

750
750 MG

NAPROXEN

NAPROSYN
SYNTEX LABORATORIES

NAPROSYN 250
250 MG

SYNTEX
375 MG

NAPROSYN
500 MG

NAPROXEN SODIUM

ANAPROX
SYNTEX LABORATORIES

275 MG

ANAPROX® DS
SYNTEX LABORATORIES

550 MG

NITROFURANTOIN

MACRODANTIN
PROCTER & GAMBLE

25 MG

50 MG

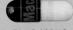

100 MG

NITROFURANTOIN MONOHYDRATE/ NITROFURANTOIN MACROCRYSTALS

MACROBID
PROCTER & GAMBLE

75 MG / 25 MG

NORFLOXACIN

NOROXIN
MERCK

400 MG

NORTRIPTYLINE HCL

PAMELOR
SANDOZ PHARMACEUTICALS

10 MG

PAMELOR
SANDOZ PHARMACEUTICALS

25 MG

50 MG

75 MG

OFLOXACIN

FLOXIN
MCNEIL PHARMACEUTICAL

200 MG

300 MG

400 MG

OXAPROZIN

DAYPRO
G. D. SEARLE & CO.

600 MG

OXAZEPAM

SERAX
WYETH-AYERST

10 MG

15 MG

15 MG

30 MG

PAROXETINE HCL

PAXIL
SMITHKLINE BEECHAM

20 MG

30 MG

PERPHENAZINE/ AMITRIPTYLINE HCL

TRIAVIL
MERCK

2 MG/ 10 MG

2 MG/ 25 MG

4 MG/ 10 MG

4 MG/ 25 MG

4 MG/ 50 MG

PHENAZOPYRIDINE HCL

PYRIDIUM
PARKE-DAVIS

100 MG   200 MG

PHENELZINE SULFATE

NARDIL
PARKE-DAVIS

15 MG

PHENTERMINE HCL

FASTIN
SMITHKLINE BEECHAM

30 MG

PIROXICAM

FELDENE
PFIZER LABS

10 MG

20 MG

PRAZEPAM

CENTRAX
PARKE-DAVIS

5 MG

10 MG

20 MG

PROPRANOLOL HCL

INDERAL
WYETH-AYERST

10 MG   20 MG

40 MG   60 MG

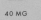 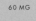

80 MG

INDERAL® LA
WYETH-AYERST

60 MG

80 MG

120 MG

160 MG

SERTRALINE HYDROCHLORIDE

ZOLOFT
ROERIG

50 MG

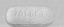

100 MG

SULFISOXAZOLE

GANTRISIN
ROCHE LABORATORIES

500 MG

SULINDAC

CLINORIL
MERCK

150 MG   200 MG

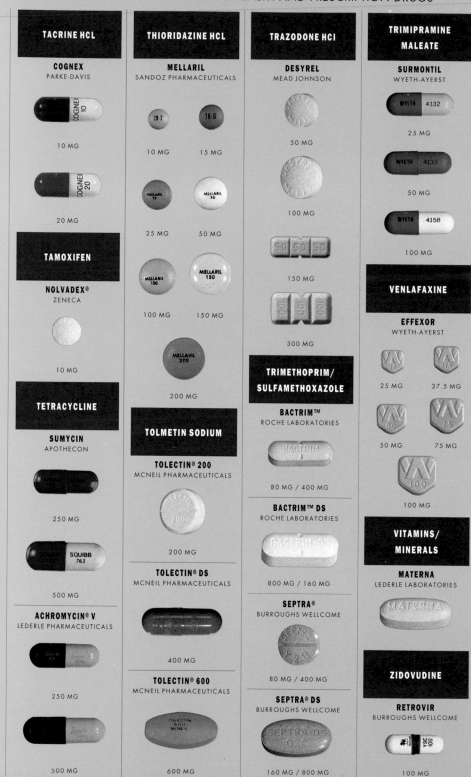

TACRINE HCL

COGNEX
PARKE-DAVIS

10 MG

20 MG

TAMOXIFEN

NOLVADEX®
ZENECA

10 MG

TETRACYCLINE

SUMYCIN
APOTHECON

250 MG

500 MG

ACHROMYCIN® V
LEDERLE PHARMACEUTICALS

250 MG

500 MG

THIORIDAZINE HCL

MELLARIL
SANDOZ PHARMACEUTICALS

10 MG   15 MG

25 MG   50 MG

100 MG   150 MG

200 MG

TOLMETIN SODIUM

TOLECTIN® 200
MCNEIL PHARMACEUTICALS

200 MG

TOLECTIN® DS
MCNEIL PHARMACEUTICALS

400 MG

TOLECTIN® 600
MCNEIL PHARMACEUTICALS

600 MG

TRAZODONE HCl

DESYREL
MEAD JOHNSON

50 MG

100 MG

150 MG

300 MG

**TRIMETHOPRIM/
SULFAMETHOXAZOLE**

BACTRIM™
ROCHE LABORATORIES

80 MG / 400 MG

BACTRIM™ DS
ROCHE LABORATORIES

800 MG / 160 MG

SEPTRA®
BURROUGHS WELLCOME

80 MG / 400 MG

SEPTRA® DS
BURROUGHS WELLCOME

160 MG / 800 MG

**TRIMIPRAMINE
MALEATE**

SURMONTIL
WYETH-AYERST

25 MG

50 MG

100 MG

VENLAFAXINE

EFFEXOR
WYETH-AYERST

25 MG   37.5 MG

50 MG   75 MG

100 MG

**VITAMINS/
MINERALS**

MATERNA
LEDERLE LABORATORIES

ZIDOVUDINE

RETROVIR
BURROUGHS WELLCOME

100 MG

PART ONE

A Woman's Special Health Concerns

CHAPTER 1   **COMMON DISORDERS OF THE REPRODUCTIVE SYSTEM**

Guide to Typical Symptoms and Their Meaning

When you feel sick, sometimes the most troubling part is not knowing what's wrong, fearing what might be wrong, and not wanting to hear the worst. Some women worry about what the doctor might do, whether the examination will be painful, and whether any help is available. Others view feeling sick as an annoyance and hope the symptoms will go away.

Symptoms as Clues

Physical discomforts are your body's way of telling you something. Unfortunately, the body's language is often quite vague and symptoms can mean many things. Pelvic pain can be a troublesome but harmless part of ovulation or a sign of serious infection. Breast lumps could mean cancer, but many are benign. The best way to learn what's wrong is to consult your doctor who can use other clues to decode the body's messages and diagnose the underlying problem. Even if you think the problem is small and will go away, you should call your doctor. Many illnesses, both major and minor, are easier to handle if caught early. And a diagnosis gives you the comfort of being certain what's wrong.

For many women, something out of the ordinary about their sexual organs, reproductive system, or urinary tract has the added complication of being embarrassing and difficult to discuss. Furthermore, the possible explanations for gynecologic symptoms may be more upsetting than the cause of, say, muscle pain. A monogamous woman who thinks the changes in her vaginal mucus are caused by a sexually transmitted disease (STD) may fear that her partner has been seeing other women. The possibility of pregnancy or cancer may be frightening enough to keep a woman out of a doctor's office where she might hear bad news.

Like everything else in life, however, it's better to face a potential problem than to deny it. You may prefer to ignore an annoying symptom. But an illness that requires treatment will only worsen without care. And most doctors want to find out what's wrong and help you, not judge you. Most women experience problems at some point in their lives with menstruation, their vulva or vagina, uterus, ovaries, fallopian tubes, breasts, or urinary tract. Gynecologic and urinary symptoms are common — your doctor has almost certainly seen women with similar problems many times before. It will not be nearly as alarming to a doctor as it may be to you.

This chapter is designed to allay unfounded or exaggerated worries by identifying common gynecologic and urinary tract symptoms and explaining possible causes. It also briefly discusses what to expect at the doctor's office. Keep in mind that your doctor's evaluation may differ from what you read here based on your description of your symptoms, medical tests and your personal history. The medical terms for some problems are included so that you'll know what they mean if your doctor uses them.

The areas to be covered are:

- Excessive or abnormal vaginal bleeding
- Abnormal vaginal mucus or discharge
- Genital warts
- Pain during menstruation
- Menstruation stopping (or never starting at puberty)
- Pain during intercourse
- Pelvic pain
- Discharge from the breast (other than postpartum)
- Breast lumps
- Painful urination
- Blood in the urine
- More frequent urination

Excessive or Otherwise Abnormal Vaginal Bleeding

Many women experience this problem at some point in their lives. It is defined as bleeding from the vagina that is not part of your monthly periods or bleeding that occurs during monthly periods but is heavier than usual.

Some common causes in women of reproductive age are the birth control pill, which can cause bleeding between periods; problems with hormones produced by the thyroid, ovaries, pituitary, or adrenal glands; infections, such as sexually transmitted diseases, of the vagina, cervix, uterus, fallopian tubes, or ovaries; and miscarriage or problems with pregnancy. A miscarriage of an early pregnancy can resemble a heavy period that occurs after the woman has missed at least one period.

Bleeding between cycles that does not last long is often due to scars, tumors, fibroids, or other abnormal tissue on the cervix or uterus. Ovarian cysts are another possibility. Regular, prolonged, heavy bleeding is often caused by growths in the uterine lining, or endometrium. These growths may or may not be cancerous.

Perimenopausal women may bleed off-cycle as part of the gradual onset of menopause. Postmenopausal women should see a doctor immediately if they experience vaginal bleeding since benign or cancerous tumors of the ovaries or uterus are more likely causes.

Other potential culprits are injury to the vagina or reproductive tract during rape or surgery, and the presence of objects such as a tampon stuck in the vagina. Bleeding disorders that affect the whole body, such as leukemia and clotting problems, can cause abnormal vaginal bleeding just as they

UNWANTED PASSAGEWAYS

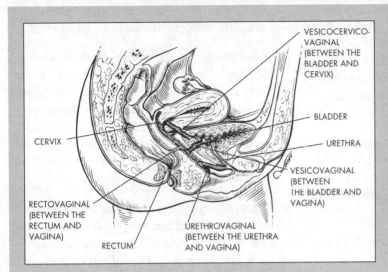

VESICOCERVICO-VAGINAL (BETWEEN THE BLADDER AND CERVIX)

BLADDER

CERVIX

URETHRA

VESICOVAGINAL (BETWEEN THE BLADDER AND VAGINA)

RECTOVAGINAL (BETWEEN THE RECTUM AND VAGINA)

RECTUM

URETHROVAGINAL (BETWEEN THE URETHRA AND VAGINA)

Fistulas—abnormal passages between organs—are usually the result of injuries sustained in accidents, childbirth, or surgery. These unwanted openings can divert urine into the vagina from the bladder or the urethra (the tube that normally empties the bladder), causing vaginal discharge. They can also develop between the rectum and the vagina. The only remedy is surgery to close the passage.

produce bleeding elsewhere. Vaginal bleeding along with fever, abdominal pain, or unusual mucus or other substances coming from the vagina (known as vaginal discharge) may indicate an infection.

Your doctor is likely to ask you about your recent menstrual periods and if you've noticed anything unusual about them. You will probably have an abdominal and pelvic exam and, if you are of reproductive age, your doctor will also do a pregnancy test.

Vaginal Discharge

Unusual mucus or other substances coming from the vagina is a common problem. The discharge is often due to infection, and frequently associated with pain, burning, itching, and painful urination. Not all infections are sexually transmitted, so don't assume that vaginal discharge means that you have an STD. There are a number of possible causes:

Inflammation of the vagina. Called vaginitis, this is the most common reason for discharges and is usually caused by infection. There are three main types of vaginal infections, all of which can be treated with oral or vaginal medications. Each infection tends to produce a distinct discharge:

- Thick, white cottage cheese-like discharge, itching, irritated skin—yeast infection, or candidiasis. Women with diabetes and those taking antibiotics are more likely to develop this type of infection. Most women will have at least one yeast infection at some point in their lives.
- Thin, yellow, foul-smelling discharge—*Trichomonas*, which is usually transmitted sexually.
- Thin, gray or white, foul-smelling discharge—bacterial vaginosis.

Pelvic inflammatory disease (PID). Frequently caused by STDs that infect the cervix, uterus, ovaries, or fallopian tubes, this is the most common and serious complication of an STD and occurs in 1 million women every year. Symptoms include vaginal discharge or bleeding, lower abdominal pain, and fever. Chronic PID can result from one or more infections. The most common identifiable causes are gonorrhea or chlamydia, both of which are sexually transmitted. About 20 percent of women with PID become infertile.

Genital herpes. This infection can produce vaginal discharge if it affects the cervix. The first episode of genital herpes also features fever, itching, headache, and general muscle aches.

Infection of the inside of the uterus. This condition, known as endometritis, is usually caused by STDs, fibroid tumors, cancer, giving birth, or intrauterine devices (IUDs).

A hole in the vagina (connecting the vagina to the rectum or bladder). Because of this passageway, called a fistula, stool or urine can pass through the vagina. The problem can develop after surgery or injury to the area, infection, inflammation, or radiation.

Inflammation of the vagina due to lack of estrogen. As a woman enters menopause, her body produces increasingly erratic amounts of estrogen. This often causes the vagina to dry out and become irritated. The condition is known as atrophic vaginitis and is treatable by estrogen replacement therapy, vaginal creams, and vaginal suppositories.

Other, less common causes of vaginal discharge include pregnancy, genital warts, cancer, and foreign objects in the vagina, such as a tampon that could not be removed.

Your doctor will ask you about the type of discharge and whether it occurs immediately before, after, or during menstruation or sexual activity. You should also expect to undergo a pelvic exam.

A DANGEROUS — AND GROWING — PROBLEM

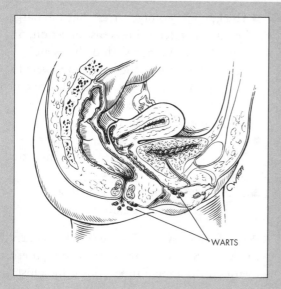

WARTS

Cases of genital warts, caused by the sexually transmitted human papillomavirus (HPV), have been increasing at twice the rate of the more widely publicized genital herpes. And these warts can be much more than a minor annoyance: They've been implicated in several types of genital cancer.

Following infection, the warts can take up to 6 months to make their appearance. First seen as small, soft, moist, pink or red swellings, the warts then grow rapidly, often developing stems and clustering together to form a cauliflower-like growth.

Standard wart medications will sometimes clear up the infection. Frequently, however, the growths must be burned off or surgically removed. For more information on this increasingly common problem, turn to chapter 11, "Coming to Terms with Sexually Transmitted Diseases."

Genital Warts

Human papillomavirus (HPV), a sexually transmitted disease, is a frequent cause of genital warts. It can also cause outbreaks in the vulva, vagina, cervix, or anal area and is sometimes accompanied by other infections and STDs. HPV is also believed to be a factor in causing cancer of the cervix, vagina, and vulva. About 50 percent to 70 percent of the sexual partners of women with HPV have, or will develop, genital warts.

If you have had several episodes of yeast infection, you should consider being tested for HPV, as HPV may make a woman more vulnerable to this problem. Gonorrhea, chlamydia, and syphilis can accompany genital warts.

Pain During Menstruation

This is a very common problem. Known as dysmenorrhea, it is often severe enough to cause absences from work or inability to perform other responsibilities. Symptoms include lower abdominal cramping, nausea, vomiting, and headache during menstruation.

In one type of painful menstruation, called primary dysmenorrhea, doctors cannot find any problem with the reproductive organs. This disorder tends to affect young women fairly soon after they first begin to menstruate. Painful contractions may occur as the uterine walls release natural substances called prostaglandins. Psychological factors may play a role.

Primary dysmenorrhea can be treated with ibuprofen (Advil, Nuprin, others) or aspirin, both of which help block production of prostaglandins. In severe cases, birth control pills or other medications containing hormones can help. Exercise, good nutrition, and reducing stress also are important.

Secondary dysmenorrhea develops after years of normal menstruation and results from disease of the uterus, fallopian tubes, or ovaries. Among the possible causes are tumors and other abnormal growths, pelvic infection, uterine cancer, and endometriosis (in which uterine tissue is found outside the uterus, in the fallopian tubes, ovaries, and abdominal organs). Endometriosis is a serious disease that can cause infertility.

When you see your doctor, he or she will ask you about your periods and the timing and severity of the pain. The doctor will also do a pelvic exam. Since treatment for secondary dysmenorrhea depends on its cause, he or she may do additional tests or refer you to a specialist.

Menstruation Stopping (or Never Starting at Puberty)

Women who have had normal periods that stop for 6 months or more are said to have amenorrhea, or the absence of menstruation. This is called secondary amenorrhea. Girls who have not begun to menstruate by the age of 16 have primary amenorrhea.

The definition of secondary amenorrhea clearly excludes minor lateness of a period and it's important to remember that 5- or 6-week cycles are normal for some women. Stress — including worrying about whether you will get your period or whether you are pregnant — can cause your period to be 1 or 2 weeks late. Severe physical or emotional stress or mental health problems can cause periods to stop for a longer time.

Full-blown amenorrhea is most commonly due to problems with the hormones that regulate menstruation. The glands that produce the hormones that affect menstruation include the pituitary gland at the base of the brain, the adrenal glands on top of the kidneys, the thyroid gland in the neck, and the ovaries.

It can take 6 months to a year for normal periods to resume after a woman stops taking birth control pills. This is because the pill blocks certain hormones involved in menstruation and it can take that long for those hormones to return to normal. Menstruation also stops during pregnancy.

In some women, menstruation stops or never starts because their ovaries do not respond properly to the hormones that normally trigger release of an egg. These women cannot ovulate on their own and menstruation is not possible without ovulation. Some women do not produce enough estrogen to ovulate. Other causes of amenorrhea are ovarian cysts and obstructions or other problems in the reproductive tract.

A variety of other factors can cause menstruation to stop, including:

■ Vigorous exercise (sometimes not the only cause—periods should return as the training schedule is reduced)
■ Obesity
■ Poor nutrition (including anorexia)
■ Diabetes
■ Chronic, nonalcoholic liver disease
■ Any chronic illness
■ Tuberculosis
■ Medications such as birth control pills, narcotics, major tranquilizers, and cancer chemotherapy drugs

In rare cases of primary amenorrhea, there is no opening in the hymen through which blood can flow. About one-third of girls with primary amenorrhea have a genetic disorder or a congenital problem with their reproductive tract.

Pain During Intercourse

This problem is so emotional and sensitive that many woman find it difficult to consult a physician. But it's important to seek treatment, and in many cases the cause is a physical illness that can be treated.

Painful intercourse, which a doctor may call dyspareunia, is a burning, tearing, ripping, or aching sensation associated with penetration. The pain can be at the vaginal opening, deep in the pelvis, or anywhere in between. It also may be felt throughout the entire pelvic area and the sexual organs, and may occur only with deep thrusting.

The most common explanation is irritation of the vagina caused by having intercourse without sufficient arousal and lubrication. This experience can create a vicious circle, leading a woman to fear intercourse which in turn makes it more difficult to become aroused. Women who have had a hysterectomy or mastectomy may have problems with arousal because of feelings of incompleteness. Stress or problems in your relationship with a partner can also block arousal. Counseling can help address these psychological issues, and over-the-counter lubricants (consult your doctor or pharmacist) can increase lubrication and reduce discomfort.

Another frequent explanation for painful intercourse is thinning and drying of the vaginal tissue as menopause begins. This happens because the body is producing less and less of the estrogen that is needed to maintain moist vaginal tissue. As the vagina's ability to make its own mucus declines, it becomes dry, itchy, and painful, leading to discomfort during intercourse. Estrogen creams and lubricating gels can help restore moisture, as can estrogen replacement therapy taken in pills or through a patch on the body.

Unintentional muscle spasms of the thighs, pelvis, and vagina can make penetration impossible. This condition, called vaginismus, can develop along with any of the other causes of painful intercourse described here or can result from psychological factors. A traumatic sexual experience, rape, or an irrational fear of genital injury can lead to vaginismus. Counseling can be helpful.

Other causes of painful intercourse include:

- Infection—vaginal, pelvic, herpes, infected cysts or boils
- Scars, tumors, or anything that narrows the vagina
- Endometriosis (uterine tissue growing outside the uterus with bleeding, pain and scarring)
- Intact hymen (in virginal young women)
- Complications of surgery
- Diseases that interfere with the physical process of arousal or orgasm (such as diabetes and multiple sclerosis)

Pelvic Pain

Many women experience pain in the lower abdominal area during ovulation, around the middle of the menstrual cycle. It usually lasts a few minutes to a few hours and is rarely severe. This does not necessarily indicate that there is any underlying problem.

Pelvic pain may also be part of premenstrual syndrome (PMS). In this case, your breasts and abdomen may swell and you may become irritable, depressed, and fatigued for a few days before your period begins.

Pain in the area of the ovaries and fallopian tubes is often due to infection. Lower abdominal pain, fever, and chills that begin a few days after a menstrual period may be caused by gonorrhea or chlamydia. Pelvic pain that is present most of the time but worsens during menstruation and intercourse may be due to chronic pelvic inflammatory disease. Chronic PID is caused by one or more episodes of pelvic infection, usually from gonorrhea or chlamydia and can lead to infertility.

Other causes of pelvic pain include ovarian cysts and endometriosis. Pain due to endometriosis usually increases during menstruation and, sometimes, during intercourse. Problems with pregnancy, such as cramping before a miscarriage or a pregnancy in the fallopian tubes rather than in the uterus, can also cause pelvic pain.

Your doctor will probably ask about the type of pain and when and where it occurs; He or she will also do a pelvic exam, and if you could possibly be pregnant, a pregnancy test.

Possible causes of pelvic pain that occurs only during menstruation or intercourse are discussed in the earlier sections.

Breast Discharge

Breast discharge is normal soon after giving birth and continues if a woman is breastfeeding. In other circumstances, however, release of breast milk can mean that the hormones causing milk production are out of balance. This condition is called galactorrhea. Release of a liquid other than breast milk can be a sign of infection, inflammation, or a tumor in the breast.

The pituitary, thyroid, adrenal, and ovarian glands all release hormones that govern production of breast milk. If the thyroid gland is not producing enough hormone it can lead to untimely release of breast milk. Another explanation is a benign (non-cancerous) growth on the pituitary gland. In these cases, menstruation usually stops as well. Diseases of the part of the brain that controls the pituitary gland are a third possibility. Other causes are stress, sexual stimulation, and drugs, including birth control pills, marijuana, narcotics, anesthetics, reserpine (Diupres, Hydropres, others), methyldopa (Aldomet), antidepressants, and other medications prescribed for mental and emotional problems.

In half of all cases, no cause is found. Your doctor may order blood tests, breast x-rays, and analysis of the fluid. If the liquid from the breast is not milk and is bloody, thin, white, green, or yellow, the cause is more likely to be a breast infection or tumor. If blood levels of a hormone that controls breast milk, called prolactin, are high, or your menstrual periods have changed, your doctor may look for a growth on the pituitary gland. An underactive thyroid can be identified through blood tests and can be treated by taking hormones in pill form. One drug, called bromocriptine (Parlodel), lowers prolactin production and may be helpful. Pituitary tumors may be removed surgically.

Breast Lumps

Finding a lump in the breast strikes fear into the heart of most women, and justifiably so. Depending on which estimate you use, breast cancer affects as many as 1 in 9 women throughout their lifetime until age 90. However, this statistic is a bit misleading. At any one point in time, your risk may be higher or substantially less. Risk increases with age, and, all other factors being equal, is highest from 80 to 90. Nonetheless, breast cancer is common and lumps are often its first sign. Because early diagnosis and treatment greatly increases chances of survival, see your doctor immediately if you find a lump in your breast. He or she will discuss with you the steps to be taken to determine if it is cancerous. Monthly breast self-examinations, following your period, are the best way to know what your breast normally feels like and to detect any changes at an early stage.

It's also important to remember that most breast lumps are NOT cancer. The most common cause of non-cancerous breast lumps is a condition called fibrocystic breast changes. About 20 percent of women have symptoms of this problem. It is so widespread that some experts consider it a variation of normal rather than a disease. These lumps are filled with fluid and become painful and swollen 5 to 7 days before each menstrual period. They shrink after menstruation is over and enlarge again before the next period. Reducing your caffeine intake can help relieve the symptoms. If the lumps do not go away after a month or two, your doctor may insert a needle into one of them and remove some fluid for analysis.

Other non-cancerous lumps can be caused by:

- Blood clots in the breast
- Breast infection (usually during breastfeeding)
- Fibroadenoma (benign tumors more common in women under 25)
- Intraductal papilloma (lumps in breast ducts; symptoms include bloody liquid from the nipple)
- Mammary duct ectasia (inflammation of tissue beneath the nipple due to a hole in the duct; symptoms include burning pain, thick liquid from the nipple, and nipple swelling)

Painful Urination

The medical term for painful urination is dysuria and the most common causes are easily treatable. They include irritated areas that the urine passes over, vaginal infection, STDs, urinary tract infections (UTIs), and changes in vaginal tissue due to menopause. About 20 percent of women will have a urinary tract infection at some point in their lives. The chances of having a UTI increases with age; this risk is still greater if you are sexually active. Infections are also a common problem in pregnancy.

People with pain during urination may also need to urinate more often or may release more or less urine than usual.

Possible causes of urinary tract pain and accompanying symptoms:

- Vaginal infection—vaginal discharge, burning, itching, pain feels like it is on the outside of the body as urine passes over irritated areas

- STDs—herpes, genital warts; pain feels like it is on the outside of the body as urine passes over irritated areas
- Urinary tract infections—may cause blood in the urine; pain feels like it is inside rather than on the outside of the body

If you also have fever, back pain, and an upset stomach, you may have a serious kidney infection and should see a doctor at once.

Less common causes of painful urination include bladder tumors or spasms, kidney stones, and scarring or narrowing of the urethra (the tube through which urine leaves the body).

A lab test of the urine can detect a urinary infection; and your doctor may do a pelvic exam as well. Treatment for an infection usually includes antibiotics or anti-infective drugs and advice to drink a lot of water.

Blood In The Urine

Even a small amount of blood in the urine can be a sign of a serious condition. Therefore, it should never be ignored. The most common explanation for this problem, called hematuria, is a urinary

BAD SIGN: BLOOD IN THE URINE

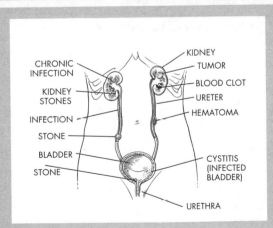

CHRONIC INFECTION
KIDNEY STONES
INFECTION
STONE
BLADDER STONE
KIDNEY TUMOR
BLOOD CLOT
URETER
HEMATOMA
CYSTITIS (INFECTED BLADDER)
URETHRA

Bleeding can start anywhere in the urinary tract; but no matter the source, it's a cause for concern. Fortunately, the most common cause, an infection, is easily remedied. Among the other possible causes: kidney stones caught in the kidney itself, the bladder, or the ureter leading to the bladder; blood clots or tumors in the kidney; or a hematoma (a pool of blood collecting around a broken vessel). Whatever the cause, this is one condition that definitely needs a doctor's attention.

tract infection. Blockage of or damage to the urethra or other problems with the bladder, can produce bloody urine as well.

Several problems in the kidneys can also cause hematuria. Possible conditions and other associated symptoms are:

- Kidney stone (symptoms: sudden pain in side and groin)
- Blood clots in the kidney
- Infection (symptoms: fever, back pain, nausea, painful stomach or abdomen, and painful urination)
- Tumor (symptoms: abdominal pain, fever, weight loss, and high blood pressure)
- Toxic medications or poisons (symptoms: drugs or chemicals processed out of the body through the kidneys can damage the tissue if taken in dangerously high amounts; symptoms of overdose will vary)

Problems elsewhere in the body that can cause blood in the urine include internal bleeding, hemophilia, leukemia, and other blood disorders. In about 5 percent of patients, no explanation is found.

Frequent Urination

The need to urinate more often than usual may or may not be accompanied by an increase in the amount released. Common causes of frequent urination without an increase in the amount include urinary tract infection; STDs such as herpes, chlamydia, and gonorrhea; pregnancy; changes in the vagina due to menopause; and in women who've had more than one preg-nancy, inability to completely empty the bladder and poor bladder support.

Stress can also make one feel the need to urinate more often, as can drinking beverages containing caffeine. Some people simply have small bladders that fill up more quickly.

Strokes or problems with the nerves that control the urinary system can affect the need to urinate. In adolescents, frequent urination can be a first sign of an overactive thyroid gland.

If the need for frequent urination is accompanied by an increase in the amount, possible causes include drinking more water than usual, diabetes, alcohol, diuretics ("water pills") for high blood pressure and other heart conditions, kidney disease, and high levels of calcium in the blood.

As you can see, frequent urination is not necessarily a cause for alarm, but if you see no simple explanation for it, a medical check-up may be in order. No matter how harmless a symptom may turn out to be, you can't be certain of your health without a visit to the doctor. If you suspect you have any of the conditions mentioned here, you'll find more information in the chapters that follow. Since no amount of knowledge can replace the certainty and relief that comes with a definite diagnosis, if you feel the slightest cause for concern, do call your doctor. □

CHAPTER 2   **COMMON DISORDERS OF THE REPRODUCTIVE SYSTEM**

What a Menstrual Problem Could Mean

There's as much variation in menstruation as there is in women. One sister has her first period at 11, the second at 14. One woman is "as regular as clockwork," another's cycles fall randomly across the calendar.

There seems to be no rhyme or reason to it. Yet in most cases, this is all perfectly normal.

But when any menstrual symptom — pain, heavy bleeding, spotting, missed periods — begins to interfere with your life, it's time to seek medical attention. Most problems are relatively uncomplicated and respond well to medication or simple surgical procedures. Others could have more dangerous consequences if the underlying cause is not treated promptly. If you have any doubts about your menstrual problems, see your doctor.

The Menstrual Cycle

Most women begin to menstruate between 11 and 13 years of age and continue until they reach menopause some 40 years later. Although the "normal" cycle is 28 days, there is no cause for concern if periods are spaced 25 to 34 days apart, since precise regularity is rare.

During the "typical" 3-to-5 day menstrual period, the average woman loses less than 2 ounces of blood.

The first menstrual period separates childhood from adolescence. Along with breast enlargement and the growth of pubic hair, it signals a young woman's sexual maturity. This monthly vaginal discharge of blood, secretions, and cells from the surface of the uterus is the final step in a complex cycle that prepares the body to conceive a child.

Each cycle begins when, responding to a cascade of hormones, a dormant egg cell within one of the ovaries begins to ripen. Cells around the maturing egg release the female hormone estrogen, prompting the lining of the uterus (the endometrium) to thicken in preparation for receipt of a fertilized egg.

When it reaches maturity, the developing egg bursts from the ovary and begins its trip down the fallopian tube to the uterus in a process called ovulation. The supporting cells left behind after ovulation then begin to manufacture another hormone, progesterone, in addition to estrogen. This second hormone fosters further growth in the lining of the uterus.

If fertilization does not take place, the ovum dies and production of estrogen and progesterone stops. Robbed of its sustaining hormones, the thickened lining of the uterus begins to break down. The dead endometrial cells, along with a little blood, are then discharged in the menstrual flow.

Normal menstruation depends on the delicate orchestration of the hormones that govern development of the egg. The menstrual cycle can also be affected by disease, diet, emotions, and defective development of the reproductive organs.

Major Menstrual Disorders

Many women experience discomfort (sore, swollen breasts, minor pain in the lower abdomen, nervousness) before their periods. They may also have mild cramps when the menstrual flow starts. In most cases, these symptoms do not interfere with their normal activities and can be alleviated by diuretics ("water pills") and salt reduction to reduce bloating; plus pain relievers such as aspirin, acetaminophen (Tylenol) and ibuprofen (Advil, Motrin).

For some women, however, symptoms can be more severe, signaling a condition that needs medical attention. These problems include:

- Premenstrual irritability and mood swings (PMS),
- Very painful periods
- Heavy bleeding
- Unusually short or long cycles
- Failure to menstruate
- Early menstruation
- Toxic shock syndrome

Should you or your daughter experience any of these menstrual abnormalities, consult your doctor. He or she will take a complete medical history, perform a thorough physical examination, and conduct tests to diagnose the cause of the menstrual problems and determine the best course of treatment.

Premenstrual Syndrome

Between 70 and 90 percent of menstruating women experience some degree of physical and mental changes before their periods, but only 10 to 20 percent suffer from Premenstrual Syndrome (PMS), a condition that seriously affects their home life, job performance, and personal relationships.

Most PMS sufferers have mood swings, irritability, and bursts of temper four to five days before menstruating, during or following ovulation, or from ovulation through the first days of their period. Other signs of PMS include bloating, sore breasts, weight gain, extreme depression, confusion, and insomnia. These symptoms usually disappear with the onset of the menstrual flow.

There is no agreement on the cause of PMS. Physicians usually concentrate on alleviating the most severe symptoms. Your doctor will probably recommend eliminating or reducing the salt and sugar in your diet and tell you to get regular exercise. If necessary, he or she will prescribe a diuretic for water retention and an analgesic for pain and headache. Tranquilizers and antidepressant medications can help alleviate mood swings and depression. For more about PMS, see chapter 3.

Painful Periods

The medical term for this problem is dysmenorrhea. It's a common complaint, especially among young women who have never borne children. Fifty percent of menstruating women have pelvic pain before or during their period, and 10 percent of them have cramps severe enough to incapacitate them one to three days each month. In the United States dysmenorrhea sufferers lose 140 million working hours each year. There are two types of dysmenorrhea, primary and secondary.

Primary Dysmenorrhea

In this form of the problem, there is no underlying physical abnormality. Symptoms may include sharp cramps in the lower abdomen immediately before the menstrual period or when bleeding begins. The pain, which is sometimes accompanied by nausea, vomiting, diarrhea, dizziness, headaches, a feeling of tension, and occasionally fainting, may spread to the upper legs and lower back.

The majority of women who suffer from primary dymenorrhea do not experience severe pain until the beginning of ovulation. Their menstrual cycles are usually regular,

HOW HORMONES TRIGGER YOUR PERIOD

In a slow, steady, 4-week cycle repeated over and over between pregnancies, a woman's body gradually prepares for conception, then discards its work and begins again.

For most of the cycle, the lining of the uterus, (the endometrium, shown here at the bottom of the 28-day chart) grows steadily richer and thicker in preparation for the advent of a fertilized egg. This growth is spurred by increasing levels of estrogen, a hormone produced as an egg ripens to maturity. Once the egg is released (see center of chart), a second hormone, progesterone, kicks in to boost the endometrium to full readiness.

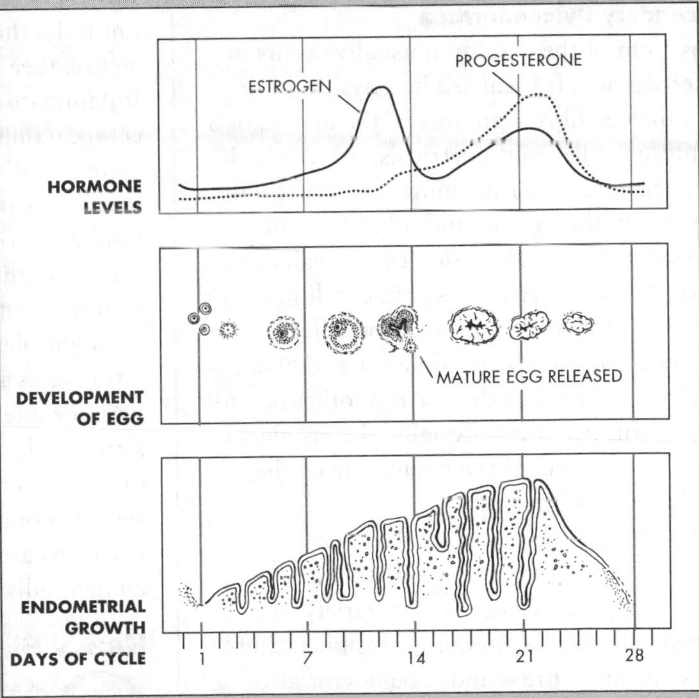

If conception doesn't occur, production of both hormones drops simultaneously (see days 21 to 28 of the chart). The enriched lining then breaks down and sloughs off, exiting the body in the monthly menstrual flow. Cued by this end-of-cycle trough in estrogen and progesterone levels, the body then begins the process anew. (For more information on the monthly ebb and flow of hormones, turn to chapter 17, "How the Reproductive System Works" .)

HORMONE LEVELS — ESTROGEN — PROGESTERONE

DEVELOPMENT OF EGG — MATURE EGG RELEASED

ENDOMETRIAL GROWTH

DAYS OF CYCLE   1   7   14   21   28

and a pelvic exam reveals no physical problems. Laboratory tests, however, usually show high levels of prostaglandins, substances which can cause both painful cramps and uterine contractions.

To relieve the cramps, most doctors prescribe prostaglandin-inhibiting medications. Aspirin is the weakest of these drugs. Motrin, Naprosyn, Anaprox, and Ponstel have proved more effective. Oral contraceptives are another alternative. By stopping ovulation and decreasing prostaglandin levels they can usually be relied on to eliminate cramps. In addition, recent research both in the United States and abroad has shown that magnesium, and even electrical nerve stimulation may reduce prostaglandin-induced menstrual pain.

Secondary Dysmenorrhea

This form of the condition usually occurs in older women. It is caused by physical disorders such as fibroid tumors of the uterus, or a condition called endometriosis, in which tissue from the uterine lining (endometrium) is found in the ovaries and other locations outside the uterus. Invasion of the wall of the uterus by endometrial tissue (a condition called adenomyosis) also may be at fault. Endometrial polyps are sometimes to blame. Pelvic inflammatory disease is another potential culprit. And occassionally, the problem is due to narrowing of the opening from the cervix into the vagina.

To identify the source of the problem, your doctor will take a case history and perform a pelvic exam using a variety of instruments and techniques, possible including x-ray and ultrasound. The doctor also may perform *dilation and curettage,* also called *D&C,* a minor procedure in which the cervix is opened so that a sample of endometrial tissue can be removed from the uterus for microscopic examination.

Endometriosis is the most common cause of secondary dysmenorrhea, especially in women over 37 years old who have had no babies for five years. For a full discussion of this disorder, turn to the chapter on "Keeping Endometriosis at Bay" later in this section.

If the problem is adenomyosis, surgical removal of the uterus (hysterectomy) may be necessary, though prostaglandin inhibiting drugs can alleviate the pain.

If fibroid tumors or endometrial polyps are at fault, surgery may be needed. (For more on this, see chapter 7, "Your Treatment Options for Fibroids," later in this section.) In milder cases, prostaglandin inhibitors may suffice. If pelvic inflammatory disease turns out to be the culprit, antibiotics may provide a cure. (See chapter 6, "The Dangers of Pelvic Inflammatory Disease"). Narrowing of the cervix requires corrective surgery. Occasionally, an IUD may be the cause. If so, the doctor may prescribe prostaglandin inhibitors, or, if necessary, recommend removing the device and using another form of birth control.

Slight bleeding from the ovary during ovulation causes some women to experience light pain for a few days in the middle of the menstrual cycle. In contrast to most forms of secondary dysmenorrhea, this pain is rarely severe enough to require medical attention. In extreme cases the doctor may prescribe birth control pills to stop ovulation.

Heavy Bleeding

Occasionally menstrual flow seems heavier than usual, or a period lasts longer than normal. In general, there is little cause for concern unless you find it necessary to use at least two extra sanitary pads or tampons a day. That means you have lost almost 3 ounces of blood over the course of a period. You should also see your doctor if a period lasts more than seven days, or two periods are spaced less than 21 days apart. Heavy or lengthy uterine bleeding occurring at regular intervals is usually a sign of an underlying physical problem.

When you go to the doctor, he or she will want to know about the frequency and amount of the bleeding, whether it's accompanied by pain or blood clots, what type of contraception you use, and whether you bruise easily or bleed often from places other than the uterus. The doctor will also do a number of tests. Urine and stool testing can detect possible problems in the urinary tract, stomach, and intestines that might cause the bleeding. If you are in your childbearing years, you should also have a pregnancy test, a Pap smear (if you haven't had one in 12 months), a biopsy of the endometrium, and a test for ovulation. If you are not ovulating, the doctor will usually perform a D&C of the endometrium .

In addition, if the physician suspects the bleeding stems from inflammation of the vagina, cervix, endometrium, or fallopian tubes, he or she will perform an internal exam, take a blood count, and may take tests for sexually transmitted diseases.

Causes and Cures

Tumors of the pelvic organs could be at fault. Fibroid tumors in the uterus are rarely cancerous but may cause heavy periods. Although small fibroids usually need no special treatment, your doctor may want to remove them. Removal of the entire uterus may be necessary if the fibroids are large or rapidly growing.

Endometrial cancer is another possible cause. Although this disease usually strikes after menopause, every women over 35 with heavy bleeding should be tested. If the test is positive, a complete hysterectomy (removal of the uterus, ovaries, and fallopian tubes) followed by radiation is the usual treatment.

Polyps, small growths attached to the wall of the uterus, can also cause excessive bleeding. Because there is a slight risk that the polyps will become malignant, especially after menopause, they are often removed.

Excessive estrogen production, combined with lack of progesterone, can cause continuous stimulation and overdevelopment of the endometrium, leading to heavy bleeding in both adolescence and the premenopausal years. To correct the condition, your doctor may prescribe progesterone to stop the bleeding. When periods become normal, one or two weeks on Provera each month for two or three months should promote shedding of the endometrium. If the problem stems from imbalance of other hormones, such as those in the thyroid, pituitary, or adrenal glands, the doctor will correct it with medication.

There are several other diseases that could be at fault. Both underactivity of the thyroid (*hypothyroidism*) and advanced liver disease can cause heavy bleeding. Women with leukemia (cancer of the white blood cells) and certain other blood disorders may also develop the problem.

Some medications can promote heavy bleeding. Among the offending drugs are steroids, digitalis (Digitoxin, Digoxin), and blood thinners such as Coumadin. Withdrawal of estrogen or progesterone medication can also be a cause.

A woman who menstruates normally loses little iron during her period, but if you bleed heavily, you may develop *anemia* (iron deficiency). In that case, the doctor will usually stop the bleeding with hormones and advise you to take an oral iron preparation.

Unusually Long or Short Cycles

Although few women menstruate exactly every 28 days, extremely short (under 25 days) or long (over 34 days) cycles can be a cause for concern, especially if you plan to have children.

Short cycles often signal low levels of estrogen and progesterone in the system, possibly resulting from an undersupply of certain precursors. Lacking these hormones, the endometrium cannot develop properly, and infertility may result. Short cycles also develop as some women approach menopause. They can also result from over- or underactivity of the thyroid gland.

Irregular periods can be a sign of appproaching menopause. But they can also arise from an increase in the number of cells in a section of the endometrium. Endometrial hyperplasias are caused when too much estrogen is produced by a women who does not ovulate. To diagnose the problem, your doctor will probably perform a D&C, scraping cells from the endometrium and doing a biopsy. Mild hyperplasias are usually treated with monthly doses of progesterone. More serious hyperplasias require long-term progesterone therapy or even removal of the uterus.

Long cycles are not necessarily a problem. Many women with long cycles produce eggs and are fertile. Their ovaries are normal, and the eggs just take a long time to mature. By far the most common cause of an unexpectedly long cycle is simply pregnancy! However, some women with regular periods

two to five months apart may have ovarian cysts. Also, when a very long cycle is accompanied by a sudden increase in body hair, a decrease in breast size, and enlargement of the clitoris; and menstruation eventually stops altogether, the problem could be a growth or tumor of the adrenal gland. To make a diagnosis, the doctor will take urine, glucose tolerance and other tests. A CT scan or Magnetic Resonance Imaging (MRI) might also be ordered.

Long cycles can also develop from over or underproduction of thyroid hormone.

Failure to Menstruate

When periods fail to start by the age of 16 or 17, a young woman has the condition that doctors call **primary amenorrhea.** For most of these girls, the problem is nothing more serious than an unusual delay. But for a few, there may be a more important underlying cause. Doctors divide young women with a significant problem into four groups.

Group 1: Girls in this group have flat enlarged breasts and an undeveloped uterus. Sometimes they have no uterus at all. Causes of their lack of menstruation range from low hormonal levels to diseases like tuberculosis, meningitis, and encephalitis. If the girl has some development of the uterus, treatment with gonadotrophic releasing hormone may make future pregnancy possible. If no pregnancy is desired, the doctor will prescribe estrogen to promote breast development. A few girls in this group are genetically male, and require other more specialized therapy.

Group 2: These young women have normal breast development but no uterus; and some may have testes (male sperm-producing organs). Although these girls can never have children, there are measures the doctor can take to correct other problems. If testes are present, they can be surgically removed after puberty and the doctor can prescribe estrogen. If the girl has a short vagina, it can be surgically lengthened to allow for intercourse.

Group 3: There are few girls with neither a uterus nor breast development Available treatments are similar to those recommended for girls in Group 2. Estrogen is prescribed to promote breast development.

Group 4: If a girl has both breast development and a uterus, the failure to menstruate may be due to an imbalance in hormone secretion. Treatment is similar to that for amenorrhea developed later in life.

If Menstruation Stops

When periods stop in a sexually active, regularly menstruating woman, the first thing that comes to mind is a possible pregnancy. If she is past 40, menopause may be the cause. But when the doctor has ruled out both pregnancy and menopause, it's time to look for other reasons.

This condition bears the medical name **secondary amenorrhea.** It is defined as the lack of a period either for six months or for at least three times as long as the length of a menstruating woman's normal cycle. Causes range from tumors and cysts to weight gain or loss, and emotional factors.

Chronic failure to ovulate is one of most common causes. A lack of ovulation is normal during the first couple of years after menstruation begins and again before menopause. But at other times it may be due to low levels of a key reproductive hormone called GnRH (gonadotrophic releasing hormone). Levels of this hormone often drop when a woman is under stress, has been on a "crash" diet, has had a head injury or serious infection such as encephalitis or meningitis, or has stopped using birth control pills.

If the doctor suspects that lack of ovulation is the culprit, he or she will ask you to record your temperature upon waking . The doctor will study samples of your cervical mucus and vaginal secretions and examine a piece of tissue from the endometrium. He or she may also need to determine whether your progesterone level rises over the course of a month.

If failure to ovulate is indeed the problem and you don't want to become pregnant, the doctor will prescribe estrogen and progesterone or an oral contraceptive. This promotes shedding of the endometrium and discourages development of growths in the uterus that can occur when estrogen levels remain high for a long period of time. If you do want to have a baby, a medication called Clomid is usually prescribed.

Several problems with the ovaries can also cause periods to stop. To check the ovaries, your doctor may ask you to begin taking progesterone. If you fail to menstruate after seven days it's an indication of inadequate estrogen levels, a possible pregnancy, or a disruption in the ovarian cycle. The doctor may also study vaginal secretions, which can show whether the ovaries are wasting away, hardened, or are able to function normally. Other tests can tell whether development of the ovaries is normal and whether they are producing estrogen properly.

Often, ovarian cysts are at fault. Together with a thickened endometrium, they are the hallmark of a condition called the Stein-Leventhal syndrome. Women with this problem fail to menstruate, may fail to ovulate (or ovulate only occasionally), have a great deal of facial and/or body hair, and may have episodes of heavy bleeding between bouts of amenorrhea. Many of these women have increased levels of testosterone, a male sex hormone normally present in small quantities in the female as well.

To diagnose the problem, the doctor will determine the levels of androgen and estrogen through laboratory tests. He or she will also examine the pelvic area to see whether the ovaries are enlarged due to the presence of cysts.

If the doctor finds a number of cysts, and you do not want to become pregnant, he or she will prescribe Provera, or birth control pills to cause the endometrium to shed. A combination of estrogen and progesterone will suppress ovarian function, and thus decrease the risk of cancer of the endometrium. If you want to conceive, the doctor may give you Clomid or Pergonal to induce ovulation.

Problems in the uterus and fallopian tubes may be to blame for amenorrhea. In some cases the lining of the uterus continues to grow unchecked for many weeks or years. Women with this condition may have one or two months without a period preceded and followed by excessive bleeding. A D&C

(scraping of the uterus) and biopsy of the lining may be necessary for diagnosis. To treat the problem, the doctor will prescribe Provera or estrogen-progesterone therapy.

Malfunctioning adrenal glands that secrete excessively high or low levels of adrenal hormone can also lead to amenorrhea. Tumors, steriod therapy, and even weight loss can all affect adrenal performance. Prednisone, dexamethasone, and hydrocortisone can often clear up the problem. Girls who are born with malfunctioning adrenals must have lifelong treatment. In most other cases, the condition clears up and treatment can be discontinued after several months.

Other glandular disorders can also be at fault. Cysts, tumors, serious infection, and eating disorders can disrupt the pituitary gland and lead to amenorrhea.

Overactivity or underactivity of the thyroid gland can cause the problem, too. To correct specific glandular imbalances, there are a number of medications your doctor can prescribe.

Anorexia nervosa, the loss of more than 25 percent of one's ideal body weight, is another potential cause of amenorrhea—as well as other serious physical and emotional problems. Almost all anorexic women stop menstruating, and many have glandular disorders leading to low levels of estrogen. If anorexia is the culprit, you'll need treatment for the underlying problem as well as the lack of periods.

Breastfeeding women may fail to menstruate for 10 or more months. Their high levels of prolactin, a hormone necessary to produce breast milk, may suppress the hormones that trigger the menstrual cycle. Since ovulation is still a possibility, all breastfeeding women should use "barrier" birth control such as a diaphragm or vaginal sponge if they want to prevent conception.

There is no substantial proof that either prolonged use of an oral contraceptive (the "Pill,") or use at an early age causes amenorrhea. Close to 95 percent of nonmenstruating users of oral contraceptives resume normal cycles spontaneously after discontinuing the medication. The one percent who fail to menstruate for more than six months after stopping the pill generally have a glandular or ovarian disorders.

Some women stop menstruating permanently before they reach the age of 35 and begin to experience the typical symptoms of menopause. Their ovaries secrete insufficient estrogen to maintain the menstrual cycle and become small and wasted away. There is no effective treatment for this condition. Progesterone will not cause a return of menstruation, and in all but a few instances, drug therapy will not restart ovulation.

Early Menstruation

Although the average age for the beginning of menstruation is between 11 and 13, a few girls develop breasts before they are eight or have their first period by nine. This condition is called **precocious puberty.**

About 90 percent of girls who menstruate early have "true" precocious puberty, that is, their reproductive system functions exactly like that of an adult. These youngsters secrete the hormones necessary for menstruation. They ovulate, are fertile, and have secondary sex characteristics. Most become short women because their higher-than-normal estrogen level stops their growth at an early age. The underlying cause is an abnormality in the brain.

Girls with "pseudo" precocious puberty do have increased estrogen levels, but do not produce the other reproductive hormones as adults do. Because of the increased estrogen, they develop secondary sex characteristics, but they are not fertile. Causes range from ovarian or adrenal tumors that produce estrogen, to an underactive thyroid, or use of certian cosmetics and estrogen-containing foods and medications.

To make a diagnosis, the doctor will check estrogen levels, inquire about birth injuries or a family history of brain disease and perform various other tests. Treatment focuses on medications which prevent the release of reproductive hormones such as GnRH. Injections of the birth-control drug Depo-Provera reduce the amount of estrogen, stop menstruation, decrease breast development, and allow growth to develop normally. However, its long-term effects may be serious. Girls who menstruate early may also need psychological counseling.

Toxic Shock Syndrome

In 1978 medical journals reported that a small number of menstruating women were developing an illness characterized by high fever, sore throat, headache, a sunburn-like rash, vomiting, nausea, diarrhea, extremely low blood pressure, fainting, peeling skin, muscle pain, kidney or liver problems, disorientation, and even shock. They named the new disease "toxic shock syndrome" (TSS).

By 1980 they had pinpointed the major culprit: superabsorbent tampons—although in a few cases, staph infection following an injury, or trauma was given the blame.

TSS is caused by toxin-producing staphylococcus bacteria. According to one theory, inserting a tampon into the vagina can produce small tears or ulcerations that allow the bacteria to enter the rest of the body. A second theory holds that extra-large tampons contain more air spaces than small sizes, and that these pockets provide the oxygen that the bacteria need to multiply.

If you suspect you are developing TSS, you should remove your tampon immediately. In eight out of ten tampon-related cases, this will stop the growth of the bacteria. Your doctor will check for the presence of staph by testing blood samples and vaginal and cervical smears. If the bacteria are at fault, antibiotics such as erythromycin will usually clear up the problem.

Superabsorbant tampons such as Rely were taken off the market soon after they were implicated in toxic shock syndrome. Since then, the number of cases has dropped dramatically. However, it's still wise to change tampons frequently, alternate tampons with sanitary napkins, especially at night, and wash your hands before inserting a tampon.

Exercise And Menstrual Problems

Controversy surrounds the role of exercise in the development of menstrual problems. Researchers have noted that more female athletes have amenorrhea, prolonged cycles, or delayed menstrual onset than do other women, but there is no general agreement on the reasons.

According to one theory, the lack of menstruation among athletic women stems from loss of weight and body fat. Glandular problems have also been blamed. Low estrogen levels, vitamin deficiency, and the stress of rigorous training and competition are other proposed causes.

On the positive side, many athletes do have regular menstrual cycles—and they have milder cramps, less PMS, shorter-lasting periods, and fewer headaches than their sedentary sisters. On balance, most doctors recommend regular, reasonable exercise. □

CHAPTER 3　　　　**COMMON DISORDERS OF THE REPRODUCTIVE SYSTEM**

PMS: Sorting Fact from Fiction

There is probably not a woman in the country who does not know what the initials PMS stand for; and few are the women who have been completely spared the physical and behavioral changes that characterize Premenstrual Syndrome (PMS). Estimates of the number of women affected by PMS vary widely. The American College of Obstetricians and Gynecologists suggests that 20 percent to 40 percent of women experience some premenstrual difficulties, with 5 percent affected significantly. Some medical experts maintain that up to 90 percent of American women experience one or more symptoms. Whatever the actual figures, women and their doctors agree that PMS is real.

PMS symptoms can begin anytime after ovulation, which occurs approximately 2 weeks before the start of your period. During the last three to 14 days of your cycle, you may notice a variety of changes in your body or disposition that can cause some degree of distress. These include:

- swelling and tenderness in the breasts;
- a "bloated" feeling or temporary weight gain of a few pounds;
- skin blemishes or acne;
- swelling of hands and feet;
- headaches;
- nausea or constipation, followed by diarrhea at the onset of menstruation;
- increased thirst or appetite;
- a craving for certain foods—especially sweets and items high in salt;
- increased irritability or mood swings;
- insomnia or fatigue;
- forgetfulness or confusion;
- feelings of anxiety or loss of control;
- sadness or uncontrolled crying.

Overall, more than 150 physical and behavioral symptoms have been associated with PMS. This complicates diagnosis and makes it difficult to classify the condition as a specific disease. And the mild premenstrual changes that many women experience have added to the confusion over PMS. Multiple severe symptoms that persist over a period of days, month after month, are more likely to be recognized as PMS than a single symptom or infrequent complaints. In addition, because the variety of symptoms and their causes are not well understood, doctors have no reliable method to determine who is susceptible to PMS, and why.

Unrelated medical problems can also mimic PMS and mislead you and your doctor. These include:

- fibrocystic breast changes, in which noncancerous lumps in the breast become swollen and painful;
- endometriosis, in which tissue from the lining of the uterus can cause pain elsewhere in the lower abdomen;
- unrecognized pelvic infections such as chlamydia;
- dysmenorrhea, or painful menstrual cramps, that can also prompt nausea and diarrhea;
- diabetes, which can cause excessive thirst or hunger;
- endocrine disorders such as an overactive thyroid;
- emotional disorders, which can be confused with the mood changes of PMS;
- allergies.

In recent years, PMS has generated a great deal of controversy in the media. While some physicians and researchers have portrayed nearly all women as suffering from PMS, generally the medical community acknowledges a significant difference between the more serious "syndrome" and the PMS "symptoms" experienced by many women.

Unfortunately, the politics of the debate have deflected attention from the very real difficulties caused by PMS. While some of the outbursts attributed to PMS have been casually dismissed as "raging hormones," family, social, and work relationships may, indeed,

suffer when a woman experiences the physical discomfort and emotional peaks and valleys of PMS. Truly violent tendencies, however, are usually caused by psychological or medical problems completely unrelated to PMS.

In fact, the most convincing evidence of PMS is its cyclical nature. All symptoms—both physical and behavioral—should disappear rapidly once menstruation begins. If physical changes continue for more than a few weeks or fail to subside once your period begins, it's important to contact your doctor to rule out other possible medical causes. Likewise, if you feel depressed premenstrually and your mood doesn't lift when your period starts, you should bring this to your doctor's attention.

No Explanation Yet

The term premenstrual syndrome was coined in 1931, when researchers first suggested that the condition was due to a hormonal imbalance related to the menstrual cycle. More recent studies have documented that PMS does, in fact, occur only during the childbearing years between puberty and menopause and subsides during pregnancy. PMS can also affect women who have had their uterus removed leading researchers to conclude that the uterus is not part of the problem.

Despite these clues and the recognition of PMS as a legitimate medical concern, researchers have been unable to find a cause. Even today, no one knows for certain what triggers PMS, though a number of theories have been advanced.

Much of the research has focused on the hormones estrogen and progesterone, which are produced by the ovaries and are known to interact with certain brain chemicals. At about day 5 of the menstrual cycle, estrogen signals the lining of the uterus to grow and thicken, in preparation for receipt of a fertilized egg. Once an egg is released from one of the ovaries at mid-cycle, about day 14 of a 28-day cycle, progesterone production begins, causing the release of nutrients and the swelling of blood vessels to prepare for pregnancy. If the egg is not fertilized, the uterine lining and the egg are shed in menstruation.

Thus, estrogen, which interacts with important brain chemicals affecting your mood and energy, dominates the first half of the menstrual cycle, while progesterone, which tends to suppress the actions of these brain chemicals, is more prevalent during the second half.

Despite this, levels of the hormones themselves appear to be normal in women with PMS. To confound the issue further, one major study found that women with PMS continued to show symptoms even after their menstrual cycles were artificially "reset" with medication. Researchers are studying the possibility that some unknown outside factor

THE PROGESTERONE CONNECTION

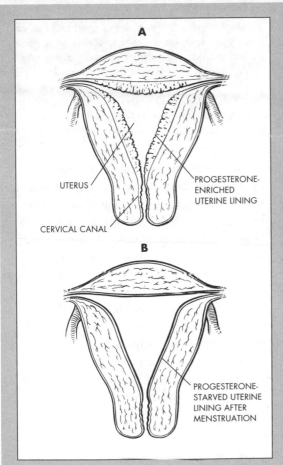

A

UTERUS

PROGESTERONE-
ENRICHED
UTERINE LINING

CERVICAL CANAL

B

PROGESTERONE-
STARVED UTERINE
LINING AFTER
MENSTRUATION

PMS coincides with the final enrichment of the uterine lining in preparation for arrival of a fertilized egg (see "A" at left). Not coincidentally, this phase of the lining's growth depends on increased levels of the hormone progesterone, which begins to appear as soon as an ovary releases its egg.

In addition to its effect on the uterus, the extra progesterone is thought to have a damping effect on certain chemicals in the brain, possibly accounting for the agitation and mood swings that often accompany PMS. But the connection--if there is one--is still far from clear. Many doctors find that additional progestrone, taken as a daily shot or suppository, helps to reduce symptoms of PMS.

Whatever the truth of the matter, this much is certain: If conception fails to occur, progestrone levels decline precipitously, and the hormone-starved uterine lining sloughs off in the monthly menstrual flow. During the following 2 weeks, when progesterone levels are low and the lining is relatively lean (see "B" at left), PMS symptoms generally abate.

disrupts the normal interaction of estrogen and progesterone with chemicals made in the brain to cause some PMS symptoms.

One theory links fluctuations in the levels of serotonin with PMS. Serotonin (a byproduct of L-tryptophan, an essential amino acid found in many foods) plays several important roles in the body: it helps regulate sleep and menstrual cycles as well as the appetite. Some researchers speculate that low levels of serotonin may underlie PMS, throwing off the delicate timing of ovulation and prompting the restlessness and food cravings so often experienced by women with PMS.

Other theories proposed by researchers include: a deficiency of endorphins, the chemicals in the brain that create a "natural high"; defects in the metabolism of glucose or vitamin B_6; low concentrations of zinc in the blood; fluctuations in prostaglandins, a family of hormone-like compounds found in most body tissue; low magnesium levels; an imbalance in the body's level of acidity; and chronic candidiasis, a vaginal yeast infection.

As of yet, there is no conclusive evidence to support any of these theories, making a definitive cure difficult, if not impossible. But research has shown that PMS responds well to a variety of treatments and that most women can minimize its effects by understanding and carefully managing their symptoms.

Deciding Whether You Have It

The first step toward effective treatment is to confirm that your symptoms actually are caused by PMS. This is usually done by process of elimination, as there are no reliable tests to diagnose the condition.

Your doctor may first recommend some simple laboratory tests, such as blood tests or urinalysis, to rule out other conditions with

COLLECTING THE EVIDENCE

Mark your calendar on the day your period starts as Day 1. Number each subsequent day and use a letter code such as "A" for anger, "B" for breast tenderness, "C" for cravings, or "F" for fatigue to record any symptoms on the days they occur. You can use capital letters if the symptoms are severe and small letters if they're moderate, or use letters in combination with a rating scale of 1 to 10 to indicate mild to severe. Additional details to record include your daily weight and, to pinpoint when ovulation occurs, your basal temperature, taken after you wake up but before you get out of bed. Your local pharmacy should stock a basal thermometer.

Alternatively, design a simple chart that lists all of your symptoms down one side of a page and the days of your menstrual period across the top. Fill in the boxes that correspond with a given symptom and the day of your cycle in which it occurs. On days that you experience only mild symptoms, color in half the box.

similar symptoms, particularly diabetes or thyroid problems. If you regularly experience pelvic pain, your doctor may check for the presence of sexually transmitted diseases such as gonorrhea or chlamydia. You should also receive a thorough physical examination, including breast and pelvic exams, to rule out other undiagnosed medical conditions.

The next step in establishing a diagnosis is to record your symptoms over a period of time to verify their appearance, severity, and duration. In fact, the only way PMS can be accurately diagnosed is by keeping a careful record of when each symptom appears each month. Simple record-keeping can be done with an ordinary calendar. See the nearby box on "Collecting the Evidence" for two methods.

It also helps to keep a diary that describes not only your symptoms but also their effect on your daily activities. Feelings of social withdrawal, outbursts at family members or co-workers, or difficulties in coping can be more thoroughly described in such a journal.

It's important to maintain your records for at least three menstrual cycles. Record your entries every day, while the symptoms and their effects are fresh in your mind. You and your doctor can then review the charts and journal to help determine whether you have PMS and the extent to which it affects your life.

Simple Steps
You Can Take Yourself

After you've been able to document the cyclical nature of your symptoms and their severity, you and your doctor can develop a treatment plan. Your doctor may first recommend simple lifestyle changes, since PMS often responds remarkably well to modifications in eating habits, stress management, and increased amounts of sleep or exercise.

Caffeine is a major culprit of PMS symptoms. Found in a variety of substances—coffee, tea, soft drinks, chocolate and some over-the counter medications—caffeine is a stimulant that is often consumed precisely for the "lift" it provides. Nevertheless, caffeine can exaggerate PMS-related problems such as anxiety, insomnia, nervousness, and irritability, and it can interfere with carbohydrate metabolism by depleting your body of vitamin B. Reducing your caffeine intake is a smart move to counteract PMS symptoms and can provide almost instant relief. In fact, some doctors routinely advise eliminating

caffeine from the diet before every menstrual period as a first step in coping with PMS.

Many women with PMS gain several pounds during the two weeks preceding their period, much of this in fluid weight. Avoiding salty foods can dramatically reduce bloating and water buildup, resulting in less breast and abdominal tenderness and less swelling in the hands and feet. Since brain cells also have a tendency to retain fluid, you may find that a salt-free diet eliminates or curbs headaches and allows you to concentrate better.

Sugar can also play havoc on your body, especially in the days preceding your period.

PMS OR PMDD?

PMS has been linked to serious psychological problems in a small group of women. In Great Britain, women have been acquitted of various crimes on the grounds that the PMS from which they were suffering at the time of their action caused a temporary psychiatric disturbance. Though PMS is not recognized as a valid legal defense in the United States, the American Psychiatric Association (APA) recently recognized the possible psychiatric implications of PMS when it classified the related Premenstrual Dysphoric Disorder (PMDD) as a "depressive disorder not otherwise specified," and included it in the appendix of the APA's *Diagnostic and Statistical Manual of Mental Disorders,* or DSM-IV.

PMDD, which is thought to affect fewer than 5 percent of menstruating women, is described by the APA as a pattern of severe, recurrent symptoms of depression and other negative moods that occur during the last week of the menstrual cycle and markedly interfere with daily living. While PMDD is not an official diagnostic category, the APA hopes its inclusion in DSM-IV will encourage further psychiatric research into the condition. (See "Spelling out PMDD.")

Eating sugary foods often initiates a vicious cycle of additional sugar cravings, as an increase in your body's need for B-complex vitamins prompts even more craving for sugar-laden simple carbohydrates. Although a link between PMS and difficulties in metabolizing sugar has not been proven, consuming sweets can put your body on a roller coaster between feeling weak and feeling high strung and jittery—your body's response to low sugar levels at one extreme, and elevated sugar levels at the other.

Nicotine, a brain stimulant, can magnify PMS symptoms much like caffeine, so reducing or eliminating smoking should be part of any treatment program. Alcohol can also intensify symptoms because it depletes the body of vitamin B, disrupts the metabolism of carbohydrates, and affects the liver's ability to process hormones.

Some foods may genuinely relieve PMS symptoms. Complex carbohydrates such as whole grains, beans, fresh fruits, and vegetables help to maintain your body's essential vitamins and minerals. Eating a low-fat diet based on grains and vegetables while reducing your intake of red meat—especially during the two weeks prior to the beginning of your period—may help to control your PMS symptoms. And at least one study has suggested that a modest increase in calcium, to 1,300 milligrams per day, may reduce irritability and physical symptoms such as backaches.

Many women also find that exercise produces positive benefits in moderating PMS symptoms, while improving their general health. Consider a monthly workout plan that rotates activities designed to strengthen your muscles, reduce fat, and relieve tension. Vigorous exercise—running, biking, swimming, aerobics, racquet sports and the like—has been shown to elevate your mood and improve alertness, while calisthenics and body-building tone muscles and improve strength. Contrary to popular belief, exercise helps to control—not increase—your appetite.

With your doctor's approval, try a program that mixes more vigorous cardiovascular exercises during the early days of your menstrual cycle with stretching, flexibility exercises, and less vigorous cardiovascular work such as walking on the days when you're most prone to PMS symptoms. This regimen can increase your heart-lung capacity and improve your overall physical condition while reducing the strain on your breasts, thighs, and abdomen during the latter phase of your cycle.

PMS is also associated with disruptions in a woman's normal sleep patterns. Women with moderate to severe PMS symptoms are more likely to complain of insomnia and are known to spend less time in deep sleep than those who are symptom-free. Reducing caffeine intake can help. You may also benefit from short naps on certain days. In any event, try to get at least eight hours of uninterrupted sleep each night, especially during the latter half of your cycle.

You may also benefit from some stress management techniques. Unlike diet, exercise, and sleep, outside stress is the one factor of daily life that no one can control. How you approach and handle stress, however, can have a tremendous impact on your behavior and mood.

The causes of stress can be physical, such as chronic or episodic illness or injury; psychological, such as fears, anxieties, or frustrations; and social, such as crying children, rush-hour traffic, and even holiday preparations. These everyday aggravations are particularly annoying during the days you're experiencing PMS symptoms.

A stress management class can help you channel the tension caused by stress so you are less likely to lose control, a common complaint of women with PMS. Whether they emphasize breathing exercises, visualization, biofeedback, or other stress management techniques, a common theme is to help you maintain a positive attitude and develop realistic expectations.

How much improvement you can expect from these remedies—and how quickly—depends largely on your commitment to them and your willingness to change your habits. You may notice dramatic improvements almost immediately, or gradual improvement over several menstrual cycles. As you continue to record your symptoms, you may observe that more sleep or a brisk walk helps during certain premenstrual days, while modifying your diet helps during others. The bottom line is to focus on continual improvement rather than dwell on the symptoms.

Even though you can make many of these lifestyle and dietary changes without seeing a physician, it's better to enlist your doctor's expertise in developing a program tailored to your particular PMS symptoms and other health factors. Since no single treatment is uniformly effective for PMS, you can benefit from your physician's experience with other women who are successfully managing their condition.

Available Medical Treatments

Lifestyle and dietary changes generally provide some degree of relief to all women who experience PMS-related distress. If your condition improves only modestly, however, your doctor may suggest a medical approach. Since there are many claims made for the benefits offered by vitamins, food supplements, and some over-the-counter medications, *you should not use any of them without consulting your physician.* It is important to remember that while some physicians support the use of certain vitamins and supplements and believe in their possible effectiveness, others cite the lack of scientific evidence of any benefit, and warn of possible harm if the products are consumed in large doses. Among the many "PMS formulas" on the market are a number of multivitamins containing some combination of vitamin B_6, magnesium, zinc, and vitamin A. The use of vitamin B_6 for PMS dates back to the 1940s. For those who believe in its effectiveness, the connection is thought to be in the vitamin's interaction with certain brain chemicals. However, its effectiveness has not been clinically proven and large amounts have been shown to be harmful. As little as 200 to 300 milligrams a day has been reported to cause toxic reactions resulting in pain or numbness in the hands or feet, awkwardness in walking or general clumsiness and nerve damage.

Some physicians have claimed that oil of evening primrose (Efamol), which contains linoleic acid and gamma-linoleic acid, helps relieve breast tenderness. However, this finding has not been confirmed in scientific studies; and the U.S. Food and Drug Administration has not approved the product as a food additive. Nevertheless, it remains widely available through health food stores and mail-order houses.

The benefits of some vitamins and food supplements, though still unproven, seem a bit more promising. In one study, vitamin E in dosages of 150 to 300 milligrams daily was reported to reduce PMS symptoms. Another study suggested that magnesium supplements may counter some of the behavioral changes associated with PMS, though magnesium can also be toxic in high doses and can impair calcium absorption. Finally, the amino acid L-tryptophan, classified as a food supplement and sold over the counter, has seemed to help some women. It may raise the serotonin level, allowing for a more restful sleep and reducing restlessness and food cravings.

Your physician may also choose from an array of prescription medications, though no "PMS drug" has yet been developed, and the effectiveness of pharmaceuticals in treating PMS has generated considerable debate. In fact, some of the medications used for PMS are potentially harmful, so you and your doctor should plan a conservative course of symptom management rather than generalized drug therapy.

Diuretics, or "water pills," help the body eliminate excess fluid through the kidneys. Your doctor may prescribe a diuretic to reduce bloating if restricting your salt intake does not help. Although studies on the benefits of diuretics for PMS have shown mixed results, they have been used longer in PMS treatment than any other medication, and have been shown to ease other symptoms, such as fatigue and depression.

Because it inhibits the action of the hormone that causes water retention, spironolactone (Aldactone) is also selected to treat PMS symptoms. Physicians typically prescribe 25 milligrams of spironolactone four times a day from the time of ovulation to the onset of menstruation.

Bromocriptine (Parlodel), a drug that suppresses lactation after childbirth, is some-times used to reduce PMS-related breast discomfort, though there is no evidence that women taking this medication show greater improvement than those who don't. The usual dosage is 2.5 milligrams once or twice daily from the date of ovulation until your period begins. Because there is a risk of side effects, your doctor will probably start this drug cautiously at low doses.

Mefenamic acid (Ponstel) is a nonsteroidal, anti-inflammatory drug that is sometimes used to relieve premenstrual pain. The usual starting dose is 500 milligrams when symptoms appear, followed by 250 milligrams twice a day for two to three days. A major risk with this medication is its uncertain effect on a developing baby. Since PMS follows ovulation, you may not know you are pregnant until your period is late. Therefore, your physician may advise you to use a barrier contraceptive before prescribing mefenamic acid or other medications used to treat PMS symptoms. A variety of nonsterodial anti-inflammatory drugs are available, including such over-the-counter products as ibuprofen (Advil, Motrin). However, all carry a risk of stomach inflammation with habitual use.

Progesterone therapy has also gained many advocates, despite the fact that neither natural progesterone or synthetic progestins has been shown to be effective in scientific studies. In fact, the use of progesterone to treat PMS has not been approved by the FDA, and some scientists question the long-term safety and consequences of this therapy. Nevertheless, because some physicians claim

SPELLING OUT PMDD

Listed below are the official criteria for a diagnosis of "premenstrual depression." "Luteal phase" refers to the second half of the menstrual cycle, following release of an egg. "Follicular phase" refers to the first half of the cycle. "Dysphoric" is medical jargon meaning "unhappy."

Criteria for Late Luteal Phase Dysphoric Disorder

A. In most menstrual cycles during the past year, symptoms in B occurred during the last week of the luteal phase and remitted within a few days after onset of the follicular phase. In menstruating females, these phases correspond to the week before, and a few days after, the onset of menses. (In nonmenstruating females who had a hysterectomy, the timing of luteal and follicular phases may require measurement of circulating reproductive hormones.)

B. At least 5 of the following symptoms have been present for most of the time during each symptomatic late luteal phase, at least one of the symptoms being 1, 2, 3 or 4:

1. Marked affective lability, e.g., feeling suddenly sad, tearful, irritable, or angry.
2. Persistent and marked anger or irritability.
3. Marked anxiety, tension, feelings of being "keyed up" or "on edge."
4. Markedly depressed mood, feelings of hopelessness, or self-deprecating thoughts.
5. Decreased interest in usual activities, e.g., work, friends, hobbies.
6. Easy fatigability or marked lack of energy.
7. Subjective sense of difficulty in concentrating.
8. Marked change in appetite, overeating, or specific food cravings.
9. Hypersomnia or insomnia.
10. Other physical symptoms, such as breast tenderness or swelling, headaches, joint or muscle pain, a sensation of "bloating," weight gain.

C. The disturbance seriously interferes with work or with usual social activities or relationships with others.

D. The disturbance is not merely an exacerbation of the symptoms of another disorder, such as major depression, panic disorder, dysthymia (chronic mild depression), or a personality disorder (although it may be superimposed on any of these disorders).

E. Criteria A, B, C, and D are confirmed by prospective daily self-ratings during at least two symptomatic cycles. (This diagnosis may be made provisionally prior to this confirmation.)

Source: *American Psychiatric Association,* Washington, DC.

to have seen improvements in their own patients, the use of progesterone to treat PMS symptoms remains common. According to the American College of Obstetricians and Gynecologists, the standard dosage for treating PMS is 50 to 100 milligrams of progesterone administered daily by intramuscular injections or 200 to 400 milligrams twice a day by vaginal or rectal suppositories. Treatment is started several days before symptoms are expected and is continued through the onset of a woman's period.

A few studies indicate that medicines used to block ovarian function, known as "medical ovariectomy," can halt the symptoms of PMS. In clinical trials, this has been accomplished by using Lupron as an injection or Synarel as a nasal spray to block the action of GnRH, the hormone that starts the menstrual cycle with stimulation of the ovaries.

However, blocking ovarian function essentially creates an artificial menopause, which can lead to osteoporosis and other post-menopausal medical problems. As a result, this approach is considered only in severe and disabling cases of PMS: the 5 percent to 10 percent of women whose PMS symptoms cause incapacitating disruptions to their jobs or family life. Therapy is generally discontinued after six months.

Some physicians prescribe tranquilizers or antidepressants, including fluoxetine hydrochloride (Prozac) for patients diagnosed with PMS. However, these medications can cause serious, even fatal, reactions in combination with other drugs and can lead to a wide range of side effects. They are generally reserved for serious illnesses such as major depression; and you should question any PMS treatment plan that seems to rely on these types of drugs without evidence of an underlyng emotinal disorder.

Other Treatment Approaches

Nontraditional approaches to PMS treatment, such as acupuncture, chiropractic adjustment, and therapeutic massage have, in the past, been ignored by the medical community although this is slowly changing. Some women experience symptom relief, although no studies have documented the effectiveness of nontraditional approaches and any benefits are considered speculative.

On the other hand, many women unquestionably benefit from joining a PMS support group. This can be particularly helpful when you are trying to modify certain behaviors, such as dietary habits. Meeting and talking with other women who share the condition, and having access to current PMS research are important benefits of support groups, as are the empathy and reassurance.

It's also possible that even the most classic cycle of PMS symptoms is masking an unrelated psychological or psychiatric problem. A skilled therapist can help uncover the presence of any hidden conditions. In general, psychotherapy can also help a woman explore the specific emotional issues that affect her premenstrually and learn healthy ways to express anger and frustration—common manifestations of PMS.

In any event, it's important to collaborate with your doctor while finding a treatment that works for you. Remember that even with your doctor's help, you may have to try several different approaches before you find relief. Keep charting your symptoms and remember that no single treatment for PMS is a one-step or permanent cure. If after a month or two of treatment, there is no change in your symptoms, you and your doctor can modify your action plan.

Taking Control

If left undiagnosed or untreated, PMS can have a major impact on a woman's life. Whether at home or on the job, you may have to struggle to function normally when symptoms occur. Emotional distress caused by PMS may trigger marital or family conflicts. You may feel an increased desire for intimacy with your partner yet feel sexually unattractive. You may even notice that PMS prompts you to withdraw socially.

Recognizing these changes in your body and mood and planning strategies to accomodate them is half the battle. The more you understand yourself and your monthly menstrual cycle, the better you can manage your PMS symptoms.

Follow your treatment program faithfully and learn to communicate your feelings with others. On the days you feel most anxious or tired, enlist the help of family members to prepare meals or run errands so you can reduce the pressure on yourself. While the goal of PMS management is to maintain a normal lifestyle even during your most difficult days, don't create needlessly difficult targets for yourself by adopting the standards of a superhero.

Many women find that there are days when PMS interferes with productivity or relationships at work. Though some physicians still advocate avoiding or postponing extra tasks on days when PMS symptoms are the most challenging, many women find that taking charge of their health and moving forward with planned schedules and tasks helps them get through their PMS symptons. As you undertake some of the strategies in this chapter and reduce the overall impact of PMS on your life, you may discover that your job, too, seems more manageable.

Although much work remains to be done before PMS is fully understood, the good news is that millions of women successfully manage their homes, jobs, academic pursuits, and creative endeavors at every phase of their menstrual cycle. Until the cause of PMS is finally established and a standardized treatment is developed, your best tactic is to understand your own PMS symptoms and take the initiative to control them. □

Curing Vaginal Infections

If you've ever been troubled with inflammation and infection of the vulva and vagina, you are far from alone. This problem, known as *vulvovaginitis,* is the most common gynecological disorder in the United States today. Fortunately, vulvovaginitis, while uncomfortable, is essentially harmless and usually responds promptly to simple treatment. Its symptoms include itching, irritation, or pain in the external genital area (the vulva) and pain in the vagina during intercourse. The vaginal discharge is often heavier than usual. It is frequently discolored (yellow, gray, or greenish), and may have an unpleasant odor.

Healthy vaginal discharge is made up of aging cells cast off from your vaginal walls, secretions from the cervix that help protect your uterus from infection and aid in fertility, and chemicals produced by vaginal bacteria and fungi ("yeasts"). Normally the discharge has no odor.

Some changes in vaginal discharge are normal, and bear no relation to a possible infection. These changes are governed by your menstrual cycle and the shifting hormonal patterns of puberty and menopause.

Relatively high levels of sexual hormones are necessary to produce vaginal discharge. So, during both childhood and menopause when hormone levels are low, discharge is minimal. Because girls have little or no vaginal secretion before puberty, parents who note a discharge in their child's diaper or underwear should consult a pediatrician.

During the reproductive years, your discharge changes in response to your monthly cycle. As your hormone levels drop after a menstrual period, the discharge becomes light. Then, as new eggs begin to develop in your ovaries, estrogen and progesterone levels increase, stimulating production of a white, milky or creamy discharge. At ovulation (approximately two weeks before your next menstrual period), this discharge changes abruptly and dramatically, becoming transparent and stretchy rather like egg white. This "fertile mucus" announces peak fertility of your monthly cycle. Fertile mucus generally lasts for only a day or two. Your

VULVOVAGINITIS: THE BASIC ANATOMY

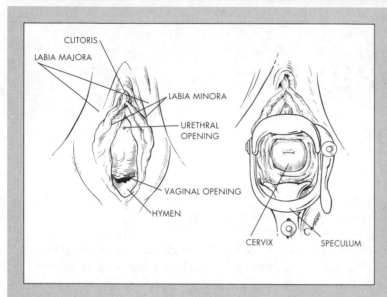

CLITORIS
LABIA MAJORA
LABIA MINORA
URETHRAL OPENING
VAGINAL OPENING
HYMEN
CERVIX
SPECULUM

When your doctor checks for possible infection, he or she will examine the whole genital area, including the vulva (bounded by the labia majora and minora, or outer and inner lips, enfolding the urinary and vaginal openings), the vagina itself, and the cervix (shown here with the aid of a speculum, an instrument used to dilate the vaginal walls). If the problem is bacterial vaginosis, there may be little visible evidence of infection. If yeast has taken hold, the vulva may be red and inflamed. When "trich" is the culprit, the vulva is sometimes swollen.

discharge then turns white and creamy again and may be slightly heavier than earlier in the cycle. With your next menstrual period, the entire process begins once more.

Best Ways to Fend Off Infection

The healthy vagina is home to a variety of microscopic organisms. Normally they live harmoniously in an acidic environment that prevents the overproduction of any one species and repels foreign invaders.

A number of factors can upset this balance: sexually transmitted disease organisms, pregnancy, menopause, certain medications, chronic illness, excessive douching, severe emotional stress, and clothing that holds in body heat and moisture. Diet may also play a significant role.

The best way to prevent vaginal infection is to take good care of yourself. Be sure to eat a healthy, varied diet and maintain your proper weight. Alleviate stress through exercise, meditation, and other tension-relieving activities. Be sure your clothing "breathes;" avoid tight garments and fabrics containing a high percentage of synthetic fiber. Use condoms and a spermicide to prevent sexually transmitted infections.

Odor-producing bacteria can thrive on the vulva and must be cleaned off. Most women find that washing the genital area daily with a simple, fragrance-free soap keeps them feeling fresh. Heavier women, frequent exercisers, and those who wear pantyhose may need to wash more often to keep the number of vulvar bacteria low.

Since your vagina is essentially self-cleaning, douching is unnecessary. Never douche more than once or twice monthly, and use plain water or a water and vinegar mixture when you do. Feminine hygiene sprays are both a waste of money and a source of skin irritation; healthy vaginal discharge has no unpleasant odor. However, tampons and diaphragms left too long in the vagina can create a terrible smell. If this happens, simply remove the forgotten object, douche once with vinegar and water or Betadine solution (both are available without prescription), and save yourself a trip to the gynecologist!

When You Turn to a Doctor

When you do visit a gynecologist, the doctor will need to know your "history" in order to make a diagnosis and prescribe treatment. Report all of your symptoms. Try to recall when you first noted them. Be frank about new sexual partners, sexual practices, or suspected infidelity by your partner. Physicians know that this information is personal and sensitive and will keep everything you tell them confidential.

The doctor will examine the skin of your vulva, vagina, and cervix for signs of infection; check the appearance of your vaginal discharge; and note any tenderness in your uterus and ovaries. (In simple vulvovaginitis, there is usually no tenderness.)

Your vaginal discharge can be examined microscopically right in the doctor's office. If cultures are necessary, a medical laboratory can usually perform the necessary tests and return the results to the doctor within 48 hours. Most of these procedures are completely painless; the worst of them is only mildly uncomfortable.

Treating Bacterial Vaginosis

Despite the fact that bacterial vaginosis (known as BV) accounts for 40 percent of all vaginitis-related office visits, this common disorder is still not well understood. Indeed, as researchers have attempted to sort out the causes, it has been renamed several times. Originally called "non-specific vaginitis," it was later redubbed "*Haemophilus vaginalis vaginitis*" and then "*Gardnerella vaginalis vaginitis.*"

For most women, BV is more a nuisance than a significant health threat. However, there is some evidence linking it to an increased risk of pelvic inflammatory disease (a bacterial infection of the uterus, fallopian tubes, and ovaries). In pregnancy, BV appears to markedly increase the risk of premature rupture of the membranes (bag of waters) and premature birth. Most doctors now routinely test and treat pregnant women for this vaginal infection.

The most common symptom of BV is a thin, white/gray vaginal discharge with an unmistakable, offensive "fishy" odor. Because the odor is strongest when the discharge is exposed to an alkaline substance such as soap or semen, it may be most apparent in the shower or after intercourse. Itching and irritation are absent or mild.

BV is so common that many people wrongly believe vaginal odor to be normal in adult women. This misunderstanding has given rise to a host of "put-down" jokes and has inspired the manufacture of many useless "feminine hygiene products."

One of the major players in BV is the bacteria *Gardnerella vaginalis*. This organism appears to be present in 30 to 40 percent of all women. But in order to cause infection, it must interact with at least three other bacteria, and the entire group must proliferate sufficiently to wipe out healthy organisms such as the *Lactobacillus*. Although we do not yet know the cause of this burst of growth,

YEAST INFECTIONS: YOUR TREATMENT ALTERNATIVES

Medication	Dosage
Femstat Cream	5 grams in the vagina every night for 3 days
Gyne-Lotrimin	One 100 milligram vaginal tablet every day for 7 days
Mycelex-G	One 500 milligram vaginal tablet 1 time, or 5 grams of vaginal cream every day for 7 to 14 days
Monistat	One Monistat 7 vaginal suppository every night for 7 days, or One Monistat 3 vaginal suppository every night for 3 days, or 5 grams of Monistat 7 vaginal cream every night for 7 days
Nizoral	One 200-milligram tablet taken orally once or twice daily for 7 to 14 days
Mycostatin	1 vaginal tablet every day for 7 to 14 days, or 1 gram of cream twice daily for 7 to 14 days
Terazol	1 vaginal suppository every night for 3 days, or 5 grams of Terazol 3 Cream in the vagina every night for 3 days, or 5 grams of Terazol 7 Cream in the vagina every night for 7 days
Boric Acid	One 600-milligram vaginal capsule every day for 14 days

researchers suspect it has something to do with sexual intercourse.

When BV is suspected, your doctor will take your history, examine your pelvic organs, and study a few drops of the your vaginal discharge under the microscope. If the diagnosis is uncertain, or if you are pregnant, a vaginal culture may be necessary.

Treatment involves five to seven days of antibiotics taken orally or inserted in the vagina. Oral metronidazole (Flagyl) is the best known and most effective medication currently prescribed. It is also available in a vaginal gel (Metrogel). If you are allergic to metronidazole or have active liver disease, bleeding or seizure disorders, several other antibiotics work reasonably well.

Most authorities recommend treating a male sexual partner only if the female becomes re-infected after completing her medication and resuming intercourse. Many doctors, however, are now treating couples simultaneously at the outset in order to avoid the need for a second course of antibiotics. There is currently no test available to detect BV in men. Although they may carry the infection, they often show no symptoms. In any case, BV presents no danger to their health. For lesbian couples, a test of the partner is recommended. If she is positive, both women should be treated to avoid reinfection.

Curing Yeast Infections

Although yeast infections are probably the most common type of vulvovaginitis, they rank second in office visits because many women never go to their doctor for this type of infection. Some recover spontaneously, others treat themselves with anti-fungal vaginal creams or suppositories available without prescription.

Classic symptoms of yeast infections include vulvar itching, redness, and irritation. If your urinary opening is inflamed, you may have to urinate somewhat more frequently than usual, and urination may be uncomfortable. If your infection is severe, your vulva may swell and fine breaks, called fissures, may appear. Your vaginal discharge will become thicker, whiter, and curd-like (similar to cottage cheese in texture and appearance). Inflammation of the vulva and vagina, combined with the dryness of your discharge, makes intercourse painful.

Yeast infections are the result of excessive growth of a family of fungi that normally live and thrive in the vagina. The most common of these is *Candida albicans*. Certain factors such as recent use of oral or vaginal antibiotics, clothing (such as nylon and lycra) that traps heat and moisture, obesity, pregnancy, and diabetes tend to disrupt the normal balance of vaginal organisms, causing the fungi to reproduce rapidly and leading to the uncomfortable symptoms we associate with yeast infections. Other possible causes of these infections include suppression of the immune system during such chronic illnesses as AIDS, the use of oral contraceptives, and eating large amounts of sugars, starch, and yeasts.

Because yeasts also normally inhabit the intestine, it's important always to wipe front to back (vaginal area first; rectal area second) after a bowel movement. During sex you must take care to prevent your vagina from becoming contaminated with organisms from your bowel and rectum.

Your chances of catching a yeast infection from a male sexual partner are quite low. The fungus does not fare well on a man's sexual organs, where exposure to the air can dry it out. However, men can develop the disease through frequent sexual contact with an infected female partner. In this case, tiny tender, itchy red bumps appear on the penis. Among lesbian couples, sexual transmission is more common. In all cases, treatment is the same.

To diagnose these infections, the doctor will take a case history, perform a pelvic

ANOTHER POTENTIAL CULPRIT

Not all vaginal irritation is the result of infection. Especially if you've passed menopause, the problem may be a condition called atrophic vaginitis. This disorder results from lack of hormonal stimulation to genital tissue. Deprived of hormones, your vulva and vagina take on a paler, smoother appearance and become drier and more easily injured or irritated by sexual activity. These changes are called "atrophy".

Atrophy occurs normally after menopause due to a fall in hormone production by the ovaries. Breastfeeding and the use of anti-estrogen medications to treat endometriosis, uterine fibroids, and other conditions can also reduce your ovarian activity and result in atrophic changes. Birth control pill users may experience mild atrophic changes, too.

The problem is easily remedied with a good personal lubricant (such as Astroglide, Replens, or KY Lubricating Jelly), and through hormone replacement therapy. For more information turn to the section on menopause.

examination, and examine a few drops of vaginal discharge under the microscope. When the diagnosis is unclear, a vaginal culture may be taken. A good response to an antifungal medication confirms the physician's diagnosis.

If you do have a yeast infection, your doctor will ordinarily treat you with either prescription or nonprescription antifungal vaginal creams and suppositories. These preparations usually provide substantial relief in a few days. You must finish all your medication even if you're feeling better. Otherwise, you run the risk of relapse. If you still have symptoms after you complete your medication, see your doctor. Several other skin conditions can mimic or coexist with yeast infections.

If you have frequent yeast infections (three or more per year), the first line of attack is elimination of any predisposing factors. If the problem persists, the doctor may prescribe preventive doses of antifungal creams or suppositories. For example, inserting a suppository one or more times per menstrual cycle has proven effective for some women.

Recently there has been substantial interest in the anti-yeast activity of boric acid. You can buy boric acid powder in the "eyecare" section of most drugstores. Pack it loosely into size "0" capsules (available at some pharmacies and most health food stores). For a current yeast infection, insert 1 capsule as deeply into your vagina as possible in the morning and again at bedtime for five to seven days. To prevent recurrent infections, use 1 capsule vaginally at bedtime twice weekly beginning one week after menstruation and ending when the next period begins. The capsules cause a very slight watery dis-charge, but are far less messy than either creams or suppositories. They may also cause mild vaginal irritation. This can be eliminated by not using them for a day or two.

Dealing with Trichomoniasis

Trichomoniasis, or "trich," is a sexually transmitted vaginitis suffered by at least 2.5 million American women yearly. In men, this infection rarely produces any symptoms; approximately 40 percent of infected women are also asymptomatic. Since they are unaware of their infection, these people unwittingly spread the infection throughout their communities.

Like most organisms responsible for causing sexually transmitted diseases (STDs), the trichomonad is fragile and cannot survive long outside the body of its host or hostess. However, infections have occasionally been traced to the use of shared washcloths or towels. Since the trichomonad dies promptly when exposed to drying, it cannot be caught from toilet seats, saunas, or dry linens.

Chemical purifiers in swimming pools and hot tubs will also kill it.

While infection with trichomoniasis can be intensely uncomfortable, it is not a serious threat to your overall health. Antibiotic treatment cures the infection more than 90 percent of the time.

The most striking symptoms are vulvar and vaginal burning and itching. The burning may be most apparent after intercourse and can affect the skin of the penis as well as that of the vagina. In addition, there may be vulvar swelling and frequent and uncomfortable urination. There is a heavy vaginal discharge, usually yellowish or green, which may or may not have an offensive odor.

The trichomonad is a tiny teardrop-shape, one-cell parasite. It has three tails at its narrow end. By whipping these tails back and forth the organism can swim about in a brisk, if rather jerky, fashion. As it swims, the host's white blood cells follow in hot pursuit. These blood cells, critical to the human immune defense system, can literally surround a trichomonad and digest it. Presumably, symptoms occur only when the body's defense forces cannot keep up with the numbers of rapidly reproducing trichomonads.

Trichomoniasis is usually easily diagnosed by a case history, pelvic examination, and microscopic examination of a sample of vaginal discharge. Your doctor may take a vaginal PAP smear or trichomonas culture if the diagnosis is unclear.

Metronidazole (Flagyl) is the most effective treatment for trichomoniasis. A single 2000 milligram dose (four 500 milligram tablets taken by mouth all at once) usually works well. If not, the treatment is generally extended over 7 days (either 250 milligrams 3 times daily or 500 milligrams twice daily). To prevent re-infection, your sexual partner must be treated as well.

The use of metronidazole in pregnancy is controversial. Many doctors avoid prescribing this medication at least until the second or third trimesters. If you are pregnant and have trichomoniasis, anti-yeast vaginal creams, which also affect trichomonads, will provide significant relief. If you are unsure whether you are pregnant, you should either have a pregnancy test taken at least 2 weeks after your last intercourse or simply delay starting treatment with metronidazole until your menstrual period begins.

This drug interacts with alcohol, causing abdominal cramps, nausea, and vomiting. Therefore, it is important not to drink alcoholic beverages while taking this medication. If you have active liver disease, certain blood disorders, current or past seizures, or a history of metronidazole allergy, you should avoid using this medication.

As with all STDs, the only certain way to avoid infection is to refrain from all sexual activity. Condoms with a spermicide offer excellent protection for those who remain sexually active. Remember that most men and nearly half of all women with trichomoniasis have no symptoms! Even if your partner is the picture of health, **use a condom!**

Remember, too, that if you find you have one STD, there's a chance you may have others as well. For more information on this and other STDs, turn to the chapter on them later in this section.

Whatever you do, if vulvar irritation or itching fails to go away be sure to check with your doctor. Especially in menopausal women, these symptoms could mean the presence of a precancerous condition or a cancer. □

CHAPTER 5   **COMMON DISORDERS OF THE REPRODUCTIVE SYSTEM**

Cervicitis: Causes and Cures

Cervicitis is probably the most common of all gynecological disorders, affecting half of all women at some point in their lives. Any woman, regardless of age, who has had even one sexual encounter and who is experiencing abdominal pain or an unusual vaginal discharge may have it. Despite the fact that it is so common, cervicitis does not yield to self–diagnosis, because its symptoms—if any—can easily be confused with those of other common ailments, including vaginitis. (See the preceeding chapter, "Curing Vaginal Infections. ")

Untreated, cervicitis can lead to problems conceiving or delivering a healthy baby. But there is good news: Cervicitis can be readily diagnosed by your doctor and successfully treated with a wide variety of drugs and procedures.

What Is Cervicitis?

Cervicitis is an inflammation of the cervix—the lower part of the uterus extending about an inch into the vaginal canal. Most commonly, cervicitis is the result of an infection, although it can also be caused by injury or irritation (a reaction to the chemicals in douches and contraceptives, for example, or a forgotten tampon).

The first symptom of cervicitis is likely to be a vaginal discharge that becomes more pronounced immediately following your menstrual period. Other signs include bleeding, itching, or irritation of the external genitals; pain during intercourse; a burning sensation during urination; and lower back pain. In its mildest form, you may not notice any symptoms at all, but a more severe case of cervicitis can cause a profuse, almost pus–like, discharge with an unpleasant odor, accompanied by intense vaginal itchiness or abdominal pain. If the infection gets into your system, you may also have fever and nausea.

Prolonged cervicitis can make it difficult—even impossible—to become pregnant. Not only does abnormal mucus production interfere with the sperm's ability to enter the cervical canal, but the infection can also spread to the uterus or the fallopian tubes leading to

A CLOSER LOOK AT THE SITE OF THE PROBLEM

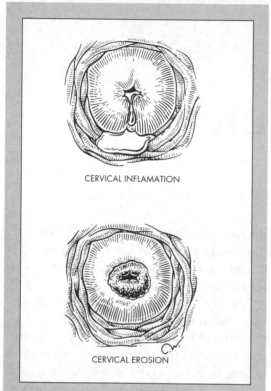

CERVICAL INFLAMATION

CERVICAL EROSION

The cervix, or neck of the uterus, encompasses the cervical canal, the normally tiny passage through which a newborn must pass on its way into the world. Located at the inner end of the vagina, the cervix is vulnerable to a variety of sexually transmitted diseases, including chlamydia, gonorrhea, trichomonas, and herpes. The delicate covering of the outer cervix is also prey to injury, which can strip off the surface layer of cells, resulting in cervical erosion. The cells lining the cervix are sometimes subject to abnormal growth as well, starting as cervical "dysplasia" and possibly progressing to cancer. For more on this problem, turn to chapters 38 and 39, "Cervical Cancer: The One That's Preventable," and "Making Sense of Your Pap Test."

the ovaries. A pregnant woman with untreated cervicitis risks miscarriage, premature delivery, or infection of her newborn during delivery, leading to pneumonia, a severe eye infection, or blindness.

Because many of the symptoms of cervicitis can be confused with signs of other disorders, it's important to see a doctor whenever you experience pain or an unusual discharge. The problem could be an infection of the vulva, uterus, fallopian tubes, or urinary tract. It could also be a sign of another cervical condition called cervical erosion. Erosion or ulceration of the cervix means that the cervical surface layer (consisting of flat, shiny cells called squamous epithelium) is partially or completely missing. An eroded area looks raw and red and may cause spotting. Injury from intercourse, the insertion of a tampon, or certain chemicals can lead to erosion.

Diagnosing Cervicitis

Inflammation of the cervix is the result of the body's normal defense system. Whenever there is injury, irritation, or infection, white blood cells are mobilized, and blood circulation within the area increases. The cervix, which is normally pale pink and smooth, becomes red and swollen.

Your doctor will identify the true nature of your problem by examining all available evidence: your symptoms, your medical history, and the results of a physical exam (including a Pap smear, a "wet smear," and tests to culture infectious organisms).

A biopsy may be recommended if your cervix appears abnormal. In this procedure, the doctor removes a small piece of tissue for microscopic examination by a pathologist, a type of specialist who focuses on studying and identifying the effects of disease.

Removing the tissue sample is usually an office procedure, customarily performed without anesthesia, or at most with a local painkiller. Discomfort is generally minor, since there are relatively few pain nerves in the cervix. After a biopsy, you should avoid intercourse, douching, and the use of tampons for at least a week, until your cervix has healed. It is normal to experience some spotting, but if heavy bleeding occurs, or if you experience pain, unusual vaginal discharge, or fever, you should contact your doctor immediately.

Colposcopy, another diagnostic technique, involves using a binocular–like instrument called a colposcope to get a magnified view of the surface of the cervix. The examination can be done during a routine pelvic exam, but if your doctor lacks the equipment or special training to do a colposcopy, he or she may refer you to another doctor for this particular exam.

Cervicography, a relatively new technique, allows the doctor to take photographs of your cervix, then send them to an expert for interpretation. The results are sent back to the doctor, who will then discuss them with you.

The Leading Causes

Successful treatment of cervicitis begins with proper identification of the cause. If some irritant is causing the cervicitis, your doctor will remove it or advise you to avoid it. If the cause is an infection, your doctor will attempt to diagnose the responsible organism.

The three most common causes of cervicitis are chlamydia, gonorrhea, and trichomonas. All three, it should be noted, are considered sexually transmitted diseases or STDs. (Cervicitis is only one of the many problems these diseases can cause. For more information, see chapter 11, "Coming to Terms With Sexually Transmitted Diseases.") If cervicitis is caused by an STD, treatment for your partner is also crucial.

A number of other organisms—including herpes simplex, streptococcus, staphylococcus, enterococcus, and *Gardnerella vaginalis*—can also cause cervicitis.

You should always avoid intercourse or have your partner use condoms while you are being treated for cervicitis, regardless of the specific cause.

Chlamydia

Chlamydial infections are caused by the *Chlamydia Trachomatis* bacteria, a parasitic microorganism that can survive only in a host cell. It is estimated that between 3 and 4 million cases of chlamydial infection occur each year, making it one of the most common sexually transmitted "bugs" in the United States.

There may be no symptoms for weeks or months following infection with chlamydia. In women, when symptoms do occur, they can include discharge, pelvic pain, bleeding, fever, and frequent or uncomfortable urination. It is important to treat a chlamydial infection promptly and aggressively to keep it from spreading to the uterus and fallopian tubes. In men, a chlamydial infection may be diagnosed as nongonococcal urethritis (NGU), with symptoms such as pain or a burning sensation during urination or a thin discharge from the penis.

If the diagnosis is chlamdydial cervicitis, your doctor will probably prescribe a broad–spectrum antibiotic. Among the most commonly prescribed treatments for chlamydia are:

■ doxycycline (Doryx, Vibramycin, others), one 100–milligram capsule taken twice daily for 7 days, *or*

THE GYNECOLOGICAL EXAM

One of the most important things you can do to ensure your continued good health is to become an active member of your health care team.

Many women find their annual visits to the gynecologist embarrassing at best and, at worst, extremely uncomfortable. But once you understand the procedures involved and actively participate in the process, you will find that discomfort and embarrassment diminish. And it always helps to remember that problems that are detected early are generally more responsive to treatment.

The first thing to do, before you even arrive at your doctor's office, is **make a list** of any symptoms you have noticed or questions you want to ask. Many women find that the anxiety surrounding the exam causes them to forget everything they had wanted to talk about. Making notes ahead of time will be a big help to both you and your doctor.

The gynecological exam usually begins with a careful **medical history** and a general physical exam. Your doctor will ask you to describe signs or symptoms, any past problems, family history of disease, your sexual activity, last menstrual period, and the contraceptives and medications you may be using. Be frank. Your physician is there to treat you, not to judge you.

Next, your doctor will probably take your height, weight, and blood pressure; listen to your heart and lungs; take your temperature; examine your thyroid gland and breasts; and take blood and urine specimens.

The **pelvic exam** provides your doctor—and you—with essential information about the health of your reproductive system. For the exam, you will be placed in that indelicate posture called the dorsal lithotomy position: on your back, with your bottom at the edge of the table, and your legs elevated and supported.

The first thing your doctor will do is inspect your external genitalia for redness, swelling, or any signs of irritation or injury.

The next step will probably be the **speculum examination.** Here, the doctor inserts an instrument called a speculum into the vagina to hold the vaginal walls apart, permitting an examination of the cervix and vaginal lining for redness, irritation, unusual discharge, or lesions.

During the speculum exam, your doctor will collect specimens for lab tests. These typically include a **Pap smear** specimen, gonorrhea and chlamydia test samples, and a slide preparation for diagnosing other infections.

Because gonorrhea and chlamydia are so common—and because both women and men can have these infections without any symptoms—your doctor may routinely test you for sexually transmitted diseases (STDs), especially if you report pain or an unusual discharge, or if you (or your partner) have multiple sexual partners.

The primary purpose of a Pap smear is to detect the presence of abnormal cells on the surface of your cervix. It is a fairly sensitive and reliable test. For a detailed discussion of this test, turn to chapter 39, "Making Sense of Your Pap Test."

The next part of the exam involves **bimanual (two-handed) examination** of the reproductive organs, with two fingers of one hand in the vagina and the other hand pressing downward on the abdomen. This procedure helps your doctor determine the size, location, and shape of the uterus and check for pain and tenderness. Typically, your doctor will also examine the internal organs by inserting one finger in the rectum while the other remains in the vagina.

Remember that the exam should not be painful. The more you can relax the muscles of your abdomen, the easier the procedure will be. And if you are experiencing any pain or tenderness, tell your doctor where it is before the exam begins, so that he or she can be extra gentle during the examination.

- azithromycin (Zithromax), four 250–milligram capsules taken in one dose, *or*
- ofloxacin (Floxin), one 300–milligram tablet taken twice daily for 7 days, *or*
- erythromycin base (ERYC, others), two 250–milligram capsules taken 4 times a day for 7 days.

Doxycycline is often the preferred medication for Chlamydia because it only needs to be taken twice a day; it is less likely to cause intestinal upset; and it stays at higher levels in the blood than tetracycline. However, if you are allergic to tetracycline drugs like doxycycline or if you are pregnant, your doctor might prescribe erythromycin. The most common side effect of erythromycin is gastrointestinal discomfort (abdominal distress, nausea, or diarrhea).

Be sure that your partner is also treated and schedule follow–up exams for both of you if the symptoms fail to disappear. You should avoid intercourse until are certain that both of you are disease–free. Your partner should use condoms if there is any doubt that he has been thoroughly treated and cured.

Gonorrhea

Caused by the *Neisseria gonorrhoeae* bacterium, gonorrhea is also transmitted through sexual intercourse. It is not unusual to be infected with gonorrhea and yet have absolutely no symptoms. Many cases of gonorrhea are first detected in the course of a routine examination from a cultured specimen of vaginal discharge. When there are symptoms, they may include unusual discharge, painful urination, pelvic pain, unusual bleeding, or fever.

Because it is common for people with gonorrhea to be cross–infected with chlamydia,

treatment is generally designed to cure both infections. The initial dose of medication is often given right in the doctor's office, *either*:

- ceftriaxone (Rocephin), 125 milligrams in an intramuscular injection, *or*
- Cefixime (Suprax), one 400–milligram tablet *or*
- Ciprofloxacin (Cipro), one 500–milligram tablet *or*
- ofloxacin (Floxin), one 400–milligram tablet

Be sure to tell your doctor if you are pregnant, allergic to penicillin or tetracycline drugs, or if you have ever had asthma, hives, hay fever, or other allergies.

The initial large dose of antibiotic for treatment of gonorrhea is followed with one of the broad spectrum antibiotics prescribed for chlamydia.

Untreated gonorrhea can cause fertility problems, birth defects if a woman is pregnant, and if allowed to spread, skin problems, arthritis, blood poisoning, and heart and brain infections.

Both you and your partner must be treated and should be tested again if symptoms fail to subside. It is important to ensure that you are both cured because new strains of penicillin–resistant gonorrhea have recently developed, and additional treatment may be necessary to completely eradicate the infection.

Reinfection is quite common, so it is wise to avoid intercourse until you and your partner are both certain of a clean bill of health.

Trichomonas

Trichomonas (frequently referred to as "trich," pronounced "trick") is caused by a one–celled microscopic organism that produces a frothy vaginal discharge. There may be no symptoms, or the infection can cause intense itchiness, redness, an objectionable

BIMANUAL EXAMINATION

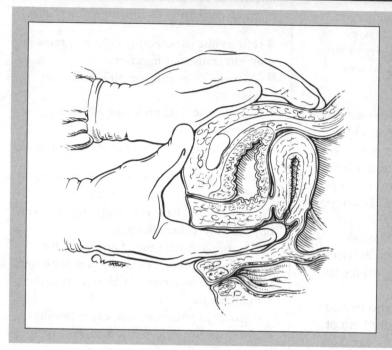

This standard gynecological technique enables the doctor to feel any abnormality in the size, shape, or position of the uterus. If the doctor detects a problem, it's possible to make a visual inspection of the uterus, ovaries, and other organs through a minor surgical procedure called laparoscopy.

odor, frequent urination, or pain. With a trichomonas infection, your vagina is likely to be more alkaline than normal, so your doctor, as part of the examination, may test the acid/alkaline balance with a strip of pH paper.

Men infected with trich rarely have symptoms. When they do, the symptoms can include irritation, discharge, or a burning sensation during urination.

Your doctor will identify the parasite responsible for the infection by smearing a sample of your discharge and a drop of salt solution on a slide, then examining it under a microscope. Trichomonas organisms are easily identifiable because they are rapid swimmers that propel themselves with flicks of their whip–like tails.

The most effective treatment for trich is anantibacterial drug called metronidazole (Flagyl, Protostat, others) given in pill form, *either*:

- 2,000 milligrams in a single oral dose, *or*
- 500 milligrams twice daily for 7 days.

Do *not* drink alcoholic beverages while you are taking metronidazole and for at least 24 hours after having taken the last dose. Mixing alcohol with metronidazole can cause cramps, nausea, vomiting, headache, and flushing. The most common side effects of this drug are stomach upset, cramps, constipation, diarrhea, and headache. More serious side effects include seizures and numbness or tingling in the arms, legs, hands, or feet. If you experience any of these symptoms, call your doctor immediately and stop taking the drug.

Be sure to tell your doctor if you have liver disease or if you are breastfeeding, pregnant, or planning to become pregnant. In any of these cases, metronidazole may not be the right drug for you. Antibiotic douches or antifungal suppositories like clotrimazole (Gyne–Lotrimin, Mycelex G, others) may help relieve symptoms; they will not, however, cure the disease.

As with all STDs, if you have trichomonas, your partner should also be treated, and you should both avoid intercourse or use a condom until follow–up tests indicate that you are both cured.

Herpes Simplex

Your doctor will suspect herpes if there are visible blisters or open sores on the cervix. Further tests (including a Pap smear or culture) can confirm the diagnosis. Because herpes simplex is a virus, antibacterial treatments such as those for other STDs will not work against it.

While there is no known cure for herpes, 200 milligrams of acyclovir (Zovirax) in pill form, taken 5 times a day for 7 to 10 days— or until symptoms subside—can be helpful in limiting the length and intensity of the first attack. Treatment should be started within 6 days after the appearance of the first symptoms, which are often tingling and itchiness. For recurrent attacks, your doctor may prescribe acyclovir in dosages such as 200 milligrams 5 times daily for 5 days; you must begin this treatment within the first 2 days after onset. You can also take acyclovir to suppress future attacks. The dosage is 400 milligrams twice daily for a year. This has been found to cut the frequency of the attacks by 75 percent.

Herpes simplex virus is highly contagious in its active stage, so you and your partner should avoid sexual contact at the first signs of an attack. If you or your partner has had a herpes simplex outbreak in the past, it is wise to use condoms routinely because the virus can be passed back and forth even when there are no symptoms.

If you have herpes, you should see your doctor and have a Pap test regularly—at least once a year—without fail, since the virus is under suspicion as a possible cause of cervical cancer.

While it *is* possible to have a normal pregnancy and a healthy baby with herpes, special care must be taken to avoid infecting the baby.

Nonspecific Bacterial Infections

Once tests have ruled out chlamydia, gonorrhea, trichomonas, and herpes, your doctor may not be able to identify the specific bacteria responsible for your condition. He or she may therefore prescribe "nonspecific" medications, such as a sulfa vaginal cream or a

TO PREVENT CERVICITIS...

- Limit your sexual contacts; know the history of your partner; and make condoms a routine part of sex.
- See your doctor immediately if your partner has been diagnosed with urethritis or if he has symptoms of the condition (pain or burning during urination, a thin discharge from the penis, or a stain on his underwear).
- See your doctor immediately if you notice a vaginal discharge or any kind of lower abdominal pain.
- See your doctor for a complete physical exam annually, regardless of whether or not you are experiencing any symptoms.
- Treat vaginal infections immediately–before they have a chance to spread to your cervix.
- Avoid chemical irritants in deodorized tampons, douches, or sprays.

douche that kill bacteria in the vagina and cervix. As the general bacterial population is reduced, your body's own defenses may be able to overcome the infection. Your doctor may also suggest creams or douches to readjust the acid/alkaline balance in your vagina, and make it less hospitable for bacteria.

Conquering Chronic Cervicitis

If you have prolonged or repeated bouts of cervicitis, your doctor may recommend a procedure designed to destroy the abnormal cells on the surface of your cervix. The most common of these procedures are cautery (also known as heat cautery), cryosurgery (also known as freezing, or cold cautery), and laser treatment. After therapy, cells from untreated normal tissue naturally grow into and replace the area of destroyed, abnormal tissue.

Cautery

Cautery is the oldest of the three treatment methods for chronic cervicitis. Electricity is used to produce a controlled current at the tip of a cautery probe. The hot tip of the probe is touched to the area of abnormal tissue and burns away the damaged cells. Cautery, which typically causes mild to moderate pain, is less likely to be recommended than the other two newer techniques, if they are available.

Cryosurgery

Cryosurgery has several advantages over cautery. It is less likely to be painful and it produces a more controlled and uniform area and depth of tissue destruction. It also causes less scarring and is therefore less likely to cause cervical stenosis (a narrowing of the cervical canal).

In cryosurgery, an intense cold source (usually compressed nitrous oxide or carbon dioxide gas) is used to freeze any tissue it touches. The cold source is administered through a hand–held instrument that looks like a gun. It takes about 2 minutes for the tissue to be thoroughly frozen. During this time, you may experience a vague sensation of coldness and mild cramping. However, the discomfort usually subsides fairly rapidly.

Laser Treatment

With laser treatment, the doctor uses an intense, focused beam of light to evaporate one tiny, precise area of surface tissue at a time. You may have a sensation of warmth or crampy pain during the treatment, very much like the typical reaction to cautery or cryosurgery.

Overall success rates are similar for laser and cryosurgery. Laser treatment is preferred when there are large areas of abnormal tissue.

Both cautery and cryosurgery can cause swelling in the cervix that can temporarily narrow or obstruct the cervical canal, so it is best to schedule either procedure for immediately after your menstrual period. The swelling should be over by your next period.

After any one of these three treatments, you may experience a profuse, watery vaginal discharge lasting as long as a week or two. You may also have spotting or bleeding, especially if your cervix was touched or bumped. Given the sensitivity in the cervical area, it is best to abstain from intercourse and to avoid tampons and douching for at least 2 weeks after treatment. Complete healing takes 6 to 8 weeks. When you resume intercourse, use a condom until a follow–up Pap smear shows that your cervix is completely healed and all traces of the abnormalities are gone. □

The Dangers of Pelvic Inflammatory Disease

Insidious and often dangerous, Pelvic Inflammatory Disease (PID) is a major health problem in the United States. More than 1 million women experience an episode of PID every year, which translates into an annual price tag of more than $4 billion. If present trends continue, by the turn of the century PID will cost Americans more than $10 billion annually in lost work time and medical bills.

For every four women who have PID, one will develop complications such as infertility or an ectopic pregnancy in one of the fallopian tubes between the ovaries and uterus—a potentially fatal condition.

Pelvic inflammatory disease is not really a single illness. It's actually an umbrella term for a variety of infections of the inner reproductive organs, including the ovaries, the fallopian tubes, the endometrial lining of the uterus, the uterine wall, the ligaments that support the uterus, and even the lining of the abdomen.

Silence Versus Symptoms

Unfortunately, PID isn't always accompanied by obvious symptoms such as fever, abdominal pain, or a vaginal discharge. Sometimes the disease is "silent" and has mild symptoms or none at all, especially in women whose PID is caused by a germ called *Chlamydia trachomatis*, the most common cause of sexually transmitted disease. In women who have been rendered infertile by an infection in their fallopian tubes (the medical term is salpingitis), roughly half don't remember having any symptoms at all!

For those who do have symptoms, the most common is a dull, constant pain in the lower abdomen. This pain may be aggravated by movement or sexual activity. The hallmark of the condition is pain or tenderness as the doctor probes during a physical examination.

Since PID is often associated with a coexisting infection of the cervix, or birth canal, some women may notice a vaginal discharge. In fact, this is often one of the first symptoms of the disease. Only about 1 in 3 women

INFECTION LURKS HIDDEN FOR MANY WITH PID

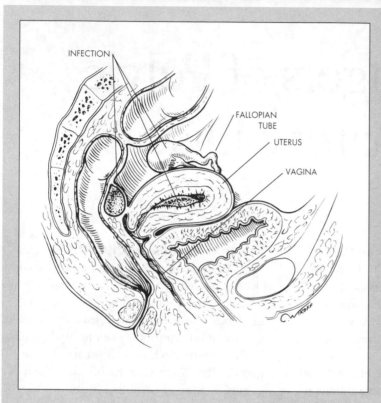

INFECTION

FALLOPIAN
TUBE

UTERUS

VAGINA

Though it can easily render you infertile, your first warning of PID might not come until you have a physical exam. As shown here, PID can attack the uterus, the fallopian tubes leading from the ovaries, even the nearby abdominal lining; yet until the infection becomes very serious, you may feel nothing. If you have an active sex life, you owe it to yourself to get regular checkups for this if no other reason.

who are diagnosed with PID has a fever. Nausea and vomiting may also signal PID, but they usually occur when the disease has progressed to peritonitis, in which the infection spreads to the lining of the abdomen.

Although some of the symptoms of PID, such as abdominal pain, vaginal discharge and fever, can signal a variety of diseases, it's wise to consult a physician promptly if you have one or more. If you do turn out to have PID, the earlier you start treatment, the better will be your chances of avoiding infertility.

The Leading Culprits

PID is usually caused by more than one kind of bacteria. The bugs most commonly involved are *Neisseria gonorrhoeae* and *Chlamydia trachomatis*, both transmitted by sexual intercourse. However, other kinds of bacteria generally accompany them. The infection usually starts in the vagina, then moves up the reproductive system through the cervix, into the uterus, up the fallopian tubes, and finally into the ovaries.

Generally, gonorrhea-associated infections start quickly with more severe symptoms than the ones caused by chlamydia. When chlamydia is the major culprit, symptoms tend to be milder and fewer, developing slowly over a period of months or years. In either case, abdominal pain frequently begins during or shortly after a menstrual period.

Risk Factors

Because its two most common causes are both sexually transmitted, sexual activity is by the far the greatest single risk factor for PID. Youth also increases the odds; roughly 75 percent of all cases of PID occur in sexually active women under 25 years of age. For reasons not yet understood, younger women are more susceptible to chlamydial and gonorrhea-associated infection than older women are. Also, the disease rarely occurs in non-menstruating women such as girls who have not yet reached sexual maturity as well as pregnant and postmenopausal women.

Clearly, there is a direct relationship between the number of sexual partners a woman has and the risk of PID—the more partners, the greater the risk. A woman who has only one partner does not have an increased risk. If he has had a vasectomy, the risk of PID is actually lowered.

Contraceptive Choices and the Risk of PID

It used to be thought that use of an intrauterine device (IUD) increased the risk of pelvic inflammatory disease. However, having a variety of sexual partners appears to be the real culprit. Women who use an IUD with a single partner are at no increased risk of the disease.

For those with multiple partners, certain other kinds of contraceptive devices—condoms, diaphragms, and spermicides—provide greater protection against the bacteria that cause PID than does an IUD. Barriers such as condoms or diaphragms physically prevent the bacteria from moving up the reproductive tract just as they prevent the passage of sperm. Spermicides used with these barrier methods, especially one called nonoxynol 9, can kill the bacteria that cause PID infections. On the other hand, frequent douching after sex can increase the risk of PID by pushing bacteria further up into the reproductive system.

Oral contraceptives don't block the passage of bacteria, but they do hinder them, lowering the risk of contracting PID and often keeping the infection milder. They accomplish this by

HARBINGER OF TROUBLE TO COME

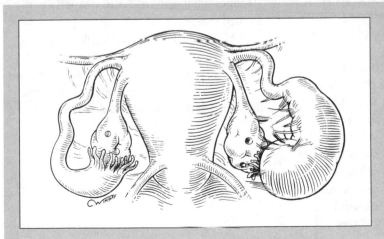

If a pelvic infection takes hold in the critical corridor between the ovary and the uterus, the resulting inflammation and swelling (see tube on right) can totally block the passage, while pus building up outside the tube can cement it to other organs and spread the infection elsewhere in the abdomen.

THE DIRE AFTERMATH OF INFECTION

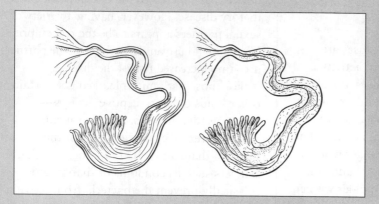

Compare the normal fallopian tube on the left with the victim of PID on the right. Even after the disease has cleared up, it's impossible for an egg to make its way through the scarred, unnaturally narrow channel the infection leaves behind. If PID effectively closes both fallopian tubes, the result is sterility.

increasing the thickness of cervical mucus which makes it more difficult for bacteria to move up the reproductive system. They also decrease menstrual flow, which presumably limits the opportunity for bacteria to grow in the upper reproductive tract.

Why Pid Is Dangerous

If PID were merely an annoying infection that could be cleared up by antibiotics with no lingering or long-term effects, it wouldn't deserve a chapter in this book. But PID is much more than an annoyance. If the infection moves up the reproductive tract to the fallopian tubes, it can cause permanent damage to these critical reproductive organs, resulting in infertility.

Gonorrhea causes an inflammation that can permanently scar the delicate fallopian tubes, decreasing their width, and making them unfit to transport eggs to the uterus. While chlamydia produces a milder form of infection than does gonorrhea, it can linger in the tubes for months prompting a violent immune response that can damage the tubes just as thoroughly as a sudden bacterial onslaught. Whether it is due to a direct

gonoccocal attack on the tubes or the more insidious chlamydial assault, the end result is the same—infertility.

In addition to destroying reproductive capacity, just one episode of PID can greatly increase your chances of having an ectopic pregnancy in which an egg begins to grow in the fallopian tube rather than in the uterus where it belongs. Ectopic pregnancies can be a life-threatening emergency requiring hospitalization and surgery. Experts estimate that the risk of death due to ectopic pregnancy is 10 times greater than it is in childbirth and 50 times greater than it is in properly performed surgery.

A bout of PID also quadruples your chances of suffering chronic (long-term) pelvic pain. If you develop this problem, surgical exploration is necessary to determine the cause and extent of the disease.

How PID Is Diagnosed

Since PID can range from the "silent" variety (no symptoms) to a full-blown infection complete with pain, fever, and abnormal blood tests, there is no "standard" diagnostic procedure. If your doctor suspects that you may have PID, he or she must be able to distinguish between the disease and emergency conditions such as an ectopic pregnancy and appendicitis. For every 100 women suspected of having PID, about three or four will actually have an ectopic pregnancy and another three or four will turn out to have appendicitis.

Most women who develop PID have abdominal pain, pelvic tenderness, and some symptoms of a lower genital tract infection such as cervicitis. To help confirm the presence of infection, your doctor will probably do a couple of blood tests. There may also be a test for human chorionic gonadotropin, a hormone that rises during pregnancy and can signal that the pain is due not to PID but to an ectopic pregnancy. You will also probably be checked for gonorrhea and chlamydia. Samples swabbed from your cervix, or birth canal, will be taken with a cotton swab and sent to a lab for examination.

If your doctor suspects the infection may be due to an adnexal abscess—a pus-filled pocket of fluid and bacteria around the ovary or fallopian tube—you may have to undergo an ultrasound examination, in which sound waves beamed into the body are used to build an image of internal organs on a computer screen.

The only completely conclusive way to diagnose PID is a surgical procedure called laparoscopy in which a special kind of viewing instrument called a laparoscope is inserted through a small incision below the navel. This type of surgery usually involves general anesthesia that puts you to sleep, but it can often be performed on an out-patient basis and does not usually require

THE WORST THAT CAN HAPPEN

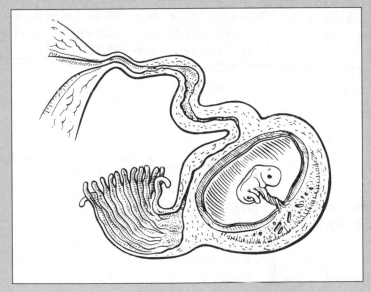

With its exit to the uterus blocked by scarring in the fallopian tube, a fertilized egg may become implanted and develop within the tube instead. Such an ectopic (outside the uterus) pregnancy can be fatal if left uncorrected. Cramps and spotting shortly after the first missed period are the major warning signs. Surgery is invariably needed.

overnight hospitalization. By examining the affected organs with the laparoscope, your doctor can make a definite diagnosis. You'll usually be given antibiotics to protect you from further infection by the operation itself. The procedure generally takes less than 45 minutes and most patients can return home after resting from 2 to 6 hours.

Although laparoscopy is necessary for a definitive diagnosis of dangerous conditions such as adnexal abscess or ectopic pregnancy, most cases of PID do not call for it; and most doctors will start treatment for PID immediately if they even suspect the problem. If you have gonorrhea or chlamydia, delaying even a few days can greatly increase your chances of complications such as ectopic pregnancy or infertility. The risk of taking some unnecessary antibiotics is far less than the risk of letting PID go unchecked.

Treatment Options

Since PID infection is almost always caused by more than one kind of bacteria, your doctor will most likely prescribe a combination of antibiotics. Only one woman in four is hospitalized for PID; so unless your infection is severe enough to need hospitalization, you will not receive intravenous (IV) medication.

The Centers for Disease Control and Prevention recommend the following antibiotic treatments for PID outpatients:

- An injection of cefoxitin (Mefoxin) plus
- Probenecid (Benemid) tablets
  or
- An injection of ceftriaxone (Rocephin) plus
- Doxycline (Vibramycin or Doryx) orally for 14 days or tetracycline (Achromycin V or Sumycin) orally for 14 days
  or

- Ofloxacin tablets (Floxin) plus
- Clindamycin (Cleocin HCl) orally for 14 days or metronidazole (Flagyl) orally for 14 days

Whichever regimen your doctor chooses, you should be checked two or three days after the antibiotics have been started to ensure that they are working. If the antibiotics don't seem to be working, your doctor may suggest hospitalization. If you are hospitalized, you can receive IV antibiotics that can work more quickly and more powerfully than ones you can take on an out-patient basis.

Since the great majority of PID cases are the result of sexually transmitted disease, it's not enough to be cured yourself. You need to make sure your partner also gets treatment. Otherwise, he'll reinfect you as soon as you resume having sex.

Preventing Recurrence

As is the case with so many illnesses, "an ounce of prevention is worth a pound of cure," because once you've had PID, it can recur, especially if you're a younger woman. In fact, roughly one of every four women with PID will suffer future episodes, and women who are hospitalized for PID have an even greater chance of entering the hospital again with PID or some related condition.

Perhaps even more alarming, recent studies suggest that silent or symptomless PID may be even more common than the classic kind in which acute abdominal pain warns you that something is wrong. However, there is also good news of sorts. Experts believe that symptomless PID is sexually transmitted, probably through germs such as chlamydia and others called trichomonas and mycoplasma. This means that you can avoid PID by sticking with a single partner, using protection, or refraining from sex. □

CHAPTER 7   **COMMON DISORDERS OF THE REPRODUCTIVE SYSTEM**

Your Treatment Options for Fibroids

The good news about fibroids is that these tumors are almost always benign—they do not cause cancer. Although fibroids do have the potential to cause problems if they grow especially large, most women, about 75 percent, manage to live with their fibroids fairly well and never have any trouble with them. In fact, many women—even some who have really large fibroids—aren't even aware they have them.

The bad news is that women are most likely to develop fibroids when they are in their 30s and 40s—a time when many women are trying to become pregnant. The traditional treatment—surgical removal of the uterus in the operation called hysterectomy—is becoming less and less acceptable to women who have not yet completed their families. Fortunately, there are now other options, with still more alternatives in development.

What Is a Fibroid?

A fibroid is the most common tumor (abnormal mass of tissue) found in the pelvis. Such a tumor develops most often between the ages of 35 and 45 years, seldom before age 20. Fibroids do not occur at all before puberty. After a woman completes menopause, they generally stop growing and may even disappear.

Usually a fibroid is found in the uterus where it is the most common form of uterine mass. A fibroid can also develop on another structure that contains smooth muscle cells. In vary rare cases, it can even "invade" another organ when it grows too large to confine itself to its original location.

A fibroid is a solid tumor that contains mostly smooth muscle held together by fibrous tissue. (That's how it came by its popular name.) Other names for fibroids are *leiomyomas, myomas, fibromas,* and *fibromyomas.*

Fibroids usually occur as multiple tumors that tend to grow very slowly. Sometimes, however, a woman may have a single fibroid the size of a grapefruit or even one so large that it fills the entire abdomen. On the other hand, a fibroid tumor may be so small that it can be only seen under a microscope. It can weigh as much as 25 or 50 pounds, with the largest fibroid tumor ever reported weighing more than 140 pounds.

It is difficult to know just how many women have fibroids, since unless they cause a problem, a woman may never realize she has them. It is, however, estimated that fibroids occur in up to 25 percent of women over the age of 30 and in nearly 40 percent of women after the age of 40.

For some reason, black women seem more likely to develop fibroids. Almost half of all black women more than 30 years of age have fibroids compared with 20 percent of white women of the same age-group. Interestingly, studies have found a low incidence of fibroids among women in Africa. Overall, however, fibroids tend to occur earlier and grow faster in black women.

Why They Develop

Even though fibroid tumors are common, no one is really sure how or why they develop, or why fibroids occur again and again in one woman and not at all in another.

Although the cause of fibroids is unknown, many physicians believe that these tumors grow when the body responds abnormally to the female hormone estrogen. Others disagree. What definitely is known is that fibroids:

■ Do not occur before puberty, when the body does not release estrogen
■ Grow bigger when women take oral contraceptives, which contain estrogen
■ Grow rapidly during pregnancy, when the body produces extra estrogen

■ Shrink and even disappear as menopause approaches and the body gradually stops making estrogen
■ Rarely appear after menopause
■ Grow when women take estrogen supplements to make up for the lack of the hormone

Still, there are many who doubt that estrogen is solely responsible for fibroid tumors. Although fibroids develop in some women who have high levels of estrogen, laboratory tests performed for many women with these tumors show completely normal estrogen levels.

In addition, while fibroids tend to grow larger when a woman is pregnant, there is little scientific evidence to show that these tumors multiply during pregnancy. Some physicians believe that the increased blood supply that occurs during pregnancy may be the cause, since fibroids require a lot of blood to survive.

Types of Fibroids

The type of problems that fibroids cause depends on their location. Therefore, your doctor's first concern will be to pinpoint the exact location of the tumors. It is this information that determines the best course of treatment.

Fibroids are categorized by their location. The various types include:

Submucous fibroid. This type occurs just beneath the lining of the uterus and can displace the lining as it grows. This displacement can lead to menstrual irregularities and discomfort. After a while, this fibroid may develop a thin stalk called a pedicle. The stalk remains attached to the uterine wall, but the fibroid is able to "travel." When this happens, the tumor may protrude into the uterus, which will then contract in an attempt to rid itself of this foreign body. The fibroid may also enter the vagina. As the fibroid moves around, the stalk may become twisted and lose blood, causing bleeding between periods. Infection may also occur.

Intramural fibroid. This round tumor is most commonly found within the uterine wall. The uterus can become enlarged as the intramural fibroid grows.

Subserous fibroid. This type grows on the outer wall of the uterus, sometimes jutting out from the lining. A subserous fibroid can grow overly large without causing any recognizable symptoms—until it interferes with other organs, creating problems there.

Pedunculated fibroid. Such a tumor develops when a subserous fibroid grows a stalk called a peduncle. As these tumors get bigger and bigger, the original blood supply may not be sufficient to feed the fibroid. If the tumor becomes twisted or begins to degenerate as the blood supply diminishes, it can cause severe pain.

Interligamentous fibroid. This tumor, which grows sideways between the layers of the broad ligament (band of fibrous connective tissue) supporting the uterus, is extremely difficult to remove without interfering with important organs or the blood supply to the uterus.

Parasitic fibroid. When a fibroid attaches itself to another organ, it transforms itself into the rarest of all types, the parasitic

FIBROIDS: THE FIVE MAJOR TYPES

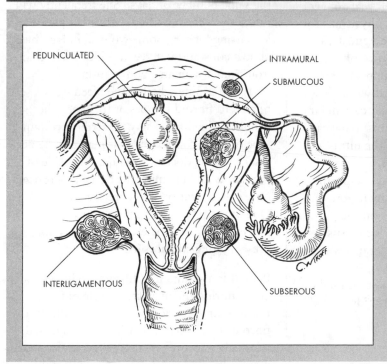

PEDUNCULATED

INTRAMURAL

SUBMUCOUS

INTERLIGAMENTOUS

SUBSEROUS

Classified by their location within and around the uterus, the non-cancerous growths known as fibroids can grow for years without causing a problem—and may vanish after menopause. *Submucous* fibroids lie just below the inner lining of the uterus, *subserous* below the outer lining, and *intramural* deep within the uterine wall. If one of these growths develops a stalk, it's called a *pedunculated* fibroid. When found in the ligaments that support the uterus, it's an *interligamentous* fibroid. If a fibroid causes any symptoms at all, the first one is likely to be excessive menstrual bleeding.

fibroid. As the tumor establishes a new source of blood, its uterine stalk gradually degenerates until the fibroid is no longer attached to the uterus at all.

Reaching a Diagnosis

A fibroid tumor, one of the masses a physician most frequently feels during a pelvic examination, is easily recognized during exploratory surgery. Many, many fibroid tumors, however, are discovered while a physician is looking for something else—or simply are not discovered at all. If a woman experiences no unpleasant symptoms, there may be no reason to look for them.

On the other hand, the mere presence of fibroid tumors can interfere with the doctor's general assessment of your health. Fibroid tumors that grow near the ovaries can make it impossible for the doctor to feel the ovaries and determine whether they are healthy—a big concern for women older than 40 years of age.

Ultrasound scanning enables physicians to distinguish these tumors. This diagnostic procedure can confirm the presence of fibroids when a woman has symptoms that raise suspicion of the tumors. However, because certain types of fibroids look similar to ovarian tumors, and the fibrous tissue can interfere with the sound waves, the ultrasound reading can be inaccurate.

Sometimes the only way a physician can be sure is to look inside via an operation. The decision to operate depends on the particular symptoms, on what the doctor suspects is the cause, and on considerations such as a woman's likelihood of developing ovarian cancer or other disorders that might be overlooked because of the fibroids.

The Classic Symptoms

Though most fibroids do not produce any symptoms, when they do cause problems—as happens in about 25 percent of those with fibroids—women are most likely to complain of (1) excessive bleeding, (2) pain, and (3) a swollen abdomen. (Actually the stomach isn't any bigger—the problem is the uterus, which stretches as the fibroids grow, pushing the intestines upward.)

Excessive bleeding occurs in about 30 percent of the women with fibroids. Most often the bleeding is caused by a type of fibroid tumor that grows underneath the endometrium, or lining of the uterus. As the tumors grow, the lining stretches, thins, and becomes distorted, all of which produce bleeding.

When a woman develops abnormal bleeding, she notices that her menstural flow is heavier, but that it lasts—at least at first—for the same number of days. She frequently will find, however, that after a while her periods are lasting longer. Some women, in fact, bleed almost constantly. Excessive blood loss drains iron from a woman's body causing anemia.

To determine whether the bleeding is related to fibroid tumors or to some other problem, the doctor may prescribe a certain type of birth control pills. It may also be necessary for the doctor to scrape the inside of the uterus and examine the tissue in a procedure called dilation and curettage or a D & C. One of the physician's major concerns is to make sure that a cancerous growth is not present alongside fibroids.

Pain, if it accompanies fibroids, will generally occur during the menstrual cycle but, more commonly, will not occur at all. With fibroid-related pain, women who have had relatively pain-free menstrual cycles for years may suddenly become very uncomfortable.

They experience painful spasms or cramps similar to those felt during labor. Indeed, the fibroid may act like a foreign body, and the uterus responds by contracting, trying to get rid of it.

If a fibroid presses on the pelvic nerves, the woman may feel hip or back pain. If the tumor becomes twisted or begins to deteriorate, the pain may be felt as a sudden severe stabbing in the lower abdomen. Sexual intercourse may also become uncomfortable.

Pain that occurs between menstrual periods is seldom caused by uncomplicated fibroid tumors. When this kind of pain is the problem, the doctor needs to seek another cause. There could be a problem with a previously undiagnosed pregnancy or with a nonfibroid tumor.

Swollen Abdomen. As fibroid tumors grow, they can push other organs out of the way resulting in all kinds of discomfort. A growing fibroid can flatten the bladder, making it necessary to go to the bathroom more frequently and creating a constant feeling of urgency. A woman may also find that she is suddenly unable to control her bladder. In severe cases, the fibroid may push on the urethra or urinary canal so hard that she cannot urinate at all and has to be catheterized. If the tumor extends towards the back and leans on the lower bowel, a woman is likely to develop a backache, become constipated, and find it difficult to have a bowel movement.

Infertility. Fibroids can make it difficult for a woman to become pregnant or, if she does become pregnant, to carry the baby for the full nine months. Many things can happen to interfere with conception, with the fertilized

egg's implantation in the uterus, and with the baby's growth. Tumors can block the sperm's pathway to the egg by distorting the uterus or pushing the cervix, or opening of the birth canal, out of alignment with the uterus. Large tumors can pinch the fallopian tubes, interfering with the egg's journey to the uterus.

Most fibroids are found underneath the lining of the uterus. As they grow, the lining above them stretches and may not receive enough nourishment. A fertilized egg may not be able to implant itself properly on the fibroid-distorted lining; and even if the egg does manage to attach itself to the thinned out lining, it may not hold on for the full nine months. The pregnancy will then end in a miscarriage. It is also difficult for the egg to attach itself to the lining if the woman constantly suffers bleeding.

As the pregnancy progresses, fibroids may occupy space meant for the baby. The tumors may also keep the uterus from expanding to accommodate a growing baby. Either of these situations could result in miscarriage or premature labor.

Fibroids may also interfere with the baby's birth, making it necessary for delivery by cesarean section. For example, the uterus may not be able to contract sufficiently, resulting in ineffective labor. Or the baby may not have enough room to assume the proper position for a normal birth. Tumors in or near the birth canal can block the baby's progress. After the baby is born, fibroids may also increase the amount of maternal bleeding.

Fibroids do not prevent most women from conceiving and delivering healthy babies. But when fibroids do cause problems, they are likely to be serious. There are many causes of infertility; only a thorough evaluation can determine whether fibroids are the culprit. If they do prove to be the reason, surgery to remove them will take care of the problem for many women.

Treatment of Fibroids

The decision to actively treat fibroids can only be made on an individual basis. Most women require no treatment at all. If the tumors are small and cause no problems, most physicians will simply schedule an examination every six months to make sure the fibroids aren't growing.

Reasons for Treatment

Your doctor may decide to treat fibroids if they start growing rapidly, cause serious pain or discomfort, or may interfere with your ability to become pregnant. In the following situations, physicians are likely to proceed more aggressively:

Bleeding. This is often the primary indication for surgery particularly if the woman is experiencing an extremely heavy flow during her menstrual period and notices blood clots. Persistent bleeding greatly reduces the amount of iron in the body, producing anemia that does not respond well to treatment.

Sudden enlargement of fibroids. Rapid growth of fibroids at any age is cause for concern, but this is particularly so after menopause, when the tumors should be shrinking due to decreased estrogen production. The doctor must make sure that not one of the tumors is malignant. Although almost all fibroids are benign, a malignant tumor could be hidden among them.

It is important to note that malignancy is not the only explanation for sudden enlargement of fibroids. This often happens during pregnancy. In women who are not pregnant, bleeding and deterioration inside the tumor are commonly at fault.

Pain, pressure and other discomfort. If the symptoms caused by fibroids become intolerable, the fibroids must be treated. Each woman must decide for herself whether she has reached this stage.

If the fibroids interfere with other organ systems, surgery may clearly be necessary. For example, fibroid tumors that encroach on the urinary system may cause so much pressure and crowding that a woman is almost unable to urinate.

Location of the tumors. Sometimes fibroids must be removed because their location is likely to cause serious problems sooner or later, as with tumors that obscure the ovaries. In addition, certain types of fibroids resemble ovarian tumors—a fact of particular concern for women over the age of 40, when the danger of ovarian tumors increases.

Surgery

When the problems caused by fibroids are severe enough to require treatment, it may be necessary to remove not only the tumors, but also the uterus. The type of surgery performed depends on the woman's age, the type of symptoms she is experiencing, and whether she plans to have children in the future. Following are descriptions of two forms of surgery—myomectomy and hysterectomy.

Myomectomy. Understandably, the prospect of any type of gynecologic surgery is upsetting to a woman who hopes to become pregnant. Yet continued presence of fibroids may in itself make pregnancy impossible. For women faced with this dilemma, a myomectomy is the procedure of choice.

A myomectomy is the surgical removal of each tumor separately without damaging or disturbing the uterus. The procedure is successful in almost all women who choose to have it performed. Generally, it doesn't matter how numerous or how big the fibroids are or where they are located.

When performing a myomectomy, the surgeon tries to remove as many tumors as possible while making as few surgical cuts as possible. It is sometimes feasible to remove certain tumors through the vagina, but in most cases the surgeon has to make an abdominal incision. During the operation, the surgeon closes up the spaces in the uterine lining where the fibroids used to be so that blood will not collect there afterward.

The possibility of blood loss is a major concern during surgery, but there are procedures and drugs that allow surgeons to limit bleeding during and after the operation. Because the fibroids are removed one at a time, surgery can take several hours—much longer than removal of the entire uterus.

It is important to remember that women who have had fibroids once are likely to have them again. The likelihood of a recurrence depends on a woman's age, race, and whether most of her tumors were removed during the procedure. Estimates vary, but one quarter to half of the women who have a myomectomy can expect to eventually develop additional tumors.

While a second—or even a third— myomectomy is an option if the tumors return, multiple myomectomies can lead to

problems. The walls of the uterus, for example, can stick together due to scarring. Or the bowel may become blocked. Unfortunately, many, if not most, of the women who develop additional fibroids eventually have to undergo a hysterectomy.

Despite these possible drawbacks, the improved outlook for preserving a woman's fertility makes myomectomy an increasingly popular choice for younger patients.

Hysterectomy. When fibroids cause severe complications, a hysterectomy, or removal of the uterus, will probably be necessary. Removing the uterus effectively removes the fibroids, because most of these tumors are attached to the uterus. Hysterectomy is generally considered the procedure of choice when:

■ A woman who has completed her family and whose uterus has grown to the size that would accommodate a 12-week old fetus suffers from severe symptoms
■ There are extensive or especially large tumors
■ The bleeding caused by fibroids is debilitating
■ The fibroids are creating problems with other organs in the body

Because a hysterectomy leaves the ovaries intact, a woman does not automatically face menopause after the operation. The decision to preserve or remove a woman's ovaries generally depends on her age at the time of surgery. The current practice is to preserve normal and healthy ovaries in women younger than 40 to 45 years of age.

There has been much criticism of unnecessary hysterectomies; and fibroids are the justification in an estimated 30 percent of cases. Limiting this surgery to older women who do not plan to become pregnant and who have serious symptoms should naturally reduce the number of hysterectomies performed.

Other Options

Physicians are starting to evaluate ways to treat fibroid tumors without surgery. A few have begun using lasers to remove them or reduce the size of fibroid tumors. Several scientific studies are underway to test a new drug treatment that shrinks fibroids. Most of the women who have used the drug had their fibroids shrink to half their starting size. The drug is leuprolide acetate (Lupron), a synthetic form of the naturally occurring substance known as gonadotropin-releasing hormone (also called GnRH).

One drawback is that the drug has to be taken regularly. Another drawback is that women have to inject themselves or use a nasal spray. Furthermore, once treatment stops, the tumors grow back rapidly.

The drug does shrink the fibroids, however, and may help women who are trying to become pregnant or plan to have surgery. The treatment might also be especially useful for women who are nearing menopause—when the fibroids will shrink on their own. It will effectively delay surgery until it becomes unnecessary. Studies of the drug's side effects and long-term consequences are still continuing. □

CHAPTER 8   **COMMON DISORDERS OF THE REPRODUCTIVE SYSTEM**

Keeping Endometriosis at Bay

Elusive, painful, and unpredictable, endometriosis can be an unrelenting scourge, ruining the life of a woman who develops it. That is, if she allows it to. With the broad range of treatments available to doctors today, there's no longer any reason to put up with the suffering and damage endometriosis can cause.

Tip-offs of Endometriosis

Painful menstrual periods with heavy, irregular flow, so common in a variety of reproductive disorders, are a hallmark of endometriosis. Pain may begin before the period and go on even after it ends, and may be accompanied by pain in the lower back. However, the problem that first sends most women with endometriosis to their doctors is a chronic pain in the pelvis (the area below the navel, above the thighs, and between the hips).

Other signs of possible endometriosis include diarrhea and painful bowel movements during periods, consistently painful intercourse, and long-standing infertility. For some women, however, the only symptom may be tenderness of the abdomen, sometimes in a particular spot. For others there may be no symptoms at all, even when the disease is well advanced.

What It Is

You can see from this description that endometriosis appears to be related to the menstrual cycle. In fact, it is a benign (not cancerous) condition that, in 95 percent of the cases, affects women only during their child-bearing years. The endometrium, a layer of tissue that lines the uterus, normally thickens with blood, shreds, and is shed through the vagina as the menstrual period arrives. Sometimes however, this tissue is found outside the uterus attached to or imbedded in other body tissues. The name given this condition, endometriosis, comes from the Greek words, *endo* (within), *metra* (uterus) and *osis* (abnormal or diseased condition).

Obviously, that's a misnomer. For in endometriosis, fragments of endometrial tissue appear almost anywhere in the body, except "within" the uterus. Most often affected are the ovaries, the fallopian tubes between the ovaries and uterus, the vagina, and the uterine wall, followed by the abdomen, intestine, bladder, and kidney. In rare cases, endometrial tissue is even found in the lungs, skin, surgical scars, certain nerves, the brain, and the lymphatic system (a connected group of glands that produce and circulate infection-fighting cells). Only in the spleen (largest organ of the lymphatic system) has the endometrial tissue never been found.

What It Does
The endometrial tissue that develops outside the uterus appears normal and, stimulated by estrogen, continues to perform its normal function—swelling to accept a fertilized egg, disintegrating when conception does not occur, and sloughing off in preparation for the next cycle. During each menstrual period, the tissue bleeds just as the endometrium does. The trouble is that the tissue is no longer in the uterus where it belongs, but elsewhere in the body. The bloody debris formed by the breakdown of this misplaced tissue has no way to escape. Accumulating in the tissues in which it has become lodged, the debris produces irritation, inflammation, and pain that can continue period after period. Unchecked, the bleeding may create scar tissue that can spread through the pelvis, twisting and attaching organs to each other, interfering with their proper function, filling

RIGHT TISSUE, WRONG PLACE

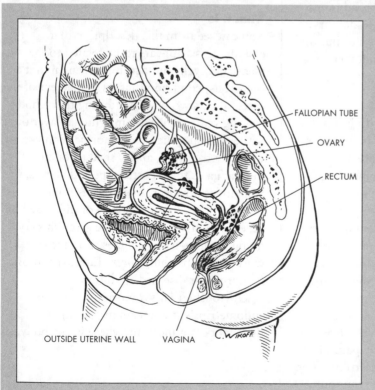

FALLOPIAN TUBE

OVARY

RECTUM

OUTSIDE UTERINE WALL   VAGINA   C. WIKOFF

Not a cancer, endometriosis develops when normal tissue from the uterine lining begins to appear in abnormal places. Favored sites are the vagina, the ovaries, and the fallopian tubes that connect the ovaries to the uterus. Patches of misplaced tissue sometimes even settle in the lungs! The vagrant tissue causes cyclical pain because it swells and sloughs off in concert with the normal lining inside the uterus.

the entire cavity, and eventually producing a tumor-like mass.

The spread of fragments of endometrial tissue outside the uterus helps explain a number of the symptoms mentioned earlier, such as chronic pelvic pain, painful intercourse, and infertility. Pain can come back with each period wherever dislocated endometrial tissue is attached in the pelvis—to the uterine wall, ovaries, bladder, or intestine, for instance. And it can get worse, remaining constant except for a few days after menstruation. A deep-seated ache from the front to the back of the pelvis is typical. If nodules of endometrial tissue have formed on the ligaments that hold the uterus in place, the result will be pain during intercourse, when the ligaments are stretched. Infertility, long considered almost synonymous with endometriosis, can result from distortion of the reproductive organs or interference with their function by misplaced endometrial tissue.

What Else It Might Be

Menstrual and pelvic pain is not limited to endometriosis. There are several other explanations your doctor must consider.

Pelvic Inflammatory Disease (PID) is a leading possibility because so many of its early symptoms are similar to those of endometriosis. PID is the result of bacterial infection. It can be cleared up with antibiotics; and in fact, a course of antibiotic therapy is one way doctors establish a diagnosis. However, there are other distinguishing clues. Women with PID often also have fever, chills, a pus-containing vaginal discharge, and fallopian tube blockage. The combination of a pelvic examination and medical history is an important way of differentiating the diseases. The doctor may also need to perform a laparo-scopy, a routine diagnostic procedure in which a tiny viewing instrument is inserted through the wall of the abdomen.

Fibroids (benign tumors of the uterus) are another possibility. These growths develop in the uterine wall, occasionally between the muscle and the endometrium. They are very common, ranging in size from a pea to a football. Like endometriosis, they can cause heavy menstrual bleeding, painful periods, and abdominal and lower back pain, though they usually have no symptoms at all. Stimulated, as endometrial tissue is, by estrogen and sometimes seen with endometriosis, fibroids can interfere with fertility.

Cervical polyps (small non-cancerous growths that project from the inside surface of the neck of the uterus, called the cervix) can also bring on bleeding after intercourse and between periods.

Cysts (fluid-filled sacs) can form in the ovaries when, for example, hormonal communication with the brain breaks down and no eggs can be released. Besides infertility, ovarian cysts can cause abdominal pain, irregular periods, and, if a cyst ruptures, internal bleeding. This could create a medical emergency.

Cervical, ovarian, and uterine cancers may also be responsible for some signs similar to those of endometriosis, including mild or acute chronic abdominal tenderness, pain and pressure, uterine bleeding, and development of an abdominal mass. Since these cancers are most responsive to early treatment, it's particularly urgent for you to get an accurate diagnosis.

Structural abnormalities in the reproductive organs, including the uterus, can lead to infertility, just as endometriosis does. They may result from weakened or stretched supporting muscles and tissues or hereditary variations in organ position and shape, as well as from scar tissue formed by endometriosis.

Uterine infections, like endometriosis, can account for painful intercourse, irregular menstrual bleeding, and lower pelvic pain. They can leave scars on the uterine wall that prevent the endometrium from accepting an egg.

Factors That Increase
the Odds of Endometriosis

Not surprisingly, distortion and obstruction of reproductive organs because of congenital defects and lifetime developments predisposes affected women to endometriosis. For example, if you have chronic pain in the pelvis from a uterus tipped out of position the risk of endometriosis is greater.

The chances of disease appearing in a woman whose mother, aunt, or sister have it are seven to 10 percent greater than in other women—so is the likelihood that it will appear earlier in life and be more severe.

The old stereotype of the typical endometriosis candidate as white, in her late thirties, and not yet a mother has now been generally discarded. The disease occurs twice as often in Japanese as in Caucasian women and it is common in American blacks. More research is needed to determine disease rates in women of other races.

Who Gets It?

From 10 to 20 percent of American women develop endometriosis some time in their lives. Currently, between 5 million and 12 million are estimated to have the disease. It has been found in girls and women aged 10 to 70, though a large majority of cases are in the childbearing years. In any case, both those who have borne children and those who have not are targets. The disease is also now recognized as more common in teenagers that once thought.

And Why?

No single cause for endometriosis is universally accepted. As one authority puts it, "there is no simple explanation"—probably because it is often accompanied by diseases with similar symptoms and effects. It varies in intensity from one person to another and is sometimes unaffected by or returns after "definitive" treatment, including hysterectomy (surgical removal of all or most of the reproductive organs).

No fewer than 12 theories have been proposed since 1921 to explain how and why endometriosis occurs. Of the three best known, the oldest is based on the fact that blood flow during menstruation can back up into the fallopian tubes, possibly carrying endometrial tissue fragments into the ovaries and abdomen. This theory does not, however, explain why only some of the nine out of 10 women who experience this backward flow develop endometriosis. Nor does it tell why some women still have endometriosis even though they have had their fallopian tubes tied, blocking access to the abdomen.

Another suggestion is that, since all tissues in which endometriosis is found originate from the same part of the embryo, some of these tissues such as the peritoneum (which covers the organs inside the abdomen), may gradually change into functioning endometrial tissue in response to chronic irritation by wandering menstrual blood. This could also account for the widely separated sites such as lungs, arms, and legs, where endometriosis has been found. However, there is no conclusive evidence that tissues with a common embryonic source can be transformed in this way.

A third idea, the "immune defect" theory, is based on the high levels of antibodies (disease-fighting proteins) found in endometriosis patients' blood, plus observation of spontaneous development of endometriosis in monkeys and the fact that women whose close relatives have the disease are at increased risk. In some women a hereditary tendency toward endometriosis, together with an immune reaction against their own tissues, might bring on the disease. Research into this theory is on the rise. Among other mysteries it might help clear up is why endometriosis is so rare in the cervix, despite its regular exposure to menstrual fluid.

Finally, environmental factors that possibly contribute to endometriosis may be uncovered by current studies of levels of the pesticide dioxin and similar chemicals in the blood of women with the disease. These studies stem from the unexpected finding of endometriosis in 80 percent of female rhesus monkeys exposed to very small amounts of these chemicals over four years. More of the monkeys on the highest doses had moderate to severe disease than those on the lowest doses. Monkeys not receiving dioxin did not develop either moderate or severe disease.

How the Disease Plays Out

While the search for causes continues, a cure for endometriosis has yet to be found. Though the disease is seldom life threatening, the damage it can do to the quality of a woman's life is immense. There is no easy way to "live with" severe pain that can return month after

THE "OTHER" ENDOMETRIOSES

Though endometriosis develops when endometrial tissue grows and functions *outside* the uterus, endometrial tissue *inside* the uterus can also grow abnormally—invading the muscular wall of the uterus on which the endometrium lies.

For many years both conditions were considered forms of the same disease and were called *endometriosis externa* and *interna*. Now they are considered two different diseases. Though both can be found in the same person 20 percent of the time, *adenomyosis*, as it is now termed, usually affects women in their 30s and 40s who've already had several children. It is thought to result from the trauma and damage to the uterine wall produced by repeated pregnancies, deliveries, and subsequent return of the uterus to normal size. Unlike the isolated tissues of endometriosis, the islands of endometrial glands formed by adenomyosis always maintain a connection with the endometrium, even when buried in the uterine wall. The disease is associated with a greater chance of developing fibroids, polyps, and endometrial cancer than is endometriosis itself.

Finally, there is *stromal endometriosis,* which doesn't look or behave like endometriosis, but instead like an abnormal growth in the uterus. Independent growths have never been found outside the uterus, though extensions of the intrauterine growth can make their way out of the uterus and involve other organs. The disease is termed stromal (supporting tissue) endometriosis because no endometrial glands are found in the lump of endometriotic tissue it forms. It is often highly malignant, and is treated as an endometrial cancer.

month and often progresses to involve major organs and other areas of the body. Symptoms can interfere with building a career or even holding a job, bearing children and caring for them, having sex, or simply enjoying life. It is not surprising that phone "help" lines for women with "Endo" (as its sufferers have dubbed it) are to be found in many communities. The psychological effects on personal relationships and feelings of self-worth can be devastating.

Though many women have a mild form of endometriosis that passes with vague and minor soreness in the lower abdomen, the adhesions and scar tissue that build up in others can eventually "freeze" the reproductive and other pelvic organs in place and, along with internal bleeding and other progressive effects, destroy them. A rating system that ranks severity of a woman's endometriosis in five stages has been established. In the first stage, pain is minimal and there is no abnormal bleeding. In the second, the pain is greater and accompanied by internal bleeding. In the next stage the disease progresses, with hemorrhaging and adhesions in which tissues covering various organs, inflamed by the endometrial growths bleeding into them, begin to stick together. The adhesions grow thicker in the next stage and destruction of organs begins. In the final stage there is total loss of reproductive function, extensive organ destruction, and a "frozen pelvis" produced by dense adhesions.

Probably the most "pain" women experience next to the severe pain of the disease itself, is the threat endometriosis presents to fertility. Nearly half of women with the disease have reported infertility problems. Severe endometriosis can, of course, block and bend reproductive organs into abnormality, yet no direct causal link has been found between endometriosis and infertility. Though pregnancy often reduces or eliminates symptoms, at least temporarily, it is not a cure. The disease can progress while the baby is developing and bring back symptoms after the child is born. If you have a family history of endometriosis, your doctor may encourage you to have children early, before the disease arrives and brings progressive complications. Of course, this advice can't help the increasing number of women who develop the disease as teenagers, especially since research seems to indicate that women with endometriosis in the family develop serious cases earlier than others.

Helping Yourself

What can you do to help yourself? Pain relief is a principal concern of anyone with the difficult and painful menstrual flow that so often is a symptom of endometriosis. Several medications that attack this pain are available without a prescription. Aspirin is the original, but ibuprofen (Advil, Motrin, others) is considered more effective. However, allergies to these drugs and too frequent use at too high doses can cause side effects. These medications reduce the effects of prostaglandins (hormone-like compounds involved in the production of pain and inflammation) that increase rapidly as menstruation approaches. They are therefore often most effective when taken just before, as well as during, your period.

Good nutrition helps fight any disease, but its value against endometriosis is somewhat limited. Most approaches are designed to reduce the effect of estrogen on endometrial tissue. B vitamins, especially B6, promote the liver's ability to change estrogen to estradiol, a form of the hormone less prone to promote endometrial growths. Vitamin E has been called an estrogen antagonist and may break down the hormone when it is present in excessive amounts. Whole wheat, citrus fruit, and yams are reported to raise estrogen levels and perhaps should be avoided. Fish oils are said to reduce prostaglandin production. Before making any of these dietary adjustments, it's wise to check with your doctor, and none should be made too radically. Remember, too, that diet cannot repair damaged tissues and organs and is probably useful only in early endometriosis.

One nutritional supplement that you should definitely keep in mind is extra iron. Excessive bleeding at menstruation can reduce this essential component of the blood. Exercise is also advisable, since it tends to reduce menstrual flow and, therefore, the irritation and inflammation where foreign endometrial tissue is growing.

None of these remedies get at the underlying problems of endometriosis, but they can make the symptoms more bearable. However, when symptoms begin to interfere with daily living, it is important to consult your doctor. Remember that the severity of the disease is not necessarily reflected by the severity of the symptoms.

Getting a Diagnosis

An accurate and complete medical history as well as a thorough pelvic examination can often go a long way towards identifying endometriosis. In fact, if you believe your symptoms may mean endometriosis, it is a good idea to write down what they are and where and when they occur. Don't leave anything out. Spitting up blood may seem unrelated to endometriosis, for example, but if it happens regularly during menstruation, it suggests a case of endometriosis in the lung (where endometrial tissue sometimes has been found). Another positive indication of endometriosis is pain

that specifically effects an unusual location in your body and happens only when your period arrives. This helps separate it from the menstrual pain that centers on the reproductive organs.

During the physical exam your doctor may find nodules formed by endometriosis in the back of the vagina, in the rectum, and on the ligaments supporting the uterus, as well as tender and enlarged ovaries, lumps in the abdomen, or a uterus drawn back and attached to the rectum.

Magnetic resonance imaging (MRI) which produces three-dimensional images of the body's interior structures, can sometimes spot endometriosis implants in soft tissue.

Ultrasound, which also produces interior images, has been used to examine tissue masses attached to the uterus and the ovaries. However, neither technique is definitive for diagnosis, nor are there any reliable laboratory tests yet available.

Several studies on basal (resting) body temperature, often used to confirm ovulation, report that in women with endometriosis this temperature remains high as their period begins—rather than dropping as it does in women without the disease. One U.S. research group reports that in their studies two out of three women with endometriosis, had temperatures above 97.8 for the first three days of their periods. This contrasts sharply with the one in 16 among those who did not have endometriosis. A combination of basal body temperature charts and a blood test may one day be able to detect if a woman has the disease.

Laparotomy, a technique that requires a substantial incision in the abdominal wall, is now seldom performed just to diagnose endometriosis. If this major operation is required to reach and attack some other disease of the pelvis, it provides an opportunity to identify and evaluate potential endometriosis.

However, most authorities now agree that the only safe, reliable way to distinguish between endometriosis, PID, pelvic growths, and other disorders that produce symptoms similar to those of endometriosis is a technique called laparoscopy. With the tiny lighted lens of a laparoscope inserted through the navel, the doctor is able to see into the abdomen and examine the organs. Implants of endometrial tissue outside the uterus can be seen and distinguished from cysts, tumors, fibroids, and adhesions in the pelvic area. So can any existing fallopian tube obstruction and pelvic inflammatory disease.

An Array of Treatments

Once a diagnosis has been made, your doctor may recommend surgery or medication or a combination of the two approaches. Surgery, of course, aims to remove the source of pain and interference with the normal functioning of affected organs. Surgical treatments range from burning up endometrial implants with a laser beam to removing the affected organs themselves. For advanced endometriosis, the doctor may consider hysterectomy and bilateral oophorectomy, in which the uterus and both ovaries are removed. This radical surgery, reserved for the most extensive and resistant cases, suppresses hormonal stimulation of endometriotic tissue growth by removing the main sources of the hormones.

Treatment with drugs also revolves around the connection that appears to exist between the hormonal variations of menstruation and the development of endometriosis. These medications moderate or suppress ovulation (the ripening and release of an egg for fertilization) to create a temporary pseudo-menopause (in contrast to the permanent menopause achieved by radical surgery). Alternatively, your doctor may decide to use hormonal medications to produce a pseudo-pregnancy. Either way, the goal is the same: elimination of the long periods of estrogen production that stimulate endometrial tissue growth. Hormonal therapy can reduce both the size and number of endometrial tissue even causing some to waste away. These treatments, however, may cause a temporary failure to menstruate, along with vaginal dryness, a near-menopausal state, and estrogen deficiency problems. What works best for one woman may not help another. Usually a combination of medication and surgical treatments tailored to the individual keeps endometriosis in check, maintains or improves fertility, and avoids serious medication side effects.

Keep in mind that no treatment can absolutely prevent endometriosis from re-appearing. Even the most extensive and complete destruction and removal of endometrial tissue that has established itself outside a woman's uterus does not guarantee permanent freedom from pain or progression of the disease. Among women whose endometrial tissue implants are destroyed by lasers or electrocautery, 40 percent are estimated to face endometriosis again within five years, and 10 percent of those who have undergone total hysterectomy will have recurring pain.

FOR MANY, PINPOINT SURGERY SOLVES THE PROBLEM

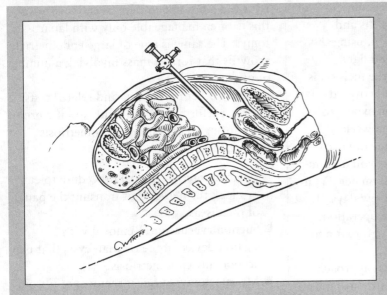

A high-tech surgical technique called laparoscopy now allows doctors to locate and remove misplaced patches of uterine tissue without leaving a major scar. Working through a inch-long incision, the surgeon can search the reproductive organs for unwanted growths, then snip, burn, or vaporize them away. Impossible until the development of fiber optics and high-resolution video, the whole procedure often takes less than a day, from admission to discharge.

Surgical Approaches

Laparoscopy, as well as providing an accurate diagnosis without major surgery, has also changed surgical treatment for the disease, especially with the added development of laser surgery. A surgeon using a laparoscope to see and diagnose endometriosis can also use it to aim an obliterating laser beam at unwanted tissue growths, adhesions, and other obstructions to normal functions. Cutting and cauterizing (tissue burning) instruments can also be used with the scope. This makes it possible to diagnose and surgically treat endometriosis in the same visit, if you and your doctor agree.

Depending on what is found during laparoscopy, and the surgical repairs needed, the operation can range from 15 minutes to several hours. You can usually be discharged from the hospital the same or next day. Since the operation requires an empty stomach, don't eat for at least eight hours before the procedure is scheduled. Patients are usually put to sleep during the operation itself.

At the beginning of the operation, a cannula (probe) is placed in the uterus and an incision made in or near the navel. (See nearby illustration.) Gas, usually carbon dioxide, is then pumped into the abdomen through the incision to inflate the cavity so the organs inside can be separated and more easily viewed. To shift the intestines away from the lower abdomen so that other organs can be seen more clearly, you are tilted head downward. The scope, inside a hollow tube, is inserted through the small incision at the navel. The scope's flexible fiber optics, which transmit light along thin threads of glass, let the doctor look all around the organs, photograph their surfaces, and collect tissues for study in the laboratory.

Sometimes the laser is inserted through the same tube as the scope; sometimes it is introduced through another small incision. It cuts, coagulates, and vaporizes cells and tissues with microscopic precision, using the heat produced by its concentrated light.

At the end of the operation, the incision is closed with a pair of stitches and covered with a plastic bandage. You can expect to have tenderness there for about a week. Trauma from manipulation of the organs, plus any left-over gas, may cause you discomfort in the abdomen, neck and shoulder. You may also feel some nausea for a few days. If you were put to sleep during the operation, you may briefly experience a sore throat and difficulty concentrating.

The advantages of this surgical approach, besides a shorter and less expensive hospital stay, include less likelihood of complications; reduced tissue injury, bleeding, and scar tissue formation; rapid diagnosis and treatment; and an easier, swifter, less painful recovery. The risks it carries are mainly those of instrument insertion and heat injury plus potential anesthetic complications. Meanwhile, it directly attacks the causes of pain and infertility, the most important concerns of women about endometriosis.

Laparotomy, on the other hand, is an operation that can keep you in the hospital for a week. Recovery is also slower and more painful, and there is a greater danger of post-op infection. The operation, which involves opening up the abdominal cavity, is called for when endometriosis is so widespread (and perhaps accompanied by other related diseases) that it can't be handled through the tiny incision used in laparoscopic surgery. Appendix, bladder, bowel, and kidney involvement, for example, may require

special surgical techniques only practical with laparotomy. If there are large cysts to be removed—not uncommon in endometriosis—this is often manageable only with laparotomy. The same is true of large endometrial growths that form a mass involving a number of organs.

Many other operations and related tests may be performed to deal with specific problems during treatment for endometriosis. Among them are:

- **Neurectomy:** A surgical procedure to cut or block the nerves that transmit the pain of the disease.
- **Suction evacuation:** Removal with a suction device of the ovarian cysts that may accompany endometriosis.
- **Myomectomy:** Surgical removal of fibroid growths from the uterus.
- **Salpingectomy:** Surgical removal of a fallopian tube.
- **Renogram:** A study of kidney function done by externally monitoring radiation levels in the bladder as a radioactive chemical enters it from the kidney.
- **Intravenous pyelogram:** an x-ray examination of the kidneys, bladder, and ureters (the tubes between the kidneys and bladder) using a dye injected through a vein in the hand or arm.
- **Cystoscopy:** Examination of the wall of the bladder with a thin, lighted probe inserted through the urinary opening.
- **Thoracentesis:** A search for endometrial blood in the lungs through a small puncture in the wall of the chest.

- **Proctosigmoidoscopy:** Insertion of lighted tube to search for tumors, polyps, or endometrial tissue in the lower bowel.
- **Barium enema:** An x-ray of the lower bowel to check for obstructions, deformities, tumors, and polyps.

Hysterectomy, either partial or complete removal of the uterus, is the final major surgical approach to endometriosis. Normally, your doctor will try to keep disease in check while preserving the uterus and at least one ovary and fallopian tube, so you can still become pregnant. However, if recurrent endometriosis is a major threat to your organs and general health and repeated surgery has made "living with" the disease intolerable, you need to consider this "radical" surgery. It is clearly a serious decision, taking into consideration your lifestyle, your age, and your psychological and physiological responses to bodily changes. You need to weigh the long-term consequences of the premature menopause that results from the operation against the option of waiting for natural menopause, when the higher levels of hormones found with fertility will gradually fall. Surgical menopause in younger women puts them at greater risk of developing coronary heart disease and osteoporosis (brittle bones).

Once the decision has been made to go ahead, you will want to be prepared for a long convalescence that could take as long as two months. The operation will be performed under general anesthetic and usually lasts several hours. The uterus will be removed through an incision in the lower abdomen or at the top of the vagina. All endometrial tissue found outside the uterus will also be removed and adhesions repaired. Usually, the operation is combined with a bilateral oophorectomy, in which the ovaries and fallopian tubes are removed, so that this source of hormonal stimulation of endometrial tissue growth disappears. You will be encouraged to get out of bed the next day and walk a little, with the prospect of going home in a week or possibly two. There may be some vaginal bleeding and discharge for a day or two.

Estrogen replacement therapy may be started within days, weeks or months, depending on whether you are experiencing any menopausal symptoms such as hot flashes and whether you and your doctor are convinced all endometrial tissue is gone. Micronized estradiol (Estrace), in small doses, by mouth or skin patch (Estraderm), can be balanced with the hormone progesterone to control any flare-up of endometriosis.

Surgery and Medication Combined

This example of using medications along with surgery, even radical surgery, illustrates how combined therapy works. In another instance, androgen, a male hormone modified in the laboratory as Danazol (danocrine) is taken for six weeks before surgery to shrink endometrial tissue and ease its surgical removal. Because the surgery follows the hormonal treatment, it's possible to get rid of adhesions formed while the hormone heals the disease. Following surgical removal of a moderate amount of endometriotic tissue, your doctor may prescribe birth control pills that contain the two female hormones, estrogen and progesterone, to be taken continuously for up to nine months. The idea, of course, is to fool the endometrial tissue outside the uterus into reacting as though the body were pregnant, so that the tissue does not grow, shed or bleed. Since the hormones achieve this in the same way they prevent conception—by producing a state of pseudo-pregnancy in which ovulation and menstruation are suppressed—the endometriosis remains inactive.

Likely Medications

Any birth control pill will do the job, but those with a high progesterone level are preferred. Potential side effects are the same as those that may be encountered when the pills are taken for contraception. (For further information see chapter 21, "Hormonal Options: Pills, Shots, and Implants.")

Progesterone-only medications also may be prescribed. Oral forms include Provera and Micronor. Quarterly injections of Depo-Provera are another alternative. These medications bring relief by shrinking endometrial tissue. Among their side effects are water retention, weight gain, and acne. As with the birth control pills, this treatment usually lasts 6 to 9 months until the problem abates. Endometriosis recurrence rates with any of these pseudopregnancy treatments are 5 to 10 percent annually. Pregnancy rates after stopping the medication are highest for progesterone-only medications.

The pseudomenopause approach to endometriosis treatment relies on medications that prevent the release of two hormones that govern production of estrogen and progesterone. This pair of hormones—called luteinizing hormone (LH) and follicle-stimulating hormone (FSH)—originate in the pituitary gland at the base of the brain. Together, they stimulate the ovaries to release eggs and produce the estrogen and progesterone that prepares the endometrium to receive an egg.

Drugs called gonadatropin-releasing hormone (GnRH) analogs, shut down secretion of LH and FSH by overloading the pituitary's production facilities. In effect, the GnRH analogs create a "reversible oophorectomy." That is, they put an end to ovulation without removing the ovaries. The near menopausal state that results stops menstruation and the growth of endometrial tissue, and reduces the pain of endometriosis. Of course, it also brings with it the problems of estrogen deficiency, ranging from hot flashes and headaches to increased risk of osteoporosis. These problems can be halted by going off these medications, and fertility then appears to be regained. In fact, these drugs are not reliable contraceptives, and your doctor will usually advise you to use barrier contraceptives if you have intercourse while taking them. Treatment is not started if you are pregnant and is stopped if you become pregnant.

GnRH analogs can be taken as a nose spray (Synarel), as a daily or monthly injection (Lupron), or as a monthly implant beneath the skin (Zoladex). A course of treatment lasts 6 months.

The drug Danazol, also stops the pituitary from secreting LH and FSH hormones, in turn drastically reducing the ovaries' production of estrogen and progesterone to an amount too small to support monthly periods. Deprived of the regular hormonal surges on which they depend, implants of endometrial tissue in the pelvis begin to shrink, and pain, both pelvic and menstrual, declines. Treatment, which may last 3 to 9 months, can be adjusted for mild, moderate, or severe endometriosis by modifying dosage. Side effects include mood, skin, hair, voice and sex drive changes. Some women gain weight; some may experience vaginal dryness, bloating, and sporadic menstrual bleeding. Levels of HDL (the good cholesterol) may fall, but gradually return to normal after treatment is stopped. Cases of high blood pressure and stroke have been reported.

As with GnRH analogs, there is no guarantee that this drug will prevent pregnancy, and the same contraceptive precautions apply. Two or 3 months after the drug is stopped periods usually return and pregnancy becomes possible. If endometriosis comes back, treatment can be resumed, provided you have not become pregnant.

All medications that change your hormonal balance need to be monitored closely by both you and your doctor. They are powerful and can be dangerous in women who have conditions that the drug may aggravate. On the other hand, most of their side effects can be controlled without giving up the medications' beneficial effects on endometriosis. It's wise to consult your doctor before starting, stopping, or resuming treatment with any of these drugs.

In addition to pain-relief medications available over-the-counter, a number of prescription products can be used to reduce the pain of endometriosis. These drugs, called non-steroidal anti-inflammatories include Naprosyn, Feldene, Ponstel, Rufen, Clinoril, Motrin, Nalfon, Dolobid, Meclomen, Tolectin, and Indocin. Narcotic pain-killers such as codeine, oxycodone, meperidine and morphine, as well as narcotics combined with other pain relief drugs, may also be prescribed.

What Treatments Cost

Though prices do change rapidly and vary from one part of the country to the other, here are some "ball-park" figures: Laparoscopy: $1,000 to $3,500, depending on the extent of the disease, plus hospital or out-patient charges. Laparotomy: $2,500 to $4,000 plus the additional cost of a longer hospital stay. A hysterectomy with a bilateral oophorectomy averages $2,200, more if extensive repair is required for endometriosis-damaged organs and tissues.

Treatment with hormonal medications (usually 6 to 9 months) runs $225 to $350 a month, not including the cost of monitoring tests and physician charges. Oral contraceptives, when they can be used, are less expensive.

Looking Ahead

The medical approach to endometriosis is long past the "it's all in your mind" stage. Doctors realize that the disease's severe, often incapacitating pain, sometimes repeated monthly for years while the disease progresses to destroy tissues, organs, and hopes of pregnancy, can devastate a woman's life. Worse yet, the disease can come back and continue even beyond the childbearing years, its unpredictable course varying from person to person.

But now, with recognition and diagnosis better than ever before, the disease is controllable in a large majority of cases. Most women can find relief through the combination of sophisticated treatments now available. The most important step is to see your doctor for a full review of the risk factors and treatment options open to you. There is no need to suffer this disease in silence. Early diagnosis and the right treatment can literally change your life. □

CHAPTER 9　　　　**COMMON DISORDERS OF THE REPRODUCTIVE SYSTEM**

What You Need To Know About Ovarian Cysts

More than any other organ in the body, the ovary has the capacity to form a large number and variety of cysts. In fact, the ovarian function of producing hormones and releasing eggs is directly linked to the formation of cysts. An ovarian cyst is a sac or pouch that develops in or on the ovary, often during ovulation. The contents of the cyst are usually liquid, but can also be solid or a mixture of liquid and solid materials. Although ovarian cysts are usually small (about the size of a pea or a kidney bean), they can become the size of a softball—or even larger. Large ovarian cysts are quite remarkable considering that the ovary itself is only about the size of a walnut.

Ovarian cysts are very common, and because most of them do result from changes in the normal function of the ovary, rather than from "new growths" or tumors, the vast majority are non–cancerous. Although they are most prevalent in women of childbearing age, ovarian cysts can occur in girls and women of all ages, from newborns to the elderly. You can develop a single cyst or multiple cysts.

Warning Signs of An Ovarian Cyst

Because there are many different kinds of ovarian cysts, and because their size and number may vary, they can cause a variety of symptoms. On the other hand, many cause no symptoms at all and may first be discovered during a routine gynecological exam, as your doctor examines the size and shape of your ovaries.

Pain

Abdominal pain is often the first indicator of an ovarian cyst. If the cyst is large, you may have pain, or a feeling of pressure or heaviness in the lower abdomen. Ovarian cysts can often bring on lower abdominal pain during intercourse. Another possible cause of pain is a process called "torsion," in which the stem that forms on some cysts becomes twisted, stopping the normal flow of blood and causing intense bursts of pain. If a cyst ruptures, this too can cause severe lower abdominal pain along with weakness, nausea and vomiting. Any of these pains may be severe enough to bring you to the emergency room or to your doctor, and may be the first time you learn you have a cyst.

Cysts can cause other, less daunting symptoms. For example, a cyst can press on the rectum, causing constipation, or on the bladder, creating an urge to urinate. Don't ignore these lesser symptoms. They could also be signs of a gastrointestinal disturbance or a bladder infection. Severe abdominal pain itself could also be due to appendicitis, an infection in the uterus or fallopian tubes, or an ectopic pregnancy.

Irregular Periods and Infertility

Occasionally ovarian cysts do cause irregular periods, particularly in a condition called poly-cystic ovaries in which the hormonal system that regulates the ovaries is disturbed, causing them to form a large number of cysts. More frequently, however, menstrual irregularities are due to other conditions, such as pregnancy, menopause, or thyroid problems.

Some women who have trouble becoming pregnant also have polycystic ovaries, but this problem is only one of many possible reasons for infertility. If you are having difficulty becoming pregnant, speak with your regular ob–gyn or with an infertility specialist. (For more information see chapter 18, "Overcoming Infertility: Tactics and Techniques.")

A Close Look at the Most Common Types

Once a month, your body produces what is, in effect, an ovarian cyst. It is part of ovulation, the process during which an egg ripens and is released from the ovary. The ovary contains follicles,

sacs containing immature eggs and fluid. Each month during your childbearing years, the ovary produces hormones that cause a follicle to grow, and the egg within it to mature.

Once the egg is ready, the follicle ruptures and the egg is released. Thus the follicle is a fluid–filled cyst that ruptures when you ovulate. Many women experience pain or cramping when this occurs. This pain is known as *mittleschmerz*, the German word for "middle (mid–cycle) pain."

Once the egg is released, the follicle changes into a smaller sac called the *corpus luteum*, or "yellow body," named for the yellowish fatty material it contains. If the egg is not fertilized, the corpus luteum gradually disintegrates and a new follicle begins growing during the next menstrual cycle. If the egg is fertilized, the corpus luteum will remain for a few months, secreting estrogen and progesterone to support the developing embryo.

Functional Cysts

Cysts that develop as part of the natural function of the ovary are dubbed "functional cysts." There are two types, the follicle cyst and the corpus luteum cyst.

Follicle Cysts can develop in two ways: during ovulation when the follicle ruptures to release the egg, or when a developing follicle fails to rupture, leaving the follicle, or sometimes several follicles, to continue to enlarge. Follicle cysts rarely grow larger than one–and–a–half to two inches in diameter, and usually rupture or shrink after one or two menstrual cycles.

Because these cysts are usually painless, most women are unaware of them. However, when one ruptures, perhaps during sexual intercourse, you may experience intense abdominal pain that is often worsened by physical activity. The pain usually subsides

TWO LEADING OFFENDERS

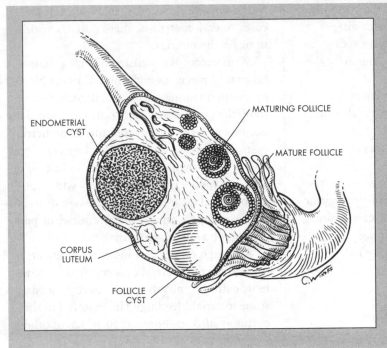

ENDOMETRIAL CYST

MATURING FOLLICLE

MATURE FOLLICLE

CORPUS LUTEUM

FOLLICLE CYST

In this cutaway view of the ovary, a follicle cyst has developed alongside an endometrial cyst. Usually painless, follicle cysts often develop when a follicle fails to release a mature egg and continues to grow instead. This type of cyst generally subsides on it own.

Endometrial cysts, however, continue to grow, frequently requiring surgical removal. They form when, in pace with the regular menstrual cycle, a misplaced patch of tissue from the uterine lining bleeds and sloughs off inside the ovary. As the blood builds up over months and years, it turns brown, giving rise to the nickname "chocolate cyst."

after a day or two but quite often is severe enough to bring you to the emergency room. You may also experience abdominal discomfort if, in response to fertility drugs, several follicle cysts begin to grow.

Corpus Luteum Cyst. The corpus luteum that forms after ovulation is also a cyst–like structure, and it is very prone to the development of fluid or blood–filled cysts that can grow from the size of an egg to the size of a softball.

Unlike follicle cysts, corpus luteum cysts usually cause pain on only one side of the lower abdomen. If you have a corpus luteum cyst, you may be experiencing menstrual changes such as late periods or bleeding between periods. Because this set of symptoms is also associated with the dangerous condition known as tubal or ectopic pregnancy, you should be sure to go to a doctor.

Polycystic Ovaries

In some women, the ovaries tend to develop numerous follicle cysts. You may hear this condition referred to as polycystic ovarian syndrome or "disease" (PCO), Stein–Leventhal Syndrome, or sclerocystic ovarian disease.

Actually polycystic ovaries are not a "disease" at all, but the result of a hormone imbalance that causes the persistent growth of follicular cysts accompanied, usually, by failure of one follicle to mature and succeed in ovulating. The condition is fairly common and usually occurs in adolescents and young women. Many women with polycystic ovaries have no symptoms, but the condition can cause fertility problems, due to infrequent ovulation, and can result in excess body hair and weight problems, due to hormone imbalances.

Because women with polycystic ovaries rarely or never ovulate, their menstrual periods are generally irregular, often with many months between periods. When they do have a period, it may be quite heavy, since the lining of the uterus has continued to grow during the months since their last period. While polycystic ovaries do not themselves become cancerous, excessive growth of the uterine lining, or endometrium, is thought to increase risk of cancer of the uterus (endometrial cancer).

Endometrial Cysts

Endometrial cysts are also known as endometriomas or "chocolate cysts," because they are filled with dark blood that resembles chocolate syrup. These cysts form as the result of endometriosis, the disease in which patches of tissue from the uterine lining are found outside the uterus. In about half the cases of endometriosis, these patches appear in or on the ovaries.

With successive menstrual cycles, these misplaced pieces of endometrial tissue bleed, gradually forming endometrial cysts. Over time, the cysts grow, and some can eventually become as large as a grapefruit. Endometrial cysts can cover a large part of the ovary and prevent ovulation, resulting in infertility. Some women have no symptoms with an endometrial cyst; others have severe menstrual cramps, pain with intercourse, or pain during a bowel movement.

Although complications are infrequent, if a sizeable endometrial cyst ruptures, its contents can spill into the pelvic cavity, causing some internal bleeding. The material in the cyst may also spill onto the surface of other

IF CYSTS KEEP COMING

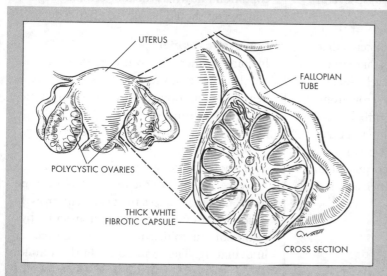

UTERUS

FALLOPIAN TUBE

POLYCYSTIC OVARIES

THICK WHITE FIBROTIC CAPSULE

CROSS SECTION

When, cycle after cycle, the hormonal system fails to trigger release of an egg, the resulting follicle cysts can build up inside the ovary, producing a condition called polycystic ovarian syndrome. While polycystic ovaries are not dangerous in themselves, the hormonal imbalance that causes them can produce infertility and, because menstrual periods are delayed, lead to excessive growth of the uterine lining.

organs in the pelvis, such as the uterus, fallopian tubes, bladder, and intestines. This can cause the formation of scar tissue (adhesions), which in turn can cause pain and fertility problems.

Cystadenomas

Unlike functional ovarian cysts, which develop from variations in the normal function of the ovaries, or endometrial cysts, which are a consequence of endometriosis, or even polycystic ovaries, which result from hormone imbalance, cystadenomas are known as neoplasms, meaning "new growths." Ovarian neoplasms are new and abnormal formations that develop from the ovarian tissue. Cystadenomas are the most common type.

Cystadenomas are classified according to the type of fluid they contain. A *serous cystadenoma* is filled with a thin watery fluid and is relatively large, between 2 and 6 inches in diameter. This type most frequently appears in women in their 30s and 40s, but may occur in women between the ages of 20 and 50.

A serous cystadenoma usually causes no specific symptoms, unless it grows to be so large that it results in weight gain and a large abdomen. Generally, these cysts are discovered during a routine gynecological exam. Although considered a benign growth, they do have the potential to become malignant.

A *mucinous cystadenoma* is filled with a sticky, thick gelatinous material and can become enormous. While most are between 6 and 12 inches in diameter, there have been rare cases of gigantic tumors measuring up to 40 inches and weighing over 100 pounds. Mucinous cystadenomas develop most often in women between the ages of 30 and 50.

Although cystadenomas are almost always benign, complications may develop. If they grow very large, they can interfere with other abdominal organs, disturbing the normal functioning of the stomach, intestines, and bowel. They may also twist, rupture, or bleed. Keep in mind, though, that if you have regular gynecological exams, your doctor would probably discover a cystadenoma long before it could grow to its potentially enormous size.

Dermoid Cysts

Dermoid cysts are also ovarian neoplasms. They are so named because they contain skin or related tissue such as hair, teeth, or bone. They are also known as benign cystic teratomas, teratoma meaning a tumor consisting of skin and hair tissue. Dermoid cysts contain this unusual type of tissue because they develop from the ovary's germ cells, the cells that normally produce the egg and contain the forerunner of all human tissues. Dermoid cysts may be present from birth, but rarely grow large enough to be noticed until adulthood.

Dermoid cysts are quite common, and although they can occur in women of any age, they most frequently affect women between the ages of 20 and 40. They generally measure between 2 and 4 inches in diameter, and usually cause no symptoms unless they become so large that they press on the intestines, bladder, or rectum. While these growths are almost always benign, there is about a 1 percent chance that a malignancy could develop. As is true of most types of cysts, the dermoid may be prone to bleeding, rupture, or twisting on its stem.

When To Seek Medical Attention

Because functional ovarian cysts usually remain quite small, often cause no symptoms, and may disappear on their own, treatment of them is not always necessary. However, since there are so many other types of ovarian cysts, you should see your doctor if you experience any of the following:

- Abdominal pain or pressure that is severe or frequent
- Pain with intercourse
- Unusual vaginal bleeding or any vaginal bleeding after menopause
- Unexplained weight gain or abdominal bloating
- Irregular periods for several months or no period with a negative pregnancy test
- Inability to become pregnant after 12 months of intercourse without using birth control

How Your Doctor Goes About a Diagnosis

The doctor will first ask about your symptoms, your medical history, and your family's medical history. If you are having irregular periods, it may be helpful to keep track of vaginal bleeding on a calendar and bring the information with you to your appointment.

Physical Exam and Lab Tests

Next, your doctor will give you a physical exam, including a pelvic examination. The pelvic exam involves inserting a speculum in the vagina to see the vaginal walls and cervix and to obtain a Pap smear or samples of vaginal discharge to check for possible infection. Once the speculum is removed, your doctor will do a "bimanual exam," (two fingers in the vagina, with the other hand pressing on your abdomen), during which he or she can feel the size and shape of the uterus and ovaries.

If you have an ovarian cyst, your doctor may find that your ovaries feel larger than normal, and you may have more discomfort during the bimanual exam than you normally do. In this case, the doctor may recommend additional laboratory tests to help make a diagnosis.

If you are of childbearing age, a pregnancy test is very important. If the doctor suspects you have polycystic ovaries, he or she may also want to check certain blood hormone levels that could be affected. The doctor may also draw blood for a "complete blood count" (CBC) to help identify a possible pelvic infection or to see if you have developed anemia due to excessive bleeding.

Ultrasound

Ultrasound, also called a sonogram or sonography, is one of the most frequently used methods of diagnosing ovarian cysts. This technology uses sound echoes to provide a picture of the tissues and organs inside the body. A sonogram can help determine the size of the ovaries; the number and size of any ovarian cysts; and whether a cyst is filled with solid or liquid material, or a combination of the two. Ultrasound may also show whether fluid has collected in the pelvis, which could be a sign of a recently ruptured cyst. If a pelvic ultrasound exam reveals that you have a functional ovarian cyst, there may be no need for further diagnostic procedures.

Ultrasound is a painless procedure performed in a radiology laboratory or doctor's office. For an abdominal ultrasound you will be asked to drink several glasses of water about an hour before the exam and to refrain

DIAGNOSTIC "RADAR"

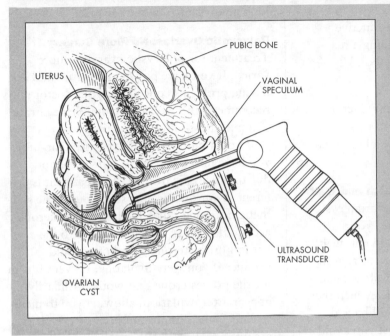

UTERUS

PUBIC BONE

VAGINAL SPECULUM

ULTRASOUND TRANSDUCER

OVARIAN CYST

Using sound instead of radio waves, ultrasound works much like radar, building images of the internal organs from the echoes they produce. In the transvaginal ultrasound procedure shown here, the device is placed inside the vagina, providing particularly accurate pictures. The technique is painless and free of radiation.

from urinating until the exam is completed. It is important to have full bladder because it enables the technician or radiologist to see all the pelvic organs. The technician will place the ultrasound transducer, a small hand–held device which receives and transmits the images, on your lower abdomen, move it around to get various views, and at certain points, capture these views on film for further review by a radiologist.

The most accurate pictures can be obtained by doing a transvaginal ultrasound, using a specifically designed transducer that is placed in the vagina. Because of the accuracy of the transvaginal ultrasound, some doctors skip the abdominal ultrasound and go directly to this method. The other advantage is that you do not have to have a full bladder.

If your ultrasound results show that your ovarian cyst could be composed of solid mate-

rial or a combination of solid and liquid material, your doctor may recommend an x–ray (or occasionally a CT scan or MRI). The x–ray is important because it can reveal the pieces of bone or teeth that are sometimes seen in dermoid cysts and because solid growths on the ovaries are more likely to be malignant.

Diagnostic Laparoscopy

Although the technologies of ultrasound and x–ray have helped to simplify the diagnosis of ovarian cysts, in certain cases more investigation is necessary. Sometimes your doctor will want to take a direct look at your pelvic organs in order to make a diagnosis. For example, if you have endometriosis, conventional tests and ultrasound are not very useful. Or, if your cyst is quite large, or not simply fluid–filled, or if you are over the age of 40 when the risk of cancer begins to increase, your gynecologist may wish to look directly at the cyst and the reproductive organs. This is done by performing a diagnostic laparoscopy. (See nearby box.)

Treating Ovarian Cysts

Treatment depends on many factors, including the type of cyst, its size, its precise location, the type of material it contains, and your age.

Functional Ovarian Cysts: "Watch and Wait"

If you have a small functional ovarian cyst that is not causing any problems, your doctor may recommend a "watch and wait" approach. That is, you may need to return for a follow–up examination or ultrasound after one or two menstrual cycles, when there is a good chance that the cyst will have dissolved. Your doctor may suggest you avoid intercourse during this time, since it can cause a cyst to rupture. If the cyst grows, especially if it becomes larger than about 2 inches, it may need to be removed surgically.

While small functional ovarian cysts generally disappear over time, they also tend to recur with subsequent menstrual cycles. In most cases, functional cysts can be controlled with the use of birth control pills, which reduce the hormones that promote growth of cysts and prevent formation of large, mature follicles that can turn into cysts. If you are already taking birth control pills for contraception, and think you may have an ovarian cyst, see your doctor because it is unlikely to be a functional cyst.

It may take a few months of using birth control pills before your cysts clear up. Your doctor can determine if the pills have been successful by repeating the pelvic exam, the ultrasound, or both. Your cysts may or may not return once you stop taking birth control pills. You can decide with your doctor how long you wish to stay on the pills.

Polycystic Ovaries: No More Surgery

Treatment for polycystic ovaries is more varied. If you have polycystic ovaries and are having problems conceiving, your doctor may recommend that you take clomiphene citrate (Clomid) to stimulate ovulation.

If you are not trying to get pregnant, and you have infrequent periods or no periods due to polycystic ovaries, the treatment is different. Your doctor may start you on the synthetic hormone called medroxyprogesterone acetate (Provera), which is similar to the natural progesterone your body would produce if you were ovulating. Provera fills in for the progesterone that would ordinarily appear after ovulation, allowing you to menstruate. This is important because even if you are not ovulating, your ovaries are still producing the estrogen that causes the uterine lining to grow. Without sufficient progesterone, the lining won't be shed during the menstrual period, and can grow too much. Although you probably feel fine and may not be eager for your periods to return, if your body is exposed only to estrogen without progesterone for long periods of time, the overgrowth of the uterine lining may increase the danger of cancer developing in the uterus.

There are several different schedules used for taking Provera tablets. Most experts agree that one good option is to take one 10–milligram tablet of Provera for 10 days each month. Taking the tablets on the first 10 days of the month makes it easy to remember. You should expect some menstrual bleeding approximately 3 to 5 days after you stop

WHAT HAPPENS DURING LAPAROSCOPY

During laparoscopy, the doctor inserts a narrow tube with a fiberoptic light at one end into the lower abdomen through a small incision just below the navel. This minor surgical procedure is used to diagnose many gynecological problems that may not be identifiable with less invasive methods, such as ultrasound or x-ray. For example, laparoscopy can help identify particular types of ovarian cysts, or determine the cause of pelvic pain or fertility problems.

Laparoscopy can also be used to treat your cyst. If it's small enough, the surgeon may be able to either drain the fluid from it or remove it through the laparoscope. Use of the laparoscope has eliminated the need for much major abdominal surgery.

Though laparoscopy is generally an outpatient procedure, it is usually performed under general anesthesia. This means that you will be required not to eat or drink for at least 8 hours prior to your surgery. You will also have a physical exam and routine blood and urine tests to be certain that you have no underlying illness or infection.

Often, using a vaginal speculum, the surgeon will attach a small instrument to the cervix that will allow movement of the uterus as needed during the procedure. The surgeon will then make a one-inch incision just below the navel and insert a small needle to deliver harmless carbon dioxide gas into the abdomen. The gas serves to lift the abdominal wall away from the internal organs and create a space so that the surgeon can see them. The needle is then replaced with the illuminated laparoscope. When the operation is finished, usually after 30 to 60 minutes, the gas is removed through a thin tube placed in the same incision. A few stitches close the incision which will probably be covered with a Band-Aid® type of dressing.

After your laparoscopy you will stay in the recovery room until you are feeling awake and alert and until your vital signs (temperature, pulse, blood pressure) are normal. Before you are sent home (usually within 2 hours after your surgery), you will receive instructions on follow-up care from your doctor and nurse. Postoperative pain should be minimal, but your doctor will probably give you a prescription for a mild painkiller.

It is not unusual to have some abdominal cramping or shoulder discomfort due to the carbon dioxide gas that filled your abdomen but this should gradually subside over a few days. You will probably be able to bathe and shower as usual, but you may need to avoid strenuous physical activity as well as sexual intercourse for a day or two.

Postoperative complications are rare, but be sure to call your doctor if you have bleeding from your incision, severe abdominal cramping or pain, or a fever over 100 degrees. Your doctor will probably want to see you a week or two later to check how you are doing, and to remove any stitches that are not the absorbable type.

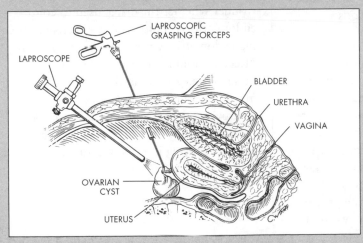

LAPROSCOPIC GRASPING FORCEPS

LAPROSCOPE

BLADDER

URETHRA

VAGINA

OVARIAN CYST

UTERUS

Though laparoscopic incisions are truly Band-Aid sized, the operation frequently requires more than one puncture. Shown here, the surgeon views an ovary through one incision while manipulating it through another.

taking the tablets. Don't forget that even though you have polycystic ovaries, you may ovulate occasionally, and it is possible to become pregnant. Provera is not a contraceptive pill. In fact, it is not recommended for use during pregnancy. If you need contraception, you should continue to use your preferred method during your treatment with Provera.

Some doctors treat the symptoms of polycystic ovaries with low–dose birth control pills. When you take birth control pills your normal periods will resume, and you'll be protected against pregnancy if that is a concern. Another advantage of birth control pills over Provera is that they decrease the production of the male hormone androgen. Not only does this help control excess hair growth, sometimes a symptom of polycystic ovaries, but it also may reduce the risk of heart disease in women with polycystic ovaries.

The original cure for polycystic ovaries was a surgical procedure called ovarian wedge resection. This involved removing at least one–third to one–half of each ovary in order to return it to normal size. In most women, this operation resulted in resumption of normal periods and normal fertility. The wedge resection is rarely done anymore thanks to the availability of drugs that induce ovulation and restore normal periods.

When Surgery Is Needed

Sometimes, however, surgical removal of a cyst is the only option. Doctors take several factors into account when deciding whether surgery is advisable. One of the most important considerations is the size of the cyst. Because there is a very slight risk of a large ovarian cyst becoming cancerous, the larger your cyst, the more likely the surgery. Although gynecologists differ on the precise "cut–off point," in most cases if a cyst is at

least 2 to 2.5 inches in diameter (about the size of a tennis ball), it will be surgically removed. If your cyst is less than 2 inches, your doctor may want to track it with ultrasound examinations over a period of a few months to see whether it grows to a size that requires surgery.

Another factor doctors consider is your age. Because ovarian cysts are less likely to become cancerous in a woman in her 20s than one in her 40s, or in a woman who has passed menopause, your chance of needing surgical removal of an ovarian cyst increases with age.

The type of cyst is also an important consideration. A "simple cyst," containing only liquid material, is less likely to require surgery than a "complex cyst," containing a mixture of materials. However, if a "simple" functional cyst grows quite large or bleeds, surgery may be necessary. Once your doctor has determined the size and type of cyst you have, he or she will discuss with you the advisability of surgery. The common types of cysts that almost routinely demand surgical removal are endometriomas, cystadenomas, and dermoid cysts.

Endometriomas. Because endometrial cysts are caused by endometriosis, you may wonder whether the drugs used to control endometriosis could also be effective in treating endometrial cysts. (See the chapter on "Keeping Endometriosis at Bay" for more on these drugs.) And indeed, these medications may help control the growth of cysts. However, because endometrial cysts can grow quite large and are prone to rupture, perhaps causing internal bleeding, these cysts are often treated surgically.

Cystadenomas. Since cystadenomas are almost always benign, it would seem reasonable to leave them alone unless they are large or cause complications. The problem is that cystadenomas often do become enormous, causing complications simply due to their size. An additional concern is that cystadenomas are "neoplasms," or new growths of abnormal tissue, and evaluation of neoplasms can be tricky. It is difficult to determine whether a neoplasm is benign or malignant simply by looking at it. Instead, tissue from most types of neoplasms needs to be analyzed under a microscope, and the only way to get a tissue sample is through surgery.

Dermoid Cysts. Dermoid cysts are also neoplasms, and therefore candidates for surgical removal. You may know before surgery that your cyst is a dermoid because if it contains teeth as one–third to one–half of them do, your doctor may have seen them on an x–ray.

What to Expect
When the Doctor Operates

Once surgery is decided upon, you'll have a meeting with your surgeon to discuss the operation and have a physical exam.

Before Surgery

Your surgeon will review the reason for your operation, the possible risks, no matter how small, and any possible aftereffects. You may find it helpful to bring a written list of questions to the meeting. Feel free to ask your surgeon to explain the operation by drawing a simple diagram of what will be removed.

Although at this point you will probably feel there are no lab tests you have not already undergone, a few basic studies may be ordered to establish that you are healthy enough for surgery:

- A complete blood count (CBC), to make sure that you have no underlying infection and that your body can tolerate loss of a small amount of blood during surgery
- A urinalysis to screen for infection and diseases such as diabetes or kidney problems
- A blood sample to check your blood type, in the unlikely event that you need a transfusion
- A recent chest x–ray or recent electrocardiogram (ECG) if you are over 40 years old

In Surgery

If you have a large cyst, your surgeon will probably remove it through an incision in your lower abdomen. The general term for any operation through the abdomen is *laparotomy*. If the cyst is small enough, your doctor may be able to remove it with a laparoscope, which requires only a small incision.

The type of operation you will have will depend on the size and nature of your cyst. The goal is to remove only the cyst, leaving the ovary intact. When the cyst alone is removed, the operation is called an *ovarian cystectomy*. If a portion of the ovary is also removed, the operation is a *partial oophorectomy*. Occasionally, the large size of the cyst or complications such as bleeding, twisting, or rupture, may require removal of the fallopian tube with the ovary. This operation is called *salpingo–oophorectomy*. Surgeons make every attempt to preserve the reproductive organs, especially if you have not yet reached menopause since it's still possible to have children when only a small portion of one ovary remains. Removal of the uterus, fallopian tubes, and ovaries (*total abdominal hysterectomy* with *bilateral salpingo-oophorectomy* or TAHBSO) is very rarely used to treat the types of ovarian cysts described in this chapter, unless there is a reasonable chance that your cyst is cancerous.

After Surgery

If you have a laparatomy, you will probably be in the hospital for a few days after the surgery. During the early recovery and post-operative period, you will receive fluids and medication through your intravenous (IV) line, but you should be eating solid foods fairly quickly. You will receive medication for pain, and you can expect to be walking around the day after surgery. Your wound should heal quickly, and if your incision was closed with staples, the staples and bandage will probably be removed before you leave the hospital. If you have non–absorbable stitches, they will probably be removed 5 to 7 days after your operation.

Before you leave the hospital, you will receive a summary of the type of operation that was performed and the type of cyst that you had. You may wish to ask for a copy of the surgery report for your records. You should also receive complete instructions from your doctor or nurse regarding what to expect in the postoperative period.

You should expect to have some abdominal discomfort for a few days after you return home. You may be given a prescription for a mild pain reliever. You should call your doctor if the medication doesn't help, or if the pain does not improve after a week. You should also contact your doctor if you develop a fever of over 100 degrees, or if vaginal bleeding is heavier than a normal period.

You should expect your incision to look quite red and feel uncomfortable for a few weeks. It is normal to notice some dried blood around the incision, but call your doctor if you see pus oozing from the wound. It's fine to bathe and shower; don't worry about getting the incision wet as long as it's not oozing. The red color of the incision will gradually fade, and eventually the scar will barely be visible.

You may be able to start some non–strenuous physical activity after a week or two. Be sure not to resume intercourse or to use tampons or anything else in the vagina until you have had your postoperative checkup (usually about 2 weeks after surgery). You will probably be able to resume all your normal activities and return to work about 6 weeks after surgery.

Unless you have had both of your ovaries removed, your periods will return to normal, usually by about 4 to 8 weeks after surgery. Remember that if even a portion of one ovary remains, you can still become pregnant if you're of childbearing age. That's one of the many reasons it's important to discuss the specifics of your surgery with your doctor.

Chances are that once the ovarian cyst has been removed, it will not recur. However, the operation does not always guarantee that you'll be cyst–free in the future. As long as you have ovaries, you can have ovarian cysts. It's a good idea to continue any medical treatments your doctor has prescribed to control the cysts and, of course, to have regular gynecological exams. □

Putting an End to Urinary Tract Infections

If you are among the many women who have had an infection of the urinary tract, you know what a painful nuisance it can be. The usual mild urge to urinate becomes a pressing matter as the nerves that tell you it's time to go to the bathroom send their signal with alarming frequency. This sudden urge can wake you up from a sound sleep several times a night. Yet after you dash to the bathroom, only a few drops come out, perhaps accompanied by a burning or stinging sensation and a strong urine smell. You may also feel a dull pain in your lower abdomen. The urine itself may look cloudy or contain blood, even if you are not having your period.

Such symptoms can be frightening. And left untreated, the infection can spread to the kidneys, causing permanent, even life-threatening damage. Fortunately, this is rare, especially if you get prompt treatment.

When you see your doctor, the first thing you'll be asked for is a urine sample, which will be cultured for bacteria. The doctor may also give you a prescription, based on your description of the symptoms, without waiting for lab results, since a fast dose of antibiotics eliminates the vast majority of urinary tract infections (UTIs). Doctors are also now starting to give their patients, particularly those plagued by repeated UTIs, prescriptions to keep at home, teaching them to treat themselves at the first sign of infection.

If you have been distressed to find the painful symptoms of a urinary tract infection returning, you are far from alone. Up to 90 percent of women will have a recurring episode at least once in their life. The chance of having repeat infection within 6 months of the first, or 3 infections within 1 year, is 15 percent. Most of the time, subsequent infections are caused by different bacteria than the first. If the original bacteria, never eliminated in the first place, are the cause, the infection will usually come back within a week or two after you have finished taking your medication.

Types of UTI

The urinary tract is divided into two sections. The upper tract includes the two kidneys and their accompanying ureters, tubes that connect each kidney to the bladder. The lower tract is made up of the bladder and the urethra through which the bladder is emptied. Infections of the lower tract are by far the more common.

Lower UTI

If you feel a burning sensation while urinating, but no other symptoms, you probably have urethritis, an infection of the urethra. Possible causes include sexually transmitted diseases, especially gonorrhea; trauma from childbirth, surgery, or catheterization; irritation from a diaphragm; or an allergic reaction to soap, vaginal cream, spermicide, bubble bath, or some other chemical substance.

Cystitis occurs when bacteria work their way up from the urethra to infect the bladder. This is the most common UTI and it is most often found in women who have repeated infections. Urethritis and cystitis frequently occur together.

Upper UTI

If a lower UTI is left untreated, the bacteria can spread beyond the bladder, through one of the ureters, and into a kidney. This infection, known as *pyelonephritis,* requires immediate medical care. Symptoms are stronger than a lower UTI: back pain (since the kidneys are located there), fever, chills, nausea, and vomiting as well as the typical complaints associated with cystitis. If allowed to persist, this condition can become chronic and eventually lead to kidney damage or even kidney failure. Multiple kidney infections can cause high blood pressure.

Why Women Are Susceptible

Urinary tract infections occur 25 times more often in women than in men. Between the ages of 20 and 50, women have UTIs 50 times more often than men. Each year, UTIs are the reason for more than 5 million visits to the doctor in the United States. By the first few years after menopause, 1 out of 10 women can expect to have had a bladder infection or worse. Why is this so?

Anatomy

One reason women are so suseptible can be found in the physical makeup of the human body. Infections in the urinary tract generally start when bacteria enter from outside. The bacteria that cause about 9 out of 10 urinary tract infections, *Escherichia coli* (abbreviated E. coli), are normally found in the lower intestine, their natural home. The trouble starts when they move into the urethra and up into the bladder.

In both men and women, E. Coli leaving the body through the rectum can sometimes re-enter through the urethra. If they succeed in reaching the bladder, they then find a warm, moist environment in which to settle and multiply rapidly. However, because a woman's urethra, at 1 inch long, is far shorter than a man's (which runs the full length of the penis) bacteria invading a woman's urinary tract have a much shorter trip and a far better chance of getting established.

Toilet Habits

After urination or a bowel movement, bacteria can enter the urethra through the vagina in two ways. First, wiping from back to front with toilet tissue can bring bacteria directly into the entrance of the urinary tract. Second, even if you keep your rectal area very clean,

E. coli can reside in your underwear and work their way around to the vaginal area during excercise.

Sex

The thrusting of sexual intercourse, especially with both anal and vaginal entry, can spread bacteria throughout your genital area while temporarily traumatizing the urethra. The more prolonged or vigorous the thrusting, the more it is likely to open the door to infection. In fact, many women who suffer from repeated bouts of urinary tract infection start to realize that the pain begins within 12 to 24 hours after sex.

Sexual activity doesn't have to be unusually forceful to induce an infection. Women who have recently embarked on an active sex life, either for the first time or more intensively than usual—as newlyweds, for example, or on vacation—frequently find themselves with UTIs, specifically, with bladder infections. That's where the term honeymoon cystitis comes from.

Barrier methods of contraception can irritate sensitive vaginal and urinary tissue as well, and irritated tissue helps create an environment where bacteria can thrive. In addition, the active ingredient in most spermicidal foams and jellies, nonoxynol 9, kills some of the vagina's beneficial bacteria, allowing the bacteria that cause cystitis to colonize. Furthermore, a diaphragm can also press against the urethra, and cause irritation. Some women are allergic to the latex in condoms or to the spermicides contained in some condoms. (Oral contraceptives have also been found to predispose women to UTIs. Fortunately, today's low-dose pill is less likely to do this than the higher-dose pills of the past.)

What's a woman to do? Two very easy steps are ensuring cleanliness and minimizing irritation. Be sure you and your sex partner keep your genital and anal areas clean at all times and wash your hands (and under your fingernails) before foreplay and sex. If your partner is uncircumcised, he should always clean under the foreskin before sex. A circumcision would eliminate that problem, and men do have them. If you include anal

WHY UTIs HIT WOMEN HARDEST

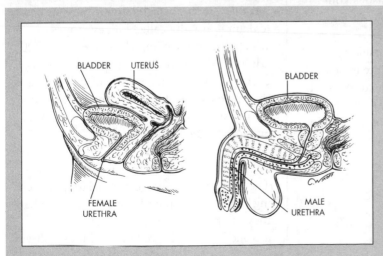

BLADDER   UTERUS

BLADDER

FEMALE
URETHRA

MALE
URETHRA

It's simply a matter of distance: Bacteria travel no more than a few inches to reach the friendly environment of a woman's bladder, while they must navigate a urethral canal four times as long in a man.

penetration in your lovemaking, be sure your partner uses a condom, discards it, and washes his penis before vaginal entry.

Vary your sexual positions, too, to avoid bruising the urethra. Keep a tube of sterile lubricant, such as K-Y Lubricating Jelly, handy. If recurring UTIs are a serious problem for you, and you think your contraception is the cause, consider changing your method.

You may also want to consider sterilization if your family is complete and you can't get rid of your UTIs after taking other preventive measures. Alternatively, your partner might consider having a vasectomy.

Pregnancy and Childbirth

The hormonal changes of pregnancy cause the muscles in the urinary system to relax. This allows urine to be retained in the ureters and bladder. Fifteen percent of pregnant women have bladder infections without even knowing it. If you get a UTI during pregnancy, it's important to treat it right away because kidney infections, dangerous enough to you, can also lead to premature ruptures of the membranes and thus premature delivery of your baby. Your doctor will know which antibiotics are safe to take during pregnancy. This is one of the reasons your doctor will ask for a urine sample during your pregnancy checkups.

Many body fluids can mix outside the body and re-enter it during the intense activity of childbirth. This, too, can lead to a UTI. In addition, the hemorrhoids that frequently disturb women after delivery provide sites for potential infection.

Menopause and Old Age

As your body ages, your bladder becomes less elastic and may not empty completely. That allows urine to collect, and create a hospitable environment for bacteria, thereby encouraging infection. Older people tend to be less active, which adds to the problem, restricting the movement of bladder muscles and thus impeding emptying. A clean, flushed bladder also requires a nutritious diet, which the elderly don't always maintain. And diabetes, which affects many parts of the body, including the urinary system, becomes more common as people age.

Other Causes of UTI

The entrance of bacteria into the urethra is not the only way a urinary tract infection can start, and plenty of people who are not sexually active get UTIs. Sometimes, a physical condition may be the cause. When it is, antibiotic treatment alone won't resolve it. Your doctor may refer you to a urologist (a specialist in the urinary tract) if he or she isn't sure of the precise cause of your symptoms.

Kidney Stones

UTIs can result from physical blockage. The most common obstacles are urinary stones (calculi)—usually called kidney stones— which send approximately 1 of every 1,000 adults to the hospital in the United States each year. Consisting mostly of calcium, and therefore as hard as a rock, these stones can be any size from tiny to large enough to fill an entire kidney.

Kidney stones travel with the urine and can be found anywhere in the urinary system. They may be painless or excruciating, depending on their size, their location, and whether they are blocking the passage of urine. If a stone becomes lodged in the thin, sensitive

AN INVITING NOOK FOR BACTERIAL GROWTH

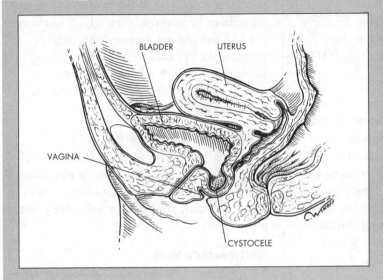

BLADDER UTERUS

VAGINA

CYSTOCELE

From its position immediately overhead, the bladder can push into the vaginal area when surgery, menopause, or multiple deliveries weaken the vaginal wall. The resulting pocket, called a cystocele, allows urine to collect, providing especially hospitable conditions for invading microorganisms.

ureter, pain is notoriously great. X-rays will show their location. You will need surgery or lithotripsy, in which the stone is "blown up" with ultrasound, if the stone is in a particularly painful or dangerous place and won't pass through the system of its own accord.

Cystocele

Another cause of a UTI is a cystocele. When the vaginal wall next to the bladder has become weakened for any reason, the bladder can protrude directly into the vagina, holding back small pools of urine. Such tissue weakening is common after several vaginal deliveries, menopause, or gynecologic surgery. Cystoceles may require surgery themselves.

Diverticula

Diverticula are crevices (abscesses) that develop on the inside wall of the urethra. If several of these small pockets merge to form a larger one, urinary debris can accumulate in

it. When diverticula become swollen or inflamed, urine may not drain well, leading to chronic infection. Surgery may be required. Suspect diverticula if you feel burning on urination between bladder infections.

Urethral Stenosis

A narrowing of the urethra, called urethral stenosis, can be present at birth or result from a number of conditions or activities. These include having had a UTI in childhood; infection of the vagina or vulva; previous infection, such as gonorrhea; a sudden increase in your sex life; childbirth; catheterization after surgery; the physical changes of pregnancy; and changes related to a deficiency of estrogen during and after menopause.

Related Conditions

Pain on urination is not always caused by a UTI. While the conditions described below are rare, your doctor may want to make sure they are not the problem before treating you for a repeat UTI.

Interstitial Cystitis

A condition caused by scarring or ulcers in the bladder lining is called interstitial cystitis. When the bladder fills, the sore areas are coated with urine. Over the course of several years, these sores cause the bladder lining to disintegrate and finally, to stop functioning altogether. Researchers are looking for ways to treat this painful and frustrating condition. Two methods are currently used: inserting dimethyl sulfoxide (Rimso 50) into the bladder through a catheter, or physically stretching the bladder under anesthesia.

Bladder Cancer

This rare condition causing tumors in the bladder is more common in men than in women. Blood in the urine, frequent and painful urination, and waking at night to urinate are typical symptoms A small tumor that is not attached to the bladder wall can sometimes be removed through an instrument called a cystoscope. Inserted through the urethra, the cystoscope works like a long, thin telescope with a light at the end. However large, deeply embedded tumors usually require major surgery.

Getting a Diagnosis

Most UTIs can be treated by your gynecologist or family physician. If the diagnosis is difficult or the treatment fails, your doctor will refer you to a urologist.

First Doctor's Visit

You will be asked to provide a urine specimen that will either be analyzed in the doctor's office or sent to an outside laboratory. A large number of white blood cells indicates that your body has made an effort to fight some kind of infection. The presence of bacteria

DIVERTICULA: A LONG-TERM SOURCE OF TROUBLE

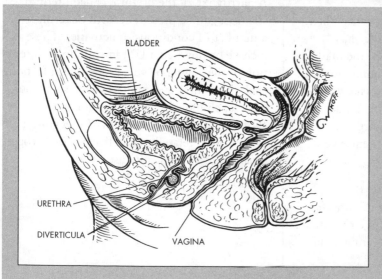

If a pouch develops at weak point in the wall of a tube such as the urethra, it's called a "diverticulum." A trap for all sorts of debris, it can become a permanent reservoir of chronic infection. Diverticula in the urethra can become inflamed, causing discomfort whenever you urinate. Diverticula can also develop in the lower intestine, leading to inflammation, bleeding, obstruction, and even life-threatening abdominal infection.

can also be directly confirmed. This is done quickly in a process called urinalysis.

If the doctor wants to find out exactly which bacteria have invaded, he or she will order a urine culture, which takes 24 to 72 hours. The laboratory may also be asked to determine which antibiotic will destroy those bacteria most effectively, so that your doctor can prescribe the most beneficial medication. (You will probably already have been given a small prescription for a broad-spectrum antibiotic— one that works against most bacteria—and for a painkilling medication to get started fighting the infection and discomfort right away.)

Other reasons for a urine culture are:

■ Suspicion of a more serious infection, such as gonorrhea;
■ Pregnancy or diabetes;
■ An infection that returns within 3 weeks;
■ Symptoms that continue for more than 7 days despite taking medication;
■ Recent surgery of the genital or urinary tract or insertion or removal of a catheter.

If you could be pregnant or your doctor suspects an anatomical problem, such as a cystocele or a tumor, your doctor will also do a pelvic exam.

More Complex Tests

If your medication doesn't work or the doctor suspects a physical abnormality that cannot be seen, you will probably be referred to a urologist for more complex procedures.

They may be performed at the doctor's office or a hospital.

A cystoscope, allows the doctor to look directly into your urethra and bladder to check for irritation or a small tumor. First you will be given a local or general anesthetic. Then the scope will be passed through your urethra and into your bladder. Through the scope, the doctor can insert tiny instruments to collect small samples of urine and tissue for the laboratory to analyze. This procedure takes about 10 minutes once the cystoscope is in place.

With cystourethrography, a chemical is inserted into the bladder through the cystoscope. X-rays are taken as you urinate. The doctor watches to see if urine is backing up instead of flowing out.

Cystometry measures how well your bladder is functioning by gauging its ability to expand and contract. After introducing water or carbon dioxide into the bladder through a catheter, technicians note the amount you urinate each time you report the urge. The test takes about 30 to 60 minutes and is usually done in a hospital. Local anesthesia will prevent pain during the procedure.

An intravenous pyelogram (IVP) is performed by a radiologist and an x-ray technician in the outpatient department of a hospital. They will take a preliminary x-ray of your abdomen. Then you will lie down and a needle will be inserted into a vein in one arm. Special dye, called contrast material, is injected through the needle. Within a few minutes, the dye is carried by the blood to the kidneys and then through the urinary tract.

The goal is to find any blockage, such as kidney stones, or slight anatomic variations in the urinary tract, that might make it easier for an infection to take hold. X-rays are taken at regular intervals, such as after 1, 5, 10, and 15 minutes. After about an hour, the radiologist should have a good idea of what's going on in your urinary tract. This test is not suggested for women who are pregnant or those who have ever had an allergic reaction to x-ray contrast material.

Treating UTIs: Many Good Choices

The drugs available to treat UTIs today are extremely effective. However, because not all medications work equally well against all bacteria or for all women, you and your doctor may have to experiment, especially if you have recurring infections.

Drug Therapy

Eighty percent of the time, cystitis can be cured with a single dose of trimethoprim (Trimpex) or 3 to 5 days of trimethoprim/sulfamethoxazole (Bactrim, Septra, others) or sulfisoxazole (Gantanol, Gantrisin, others). If you are allergic to sulfa drugs, you may be given one of the new quinilone antibiotics such as ciprofloxacin (Cipro), norfloxacin (Noroxin), ofloxacin (Floxin), enoxacin (Penetrex), or lomefloxacin (Maxaquin). Sulfa drugs should not be taken during the last 4 weeks of pregnancy because they can cause jaundice in the newborn. Other popular antibiotics are cephalexin (Keflex), cefixime (Suprax), and cefuroxime (Ceftin, Kefurox, Zinacef).

The short-term therapy that is commonly used today is far better than the former standard of 7 to 14 days of antibiotics. That regimen was somewhat self-defeating, since vaginal yeast infections are one side effect of long-term antibiotic therapy—and yeast infections can trigger UTIs! Other side effects included diarrhea and allergic reactions.

Treatment will be longer and require different or additional drugs if the urine culture shows tougher bacteria than E. coli, such as Staphylococcus, Chlamydia, or Mycoplasma. More than one kind of bacterium may be present; if so, they must all be eradicated.

Some doctors prefer to prescribe other drugs. Amoxicillin (Amoxil, Trimox, Wymox) and ampicillin (Omnipen) are less effective for some women, but might work well for you. Nitrofurantoin (Macrodantin) and cephalosporins antibiotics such as Ancef and Kefzol can be used as well.

To relieve pain almost immediately, you may also be given a prescription for an antispasmodic, such as methenamine (Prosed, Urised) or flavoxate (Urispas). These drugs relax the bladder muscle, reducing the constant urge to urinate. Also commonly prescribed is a local anesthetic, phenazopyridine hydrochloride (Pyridium).

Be sure to do your part to make your treatment work. Finish all prescribed antibiotics, even though your symptoms will probably stop within hours. Painkillers kill pain but not the bacteria that cause them. Your doctor may ask you to make an appointment to return for a repeat urine culture in a week or two—and keep the appointment even if you feel fine. Remember that UTIs can come back quickly and with a vengeance.

Hospitalization

Urinary tract infections rarely send anyone to the hospital. Hospitalization is necessary for surgery to correct certain physical conditions, such as a large cystocele protruding into the vaginal wall. If a kidney infection develops, hospitalization is often required to supply strong drugs or pain relief through an IV line.

Since the nausea and vomiting that frequently accompany a kidney infection can lead to dehydration, an IV line can also supply fluids to prevent that from happening.

Controlling UTIs Yourself

So many women are pestered by chronic cystitis that some doctors are now teaching some of them to treat themselves. Starting treatment at home without waiting for an office visit reduces pain at the first sign of infection, and taking antibiotics right away will begin to kill bacteria before they have a chance to proliferate. Self-treatment can save money as well.

If you have had cystitis several times in the past year and believe you can follow directions carefully, ask your doctor about self-treatment; he or she will tell you exactly what to do. In the meantime, here are some temporary measures you can take.

Tips for Self-Care

- If you feel pain, don't suffer. Unless your doctor has instructed otherwise (and if you don't have your prescribed painkillers on hand), take one or two extra-strength non-aspirin painkillers (Tylenol, Advil, others) until you can have your urine tested.
- As soon as you can, relax and put your feet up. Hold a heating pad or hot-water bottle against your abdomen or even directly in the urethral area (don't let it get too hot). If your genital area is warmer than the urine waiting to be excreted, it won't burn as much when you urinate.

The Cranberry Connection

Should you drink gallons of cranberry juice for a UTI? Like any citrus juice, cranberry juice keeps the urine in an acid state, which

WHEN IT FEELS LIKE A UTI, BUT ISN'T

Symptom: Frequent Urination
Potential Culprits:
- Drinking a lot of liquids
- Drinking alcohol or beverages containing caffeine (coffee, tea, cola)
- Taking "water pills" (diuretics)
- Stress and anxiety
- Physical changes of pregnancy or menopause
- Pressure on the bladder by a pelvic mass

Symptom: Painful Urination
Potential Culprits:
- Vaginal infection
- Active genital herpes infection or other sexually transmitted disease
- Bruising from sexual intercourse, bicycling, horseback riding
- Chemical irritation from:
  - Tight jeans
  - Non-cotton underwear, tights, pantyhose
  - Laundry soaps used to wash underwear or nightwear
  - Bath oils
  - hygiene sprays or similar products
  - Talcum powder
- Gynecologic surgery
- Having a catheter (tube for urine) inserted after surgery
- Interstitial cystitis (rare)
- Bladder cancer (rare)

Symptom: Blood in the urine
Potential Culprits:
- Many diseases, including sickle cell anemia
- Long-distance running ("jogger's hematuria")

discourages bacterial growth. An extra attraction of cranberry juice—and blueberry juice as well, one group of researchers found— is that it contains compounds that seem to make the walls of the bladder slippery. As a result, bacteria slide off (and out) instead of sticking around to cause infection.

However, it takes a tremendous volume of unsweetened, undiluted cranberry juice to keep urine acidic, especially if you are drinking and urinating a lot anyway, as you should be. One alternative is to grind fresh cranberries with honey and eat them with plain yogurt every night. Some cystitis sufferers take a 250-milligram tablet of vitamin C every 4 hours (or 1,000 milligrams of the time-release type once a day) to prevent recurrent infections.

The downside of highly acidic urine is that it stings badly when passing through an inflamed urethra. Some women who have rejected cranberry juice and other acidic drinks after just that experience recommend the opposite: that you *neutralize* (alkalinize) your urine, making it less acidic, and therefore, *less* painful when you urinate.

Thus, if cranberry juice has proved unbearable, you might try the opposite route. At the first sign of a UTI, drink a pint of hot or cold water mixed with 1 teaspoon of sodium bicarbonate (baking soda). Follow this with a large glass of water every 20 minutes for 3 or 4 hours. Once an hour, stir another teaspoonful of bicarbonate into the water you're about to drink. (If you have a heart condition or high blood pressure, ask your doctor first.) The bicarbonate can be mixed with jam instead. If bicarbonate makes you queasy, try potassium citrate. Alternatively, some women chew or swallow commercial antacids, such as Rolaids and Tums, to relieve the burning of urination. The "best" method is whatever works for you.

Other dietary changes that have helped some women are avoiding citrus fruits and spicy foods, and decreasing intake of refined starches and sugars, vegetable fats, onions, beans, and chocolate.

There are also some age-old home remedies you can try, such as tea made from yerba buena, uva-ursi, comfrey, or lemon balm (available at health food stores). Another non-drug remedy that works for some women is six to eight tablets of dolomite every few hours. You should, however, consult your doctor before trying any remedy.

Preventing UTIs— the First or the Tenth

While antibiotics and self-treatment remedies take care of an infection once you have it, there are also many ways to try to prevent recurring urinary tract infections. Experiment to see what works for you.

Diet

As part of any healthy diet, you should drink six to eight glasses of water a day and minimize your intake of alcohol and caffeine. If you do drink alcohol or caffeinated drinks, try to counteract their effects by drinking plenty of water.

Some of the dietary changes that relieve the pain of UTI may also help prevent them. Try to cut back your intake of refined starches and sugars, vegetable fats, onions, beans, and chocolate.

Toilet, Bathing, and Menstrual Habits

Try to urinate every two to three hours rather than "holding it in." After the flow of urine has stopped, lean forward on the toilet and gently press out the last few drops. This is known as double emptying. Most important though is to keep your genital area clean by wiping from front to back after bowel movements and cleaning the urethral area with moist cotton balls. You should wash your entire genital area every day with mild, unscented soap, then rinse and pat dry with a clean, soft, cloth.

Some doctors believe that women with frequent UTIs should always take showers rather than baths. Others believe a hot bath during a bout of UTI will help kill the bacteria. If you decide on baths, do not use bath oils or bubble bath and limit them to one or two a week, with no more than five minutes of soaking time. Hot water can excite the urethra.

Do not use oils, feminine hygiene sprays, or talcum powder in your genital area and don't douche with any chemical substances. All of these agents irritate the skin.

When you have your period, frequently change whatever form of sanitary protection you use. Both sanitary napkins and tampons have been known to provide a route for bacteria. In addition, tampons may put pressure on the urethra, encouraging infection. If you think your brand is the problem, switch to a different product.

While at home, wear long skirts without underwear for several hours a day if you can. This can increase circulation while eliminating genital contact with potential infection-bearing material.

Clothes and Laundry

Avoid nylon-crotch underwear and tight jeans, both of which create a moist environment in which bacteria can grow. Instead, it's best to wear only cotton-crotch underwear and pantyhose and to change them at least once a day. Similarly, if you've been swimming, change into a dry suit after you come out of the water, particularly if you were in a chlorinated pool. Use a mild laundry detergent and make sure that your clothes, nightwear, and sheets are well rinsed. Do not use a public laundry to wash your underwear since soap and detergent deposits can accumulate in the washers. If you don't have your own washing machine, the best and oldest method of sterilizing underwear is boiling it in a pot.

Sex

Urinate and drink a glass of water before having intercourse. Within 10 minutes after sex, urinate again to flush out any bacteria that may have entered the vagina. If you find that UTIs are a constant problem, try washing your vaginal area with a hand-held shower attachment after sex.

If you use a diaphragm, make sure it is the correct size with a snug but comfortable fit. Pressure from the rim of the diaphragm can lead to UTIs. If you've lost or gained more than 10 pounds, have your diaphragm refitted. Remember that many forms of birth control can create situations that encourage a UTI. If necessary, talk to your doctor about alternatives.

A Healthy Future

In the great majority of cases, the prognosis for urinary tract infections is excellent. Improved drugs now provide fast relief of symptoms as the infection is cleared up. Also remember that even if you're plagued with recurrent infections, there are plenty of measures you can take to fight back. Between your own efforts and your doctor's treatments, you *can* keep this painful problem at bay. □

CHAPTER 11   **COMMON DISORDERS OF THE REPRODUCTIVE SYSTEM**

Coming to Terms with a Sexually Transmitted Disease

The microbes that cause sexually transmitted diseases are equal opportunity bugs. They don't care if you are white or black, rich or poor, educated or illiterate, happy or sad. If you're a warm body, you'll do. STD germs settle in an estimated 12 million Americans each year. Worldwide, they find 250 million new hosts a year.

These numbers reflect men and women, young and old. STD germs love everybody who loves, because they are spread by intimate body contact. The word "venereal," as in venereal disease, comes from the name of the Romans goddess of love, Venus.

Germs can, however, be biologically sexist in the damage they do. Women suffer more adverse consequences from STDs than do men because, generally, it is easier for an STD to be transferred from a man to a woman. More harm can be done to a woman's reproductive organs if an infection is left untreated — and, women's infections do, in fact, go untreated more often, since women are less likely to show symptoms of an STD. The absence of symptoms in the presence of an infection is known medically as being "asymptomatic".

Two-thirds of all STDs occur in people under the age of 25. This isn't necessarily because this age group is more vulnerable to STDs. It's simply that these people are more likely to expose themselves to the number one risk factor for STDs: having sex with multiple partners without adequate protection from germs.

Bacteria, Viruses and Bugs

Over a lifetime, the body can host many different kinds of germs including those that cause sexually transmitted diseases. There are three types of STDs — bacterial, viral, and bugs.

Bacterial STDs are transient which means they will respond to medication and can be kicked out of your system. However, if they remain untreated they can cause very serious damage.

Bacterial STDs include gonorrhea, a bacteria which can cause infertility, heart disease, blindness, damage to the urinary tract, arthritis, and damage to an unborn child; chlamydia, which has been implicated as a risk factor for cervical cancer and is a major cause of infertility; syphilis, which can affect the nervous system, cause blindness, deafness, heart disease, insanity, and result in the birth of a stillborn or crippled child; and chancroid, which causes genital sores and enlarged lymph nodes.

Viral STDs are permanent. Once you acquire one, it stays in your system forever. You will not be troubled by a viral STD as long as it remains dormant, but they do act up now and then. Human Papilloma Virus (HPV) generally hides in the genital tract, and causes genital warts from time to time over the years. Some strains can lead to cervical cancer. Herpes Simplex Virus (HSV) lives in nerves at the base of the spine and causes painful blisters to form, mostly on the vulva and in the mouth. Human Immunodeficiency Virus (HIV) can also remain in the system but once it manifests itself, it becomes a deadly disease with no cure and limited treatment options. HIV is discussed in detail in chapter 13, "The Growing Danger of AIDS."

Sexually transmitted skin infestations are caused by tiny bugs called arthropods. Using pesticides will easily rid you of them. The two most common are pubic lice, a.k.a. "crabs" and scabies. Pubic lice attach themselves to the base of pubic hairs where they bite the skin and lay their eggs. Scabies burrow into the skin to lay eggs. They are much tinier than pubic lice and cannot be seen with the naked eye.

Best Ways to Prevent Infection

The only way to avoid these germs, is to abstain completely from vaginal, oral, or anal intercourse. Since this is not a desirable option for most women, you can reduce the chance of getting an STD by:

- Having sex with only one uninfected partner who only has sex with you
- Limiting the number of your sexual partners if you do have more than one
- Using latex condoms during any kind of intercourse
- Using spermicides like nonoxynol-9 which can kill some of the germs
- Having regular checkups to make sure you aren't infected with an STD that may be asymptomatic

Taking Action

Different types of sexual activity carry different kinds of risks. Knowing your risk level can help you determine how often you should be checked for STDs. You can decide whether you are at high, moderate, or low risk (and thus how often you should be checked) based primarily on the number of partners you have had and the number of partners your partner has had. For additional pointers, see the box on checkups.

Where to Go For Help

If you suspect you have a sexually transmitted disease, or you've recently been told by a sex partner that he has been diagnosed with one, you'll want to seek medical attention as soon as possible. There are a number of different options.

- *Schools and universities* generally provide care to enrolled students at the school or campus clinic for free, or, at reasonable rates. The clinic may or may not offer comprehensive care, including testing, counseling, and education.

- *Hospital clinics* sometimes offer STD screening and treatment. Costs and services will vary by hospital.
- *Community clinics* offer free or low-cost health services. They may be non-profit organizations, such as Planned Parenthood affiliates, or be related to the state or county health department. Rates are sometimes on a sliding scale depending on income. Some community clinics may not offer comprehensive care.
- *State clinics* treat patients regardless of their ability to pay. The state health department's STD clinic is most likely to offer comprehensive services because it is mandated by the federal government to control STDs in the state. The state public health department can be a wealth of information about services in your area if you are too far away to attend the state clinic.
- *Private doctors* vary in their interest and knowledge of STDs and might not offer comprehensive care. However, if you have an ongoing relationship with an ob-gyn who knows your history, or you can get a referral, this can be a good option, although it is also probably the most expensive.

The level of privacy and confidentiality can vary by state due to different reporting laws, and even by clinic and doctor. Your best bet is to ask your doctor or nurse about their accommodations for keeping information private. Ask these questions: (1) What precautions do you take to ensure that no one can find out why I was here? (2) What will be done with my records? and (3) Do I have a right to keep my records from being sent to others, such as future health care providers or insurance companies?

CHECKUPS: HOW OFTEN IS RIGHT FOR YOU?

You are at high risk and should be checked every one to three months if...
- You currently have many sexual partners
- You currently have casual sex with partners you know nothing about
- Your sexual partner currently has many partners
- You or your nonmonogamous sexual partner live in a city with high STD rates

You are at moderate risk and should be checked every three to six months if...
- You exchange body secretions or make contact with the oral or anal mucous membranes of others during sexual intercourse
- You or your partner sustain slight damage to the tissues of the vagina or anus during sex

You are at low risk and should be screened every 12 months for two years if...
- You and your partner have been monogamous for a long time.

Prepare for questions

You and your doctor will try to match your symptoms with an STD. You should also expect to be asked what may seem like very personal questions. This is called "taking a sexual history." Here are some questions that doctors and nurses often ask in order to know what infections to test for, plus the reasons they ask them:

Q: *Have you had a sexual experience with another person in the past year?*
R: Gives your doctor or nurse an idea of what else to ask you.

Q: *(If yes) With how many different people in this year?*
R: Your doctor needs to know because the more partners you've had, the greater your risk for having contracted any STD. There is no wrong answer.

Q: *(If yes) What kind of sex have you had, vaginal, oral, or anal?*
R: Different kinds of sex can cause trauma to different parts of the body. Knowing this can help your doctor make his or her diagnosis.

Q: *Can you tell me about your sexual life before this last year?*
R: You may be married or monogamous now, but might have put yourself at risk a year ago.

Q: *Have you ever had a sexually transmitted disease of any kind?*
R: People who've had an STD before are often at higher risk for other infections.

Q: *Have you ever shared a needle or injection equipment with another person for any reason?*
R: Sharing needles can infect you with someone else's blood. It is a main mode of transmission for Human Immunodeficiency Virus (HIV).

Q: *What do you do to protect yourself from STDs?*
R: Your answer will help your doctor or nurse understand how much you know about the infection process.

What's next?
After you are diagnosed with an STD, your doctor will either let you know your treatment options or simply give you a prescription. **It is extremely important that you finish all medications completely, even if you're** feeling better in a day or two. Incomplete drug treatments are responsible for the "super bugs" — those germs that don't respond to the treatment that once knocked them out. Being exposed to a small amount of the medication instead of all of it allows germs to mutate and become stronger.

As far as sexual activity, it's best to avoid any type of contact that could infect your partner or delay your healing. Check with your doctor about what to avoid and for how long.

If you are asked to return to your doctor or the clinic for follow-up, plan to do so. Even if you feel well, they will want to ensure that you are completely cured or at least, that you were properly treated. This follow-up could save you from pain and suffering later if they find that further treatment is needed.

You may be asked how you plan to notify past sexual partners about your infection. Partner notification is essential in stopping the spread of STDs. If you can't bear to tell past partners yourself, many health workers (especially those working at the state health department) will do it for you without using your name. For guidance in telling current and potential partners, see "Finding the Support You Need," later in this chapter.

Common Sexually Transmitted Diseases

The following section discusses the eight most common STDs in North America, grouped by symptoms. Information on other sexually related diseases can be found in chapter 4, "Curing Vaginal Infections" and chapter 13, "The Growing Danger of AIDS." The first group discussed here, Human Papilloma Virus (HPV), Herpes Simplex Virus (HSV), syphilis, and chancroid, is characterized primarily by lumps, bumps and sores. The second group, chlamydia and gonorrhea, is characterized mainly by vaginal discharge. The last section covers pubic lice and scabies, the hallmark of which is itching. Each disease has more than one symptom, but this arrangement will get you started. You can also check for additional details in the box on "Matching Your Symptoms to an STD."

MATCHING YOUR SYMPTOMS TO AN STD

It is important for your doctor to know as much as possible about your condition, since, if you have an STD, you will want it to be properly diagnosed. Check the following chart and read the matching sections on the infection you think you might have. Then give your doctor as many specifics as you can.

If you've noticed:	see the sections on:
Fever	Herpes Simplex Virus (HSV) Chlamydia, Gonorrhea
Flu-like symptoms	Herpes Simplex Virus (HSV) Syphilis
Hair loss	Syphilis
Itching or tingling in the genital area	Human Papilloma Virus (HPV) Herpes Simplex Virus (HSV) Pubic lice, Scabies
Itching on the body	Pubic lice, Scabies
Lower abdominal or rectal pain	Chlamydia, Gonorrhea
Painful urination	Herpes Simplex Virus (HSV) Chlamydia, Gonorrhea
Rash	Syphilis Gonorrhea Scabies
Sore vulva	Herpes Simplex Virus (HSV) Gonorrhea
Sores or blisters	Herpes Simplex Virus HSV) Syphilis Chancroid
Swollen glands	Herpes Simplex Virus (HSV) Syphilis Chancroid
Unusual vaginal bleeding	Chlamydia, Gonorrhea
Vaginal discharge	Chlamydia, Gonorrhea
Warts or other growths	Human Papilloma Virus (HPV)

Lumps, Bumps and Sores:
Human Papilloma Virus (HPV)

HPV refers to a group of more than 60 viruses. They are responsible for warts anywhere on the body, but only certain types are sexually transmitted. These are called condylomata acuminatum, better known as genital warts or venereal warts. Like other warts, they can not be cured but they can be treated.

Warts are the "clinical" version of this infection; that is, they can easily be seen and diagnosed. However, there is a much more common version, referred to as "subclinical," in which the virus resides under the skin and cannot be seen. Some experts believe that HPV causes warts in about 30 percent of infected people and subclinical infections in the other 70 percent. The subclinical varieties have been linked to cancer, so it is important for women to have yearly checkups including Pap smears to detect precancerous cervical changes.

HPV is coming close to being considered an epidemic in the United States, with a 1,000 percent increase in the number of HPV patients since 1987. Since it is a nonreportable disease, accurate figures aren't available, but it is believed that 48 million to 50 million Americans currently live with this virus. Almost one million Americans are newly infected with the HPV virus every year.

■ *Risk factors:* You are more likely to get genital warts if you are between the ages of 20 and 24, if you or your partner have multiple or casual sexual partners, and if you have another STD, such as chlamydia or herpes simplex virus (HSV). If you are pregnant, using oral contraceptives, or have a condition that suppresses the immune system such as Hodgkin's disease or leukemia, you are also at higher risk for viruses such as HPV. Researchers have also found that white

GENITAL WARTS: DON'T JUDGE BY APPEARANCES

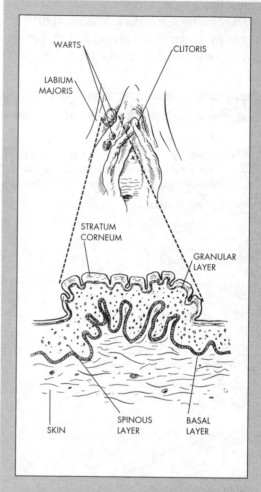

Although these warts signal the presence of the human papilloma virus (HPV), they show up in as few as 30 percent of infections. The cases in which the wart doesn't appear are actually more dangerous, since this type of HPV has been linked to the development of cervical cancer. The danger of cancer resulting from undiscovered infection makes the need for regular checkups all the more urgent. When discovered early enough, cervical cancer can usually be cured.

people have higher rates of HPV than do others. People who smoke put themselves at higher risk as well.

■ *Signs and symptoms:* Many people with HPV have no signs or symptoms. If and when warts appear, they can be on the vulva, in or around the vagina or anus, on the cervix, or anywhere on the groin or thighs. They may also be found in the mouth. Warts on men usually show up on the penis or scrotum. The warts can appear as raised or flat, small or large, and single or clumped in a group that sometimes looks like cauliflower. Normally, the warts are flesh-colored and painless. They can also appear as slightly pink or grey. Rarely, they cause itching, pain, or bleeding.

■ *Cause:* HPV is spread by skin to skin contact, especially during vaginal, anal, or oral intercourse. It is thought that the virus enters the body through tiny breaks in the skin, which could be caused by the friction of sex or even by using tampons incorrectly. Once it is in the skin, the virus makes its way into the lower layers of skin. It can stay there for months or years, and may never come back up to the surface at all. For this reason, it is important to understand that if you are diagnosed with HPV, you could have gotten it at any time in your past sexual life.

■ *Incubation period:* Viral infections are harder to get than bacterial ones. It can take from four to six weeks to infect a partner with HPV. In two-thirds of infected people, it can be up to nine months before any warts appear.

■ *Possible health affects:* Although the reason is unclear, women with HPV are at increased risk for cancer of the vulva and cervix. However, only a few strains have been linked to cancer (types 16, 18, 31, 33, and 35) , and the potential for malignancy is low. These strains usually cause subclinical infections. The strains that cause growths (types 6 and 11) do not lead to cancer. Annual pap smears, are particularly important for women with malignant strains, and for women at high risk for exposure to any type of STD. In addition, women with HPV should periodically have an examination of the cervix, vagina, and vulva.

■ *Diagnosis:* HPV remains a mystery because it can not be grown in the lab and there is no blood test for it. For the 30 percent of people with the clinical or outward expression of the virus — the warts — diagnosis is made just by looking at them. Some warts are very hard to see because they are flat and look like normal skin, so your doctor will look at them through a magnifying lens called a colposcope. Also, your doctor or nurse will probably put a vinegar-like substance called acetic acid on your cervix and on the skin of your vagina. If the area then turns white, it is possible you have HPV. If the diagnosis is still unclear, several more sophisticated tests are available.

■ *Treatments:* Treatment of HPV should be considered cosmetic rather than curative. Like other viruses, no therapy has been shown to cure HPV. Many treatment regimens are available and the choice is based on factors, such as the size and number of warts, as well as the expense, convenience, and potential adverse effects of the treatment.

Regardless of treatment, one in four HPV-infected people will have a recurrence within three months. Many studies have shown that small warts and warts that have been present for less than one year are the ones most amenable to treatment. In any case, never

SPORADIC SIGNS OF A PERMANENT INFECTION

The hallmark of a herpes infection, these tiny blisters may break out for up to three weeks, then disappear on their own—only to return at unpredictable moments later on. Treatment with the drug Zovirax can ease the severity of an outbreak, but won't eradicate the infection. Because the herpes virus can be passed along even when there are no blisters in evidence, chances of contracting it are comparatively high: 200,000 new cases are reported each year.

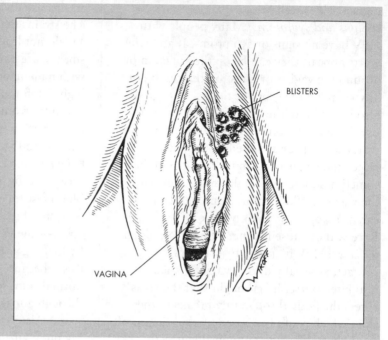

use an over-the-counter wart remedy for genital warts.

Here is a list of available treatments, along with their best use and potential side effects:

Nothing. Letting the warts go away by themselves is actually a common treatment. Within three months, 20 to 30 percent of patients' noncervical warts will have cleared up on their own.

Cryotherapy. The warts are frozen with liquid nitrogen. This relatively inexpensive treatment is best used for small, single warts. There may be pain at the site where the liquid is applied.

Podofilox (Condylox). This prescription drug is applied at home with a cotton swab, twice daily for three days, followed by four days of no treatment. You can repeat this cycle up to four times. This safe and rela-

tively inexpensive drug is for external warts only, not those that might be in the vagina or on the cervix. You will probably feel burning and experience some irritation. Do not use this drug if you are pregnant.

Podophyllin (Pododerm, Podocon-25). This chemical, applied by a doctor or nurse, is best used on small, external warts. It too is safe and relatively inexpensive, but causes mild to moderate pain and discomfort at the site. It should not be used on large vulvar surfaces. Podophyllin needs to be washed off after one to four hours and you will need to be treated weekly for up to six weeks. Very large amounts can cause harmful side effects, including nerve damage. Do not use this treatment if you are pregnant.

Trichloroacetic acid (TCA). TCA is absorbed by the wart and causes it to slough off. You will feel some burning at the site of application. Application is repeated weekly for up to six weeks. It is also best used for external warts.

Electrocautery. Warts are destroyed with an electric current. Local anesthesia is required, and discomfort is moderate.

Laser vaporization. Intense light is used to destroy the wart. This procedure is useful for extensive warts on the genitals or vocal cords and should be tried only after other regimens have failed. Local anesthesia is required, scarring and infection are possible, and you will probably need analgesic for the pain for about three weeks. Laser treatment is also expensive.

Interferon therapy. Injected into the wart itself, this antiviral drug is not generally recommended because it is expensive, time-consuming, produces adverse effects in many people, and has not proven to be any more effective than other treatments.

■ *Follow-up:* If either you or your partner are being treated with medication, it is advisable to abstain from sex, due to the possibility of reinfection and because the friction caused by sex could impede healing. Once the warts are gone, you do not need to return to your clinic. If your partner does not have obvious warts, there is no need for him to be treated.

■ *Prevention:* Most experts believe that recurrences of warts are caused by the virus being reactivated rather than by reinfection. Condoms do offer some protection from reinfection, though. Obviously, areas not covered by the condom, like the vulva and scrotum, are vulnerable to repeat infection. Spermicides have not proven to be effective against HPV.

You can help protect yourself from HPV by trying to prevent the tiny skin abrasions through which the virus can enter the body. For example, the tender lining of the vagina can tear easily when it is dry. Since sexual intercourse can cause lacerations of the vagina, use a lubricant if dryness is a problem. Also, don't use tampons at the beginning or end of your period when the vagina is dry; use a sanitary pad instead, until your period is well underway and again towards the end.

■ *Pregnancy:* Pregnant women should not use podophyllin and podofilox. Other treatments should be discussed with your doctor. Infants born to HPV-infected mothers can be born with warts in and around their larynx (voice box) although this is very rare. Cesarean deliveries are not necessary unless warts are so extensive that they block the birth canal.

Lumps, Bumps and Sores: Herpes Simplex Virus (HSV)

HSV is a member of the family of viruses responsible for chicken pox, shingles, and infectious mononucleosis. The strain HSV-1 of this common virus is also responsible for cold sores, canker sores, and fever blisters that appear on the mouth. HSV-1 may be responsible for the genital sores we think of in relation to herpes, but more often the strain HSV-2 is the cause of sores and blisters below the waist. Like other viruses, there is no cure for HSV, but there are drugs to help manage most infections.

The virus which causes herpes lives in nerve cells at the bottom of the spine, and "creeps" to the surface once in a while to cause sores and blisters. In fact, herpes is named after the Greek word for "creeping". Recent studies have shown that most people with a herpes infection — probably as many as three-quarters — don't even know they have the disease because they have no symptoms: they never have any sores or blisters to alert them to the infection.

People who are unaware that they are infectious can unwittingly spread the disease. But even people who are aware of their infection can unknowingly spread it because viral particles are "shed," meaning they are present on the skin of the genitals, even when no sore or blister is apparent. This "asymptomatic" shedding happens prior to reappearance of the sore.

Because of its ease of transmission, the virus has become extremely common. HSV is not a reportable disease, but an estimated 30 million Americans or more are thought to have it. More than 200,000 new cases are expected each year.

■ *Risk factors:* You are more likely to get herpes if you or your partner have multiple or casual sexual partners. Rates are high among all racial groups. Approximately one in every five 30-year-old white females has HSV.

■ *Signs and symptoms:* Many people with HSV have no signs or symptoms. If and when trademark sores appear, they can be on the vulva, in or around the vagina, in the anus, or on the cervix. Many women notice itching or a tingling sensation in the genital area before the sores appear. These are known as "prodromal symptoms."

The first "outbreak" of a herpes infection is always the most severe, often lasting for three weeks or longer. The average length of time for a first episode is 12 days. Fever, headaches, swollen lymph glands, and sore muscles (especially in the legs) are common, in addition to the painful blisters. Some people will have one blister during an outbreak, while others will have many. Blisters deep in the vagina or cervix may not cause any pain. Recurrent episodes, during which the virus is reactivated, are milder and usually last about five days. For many people, the recurrences will occur less frequently over time.

■ *Cause:* HSV is spread by skin to skin contact, especially during vaginal, anal, or oral intercourse. HSV-1 and HSV-2 are almost identical, so someone with a cold sore performing oral sex can give his or her partner genital herpes. It is thought that 20 percent of genital herpes is transmitted during oral sex.

Once the virus enters the genital area, it quickly camps out in clumps of nerves at the base of the spine. It can lie dormant there for the rest of one's life, as it does in about 10 percent of all cases, or it can reappear sporadically. Many things can trigger recurrence of symptoms: surgery, illness, stress, fatigue, skin irritation (such as sunburn), dietary imbalance, menstruation, hormonal imbalance, or vigorous sexual intercourse.

■ *Incubation period:* Symptoms usually start appearing within a week after infection if they are going to appear at all (remember, as many as 75 percent of people with HSV may be asymptomatic.) However, symptoms have been known to start one day to 26 days after exposure to the virus.

■ *Possible health affects:* One complication from HSV is very rare and easily avoided: accidentally spreading the infection to the eyes. This can occur if you should happen to rub your eyes or put in contact lenses after touching an HSV sore. The herpes virus is easily killed with soap and water, though, so

HELP WITH HERPES

Having trouble paying for acyclovir treatment? Burroughs Wellcome Co., the makers of Zovirax, offers a patient assistance program for hardship cases. Request an application by calling 1-800-722-9294.

an eye infection can be avoided through stringent hygiene during outbreaks.

Although an association between herpes and cervical cancer has not been established, women with the virus should have regular Pap tests because of their increased risk of other infections such as HPV.

■ *Diagnosis:* It is important to see your doctor while symptoms are still present, because diagnosis is made by viewing sores and by taking a sample from the sore to look at under a microscope. Blood tests that detect antibodies to HSV are also reliable. You can request a specific culture for HSV, but it is fairly expensive and takes about a week to give results.

■ *Treatments:* Although nothing is available to rid the body of a virus, acyclovir (Zovirax) can alter the herpes virus' ability to cause damage once it comes out of its hiding place in the nerve ganglia.

Zovirax is the most frequently prescribed drug for an initial herpes outbreak. Duration of symptoms can be reduced from nine days to about five; healing time is reduced from about three weeks to about two weeks; and viral shedding can be cut down from 10 days to about two.

The topical cream form of Zovirax can be effective for the initial outbreak, but rarely works well for recurrences. Taking oral Zovirax for recurrent outbreaks, while it can

still be effective, has a less significant impact for some people.

The recommended regimen for an initial herpes outbreak is 200 milligrams orally five times a day for seven to 10 days or until symptoms disappear. If you are aware enough of your body and can know when a herpes attack is about to strike, taking Zovirax within two days of onset can help lessen the severity of recurrences. Usually the initial warning symptoms — muscle aches, genital itching and tingling — will alert you. For recurrent outbreaks, you will probably take Zovirax for five days, at a dose of either 200 milligrams five times a day, 400 milligrams three times a day, or 800 milligrams twice a day. This conservative therapeutic approach can reduce shedding time by almost half, from nearly four days to slightly over two days.

Taking Zovirax only at the onset of an outbreak is referred to as "episodic" therapy. If you suffer from many outbreaks a year — once every month or two — or if having herpes is causing you great psychological distress, you might consider "suppressive" therapy. Taking the drug suppressively (400 milligrams twice a day, every day), reduces outbreaks by at least 75 percent among patients with frequent outbreaks. It has not, however, been shown to cut down on viral shedding, so you could still pass the disease to a partner, and the outbreak will resume when therapy stops.

There is varying opinion on how long a person should stay on suppressive therapy. The U.S. Food and Drug Administration currently recommends only one year, although studies have shown that patients do well with three or even seven years. Additionally, suppressive therapy's expensive, costing between $2 and $4 a day. Talk with your doctor to decide what is best for you.

Drug companies are working hard to come up with new drugs to fight herpes outbreaks. Zovirax was a breakthrough that helped many people, but it has its flaws. Only 15 percent of the drug is actually absorbed into your body for use against the virus. For this reason, it is important to understand that if your bowels are moving more quickly than normal (as with gastrointestinal problems), you may not be getting a high enough level of the drug.

A new drug called valacyclovir is being studied, and researchers believe it will have an absorption rate of about 80 percent. Neither valacyclovir, or another drug, famcyclovir, will be available until clinical studies are completed and the drugs have received FDA approval.

■ *Follow-up:* If an initial outbreak warns that you have herpes, tell all sex partners from the prior three weeks. If you find out some other way, from a blood test for example, you may not know when you were infected. It is up to you and your doctor to decide which partners to tell. It is also up to you to decide when and if to tell a new partner about your infection.

■ *Prevention:* People with herpes are most likely to shed the virus asymptomatically for up to three months after the initial outbreak. It is not known exactly how often asymptomatic shedding occurs, though researchers believe it is a major cause of the high numbers of herpes cases. However, in long-standing marriages where one partner is

infected and the other is not, the uninfected partner often stays herpes-free. Use of condoms and spermicides (which kill the herpes virus) is an important part of any prevention strategy.

HSV-1 and HSV-2 can easily migrate through the body, so oral sex should be avoided when there is an active sore on the mouth or genitals.

■ *Pregnancy:* The most serious known complication of herpes threatens infants born to HSV-infected mothers. An HSV-infected baby is at risk for blindness, brain damage, and even death. Fortunately, the risk of transmitting the infection to a newborn at birth is low, even for women who have long-standing, recurrent outbreaks. If the baby does get infected (a less than 3 percent chance for women with recurrent infections), Zovirax will probably be used as treatment. HSV also increases the risk of miscarriage or premature labor and delivery.

The group at highest risk are women who acquire HSV late in their pregnancy, particularly those who have no immune defense to the virus (developed from having had diseases like chickenpox, or cold sores, etc.). Women with immune defense, which can be measured by antibodies to HSV in the blood, pass immunity to the baby through the placenta during the third trimester of pregnancy. Infants born to HSV-infected and antibody-carrying mothers are thus protected from the disease should they come into contact with it as they pass through the birth canal. Most HSV-infected women can have normal, vaginal deliveries. Having an active sore at the time of delivery will warrant a cesarean delivery.

If you are pregnant and either have HSV or have sex with an infected partner during your pregnancy, or if you or your partner have sex with more than one partner during your pregnancy, be sure to tell your doctor. He or she will then test to see if you are shedding the virus when it comes time to deliver the baby.

Zovirax has not been thoroughly studied for use by pregnant women, so your doctor will probably advise stopping suppressive or episodic therapy during pregnancy.

Lumps, Bumps and Sores:
Syphilis

This is an ancient disease, described in Chinese medical texts as long ago as 2,000 B.C. Yet it is still with us today. As a matter of fact, the United States sustained a syphilis epidemic from 1986 to 1990.

Since the latest epidemic, rates of syphilis have been falling but are still high, especially in the southern United States. In 1990, more than 50,000 cases were reported to the Centers for Disease Control and Prevention (CDC). By 1992, the number of reported cases had fallen to about 30,000; in 1993, the number of reported cases was less than 23,000.

■ *Risk factors:* You are more likely to get syphilis if you or your partner have multiple or casual sexual partners. From one act of unprotected sex with an infected partner, you have a 30 percent chance of getting syphilis.

■ *Signs and symptoms:* Syphilis is marked by three stages:

Stage 1 (Primary syphilis): This stage is characterized by a painless sore with hard, cartilage-like edges. It can appear anywhere on the body where there has been sexual contact, such as the vulva, vagina, cervix, anus, tongue, or on a man's penis or scrotum. If untreated, the sore(s) will disappear in three to eight weeks. This chancre sore is highly infectious.

Stage 2 (Secondary syphilis): Six to eight weeks later, syphilis in the blood can cause a non-itchy rash, swollen lymph nodes, sore throat, weight loss, headaches, hair loss, and general feeling of unwellness. Sores which can look like herpes sores or genital warts, can also appear in moist areas. If left untreated, these symptoms will disappear in two to six weeks.

Stage 3 (Latent syphilis): Years to decades later, 20 percent to 30 percent of people infected with syphilis will experience complications such as damage to the eyes, ears, heart, and bones; paralysis; mental derangement, and death.

■ *Cause:* A spiral-shaped bacterium, *Treponema pallidum,* is responsible for syphilis infections. It is most often spread during sexual intercourse, but can also be spread through transfusions if the tainted blood has not been properly screened.

■ *Incubation period:* Although the first stage of syphilis can show up three weeks after infection, it has been known to take up to 90 days.

■ *Possible health affects:* Syphilis can damage the eyes, liver, kidneys and other organs. The open sores are also ideal ports of entry for organisms that cause diseases such as Acquired Immune Deficiency Syndrome (AIDS), Herpes Simplex Virus (HSV), and Human Papilloma Virus (HPV).

Within 24 hours after treatment for early stages of the disease, 60 percent of patients experience what is called a "Jarisch-Herxheimer reaction" which can cause headache, flu-like symptoms and flushed lesions. There is no proven way to prevent this reaction, and it usually goes away without complications within 24 hours.

■ *Diagnosis:* Diagnosis is made by taking a fluid sample from a primary or secondary sore, or from a nearby lymph node, and examining it under a microscope. Blood tests are also used to detect syphilis.

■ *Treatments:* Although many diseases have become resistant to the drugs first used against them, syphilis still responds to the old standby, penicillin. It is 98 percent effective at all stages of the disease, but the dosage and length of treatment will depend on the disease stage and the symptoms.

People allergic to penicillin are often treated with doxycycline (Doryx, Vibramycin, others), 100 milligrams orally twice a day for two weeks, or tetracycline (Achromycin), 500 milligrams orally four times a day for two weeks. These drugs are not as effective as penicillin, but do cure over 90 percent of cases.

■ *Follow-up:* Blood tests are done after three months and then at six months. A spinal tap to test cerebrospinal fluid for secondary syphilis is recommended one year after treatment. Relapses of syphilis are more often due to reinfection than to failure of treatment, which is rare.

■ *Prevention:* Because of the seriousness of untreated syphilis infections, all sex partners exposed must be notified. Here is a guideline for identifying at-risk partners:

—If you have primary syphilis, contact all partners you've had during the three months prior to first noticing your symptoms;

—If you have secondary syphilis, contact all partners you've had during the six months prior to first noticing your symptoms;

—If you have latent syphilis, contact all partners you've had during the year prior to first noticing your symptoms.

Abstain from sex until tests show you can no longer spread the infection. To avoid infection or reinfection, use latex condoms for each act of penetration (vaginal, anal, or oral).

■ *Pregnancy:* Congenital syphilis (infection before birth) can be fatal for the developing baby. If the baby survives, deafness, anemia, and permanent damage to bones, liver, and teeth are all possibilities. Sometimes these symptoms do not appear until the child is a teenager.

If a woman has had syphilis for more than four years, chances are low that the baby will be infected. If she has been infected more recently, especially during her pregnancy, congenital syphilis is likely.

The reaction to treatment, the Jarisch-Herxheimer reaction, may induce early labor or cause fetal distress. It's more important to get treatment than to avoid this possibility.

Lumps, Bumps and Sores: Chancroid

This is a very common sexually transmitted disease in underdeveloped countries, where its incidence far exceeds that of syphilis. It is included here because experts at the Centers for Disease Control and Prevention believe that rates of chancroid in the United States are under-reported.

In 1990, 4,223 cases were reported, down only slightly from the 5,035 cases reported in a 1987 epidemic. Researchers say that as many as seven outbreaks may have gone unreported in the U.S. since 1987, due to a lack of standardized reporting procedures.

■ *Risk factors:* You are more likely to get chancroid if you or your partner have multiple or casual sexual partners. Risk factors, like prevalence rates, are not well understood.

■ *Signs and symptoms:* Chancroid is characterized by soft, gray, painful ulcers containing

CHANCROID OR CHANCRE SORE?

If it's a chancre sore, you can expect a diagnosis of syphilis. The sore itself is painless and will disappear on its own in three to eight weeks—but if untreated, the underlying syphilis infection will remain to ravage the body in later years. Of the two kinds of sores, this is the more insidious one: easy to ignore, yet ultimately life-threatening.

Chancroid, on the other hand, is much more likely to send you to the doctor in a hurry. The sores are painful, tend to merge into large patches of damaged tissue, and are often accompanied by an infected abscess in the groin. If left untreated, they can spread to new locations; and they provide an ideal entryway for HIV, the cause of AIDS.

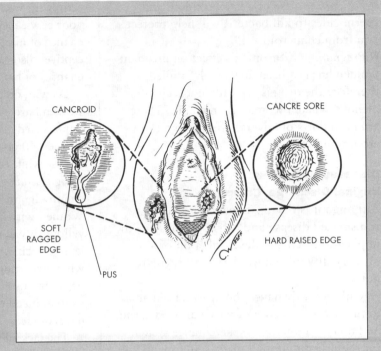

CANCROID

CANCRE SORE

SOFT RAGGED EDGE

HARD RAISED EDGE

PUS

pus. The ulcers often have ragged edges and bleed easily when touched. Another symptom is markedly enlarged lymph nodes in the groin.

■ *Cause:* Chancroid is caused by a bacterium known as *Haemophilus ducreyi* which is transmitted by sexual contact.

■ *Incubation period:* Ulcers appear within two to seven days after infection.

■ *Possible health affects:* Chancroid is associated with human immunodeficiency virus (HIV). The open sores on the genitals facilitate HIV transmission.

■ *Diagnosis:* Chancroid is often misdiagnosed as genital herpes (HSV) or syphilis by doctors unfamiliar with the disease. Since a precise diagnosis requires a culture with a substance that is not readily available, many doctors or clinics are unable to make a definitive diagnosis. They, therefore, start by ruling out syphilis and HSV through tests for those infections. If the tests come back negative, they then diagnose chancroid.

■ *Treatments:* The recommended treatment regimens are either azithromycin (Zitromax), 1 gram orally in a single dose, ceftriaxone (Rocephin), 250 milligrams intramuscularly in a single dose or erythromycin (PCE, ERYC, others), 500 milligrams orally four times a day for seven days.

■ *Follow-up:* You should be re-examined within a week after you begin taking medication. All sex partners during the 10 days before your symptoms started should be notified and treated.

■ *Prevention:* Use of a latex condom and spermicides to kill bacteria will help protect you from chancroid.

■ *Pregnancy:* Zithromax's effect on pregnant women has not been adequately studied; therefore the drug is typically not recommended when a woman is pregnant. There are no reports of adverse effects from chancroid in infants.

Diseases that Cause
Vaginal Discharge: Chlamydia

Although it is the most common sexually transmitted disease and carries serious health implications, chlamydia is still a bit of a mystery. If you've never heard of it, you're not alone.

Only recently have laboratories been able to prove the existence of the chlamydia germ; and there is no national surveillance system for the disease, though many states mandate doctors to report cases they find to the Centers for Disease Control. Based on information from these states, experts estimated that there are between three and four million cases of chlamydia in the U.S. each year. The American Social Health Association, an organization dedicated to researching STDs and their effects, predicts that by the year 2000, there will be 40 million cases.

■ *Risk factors:* You are more likely to get chlamydia if you are under the age of 20, if you or your partner have had many other partners, if you are using oral contraceptives, and if you have an inflamed cervix (cervicitis). Statistics show that people under age 20 more often have multiple sex partners, and that teenagers are more likely to experience a form of cervicitis called cervical ectopy. Having cervical ectopy means that thin and vulnerable layers of your cervical cells are exposed, increasing your chance of infection there. Taking oral contraceptives also causes some increase in your chances of having cervical ectopy.

As with other STDs, chlamydia strikes women harder than men. From one act of unprotected intercourse with an infected partner, 40 percent of women will contract the disease while only 20 percent of men will do so.

■ *Signs and symptoms:* The symptoms of chlamydia are similar to those of gonorrhea. Women with symptoms usually experience a yellowish vaginal discharge called mucopurulent cervicitis. Other symptoms include pain when urinating, lower abdominal or rectal pain, mucus-covered stools, intermittent vaginal bleeding, and pain or bleeding during intercourse.

The lack of symptoms in many people is what makes chlamydia such a dangerous and mysterious disease. Up to 25 percent of infected men and 75 percent of infected women are usually asymptomatic, that is, they have no signs or symptoms of the disease, and can therefore spread it unknowingly.

■ *Cause:* Although chlamydia is caused by a bacteria, the germ shares properties with viruses, including dependence on the host cell for energy and division. This combination of characteristics has made the Chlamydia trachomatis bacterium elusive to researchers, and is the reason diagnostic tests are difficult and expensive.

■ *Incubation period:* Signs of the disease, if any, usually show up between one to two weeks after infection.

■ *Possible health affects:* Public health experts believe that one-quarter to one-half of the one million yearly cases of Pelvic

Inflammatory Disease (PID) are due to chlamydia. PID can lead to tubal infertility and ectopic pregnancy, a potentially dangerous situation in which the fertilized egg implants in the fallopian tube instead of in the uterus. Reports from the Centers for Disease Control and Prevention show that 30 percent of women with untreated chlamydia infections will become sterile.

Recent research on chlamydia-caused PID points to either an allergic response to the proteins of the bacteria or an immune response. Since chlamydia proteins and human proteins look alike, the body could mistake its own normal cells as foreign and attack them. Either reaction would cause the scarring and tubal obstruction that are the hallmarks of PID.

■ *Diagnosis:* Your doctor will suspect chlamydia if your cervix is red and swollen and bleeds easily. He or she will confirm the diagnosis with either a tissue culture, a test called an enzyme-linked immunosorbent assay (ELISA for short), or a process called immunofluorescence.

■ *Treatments:* The recommended treatment is either doxycycline (Doryx, Vibramycin, others), 100 milligrams orally twice a day for seven days, or azithromycin (Zithromax), in a new single-dose treatment of 1 gram orally. The effectiveness of the two drugs is the same. You should decide what's best for you: Doxycycline is four times less expensive, but azithromycin is much more convenient.

Other treatments include ofloxacin (Floxin), 300 milligrams orally twice a day for seven days, erythromycin (PCE, ERYC, others), 500 milligrams orally four times a day for seven days, or sulfisoxazole (Gantrisin), 500 milligrams orally four times

a day for 10 days. Sulfisoxazole treatment is not as effective as the other regimens.

■ *Follow-up:* You won't need to be retested for chlamydia after you have finished your medication unless your symptoms continue or you have been re-exposed to the disease. If you do need retesting, it should be at least three weeks since you have finished the medication.

Since chlamydia can also cause infertility in men, it is important that all your recent sexual partners receive treatment as well. If you are symptomatic, all partners from the last 30 days should be notified. If you are asymptomatic, it's harder to be sure who might have been infected, but you should at least notify all partners from the last 60 days.

■ *Prevention:* Condoms can protect you from the chlamydia bacteria. Other methods, such as the diaphragm, cervical cap and spermicides may also help protect you. It is advisable not to have sex during your treatment.

■ *Pregnancy:* Pregnant women who also have chlamydia have been known to get postpartum endometriosis. Endometriosis is a condition in which pieces of the lining of the uterus are found in abnormal locations outside the uterus, such as the lining of the pelvis or the ovaries, bowel, fallopian tubes, and even the lungs.

Pregnant women with chlamydia are also at increased risk for spontaneous abortions and stillbirths. Infants born to chlamydia-infected mothers are at greater risk for conditions such as eye infections, pneumonia, and bronchitis.

Diseases that Cause Vaginal Discharge: Gonorrhea

This is the oldest known sexually transmitted disease. In the 14th century it became known as the clap, a name we still use today. It is also referred to as "the drip" or "the dose."

Until 1991, gonorrhea was the most commonly reported STD in the United States, even though rates have been steadily decreasing since the mid 1970s. The number of cases reported to the Centers for Disease Control and Prevention in 1992 was 433,949; by the end of November 1993, the number of cases was 336,169. Some experts believe many cases go unreported, and they estimate the actual number to be about two million a year.

■ *Risk factors:* You are more likely to get gonorrhea if you or your partner have casual sexual contacts with others and if you are under the age of 20. From 1981 to 1991, adolescents were the only group of Americans showing an increase in the number of cases; people aged 15 to 19 have twice the number of infections as those aged 20 to 24. People living in the South Atlantic region of the U.S. (from Delaware down the eastern seaboard) may be at higher risk because this region has the highest number of reported cases.

People with limited access to health care also seem to have a higher risk for getting gonorrhea. Other groups at high risk of this or any other STD include people living in large cities, singles, those who have had past gonorrhea infections, drug users, and prostitutes.

A man having unprotected sex once with a woman infected with gonorrhea has a 20 percent to 25 percent chance of catching the disease. A woman having unprotected sex once with an infected man has an 80 percent to 90 percent chance of catching it.

■ *Signs and symptoms:* The symptoms of gonorrhea are similar to those of chlamydia. Women with symptoms usually experience increased vaginal discharge. Other symptoms include pain when urinating, lower abdominal or rectal pain, intermittent vaginal bleeding,

TUBAL INFERTILITY AND GONORRHEA

A recent study suggests that women who've had gonorrhea are much more likely to be infertile because of obstructions in or adhesions on their fallopian tubes. The risk is also twice as high for women who've had past trichomoniasis infections. (See chapter 18, "Overcoming Infertility: Tactics and Techniques.") Women who reported having herpes, genital warts or yeast infections were at no higher risk than any other women.

The researchers also found some other risk factors for tubal infertility. The women they studied were older, more likely to be smokers, had higher rates of pelvic inflammatory disease (PID), and were more likely to have used an intrauterine device (IUD) for contraception in a monogamous relationship.

pain or bleeding during intercourse, and fever. Half of all women with gonorrhea infections also have a gonococcal rectal infection and may have discomfort in the anal area.

Up to 70 percent of infected women are asymptomatic. Only 10 percent of infected men are without symptoms. Therefore, your first warning of infection may be from your partner. He will experience painful urination and have a milky discharge from his penis. He may feel the need to urinate frequently.

■ *Cause:* Gonorrhea infections are caused by a kidney bean-shaped bacteria scientists call *Neisseria gonorrhea.* These germs live in the cervix in women and inside the urethra (the tube that carries urine) in men.

■ *Incubation period:* Symptoms usually develop within 10 days of infection.

■ *Possible health affects:* Untreated infections can lead to Pelvic Inflammatory Disease (PID), which increases by 40 percent your chance of having a tubal (ectopic) pregnancy or becoming infertile. You also become susceptible to septicemia (blood poisoning), arthritis, or problems related to the skin, heart, or brain.

■ *Diagnosis:* For men, a simple test called a gram stain is sufficient for diagnosis, but for women a tissue culture is often needed, since many organisms in the cervix look similar to the gonorrhea bacteria. A blood sample may be taken to test for syphilis, and a test for chlamydia may be done. Your tissue culture should be ready within 48 hours.

■ *Treatments:* Many strains of gonorrhea are now resistant to standard drugs such as penicillin and tetracycline. However, two new types of drugs, the cephalosporins and the quinolones, are highly effective in treating gonorrhea. The cephalosporins include ceftriaxone (Rocephin) in a single 125-milligram intramuscular injection, and cefixime (Suprax) 400 milligrams orally in a single dose. The quinolones include ciprofloxacin (Cipro) 500 milligrams orally in a single dose, and ofloxacin (Floxin) 400 milligrams orally in a single dose. Ceftriaxone is expensive but offers higher and more sustained activity against infection than does cefixime. Ciprofloxacin is less expensive than ceftriaxone and has proven to be highly effective.

For those who are allergic to or who can not tolerate the cephalosporins and the quinolones, an injection of spectinomycin (Trobicin), is given in a single 2-gram intramuscular injection. Though spectinomycin is expensive, it will cure gonorrhea infections of the throat.

Your doctor may also suggest treatment for chlamydia since the two infections frequently occur together and chlamydia is often asymptomatic. For information on chlamydia treatment, see the previous section.

There are many other drugs available to treat gonorrhea. You can discuss them with your doctor.

■ *Follow-up:* You won't need to be retested for gonorrhea after you have finished your medication unless your symptoms continue or you have been re-exposed to the disease.

If you received treatment because you had symptoms, all sex partners from the prior 30 days should also get treatment. If your infection was found incidentally, all sex partners from the last 60 days should be treated.

■ *Prevention:* Latex condoms can protect you from the gonorrhea bacteria. Other methods, such as the diaphragm, cervical cap and spermicides also offer some protection. It is advisable to abstain from sex during your treatment, and until all tests are negative.

■ *Pregnancy:* Pregnant women with gonorrhea can not be treated with quinolones or tetracyclines. If you are pregnant, you may be given a cephalosporin or a single injection of spectinomycin.

Diseases that Cause Itching: Pubic Lice

These lice are wingless insects with six legs and a square body. They look like sea crabs, which is why they are often referred to as "the crabs." The lice cling to pubic hair and feed on blood. The female of the species lays about 50 eggs, called nits, and attaches them to the base of a hair strand. The average lifespan is 25 to 30 days.

There has been a resurgence of pubic lice that parallels increasing rates of other sexually transmitted diseases.

■ *Risk factors:* You are more likely to get pubic lice if you or your partner have multiple or casual sexual partners. It's easier to get

THE MOST CONTAGIOUS STD

Named for their crab-like appearance, pubic lice are large enough to be visible, and leave little bluish marks where they bite. If your sexual partner has lice, you have a 95 percent chance of picking them up. Some of the old wives' tales are true, too. You *can* catch lice from dirty sheets and towels, though not from toilet seats.

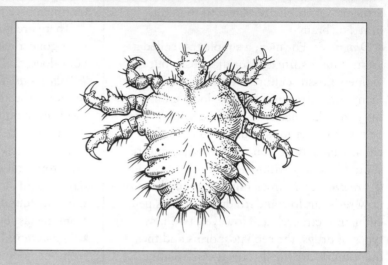

lice than any other STD. From just one sexual encounter with an infested person, you have a 95 percent chance of picking them up.

■ *Signs and symptoms:* You will know if you have contracted pubic lice because you can see them. You may also see little bluish marks in the pubic area or thighs where they've bitten you. The lice often cause itching, which is thought to be from an allergic reaction to their bites. Although crabs are found most often in the pubic area, they can be found on any other hairy part of the body, such as the chest, armpits, beard, and eyelashes. They normally leave the hair on the head to their cousins, body lice.

■ *Cause:* Pubic lice is caused by a parasite known as *Phthirus pubis* that is transmitted by close body contact, most often by sexual intercourse. Since the lice can live away from their host for 24 to 48 hours, there are other possible modes of transmission such as sheets and towels (but not toilet seats).

■ *Incubation period:* Eggs hatch in seven to

10 days. But depending on the number of lice transmitted, it could be two to four weeks before you notice anything.

■ *Possible health affects:* Having pubic lice raises the suspicion of other STDs.

■ *Diagnosis:* You can tell if you have pubic lice just by looking for them. This is how your doctor will diagnose them.

■ *Treatments:* Shaving the hair is unnecessary. Recommended treatment regimens are either a 1 percent lindane shampoo (Kwell), applied for four minutes and then washed off, or a 1 percent permethrin cream rinse (Rid) which is washed off after 10 minutes. Both of these pesticide treatments require a prescription, with lindane being the less expensive. Lindane should not be used by people with extreme dermatitis because it could cause seizures.

You can buy other pesticide treatments, containing pyrethrin with piperonyl butoxide

(A-200, Rid), without a prescription. They are applied for 10 minutes and then washed off. If you are allergic to ragweed, you should avoid these products. There are also products for inanimate objects such as furniture. These should not be used on humans or animals.

If you have lice clinging to your eyelashes, do not use any of these pesticide treatments to get rid of them. Instead, put some Vaseline on the edges of your lids twice a day for 10 days, which will smother the lice. You can also pluck them and the nits off with tweezers.

■ *Follow-up:* You should be re-examined after a week if the lice do not disappear. It is normal to still feel itchy for several days after treatment. All sex partners from the last month should be notified and treated. Avoid sexual contact until the lice and nits are gone. Clothing and bed linen used in the two days prior to treatment should be washed and dried, or dry cleaned.

■ *Prevention:* There is no certain prevention, but since lice are mostly spread in environments where there is lack of good hygiene, avoid using unclean towels, bedding, or clothing. Using a latex condom will not protect you from pubic lice because it does not cover the pubic hair

■ *Pregnancy:* Pregnant or breastfeeding women should not use lindane shampoo or a pesticide containing pyrethrin with piperonyl butoxide.

Diseases that Cause Itching: Scabies

Scabies has been around for a long time and is probably responsible for the term, "Seven Year Itch." These bugs have three pairs of strong, stubby legs, which the female uses to burrow under the skin.

This extremely common skin infestation has been on the rise in the United States since 1973. Actual prevalence rates are unknown, but epidemics appear to be associated with wars. Unlike other parasitic infestations such as pubic lice, scabies is hard to contract. It

MICROSCOPIC SOURCE OF "THE SEVEN YEAR ITCH"

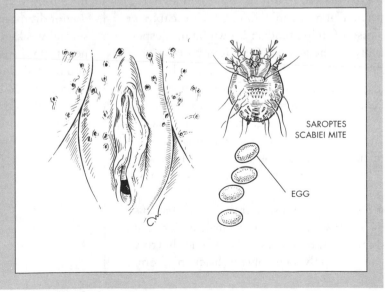

You'll never see the tiny bugs called scabies. Instead, their presence is announced by the severe itching they cause as they burrow under the skin. Unlike crabs, they are picked up only through prolonged contact with an infected person. Though they do not pose a serious threat to your health, you'll want to get rid of them as quickly possible, using a preparation such as Elimite, Eurax, or Kwell.

SAROPTES SCABIEI MITE

EGG

requires prolonged contact with an infected person or infected belongings such as bedding.

■ *Risk factors:* You are more likely to get scabies if you or your partner have multiple or casual sexual partners. Overcrowded living conditions, poor hygiene, and malnutrition probably contribute to the problem.

■ *Signs and symptoms:* Itching, which gets worse at night, after exercise, or after hot baths or showers, is the main complaint with scabies. Hands, arms, feet, ankles, armpits and buttocks, as well as the genitals, can all be affected.

Scabies are so tiny, they can not be seen with the naked eye. However, you can often see the burrows under the skin made by the female when she lays her eggs, particularly in the spaces between your fingers.

■ *Cause:* Scabies is caused by the mites *Sarcoptes scabiei var hominis*. It is passed from person to person through close contact, including sexual activity. It can also spread through sheets, clothes and furniture.

■ *Incubation period:* The typical incubation time is five weeks, but since symptoms are due to an allergic reaction, if you've had scabies before, you'll notice symptoms sooner.

■ *Possible health affects:* Approximately 7 percent of all people infected with scabies get a rash of itchy, reddish-brown bumps, especially on the genitals. This is just a more severe allergic reaction than normal but it may take weeks or months to disappear. People whose immune systems are working overtime—for example, those who've had another illness for a long time—may notice thick, flaky lesions on their skin. This is called Norwegian scabies, and it is extremely contagious.

■ *Diagnosis:* You will probably be able to see the burrows made by the female under your skin. If you're not sure it's a scabies burrow, you can apply some blue or black ink from a

pen or marker to the suspect area. Soak a cotton swab with alcohol and rub off the excess ink. If you're dealing with a burrow, the ink will be sucked into it and you will be able to see a thin line of ink under your skin. For an exact diagnosis, your doctor can scrape off some affected skin and examine it under a microscope.

■ *Treatments:* There are several recommended treatment regimens. One is 5 percent permethrin cream (Elimite) applied all over the body, and washed off eight to 14 hours later. Another treatment is a one ounce application of 1 percent lindane lotion or 30 grams of lindane cream (Kwell) applied thinly all over the body and washed off eight hours later. Both of these treatment are effective, but lindane is less expensive. Lindane should not be used by people with extreme dermatitis because this could cause seizures.

Crotamiton 10% (Eurax) can also be used. It is applied after a bath or shower, with a second application 24 hours later. A cleansing bath should be taken 48 hours after the last application.

■ *Follow-up:* You might be asked to come in for a follow-up after a week if the symptoms do not disappear. It is normal to feel itchy several weeks after treatment. All sex partners from the last month should be notified and treated, and family members should be checked too. Clothing and bed linen used in the two days prior to treatment should be washed and dried, or dry cleaned.

■ *Prevention:* There is no certain prevention, but since scabies are mostly spread in environments where there is a lack of good hygiene, avoid using unclean towels, bedding, and clothing.

■ *Pregnancy:* Pregnant or breastfeeding women should not use treatments containing lindane.

Finding the Support You Need

Do any of these emotions sound familiar: depression, anger, isolation, disillusionment, turmoil, fear, hopelessness? If so, you aren't alone. Most people who find out they have a sexually transmitted disease share some or all of these feelings.

Such non-medical aspects of diseases — both curable and chronic — can be more devastating than the physical symptoms. They may even interfere with the healing process; stress often makes us more susceptible to illnesses of all kinds, and can be blamed for many recurrences of chronic STDs like HPV and HSV.

Hundreds of studies have shown that the most important help in coping with a disease is social support. But when you tell someone that you have an STD, you risk social rejection, or at least an altered reputation. Recent surveys of people with HPV and HSV confirm that most people have these fears. They aren't totally unfounded either; about one-quarter of respondents said they were rejected by a sex partner after telling them they had a sexually transmitted disease.

Still, most respondents did tell current and previous partners about their infections. They also confided in friends and family. Many psychologists believe that talking to people you trust is the most important thing you can do in coming to grips with having an STD.

Stages of Coping

Having any kind of STD is difficult to face. Most people have more problems dealing with the incurable viral diseases than they do with the easily treatable infections like chlamydia, syphilis, and gonorrhea.

Some doctors have noticed that HPV and HSV patients go through a four-stage psychological healing process: denial, resistance, adjustment, and integration. Not everyone will have these same experiences, or even in this order and recurrences of the infection can start the whole process over again. Whatever you feel, the underlying concept is that your mind will let you handle only as much as you can at a given time. Knowing about the stages can help you understand where you are in the coping process.

Stage 1: Denial. This comes with the shock of being told that you have an STD. "It simply can't be true," is your most likely thought. This is a normal reaction to emotional overload. If you are in this stage, try at least to avoid unprotected sex, because you don't want to infect anyone else.

Stage 2: Resistance. Now you are going to fight this disease. You are very goal-directed, and ready to try all different types of remedies, no matter how offbeat they are. Here is where a support group may be helpful for coming to terms with an STD and for learning about treatment options.

Stage 3: Adjustment. You're starting to realize you are one of many people who have an STD, but, you are still grieving for your lost, "clean," innocent self. This is normal and in fact is considered to be a a positive attitude even though it doesn't feel like it. You will probably begin to rearrange your priorities and change your life in appropriate ways.

Stage 4: Integration. Now you're at peace with the situation and ready to go on with your life. It is easy to talk about the disease with others.

Hopefully, the outcome of this process is that you will be able to think of your disease in a positive way. This does not mean that having an STD is a good thing but rather that you are able to take something positive from it. Perhaps it has changed your perspective on life, brought you closer to family and friends, or offered the opportunity to look for more meaningful sexual relationships.

Telling Your Partner Isn't Easy

If you ask most people who have an STD, especially an incurable one, which is harder, coping with their infection or telling their partner, they might have difficulty deciding. For past sexual contacts, the burden can often be handled for you anonymously by public health workers whose job it is to trace sex partners of people infected with STDs. But when it comes to telling current or prospective partners, you're on your own.

Some people decide not to tell their current or potential partners about past or latent infections. They may feel no harm will come to their partners because the infection has been successfully treated or is safely dormant. Since they don't want to lose the relationship, they keep their infection a secret. However, these people appear to be a minority. In the

surveys conducted among people with HPV and HSV, 69 percent reported that they told their current partner about their infection, and 49 percent said they always told potential partners, while only 6 percent said they never told potential partners.

The decision is a personal one and depends on several factors, including whether you value trust and honesty in a relationship, and whether you can live with any guilt that would arise. But basically it comes down to one simple question: would you want to know about something that could affect your health, or would you rather have someone decide that for you?

If you decide to discuss this deeply personal matter with a prospective partner, here are a few things to keep in mind:

It's best if you have already come to grips with the situation yourself. If you are unsure and depressed because you have an STD, you won't sound confident. It is unlikely that your partner will feel comfortable with the situation if you aren't, so make sure you have all the facts. Be ready to answer questions with correct information. Prepare your partner as much as possible, instead of dumping the news on him all at once. You might even want to rehearse some lines ahead of time. Whatever your state of mind, however, don't forget the importance of early treatment should your partner require it.

Pick a good time and place. There may not be a really good time to tell someone about an STD, but there are definitely bad times. Don't pick a time when you are likely to be interrupted. Don't wait until you're in bed together. And especially don't wait until after you've had sex, which will only get the issues tangled up in emotions and distrust.

Give him time to think about it. You may think that this should be easy to handle for someone who is not infected, but he has to weigh the risks of going through exactly what you did. Deciding to take a risk is not easy for a lot of people.

If the reaction is negative, you are not to blame. Most people respond well to the news. In fact, with the alarming rates of STDs in the United States, there's a reasonable chance that he's already heard a similar disclosure. Remember too, that if he can't cope with the situation, he is not rejecting you as a person; he is rejecting the risk involved. This is a difficult concept for many people, and it still hurts if someone rejects the risk you pose. But remember, you are far from alone.

For More Information...

Contact the American Social Health Association (ASHA), an organization dedicated to researching and providing information about STDs. They can send you pamphlets on various STDs. They also operate a Herpes Resource Center with ties to over 100 local self help groups for people living with herpes, and they maintain a herpes hotline. ASHA also publishes two newsletters called The Helper and HPV News.

Your local or state health department's STD clinic can provide you with care, counseling and information. Here are some other resources that may be helpful to you:

The National Herpes Hotline: 919-361-8488 (Monday through Friday, 9 AM to 7 PM Eastern time)

The Herpes Resource Center: HRC, ASHA, PO Box 13827, Research Triangle Park, NC 27709. Phone: 919-361-8488.

National STD Hotline: 1-800-227-8922 (Monday through Friday, 8 AM to 11 PM Eastern time) □

CHAPTER 12   **GENERAL HEALTH CONCERNS**

Heart Disease: The Greatest Threat of All

Think of a heart attack victim and you'll probably picture a middle-aged man, perhaps a little paunchy, most likely a workaholic executive type. It's a stereotype that has been reinforced by the media and by the medical profession itself, which in the past has focused much of its research into heart disease on this type of patient.

Not Just a Man's Disease

The facts, however, tell quite a different story. Heart disease is more than just a man's disease—much more. One in 9 women between the ages of 45 and 64 has some form of cardiovascular disease, ranging from coronary artery disease to stroke or renal vascular disease. By the time a woman reaches 65, she has a 1 in 3 chance of developing cardiovascular disease. And a number of studies show that African–American women are at even greater risk than these averages.

Heart disease, in its various forms, is the leading killer of American women. The following statistics paint a graphic picture:

- One–third of all deaths of American women each year are attributable to heart disease. Heart disease kills more women each year than cancer, accidents, and diabetes combined.
- All forms of cardiovascular disease kill nearly 500,000 American women a year. Stroke alone kills 88,000.
- Myocardial infarction, commonly known as a heart attack, kills 244,000 women a year.
- Forty percent of women with heart disease will eventually die of it.

The reason that so much more attention has been focused on men is that they are much more likely to be stricken with heart disease in their prime middle years, whereas women tend to get it 10 to 20 years later. For most women, it is only after menopause that heart disease becomes a problem. But a woman of 60 is about as likely to get heart disease as a man of

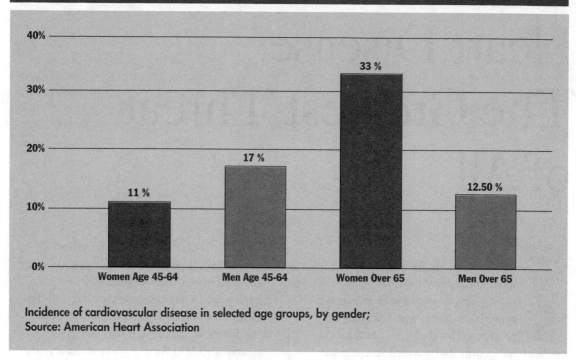

CARDIOVASCULAR DISEASE: THE FATE OF EVERY THIRD WOMAN

Incidence of cardiovascular disease in selected age groups, by gender;
Source: American Heart Association

50, and by time they are in their 70s, men and women get heart disease at equal rates.

The significance of these facts is clear when you consider the aging of the American population. By the year 2000, 38 percent of American women will be 45 years of age or older. By 2015, that percentage will rise to 45 percent. This means that heart disease in women will be an even bigger problem in the future than it is now.

Until now, treatment of women with heart disease has been based primarily on what is known about men. Given the many factors unique to a woman's health, this is not satisfactory. Treatment cannot adequately take account of these factors until they have been systematically studied and evaluated.

Until that happens, it is likely that women will continue to pay with delayed diagnosis,

inadequate treatment, and a toll that can be counted in disabilities and deaths. In fact, some studies have shown that despite the fact that women with heart disease are often sicker than men with the same disease, they are frequently treated less aggressively.

The good news is that things are changing. Greater attention to women's health in general and a growing awareness of the risks of heart disease in women are replacing the disregard of the past. An increasing number of scientific studies are focusing on how heart disease affects women. Gradually, doctors are becoming better informed about the dangers to women from heart disease, so that they are less likely to attribute chest pain to anxiety or other non-heart-related problems. And women themselves are learning that their own attention to their health must not be limited to an annual visit to the gynecologist.

So why is this important? If nothing could be done about heart disease, all of this attention might be academic. However, heart disease is both preventable and treatable; and as doctors learn more about what causes the problem, it is becoming increasingly apparent that there is much that you can do to prevent it from ever occurring. Diet and lifestyle changes can be very effective preventive efforts for some forms of heart disease. To work best, these efforts should begin early in life, long before you perceive yourself to be at risk. And if heart disease does strike, modern science and technology have an ever–growing arsenal of weapons available to successfully fight it and restore its victims to healthy and productive lives.

Statistics reflect an encouraging trend. Better understanding of preventative measures and increasing sophistication in diagnosis and treatment have resulted in decreasing rates of heart disease in both men and women. For example, in the 1980s, death rates from heart disease went down 27 percent for white women and 22 percent for African–American women.

Inside the Circulatory System

When we talk about heart disease we are talking about not just disorders of the heart itself but of a variety of conditions that affect the body's circulatory system. To understand heart disease, and the confusing jargon that describes it—cardiovascular disease, coronary artery disease, myocardial infarction, heart failure, and so on—it helps to have some knowledge of the basic components of this system, and how they work.

A quick lesson in anatomy can help. The heart is the central organ of the circulatory system, a muscular pump a little larger than your fist that continuously forces blood through the lungs, where it takes on oxygen, and then through the arteries, capillaries, and veins that make up the rest of the circulatory system. The expansion and contraction of the heart as it sends blood through the body is your heartbeat. To get an idea of what a tireless workhorse the heart is, consider this: the average heart beats about 100,000 times every day, pumping about 2,000 gallons of blood.

The heart is made up primarily of muscle tissue, called myocardium, and is divided vertically by the septum. It consists of four chambers: two atria in the upper half and two ventricles in the lower half. The pumping of blood through the chambers is aided by four valves that open and close, allowing blood to flow through the heart in only one direction when it contracts. The four heart valves are:

- The tricuspid valve, located between the right atrium and the right ventricle.
- The pulmonary or pulmonic valve, between the right ventricle and the pulmonary artery leading to the lungs.
- The mitral valve, between the left atrium and the left ventricle.
- The aortic valve, between the left ventricle and the aorta, the main artery from the heart to the rest of the body.

It is important to be familiar with these valves because women are more likely than men to have valvular disease, particularly mitral valve prolapse, which is discussed in greater detail below.

The healthy heart operates in a highly organized fashion, triggered by electrical signals. Oxygen-depleted blood comes into the right atrium through the superior and inferior vena cava, the body's largest veins. It is pumped into the right ventricle, then into the pulmonary artery and on into the lungs, where it receives fresh oxygen. Oxygenated blood, a brighter red in color than before, flows back to the heart, entering the left atrium, then moving into the left ventricle, and finally pushing through the aorta into the network of arteries that branches out through the body. The first two arteries that branch from the aorta are the major coronary arteries, which supply blood to the heart muscle itself, enabling it to continue pumping.

The veins, arteries, and tiny capillaries that connect them are the blood vessels that make up the vascular system. These blood vessels are more than just tubes through which the blood flows as it circulates throughout the body. The muscular walls of the arteries act as mini– pumps themselves, expanding with every heartbeat to help push the blood along, while veins are equipped with a type of one–way valve, to prevent blood from flowing backwards.

THE GEOGRAPHY OF THE HEART

Surprisingly small given its importance, the heart is a fist-sized mass of muscle that pumps blood first through the lungs to pick up oxygen, then on through the rest of the body to deliver that oxygen to the body's cells.

The heart lies at the center of an elaborate circulatory system that branches out in an intricate network of ever smaller vessels, ending in microscopic capillaries throughout all the body's tissues. The arteries, which conduct blood out from the heart, give the circulation an added boost, expanding with every heartbeat and contracting while the heart is at rest. The

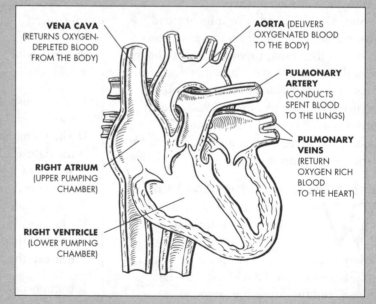

VENA CAVA (RETURNS OXYGEN-DEPLETED BLOOD FROM THE BODY)

AORTA (DELIVERS OXYGENATED BLOOD TO THE BODY)

PULMONARY ARTERY (CONDUCTS SPENT BLOOD TO THE LUNGS)

PULMONARY VEINS (RETURN OXYGEN RICH BLOOD TO THE HEART)

RIGHT ATRIUM (UPPER PUMPING CHAMBER)

RIGHT VENTRICLE (LOWER PUMPING CHAMBER)

veins, which return blood to the heart, are equipped with a series of valves designed to keep the blood from flowing backward as it finishes its round trip through the system.

Of all the vessels in the body, the coronary arteries are the most important, for it is their job to supply life-sustaining oxygen to the heart muscle itself.

What Can Go Wrong

With the basic features of the heart and circulatory system in mind, it's easier to sort out the different categories of heart disease.

Ischemic Heart Disease

This category includes anything obstructing the blood flow. (Ischemia comes from two Greek words meaning " keeping back" and "blood.") The most common obstruction is atherosclerosis, a buildup of fats and calcium on the interior walls of the coronary arteries. This condition is called coronary artery disease or CAD. Atherosclerosis is a progressive problem that, in some people, begins early in life. It can be the result of genetics, diet, cigarette smoking, high blood pressure, or a combination of some or all of these factors. Obstructed arteries can in turn lead to two of the most common heart disorders: angina pectoris or myocardial infarction (MI).

Angina is chest pain that occurs when the heart receives an inadequate blood supply during periods of increased demand, such as unusual exertion or emotional excitement. During such periods, the coronary arteries ordinarily expand to deliver more blood to the heart muscle. Atherosclerotic arteries, however, gradually become rigid, fail to dilate, and can't meet the demand. Usually angina subsides when the exertion stops; however, some people suffer from angina even when resting.

In the past, treatment of angina in women has typified the controversy about the perception of heart disease as a male problem. All too often doctors have dismissed chest pain in women as something benign, perhaps related to anxiety, and not requiring further testing or diagnostic procedures. As both women and their doctors are educated that chest pain that seems like angina could be heart disease, that problem should diminish. Angina is often the first symptom of more serious heart problems to come, and should not be ignored.

MI, or heart attack, occurs when the blood supply to the heart muscle, or myocardium, is severely reduced or stopped, as when a blood clot becomes lodged in a coronary artery. Deprived of its blood supply, the area of heart muscle served by the blocked artery weakens and dies. The affected area is called an infarct, hence the term "Mycardial infarction." A heart attack is also called coronary thrombosis (referring to a clot) or coronary occlusion, meaning an obstruction. A heart attack can also be the result of an unexplained temporary spasm of a coronary artery.

Silent or unrecognized MI has been found to be more common in women than men. In the Framingham Heart Study, an ongoing analysis of the health and disease of a large group of people in the town of Framingham, Massachusetts, 35 percent of MIs in women were initially unrecognized, compared with 27 percent in men. Framingham and other studies have also shown that compared with a man, a woman's first heart attack is more likely to be fatal; she will require longer hospitalization after a heart attack; and she is more likely to die in the first year after an attack.

Warning Signs. Everyone, male and female, should be aware of the warning signals of a heart attack. Shortness of breath, fatigue, nausea, and upper abdominal pain have been noted as more common in women than men. The general signs, as listed by the American Heart Association, are:

- Uncomfortable pressure, fullness, squeezing or pain in the center of the chest that lasts more than a few minutes, or goes away and comes back.
- Pain spreading to the shoulders, neck, or arms.
- Chest discomfort with light–headedness, fainting, sweating, nausea, or shortness of breath.

Valvular Heart Disease

Valvular disorders are much more common in women than men. One study, the 1987 National Hospital Discharge Survey, found that 71 percent of patients with aortic or mitral valve disease were women.

Mitral valve prolapse (MVP), the most common valvular heart disease, affects about 5 percent of all women in this country (compared with 3 percent of men). With this condition, the valve between the left atrium and ventricle does not shut tightly, allowing a partial two-way flow called "regurgitation." The cause of most cases of mitral valve prolapse is thought to be genetic. Symptoms of this can include chest pain, shortness of breath, heart palpitations, fainting, and anxiety or panic attacks. However, since these non-specific symptoms also apply to other conditions, more definitive testing is needed for a diagnosis of MVP.

Other valve disorders can result from rheumatic fever, a disease caused by a bacterial infection. Once thought to be nearly eliminated in this country, rheumatic fever has had something of a comeback in recent years. The most common consequence of rheumatic fever is mitral valve stenosis, a narrowing of the opening of the mitral valve which makes it more difficult for the blood to flow through the valve. The aortic valve can also be affected.

Connective tissue diseases such as Marfan syndrome and systemic lupus erythematosus

HOW CHOLESTEROL HURTS THE HEART

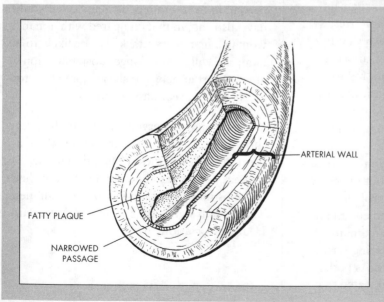

ARTERIAL WALL

FATTY PLAQUE

NARROWED PASSAGE

When fatty deposits of cholesterol and dead cells collect around minute defects in the walls of the coronary arteries, the condition is called atherosclerosis, and heart disease lies ahead. Forced through an increasingly narrow channel, blood flow to the heart muscle declines, leaving the heart starved for oxygen and leading to the pain called angina. Worse yet, if a blood clot blocks the remaining opening, part of the heart muscle will die—the crisis known as a heart attack.

(SLE) also frequently lead to valvular disorders. Nearly 90 percent of SLE patients are women.

Diseases of the Heart Muscle

Cardiomyopathy is the term used to describe any disease of the heart muscle. The problem can result from many of the conditions listed above, including heart attack, atherosclerosis, and rheumatic fever. It can also be brought on by high blood pressure which may enlarge the heart. Idiopathic cardiomyopathy is a condition for which no cause is known. In hypertrophic cardiomyopathy, heart muscle tissue grows improperly. Viral cardiomyopathy is caused by certain viruses. Ischemic cardiomyopathy is caused by numerous tiny infarctions in which destruction of heart muscle is too limited to be felt as it occurs, but cumulatively damages the heart. Hypertensive cardiomyopathy is caused by untreated high blood pressure. Preliminary research into these diseases has shown differing patterns in men and women, with men usually afflicted sooner and more severely.

Congestive heart failure occurs when the heart muscle is unable to maintain normal blood flow throughout the body. It can happen when the heart muscle or valves are damaged or the nerves governing the heartbeat are working improperly. It may also result from other diseases such as anemia (a blood deficiency disease), pulmonary emboli (blockages of the pulmonary artery), some infections, rheumatic fever, or thyroid disease. Congestive heart failure can cause swelling in body tissues and a buildup of fluid in the lungs. Swelling, particularly in the legs and ankles, is often an early sign of congestive heart failure. Shortness of breath is another.

Infections of the heart valves and heart lining can result in a condition called bacterial endocarditis. These infections are most often seen in people with structural abnormalities of the heart, valve malfunctions, or artificial valves. Bacterial endocarditis is also seen in injection drug users.

Arrhythmias

Arrhythmias are irregular heartbeats. They are caused by malfunction in the electrical signals that stimulate the heart to beat. Bradycardia is the term for heart rates of less that 60 beats per minute; tachycardia refers to more than 100 beats per minute. Arrhythmias can cause a wide range of symptoms, ranging from a barely perceptible palpitation or skipped beat to collapse and death.

Bradycardia may prevent the heart from pumping enough blood to the body, causing fatigue, light–headedness, loss of consciousness, or even death if the rate becomes so slow that the heart and brain stop working.

In the case of tachycardia, the ventricular chambers of the heart may not have sufficient time to fill with blood, thus reducing the heart's ability to pump properly. Sometimes this is accompanied by chaotic electrical signals in the upper chambers called atrial fibrillations. Tachycardia can result in shortness of breath, chest pain, light–headedness, or loss of consciousness.

Arrhythmias are common, even in healthy people, but they are seen more often in people whose hearts have been damaged by other forms of heart disease such as atherosclerosis, high blood pressure, or scarring from a heart attack. They may also be caused by problems or defects of the nervous system, which delivers the electrical signals to the heart. Certain substances can also cause arrhythmias, including alcohol, cigarettes, cocaine, and even some cardiac medications.

Noncoronary Cardiovascular Disease

This type of disease occurs in the circulatory system, but not directly in the heart. The two most common conditions in this category are hypertension (high blood pressure) and stroke.

Hypertension. Blood pressure is the measure of the force of blood traveling through the circulatory system. As blood flows through the arteries and arterioles (small arteries), their walls contract or expand, changing the resistance to blood flow. Contraction increases the resistance, reducing blood flow,

THE "FEMALE" HEART DISEASE

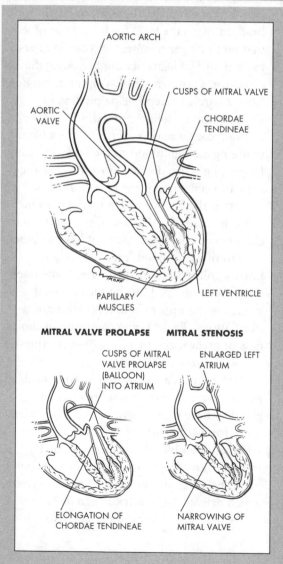

AORTIC ARCH

CUSPS OF MITRAL VALVE

AORTIC VALVE

CHORDAE TENDINEAE

PAPILLARY MUSCLES

LEFT VENTRICLE

MITRAL VALVE PROLAPSE   **MITRAL STENOSIS**

CUSPS OF MITRAL VALVE PROLAPSE (BALLOON) INTO ATRIUM

ENLARGED LEFT ATRIUM

ELONGATION OF CHORDAE TENDINEAE

NARROWING OF MITRAL VALVE

By a 2 to 1 margin, diseases of the heart's aortic and mitral valves develop more frequently in women. Often of genetic origin, the diseases are also associated with connective tissue disorders found primarily in female patients.

Positioned at the portal between the left atrium and ventricle, the mitral valve is particularly vulnerable to a condition called prolapse. Instead of sealing the portal between the two chambers when the ventricle contracts, a prolapsed mitral valve is forced backward into the atrium, allowing some of the blood that has just left there to return. As a result, each heartbeat pushes a little less blood through the aorta and onward to the rest of the body; and the heart must work just a little bit harder to keep the body adequately supplied. The culprits in this condition are stretched and weakened papillary muscles, which ordinarily hold the lips of the valve tightly in place.

The mitral valve plays a role in other problems as well. In the condition called mitral valve stenosis, the opening narrows, hindering the normal progress of blood from the atrium to the ventricle. The problem is an aftermath of rheumatic fever.

increasing blood pressure, and thereby causing the heart to work harder.

Nearly everyone is familiar with the blood pressure cuff, called a sphygmomanometer, which is strapped on during a physical examination to measure blood pressure. It takes two measures: the systolic pressure, the first number, is the force of blood flow when the heart beats; the diastolic pressure, the second number, is the pressure between heartbeats when the heart is at rest. Blood pressure goes up with age and there is a wide variation in what is considered normal, but generally a reading higher than 140/90 means high blood pressure, or hypertension.

Men are more likely to have high blood pressure than women, but African–American women have higher levels than any other group. One study that measured blood pressure in 35- to 74-year-old women found that 20 percent of white women had high blood pressure, compared with nearly 40 percent of African–American women.

The cause of most hypertension is unknown, although overweight and excessive salt in the diet seem to be contributing factors. A genetic component is also likely. Although hypertension itself is not often listed as a cause of death, it can lead to fatal conditions such as heart attack and stroke.

Stroke is a form of cardiovascular disease that affects the arteries leading to the brain. It occurs when one of these arteries bursts or becomes clogged by a blood clot. When the brain is deprived of the oxygen carried by blood, nerve cells in the affected area die. Stroke can cause disabilities, including partial paralysis and loss of speech, memory, or understanding, and frequently proves fatal.

Sometimes strokes are preceded by transient ischemic attacks (TIAs), called little strokes, which occur when an artery leading to the brain is temporarily clogged. These attacks usually last only minutes and leave no residual effects, but may be a sign that a more serious stroke will occur in the days, weeks, or months to come.

Other signs of stroke, as described by the American Heart Association, include:

- Sudden weakness or numbness of the face, arm, or leg on one side of the body.
- Sudden dimness or loss of vision, especially in only one eye.
- Loss of speech, difficulty talking, or difficulty understanding speech.
- Sudden, severe, unexplained headache.
- Unexplained dizziness.

As with hypertension, which is often linked to stroke, African–American women are as much as twice as likely as white women to suffer strokes.

Peripheral vascular disease, a narrowing of the blood vessels in the arms and legs, is another disease of the circulatory system. It is very strongly linked to cigarette smoking and diabetes and is much more common in men than in women.

How To Stave Off Disease

As these descriptions of the various forms of heart disease indicate, much is known about the causes, often referred to as "risk factors." Some—such as heredity, age, race, and gender—cannot be controlled. But many others are controllable and there are many ways you can prevent heart disease.

Basically, heart disease prevention falls into two categories: lifestyle or behavior modification; and pharmacological intervention, or use of medications.

Lifestyle

Cigarette Smoking. The single most important thing you can do to prevent heart disease is not smoke. If you do smoke, you should stop; your risk of heart disease will begin to decline, reaching the level of a non-smoker after 5 to 10 years.

The higher risk of cardiovascular disease in women due to smoking is similar to that of men. Low tar and low nicotine cigarettes seem to be no less harmful than regular cigarettes. A range of studies has shown that women who smoke are from 2 to 6 times more likely than non-smokers to develop heart disease. Statistics from the Nurses' Health Study, a large, ongoing survey of women's health, show that half of the cases of heart disease in women aged 30 to 55 can be linked to cigarette smoking.

The most dramatic increase in risk is in women who smoke and use oral contraceptives. Tests have shown that these women are 20 to 30 times more likely to suffer heart disease and stroke than women who do neither. However, most of the data on this subject came from studies done when participants were taking a much higher dose of estrogen than is currently prescribed. As a result, further research is needed on the effects of today's lower-dose oral contraceptives.

Cigarettes act in a number of ways to increase your risk of heart disease. Smoking causes thickening of the blood, which can lead to clots. It raises the level of carbon monoxide in the blood, robbing the heart and other tissues of needed oxygen. The nicotine in tobacco also constricts the coronary arteries, raising blood pressure, and causing the heart to work harder. Thus smoking increases the amount of oxygen that the heart needs, while at the same time decreasing the amount it gets.

High blood pressure contributes to heart disease because it makes the heart work harder. Controllable factors that contribute to high blood pressure include overweight, lack of exercise, excessive salt intake, and cigarette smoking. It follows logically that losing weight, exercising, limiting salt in your diet, and stopping smoking can reduce blood pressure to healthier levels. Living with continually high levels of stress is also linked to high blood pressure.

The first thing you can do to control your blood pressure is to know what it is. Although you can measure blood pressure with a sphygmomanometer at the supermarket or shopping mall, it is a good idea to discuss the implications of your blood pressure level with your doctor.

Cholesterol, a very popular topic these days, is a substance that circulates in the blood, and is essential for functions such as producing some hormones (including estrogens) and building a protective membrane for our cells. We get some from what we eat, but mostly it is manufactured in the liver.

Cholesterol travels through the bloodstream attached to lipoproteins, compounds composed of fats (lipids), proteins, and triglycerides. There are four kinds of lipoproteins, classified according to their weights: very low density (VLDL), low density (LDL), high density (HDL) and very high density (VHDL). You've probably heard about " good" and " bad" cholesterol. The good is HDL, which is associated with a cleansing effect in the blood; and the bad is LDL, which leaves deposits on the interior walls of the arteries, hampering the flow of blood and leading to atherosclerosis.

In general, a total cholesterol count of less than 200 milligrams per deciliter of blood is viewed as healthy; if that count reaches 240, the risk of heart disease doubles. However, most of the studies that have drawn this conclusion have been done on men. One study focusing on women has found that the most important factor predicting coronary artery disease in women is *not* total cholesterol, but the ratio of HDL to total cholesterol: The higher your HDL, the less likely you are to get heart disease.

Triglycerides are another kind of fat in your bloodstream, but elevated triglycerides are not necessarily associated with an increased risk of heart disease. Triglyceride levels fluctuate widely throughout the day, depending on what you eat. They may, however, be associated with high cholesterol levels.

You can do a great deal to achieve a healthier cholesterol level by controlling your diet. Reducing cholesterol and fat intake, particularly saturated fats, will lower total cholesterol levels. Monounsaturated fatty acids (such as those found in olive and canola oil) tend to raise HDL, so those are the healthiest oils to choose for cooking. Polysaturated oils (safflower, corn) lower LDL, which is good, but also lower HDL. The worst offenders are the saturated fats (meat fat, butter), which raise LDL, lower HDL, and also include cholesterol itself. (For more information, turn to chapter 15, "A Common–Sense Look at Diet and Health.")

Diet is not the only thing that affects your cholesterol level; other factors include heredity, smoking, and hormones. Estrogen plays an important role in keeping cholesterol levels down, and the hormonal changes of menopause will adversely affect your LDL and HDL counts.

Exercise and weight. Lack of exercise has been shown to be a risk factor for heart disease. Regular aerobic exercise seems to tone the heart muscle and help prevent heart disease. Again, most of the studies about exercise and heart disease have been done on men, but the effects are thought to be similar in women. Strenuous athletics are not necessary; moderate exercise such as brisk walking or stair–climbing are sufficient to benefit the heart.

Exercise also lowers cholesterol and blood pressure and is usually associated with weight loss. Being overweight also contributes to high cholesterol and high blood pressure, both factors in developing heart disease.

Body shape is another risk factor for heart disease. Women with " apple-shaped" bodies—more weight around the waistline—have a greater risk than " pear-shaped" women who carry most of their weight around their hips.

Women, especially those who have already suffered heart disease and those with high risk factors, should know that although the benefits of exercise usually outweigh the risks, there is a slight chance that strenuous exercise can contribute to heart attacks, strokes, and arrhythmias. You should plan and discuss any exercise program with your doctor, particularly if you have not been physically active for a while.

Alcohol consumption. The effect of alcohol on heart disease is a very controversial subject. On one hand, there is plenty of documentation of the negative effects of excessive drinking on not just the heart, but a number of body systems. On the other, a number of tests in recent years have indicated that moderate drinking (1 or 2 drinks a day) may protect against heart disease.

The American Heart Association has addressed this issue by advising that drinking is safe only in moderation; and that if you don't already drink, there really is no benefit to starting.

Social and psychological factors. It was once speculated that as women entered the workforce in increasing numbers and began experiencing the same workplace stresses as men, heart attack rates in middle-aged women would begin to approach those of their male counterparts. That has not happened. Women working outside the home have about the same rates of heart disease as women who don't. Twenty years of research in the Framingham study found that employment itself is not predictive of heart disease, but factors such as high demands and low control of the situation, as well as financial anxiety, are related to higher rates of heart disease.

In men, heart disease has been linked to the so-called " Type A" personality, the impatient, driven, competitive personality type. No similar link has been found in women. In fact, Framingham data have shown that women who suppress anger and hostility are more likely to suffer heart disease than those who express it in the Type A manner. Having depression or anxiety is also linked to increased rates of heart disease in women.

Research over the last 10 years has consistently found that heart disease occurs more frequently in less educated women in lower socioeconomic groups than in better educated women in higher socioeconomic groups. The reasons for this are probably related to a number of factors including poorer health care, lack of health insurance, gender discrimination, and increased stress.

Drugs

A number of different drugs can also play an important role in preventing heart disease.

Aspirin has received a lot of attention since several studies found that, in small daily doses, it helps prevent heart attacks. Unfortunately, the tests that turned up these results were done only on men, and it is not known whether the findings are applicable to women. Preliminary studies of women's use of aspirin seems to suggest that a similar protective factor may be found. Aspirin is thought to lower heart attack risk because of its blood-thinning effects. But more research is needed before aspirin's benefits for women are fully defined.

Since some women should not take aspirin because of other medical conditions (for example, clotting disorders), and because dosing is different for preventive therapy than it is for headaches or other common uses, you should consult your physician before taking aspirin to prevent heart disease.

Hormone replacement therapy has become one of the most controversial areas of women's health. When you pass through menopause, your body produces ever decreasing amounts of estrogen. And since it is after menopause that heart disease rates in women rise towards those in men, natural estrogen depletion is thought to be a major factor. (Although not the only one: Some scientists are testing the hypothesis that iron loss during menstruation also helps protect against heart disease.)

Many studies have found that women on estrogen replacement therapy during and after menopause have a lower risk of heart disease. However, the subject is still controversial because replacing estrogen also increases the risk of other diseases, particularly endometrial cancer and possibly breast cancer. The therapy has evolved over the years, and most women on hormone replacement therapy now receive a combination of estrogen and progestin, a hormone that prevents endometrial cancer. However, not much is known about whether the addition of progestin decreases estrogen's heart benefits, and a number of studies are only now underway to test that effect.

The drugs used for hormone replacement therapy are the same as those in oral contraceptives, except at much lower doses; and combining oral contraceptives and cigarette smoking compounds the risk of heart disease. It's not known whether smoking has the same effect during hormone replacement therapy. This is another area that needs further investigation. For more on the hormone replacement controversy, see chapter 31, "Hormone Replacement Therapy: Weighing the Pros and Cons."

High blood pressure medications are available in great variety if diet and behavior changes are not effective. There are five major types:

- Diuretics, which reduce the amount of salt and fluid in the bloodstream, in turn reducing blood pressure.
- Beta blockers, which reduce the force and speed of the heart's pumping action.
- ACE inhibitors, which reduce the level of angiotensin, a chemical that the body produces to raise blood pressure.
- Calcium channel blockers, which relax the arteries and reduce resistance to bloodflow.
- Vasodilators and alpha adrenergic blocking agents, which also relax the arteries.

Cholesterol lowering drugs work in several ways: They prevent the body from producing cholesterol, reduce the absorption of the cholesterol that you consume, or combine with cholesterol to remove it from the bloodstream. Some of the drugs that are used include niacin, lovastatin (Mevacor), cholestryamine (Questran), gemfibrozil (Lopid), and probucol (Lorelco).

Vitamin E, in early studies of women, has shown promising effects on the heart. Taken for a sustained period of time at high enough levels, it seems to lower the risk of heart disease. However, researchers are unwilling to make a firm recommendation until additional evidence is in.

How To Diagnose The Disease

A lot of attention is given to many of the "miracle" drugs offered by modern science. Equally impressive are some of the diagnostic tools that have been developed to detect heart disease, so that it can be appropriately treated and controlled.

Diagnostic procedures range from non–invasive tests done outside the body to invasive probes into the circulatory system. Often, positive findings on non– invasive tests like the electrocardiogram or treadmill test signal the need for more invasive procedures.

Electrocardiogram

The electrocardiogram (known popularly as the ECG or EKG) is a graphic representation of the electrical currents that run through the heart as it pumps. The ECG can be taken while you are resting or exercising (usually on a treadmill), and the only discomfort you might experience is several small electrodes attached to your skin.

Normal ECG readings in women during exercise are likely to mean that no heart disease is present; and—compared with men—abnormal readings are much more likely to be false positives; that is, not truly a sign of heart disease. One study found false positives in only 8 percent of the men tested and a whopping 67 percent of women undergoing the same test. In other words, even if stress testing is positive, there's still an excellent chance that your heart is healthy. Some doctors skip the stress test altogether, especially in a patient with clear physical symptoms (such as repeated incidents of angina), and move directly to more specific testing.

Radionuclide Studies

These studies follow radioactive substances that have been injected into the bloodstream. One common example, exercise thallium scintigraphy, uses computer imaging to track an injection of radioactive thallium through the bloodstream and assess bloodflow to the heart during exercise. This test also turns up many false positives in women because breast tissue can create a shadow that looks like a blockage. Another form of radionuclide testing is used for women who are unable to exercise strenuously enough for exercise

testing. The drugs used in these tests, dipyridamole (Persantine IV) or adenosine (Adenocard), mimic the effects of exercising.

Echocardiogram

Echocardiography is a diagnostic method that measures ultrasound waves. The waves are transmitted into the body, and the echoes that come back from the heart's surface are transformed into a video picture showing the size, shape, and movement of the heart. Like radionuclide studies, echocardiography can be combined with exercise or drug–induced stress to study the heart and blood flow under stress conditions. Dobutamine (Dobutrex) can be administered during echocardiography to simulate the effects of exercise on the heart. Doctors frequently use echocardiography to confirm a suspicion of mitral valve prolapse and other valvular disorders.

Angiogram

Angiography is a way of seeing the interior of the heart and blood vessels. In a procedure more invasive than electro– or echocardiography, a catheter (a long, flexible tube) is inserted into a large blood vessel, usually the femoral artery in the upper thigh, and threaded up to the heart in a procedure called cardiac catheterization. Contrasting die is injected through the catheter, allowing x–rays of the heart and blood vessels that can show the degree of blockage.

The angiogram is probably the most definitive tool for diagnosing heart disease, but because it carries a small risk of injury or death, it is not routinely prescribed. One of the controversies about women's health care focuses on the angiogram, which is ordered much less frequently for women than for men. One study found that 10 times as many men as women (40 percent, compared to 4 percent) were referred for an angiogram after a positive ECG stress test. This is partly because of the known high number of false positives in women's stress ECGs, but it may also reflect a pervasive pattern of less aggressive treatment of heart disease in women. Many physicians treating women with heart disease believe that this pattern is changing as the medical profession and women themselves become more aware of the true risk of serious heart disease.

Treatment Options Today

As with most other diseases, there is a broad range of treatments available for heart disease, proceeding from the minimum—lifestyle and behavior changes—to the maximum—heart transplant. Lifestyle changes to treat heart disease parallel those to prevent it. A primary difference is that if you already have heart disease, you should consult closely with your doctor as you consider which changes will be most appropriate.

There are, of course, many intermediate steps between simple lifestyle changes and heart transplant. These include a variety of drug therapies; angioplasty, in which arteries are widened with the insertion of a balloon; and several different surgical procedures including valve replacement and bypass operations.

Heart disease is really a variety of diseases that strike different parts of the circulatory system and act in different ways. They are progressive, interrelated conditions, and treatment of one problem early in the continuum—for example, coronary artery disease—can prevent more serious consequences such as heart attack.

Obviously, there is no single treatment. And there are no definitive solutions to the problem of determining which therapies—most of which have been tested primarily on men—will work best for women. But understanding the available options is an important first step in deciding, with your doctor, which treatment is best for you.

Drugs

Drugs have been used to treat heart disease for centuries. There's a wide variety; and they work in a variety of ways. Little is known about whether heart medications affect women differently than men. But so far, indications are that the drug's effects are similar, regardless of gender, although the most effective dosage levels may vary.

Digitalis. Two hundred years ago a British physician discovered that digitalis, an extract from the foxglove plant commonly grown in English gardens, strengthens the contraction of the heart muscle. This drug is still used to treat congestive heart failure, and is also useful in correcting irregular heartbeats.

Nitroglycerin. Nearly a century later, a Scottish medical student theorized that amyl nitrite, known to relax the capillaries, could relieve the pain of angina by increasing blood flow to the heart. A form of that drug, nitroglycerin, is still widely used for this purpose.

Beta blockers, often used to treat high blood pressure, are among the most valuable drugs used to treat the heart. They act to block the activity of the beta-adrenergic system, a highly integrated nerve and hormonal system that affects the heart's rhythm and strength of contractions, among other things. Propranolol (Inderal), the first and most widely used of the beta blockers, has been found effective for treating angina, high blood pressure, and migraine headaches.

PUTTING THE PRESSURE ON PLAQUE

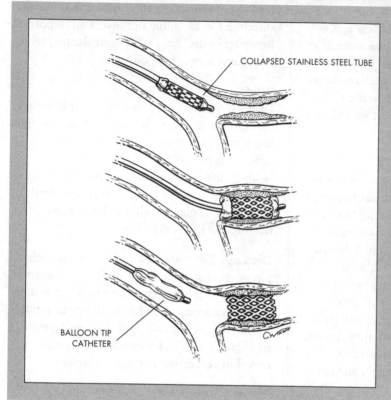

COLLAPSED STAINLESS STEEL TUBE

BALLOON TIP CATHETER

For many people with clogged coronary arteries, angioplasty now provides a less traumatic alternative to traditional bypass surgery. During this newer procedure, a balloon-tipped catheter is threaded up through the circulatory system until it reaches the diseased artery, then inflated to squeeze back the encroaching plaque. Often the balloon is surrounded by a collapsible mesh tube called a stent. When the expanded stent has been lodged firmly against the plaque, the balloon is deflated and withdrawn.

This, and related drugs, are also effective in preventing second heart attacks.

Calcium channel blockers were first approved to treat irregular heartbeat, but were found to have other uses. The flow of calcium across cell membranes in the heart muscle plays a large role in determining how hard the heart contracts: decreasing the flow of calcium across membranes can improve heart function. These drugs—the most widely used is verapamil (Isoptin, Calan)—also relieve the pain of angina by relaxing the coronary arter-

ies and helping the heart beat more easily. Calcium supplementation (either dietary or through pills) is not thought to effect the action of calcium channel blockers.

Thrombolytics, known as clot-busters, are among the wonder drugs of modern heart medications. Drugs such as Tissue-Plasminogen Activator or t–PA (Activase) and streptokinase (Streptase) dissolve blood clots when injected into the bloodstream. If administered shortly after a heart attack, they can clear the obstruction before heart tissue is deprived of oxygen and dies. Speed is critical for the effectiveness of these drugs. New federal guidelines recommend that most heart attack patients be given a thrombolytic within 30 minutes of arrival at the emergency room.

Some of the limited existing data about women and thrombolytics indicate that women are not as likely as men to get these drugs in the emergency room, and when they do, the drugs do not work as effectively. No one doubts, however, that these are important drugs to use in treating both women and men.

Angioplasty

This procedure involves attaching a tiny balloon to the tip of a catheter, threading it up through an artery until it reaches a developing blockage, then inflating the balloon to push the blockage aside and enlarge the artery opening, or lumen. The technical name for this procedure is percutaneous transluminal coronary angioplasty or PTCA. It has a high success rate, although blockage returns in many patients in about 3 months. A refinement of angioplasty is a procedure using a collapsible stent, a stainless steel tube that is inserted and opened by inflating the balloon, then left in place as a more permanent vessel opener when the balloon is removed. Valvuloplasty, a procedure similar to angioplasty, uses the balloon to open an obstructed portion of a heart valve.

Women undergoing angioplasty have lower success rates and higher complication rates than men. This may be because women are usually sicker and older when the procedure is performed, and because the generally smaller surface area of the interior of their blood vessels makes the treatment more delicate. Technological advances in designing equipment specific to the needs of women may help to eliminate these disparities.

Surgery

Women are referred for heart surgery less frequently than men and they have poorer outcomes, including a higher incidence of death. Still, surgery can be very effective, although even when successful, it is seldom the final "cure," and many heart patients continue to require some kind of daily medication thereafter.

Coronary artery bypass graft (CABG), known popularly as simply bypass surgery, is the most common form of heart surgery. In bypass surgery, a clogged portion of a coronary artery is replaced with a short piece of a blood vessel that has been removed from another part of the patient's body.

Women are probably referred less than men because their outcomes are not as good. This could be a blessing: Many think that CABG is prescribed for men more often than it should be. Women are sicker and older when they are referred for bypass surgery, which may help explain the poorer outcomes. Once a woman leaves the hospital following this surgery, however, her long term survival rate is equal to a man's.

Valve replacement surgery is used when medications are not effective in correcting the problems of damaged or congenitally malformed heart valves. The natural valve is replaced with an artificial one made of light metal or plastic, or with a specially prepared valve taken from an animal, most often a pig. Little is known about the different outcomes in men and women who receive these replacements.

Electrical Devices. Some people have an irregular heartbeat that cannot be corrected with medications. If the heartbeat is too slow, a surgically implanted pacemaker can be an

HOW BYPASS SURGERY GETS ITS NAME

When a blockage occurs in one or more of the coronary arteries supplying the heart muscle with blood, the most effective solution is often to establish a new route around the barrier—to literally bypass the site of the problem. To do this, surgeons generally snip out a small portion of the saphenous vein in the leg and graft it to the diseased coronary artery on either side of the blockage. Short of an open heart procedure or a transplant, this operation is about as major as surgery gets.

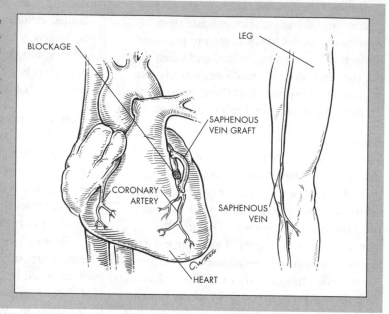

effective device to increase the heartbeat, and many people live for years with one of these devices in place. Often medications are still required after insertion of a pacemaker. Another device, the implantable cardioverter–defibrillator, automatically detects the rapid or uncontrolled beats of ventricular tachycardia or fibrillation when they occur and within seconds generates an electrical shock to correct the problem.

A heart transplant is the most dramatic of all treatments. The procedure is used most frequently in patients with severe cardiomyopathy (heart muscle disease). Heart transplants are very rare, since they depend on the advanced technological resources of a sophisticated medical center and the availability of a compatible donor heart. However, with advances in anti-rejection drugs, the operation is recognized as an option that can

prolong life by years in appropriately selected patients. Because it is still so rare, little data is available about the differences between men and women who have received heart transplants

Cardiopulmonary Resuscitation

CPR is an emergency intervention for someone suffering cardiac arrest. Designed to keep oxygenated blood flowing to the heart and brain until the heartbeat resumes or life support is started, it is a combination of chest compression and mouth-to-mouth breathing. Only people properly trained in CPR should attempt to administer it.

Other Dangers

As is the case with many illnesses, heart disease in women can be complicated by other factors. The two most important are diabetes and pregnancy.

Diabetes

Diabetes most commonly occurs after the age of 45. Depending on severity, it is treated with oral medications that lower blood sugar levels or with regular injections of insulin. More women than men have diabetes, but this may simply be because there are more women than men in the older age groups.

Ischemic heart disease is the most common cause of death in diabetics, even though diabetes itself is listed as one of the top-ten causes of death in this country. At any given age, a woman with diabetes has more than twice the risk of having a heart attack than a woman without diabetes. The increased risk of heart disease in diabetics is also greater in women than in men. Diabetics are also more likely to be overweight, have high cholesterol, and suffer from hypertension, all of which are also risk factors for heart disease.

Pregnancy

Because coronary artery disease usually strikes later in life, it is rarely a complication during pregnancy. However, a number of heart problems, such as congenital defects and valvular disease, do occur in women of childbearing age. Most of these diseases can be well-managed in pregnancy and present little danger to mother or baby. There is even a report of a woman who had a baby four years after having had a heart transplant.

Some symptoms of pregnancy are very similar to symptoms of heart disease; for example, fatigue, shortness of breath, swelling in the arms and legs, and sometimes palpitations. If you are pregnant, and concerned about such symptoms, discuss them with your doctor; usually there is little cause for alarm. Similarly, heart murmurs are commonly heard during pregnancy, but usually just indicate increased blood flow across the aortic and pulmonary valves, rather than a valve abnormality. Your blood pressure should be monitored regularly during pregnancy, because it often rises.

Most diagnostic techniques for heart disease can be used during pregnancy, but those requiring radioactive substances should normally be avoided because of possible harm to the developing baby. (Radioactive substances are sometimes used during pregnancy when the need for diagnosis in the mother outweighs the risk to the baby.) Echocardiography is not harmful to the child, and is used for diagnosis in a pregnant heart patient whenever needed. □

CHAPTER 13

The Growing Danger of AIDS

Sarah Lyons couldn't imagine what her problem was. She would awaken in the middle of the night drenched with sweat. Her glands were constantly swollen and tender. She couldn't shake a low-grade fever. Debilitating fatigue had become an overwhelming fact of her life. She knew she must have a serious medical problem, but she couldn't figure out what it was—and neither could her doctors.

It was 1986, and AIDS had become a widely publicized disease known to strike homosexual men and injection drug users. The word most often used to describe AIDS was "deadly," because there was no cure or effective treatment, and patients often died within months of diagnosis.

But AIDS wasn't something that women like Sarah Lyons (not her real name) worried about. A white, middle-class, 33-year-old telephone company worker from the suburbs of Baltimore, Sarah never thought of AIDS as she trekked from one doctor to another seeking a diagnosis for her puzzling combination of symptoms. Months of consultations,

biopsies, and spinal taps failed to provide an answer, as doctors tested her for a variety of diseases and conditions, but never even speculated that she might have AIDS.

Finally, even though she had never injected drugs, even though she was in a sexual relationship that she thought was mutually monogamous, Sarah was tested for HIV, the human immunodeficiency virus that causes AIDS. Her test was positive—she was indeed infected with HIV. Her diagnosis was ARC, or AIDS-related-complex, the name then used for the set of symptoms that is caused by HIV but is not yet fully developed or "full-blown" AIDS.

Years later, as Sarah would go on to fight the ravages of full-blown AIDS, women with symptoms like hers would still find themselves groping for a diagnosis. Because as AIDS—acquired immunodeficiency syndrome—moved into its second decade, the health care system in the United States was only beginning to see it as a disease that should concern women.

Some Sobering Statistics

The sad fact is that AIDS in women can no longer be ignored or minimized because so many women are being stricken. Currently, the number of AIDS cases is rising more rapidly among women than any other population group. According to the federal Centers for Disease Control and Prevention (CDC), which tracks cases of infectious diseases in this country, 40,702 cases of AIDS in women had been reported by October 1993, accounting for more than 12 percent of the total number of cases in adults. AIDS was the fourth leading cause of death in women aged 15 to 44, and the second leading cause of death for black and Hispanic women in this age group.

A brief glimpse at statistics over the years shows how dramatically the AIDS epidemic among women has grown in this country. In 1981, when AIDS was called "GRIDS" for gay-related immunodeficiency syndrome, six cases of AIDS were reported in American women. A year later that number was up to 52; within another year it had quadrupled. In 1986, nearly 2,000 women in the United States had been diagnosed with AIDS. By 1989, the number exceeded 10,000. And by 1993, that number had quadrupled again.

And, as with all AIDS statistics, these numbers represent only the tip of the iceberg. When AIDS was first defined, total cases numbered in the dozens and HIV, the virus, had not yet been identified. The syndrome was characterized by deficiencies in patients' immune systems that provided the opportunity for a variety of infections to set in. These infections (discussed below) were called opportunistic infections, and the AIDS diagnosis was based on their presence.

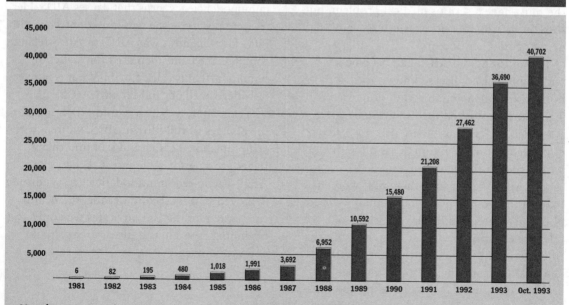

THE SOARING AIDS RATE IN WOMEN

Year by year cumulative totals; source: Centers for Disease Control and Prevention, September 1993

From HIV to AIDS

After the HIV virus was identified in 1984, a more definitive diagnosis became possible. But infection with HIV does not mean you have AIDS, which, in fact, is the final stage of HIV infection. Many less severe and less life-threatening infections often develop before full-blown AIDS sets in. Through the years, the CDC has expanded its definition of AIDS to include more diseases—including some gynecological conditions—but the number of actual AIDS cases remains only a small proportion of those infected with HIV.

The term "ARC," (Aids-related Complex) which was used to describe Sarah Lyons' condition, has largely been replaced by "HIV disease." Another commonly used phrase is simply "HIV/AIDS." Although the epidemic is too young for patterns to be completely predictable, it has become increasingly evident that most, if not all, cases of HIV infection will eventually progress to full-blown AIDS. However, it may take ten years or longer after infection with HIV for any symptoms to appear, and years longer for an AIDS diagnosis to be made.

Clearly, the more than 40,000 cases of AIDS in women in the United States represent only a fraction of the HIV/AIDS problem for women in this country. The CDC estimates that 1 million Americans are infected with HIV, and as many as 12 percent—or 120,000—are female. Moreover, the fastest growing method of transmission is heterosexual contact—the way women are most likely to get the disease.

The Spread of Aids

Although AIDS was viewed for years in the United States as a disease most likely to strike homosexual men and drug users who shared needles, the picture that was emerging world-wide had quite a different look. In Africa, where the incidence of disease also grew rapidly in the early to mid-1980s, women were and still are just as likely as men to be its victims and most cases have been spread through heterosexual contact. Many epidemiologists, scientists who track the spread of disease, have warned that the pattern in Africa is likely to be duplicated in the United States in the years to come.

The international statistics are sobering. A United Nations study conducted in 1993 estimated that 3,000 women around the world become infected *every day*. By the year 2000, some AIDS experts say, more than 40 million people worldwide will be infected with HIV and at least half will be women.

In the United States, AIDS in women is clustered in certain racial groups and geographic areas. About one-quarter of the cases are in white women, with black and Hispanic women accounting for the remaining three-quarters, even though they represent only 19 percent of the population. Cases tend to be concentrated in urban areas in the East Coast, with some studies showing focal points with alarmingly high levels of infection. For example, a survey of women attending public family planning clinics in New York found rates of HIV infection of nearly 1 percent in clinics in the Bronx, and close to that in Queens and Brooklyn.

However, as the stories of Sarah Lyons and hundreds of other women illustrate, dismissing HIV/AIDS as a problem that only affects a certain portion of the population could be a deadly mistake for any woman. The AIDS virus does not discriminate.

What AIDS Looks Like

AIDS was first observed in 1981 by physicians in New York City and San Francisco. A growing number of homosexual men were turning up in medical offices and hospital emergency rooms, with a diverse group of symptoms that could not be explained. The sickest among them often had *Pneumocystis carinii* pneumonia (PCP), a type of pneumonia that is caused by a common organism that most people readily fight off; or Kaposi's sarcoma, a skin cancer that shows up as purplish blotches on the skin, generally strikes elderly men, and is usually quite treatable.

Laboratory testing found that these patients had severely impaired immune systems. Certain white blood cells important in fighting infection, called T-lymphocyte cells or, more specifically, CD4 cells, are usually found in concentrations of about 1,000 per cubic millimeter in a healthy person. In people with AIDS, these counts were often found to be below 200.

Doctors were also seeing a growing number of patients who—like Sarah Lyons—had unexplainable symptoms that were often resistant to treatment. A list was soon developed of warning symptoms of HIV infection. These include:

- Chronic fever
- Extreme fatigue
- Diarrhea
- Unintentional weight loss
- Persistent sweating at night
- Swollen lymph glands
- Fungal infections, including thrush, a yeast infection of the mouth

Doctors also began to see that as HIV infection progressed and the immune system became less and less able to fight off infec-

tions, many more serious diseases were likely to take hold:

- Kaposi's Sarcoma
- *Pneumocystis carinii* pneumonia (PCP)
- Bacterial infections of the blood and lungs
- Other cancers, such as lymphoma
- Severe oral or genital herpes
- Cryptococcal meningitis, a fungus which infects the brain
- Cytomegalovirus (CMV) infection, which often causes blindness
- Tuberculosis
- *Mycobacterium avium-intracellulare* (MAI), a tuberculosis-like organism that causes generalized infection
- Neurological disorders, including progressive mental derangement
- Diarrhea caused by *Cryptosporidium* and other parasites

In 1993, the CDC expanded its definition of AIDS to include anyone with a CD4 cell count below 200 who was infected with HIV, and added several previously unlisted medical conditions to the roster of typical warning signs, including cervical cancer. Many female AIDS activists felt that this listing of cervical cancer was a long overdue recognition that AIDS in women often had a different look than AIDS in men.

What AIDS Looks Like in Women

PCP pneumonia is the single most common AIDS-defining infection in both men and women, and all of the conditions listed above (except Kaposi's sarcoma, which is rarely seen in women) affect women as well as men. But women with HIV/AIDS bear the burden of a range of additional complications. HIV infection can cause unique gynecological problems; it can make existing gynecological problems worse; and it can prevent normal healing.

Because it was years before HIV/AIDS was thought of as a disease that strikes women, specific problems that women experience were not associated with AIDS. For many women, this meant that they were never diagnosed with AIDS, even though they may have died of a condition associated with HIV infection. Now, women with abnormal Pap smears, pelvic inflammatory disease, persistent yeast infections, and genital ulcers have to consider the possibility that HIV is the source of their problems since all of these conditions have been associated with HIV.

Thrush (also called yeast infection) is often the first clue that a woman has HIV infection. Thrush, the commonly used name for a fungus infection caused by the *Candida* organism, is also called candidiasis. It can occur in the mouth or throat, or in the vagina. As T-cell counts decline, thrush becomes more and more likely to develop.

Women with HIV are also particularly susceptible to infection with human papillomavirus. This virus is thought to cause genital warts and has also been associated with cervical cancer and other forms of cervical disease. Women with HIV/AIDS have been found to have ten times the number of abnormal Pap smears (the test for abnormal cervical cells) as non-HIV-infected women.

Because of the high incidence of cervical abnormalities in HIV-infected women, many gynecologists now recommend that these patients have a Pap smear every six months. However, some studies have found that the Pap smear can fail to detect abnormalities.

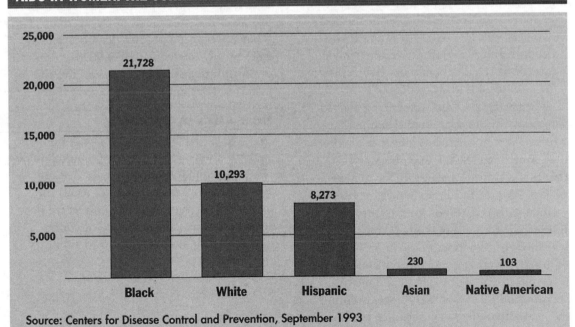

AIDS IN WOMEN: THE CURRENT ETHNIC PROFILE

Black	21,728
White	10,293
Hispanic	8,273
Asian	230
Native American	103

Source: Centers for Disease Control and Prevention, September 1993

HOW AIDS HAS SPREAD TO WOMEN

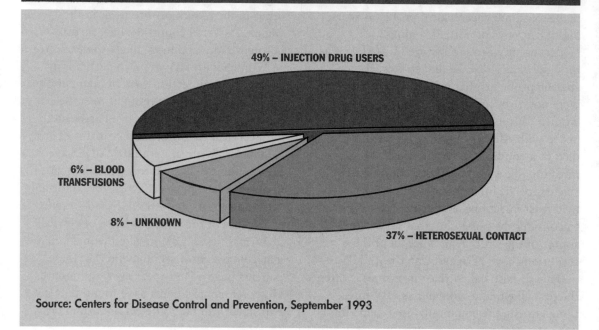

49% – INJECTION DRUG USERS

6% – BLOOD TRANSFUSIONS

8% – UNKNOWN

37% – HETEROSEXUAL CONTACT

Source: Centers for Disease Control and Prevention, September 1993

Colposcopy, a more invasive way of examining the cells of the vagina and cervix, is being used more and more for diagnostic purposes in women with HIV/AIDS. It is an expensive procedure and not routinely recommended. However, it is a diagnostic alternative that you can discuss with your doctor

When AIDS cases in women first started getting attention, some studies found that women were not living as long as men after they were diagnosed. It soon became clear that this was not because the disease was striking women harder than men, or because women were less responsive to treatment. Rather, the reason for shorter survival times was thought to be socio-economic. Women with AIDS were more likely to be poor, with less access than men to social and medical services and thus, less likely to get prompt medical attention. They were also less likely

to get a definitive diagnosis of HIV disease because of the perception of HIV as a male problem. It is now clear, however, that women who get a prompt diagnosis and are aggressively treated for HIV/AIDS and its opportunistic infections can expect to live just as long as men.

How AIDS is Spread

HIV/AIDS is spread through bodily fluids, most frequently blood, male seminal fluid, or female vaginal secretions. For transmission to occur, the infected fluid must enter the uninfected person's body through some kind of cut or opening in the skin or mucous membranes in the body.

The virus can be transmitted at any stage of infection. You need not be symptomatic, or even know you are infected, in order to pass the AIDS virus to someone else. People are most infectious within the first six months to one year following their own infection, and then six to ten years later as their immune system becomes more suppressed.

However, exposure does not necessarily mean infection. Epidemiologists are still trying to determine why some people become infected when they are exposed and others do not, and what other factors may be involved. Studies on the wives of hemophiliac men with AIDS have found some that did not become infected with HIV despite repeated sexual contacts over years. On the other hand, some cases of transmission are documented from just one sexual contact.

The CDC divides the source of existing HIV infection among women into four categories, with the following percentage of cases in each (as of September 1993):

Injection drug users ....49 percent
Heterosexual contact ....37 percent
Blood transfusion recipients ....6 percent
Unknown ....8 percent

Heterosexual contact is the fastest-growing category for both men and women. In 1992 it replaced injection drug use as the most likely mode of transmission to women. And it is quite likely that the numbers for this category are underestimated, because if a woman injects drugs, that is listed as her transmission category, even if she also has a sexual partner who is HIV-infected and may have infected her.

In explaining the transmission of the AIDS virus in women, it is helpful to look at a slightly different classification of categories:

Sexual transmission

HIV/AIDS is primarily a sexually transmitted disease. Like any other sexually transmitted disease, it can be spread through homosexual or heterosexual contact. Because AIDS was first observed in this country in the gay community, it was often perceived as a gay disease, but that is a serious misunderstanding.

Women are more at risk than men to be infected through heterosexual contact because there are still many, many more men than women who are infected. In other words, a woman has a greater chance of selecting an infected sexual partner than a man does.

The easiest way for HIV to be transmitted sexually is through anal intercourse. This is because the delicate tissue in the anus can easily tear during sex. Other reasons for the efficiency of anal transmission include the neutral pH of the anal region, which is an environment that HIV seems to like, and the existence of receptor cells in the anus to which HIV attaches itself.

HIV is also transmitted through vaginal intercourse, and again the risk is greater for women than it is for men. Studies have found that women are more than twice as likely to become infected by men, than men by women. There are several reasons for this. First, there is more virus contained in semen than in vaginal fluid; and second, semen has access to a large surface area, the vagina and cervix; and third, when a man ejaculates into a woman, the seminal fluid remains inside her for hours, giving the virus plenty of time to infect.

The presence of other sexually transmitted diseases also increases the risk of HIV infection. If you have any kind of abrasions or lesions on your vagina, there is an increased chance of infection if you are exposed to the virus. Genital ulcers increase your risk both of being infected and of infecting your partner if you are HIV-positive.

Although theoretically HIV could be transmitted through oral sex, no cases have been confirmed, and most epidemiologists think that it is unlikely.

Another form of sexual transmission is artificial insemination. If a woman is artificially inseminated with HIV-infected sperm, she can become infected. However, most sperm banks now screen for HIV.

Contaminated Blood

A second way that HIV can be spread from one person to another is through contact with blood or blood products that are contaminated with HIV. Most commonly, this occurs when users of illicit drugs share needles. After drugs are injected, the user withdraws the needle, extracting a few drops of his blood into the syringe, and this blood goes directly into the body of the next person to use it. This is an all too efficient method of transmitting bloodborne viruses. It also occurs in health care facilities in some countries where needles and syringes are reused without proper sterilization.

In the initial stages of the AIDS epidemic, hundreds of people were infected when they received contaminated blood in transfusions. Similarly infected were hemophiliacs, who rely on products manufactured from the blood of many donors. Since the discovery of HIV, screening of all blood products has become a routine part of blood collection procedures and there is now only an infinitesimal chance that HIV will be transmitted in this way. However, because AIDS was associ-

ated with blood transfusions, many Americans are confused and think that they can become infected with HIV by donating blood. In this country, blood is taken from donors with sterile needles that have never before been used, and there is no way a blood donor can be infected with HIV while donating blood.

Maternal/fetal Transmission

The third primary means of HIV transmission is maternal/fetal transmission. About 30 percent of pregnant HIV-infected women pass the virus to their babies, either during pregnancy or at the time of birth. The exact mechanism of transmission is not understood. Why as many as 70 percent of babies escape infection is also not clear. HIV is also found in breast milk, and some babies have been infected through nursing. AIDS and pregnancy is discussed in greater detail later in this chapter.

Other Means of Transmission

There is a documented case of a dentist with AIDS transmitting the disease to his patients, although how it occurred has eluded medical detectives. Obviously, it is theoretically possible for it to happen if the dentist has an open cut or sore on his hand that bleeds in the patient's mouth. However, this is extremely unlikely since dentists almost always wear gloves when they work with patients.

This is true for all dental, medical, and surgical procedures. Studies have been done of at least two surgeons who had AIDS, and it was found that *none* of their patients had been infected. In fact, the health care worker is at greater risk of being infected than the patient.

There is also a theoretical possibility that HIV could be transmitted through procedures such as haircuts or manicures, if an infected practitioner is bleeding and a client has an open cut or infected blood from a previous client is passed along on an unsterilized instrument. However, these too are very unlikely ways for the virus to be spread, and no cases have been documented.

How AIDS is not Transmitted

Unlike the common cold and flu viruses, HIV is not airborne and cannot be spread through coughing, sneezing, touching, or any other kind of casual contact. You cannot get it from toilet seats, doorknobs, or mosquito bites. People live in the same household for years with HIV-infected people without becoming infected. HIV-infected children go to school without any threat of spreading the virus to other children. Caretakers routinely change the diapers of HIV-infected babies without becoming infected.

It has become apparent through the years that HIV is a very difficult virus to transmit, unless the conditions are exactly right, as in sexual contact. Unfortunately, because of the deadly nature of AIDS, many rumors and much misinformation have grown around the subject. A properly informed person who takes appropriate precautions has little to fear.

How to Protect Yourself from AIDS

HIV is a virus that is spread through certain actions that can be controlled. However, two activities most often involved in the spread of HIV are drug addiction and sexual activity, both of which can be compulsive and difficult to control. Despite this, progress is being made.

Knowing how AIDS is spread is the first line of defense. An example can be seen in the gay community, where HIV infection rates have gone down as the impact of AIDS has been felt and procedures for safer sex have been widely publicized.

The only sure means of prevention is abstention. This applies to both drugs and sex. If you don't inject drugs, if you don't have sexual intercourse, then you will run no risk of being infected by HIV through these modes of transmission.

Short of that, there are steps you can take to reduce risk. Drug users should never share needles. Some cities have started needle exchange programs so that addicts will, at least, have uncontaminated needles. At the very minimum, a used needle should be sterilized with a bleach mixture to kill the AIDS virus.

With sexual behavior, keep in mind that you are being exposed not only to your partner, but to *every person your partner has ever had sex with*. The only way you can be sure that you are not being exposed to HIV is if you are certain that your partner is HIV-negative (which can be established by testing, as explained in the next section), and equally certain that your partner is currently not having sex with anyone else.

If you are not confident of both of these facts, the best way to protect yourself is to use a condom during every act of sexual intercourse. A latex condom in place throughout all genital and anal contact has been shown to be an effective barrier against the spread of HIV. However, no barrier method is foolproof and the tiniest pinprick in a condom could allow the passage of HIV. (Note that while the condom is also a birth control device, other methods of birth control do *not* prevent the spread of disease. Just because you are taking birth control pills, for example, does not mean that you need not use condoms to protect yourself from HIV.)

Some spermicides, particularly nonoxynyl-9, have been found to kill HIV in laboratory settings, although this effect has not been proven in actual practice. Using a spermicide may provide a second layer of prevention, but it could also have the reverse effect. Some women are sensitive to certain spermicides in which case the spermicide can cause vaginal irritation, thereby easing transmission of the virus.

For women, insisting on the use of condoms for all acts of sexual intercourse may mean employing new means of negotiation with sexual partners and taking control of relationships in a new way. Men may be resistant to using condoms; women may be reluctant to threaten a relationship by introducing the subject. These are issues that every woman must work out for herself, along with her partner.

In late 1993 a new device was marketed in the U.S.—the female condom. It is a latex sheath that is comparable to the male condom, except that it fits into the vagina rather than being slipped over the penis. It has a two flexible rings: one on the closed end that goes up into the vagina to rest against the cervix; the other at the open end that hangs outside the vagina. The female condom is a rather bulky device and market-

ing tests found many aesthetic objections to it, but it does offer protection that a woman can control. As such, it is an important first step in providing women with a protective tool that is under their own initiative.

Remember, too, that drugs play a role in the transmission of HIV apart from needle-sharing. Drugs and alcohol impair judgment and can affect your ability to make responsible decisions in sexual situations.

Getting tested for HIV

Shortly after HIV was discovered in 1984, a laboratory procedure became available to test for the presence of the virus. Today, AIDS testing is widely accessible through state and local health departments, clinics (particularly infectious disease clinics and clinics that specialize in the treatment of sexually transmitted diseases), and some private doctors and laboratories. The test requires only the drawing of a small amount of blood. It is quite reliable and may be free or inexpensive at a public clinic. In some areas it is possible to be tested anonymously under a number or fictitious name. In most settings you can expect to learn the results within a week.

The most widely used test looks not for the virus itself, but for antibodies that the immune system produces when it is infected with the virus. Actually two tests are usually performed. If the first test, called the ELISA (enzyme-linked immunosorbent assay), is positive for the presence of HIV antibodies, a confirmatory test called the Western blot is done.

Most people who are infected with HIV produce antibodies within a couple of months of infection. If you think you have been exposed to the virus and a test performed shortly after this exposure turns out to be negative, you should probably wait another couple of months and be tested again. By six months after exposure, most people will have the antibodies necessary to produce an accurate test result.

Because of the confusion and misinformation that often surround the subject of HIV/AIDS, testing for HIV should always be accompanied by counseling, both before the test is given and when the results are known. It is important to understand what a positive (infected) test result means for you and for your sexual partner(s), and what steps you can take to deal with the problem. Likewise, don't interpret negative (uninfected) test results as permission to continue irresponsible and risky behavior.

For years, AIDS testing was dismissed by many as having little value because there was not much that could be done if you knew you were HIV-positive. Also, many people feared that if it were known they were infected with the AIDS virus, they could lose their health insurance, their jobs, and even their friends and family. It is not hard to see why, for many, it seemed better not to know.

However, that situation is changing as more treatment options become available for HIV/AIDS patients. Preventive therapies are now available for HIV infection itself, as well as for some of the opportunistic infections. There is much you can do to help yourself if you know you are infected with HIV.

Another reason to know your HIV status is to prevent spreading the infection to others. This is important if you are beginning a new sexual relationship, and of particular importance if you are thinking of becoming pregnant.

How is HIV/AIDS Treated?

There is no cure for AIDS. There is no vaccine. These bleak facts are the bottom line for the disease that has become one of the biggest killers of young women in the world.

However, there are a number of treatments that are prolonging lives and improving the quality of life for infected patients. Billions of dollars are spent every year in a search of treatments and vaccines. Research trials are investigating how combinations of drugs work on the disease. Even without an actual cure, many physicians predict that one day HIV/AIDS may be a disease that can be managed with medications, much like diabetes or high blood pressure, and that patients will be able to live long and productive lives.

Most of the testing on AIDS-related drugs has been done on men, and some of these drugs may have different actions when taken by women. New studies are gradually gathering information that is specific to women. Meanwhile, doctors must rely on information gained from existing tests and their own experience and intuition in tailoring dosages and combinations for their female patients.

Treatment falls into two categories: medication that works against the AIDS virus itself, and medication that treats the opportunistic infections, including gynecological problems.

Antiviral Medication

Technically HIV is classified as a retrovirus. Such viruses contain an enzyme called reverse transcriptase, which is what they use to reproduce themselves. There are currently four drugs used to treat HIV infection, and all four work to prevent the action of reverse transcriptase. These drugs are:

- Zidovudine (AZT or Retrovir)
- Didanosine (ddI or Videx)
- Zalcitabine (ddC or Hivid)
- Stavudine (d4T or Zerit)

These compounds have been shown, both in the laboratory and in patients, to slow the progress of HIV infection and to prolong life. However, all are powerful drugs with potentially toxic side effects. AZT may cause anemia, and patients may require blood transfusions to supplement red blood cell levels. Didanosine has been associated with inflammation of the pancreas, and zalcitabine with harm to the nerves, causing, in particular, numbness in the feet. Among other side effects of these drugs are headaches, fever, and nausea.

Also, over time the virus may develop resistance to a particular drug, reducing its effectiveness after prolonged use. Switching from one drug to another is effective for some patients who develop tolerance.

Some studies have found that HIV-infected women using zidovudine have higher rates of liver disease than men taking the drug. Women taking this medication should have periodic checks of liver function.

Fighting off Opportunistic Infections
Since *Pneumocystis carinii* pneumonia (PCP) is the most common opportunistic infection in both male and female AIDS patients, special attention has been given to developing ways to prevent it. Three drugs have been found effective in preventing PCP: trimethoprim-sulfamethoxazole (Bactrim, Septra), which is taken orally; dapsone, also taken orally; and pentamidine (Pentam, NebuPent), which is taken through aerosol inhalation.

With the exception of dapsone, these drugs can be given intravenously to treat PCP after it develops.

Fluconazole (Diflucan), an oral anti-fungal medication, has been used to prevent thrush and cryptococcal infections in patients with very low CD4 counts. Rifabutin (Mycobutin), a new drug, is being used to prevent *Myobacterium avium-intracellulare* infections in these patients.

Treating Gynecological Problems
The gynecological problems of HIV-infected women should be treated promptly and aggressively. Because of the association between HIV and cervical disease, regular Pap smears are imperative, and colposcopy and biopsy are recommended following abnormal Paps. Abnormal growth of cervical cells can be treated with electrocautery or loop diathermy, procedures that burn away affected tissue; cryotherapy, which freezes it; laser vaporization; or cone biopsy, which removes the tissue surgically. Cervical cancer is usually treated with a hysterectomy to remove the entire uterus.

Pelvic inflammatory disease is sometimes resistant to treatment in HIV-infected women. Some gynecologists recommend admitting patients with PID to the hospital, so they can be treated with intravenous (IV) antibiotics. The usual course for a moderately severe case is a week's hospitalization with IV treatment, followed by two weeks on oral antibiotics.

Vaginal thrush, or candidiasis, is probably the most common gynecological problem experienced by women with HIV/AIDS. There are several simple preventive measures that may help ward off these yeast infections. For example, cotton underwear (rather than less absorbent nylon) can cut down on moisture, which promotes the growth of the *Candida* organism. Some doctors advise reducing intake of caffeine, sugar, and alcohol, which are thought to promote yeast infections, although these connections are not well established. Douching is discouraged, since it may wash out natural organisms in the vagina that prevent *Candida* infection. Antibiotics taken for other infections can increase the chances of developing thrush, but eating yogurt can help reduce the risk. Topical anti-thrush medications such as miconazole (Monistat) or clotrimazole (Mycelex-G or Gyne-Lotrimin) are effective, but often a two-week course is advised, instead of the standard seven-day treatment. If the infection is particularly stubborn, treatment with oral anti-fungals may be necessary.

AIDS and Pregnancy

AIDS in babies first brought widespread attention to women with AIDS, and the women were largely regarded not as AIDS patients themselves, but as the means of transmission to their children. Although that emphasis is changing, the fact remains that many women who are infected with HIV are first diagnosed when they are pregnant, or shortly after they give birth.

Still, pregnant HIV-infected women have not been studied systematically. Many questions remain about the effect of pregnancy on the course of the disease in the mother, about the effect of HIV on the developing baby, and about the effect of anti-HIV medications on the baby.

Pregnant women who are diagnosed with HIV need to be told of the chances of transmitting the infection to their babies so that they can make an informed choice about continuing or terminating the pregnancy.

It is also not clear whether HIV infection has a negative impact on the pregnancy. Nearly three-quarters of the babies born to HIV-infected mothers will *not* be infected themselves. However, because babies carry their mothers' antibodies, even non-infected infants will test positive for HIV for a year or longer after birth.

Although a slight decline in immune function has been observed in healthy pregnant women, it is not clear that pregnancy worsens the health of women with HIV/AIDS. Studies have shown mixed results, but a clear pattern of worsening health with pregnancy is not apparent.

Most obstetricians who treat women with HIV/AIDS recommend that these women take the same medications as those who are not pregnant. Indeed, one recent study has shown that AZT can cut the risk of transmitting HIV to the baby by fully two-thirds. Other studies have shown that AZT does not cause fetal malformations, fetal distress, or premature birth. It seems likely that a course of AZT during pregnancy may soon become accepted practice in the presence of HIV.

Whether she takes AZT or not, any HIV-infected woman who is pregnant or planning to become pregnant needs to discuss the situation with her doctor. Some of the drugs used against opportunistic infections are known to harm developing babies. Less is known about the effects of didanosine and zalcitabine; but for the sake of the baby, a woman without symptoms who still has a healthy CD4 count can probably safely delay treatment with these drugs until after the completion of pregnancy.

Because it is thought that infants may become infected with HIV during delivery, some doctors suggest that HIV-infected women deliver by Cesarian section, rather than vaginally, to lessen the chance of infection. Others point out that HIV is more efficiently transmitted through blood than vaginal fluids, so that C-section may actually increase the risk of infection for the baby.

HIV-infected women who are pregnant carry a heavy emotional load. At this time of new beginnings, they are forced to face the fact that they have a fatal disease and may not live to see their babies grow up. On top of this, they are confronted by the possibility of an HIV-infected child, with all the burdens that implies. Women in this situation need support from their loved ones, from other women who have been in a similar situation, and from health care professionals.

Hope for the Future

AIDS, since it was first identified, has posed a variety of not only medical, but also social and political problems. Until recently, the plight of HIV-infected women was totally overlooked. Now, however, the HIV/AIDS treatment community in this country has finally begun to address the problems of women with AIDS. Most large cities now have support groups for such women. More and more drug trials are enrolling women and special studies are being set up specifically for women. Gynecologists and family practitioners are increasingly likely to recognize symptoms of HIV infection in their female patients, and refer them to specialists if they do not feel capable of treating them.

Although AIDS is often viewed with despair, there is good reason for hope. As more and more people learn how to protect themselves from infection, the spread of AIDS can be slowed. And for those who are infected, research continues to show slow but steady progress. As accurate information about the spread of HIV makes its way to the public, every woman can learn that it is within her power to prevent herself from becoming infected with HIV.

In June 1993, the federal government announced the beginning of the Women's Interagency HIV Study, a four-year project that is studying what HIV/AIDS in women looks like, how it progresses, and how it is best treated. Future research will concentrate on how HIV affects the female reproductive systems and will examine more closely the mechanisms of heterosexual and maternal/fetal transmission of HIV.

In little more than a decade, we've learned a tremendous amount about HIV/AIDS. As research and education continue, they can only mean continuing progress in treatment and prevention—progress that can save and prolong lives and give valid reasons for at least some optimism about this devastating disease. □

CHAPTER 14   GENERAL HEALTH CONCERNS

Taking Control of Headache

f you're one of the 50 to 70 million Americans who have recurring headaches, you've probably learned how frustrating the search for effective treatment can be. Recurring headache may be the most common reason for seeking medical care. Headaches account for about 10 million visits to physicians' offices each year—not counting visits to nonphysicians, chiropractors, hypnotists, or other health care providers who offer headache relief. But as common as the condition is, it is still in many respects a mystery. Researchers aren't exactly sure what causes headaches or which people are more susceptible, though they believe a biological predisposition may be responsible and that overuse of pain-relievers and caffeine can make them worse. Likewise, doctors can't always tell what kind of headache an individual has and therefore what kind of medicine would be best.

You've probably heard headaches described in various ways; terms often used include tension headache, muscle contraction headache, stress headache, daily chronic headache, migraine headache, and cluster headache. Specialists also deal with posttraumatic headache and disease-related headache.

Types of Headaches

n 1988, the International Headache Society (IHS) developed the criteria most often used to differentiate these headaches from one another. Physicians from around the world took two years to outline a classification system. It is based on clinical features of the headache, including:

■ Number of attacks per month
■ Length of time per attack
■ Pain characteristics
■ Accompanying symptoms

With such an elaborate system, it seems that diagnosing your headache would be easy. Not so! The reason it's sometimes hard for a health care provider to diagnose the type of headache you have is that different kinds often have similar symptoms. Even the

Headache Society admits that its criteria have substantial diagnostic overlap.

Cluster headache, posttraumatic headache, and disease-related headache are not as confusing as the others, because they have more distinct characteristics. Diagnosis is often more difficult, when it comes to tension headache (which is the same as muscle contraction and stress headache), daily chronic headache, and migraine.

Migraine Headache

In the United States, it is estimated that 17.6 percent of women and 5.7 percent of men have one or more migraine headaches a year, with half of all the 8.7 million women who suffer from mild-to-moderate migraine saying they have more than one migraine each month.

Reports of migraine in the United States have increased dramatically since 1980, when only 25.8 people per 1,000 suffered from them. By 1989, that number had risen to the record level of 41 people per 1,000. Most of this increase was in people less than 45 years old, and the jump was greater among women than men.

The characteristic that usually distinguishes migraine from other types of headache is its unilateral quality. Writings from as early as the second century A.D. point to a syndrome affecting only one side of the head.

Although migraine can set in at any time of life, the most common age range for onset is from 10 to 30 years. After an initial attack, migraine may stay in remission for years to decades.

It is highly likely that there is a genetic factor involved in migraine headache. Ninety

TENSION AND MIGRAINE: ARE THEY THE SAME?

Scientists used to believe that muscle contractions caused tension headache and that constriction and dilation of blood vessels in the head caused migraine. They also thought that they were two separate disorders. New evidence is leading researchers to conclude that headache occurs on a continuum, that is, a continuous progression, with one type leading to the other. Tension headache is on one end and migraine on the other. This continuum means that people who usually suffer from tension headache could sometimes experience migraine-like symptoms, while people who usually suffer from migraine could sometimes experience tension headache type symptoms. Daily chronic headache falls in between the two types. Scientists are still not sure, however, whether the same biological mechanisms cause each of these types of headache.

In the simplest diagnostic model, you have:

- **Tension headache** if the pain is mild and spreads in a band across your head;

- **Common migraine** when the pain becomes more severe and throbbing, usually on one side of your head (unilateral);

- **Classic migraine** when nausea, vomiting or sensitivity to light or sound accompany the severe, throbbing, unilateral pain;

- **Daily chronic headache** when you have some aspects of both tension and migraine headaches.

percent of migraine sufferers can identify a parent, aunt or uncle, or grandparent with migraine. Family members also commonly suffer from other types of headaches.

Migraine can be classified as either **classic** or **common**. About 20 percent of migraine sufferers have the classic variety, which is distinguished by an aura – a peculiar sensation preceding the appearance of more definite symptoms. It can range from visual disturbances, to bizarre alterations in consciousness called the "Alice in Wonderland phenomenon," to loss of consciousness altogether.

Visual disturbances, the most common symptom of classic migraine, can include temporary blindness, blurred vision, flashing lights or dots, "floating" images, and glittering zigzag lines. Less common symptoms include alterations in the perception of shapes, colors, sizes, and body image and perhaps alterations in smells and tastes.

Other features of the classic migraine aura include gastrointestinal distress like nausea and vomiting (though people with common migraine can experience this, too). Diarrhea, lack of appetite, abdominal cramping, dizziness, anxiety, depression, mental cloudiness, irritability, and food cravings—especially for sweets and chocolate—can occur.

The pain from both classic and common migraine is usually in the front of the head, in the eye or temple region. It is most often a throbbing pain that lasts for less than a day in two-thirds of people with migraine. Attacks that last three or four days are not uncommon, however.

Migraine can be confused with other diseases. Before a diagnosis can be made, your doctor will consider other possible causes including stroke, low blood sugar, organ malfunction such as kidney disease, aneurysms (ballooned blood vessels), epilepsy, congenital malformations of blood vessels, tumors, excessive pressure in the eyes, excessive amounts of cerebrospinal fluid in the brain, connective tissue disease, and some forms of heart disease.

Tension Headache

Muscle contraction headache, stress headache, ordinary headache, psychomyogenic headache, and idiopathic headache are some of the many other names for tension headache. A mild to moderate squeezing or pressing pain which is steady and nonthrobbing on both sides of the head, back of the neck, and possibly the facial area characterizes a typical attack. It can last from an hour to several hours or more and may occur once or twice a week.

By IHS standards, tension headache can be either an episodic tension headache or a chronic tension headache. The problem is considered episodic if 10 such headaches have occurred any time previously. Sensitivity to light or sound may also be part of this kind of headache. To be labeled chronic the headache must occur more than 15 times a month.

Tension headache can occur at any age. It is often hereditary. Sore and contracted neck, shoulder, and/or back muscles usually accompany it.

Daily Chronic Headache

Symptoms of tension headache can be so vague that it used to be a sort of "diagnostic wastebasket" for all disorders that did not relate to blood vessel abnormalities or that could not clearly fit some other category. Recently, however, researchers have discovered many similarities between tension headache and migraine. Most now believe the two types may be on the same continuum, with tension headache just a mild form of migraine.

Many things known to trigger migraine also trigger tension headache. Both people with migraine and people with tension headache can benefit from biofeedback aimed at relaxing the muscles. Medications that work for one type of headache often work for the other.

These observations have led scientists to categorize a new type of headache called the daily chronic headache—a condition of daily or almost daily discomfort accompanied at various times by migraine-like symptoms.

This combination of tension and migraine headache shares many characteristics with both types. As with migraine, depression and anxiety accompany daily chronic headache, and it occurs intermittently throughout life until it ultimately subsides. The pain, like that of tension headache, is dull and moderate most of the time. Daily chronic headache is also hereditary and can disturb sleep patterns.

As with both migraine and tension headache, people suffering from daily chronic headache often overuse painkillers like aspirin or prescription drugs. The overuse of medication, and of caffeine, is believed to be a major causative factor in daily chronic headache.

Cluster Headache

Unlike migraine, which primarily affects women, cluster headache mainly affects men. Although the exact U.S. incidence isn't known, an estimated 500,000 to 2 million Americans experience cluster headaches.

These excruciatingly painful headaches occur in bursts every year or two, seemingly more often in the spring and autumn than any other time. The cluster period usually lasts between two and three months. The penetrating and mostly nonthrobbing pain is often felt behind the eyes or in the temples. Attacks can last from 45 minutes to 2 hours and tend to occur at night.

Individuals who smoke cigarettes or drink alcohol excessively are more likely to suffer cluster headaches. Many cluster headache sufferers also have peptic ulcers. Women who have cluster headaches may also have a history of migraine.

Posttraumatic Headache

As many as half of all people who suffer a head or neck injury will develop one or more headache patterns after the primary injury has healed. Symptoms are the same as those of migraine or tension headache. Certain areas of the head may also be sensitive to touch.

The condition seems to be unrelated to the amount or severity of damage caused by the primary injury. Symptoms usually develop 24 to 48 hours after the trauma, but can develop later.

Disease-Related Headache

Headache is a universal symptom; over 300 conditions cause it. The disease conditions include:

- Allergies
- Brain tumor
- Connective tissue diseases (temporal arteritis, systemic lupus erythematosus)
- Constipation
- Disorders of the head, neck, ear, nose, throat, and mouth
- Excessive cerebrospinal fluid in the brain
- Exertion
- General or local infection
- Heart valve disease
- Low blood sugar
- Nerve pain
- Pressure on the cartoid artery
- Sleep apnea (lapse in breathing during sleep)
- Stroke and stroke-like conditions (high blood pressure)
- Temporomandibular joint (TMJ) problems (malfunction at the hinge of the jaw)

THE TRADITIONAL CULPRITS

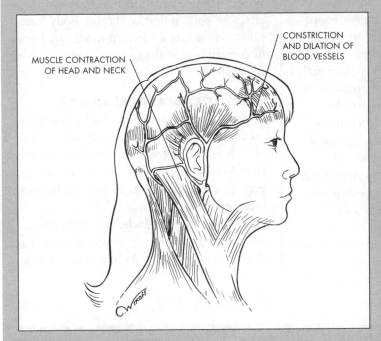

MUSCLE CONTRACTION OF HEAD AND NECK

CONSTRICTION AND DILATION OF BLOOD VESSELS

Muscle tension and constricted blood vessels have long been assigned the blame for headaches. For tension headaches, contraction in the muscles around the skull was considered the culprit. For migraine, constriction of blood vessels in the head—both within the skull and on the scalp—was assumed to be the trigger. Lately, however, this distinction has blurred; and additional suspects have come under investigation (see "A New Theory Implicates the Trigeminal Nerve" nearby).

What Causes Headaches?

Scientists have yet to completely unravel the cause or causes of headaches. It was once believed that constriction and dilation of blood vessels caused migraine headache, while muscle contraction caused tension headache. The constriction of vessels in the head was thought to cause the aura of migraine, as well as the nausea and vomiting. The subsequent relaxing, or dilation, of the vessels then brought on the pounding pain associated with migraine.

These changes are still thought to play a big role in head pain, but a much more complicated explanation is beginning to emerge from recent scientific findings. Many experts now speculate that migraine and tension headache have the same origin in the brain.

The Body's "Anti-pain" System

The brain stem—the structures of the brain located behind the eyes and nose—contains an "anti-pain" system. When this area recognizes an incoming nerve signal as painful, it responds with a powerful pain-relieving effect.

The pain of headache is thought to begin with the trigeminal nerve, which is located in the brain stem. The largest in the head, this nerve carries sensory impulses to and from the face. When stimulated, perhaps by a certain headache trigger, it releases a burst of neurotransmitters (chemicals that pass impulses from one nerve to the next). This, in turn, normally prompts release of yet another neurotransmitter called serotonin.

Serotonin acts as a filter, screening out unimportant signals—for example, weak, repetitive, or familiar background noise like music and other people's conversations—while admiting signals that demand attention, such as unusual or significant sounds like a baby's cry or your name being called. The more serotonin, the greater the screening action. High serotonin levels correlate with sleep.

Under ordinary circumstances, pain signals from the trigeminal nerve are counteracted by increased serotonin levels. But in people suffering a headache, serotonin levels often prove too low. Scientific tests have shown a clear relationship. When injected with a drug that depletes serotonin, test subjects got headaches. Likewise, when they were injected with serotonin, the headache went away.

Significantly, lack of serotonin has also been implicated in depression and sleep disorders, two problems that afflict many headache sufferers. The role of serotonin is not, by itself, a full explanation of headache. But as researchers continue to unlock the secrets of our neurotransmmitters and their effect on pain, mood, and other body functions, we can look forward to an ever better understanding of the causes—and cures—of headache.

What Triggers Headaches?

Almost everyone has had a headache some time in life. If you get them on a regular basis, you may be predisposed to headaches because of your genetics, your perception of life stress, or your body's own metabolism.

If you've had headaches for some time, you're probably already aware of some things that can trigger them. Although everyone's

A NEW THEORY IMPLICATES THE TRIGEMINAL NERVE

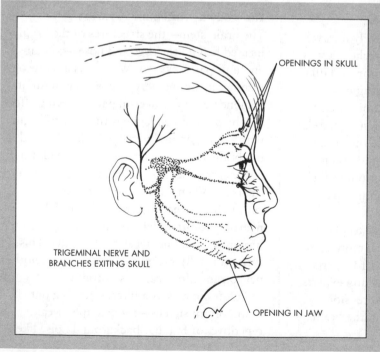

OPENINGS IN SKULL

TRIGEMINAL NERVE AND BRANCHES EXITING SKULL

OPENING IN JAW

Originating in the brain stem deep inside the head, the trigeminal nerve fans out to almost all parts of the face and skull. Ordinarily, sensitizing chemicals released by this nerve are damped down by a compensatory increase in serotonin, one of the nervous system's natural "tranquilizers." But in headache sufferers, this built-in protection appears to break down. When serotonin levels periodically decline, a headache flares up.

situation is different, there are several factors that are almost universal when it comes to bringing on a headache. In a recent study, 199 chronic headache sufferers filled out a questionnaire about the conditions that they experienced just before a headache. The results show us that the most frequently cited precipitating factors were, in order of frequency:

- Anxiety
- Glare
- Noise
- Anger

The least common factors cited were: sneezing, relaxation, pollen and sexual activity.

The best way for you to control your headaches is to determine what triggers them. Here are some other factors known to trigger headaches:

- Emotions
- Diet
- Medications
- Hormones
- Eating and sleeping patterns
- Environmental factors
- Physical exertion

Emotions

There is a link between headaches and emotional distress. Emotions can bring on headaches, keep them going, and make them worse.

Emotions don't cause your headaches; rather, they just make you more vulnerable to them. When the mind influences the body, the result is called a *psychosomatic* condition. You may have heard this term used negatively to describe people who believe they have illnesses that they really don't. This is an incorrect use of the word. Psychosomatic simply means that the state of the mind (the *psyche*) can influence the biological mechanisms of the body (the *soma*). In this sense,

SINUSES AS SCAPEGOATS

Many people who suffer from headaches erroneously blame it on their sinuses. It is estimated that as many as 95 percent of people who believe they suffer from "sinus headache" really have no problem with their sinuses at all.

Migraine and cluster headache can cause the same symptoms as sinus infection, notably pain around the eye, forehead or temple; sense of nasal stuffiness; and even nasal drainage. Adding to the confusion is the fact that many decongestant-containing sinus medications can relieve all kinds of headaches

To find out if your headaches are caused by your sinuses, get a checkup from a physician.

several other medical conditions, including peptic ulcer disease, asthma, and some irregularities of heart rhythm are psychosomatic.

Using the Minnesota Multiphasic Personality Inventory (MMPI), a psychological test to determine personality traits, scientists studying headache patients have concluded that they are exceptionally prone to depression, denial, and preoccupation with their symptoms.

Keep in mind, however, that these researchers aren't sure whether these tendencies are a cause of headache or a result. In either case it's possible that people prone to headaches may perceive stress as more overwhelming than those who don't get headaches.

It's interesting to note that these scientists found a difference between tension headache sufferers and those with migraine. Study participants who had migraine scored higher in the section of the test devoted to depression, while those with tension headache scored higher in those sections on symptom preoccupation, anxiety, and denial. This led to the conclusion that people with tension headaches might be more emotionally vulnerable than migraine sufferers. The researchers speculate that the greater impact of emotions in this group could be due to the higher *density* (the severity times the frequency of pain) of tension headaches.

Another recent study of emotions and headaches found that depression was strongly related to *disability*, defined as an individual's feelings of disruption in his or her daily life. This study of 139 patients also found that expressed anger did not produce perceived disability, but unexpressed anger did. The researchers suspect that unexpressed anger may amplify the feeling of depression among chronic headache sufferers.

Diet

One-quarter of headache sufferers say that certain foods trigger their head pain. Many foods contain substances that can provoke the release of the neurotransmitters implicated in causing headaches.

Tyramine. Foods containing this substance can trigger headaches. A member of the amines group of organic chemical compounds, tyramine may influence the release of the neurotransmitter serotonin. Common foods that contain tyramine include:

- Chocolate
- Aged cheese
- Vinegar (relish, salad dressings, sauces, catsup)
- Organ meats (kidney, liver)
- Alcohol (especially red wine)
- Sour cream
- Soy Sauce
- Yogurt
- Yeast extracts

Nitrites. Foods containing nitrites as preservatives can also trigger headaches. It is estimated that 12 billion pounds of nitrite are currently used in the United States to give meats a pink color and a cured taste. Foods containing nitrites include:

- Smoked fish
- Bologna
- Pepperoni
- Bacon
- Frankfurters
- Corned beef
- Pastrami
- Canned ham
- Sausages

Monosodium Glutamate. This food additive, frequently called (MSG), may also cause headache pain. A flavor enhancer, it is sold under the trade name Accent, among others. It is also called hydrolyzed vegetable protein (HVP), hydrolyzed plant protein (HPP), "natural flavor" or "flavoring," and kombu extract. An estimated 20,000 tons are used yearly to add flavoring to foods such as:

- Dry roasted nuts
- Potato chips
- Chinese food
- Processed or frozen food
- Soups and sauces
- Diet foods
- Salad dressings and mayonnaise

Alcohol. Alcoholic beverages, like beer, wine, champagne, and liqueurs, can cause headaches through their property of expanding blood vessels, through the tyramine that some contain, or through dehydration, which produces the infamous hangover headache. Red wine and brandy are two drinks most likely to trigger a headache

The least likely alcoholic beverages to cause a problem are blended whiskey such as scotch, vodka, and sauterne or Riesling wines.

Vitamins. High doses of vitamins can trigger headaches. Vitamins sometimes responsible for head pain include vitamin A in high doses and B vitamins (especially niacin).

Water. Simple lack of water—dehydration — is a major cause of headache, particularly migraine. Alcohol, air travel, and summer sports activities can all lead to dehydration, in turn triggering a headache. Illnesses with fever or diarrhea are other leading offenders.

Caffeine. This pervasive substance can be a friend or a foe. It is used as an ingredient in most pain relievers because it enhances intestinal absorption of the drug. But caffeine can also trigger headaches in sensitive people and in those who take too much.

You can get headaches from too much caffeine and from caffeine withdrawal. Withdrawal starts from 8 to 16 hours after the last ingestion, which explains why many people get a headache toward the end of their workday, or when they wake up in the morning.

Caffeine is a stimulant that affects the heart, lungs, blood vessels, muscles, stomach, kidneys, and overall metabolism. It can cause jitteriness, anxiety, agitation, gastrointestinal distress, sleep disturbances, and depression. Caffeine headaches are characterized by fatigue, grogginess, clouded thinking, and often throbbing pain.

Drinking 8 to 10 cups of brewed coffee (1 gram of caffeine) in a row would begin to endanger your health. You could actually die if you ingested 10 grams or more.

Other foods. A number of other items are sometimes implicated in headaches. They include: citrus fruits, dairy products, soybeans, wheat products, onions, fatty foods, seafood, and artificial sweeteners (aspartame or NutraSweet).

Medications

Some medicines used to treat illnesses may actually trigger headaches. If you are taking any of the following medications, talk with your doctor about possibly switching to another non-headache-provoking drug. **Don't, however, stop taking any of these medicines on your own!**

- Nitroglycerin (for heart disease)
- Medication for high blood pressure
- Medication used to dilate blood vessels
- Medication used to treat ulcers
- Antiseizure drugs

Oral contraceptives (the Pill) may or may not cause headaches, and may or may not make existing headaches worse, depending on the individual. Because most women who take the Pill are in the age range for headache onset, the Pill might be "guilty by association." On the other hand, headaches could be triggered by the Pill formulation itself or the varying levels of estrogen delivered by tripha-

CAFFEINE— HOW MUCH ARE YOU GETTING?

Here are a few food sources and the approximate amount of caffeine they contain:

Food	Caffeine (milligrams)
1 cup of brewed coffee	100-150
1 cup of instant coffee	85-100
1 cup of tea	60-75
1 cup of decaffeinated coffee	2-4
1 cup of cocoa	40-55
1 glass cola (8 oz.)	40-60
1 chocolate bar	25

sic oral contraceptives (those supplying different doses of hormones each week).

Studies of the Pill and headaches have shown mixed results. Some show relative increases in the frequency of headaches among Pill users while other studies show no difference. In one study, women who were told they were receiving the Pill reported high headache frequency, even though they were receiving a placebo (a dummy pill).

The Rebound Headache. Many people who suffer from headache tend to abuse either over-the-counter (OTC) or prescription drugs that can stop or control their pain. Overuse of these drugs can actually perpetuate and worsen headaches, leading to what is considered an analgesic-rebound headache. Overused OTC pain relievers (analgesics) include aspirin and acetaminophen (Tylenol, Panadol). The prescription headache drug ergotamine (Cafergot) is also often overused.

The first study to identify this problem was carried out in 1982. People who had daily chronic headache were divided into two groups. One received the antidepressant drug amitriptyline (Elavil), while the other group did not. Half of each group was allowed to use pain relievers. The group of patients taking both amitriptyline and a pain reliever showed an overall improvement of 30 percent over four weeks, but the patients taking only amitriptyline showed an overall improvement of 70 percent. Those patients taking only pain relievers improved by 18 percent and those patients taking nothing at all improved by 43 percent.

This study not only proved that eliminating pain relievers could help headache patients recover, but also showed that pain

HEADACHES AND HORMONES: WHAT'S THE CONNECTION?

There is strong evidence of a relationship between headache and hormones.

First, women get migraine much more often than men do, but it's only after puberty, when women begin to produce higher levels of female hormones, that gender makes a significant difference.

Second, 60 percent of women with migraine report that their headaches happen more often right before, during, and after menstruation, when hormone levels change. This type of headache is known as menstrual migraine.

Third, headaches tend to improve during the second and third trimester of pregnancy.

Fourth, recurring headaches may stop for menopausal women, or they may get worse.

The female hormones estrogen and progesterone can affect the amount of serotonin available in the body. Additionally, estrogen increases prostaglandins, which cause menstrual cramps. Both estrogen and prostaglandins are active in the body's anti-pain system.

relievers could actually block the effectiveness of other headache medications. Confirming the results, another researcher found that 77 percent of chronic headache patients who were hospitalized and taken off pain relievers either became headache-free or had far fewer headaches. Still another researcher was able to show that 80 percent of hospitalized patients stopped getting headaches within 2 weeks of giving up pain relievers.

Eating and Sleeping Patterns

Fasting or missing meals is a major headache trigger. Researchers found that for the majority of more than 2,000 women who experienced a migraine, the lack of food for 5 hours during the day or 13 hours overnight was a primary factor in triggering their headaches.

No one completely understands why this is so. Presumably, fasting can affect the level of neurotransmitters; and low blood sugar from lack of food can cause blood vessels to dilate, leading to headache.

Nighttime sleep and naps during the day also may play a role in the headache process. Too much sleep or too little sleep can trigger headaches in the headache prone.

Environmental Factors

What you do for a living and where you spend your time can also lead to headaches. You might have already had experience with this type of environmental trigger if you work in a place where you inhale fumes or toxins. Some environmental substances that can lead to headaches include: turpentine, carbon tetrachloride, benzine, formaldehyde, heavy metals (especially lead), and carbon monoxide.

Other workplace conditions to consider are bright lights, glare, noise, and eyestrain.

Vision-Related Headaches. Although headaches related to eye disorders occur much less frequently than is generally supposed, eyestrain and diseases of the eye can lead to headaches. Straining your eyes through excessive reading or squinting at a computer screen, for example, will fatigue muscles controlling eye movement. You also may suffer vision-related headaches if you habitually work under flickering fluorescent lights.

It's difficult to separate eyestrain headache from tension headache. Sitting in the same position for extended periods of time, while reading or typing on a computer, will cer-

tainly strain neck and shoulder muscles as well as the eyes.

Narrow-angle glaucoma, a rare eye disease, can cause pain around the eye, forehead, or temple region. Its symptoms mimic those of migraine or cluster headache, so if you have either problem it's important to get your eyes checked, both for this condition and for general vision impairment.

Other Factors. Some headache sufferers experience head pain during or after such exertion as playing tennis, jogging, jumping rope, playing handball, and sexual orgasm. Changes in the weather can change body chemistry, and have been known to trigger headaches. Heavy cigarette smoking and motion can also lead to headache.

The Headache Diary

Keeping track of your headaches could be enlightening for both you and for your doctor. It can help pinpoint the cause or causes. Keep a record by starting a headache diary in which you jot down as much information as possible about the things that could possibly have triggered your next six headaches.

In recording information, remember the five W's: Who, What, Where, When, Why. You can add a How to the list, too.

Who: Who were you with before the headache started? Someone who irritated you or made you angry? Someone who hurt your feelings?

What: What medications did you take to treat the headache? What other medications were you taking at the time? What symptoms did you experience?

Where: Where were you right before the headache started? At work under glaring lights or in the presence of loud noises or fumes? At home resting after a stressful day?

When: When did the headache start? When did it stop? When was the first day of your menstrual cycle?

Why: Why would your headache start? Some particular food or drink? (Check the lists above for foods which can cause a headache.) Did you get more sleep than usual or not enough? Did you forget to eat breakfast, lunch, or dinner? Did your headache start after some physical activity?

How: How did the pain feel? Was it throbbing, on one side of the head? Was it bandlike, stretching across the temples? How did you cope? Did you have to miss work or lie down to rest?

With your headache diary, you are on your way to coming to grips with your problem.

Getting Control

Once you have identified the things that trigger your headaches, it's time to change your life-style. Altering your daily routine is one of the best ways to control your head pain.

Most important, don't think of yourself as "stuck" with headaches or as "an emotional basket case." Headaches are a medical condition, just like diabetes or high blood pressure. As with these other conditions, some relatively simple tactics are often enough to keep the problem under control. And, luckily, we know a lot more about headache prevention and treatment than we did in the past.

You can control your headaches in many ways—some easier than others. Here are a few suggestions that have worked for others:

For Emotional Triggers ....

■ Laugh. Laughter is the best medicine for almost any ailment. It makes the arms and legs relax by reducing muscle tension. Laughing also causes beneficial reactions in the brain's anti-pain centers.

■ Get short-term or long-term counseling. A trained professional can teach you how to express anger or how to cope with stress and negative thoughts and feelings.

■ Let your family know what triggers your headaches.

■ Write a letter to someone who has made you angry. You don't have to mail it. Simply venting your feelings could relieve your stress.

■ Relax. That's not as simple as it sounds, but it is a skill you learn by practice. Migraine and tension headaches involve tension in the head and neck muscles, as well as difficulties with blood flow. Relaxation (as well as massage and biofeedback) will decrease muscle tension and increase the dilation of blood vessels, thereby increasing the flow of blood.

■ Investigate biofeedback therapy. Biofeedback is a technique for learning to relax and control emotional triggers such as stress and anger. It often involves placing

RELAXATION AT YOUR FINGERTIPS

You can relax almost anywhere, anytime, using a variety of techniques. Here are a few:

■ Take a full, deep breath; hold it for 5 to 10 seconds. Slowly blow out. Repeat this until you have done it at least 10 times or for as long as you like.

■ Close your eyes and picture a particular muscle group. Tighten that muscle for 5 seconds, then release it. Repeat this procedure until that muscle feels relaxed. Then move on to another muscle group until you have relaxed your whole body.

■ Repeat certain relaxing phrases: for example, "The muscles of my face are letting go." Try to visualize what is happening (that is, picture your facial muscles being so light they almost float away).

electrodes on the skin over specific muscles or slipping a device over the finger to detect changes in body temperature. The goal of this therapy is to teach you how to release tension and increase blood flow on your own without using the machine.

For Dietary Triggers ...

■ Try eliminating from your diet the foods known to trigger headaches.

■ Keep alcohol to a minimum.

■ Try magnesium supplements. Low levels of magnesium can bring on headaches, especially around the time of your menstrual cycle. Low levels are also associated with increased irritability and spasms of the muscles. In a study of 3,000 women, 80 percent seemed to respond positively to magnesium supplements. The recommended dosage is 200 milligrams a day; you need to try it for about two months to see if it helps. Check with your doctor before you begin; if you have a kidney problem you should avoid this supplement. You should be aware, too, that magnesium may cause diarrhea.

For Metabolic Triggers ...

■ Stop overusing substances that cause headaches, like caffeine and certain medications. You can expect mild-to-moderate headache pain while you are weaning yourself off caffeine. If you are "addicted" to aspirin and have what's called a rebound headache syndrome, you may have to live through 2 weeks of daily headaches to rid yourself of this problem. If you are overusing a prescription drug such as Cafergot, taper off slowly. You could harm yourself by suddenly discontinuing a prescription medication.

■ If you are using oral contraceptives, and suspect hormones are triggering your headaches, talk to your gynecologist about changing your formulation. Your pain may decline or disappear if you use monophasic formulations (the same dose of hormones each week of the cycle) rather than triphasic formulations (with doses increasing over each week of the cycle).

■ If you suffer from menstrual migraine, you can reduce the effects of falling estrogen levels during your menstrual cycle by using estrogen supplements. There are several ways to take supplements, one of which is a patch (Estraderm) worn on the arm that releases estrogen into your body.

For Daily Activity Triggers ...

■ Maintain consistency in your eating and sleeping patterns. Try to wake up and go to sleep at about the same time every day, even on weekends and vacations. Avoid long delays between meals.

■ Stop smoking cigarettes, or at least decrease the number of cigarettes you smoke.

■ Exercise regularly. Although exertion may trigger headaches in some people or make them worse once the headache has started, studies have shown that regular aerobic exercise can reduce the severity of future attacks. Exercise is known to stimulate pain-regulating substances in the brain.

■ Do a workplace analysis. Consider the type of lighting you use, the height of your chair, the time you spend working at an angle, placement of windows, darkness of letters on your computer screen, and any other factors that might contribute to your headaches.

■ Take regular breaks from repetitive tasks.

■ Gently stretch and flex your neck muscles regularly during the day to reduce strain on sensitive nerves. A recent study found that people with recurring headaches have a more limited range of neck motion. This reduced range of motion might be the cause of headaches, or might be part of a chronic headache complex.

Getting a Correct Diagnosis

Most headaches are primary, that is, they are not caused by some other ailment. To make the correct headache diagnosis, however your doctor will want to conduct some tests to rule out an underlying illness.

Your doctor will want to talk to you about your health in general and your usual activities. Be sure to mention any past head injury, abuse of medicines, hormonal changes, or exposure to various harmful substances as the cause of your headaches.

This is the time a thorough headache diary will come in handy. Knowing such things as the factors that trigger or relieve your headaches, when they happen most often and what your moods are usually like before a headache can assist the doctor greatly in arriving at the correct diagnosis.

Here are a few other diagnostic tools your physician might use or suggest:

■ Psychological exam: Your doctor may suggest an evaluation by a trained mental health professional to determine if psychological influences are aggravating your problem. This evaluation and any subsequent counseling should only be one component of an overall treatment plan.

■ Office tests: Simple tests to check your ears, nose, throat and jaw might reveal infections that could cause your headaches.

■ Blood tests: Changes in blood chemistry can signal early stages of some disorders, including kidney and liver disease, anemias, thyroid disease, and low blood sugar.

■ X-rays: More advanced technology has generally replaced simple x-rays; the use of x-rays determining the causes of headache is limited. They can, however, detect some conditions, such as sinus infection or excessive fluid around the brain.

■ Electroencephalography (EEG): EEG shows electrical activity of the brain. It can detect some disturbances in brain function, irregularities in rhythm, the presence of seizurelike activity, and the effects of metabolic substances on the nervous system. Experts do not always agree on the usefulness of EEG, but some use it to screen for patients who may need more expensive tests.

■ Computed Axial Tomography (CAT) Scan: This test can detect conditions inside the brain by radiographically showing "slices" of brain structures that reveal most physical causes of headaches. It can detect blood clots, for example, but not aneurysms (ballooning blood vessels). A CAT scan is a more technologically advanced form of x-ray. Most people are injected with a relatively harmless dye so that structures show up better. If you are allergic to shellfish, which contain iodine, you might be allergic to this dye, which also contains a form of iodine.

■ Magnetic Resonance Imaging (MRI): This test is more advanced than a CAT scan. It uses magnetic fields and radio waves instead of x-rays. When someone is placed inside the MRI machine, which is essentially a large (but very sophisticated) magnet, the magnetic field will orient some of the atoms of the brain in a certain direction. Radio waves then detect changes in movement of these atoms, to create a detailed picture of the brain.

Both CAT scans and MRI are somewhat controversial in headache treatment on medical, ethical, and legal grounds. Most people undergoing these tests have normal results. Many insurance companies hesitate to reimburse for these tests, perhaps because they actually diagnose so few headaches.

Treatment Options

Headaches can't be cured, but they can be controlled. There are many medications that can either stop the pain associated with headaches or stop the symptoms, like nausea, that accompany them.

Using medication should be only one part of a wellness program. Life-style changes—such as avoidance of any known headache triggers, personal and family counseling, stress management, and relaxation therapy—should accompany any drug plan your doctor prescribes.

There are two ways to benefit from available medications. You can take them either prophylactically (every day to reduce the severity and frequency of possible attacks), or abortively (once the headache begins).

Prophylactic Treatment

Your doctor probably won't suggest prophylactic treatment unless you have several attacks per month. If you take drugs this way, your physician will monitor you for side effects, such as weight gain, water retention, lethargy, memory impairment, and hallucinations. Do not try to combine any weight loss medications with prophylactic drugs, and do not stop taking the drugs suddenly.

Here are a few principles of prophylactic treatment:

- It should begin with low doses, which are increased slowly.
- Every month or two, it should be tested to see if it is working correctly.
- Your doctor should check that you are not taking any other drugs or vitamins that could interfere with the headache medication.
- You should be sure you are not pregnant.
- Medication should be tapered off and discontinued once your headaches are under control.

Although there is no set schedule for how long someone should stay on prophylactic therapy, many experts consider more than six months excessive.

The major prescription drugs used to treat tension, migraine, and sometimes cluster headaches prophylactically include: *beta blockers* such as Tenormin, Lopressor, and Inderal; *calcium channel blockers* such as Cardizem, Dilacor, and Procardia; *antidepressants* such as Elavil and Zoloft; *serotonin antagonists* such as Sansert; *anticonvulsants* such as Tegretol, Depakote, and Dilantin; and *ergot derivatives* such as Cafergot and Sansert.

Beta blockers slow down your heart rate and lower your blood pressure. They may make you feel tired and gain weight. These drugs may also upset your stomach, make you depressed, cause nightmares or insomnia, or cause you to lose some hair. All these symptoms, however, are reversible after you stop taking the drug.

Calcium channel blockers have relatively few side effects, but these may include the possibility of increasing your headaches, and causing dizziness, gastrointestinal distress, swelling of the ankles, and depression. They can also lower blood pressure and change your pulse rate.

MEDICATIONS DURING PREGNANCY

Medications could possibly affect a developing baby by way of the placenta or a newborn by way of breast milk. If you are pregnant or breastfeeding, here are several things you will want to keep in mind about medication for your headaches.

- The best course of action is to avoid medication altogether. Since headaches usually improve after the first trimester, you might try ice packs, massage, and relaxation therapy until then.

- If you can't stand the pain and need some medication, use acetaminophen (Tylenol, Panadol) instead of aspirin, because it is safer.

- Your doctor can prescribe a medication containing codeine or other narcotics. Barbiturates, ergot alkaloids, and serotonin agonists should not be prescribed.

- To minimize your baby's exposure to a medication, take it right after you complete a breastfeeding.

Antidepressants can worsen conditions like glaucoma. Other potential side effects include dry mouth, sedation, retention of urine, constipation, blurred vision, intense dreaming, weight gain, and lowering of blood pressure. They may also cause nausea, jitteriness, and flulike symptoms. These symptoms will disappear when you stop taking the drug.

Serotonin antagonists can be beneficial for 50 to 60 percent of migraine sufferers; but they are not used often because of the possible side effects, which include temporary muscle aching; abdominal, leg or chest pain; hallucinations; and a sense of swelling in the throat. When used for long periods of time (more than six months), these drugs can cause scar tissue to form in the chest and abdomen.

Anticonvulsants can cause dizziness, drowsiness, rash, and insomnia.

Ergot derivatives can cause nausea, abdominal pain, and leg pain.

Abortive Treatment

The first line of attack against a headache once it is underway is to take over-the-counter pain relievers, such as aspirin, acetaminophen (Tylenol, Panadol, others), or ibuprofen (Motrin, Advil, others). To increase the effects of these drugs, your doctor can prescribe medication that is a combination of an analgesic with one or more other components to relieve anxiety, for example, or decrease nausea.

Acetaminophen relieves pain and reduces fever, while ibuprofen acts primarily to relieve inflammation. Aspirin has all three of these properties. None of these drugs contains steroids.

In addition to aspirin and ibuprofen, there are other anti-inflammatory drugs usually classified as *nonsteroidal anti-inflammatory drugs* (NSAIDs). These are useful in treating headaches, both symptomatically and prophylactically. They are all different, so if one type of NSAID does not work, you can try another. NSAIDs include Naprosyn, Anaprox, Ponstel, Meclomen, Tolectin, and Toradol.

Side effects of NSAIDs include gastrointestinal pain, nausea, constipation, diarrhea, light-headedness, and dizziness. Ironically, they can also cause headaches in some people. Liver abnormalities could result from taking NSAIDs, and people with active ulcer disease should not take them at all.

To treat headaches that are unresponsive to standard pain relievers, physicians often prescribe *ergot alkaloids*. This group includes drugs containing ergotamine and dihydroergotamine (D.H.E.). Ergotamine is useful for both migraine and cluster headaches.

The brand names of ergot derivatives include Cafergot, D.H.E. 45, Ergostat, Sansert, and Wigraine.

Ergotamine should not be used by those who have peripheral vascular disease, liver or kidney problems, coronary artery disease, hypertension or malnutrition. It cannot be used during pregnancy and breastfeeding. Some potential side effects are nausea and vomiting, muscle cramps, stiffness, fatigue, numbness, paralysis of the extremities, and chest discomfort.

Excessive amounts of ergotamine, like analgesics, can actually induce headaches; be careful how much you rely on it.

D.H.E. has fewer side effects than ergotamine and is effective in treating even the most severe migraine. D.H.E. can cause nausea, vomiting, leg cramps, and anxiety, but these side effects are rare and usually mild. For patients with headaches so severe they have to be hospitalized, D.H.E. can be given intravenously.

New Approaches

A new drug—with the brand name Imitrex—is available to fight migraine headache once it has begun. This selective serotonin agonist known generically as sumatriptan, acts just like serotonin in the body. To use it, your doctor will show you how to give yourself a shot, because currently it comes only in injectable form.

Once taken, Imitrex starts to work in 15 to 20 minutes. Forty percent of people using it have a recurrence of their headache about 13 hours after the first dose and need a second shot. The maximum dosage is two shots every 24 hours.

Imitrex helps 70 to 80 percent of the people who have used it. In most people, it relieves not only the head pain, but the aura of migraine (nausea, vomiting and sensitivity to light and sound) as well.

Side effects of this serotoninlike drug can include tingling in the head, flushing, warm or hot sensation, chest tightness and pressure, visual disturbances, and neck and jaw tightness. Additionally, 40 percent of people have skin reactions at the site of injection.

People who have heart disease or uncontrolled high blood pressure cannot take Imitrex. Studies have not been done with pregnant women, so it should be used only if the potential benefit would justify any potential risk to the developing baby.

Imitrex is a relatively expensive drug. In fact, the manufacturer has been offering the first dose free, so that potential users can determine if it actually works for them before they spend any money.

There are many other approaches to headache treatment still on the horizon. For example, to treat cluster headache, some patients are being exposed to bright light for two hours in the evening to stimulate and reset their circadian rhythm (wake/sleep cycles). So far, results are too preliminary to draw any real conclusions about this treatment.

Capsaicin, an extract from hot peppers, also shows some potential as a headache remedy. It stimulates nerve endings and then depletes them of pain-causing chemicals. While there have been positive results when using capsaicin for some other painful conditions, studies now underway with headache are too incomplete to make a reliable judgment. □

CHAPTER 15

A Common Sense Look at Diet and Health

These days when the conversation turns to diet, the question is not so much what we *should* eat as what we *shouldn't*. Deficiency diseases are almost history. Scientists have identified 19 vitamins, minerals, and other nutrients needed for good health; and our foods are laced with supplements to make sure that we get them.

Our problem today is not *too little* but *too much*—too much fat, salt, sugar…too much of whatever the latest study has chosen to attack. We now get so much advice on what foods to avoid that it's tempting to simply throw up your hands and forget the whole thing. Unfortunately, that's not a realistic option.

Some 34 million Americans are now classified as "obese"—that is, 20 percent or more above their ideal weight. And with obesity comes increased risk of heart disease, diabetes, stroke, and some forms of cancer.

Indeed, according to the American Cancer Society, 50 percent of cancers in women and 30 percent in men may be related to diet.

Worse yet, an estimated 67 million Americans, 1 out of 4, now have some form of heart disease, and several of the leading risk factors for heart disease, including high cholesterol, obesity, diabetes, and high blood pressure, can all be aggravated by diet.

Eating a well–balanced healthy diet really can be a life–saver. But deciding what's healthy is no easy task when we're faced with an almost daily onslaught of often controversial, sometimes even contradictory, nutritional information. To help sort through the conflicting claims, here's a quick review of the basic facts we know today.

The Carbohydrate Craze

Carbohydrates, along with proteins and fats, provide the energy we need from our diets. In fact, carbohydrates provide most of the calories your body uses. As an easily available source of energy, carbohydrates are an ideal "fuel for fitness" for both the recreational and professional athlete.

Because carbohydrates yield only 4 calories per gram, they are essential to any weight control program. This idea runs counter to earlier theories about dieting, where the first things to get ousted from the diet were those "fattening" breads, potatoes, and pastas. High–carbohydrate foods are actually low in fat—unless you add fat in cooking or at the table.

Foods high in carbohydrates are a staple of diets both for diabetics and for those who want healthy hearts. High in nutrients, these foods also add fiber to the diet, which helps control both blood sugar and blood choles- terol levels.

Except for the carbohydrate found in milk, almost all carbohydrates come from plants. Unfortunately, when it comes to nutritional value, not all carbohydrates are created equal. There are two types: simple and complex. Although both provide 4 calories per gram, they have distinctly different functions.

Simple Carbohydrates

Structurally, simple carbohydrates consist of 1 or 2 sugar units linked together. This makes them an easy–to–absorb source of energy. Most simple carbohydrates, often referred to as *simple sugars*, have one appeal- ing trait in common—sweetness. Common forms of simple carbohydrates are sucrose (table sugar), glucose (dextrose), fructose (fruit sugar), lactose (milk sugar), and maltose (malt sugar). Other forms of these sugars are honey, corn syrup, maple syrup, and any type of "sugar," such as brown sugar, confectioner's sugar, and beet sugar. Simple sugars provide calories, but few vita- mins and minerals.

Is sugar, with its minimal nutrient contri- bution, really the "health culprit" it is made

THE FAMED "FOOD PYRAMID"

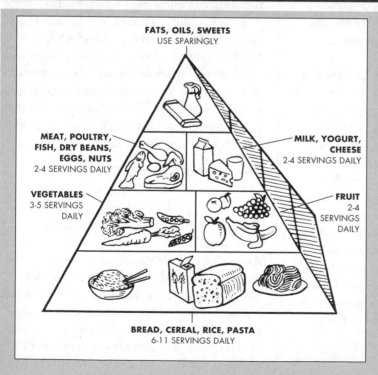

FATS, OILS, SWEETS
USE SPARINGLY

MEAT, POULTRY, FISH, DRY BEANS, EGGS, NUTS
2-4 SERVINGS DAILY

MILK, YOGURT, CHEESE
2-4 SERVINGS DAILY

VEGETABLES
3-5 SERVINGS DAILY

FRUIT
2-4 SERVINGS DAILY

BREAD, CEREAL, RICE, PASTA
6-11 SERVINGS DAILY

This government-developed diagram reflects the latest consensus on healthy diet. Carbohydrates—represented by the broad slab supporting the pyramid—are definitely in. Fat—shown in the little capstone at the peak—is unquestionably out. Not that a little fat is bad, mind you. The problem is that almost all of us get far too much of it. If you make no other change in your diet, you should at least consider cutting out most of the fat.

out to be? Throughout history, sugar has been blamed for everything from obesity and diabetes to hyperactivity in children. Yet the only disorder sugar has ever been firmly linked to is tooth decay.

Although most people believe that "sugar makes you gain weight," evidence favors fat as the main cause of obesity. Many foods thought of as "sweets" are in fact high–fat foods that happen to have sugar in them—for example, ice cream and pastries. Fat, not sugar, contributes most of the calories in these foods. Some weight watchers, however, think that sugar triggers eating binges. If it has this effect on you, you may need to limit sugar for behavioral, rather than nutritional, reasons.

Believe it or not, researchers have not conclusively linked sugar intake to the development of diabetes, heart disease, or behavioral changes. Usually other factors—fat intake, obesity, or some social or psychological situation—offer a more likely explanation. The best argument against including too much sugar in your diet is one of priority. Sugars often displace more healthful foods: a candy bar displaces a piece of fruit, soda displaces milk. But so long as it is not at the expense of more nourishing foods, there's no harm in including some sugar in your diet.

Complex Carbohydrates

The majority of calories in your diet come from complex carbohydrates, often referred to as starches. Foods rich in complex carbohydrates are grains (bread, rice, pasta and cereal), some fruits, and some vegetables, notably beans and potatoes. Unlike simple sugars, complex carbohydrates consist of long chains of sugar units linked together.

Before they can be absorbed, these sugars must be split apart, and this means they are more gradually absorbed into the bloodstream. Complex carbohydrates, therefore, provide a more lasting source of energy. This is particularly important for athletes fueling up for an event.

Fiber

Unlike the "empty calories" provided by simple sugars, the foods that contain complex carbohydrates come stocked with vitamins and minerals. If you choose whole grains and unprocessed fruits and vegetables, you will also increase your intake of another increasingly important dietary component—fiber.

While most people know that fiber is good for them, many are not sure of exactly what it is or why it's so healthy. Simply stated, dietary fiber (or roughage) is the part of a plant that cannot be digested by the human body. There are two different types: water–soluble fiber and water–insoluble fiber. Most plant foods contain varying amounts of both types. Each, according to certain health claims, has specific benefits, so you should know which foods contain each one.

Until a few years ago, the principal focus was on **water–insoluble fiber**, the type found primarily in fruits, vegetables, and whole grains (wheat, seeds, beans, and brown rice). Insoluble fiber softens the stool and stimulates the digestive tract. For this reason, it alleviates constipation, hemorrhoids, and diverticulosis, another intestinal disorder. Some studies also suggest that it may decrease the risk of colon cancer, possibly by speeding the passage of cancer–causing agents through the colon.

Water–soluble fiber has been in the spotlight lately, because it is apparently able to lower blood cholesterol levels. It is also of particular interest to diabetics; it slows the absorption of sugar into the bloodstream, thus reducing the need for insulin or other diabetes medications. Advertising campaigns of recent years would lead one to believe that oat bran is the only source of this valuable fiber, but many other foods, like barley, fruits, vegetables, and beans, can provide soluble fiber while adding variety to your diet.

How beneficial is a high–fiber diet? Since it is also typically low in fat, and because those who choose to follow it are individuals who readily modify their life–style, it is difficult to determine exactly which factor is helping them. Regardless, more and more studies point to the benefits of a high–fiber diet. At present, fiber intake among Americans is estimated at about 12 grams per day. Most experts agree that we should at least double our daily fiber intake to about 20 or 30 grams. It is not necessary to specifically target soluble or insoluble fiber sources, as both are easily included in a diet that is high in fiber overall.

As for the benefits of a high–carbohydrate diet in general, numerous studies suggest that it may help control obesity, diabetes, and cardiovascular disease. Most likely, this is due not just to the health effects of carbohydrates, but also to the presumed replacement of high–fat foods with high–carbohydrate substitutes. Carbohydrates provide about 45 percent of calories in men, 46 percent in women. About a quarter of these calories came from simple sugars. Authorities recommend that you get more than 50 percent of your calories from carbohydrates, with emphasis on the complex variety.

How Important is Protein?

Protein is necessary for the growth, maintenance, and repair of every cell in the body. It is present in countless forms throughout the body—as part of enzymes, hormones, antibodies, oxygen carriers, bones, muscle, hair, and skin, to name a few. Unlike the fuel–providing carbohydrates, proteins are the building blocks that provide structure and perform vital functions. However, when needed, proteins can break down to provide energy—4 calories per gram.

Small units called amino acids unite to form the structure of proteins. Altogether there are 20 common amino acids. They mix and match in thousands of different combinations to make up specific proteins. Since your body cannot manufacture nine of these amino acids, you must get them from your diet. Proteins in your food provide them, with the most concentrated sources coming from animal products—meat, chicken, fish, dairy products, and eggs. However, it is also possible to get protein from plants such as beans, nuts, and grains. In fact, most of the people in the world get their protein from vegetable sources for either cultural or economic reasons.

Animal versus Plant Proteins

Proteins from meat, poultry, fish, and dairy foods are called complete proteins because they furnish all the amino acids needed for growth. Most plant proteins, on the other hand, are incomplete: Except for the soy bean, no single plant provides all nine essential amino acids. (Soy, though complete, is still considered inferior to animal proteins.) You can, however, meet your daily requirements by consuming a variety of plant proteins over the course of each day. For example, the amino acids from beans taken

PROTEIN FROM PLANTS

Here are some of the plant-based foods that can provide you with protein.

Grains	Legumes
Nuts and Seeds	Whole grain bread
Dried beans	Walnuts
Pasta	Dried peas
Pecans	Rice
Lentils	Almonds
Barley	Tofu
Sesame seeds	Bulgar products
Sunflower seeds	Oats
Chickpeas	Cashews
Cornmeal	Lima beans
Peanuts	

at one meal can complement the amino acids from rice eaten at another meal that day. Other examples are peanut butter and wheat bread, or macaroni and cheese. (In the latter case, the essential amino acids from the animal product, cheese, allow the body to better use the amino acids in the macaroni.)

Dietary protein deficiencies in this country are relatively rare. When they do occur, they are usually the result of a disease that causes loss of appetite or loss of large amounts of protein from the body.

Excess dietary protein is a much more common problem. Government surveys estimate that the average American consumes about 100 grams of protein per day—almost twice the recommended daily allowance (RDA) of 50 grams for women and 63 grams for men. Excess protein taxes the body physiologically. Once it's digested and absorbed, end products of protein metabolism are excreted in the urine; so any excess places extra burden on the kidneys. Nor does excess protein build muscles. It is either burned as energy or stored—not as muscle, but as fat. Many athletes, particularly those involved in strength training, believe that to build muscle you need more protein. In fact, Americans already get more than enough; and exercise, not extra protein, is the only way to increase muscle size and strength.

Fat: The Danger in our Diet

If the media have drummed nothing else into us about diet, the message about fat is clear: It's bad for you! It causes obesity. It raises your cholesterol. It causes heart disease. It may even contribute to development of cancer.

But if it is all that bad, why is it part of our natural diet chain? Despite its bad press, fat does contribute to many important bodily functions. It provides the body with essential fatty acids (linoleic and linolenic acids) needed for normal reproduction and growth, as well as for production of prostoglandin, a hormonelike compound that helps regulate blood pressure, blood clotting, and inflammation. On a practical level, fat cushions bones and vital organs, protects the body from extreme temperatures, carries fat-soluble nutrients, and serves as an important energy reserve. Though fat reserves have become the bane of modern times, their original purpose was to sustain early humans through times of famine.

At 9 calories per gram, fat remains an important storehouse of calories to be tapped for sustained work and exercise. After a 20-minute aerobic workout, the body begins to deplete its carbohydrate stores. At this point, fat steps in to provide an almost endless source of fuel.

For those who are not physically active, however, high intakes of fat lead to obesity. Fat requires few calories for its metabolism—it "slides" right into storage at little expense to the body. With carbohydrates, on the other hand, it takes a significant number of calories to convert excess amounts into fat for storage. While we need only about 1 percent to 2 percent of our calories from linoleic acid (the most essential fatty acid) to prevent a deficiency, the average American gets about 37 percent of total calories from fat. The good news is that this is down from a high of 41 percent of calories in 1977.

So what should your fat intake be? The consensus among experts is to get no more than 30 percent of your calories from fat. Where that fat comes from also matters quite a bit. Certain types of fat are more likely to raise blood cholesterol, high levels of which are associated with an increased incidence of atherosclerosis, in which cholesterol–containing plaques build up on the inside of artery walls, causing progressive narrowing.

The term *dietary fat* really encompasses three types: polyunsaturated, monounsaturated, and saturated. Saturation refers to the chemical structure of a particular fat. In general, the more saturated a fat is, the more solid it is.

Polyunsaturated Fats

These fats are liquid at room temperature. They are found in plant oils, including sunflower, safflower, soybean, sesame seed, and corn oil. They also appear in cold–water fish like tuna, salmon, and mackerel. Polyunsaturated fats help lower blood cholesterol levels, and when found in fish oils act as a blood thinner, decreasing the risk of life–threatening blood clots forming in the arteries of the heart. Our present intake of

polyunsaturated fat averages about 7 percent of total calories. The recommended amount is up to 10 percent of total calories.

Monounsaturated Fats

These fats are also found in fish oils, as well as in olive oil, peanut oil, canola oil, and avocado. Initial interest in monounsaturated fats arose in part from research revealing that in Mediterranean countries, where olive oil is plentiful in the diet, the incidence of cardiovascular disease is low. Many experts now think that if you substitute monounsaturated fat for saturated fat in your diet, you can lower your cholesterol level. There is also a theory that monounsaturates may be even better than polyunsaturated fats at lowering blood cholesterol. Though we presently consume about 14 percent of our calories as monounsaturates, well within the recommended range of 10 percent to 15 percent, there is a possibility that higher intakes will be recommended in the future.

Saturated Fats

This type, usually solid at room temperature, comes most often from animal sources, for example, meats and whole–fat dairy products. Some vegetable fats, notably palm oil and coconut oil, are also saturated. While animal fat is usually easy to see and therefore often trimmed away, vegetable fats are more likely to be hidden in certain foods, such as baked goods and milk chocolate.

Another widely consumed, though often unrecognized, form of saturated fat is *hydrogenated vegetable fat*. Many manufacturers take unsaturated fats, like soybean oil, and solidify them through a process called hydrogenation, creating products like margarine. Unfortunately, this process reduces their polyunsaturated content.

Saturated fats have a well–earned reputation as the villains of the American diet. Studies from countries the world over show that the more saturated fat people eat, the greater their chances of developing coronary artery disease. Saturated fats may actually raise blood cholesterol levels more than dietary cholesterol itself. Why this happens is not clear. One theory is that saturated fats suppress the receptors in the liver that clear the blood of the low–density lipoprotein (LDL) cholesterol that sticks to artery walls. Another theory is that saturated fat stimulates production of LDL cholesterol in the liver.

Cholesterol

The best rule to follow with cholesterol is the less of it, the better. Like fat, some cholesterol is necessary for good health, for it is a vital component of cell membranes, nerves, and hormones. But, unlike fat, our liver produces all we require; we don't need any cholesterol at all in our diet.

Nevertheless, we get plenty. Many common foods contain cholesterol, some much more than others. Remember this: Because cholesterol is made by the liver, only animal products contain cholesterol. It is not a problem in peanut butter, margarine, or vegetable oil. Cholesterol is most abundant in eggs and organ meats (after all, cholesterol is made in the liver), but some cholesterol is found in all animal products. Even seafood, particularly shrimp, contains some cholesterol, though with its low saturated fat content, shrimp is no longer considered as "forbidden" as it was in the past.

Some people seem more sensitive to high intakes of dietary cholesterol than others. For everyone, however, experts recommend an intake of no more than 300 milligrams of cholesterol per day. Current daily intakes average about 370 milligrams, with women averaging a bit less.

As for recommended levels of blood cholesterol, the National Cholesterol Education Program (NCEP) has established guidelines to help identify those at risk of cardiovascular disease based on their blood levels of total and LDL cholesterol. Total blood cholesterol is actually made up of two components: low–density lipoprotein (LDL) and high–density lipoprotein (HDL). The more abundant form is LDL cholesterol. Excessive levels of LDL are associated with increased risk of cardiovascular disease. High levels of HDL, on the other hand, tend to prevent the disease. So, the lower your total and LDL cholesterol and the higher your HDL cholesterol, the better. According to NCEP guidelines, a desirable total blood cholesterol level is less than 200 milligrams per deciliter of blood; a desirable LDL level, less than 130 milligrams per deciliter. Your HDL cholesterol level should exceed 35 milligrams per deciliter. If your HDL is greater than 60, you're lucky—you have a negative risk factor for cardiovascular disease.

Fat and the Cancer Connection

The link between fat intake and cancer is controversial, particularly when it comes to breast cancer. Though we know little about why breast cancer develops, some have speculated that diet might initiate the disease. Breast cancer is common in countries where women have high average intakes of total and saturated fat, animal protein, and total calories. As dietary fat intake increases, so do the estrogen levels in a woman's tissues, and some studies have implicated estrogen in the development of breast tumors. For the same reason, obesity in postmenopausal women is thought to increase the risk. Excessive dietary fat has also been implicated in the development of cancer of the colon.

While we lack conclusive data on this subject, the mere suggestion of a potential link between dietary fat and breast cancer lends support to recommendations for a low-fat diet for all women. Keeping to a low-fat—particularly a low-saturated-fat, low-cholesterol—diet also helps lower LDL cholesterol. According to the NCEP, less than 10 percent of your calories should come from saturated fat, and possibly less than 7 percent. HDL—the only good cholesterol—is not found in any foods and it can't be added to your diet. The only way to get more of it is to exercise.

Despite all the bad news, who will deny that fat lends flavor, aroma, and a sense of satisfaction to meals? Fat is here to stay, and it can be enjoyed in moderation. For the best ways to work a healthy amount of fat into your diet see "The Bottom Line" at the end of this chapter.

Value Of Vitamins

Our bodies use vitamins to regulate crucial functions within the cells. Since the first vitamin was identified around the turn of the century, our knowledge of these essential dietary elements has been changing almost daily. Early treatment of vitamin deficiencies resulted in amazing—almost "miraculous"—improvements in health. Sailors, for example, no longer died from scurvy, and children going blind from vitamin A deficiency abruptly regained their

WATER

Of all the things we ingest, water is probably the most important—and the most neglected. You can live without nutrients for weeks or even months, but without water, you can survive for only days. Water accounts for 60 percent of the body's weight. Water shuttles nutrients and oxygen to cells, where it participates in the chemical reactions that produce energy. It also transports waste products out of the cells and eventually out of the body. Water cushions joints, acts as a lubricant, and keeps food moving through the digestive tract.

Water regulates body temperature. It brings heat to the skin surface in the form of perspiration, thus cooling the body and preventing heat stroke or other temperature-related illnesses.

We get some of our water from foods, which are generally 85 percent to 96 percent water, but most of it comes from fluids such as juice, milk, soup, tap water, or anything else normally liquid at room temperature. (Don't forget gelatin desserts, ice, and frozen juice bars.) Ideally, you should drink 6 to 8 glasses a day. Beverages that contain caffeine or alcohol are poor choices; they act as dehydrators by causing increased urine production.

Plan ahead to avoid the dehydrating effects of exercise. Load up with 16 ounces of cool water 10 to 15 minutes before an activity. During exercise, 4 to 6 ounces of cool water every 10 to 15 minutes will help keep sweat production up and body temperature down. Be sure to drink even more in hot weather.

sight. Except for vitamins D and K, which the body is able to manufacture, vitamins must be obtained from the diet. Though needed in only small amounts, they play an indispensable role in storage and production of energy, and assist in tissue formation.

At this time, we know of 13 essential vitamins. They are classified as either water soluble or fat soluble, depending on how they are transported and stored. This distinction is important. Because the water component of the body turns over frequently, you have to replenish water–soluble vitamins daily. On the other hand, fat–soluble vitamins are stored in fat and tend to stay with you. This makes it possible to overload on fat–soluble vitamins if you take them in large, potentially toxic, amounts. But it also means that fat–soluble vitamins do not have to be taken daily.

Water–Soluble Vitamins

Included in the water–soluble group are **vitamin C** and the **B complex vitamins.** Though deficiencies are relatively rare in the United States, recent research has brought several of these vitamins back into the limelight.

Vitamin C, also known as **ascorbic acid,** strengthens bone and blood vessels, aids in iron absorption, and promotes wound healing. Contrary to popular belief, there is no conclusive evidence that vitamin C prevents or speeds recovery from a cold. Studies done on this issue seem to be prone to the "placebo effect"—people are influenced by what they *think* helps, whether it does or not. The recommended daily allowance (RDA) of vitamin C is 60 milligrams, 100 milligrams if you smoke (smokers have lower blood levels of vitamin C than nonsmokers). From 4 to 8 ounces of orange juice will supply this amount of vitamin C. Other good sources of vitamin C are citrus fruits, strawberries, cantaloupe, tomatoes, broccoli, potatoes, sweet potatoes, and greens.

Abuse of vitamin C supplements is common; the most frequent side effects are nausea, abdominal cramps, and diarrhea. Large amounts of vitamin C can also interfere with the accuracy of certain lab tests. Theoretically, huge doses over a prolonged period could also cause kidney stones.

Niacin, thiamine, and **riboflavin** are important players in the processes that produce energy from nutrients. These B vitamins are widely available from dairy products, meats, fish, poultry, whole grain or enriched breads and cereals, and nuts. Although most people in developed countries get adequate amounts, alcoholics are an exception. They tend to have vitamin–deficient diets and, in the case of thiamine, lose too much in their urine.

Megadoses of niacin, sometimes prescribed for its cholesterol–lowering properties, can cause *niacin flush,* a hot, tingling sensation in the skin that sometimes makes the therapy intolerable. Megadoses of vitamins, defined as 10 times the RDA, act more as drugs than as nutrients. It's wise to avoid self–prescribing them.

Folic acid, another of the B–complex vitamins, is required for the formation of all new cells. Along with B_{12}, it is particularly involved in production of red blood cells. A deficiency of either of these vitamins can cause anemia. B_{12} also helps maintain the protective covering of the nervous system; a deficiency becomes apparent when nerves and muscles malfunction. B_{12} is found only in animal products: meat, fish, poultry, eggs, and dairy products, leaving strict vegetarians at risk of deficiency. Folic acid is most plentiful in liver, leafy green vegetables (like spinach, broccoli, and asparagus), beans, and seeds; it is also found in whole grains, pork, poultry, shellfish, and citrus fruits.

Recently, folic acid deficiency has been shown to play a central role in development of the neural tube defects *anencephaly* and *spina bifida*. Anencephaly is the absence at birth of all or a major part of the brain. In spina bifida, a portion of the spinal column does not completely close. Many spina bifida victims, even after surgery, have trouble walking and suffer bowel and bladder problems. Significant evidence indicates that adequate folic acid intake *before conception* and into early pregnancy can reduce the baby's chances of a neural defect. Evidence is so compelling that now the U.S. Public Health Service, recognizing the need for folic acid before a woman even knows she's pregnant, states that anyone who may become pregnant should get at least 0.4 milligram (400 micrograms) of folic acid each day. For women who have a history of a neural tube defect in a previous pregnancy and who hope for another child, physicians may prescribe an even higher dose of 4 milligrams of folic acid daily. Women on birth control pills also need higher doses, in case the pills fail.

Vitamin B6 is involved in numerous processes: red blood cell formation, release of glucose (sugar) from its storage forms, and conversion of the amino acid tryptophan into niacin. Deficiency rarely occurs alone, but usually accompanies multiple B complex deficiencies. Signs of deficiency include neurologic problems, skin rash, and anemia. B6 is widely available in meat, fish, poultry, beans, fruit, whole grains, and green vegetables.

The last two B vitamins, **biotin** and **pantothenic acid**, play important roles in the body's use of carbohydrate, protein, and fat. Since both are widespread in the food supply, healthy people with ordinary diets are not at risk of deficiency.

Fat–Soluble Vitamins

Vitamin A was the first fat–soluble vitamin to be identified. It is probably the most diverse in its functions, which include roles in vision, immune and stress responses, energy production, blood production, maintenance of the nervous system and numerous other body tissues, and normal growth and reproduction. Often, its presence in food is obvious. Its active form, retinol, is yellow and is found in butter and eggs. Other less obvious sources of retinol are cheese, fortified milk, cream, fortified margarine, and liver. Vitamin A's *precursor* (so–called because it is converted to vitamin A in the body) is **beta carotene**. A bright orange color, beta carotene is found in apricots, cantaloupes, squash, carrots, sweet potatoes, and pumpkins. Other good sources of beta carotene are broccoli and leafy greens like spinach.

Vitamin A deficiency affects the ability of the skin and the linings of the internal organs to resist cancer, particularly of the skin, lung, bladder, and pharynx. Beta carotene has other health–promoting properties linked to its antioxidant characteristics (see the next section of this chapter).

While adequate intakes of vitamin A are vital for good health, excessive use of *active vitamin A* supplements such as retinol can be dangerous. Symptoms of vitamin A toxicity are headache, vomiting, hair loss, dryness of the mucous membranes, bone abnormalities, and liver damage. Toxicity usually occurs only after long–term megadoses amounting to 15,000 micrograms of retinol (50,000 international units [IU]) in adults and 6,000 micrograms (20,000 IU) of retinol in infants and children. Such doses are not usually obtained from food alone.

Beta carotene is not known to cause toxicity, primarily because your body will stop converting it to vitamin A when needed levels are reached. Instead, the beta carotene is stored in fatty tissues, so that an accumulation under your skin can tint it orange. Although unbecoming, this condition is not harmful. It fades when you decrease your beta carotene intake.

Vitamin D ranks with calcium as crucial protection for your bones. Vitamin D helps maintain blood calcium levels by regulating the absorption of calcium in the digestive system and its excretion in the urine. Best sources of vitamin D are butter, fortified milk, fortified margarine, eggs, and liver. It is also produced by our intestinal bacteria, and is manufactured by skin exposed to sunlight. The average person needs only 10 to 15 minutes in the sun each day. Keep in mind that sunscreen blocks vitamin D synthesis.

The most obvious signs of vitamin D deficiency are bone abnormalities. In children, vitamin D deficiency causes the abnormal bone growth called *rickets*. Though no longer common, the disease has long been known to respond to treatment with cod liver oil, which we now know is high in vitamin D. Adult rickets or *osteomalacia*, is most often seen in women with low calcium intakes and little sun exposure who have repeated pregnancies and breast–feed their babies. In this instance, calcium is withdrawn from the bone but not replaced. These women can benefit from extra calcium and vitamin D. A number of studies suggest that increased intakes of vitamin D may also improve calcium absorption in elderly people and some victims of osteoporosis. Use care with vitamin D supplements, however, as it is the most potentially toxic vitamin. Avoid doses significantly above the RDA.

Vitamin E, classified as an antioxidant, is especially important to the lungs, and the red blood cell membranes. Vitamin E also protects white blood cells, which play a major role in the immune system's defense against disease.

The leading sources of vitamin E are polyunsaturated vegetable oils, followed by green leafy vegetables, wheat germ, whole grains, nuts, and seeds. If you have the typical intake of fat, you will rarely suffer vitamin E deficiency unless you have a disorder that interferes with fat absorption.

Vitamin K, the last of the fat–soluble vitamins, helps blood to clot. Without vitamin K, wounds would bleed for dangerously long periods of time, and surgery would be impossible. Bacteria in the intestine can synthesize vitamin K, and because of this, deficiencies are rare. Due to its role in helping blood to clot, those who take blood–thinning medications should avoid excessive amounts of vitamin K (primarily found in green leafy vegetables and liver.) On the other hand, people taking antibiotics may need more. Vitamin K toxicity is not a problem.

The Antioxidant Story

Recently, anitoxidants have become a media buzzword. These nutrients—mainly vitamin E, vitamin C, and beta carotene—are thought to ward off disease and slow the aging process. Along with other substances known as antioxidant enzymes and scavengers, these vitamins seem to protect the body's cells from the damaging effects of oxygen. They do this by neutralizing so–called *free radicals*,— unstable oxygen by–products that can damage cell DNA, proteins, carbohydrates, and fats. Normal body processes, such as breathing and digesting food, produce free radicals. Environmental pollutants, such as cigarette smoke, also produce them. They can cause severe damage to cell structures.

Under normal conditions, the body's own antioxidant enzymes and scavengers remove or deactivate free radicals. But if levels of free radicals get too high to handle, the body may need reinforcement with antioxidant vitamins.

While the role that free radicals play in disease and aging is not completely understood, some scientists believe they either cause or accelerate the progression of age–related diseases. In cancer, free radicals may damage DNA, thus promoting the disease. In cardiovascular disease, oxidation of LDL cholesterol may be a first step in development of arterial plaque. Some speculate that Parkinson's and other neurologic diseases are in part caused by the effects of free radicals on nerve tissue. And cataracts may result from free–radical damage to the lens of an eye.

Vitamin E is the premier antioxidant. It also supports the immune system, blocks formation of nitrosamines (suspected carcinogens), and repairs damaged cell membranes. In some research studies, it has been shown to protect against various forms of cancer.

High intakes of beta carotene are also thought to lower the risk of cancer, particularly of the lung, but also of the breast, cervix, uterine lining, gastrointestinal tract, and oral cavity. And Vitamin C is believed to defend against cancer in several ways:

- It deactivates free radicals;
- It boosts immune function;
- It may help detoxify cancer-causing substances, such as pesticides, heavy metals, and industry–produced hydrocarbons, and may prevent formation of the cancer-causing nitrosamines.

Vitamin C is most strongly associated with protection against gastrointestinal, breast, and cervical cancer. However, many studies of both vitamin C and beta carotene involved diets with numerous other nutrients and fiber, so there's a possibility that the protective effects result from a number of dietary influences working together.

In cardiovascular disease, both vitamins C and E interfere with the oxidation of LDL cholesterol, with vitamin C having the stronger effect. One large study showed that women with a daily vitamin E intake of greater than 100 IU had a 36 percent lower risk of heart attack than those with intakes of less than 30 IU daily. Beta carotene also seems to play a role in reducing the risk of heart attack and stroke. All three antioxidant vitamins affect blood platelet aggregation, which causes formation of blood clots. By reducing the platelets' "stickiness," the antioxidants make the platelets less likely to adhere to the inside of blood vessels and to each other, thus reducing the chance of life-threatening blood clots.

The Latest Cancer Fighters: Phytochemicals

Also hot in current nutritional news are the phytochemicals, naturally occurring substances in plants thought to possess disease–fighting properties. Research into phytochemicals has helped fuel the recent push to increase our intakes of garlic, broccoli, and similar vegetables classified as cruciferous.

The phytochemicals' potential role against cancer and heart disease has sparked a flurry of research. Cruciferous vegetables, notably broccoli, cauliflower, cabbage, and brussels sprouts, are rich sources of indoles, the basic components of many biologically active substances like serotonin and tryptophan. Indoles may stimulate enzymes that break down carcinogens into harmless substances. They appear to be particularly protective against stomach and intestinal cancers. Cruciferous vegetables are also high in fiber, and beneficial in preventing colon cancer.

A compound found in garlic extracts, **allyic sulfide,** is thought to protect against cancer, as well as inhibiting cholesterol synthesis and thereby reducing the risk of arterial plaque. In addition, parsley, carrots, citrus fruit, berries, cucumbers, cruciferous vegetables, peppers, squash, yams, tomatoes, eggplant, and soy products contain flavonoids, a group of substances that may act to block receptors for hormones that promote cancer. Other phytochemicals—phenolic acid, coumarin, isothiocyanates, and catechin—are also under study as disease fighters.

Questions that still need answers, for phytochemical and antioxidants alike include: "How much should I take?" and "What combinations will give me the best effect?" Although there does seem to be a role for these nutrients—possibly in amounts well above their recommended daily allowances—the jury is still out as to whether supplements are warranted and safe. Until we have answers, the most practical advice is to follow current recommendations and increase intakes of all fruits and vegetables. The National Cancer Institute is now promoting

THE CALCIUM IN YOUR FOOD

Food Item	Calcium (mg)
1 cup milk, whole, 2 percent, 1 percent, or skim	291–302
1 cup plain, low–fat yogurt	400
1 cup fruited, low–fat yogurt	314
1 oz. cheddar cheese	204
1 oz. American cheese	124
1/2 cup 1 percent low–fat cottage cheese	69
1/2 cup tofu processed with calcium	258
1/2 cup greens (beet, kale, okra, mustard), frozen, cooked	75–90
1/2 cup spinach*, frozen, cooked	139
1/2 cup broccoli, cooked	47
1 orange, medium	56
1 cup chili with beans, canned	119
1/2 cup macaroni and cheese	199
1/8 piece of 12–inch cheese pizza	116

*Not a good source of calcium; contains substances that bind it.

the "5–A–Day Plan"—eat at least 5 servings of fruits and vegetables each day, at least one high in vitamin C, one high in vitamin A, and one high in fiber; include cruciferous vegetables several times each week.

Minerals: A Woman's Special Needs

Like vitamins, minerals provide mandatory support for certain life–sustaining functions. They regulate reactions like nerve transmission, blood clotting, and oxygen transport. Most important, minerals provide structure to the body in the form of bones. There are 60 minerals in the body, but

7 predominate, namely calcium, phosphorous, magnesium, potassium, sodium, chlorine, and sulfur. All others—needed in tiny amounts—are called trace minerals. Quantity does not necessarily dictate importance, however. Iron, for example, is needed in only trace amounts, but is involved in one of the body's most vital functions—the transport of oxygen.

Four key minerals you, as a woman, particularly need to maintain your health are calcium, iron, potassium, and sodium.

Calcium

Most Americans, particularly women, do not get enough calcium. The adult body contains about 1200 grams of calcium. Only 1 percent is found inside cells and body fluids, where it plays a part in nerve conduction, muscle contraction, and blood clotting. The remaining 99 percent is stored in bones and teeth. While we think of the skeleton as a stable structure, it is actually in a constant state of turnover—calcium is deposited and withdrawn throughout our lives. In childhood and adolescence, more calcium is deposited than withdrawn. Later in life the reverse occurs. Calcium levels in the blood must remain within a certain range. Specialized hormones that regulate calcium levels will "rob" the bones of calcium if necessary. Vitamin D, and possibly lactose, the sugar in dairy products, aid the absorption of calcium in the intestine.

By far the most concentrated sources of calcium are milk, and milk products. There are smaller amounts in dark green leafy vegetables, broccoli, calcium–processed tofu, sardines, salmon (including the bones), and some fortified cereals.

THE WAY TO STRONGER BONES

Calcium does not act alone. Follow these bone–strengthening recommendations:

- Increase physical activity—it helps maintain mobility and strengthens bones by exerting pressure on them.
- Obtain adequate vitamin D through sun exposure and diet.
- Avoid eating excessive amounts of protein—too much may cause increased loss of calcium in the urine.
- Avoid cigarette smoking.
- Drink alcohol in moderation.

A word of caution: Both smoking and drinking alcohol are life–style factors associated with increased risk of osteoporosis.

Osteoporosis, a disease in which the bones become brittle and porous, strikes women more often than men, frequently causing bone fractures. Osteoporosis affects about 25 million Americans in all, and often progresses for years undetected. For the many older women who suffer fractures, the disease can mean loss of independence, and for 12 percent to 20 percent, even death.

One major risk factor for osteoporosis is continually low calcium intake. The less calcium you consume early in life, the less bone you have to spare as you get older. Bone density reaches its peak around age 30 to 35 and remains fairly stable until middle age. After menopause, bone loss speeds up for the first 5 to 10 years, with the total loss reaching 10 to 15 percent.

This bone loss results from a decline in estrogen, which prior to menopause helps to maintain proper calcium levels. Lower estrogen levels also somewhat inhibit digestion of calcium. After menopause, estrogen replacement therapy can slow this process. (For more information, see chapter 30, "Holding Back Osteoporosis.")

Calcium intake in early life builds up bone reserves before menopause. Yet even later in life, increasing calcium intake may slow the rate of bone loss, particularly in older women 5 to 20 years into menopause. The ideal amount of calcium needed is unknown and probably varies from woman to woman. Many believe the current RDA of 800 milligrams for both men and women is too low. The National Institutes of Health recommend 1,000 milligrams per day for men and premenopausal women, 1,500 milligrams for most postmenopausal women, and 1,000 milligrams per day for postmenopausal women treated with estrogen.

Calcium also appears to exert a positive effect on high blood pressure in some people. Exactly how is unknown, and it's premature to make any specific dietary recommendations concerning this. It's another good reason, however, for making sure you get at least the recommended allowance in your daily diet.

Lactose Intolerance. If you are one of the many women who suffer from lactose intolerance, eating dairy products may give you painful bloating, gas, and diarrhea. Lactose intolerance is caused by a deficiency of the enzyme lactase, which breaks down milk sugar into digestible sugars. As undigested lactose passes through the digestive tract, intestinal bacteria consume it for energy, producing gas and other intestinal irritants. The degree of lactose intolerance varies. Some people cannot eat any dairy products at all, others can tolerate small amounts taken with other foods. For some, a lactase supplement taken before consuming any dairy products solves the problem. Aged cheese and yogurt with active cultures are often easier to digest because bacteria have already broken down most of the lactose during fermentation.

If you are one of those who just will not eat dairy products, you should consider calcium supplements to make up the difference. The many calcium supplements available differ in the amount of elemental calcium they provide. Calcium carbonate, for example, is about 40 percent calcium, whereas calcium lactate is only about 13 percent, and calcium gluconate only 9 percent. Purity is another concern. Although bone meal and dolomite (calcium magnesium carbonate) are 31 percent and 22 percent calcium respectively, they may also contain lead or other toxic metals. While it is difficult to overdose on calcium from foods, the same cannot be said of supplements. The safe upper limit seems to be about 2,500 milligrams per day. Anyone at risk of developing kidney stones, however, should limit daily intake to no more than 1,000 milligrams.

Which form of calcium is best? In general, calcium carbonate seems to come closest to dietary calcium in absorbability, but, like any other supplement, it lacks the other nutrients plentiful in dairy products that help build bones.

In most people, supplements are absorbed better when taken between meals. If you are elderly, however, the stomach acid needed for digestion may be more plentiful when food is present, so it's best to take the supplements at mealtime.

Iron

Another major dietary concern for women, iron is the blood-building mineral. It plays an important role in transport of oxygen throughout the body. It is also thought to help the body use beta carotene, and aids in clearing fats from the blood. Most iron in the body is stored in the oxygen–carrying proteins hemoglobin and myoglobin, found in the blood and muscles, respectively. The less iron your body has already stored, the more dietary iron you will absorb. Other factors that govern absorption are the form of iron and the presence of other nutrients. Inadequate intake or excessive loss from bleeding can cause iron–deficiency anemia, a condition in which the body is unable to absorb enough iron from marginal supplies. Anemic red blood cells contain too little hemoglobin and therefore deliver too little oxygen to the cells. Symptoms of anemia are fatigue, apathy, lowered resistance to infection, and decreased exercise tolerance.

The principal sources of dietary iron are meat, eggs, vegetables, and iron–fortified cereals. Iron from vegetables and grains is absorbed more readily in the presence of Vitamin C or meat. You can readily meet your daily need by having orange juice with iron–fortified cereal, or a baked potato with your steak. On the other hand, substances called *phytates* (found in whole grains and beans) interfere with iron absorption, as do substances in coffee, tea, bran, calcium phosphate, and antacids.

Even under the best conditions, iron is poorly absorbed from food. In fact, a healthy woman absorbs only about 10 percent of the iron in her food, absorbing the most from meats. In the United States, iron deficiency is most likely to occur in children, women in their childbearing years, and those who are pregnant. Even if you are convinced you're anemic, however, you should not take iron supplements without the advice of a physician. Iron toxicity can be serious—even fatal; so it's important to store iron supplements well away from children. The recommended daily allowance, or RDA, is 10 milligrams for men and older women, and 15 milligrams for women during childbearing years. If you are pregnant, double your intake to 30 milligrams per day. Because women generally eat less than men, they need to pay special attention to including high–iron foods in their diets. A tip—if you use cast iron pans in cooking, you will increase your iron intake because iron from the pan leeches into the food.

Potassium

This indispensable mineral is necessary for muscle contraction, nerve transmission, and proper functioning of the heart and kidneys.

WAYS TO WORK IRON INTO YOUR DIET

Food Item	Iron (mg)
1 cup spinach, cooked	6.4
1 cup peach halves, water packed	0.77
1 cup kidney beans, cooked	5.2
3.5 oz. sirloin steak	3.36
1/2 cup broccoli, cooked	0.65
1 slice whole wheat bread	0.86
1/3 cup All–Bran cereal	4.5
1 1/4 cup Cheerios	4.45
2/3 cup raisins	2.08
3/4 cup oatmeal	8.35
1/2 chicken breast	0.89

It also helps maintain fluid balance in the cells. While more than 90 percent of potassium is absorbed in the digestive tract, changing the amount in your diet will not significantly change potassium levels in the blood. The kidneys tightly regulate how much potassium is in the blood by reabsorbing what they need and spilling what they do not in the urine. Tight control is vital, because large fluctuations in blood potassium levels affect heart rhythms.

Potassium regulation is so efficient that under normal conditions deficiency is never a problem. When it does happen, it is usually due to the excessive loss of potassium that occurs with prolonged vomiting, chronic diarrhea, laxative abuse, or use of diuretic medications. Often referred to as "water pills," diuretics are commonly prescribed to treat high blood pressure. These medications flush excess water out of the system and often potassium along with it. Because of this side effect, a diet rich in high–potassium foods is recommended to offset losses caused by diuretics. Potassium is widely available in our food, the best sources being oranges, orange juice, bananas, potatoes, dried fruits, yogurt, milk, meat, and poultry. Do not take potassium supplements without a doctor's supervision.

Although there is no official RDA for potassium, the minimum requirement is estimated at 1,600 to 2,000 milligrams per day. Some studies indicate that potassium may lower blood pressure in certain individuals; higher intakes may thus be beneficial.

Sodium

Better known as salt, sodium is the chief regulator of fluid in the body. Like potassium, sodium is eliminated by the kidney. Sodium deficiency, although unusual, can result from the kind of heavy, persistent sweating that occurs during prolonged exercise in hot weather.

Sodium is all too plentiful in our diets. The average American consumes between 4,000 and 5,800 milligrams of sodium per day. Contrast this with the recommended intake of 2,400 milligrams per day, and the minimum requirement of only 500 milligrams, and you can see that most of us consume at least twice the sodium considered healthy. One–third of this occurs naturally in foods, one–third is added during processing, and one–third is added during cooking or at the table.

Aside from table salt, the biggest contributors of sodium to our diets are cured meats, including ham, bacon, sausages, frankfurters, and luncheon meats; cheese; pickles; canned and frozen foods (unless marked "no added salt" or "low sodium"); commercial pasta, potato and rice dishes; salty snacks; and "fast foods."

The main problem with sodium is its effect on blood pressure. High blood pressure affects about 60 million Americans. It is a major risk factor for both heart attack and stroke, as it causes injury to the linings of arteries, which in turn makes cholesterol plaques likely to form. High blood pressure usually displays no outward symptoms. Because of its silent onset, many people have the condition without knowing it. From adolescence through age 45, men are more likely to have high blood pressure than women. After 45, the reverse holds true.

Blood pressure is a measure of the force that blood exerts on the inside of the artery walls. The amount of fluid in the circulatory

CONSIDER A MULTIVITAMIN/ MINERAL SUPPLEMENT IF YOU...

...Are on a diet.

...Are elderly, and don't eat enough.

...Have an illness that kills your appetite.

...Have an illness that reduces digestion (a danger for alcoholics).

...Take medications that block the body's use of nutrients.

...Are recovering from illness, or injury (your body demands extra nutrition).

...Are pregnant.

...Practice strict vegetarianism.

...Have heavy periods.

...Are at risk of osteoporosis.

---

system affects this. Sodium causes fluid retention; so the more sodium in the blood, the more fluid there will be, too.

The evidence correlating sodium with high blood pressure is not clear–cut. For years researchers have associated high intakes of salt (or sodium chloride, which is a compound of sodium and chlorine) with elevations in blood pressure. Recently it has become less clear whether the culprit is the sodium or the chlorine.

Most people get rid of excess salt by excreting it in the urine. However, some salt–sensitive individuals (people with kidney disease, those whose parents have high blood pressure, blacks, and those over age 50), definitely undergo an increase in blood pressure from eating salty foods. For these people, salt restriction is likely to help control blood pressure. Because it is hard to tell who is salt–sensitive and who isn't, everyone with high blood pressure is advised to cut back on salt.

Should You Take A Supplement?

Nearly 4 out of 10 adults in the United States take vitamin and mineral supplements regularly. We spend more than $2.5 billion on them annually. They are the third largest product category sold over–the–counter.

Supplement use, according to surveys, is heaviest among people who have one or more health problems; but some who describe their health as very good or excellent are also avid users. Supplement users tend to be especially health conscious. They also are likely to believe that marginal vitamin deficiencies are more common than generally thought.

Arguments against supplements focus not on daily multivitamins, but on the hazards of high–dose supplements. High doses of any nutrient may be dangerous; and toxic levels differ from one person to another. Indeed, since it is easily misdiagnosed, supplement overdose could be more common than we realize. Confusing the matter further is the lack of scientific data establishing a reasonable margin of safety for the average adult.

It's also true that nutrients are generally absorbed better from food than from pills. Foods contain an array of nutrients that facilitate each other's absorption, while individual supplements must go it alone. If you stick to a well–balanced diet, you can obtain all the vitamins, minerals, fiber, calories, and other substances—presently known and yet to be discovered—that you need to maintain good health.

The only people who really need to consider a supplement are those who are malnourished (dieters, some of the elderly, people with illnesses affecting their appetites), people with impaired digestion, those on medications that block the body's use of a nutrient, sick people with extra nutritional requirements, pregnant women, vegetarians, women with heavy menstrual bleeding, and women at risk of osteoporosis. If you fall into one of these groups, or decide you want a supplement to improve general health, base your choice on fact, not hype. Check with your doctor if you have any doubt, and choose a supplement that provides nutrient amounts close to the recommended allowances. Avoid megadoses (doses 10 times or more than the RDA), particularly of vitamins A and D. Opt for a brand made by a reputable manufacturer, whose production standards are likely to be well–regulated. (A recently described disorder called eosinophilia–myalgia syndrome was traced to a contaminant in an amino acid supplement, *L–tryptophan*, manufactured in Japan.) You need not buy the most expensive brand. Store brands may be just as good and cheaper. Steer clear of supplements whose advertisers make outrageous claims of benefits for a specific ailment or for "stress."

Your Changing Needs Throughout Life

Nutrient needs of men and women do not differ appreciably until adolescence. Growth accelerates in girls beginning around 10 or 11 years of age, peaking at about age 12.

Adolescence

At this stage, girls acquire a larger amount of body fat than boys in preparation for childbearing. This rapid growth significantly increases the need for all nutrients, but particularly for protein, calcium, and iron. The developing young woman needs calcium to support bone growth and to build up calcium deposits as a defense against osteoporosis later in life. She must also replace the iron lost from menstruation in order to avoid anemia. In short, this is not the moment to switch from milk to soda, as so many teenagers do.

Adolescence is also a high–risk time for anorexia nervosa, a condition 10 times more common in girls than boys. Girls with this problem starve themselves and often overexercise, all in reaction to a distorted body image that makes them overestimate their weight. A related disorder, bulimia, combines recurrent food binges with self–induced vomiting and excessive laxative use. (For more on these distressing disorders, turn to Chapter 34.)

Just as sad as a 12–year–old worrying about her weight are the social and emotional effects of **adolescent obesity.** Many teens consume a high–fat diet of "fast foods" and snacks needlessly high in calories. If you keep low–fat snack foods handy, and try to encourage exercise, you may be able to prevent an overweight child from becoming an obese adult.

Pregnancy

The nutritional demands of pregnancy are extraordinary both for healthy development of the baby, and to maintain the health of the mother–to–be. Indeed, a developing baby will get the nutrients it needs for growth at the mother's expense, if necessary. Daily calorie demands increase by 300 calories in an adult mother–to–be, more in a pregnant teen, who needs to support her own continued growth along with that of her baby. Ideal weight gain is about 2 to 4 pounds during the first 3

HOW FITNESS FITS IN

No matter how old you are, or what medical problems you may have, physical fitness is essential to your health. You don't have to become part of the fitness craze in order to stay healthy, but you do need to make a deliberate effort to get enough exercise. How much is enough? The four measurements of physical fitness are:

- Aerobic endurance
- Muscular strength
- Body composition
- Flexibility

Aerobic Endurance

This is a simple measure of how long you can keep up an activity that requires oxygen, such as running, brisk walking, cycling, rowing, dancing, cross–country skiing, stair climbing, swimming, or hiking. Aerobic exercises should be performed at a moderate intensity, enough so that the heart rate speeds up, but not so much as to fatigue the muscles before oxygen has a chance to reach them.

Some exercises are too intense to be aerobic. These "anaerobic" exercises demand more oxygen than can readily get to the working muscles. This type of exercise can be performed for only a short period of time before muscles begin to "burn" and tire out. Anaerobic exercise includes weight–lifting, sprinting, and spurts of activity during football, basketball, tennis, or soccer.

For those interested in shedding pounds, aerobic exercise is the way to go. It supplies the oxygen needed to burn off fat. If you have a choice between a high–intensity workout for a shorter period of time or a low– to medium–intensity workout for a longer period, opt for the latter. Low– to medium–intensity workouts strengthen your heart, lungs, and circulatory system, but inflict fewer exercise–related injuries to muscles and joints. You are more likely to stick with this kind of workout program, too.

How often should you work out? The American College of Sports Medicine recommends some form of aerobic activity 3 to 5 times a week. Exercising more often increases the risk of injury without providing much extra benefit. Each workout should last 20 to 60 minutes, depending on intensity (30 minutes of jogging versus 60 minutes of walking). Always include 5– to 10–minute warm–up and cool–down periods.

How do you know if you are working hard enough? Your heart rate can tell you. The target heart rate for an aerobic activity is between 60 and 90 percent of your ideal maximum heart rate. To calculate what that range is for you (let's assume that you are 40 years old), do the following:

- Subtract your age (40) from 220 to determine the maximum heart rate, in beats per minute, that's right for your age. Example: 220 – 40 = 180 beats per minute.
- Multiply this number by 0.60.
  Example: 180 X 0.60 = 108 beats per minute
- Then multiply the number again by 0.90.
  Example: 180 X 0.90 = 162 beats per minute
  These results represent your target heart rate at 60 to 90 percent of maximum. Because it's easier to check your pulse for a 10–second period, take these two numbers and divide each by 6 (there are six 10–second periods in a minute):

  108 divided by 6 = 18
  162 divided by 6 = 27

Thus, a 10–second check of your heart rate, taken on your wrist or neck, should be between 18 and 27 beats. If it is lower, pick up the pace. If it's higher, slow down.

Muscular Strength

To increase muscular strength as opposed to aerobic endurance, you need to undertake resistance training using free weights or weight/resistance machines. Lifting heavy weights or working against a heavy resistance until the muscle is fatigued (usually only a few repetitions) improves muscle strength. Lifting lighter weights and repeating it more frequently increases muscle endurance. Exercises should work all major muscle groups.

As a supplement to aerobic exercise, fitness experts recommend about 20 minutes of strength training at least 2, but no more than 3 times a week. Each session should include 8 to 12 repetitions of 8 to 10 different exercises. Because lifting heavy weights can rapidly increase blood pressure, check with your physician before starting a strength-training program if you have any form of heart disease.

When you plan your exercise program, keep in mind that any amount of exercise is better than nothing at all. Even if you do not exercise enough to improve aerobic conditioning, you may still be doing enough to burn calories, strengthen bones, raise your HDL cholesterol, and reduce your risk of cardiovascular disease.

Body Composition and Flexibility

No matter what your age, you can get the exercise you need. Older women may have to ease into an exercise program more gradually, but they can still reap the benefits. With age, we lose muscle because of inactivity. Unless checked, the result is gradual weight gain due to loss of metabolically active tissue. We call muscle "metabolically active" because even at rest it is burning calories. Regular exercise helps to maintain muscle and burn calories, thus controlling weight. Quick-weight-loss diets without exercise cause loss of muscle as well as fat and almost guarantee that the pounds will return. Keeping muscles toned also keeps the tasks of daily living easier as we get older. Stretching exercises help maintain both flexibility and mobility.

The psychological benefits of exercise are worth remembering, too. Exercise is a great stress reducer. Women who exercise regularly report improved mental capacity and outlook, better self-image and self-confidence, higher energy levels, and more restful sleep. Exercise conditions not only the body, but the mind.

months and about 1 pound per week thereafter. Women who are overweight at the beginning of pregnancy should gain less, but at least a total of 16 to 24 pounds. Underweight women should gain more. When you are pregnant, try to avoid too many high-fat, empty-calorie foods. They'll put on extra pounds that may be difficult to lose later.

Protein needs during pregnancy increase from the usual 50 grams per day to a total of 60. However, many women in the United States already get this much or more in their usual diets. You can get this amount from four 8-ounce glasses of milk (32 grams of protein) and 4 ounces of meat, fish, poultry, or cheese (28 grams of protein).

A pregnant woman's recommended daily allowance of folic acid to support both the baby's growth and her own increasing blood volume is twice the usual. Don't forget that folic acid deficiency can cause serious birth defects. At least 400 micrograms per day is now recommended for anyone even contemplating pregnancy. Prenatal vitamins easily supply this amount.

Remember, too, that if the mother doesn't get plenty of calcium, her baby will simply withdraw what it needs for its own bone and teeth development from her bones. The recommended allowance for calcium during pregnancy and while breastfeeding is 1,200 milligrams per day—hence the recommendation for 4 daily servings of milk or milk products.

The baby's development and increased maternal blood volume also boost the need for iron. With the RDA doubling to 30 milligrams per day, many pregnant women need to supplement their high-iron foods with additional iron. Pregnancy means the need for additional fluids, too—about an extra 2 quarts per day. Breastfeeding mothers continue to need extra nutrients, including calcium, to produce milk for the growing infant. Producing milk requires about 750 extra calories a day.

The Later Years

From middle age onward, your focus needs to turn to a heart–healthy diet, high in fiber, and low in fat to help with weight control. The way you eat at 30, 40, and 50 can make a big difference in your quality of life later on. While some weight gain with age may be normal, there is much you can do to stay trim. Limiting fat intake to less than 30 percent of your daily calories is an excellent start; and cutting back on fat is the easiest way of holding down total calories, too: Every gram of fat you trim from your diet saves you 9 calories. Remember that your future bone health relies on continued intakes of calcium and vitamin D, particularly after menopause. And given all the known and suspected health benefits of fruits and vegetables, plan on making them a major part of your diet—at least 5 servings per day.

Nutritional needs continue to change for women over 50, but by how much is uncertain. At present, recommended daily allowances are the same for everyone in this age group, but individual needs may differ. For example, stomach acid secretion, which aids digestion, decreases with age in some people, but not in others.

Dehydration becomes more common as we age. The elderly may have a less sensitive thirst mechanism, pay less attention to it, or simply have more trouble getting to a glass of water when they want one. The result can be lethargy, muscle weakness, and constipation, symptoms often written off as "normal" in the elderly. The standard 6 to 8 glasses of fluid per day is as important to the elderly as to anyone else.

Since older people tend to eat less, they need to make every meal count, with a highly nutritious, well–balanced diet, even if chewing problems dictate the need for softer foods. They should get as much fiber as possible to avoid constipation, plenty of calcium–containing foods to control osteoporosis, and perhaps some extra iron and zinc, both of which tend to be deficient in the elderly. (Zinc deficiency can cause taste changes and poor wound healing. Zinc is found in meat, seafood, grains, and vegetables.) If it's impossible to get a fully balanced diet, a multivitamin with minerals is in order.

The Bottom Line

For some women, food is a challenge, for others a compulsion. But food is not like cigarettes or alcohol—you cannot quit if eating gets out of control. Instead, you must strike a balance. There are no good and bad foods, only those that should be eaten more or less often. If your usual diet is rich in complex carbohydrates and low in fat, an occasional celebration will do you no harm. If you eat out daily, with a little bit of knowledge and some judicious choices, you can manage that, too. While you focus on cutting back on fat, increase your intake of health–protecting fruits, vegetables, and grains. Think of healthy eating as a life–style choice, not a diet. The changes you make should be livable enough to last a lifetime.

Here are the steps you need to take to keep your diet healthy:

(1) Put your low–fat diet into practice by pin-pointing sources of fat. Butter, margarine, vegetable oil, lard, shortening, mayonnaise, salad dressings, gravies, cream, sour cream, and cream sauces are almost exclusively fat. Other foods like meats, cheese, nuts, snack foods, ice cream, milk chocolate, and many baked and fried foods derive many of their calories from fat. Your goal is to keep total fat–derived calories below 30 percent on average. If you hit 40 percent one day, balance it out with 20 percent the next. Short of calculating out everything you eat, the best approach is to:

- Limit added fats, or substitute low–fat or fat–free alternatives, like low–fat mayonnaise or fat–free salad dressing.
- Trim visible fat from meat, and remove skin from poultry.
- Grill, roast, bake, barbecue, broil, stir–fry, microwave, or poach foods, but don't deep fry. (Frying foods drastically increases calories.)
- Use nonstick pans or nonstick spray if frying. Sauté in broth instead of oil.
- Choose lean cuts of meat like beef round.
- Use skimmed milk instead of whole milk or cream in recipes.
- Skim fat from homemade soups.
- Order fast–food burgers and grilled chicken sandwiches without their mayonnaise–based sauces.
- Opt for cereal, bagels, or English muffins for breakfast. Croissants and commercially–made muffins are usually loaded with fat.
- Try fat–free cream cheese, jam, jelly, or fruit spread on bagels or toast.
- Snack on low–fat pretzels, rice or corn cakes, animal crackers, fruit, or dry cereal.

Keep high–fat snacks out of the house. Better still, skip snacks.
- Read labels. Ingredients are listed according to quantity, from the highest to the lowest. New labeling laws require useful information, such as the amount of saturated fat in an item and the percentage of fat–derived calories it contains.
- When determining grams of fat consumed, pay attention to serving sizes. You may be eating 2 servings or more.

(2) Keep cholesterol intake to less than 300 milligrams per day.

(3) Eat 5 or more servings of fruits and vegetables per day, especially those high in vitamin C, vitamin A, beta carotene, and fiber. In general, a serving is 1 small piece of fruit, half a cup of cooked or canned fruits and vegetables, or 1 cup raw.

(4) Increase your intake of complex carbohydrates, especially whole grains. Experts recommend 6 or more servings of foods like bread, rice, pasta, cereal, and beans.

(5) Watch the size of your protein portion. Most women need a daily intake of only about 6 ounces (cooked) of meat, chicken, fish, or a substitute like cheese or eggs. Excess protein can mean extra fat, and high amounts of protein may increase calcium losses in the urine.

(6) Drink alcohol in moderation. Excessive drinking is linked to osteoporosis. If you're pregnant, avoid alcohol entirely.

(7) Limit daily salt intake to 6,000 milligrams, preferably less. Watch your intake of salty, processed foods. Season with butter–flavored granules, lemon, vinegar, broth, wine, garlic, herbs, and spices instead of salt. (Your risk of developing high blood pressure increases with age.)

(8) Adopt a high–calcium diet for life. Skim milk provides calcium and vitamin D without the fat and calories.

(9) Do not overdo supplements. Pills are no match for the nutrients found in food. Megadoses of vitamins act more like drugs than nutrients, and can even be dangerous.

(10) Keep an eye on your iron intake. Many women rely on iron–fortified cereals to contribute iron to their diets. You may need iron supplements during pregnancy, when increased needs exceed what even a high–iron diet can provide.

(11) If you're in your childbearing years, get at least 0.4 milligram (400 micrograms) of folic acid daily to reduce the risk of having a child with a neural tube defect. Excellent sources are spinach, broccoli, chickpeas, romaine lettuce, wheat germ, and fortified breakfast cereals (25 percent of the US RDA per ounce). If you're pregnant, take a folic acid supplement. □

CHAPTER 16

GENERAL HEALTH CONCERNS

Plastic Surgery: What to Expect

Is there anyone who's completely thrilled with what nature—and genes—have given them? Don't we all have a secret little wish list of body parts that could stand improvement? Today, it seems as though all you have to do is imagine a little tuck here, maybe a nice boost there, and plastic surgery makes it so.

Of course, it's not really that simple, but there has been a lot of progress in the past two decades: Procedures that were once exclusively the privilege of the rich and the famous are now being done for the rest of us. The surgery is safe and available, and can make a tremendous difference in the way you see yourself and how you face the world. You have to remember, though, that plastic surgery is a clinical procedure, not a panacea. It must be approached with realistic expectations. If you look for improvement rather than a miracle, you'll avoid a lot of disappointment. Here's a look at what's available, what it can do, and what's really involved.

Facialplasty: The Classic Facelift

Gravity and longevity are a formidable combination, leaving their mark on the skin and on all that lies beneath it. The skin shrinks here and sags there, thins out, and becomes increasingly susceptible to the damage caused by exposure to the sun.

Sad to say, our faces begin to rearrange much earlier than most of us would like to admit. "Crow's feet," those short straight lines radiating from the outer edge of the eyes, can appear any time after the age of 30. Skin in the upper eyelids loosens as well. Creases in the forehead, between the eyebrows, and around the nose and mouth suddenly seem more noticeable when a woman reaches her 40s. By the age of 50, the neck starts to wrinkle, the jawline seems to blur, and the tip of the nose may look a bit droopy. Although signs of age appear at different times in different women, facial wrinkling and sagging become hard to ignore by the sixth decade of life.

A facelift (facialplasty) can turn the clock back a few years. Such procedures have been done since the early 1900s, but the modern era of facelifting dates from the 1970s when plastic surgeons began using techniques that correct the age–related changes that occur deep beneath the skin.

While a properly performed facelift will make a woman look younger, the procedure won't work miracles. Surgery can't transform you into a "different" woman, or save a marriage. One of the toughest jobs facing a plastic surgeon is deciding who will truly benefit from the surgery and who is likely to be disappointed.

Planning and Preparing for Surgery

Careful questioning during the first appointment helps doctors identify women who expect the impossible. If you have trouble describing exactly what you want to change or seem distraught about a relatively minor "deformity," you are *not* a good candidate for a facelift, and probably won't receive one.

If the doctor thinks plastic surgery would be good for you, he or she will ask about your medical history, any allergies, previous surgery, reactions to medication, and personal habits such as smoking.

Anything that may interfere with natural blood clotting mechanisms such as high blood pressure and medicines containing aspirin, poses the danger of excess bleeding and must be avoided. Smoking causes skin sloughing, in which areas of skin literally slide off the face, leading to additional scars. Surgery may therefore be delayed for several weeks until your blood pressure has dropped to normal levels, for example. Aspirin and smoking are banned for at least two weeks before surgery.

Preparations for surgery include a comprehensive physical examination. The doctor also checks every part of the face for creases, wrinkles, lines, puffiness, and sagging. The doctor will assess your skin's thickness, elasticity, and mobility; check the jaw and neck for fatty deposits; examine the thickness of the hair and note the location of the hairline; and document any previous surgical incisions and scars. An assistant will then take a series of photographs which the surgeon will use to plan the operation and explain the procedure to you. The photographs will also remind you later of how you looked before surgery. Such photo sessions are standard before just about any kind of plastic surgery.

The doctor will explain the surgical plan feature by feature. Some trouble spots can be improved but not eliminated. Forehead lines, crow's feet, and creases around the nose and mouth can be softened, for example, but not removed altogether. Fine wrinkles can, however, be treated with a chemical face peel after the area has healed.

Facelifts involve close work around the mouth and hairline, where bacteria hide in large numbers. To minimize contamination, you will be asked to remove all makeup the night before surgery and to scrub your face and wash your hair and scalp with a medicated soap.

The Operation

Your hair will be combed away from your face. Antibiotic ointment may be combed into your hair to flatten it and prevent infection. You'll take antibiotic medication and perhaps a sedative as well.

The surgeon will place marks on your face as a surgical "blueprint" just before you receive general anesthesia.

The relatively small facialplasty incisions, next to each ear, give the surgeon full access to

THE SURGICAL REMEDY FOR SAGGING SKIN

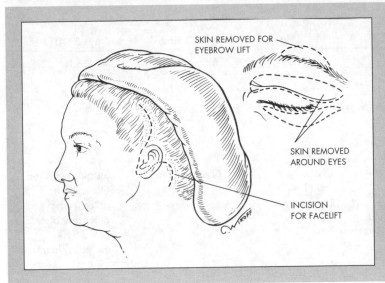

SKIN REMOVED FOR
EYEBROW LIFT

SKIN REMOVED
AROUND EYES

INCISION
FOR FACELIFT

A facelift can't produce perfection, but it can reduce the bags, wrinkles, and creases that come with advancing age. Tucked under the hairline and behind the ears, the basic incisions are almost unnoticeable. Separate invisible incisions alleviate baggy eyes. Be prepared, though, for a long convalescence: it can take up to 3 months for swelling and bruising to totally disappear.

the face, from cheeks to chin. The forehead, eyes, and nose are done with separate incisions. Electrocautery is used to singe the blood vessels and minimize bleeding. The skin is pulled tight, redraped, and tacked down in two spots above and behind the ear. The surgeon trims the extra skin and closes the incision. The procedure is then repeated on the other side of the face.

After the Operation

After the procedure, an elastic net dressing that leaves only a small part of the face and eyes exposed will cushion the skin flaps and absorb drainage from the wounds. This dramatic mummy–like dressing helps remind you to let your face rest.

Dietary restrictions are necessary after facial surgery to limit the nausea and vomiting induced by anesthesia. Furthermore, chewing can cause bleeding. You'll start out on clear liquids and quickly progress to a full liquid diet. Soft foods are added the day after

surgery. If all goes well, you can return to your usual menu the day after that.

Movement is discouraged for 24 hours. Don't talk on the phone and walk as little as possible. Keep your head still and slightly elevated at a 30–degree angle. After 24 hours, you can resume light activity. Most surgeons keep their facialplasty patients in the hospital for at least one night.

You'll wash your hair on the third day after surgery and at least every other day after that, to keep the incisions clean. The stitches will be removed on days 5 through 10 after surgery.

You can expect swelling, black–and–blue marks, and numbness for many weeks after a facelift. Most women are confident enough to venture out of the house after a few weeks although all swelling and bruising may not disappear for 3 months. Sun block is strongly recommended for the first 6 months.

AFTER A FACELIFT

	Day 1 (First 24 hours After Surgery)	Day 2 (24–48 Hours)	Day 3 (48–72 Hours)	Days 5–10
Diet	Clear liquids, then full liquid diet (to prevent nausea and vomiting due to anesthesia). No chewing (causes bleeding).	Soft foods	All foods	All foods
Activities	Overnight in hospital. No phone calls. Very little walking. Head slightly elevated. No bathing or showering.	Discharged from hospital. Light activity.	Shampoo hair.	Stitches removed. Shampoo hair at least every other day after day 3 (to keep incisions clean).

Several complications can follow facialplasty:

Hematomas. The most common problem you may encounter is the formation of a hematoma, the pooling of blood under the skin. If too much blood collects—a situation that occurs only 10 percent of the time—the surgeon pierces the skin and drains it. Most "major" hematomas appear within the first 10 to 12 hours after surgery. Another 10 to 15 percent of patients develop smaller hematomas, many of which aren't noticed until the swelling goes down.

Skin sloughing. This happens most often in the skin around the ear, where the skin is especially thin and is also geographically farthest from the circulation system that supplies blood to facial structures. Superficial skin sloughs (in the top layer of the skin) may leave little or no scarring. In the 1 to 3 percent of facialplasty patients who develop deeper, full–thickness skin sloughs, however, some amount of scarring is inevitable. The risk of skin sloughing is up to 12 times greater in cigarette smokers than in nonsmokers.

Numbness. Your face may feel numb for 2 to 6 weeks after surgery. The reason is that lifting the skin disrupts the sensory nerves that provide feeling to it. Disturbing a facial nerve branch can interfere with your ability to move parts of your face. Full movement usually returns within a few weeks to a year after the injury, but can sometimes take even longer.

Scars. Facelift scars tend to fade away, becoming virtually invisible. The scars can become more evident if the blood supply to the skin flaps was compromised during surgery or the skin was pulled too tight, causing tension on the incision.

Hair loss. About 1 to 3 percent of people who have had facialplasty lose some hair, usually around the temples, where the incision interrupted the blood supply.

Dark Spots. Patches of darker skin may appear when facial swelling prevents the diagnosis of small hematomas. In most cases, the skin gradually lightens back to normal, although the process can take 6 to 8 months. In rare cases, the darker spots become permanent.

Related Operations

Many women have other procedures performed along with facialplasty. Tightening the muscles in the neck and cheeks lifts and contours the cheeks, redefines the jawline, and eliminates "turkey neck." Some patients request cheek implants; others have fat removed from their cheeks. Silicone chin implants are another common request; a small implant can dramatically improve a formerly chinless profile. Chemical peels remove the fine spiderweb of wrinkles that a facelift can't touch. Dermabrasion smoothes deep pitting or scarring.

Chemical Peel

A chemical peel erases the wrinkles that remain after a facelift. The procedure is also used to treat discolored spots on the skin. Because the line between peeled and unpeeled skin blends more evenly in lighter skin, results tend to be best in women with fair complexions.

Chemical peeling can be performed on wrinkles in some areas, such as those around the mouth, at the same time as facelift surgery. A lower eyelid peel, on the other hand, is never done at the same time as eyelid surgery. To prevent heavy scarring extensive peeling is postponed until after the facelift heals.

The peeling procedure is simple. A small amount of a chemical solution, usually phenol, is applied to the face with a cotton-tipped swab. The skin is gently stretched to allow the fluid inside the wrinkles. The solution is applied all the way to the hairline so that no line will be visible between treated and untreated skin.

When the solution dries, the skin will have a white, frosted appearance. The face should not be washed for 24 to 48 hours. After about 10 days, the "crust" falls off to reveal the smooth, pink skin. Normal color returns to the skin within 6 to 12 weeks.

Irregular heartbeat is the most common complication associated with phenol peels. This problem can be avoided by applying the solution to small areas of the face one at a time over the course of an hour.

Chemical peels always create some redness, which generally lasts no more than 6 weeks. Some people, especially those with darker skin, notice that their skin is lighter or that they develop a blotchy sunburn. Scarring is uncommon but will occur if aggressive peeling is done in combination with an extensive facelift or if the peel is done on the neck.

Dermabrasion

When skin irregularities cannot be treated by facelift or chemical peeling, they can be "sanded off." The procedure is most effective in repairing the pits that result from deep scarring, such as from severe acne.

Dermabrasion wears down the raised areas of skin around the depression so that the difference in elevation is less noticeable. The results are permanent; once the skin has been thinned, it never regains its former thickness.

The procedure can be performed under either local or general anesthesia. There is a small amount of bleeding as the skin is scraped. Ointment is sometimes applied afterward. The deeper the abrasion, the longer it takes to heal.

Women with fair skin tend to have the best results. Those with darker skin may notice a change in skin color as they heal. The procedure causes a certain amount of redness, which can persist for several months. Because the skin is more sensitive after dermabrasion, direct sunlight should be avoided for several months.

Forehead and Brow Lift

A facelift tightens only the lower part of the face. It will not correct age–related "defects" above the cheeks. At the initial evaluation, the plastic surgeon may recommend separate procedures on the eyelids or forehead to correct such problems. These operations can be performed separately or in combination with the facelift.

A forehead and brow lift is generally recommended to counteract sagging and to reduce creases and wrinkles across the forehead and between the eyebrows. This procedure also corrects baggy upper eyelids. A forehead and brow lift can help eliminate eyelid fullness that cannot be corrected by eyelid surgery alone.

An aging forehead dramatically affects the appearance of the rest of the face. The forehead muscle is stimulated by nerves that can cause wrinkles. With time, the wrinkles gain prominence and the brow sags. As the skin pushes downward, the eyelids become puffier, and the skin on the nose may even slide down the bridge so that the tip appears to droop.

Repeated muscle contractions in the forehead create lines and creases. The scowling facial expression that results eventually pulls the forehead further downward. The contrac-

tions also pull the nasal skin upward, causing wrinkles and creases around the nose.

The operation is tailored to individual needs. The surgeon checks the position of the upper eyelids and eyebrows and gently pushes the forehead up towards the hairline. If the surplus eyelid skin "disappears," a forehead and brow lift alone will work well. If too much skin remains, eyelid surgery (blepharoplasty) will also be necessary.

In most cases, the incision for a forehead lift is made a couple of inches behind the hairline. It's not necessary to shave the hair. If facialplasty is also being done, the two procedures are performed simultaneously and the respective incisions are joined.

Before you receive anesthesia, the surgeon will mark the incision line and the forehead and brow creases. The doctor then injects anesthetic solution into the incision line, across the top of the eyes and down to the top of the nose. This solution causes the blood vessels to constrict, thus limiting the amount of blood that can escape from the incision. A plastic lens may be placed on each eye to protect them during the operation.

A sagging forehead is corrected by stretching the skin up toward the hairline. Forehead lines are eased by removing some of the muscle that causes the creases. The skin is then brought back up over the forehead and held in place with surgical staples. The extra skin is trimmed and the wound is closed. The incision is covered with gauze. The same type of elastic dressing is used as after a facelift.

Pressure and mild discomfort are the most common complaints after a forehead and brow lift. Hematomas are rare. Since your eyes may not close completely for the first day, you'll be given special ointment to keep the corneas from drying out. Swelling and bruising around the eyes are often greater on the second or third day.

If you've not had any other surgery, the dressing can be removed after the first day. If you've also had a facelift, the forehead dressing will be left in place for an extra day. Daily hair washing is allowed starting on the second or third day after the forehead and brow lift.

Although hematomas are rare with this surgery, the potential consequences in terms of hair loss can be worrisome. A patient complaining of pain will be watched very closely. Patients generally don't lose much hair unless the skin was pulled too tight when the incision was sutured. Patients with thin, fine hair are more likely to notice some hair loss, particularly where the staples were placed. When hair loss occurs during routine brushing and combing, the problem is likely to continue for as long as 3 to 6 weeks.

Muscle paralysis is rare and usually when it does occur, temporary. If you can move your forehead at all, you will eventually regain normal movement. Full recovery, however, can take as much as 10 to 12 months. You may also feel itching and numbness for 6 weeks or up to 6 months.

Eye Tuck

The first signs of aging generally appear around the eyes. When a woman reaches 30, the forehead begins its downward descent, taking the eyebrows along with it. The downward pressure bunches up the sagging skin and gives the upper eyelid a hooded appearance. These effects intensify with age. Blepharoplasty, which tightens the eyelids, is usually more effective after a forehead and

brow lift has reduced the amount of skin around the eyes.

During your evaluation, the surgeon will explain that incisions within the eyelid usually heal without noticeable scars. The surgical technique will be tailored according to your goals, the amount of muscle relaxation and sagging in each eyelid, and whether you are also getting a forehead and a brow lift. The plastic surgeon may check with an ophthalmologist about your vision and the possibility of glaucoma.

Many surgeons perform blepharoplasty with local anesthesia and a sedative. This surgery requires close work, with a very bright light shining into your eyes. The doctor may cover your eyes with ointment to protect against dryness and possible injury if an eye is scraped by gauze. Ointment is reapplied after surgery.

The surgical technique is basically the same as for facelifts and forehead lifts. The skin is freed from underlying tissue, pulled tight, trimmed, and sutured. The surgeon may also remove fat deposits to eliminate bags under the eyes. Note: If the plastic surgeon overcorrects the eyelid problem, the skin may be too tight, leaving a perpetually surprised look.

After the operation, cold compresses for the first 24 hours reduce swelling and help ward off feelings of claustrophobia from having your eyes bandaged. The eyelids will not close completely at first. This situation gradually corrects itself as swelling subsides and the eyes regain their muscle tone. If the problem persists, there are several exercises and techniques that can help return the eyes to normal. Examples include tightly closing your eyes to strengthen the eyelids and taping them shut when asleep.

Makeup is banned for 2 weeks after blepharoplasty. After that time, women are cautioned to remove their makeup as gently as possible.

Rhinoplasty: Refashioning the Nose

What is sometimes disparagingly called a "nose job" can do much more than create a smaller, cuter nose. In addition to improving appearance, it gives an opportunity to correct any breathing problems you may have.

The nose is a complex structure consisting of an outer layer that slides over the semi–rigid inner layer of cartilage and lining. The two layers work together in a delicate balance. Any manipulation of either can upset the equilibrium and lead to serious physical and aesthetic problems. An aggressive attempt to reduce the size of the nose can compromise its underlying structure. The cartilage could collapse and obstruct the airway.

Surgeons prevent this type of problem by rearranging, rather than reducing, the underlying skeletal structure, reshaping the nasal contour while preserving nasal function. The trouble is that many prospective patients don't understand that rhinoplasty is always a compromise.

Explaining what can and cannot be accomplished is a considerable challenge for the surgeon. One important point to remember is that the nose is not perfectly symmetrical; the two sides develop independently.

Removing a hump or bump on the bridge of the nose may reveal a natural curve that

DECEPTIVE ANATOMY OF THE NOSE

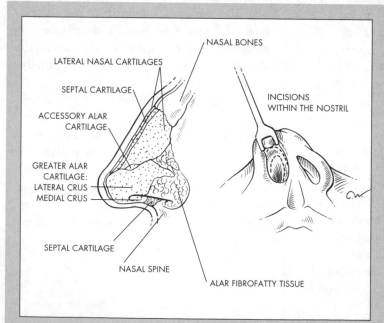

NASAL BONES

LATERAL NASAL CARTILAGES

SEPTAL CARTILAGE

ACCESSORY ALAR CARTILAGE

INCISIONS WITHIN THE NOSTRIL

GREATER ALAR CARTILAGE:
LATERAL CRUS
MEDIAL CRUS

SEPTAL CARTILAGE

NASAL SPINE

ALAR FIBROFATTY TISSUE

Underlying the smooth exterior of the nose is a hodgepodge of bone, cartilage, fatty tissue, and mucous membrane. It's no wonder, then, that rhinoplasty is a highly individual operation, and that a second operation is occasionally needed to make adjustments for the first. You can count on a protracted recovery period, too: anywhere from 3 months to a year.

must then be camouflaged by another procedure. Trimming a bulbous tip may throw off the proportions of the rest of the nose; what looks good in profile may be unattractive when seen from the front.

Planning and Preparing

At your first appointment, the surgeon will take photos from all angles and ask you to explain what you consider good and bad about your nose. The nature of your complaints will influence the surgery, too. There is a big difference between "my nose is too large" and "I can't breathe."

The surgeon will use a model of the nose to describe what will be reduced, what may need to be enlarged (augmented), and what should be left alone. If you already consider your nose too large, you may be surprised to hear the surgeon suggest augmentation. But adding a little bit here or there can make another part of the nose look smaller without interfering with the airway.

It is important to understand the finer points of rhinoplasty and to agree with your surgeon on the approach to be used. You'll also need to accept the surgeon's priorities of safety, function, and appearance, in that order, and be willing to live with the potential consequences and complications.

Sometimes a second operation is required to modify the results of the first one or to make additional changes after the nose has healed. Also, some "defects" must be corrected in stages in order to keep a passage open for air.

Rhinoplasty encompasses several procedures. As a result, it's hard to generalize. The surgeon can't always predict the complete anatomy of a nose or visualize its volume and texture until it has been opened for surgery. A standard procedure to correct a specific problem may have to be modified once surgery begins.

After the Operation

You'll wake up after rhinoplasty to find your nose packed with bandages layered around plastic tubes called suction catheters, placed to keep the nasal airway open. Many people find that they can breathe much more easily than before, catheters and all. Depending on the type of surgery and the amount of bleeding, the packing will remain in place for 24 hours to a week.

Bleeding is fairly common with certain procedures and can be frightening. The more upset you get, the more likely you are to bleed. Often, simply remaining calm will dramatically reduce the blood flow. Infection is rare. The nasal packs are sometimes covered with antibiotic ointment, especially when packing must remain in place for several days or more.

Healing can take as long as a year. The nose continues to contract for several weeks after surgery. The outer layer of skin feels hard and remains stiff for up to 3 months and maybe for as long as a year. The tip of the nose will probably rotate slightly. Swelling seen from the front disappears slowly, and the nose will look bigger than it really is until the swelling has subsided.

Sometimes subsequent surgical "rehabilitation" is necessary to fine-tune nasal function or appearance. If so, the follow-up procedure will be scheduled after healing is complete, usually in 6 months to 1 year.

A person who has realistic goals is likely to be very happy with her "new" nose. A patient who expects the impossible, however, is sure to be disappointed.

Breast Augmentation

Society's preoccupation with large breasts has caused unhappiness in quite a few women with small ones. Breast augmentation to make up for nature's "shortcomings" can give a major boost to a woman's self–esteem. Having bigger breasts won't guarantee happiness or solve emotional or psychological problems. But, when performed for the right reasons, breast augmentation can greatly improve a woman's outlook on life.

Breast augmentation surgery first gained popularity when the silicone gel prosthesis was developed in 1963. Over the years, a variety of implants became available. Today, however, for a variety of legal and regulatory reasons, only the saline–filled silicone implant is in general use. Fortunately, this implant does a relatively good job. Besides the fact that saline (salt–water solution) is considered by many to be safer than silicone gel, breasts augmented with saline–filled implants are less likely to get firm or hard. The trade–off is that saline implants are not quite as soft as those filled with silicone gel and, if they develop a leak, will quickly go flat and need to be replaced.

The controversy over silicone gel implants remains unresolved. There is no conclusive scientific evidence that this type of implant poses a significant health hazard. Nevertheless, there have been accusations that it does and there are still unanswered questions. The best guess among the experts is that when all the information comes in, silicone gel implants will be shown to be either entirely safe (if anything can truly be said to be entirely safe) or to pose a risk to only a very tiny minority of women who develop unusual reactions to them. For now, however, the best advice is to use saline–filled implants.

Planning and Preparing

The evaluation for breast augmentation begins with a complete medical and personal history. The doctor will ask whether you have ever had breast disease, cysts, or breast pain or tenderness. Information about your life-style and recreational activities will help the surgeon design breasts that look natural when you engage in your usual activities.

The next step is a thorough examination of your "old" breasts. The doctor will see whether both breasts look the same (symmetry) and evaluate the elasticity of your skin to determine whether it will be able to stretch enough to accommodate an implant. Any congenital deformities and pronounced scars are noted. The doctor will look at the angle formed by the breast against the chest to determine the possible effects of heavier, implanted breasts and whether you will be able to support them.

If a breast mass or any other abnormality is found during the physical examination of the breasts, or if the medical history reveals any worrisome or questionable condition, the doctor will order further tests.

The psychological evaluation is just as important as the physical findings. Some women have unrealistic expectations and think that new breasts will solve all their problems. Any reputable doctor who suspects that a woman expects too much from the operation or is emotionally unstable will postpone surgery and recommend counseling.

The surgeon can't promise you a specific bra cup size or measurement. A lot depends on your weight. An extremely small–breasted woman with tight skin may be able to handle

THREE ROUTES FOR IMPLANT SURGERY

Although breast implants always wind up in roughly the same position, the best route inward can vary. Here are the pros (and cons) of each major approach.

■ Inframammary:—in the fold underneath the breast. This site permits a large incision, which provides better access to the breast and makes it easier for the surgeon to avoid blood vessels and ducts while creating the pocket. The scar is concealed by the natural fold of the breast.

■ Periphery of the areola: around the edges of the areola, the area of darker skin that surrounds the nipple. The scar is naturally camouflaged by the areola. If the areola is small however, the incision may not be large enough to receive the implant.

■ Transaxillary: under the arm. The scar is hidden beneath the arm. Drawbacks: The surgeon must cut through more tissue to reach the center of the breast, and may have more difficulty controlling bleeding.

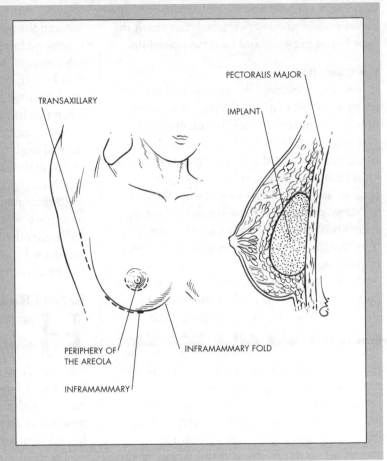

only a slight increase in breast size, followed by additional surgery after the skin has had time to stretch. A heavy woman, on the other hand, might notice only a slight change in her breasts even after receiving large implants.

It's important to agree with your surgeon about your goals for mammoplasty. While the doctor will certainly consider your wishes, final decisions regarding the size and volume of the implant must often be made in the operating room. Many surgeons favor a course of moderation to make sure the newly enlarged breasts don't overwhelm the woman's body.

As you discuss the operation the doctor will tell you about types of incisions and anesthesia, where and how the surgery will be performed, potential postoperative problems, and follow-up procedures. Photographs of both breasts are taken from the front and from each side. You will be instructed to avoid taking aspirin for 2 weeks before surgery and not to smoke for 1 week before and 1 week after surgery. Aspirin-induced bleeding could cause serious problems. Smoking leads to coughing, which places a strain on the chest. Smoking also causes blood vessels to constrict, which can result in high blood pressure and increased bleeding.

The Operation

During the operation, the surgeon will first create a pocket within the breast, then insert a prosthetic implant into it. The surgery can be performed in a hospital or in an outpatient clinic. General anesthesia is preferred, although local anesthesia can be used. The surgeon chooses an insertion site (see box nearby).

Many prefer the below–the–breast route, which provides good access, leaves a very thin scar, and usually makes a second incision unnecessary.

After forming the pocket, the surgeon decides what size the implant should be. Using a selection of sterile "sizer" implants, the surgeon literally begins trying them on for size. The temporary implants selected are placed in both breast pockets and gently manipulated to make sure the breasts appear natural. The two breasts are then compared from all angles to make sure they match. The next step is to raise the patient into a more vertical position. Overhead lights are aimed at the nipples from either side, and the surgical team moves to the foot of the table for yet another visual inspection. The woman is returned to the reclining position and the temporary sizers are replaced with permanent implants.

After the Operation

Dressings are removed after 24 hours, at which point you may bathe or shower as usual. Wearing a brassiere is optional. The ban on smoking continues for a full week after surgery. Vigorous physical exercise is inadvisable for 3 weeks. You may be asked to move the implant upwards and sideways once or twice a day. Sutures are removed 7 to 10 days after the operation.

Improved surgical techniques have greatly reduced the problems that were formerly common after breast augmentation surgery. Infection and hematomas are now rare. There may be some discomfort, numbness, and thickened scarring. The skin may be highly sensitive when touched or lack normal sensation.

Some complications occur as part of the normal healing process. For example, the skin and tissue may constrict or tighten around the prosthesis, causing the implant to feel firmer than expected. This most often happens 6 to 12 months after surgery and represents the body's natural response to a foreign substance. If necessary, the situation can be corrected surgically.

Breast Reduction

Heavy, sagging breasts often lead to neck and back pain and soreness where the brassiere straps cut into the shoulders. Rashes or sores can develop under very large breasts due to their constant contact with the chest wall. This chronic problem is aggravated by perspiration in hot, humid weather.

Tremendous breasts can cause no end of embarrassment or simply get in the way. An out–of–proportion chest makes exercise difficult and causes many women to feel that they are not taken seriously in their professional lives.

Reduction mammoplasty, which solves these problems, is not some 1990s fitness fad. This surgery is believed to date as far back as the mid–1600s. It is typically performed on young women in their late teens to early 20s, after the breasts have stopped growing. The psychological benefits of resembling one's peers during the emotionally traumatic teenage years, however, make surgery a wise choice for many young girls, even if more surgery is needed for additional growth later.

Some women in their 60s and 70s enthusiastically choose reduction mammoplasty to resolve a lifelong problem. There are physical benefits for older women as well. As a woman ages, it can become increasingly difficult for the skeletal system to support heavy breasts.

Planning and Preparing

Before reduction mammoplasty, a screening mammogram x–ray is done so that the surgeon can rule out the possibility of encountering a mass or lump during the operation. Another mammogram will be taken a few months after surgery to serve as a basis for comparison with future x–rays.

Reduction mammoplasty entails removing large amounts of breast tissue, which is full of blood vessels and capillaries. Because a considerable amount of blood may be lost during surgery, women who plan to have this operation are advised to donate 2 units of blood beforehand. If a transfusion is necessary, for safety's sake it can then be done with their own blood.

The Operation

In the operating room, you'll sit on the side of the operating table as the surgeon quickly marks your breasts to indicate what parts will be removed. The procedure itself will vary according to the methods chosen to remove the skin and tissue and the planned location and appearance of the scar. Tissue is removed on either side of a vertical strip containing the areola and nipple. This strip of skin and tissue, which runs the entire length of the breast, from top to bottom, is called a

pedicle. The pedicle protects the nerves and blood supply to the nipple and areola.

The surgeon weighs the amount of tissue removed from each breast to keep the reduction equal. The final size and symmetry, of course, will depend more on what remains than on what was removed.

Once enough tissue has been removed, the surgeon makes a cosmetic tuck at the top of the pedicle, moving the nipple and areola into their new position, and begins to close the skin around the breasts. If one breast appears to be larger or fuller than the other, the surgeon may decide to remove additional tissue and improve the match.

The marking that takes place before surgery begins is one of the most critical aspects of the procedure. If the surgeon moves the nipple and areola too high, they will seem to sit unnaturally on top of the breast instead of at the tip. The surgeon must also anticipate the "dropout" effect that will occur as the breast slowly settles into place. As gravity and time move the tissue within the breast, the breast volume can shift, leaving the nipple and areola out of place. This condition can be corrected by additional cosmetic surgery, but only with difficulty.

After the Operation

The nipple and areola area also causes concern after surgery, as the surgeon waits to make sure this important tissue has survived the procedure. The surgeon checks the color of the nipple and areola on each breast soon after surgery to make sure the blood supply is still in good shape. If the surgeon has any reason to suspect a problem during surgery, a fluorescein dye may be injected to trace the movement of blood through the breast.

You can probably leave the hospital within 2 days of this surgery. You'll be told to wear a brassiere 24 hours a day for the next 2 weeks.

Nipple Grafting

This procedure involves removing most of the breast, reshaping the remaining tissue, and grafting the nipple and areola back onto the new breast. The nipple and areola are removed quickly and placed on a moist saline sponge. The surgeon then removes much of the breast tissue, creates a pocket within the breast, and inserts the remaining breast tissue. The skin is gathered around the new breast, which takes shape as the surgeon begins to suture the skin. The nipple and areola are then sutured in place. The major concern during surgery is the possibility of amputating too much breast tissue and thus having too little left over to create the new breast.

One advantage of this free nipple grafting technique is that it enables the surgeon to fashion an attractive breast from scratch. It's especially useful when the woman has *very* large breasts. Because this type of surgery can be performed quickly, anesthesia is brief and blood loss is minimal.

Another advantage of the procedure for very large–breasted women is that it can be extremely difficult to protect the pedicle when there is extensive tissue removal. Reshaping a greatly reduced breast around a pedicle can also lead to a disappointing result in terms of the new breast's shape and form.

However, nipple grafting also has disadvantages: The nipple and areola are likely to look unnatural and may not even survive. Their color may fade, which is a particular problem for women with darker skin. The nipple will lose all sensation and fail to become erect when stimulated. Breastfeeding is no longer an option once the milk ducts have been greatly rearranged if not removed entirely.

This procedure is considered preferable to reduction when the nipple and areola must be moved up by more than 6 inches. It is also a good choice for elderly women who don't consider nipple sensation a top priority. While surgeons tend to avoid using this procedure in younger women, those with particularly massive breasts commonly have relatively little nipple sensation before surgery anyway.

Breast Lift

One of the more pleasant aftereffects of breast reduction surgery is that the remodeled breasts are higher and tighter. Mastopexy is the name of the procedure that lifts the recently reduced breast into its new position. Mastopexy can be used to counteract the effects of time and gravity even when no surgery is done to alter breast size.

Aging is not kind to the breasts. The skin stretches, the volume of the breast thins out, and the breast loses its firmness and begins to sag. Pregnancy, weight loss, breastfeeding, and menopause all speed the natural aging process. The stretch marks that may linger after pregnancy make the breasts look flabbier than they really are. Rapid weight loss can have the same effect.

Mastopexy is performed with local anesthesia in an outpatient facility. Nipple placement is the most crucial part of the operation. After selecting the new nipple site,

ARE YOU A CANDIDATE FOR CONTOUR SURGERY?

If you are...	And your problem is...	You should...
Under age 20, with firm skin and no flabbiness	Irregular fat deposits in one or more locations	Consider liposuction; you are definitely not a candidate for surgery.
Between 20 and 35 years of age, in good shape, with no flabby skin or major bulges	Fat deposits	Stick with liposuction; for large deposits, 6–month intervals between procedures will allow skin to tighten without surgical assistance.
Any age	Loose skin	Consider surgery to tighten and contour; if you have fat deposits, consider liposuction as well.

the surgeon marks the areola, which stretches with time like the rest of the breast. If this circle of tissue isn't trimmed, it will appear to cover a disproportionate amount of the newly tightened breast.

Even mastopexy can't eliminate the constant pull of gravity. Some additional sagging is expected about 6 months after surgery. The surgeon plans for the inevitable by making the lift a little tight.

If the breasts start sagging right away or if the sagging is excessive, the surgeon can do a minor revision in the office. Women who had serious sagging before surgery undergo a remodeling procedure similar to breast reduction. Other women have breast augmentation in conjunction with mastopexy.

After surgery, you'll wear a brassiere 24 hours a day for 6 weeks. The brassiere acts as a bandage while providing support. The breasts may look strange at first—somewhat flat, with the nipples pointing downward—but this situation generally corrects itself within a few months.

Although some scarring is inevitable, most of it can be hidden in the natural breast fold. Some women notice a loss of cleavage. Despite the disadvantages, mastopexy provides good–looking breasts that are tighter, firmer and back to a higher point on the chest, where they belong.

Body Contour Surgery

Body contour surgery (torsoplasty) is basically an aesthetic tune–up for the entire body. The surgical team develops a plan to lift and reshape any desired combination of the breasts, abdomen, buttocks, thighs, flanks, and upper arms.

Surgery can be performed all at once or in stages. The decision depends on many factors, including age, weight, overall health, and the amount of tissue that must be removed.

A full torso overhaul takes 5 to 6 hours. Cumulative blood loss is a concern. Women scheduled for three or more procedures as well as liposuction donate at least 2 units of their own blood before surgery. This assures an infection–free supply in case transfusion is necessary.

For women over age 50, surgery is usually done in two stages, with at least a 3 months between operations.

Liposuction, which involves removing fat deposits through a medical "vacuum cleaner," is an even more accessible form of full–body surgery. It can be done more quickly than more traditional types of surgery and is less invasive.

The various procedures used in body contouring follow the same basic protocol: The surgeon makes an incision, dissects the skin away from muscle and tissues, removes whatever needs to be removed, places the skin snugly back into position, trims any excess skin, and closes the incision.

Abdominal surgery (abdominoplasty, or "tummy tuck") restores elasticity, tightens the skin over the abdomen, and eliminates stretch marks. Flank surgery corrects flab below the waist and above the buttocks. Surgery on the buttocks makes them smaller, lifts them, removes dimples caused by years of gaining and losing weight, and improves their shape. Similarly, surgery on the thighs and upper arms tightens wobbly skin and removes excess volume with liposuction, which can create an even, pleasing contour. These operations can be performed in any combination. Work on the breasts and abdomen is by far the most popular.

Intravenous antibiotics usually are given during surgery and for up to 5 days afterward. A vacuum drain is placed in the stomach after abdominoplasty to remove fluids. The drain remains in place for most of the hospital stay, which is 3 days or longer.

After breast reduction, abdominoplasty or flank surgery, an elastic girdle and brassiere must be worn for 4 weeks. After liposuction alone, the girdle is worn for 10 days.

Once discharged, you'll stay home for the rest of the week. You may venture out during the second week until you begin to feel tired. Most women can resume their regular schedules, including driving, by the third week. They can swim and enjoy other outdoor activities 4 weeks after surgery and do moderate exercise after 8 weeks. Sunbathing is strongly discouraged for 4 months. The abdomen can develop a severe burn if exposed to direct sunlight before this time.

Making Your Decision

As you can see, plastic surgery is not something to undertake lightly. A facelift will disrupt your life for weeks or even months as you progress to full recovery. Work on your nose could take as long as a year to heal completely. In spite of it all, however, more and more women have decided that the prospect of many years of better looks and greater self–confidence outweighs the temporary pain and inconvenience they know to expect.

Is it right for you? Only you—and your doctor—can ultimately decide. □

CHAPTER 17   **FERTILITY AND FAMILY PLANNING**

How the Reproductive System Works

Human reproduction, always an object of the most intense interest, has lately become the darling of the media, the subject of innumerable television talk shows, magazine articles, and newspaper editorials. With each new medical breakthrough in fertility and family planning, the noise level grows higher. From elementary school onward we're now deluged with information—some factual, some not—on menstruation and menopause, conception and contraception.

Sorting it all out may seem impossible. But a reasonable understanding of the basics of reproduction can make the job easy. As you weigh your options, whether to encourage pregnancy or forestall it, your best resource is a working knowledge of the organs, glands, and hormones that prepare your body for motherhood.

A Quick Review of the Reproductive Anatomy

Our overview of the reproductive system begins at the external genital area— or **vulva**—which runs from the pubic area downward to the rectum. Two folds of fatty, fleshy tissue surround the entrance to the vagina and the urinary opening: the **labia majora,** or outer folds, and the **labia minora,** or inner folds, located under the labia majora. The **clitoris,** is a relatively short organ (less than one inch long), shielded by a hood of flesh. When stimulated sexually, the clitoris can become erect like a man's penis. The **hymen,** a thin membrane protecting the entrance of the vagina, stretches when you insert a tampon or have intercourse.

From this point onward, the reproductive system leads deeper and deeper into the body.

The Vagina

The vagina is a muscular, ridged sheath connecting the external genitals to the uterus, where the embryo grows into a fetus during pregnancy. In the reproductive process, the vagina functions as a two-way street, accepting the penis and sperm during intercourse and roughly nine months later, serving as the avenue of birth through which the new baby enters the world .

The Cervix

The vagina ends at the cervix, the lower portion or neck of the uterus. Like the vagina, the cervix has dual reproductive functions.

After intercourse, sperm ejaculated in the vagina pass through the cervix, then proceed through the uterus to the **fallopian tubes** where, if a sperm encounters an ovum (egg), conception occurs. The cervix is lined with mucus, the quality and quantity of which is governed by monthly fluctuations in the levels of the two principle sex hormones, estrogen and progesterone.

When estrogen levels are low, the mucus tends to be thick and sparse, which makes it difficult for sperm to reach the fallopian tubes. But when an egg is ready for fertilization and estrogen levels are high the mucus then becomes thin and slippery, offering a much more friendly environment to sperm as they struggle towards their goal. (This phenomenon is employed by birth control pills, shots and implants. One of the ways they prevent conception is to render the cervical mucus thick, sparse, and hostile to sperm.)

Later, at the end of pregnancy, the cervix acts as the passage through which the baby exits the uterus into the vagina. The cervical canal expands to roughly 50 times its normal width in order to accommodate the passage of the baby during birth.

The Uterus

The uterus is the muscular organ which holds the developing baby during the nine months after conception. Like the cervical canal, the

HOW THE SYSTEM FITS TOGETHER

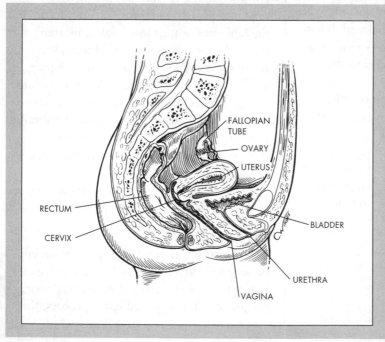

FALLOPIAN TUBE
OVARY
UTERUS
RECTUM
BLADDER
CERVIX
URETHRA
VAGINA

Deep within the pelvic region lie the specialized female organs that make conception and pregnancy possible. In this cutaway view, you can see how the cervix acts as the gateway between the vagina and the uterus, where an egg, if fertilized, will be nurtured and, over the course of nine months, grow to be a newborn child. Riding atop the uterus are the two ovaries, storehouse of all a woman's eggs. The fallopian tubes, where fertilization by a sperm will occur, are narrow conduits connecting each ovary to the uterus.

A CLOSER LOOK AT THE UTERUS

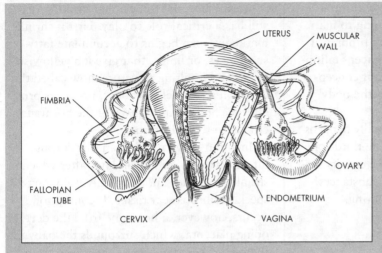

FIMBRIA
UTERUS
MUSCULAR WALL
FALLOPIAN TUBE
OVARY
CERVIX
ENDOMETRIUM
VAGINA

Note the thick muscular walls—crucial when the baby is ready for delivery—and the lush inner lining, or endometrium, which nurtures the developing egg. From this angle, you can also see how the fallopian tubes cradle the ovaries in their feathery fimbria, ready to conduct a mature egg away from the ovary and on into the uterus.

uterus expands considerably during the reproductive process. In fact, the organ grows to from 10 to 20 times its normal size during pregnancy.

Each month the uterus goes through a cyclical change, first building up its endometrium or inner lining to receive a fertilized egg, then, if conception does not occur, shedding the unused tissue through the vagina in the monthly process called menstruation.

The Fallopian Tubes

Beyond the uterus, the fallopian tubes connect the rest of the system to the ultimate source of the eggs, the two ovaries. Each of these tubes is roughly five inches long and ranges in width from about one inch at the end next to the ovary, to the diameter of a strand of thin spaghetti.

The trumpet-shaped part near the ovary has about 20 to 25 feathery projections called fimbria, one of which is attached to the ovary. It is the fimbria that each month urge an egg to exit the ovary and begin its trip towards the uterus.

The Ovaries

The ovaries are a woman's storehouse of egg cells. They are among the first organs to be formed as a female baby develops in the uterus. At the 20-week mark, the structures that will become the ovaries house roughly 6 to 7 million potential egg cells. From that point on, the number begins to decrease rapidly. A newborn infant has between 1 million to 2 million egg cells. By puberty the number has plummeted to 300,000. For every egg that matures and undergoes ovulation, roughly a thousand will fail, so that by menopause, only a few thousand remain. During the course of an average reproductive lifespan, roughly 300 mature eggs are produced for potential conception.

The egg cells remain inactive until puberty, when the reproductive system is activated by a cascade of substances called sex hormones. Then, each month about 20 egg cells, each encased in a sac called a follicle, begin to ripen. Responding selectively to the sex hormones, one follicle becomes dominant while the others shrink away. The egg within the dominant follicle continues ripening to maturity. Then, helped by the feathery fimbria, it exits the ovary and enters the adjacent fallopian tube to be either fertilized or, if conception fails to occur, expelled from the body during menstruation.

If fertilization is to occur, it usually happens when the egg's journey is about one-third complete. Once a sperm unites with the egg, its surrounding gelatinous coat releases substances that prevent more sperm from entering.

The Corpus Luteum

The fertilized egg then continues on its journey through the fallopian tube. About four or five days after fertilization, it enters the uterus and implants itself on the endometrium, which has been primed by the sex hormones to accept and nurture it.

Meanwhile, the follicle that held the egg still has a critical role to play. First it shrinks markedly, then begins to accumulate fatty substances, or lipids, that give it a yellowish tinge. The resulting structure, now called the corpus luteum (yellow body), produces progesterone and estradiol, two of the hormones critical to reproduction.

In a non-pregnant woman, the corpus luteum lasts for about 14 days, after which it shrinks and dries up, eventually becoming a speck of fibrous scar tissue. If conception occurs, however, a hormone from the developing placenta, which surrounds the baby in the uterus, stimulates the corpus luteum to maintain its production of progesterone during the first trimester of pregnancy.

FROM FOLLICLE TO "YELLOW BODY"

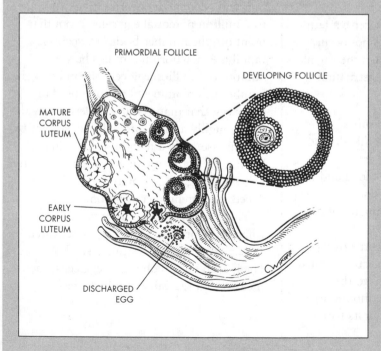

PRIMORDIAL FOLLICLE

DEVELOPING FOLLICLE

MATURE CORPUS LUTEUM

EARLY CORPUS LUTEUM

DISCHARGED EGG

Host to a lifetime supply of eggs, the ovaries each month launch about 20 contenders towards potential conception. Each ripens in a supporting follicle, growth of which is triggered by the aptly named "follicle-stimulating hormone." In turn, the winning follicle gives off increasing amounts of the hormone estrogen, which prepares the lining of the uterus for pregnancy. Once a mature egg has begun its trip through the fallopian tube, remnants of the winning follicle form the corpus luteum, or "yellow body." Progesterone from the corpus luteum halts development of the remaining follicles and brings the lining of the uterus to peak preparedness.

How Hormones Orchestrate Reproduction

Conception and pregnancy are governed by the ebb and flow of sex hormones that each month prompt crucial changes in your reproductive system. Production of these hormones depends, in turn, on the changes they themselves produce, so that an elegant cycle of feedback and response dictates their levels.

The most notable outward sign of this carefully balanced interplay is, of course, your monthly menstrual cycle or period. This cycle begins with your first day of menstrual bleeding and ends at the start of the next period. The average cycle is from 25 to 34 days and the average menstrual flow lasts from 3 to 5 days

The menstrual cycle has two distinct phases: the follicular (proliferative) phase during which the egg grows and gets ready to enter the fallopian tube; and the luteal (secretory) phase when the corpus luteum is prepared to help maintain a possible pregnancy. The endometrium, or uterine lining, starts to grow, and reaches its greatest thickness during the luteal phase. If conception fails to occur, the lining is then discarded in the menstrual flow, and the cycle begins anew. This entire circle of changes is directed by the on/off production of six key hormones.

Estrogen, Progesterone, Androgen

While many hormones interact in the reproductive process, perhaps the three most well-known are estrogen, progesterone, and androgen.

There are several forms of estrogen but the one most important for reproduction is estradiol, a substance secreted by the ovary. In addition to being responsible for the development of sexual characteristics in women, estrogen governs the monthly thickening of the endometrium and the quantity and quality of cervical and vaginal mucus so important to the successful passage of the sperm.

Progesterone, the principle hormone secreted by the corpus luteum, is chiefly responsible for preparing the endometrium to accept a fertilized egg. The corpus luteum continues to secrete progesterone during the first three months of pregnancy until the placenta can fend for itself.

Androgen is produced by follicle cells in the ovary and is converted into additional estrogen. Androgen causes the disappearance of all of the follicles not destined to produce an egg during a given monthly cycle.

Gonadotropin Releasing Hormone

Called "GnRH" for short, this is the hormone that governs the level of estrogen in your body. It is produced by the hypothalamus, a gland located at the base of the brain.

At the end of your mentstrual cycle, declining levels of estrogen in your bloodstream spark the hypothalamus into a burst of activity, doubling or even tripling productin of GnRH. Production occurs in pulses. During the first, or follicular, phase of your cycle, when production is highest, the pulses come at hourly intervals. Later, during the luteal phase, they slack off to about once every two or three hours. Finally, as the luteal phase ends and estrogen levels reach their lowest ebb, the cycle starts again.

Gonadotropins

GnRH does its work through two intermediaries: follicle stimulating hormone (FSH for short) and luteinizing hormone (LH for short). These two hormones, known as gonadotropins, are produced by the pituitary gland. When levels of GnRH rise in your

KEY PLAYERS IN THE MONTHLY HORMONAL CYCLE

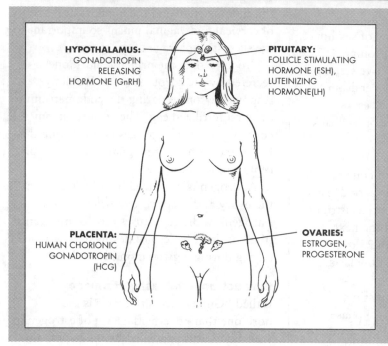

HYPOTHALAMUS:
GONADOTROPIN
RELEASING
HORMONE (GnRH)

PITUITARY:
FOLLICLE STIMULATING
HORMONE (FSH),
LUTEINIZING
HORMONE(LH)

PLACENTA:
HUMAN CHORIONIC
GONADOTROPIN
(HCG)

OVARIES:
ESTROGEN,
PROGESTERONE

Two master hormones govern all the others. **Gonadotropin Releasing Hormone (GnRH)** from the hypothalamus in the brain sparks release of follicle stimulating hormone and luteinizing hormone from the pituitary gland, which in turn prompt production of estrogen and progesterone in the ovaries. If conception occurs, **Human Chorionic Gonadotropin (HCG)** from the developing placenta takes over, perpetuating production of progesterone. High progesterone levels shut down production of GnRH, leaving HCG in control for the duration of the pregnancy.

bloodstream, the pituitary responds by increasing its release of FSH and LH. The two hormones are then free to begin working changes in the ultimate target, the ovary and the egg-containing follicles.

Here's how the process plays out.

The First Phase:
Bringing as Egg to Maturity

As estrogen and progesterone levels bottom out at the end of the menstrual cycle and a new one begins, the hypothalamus hikes production of GnRH, switching the pituitary over to higher output of FSH and LH. FSH levels are at their peak at this point, allowing this

hormone to successfully stimulate about 20 egg follicles in one of the ovaries.

Within each of these follicles, FSH fosters an increase in the number of cells that produce estradiol, the most important kind of estrogen. Meanwhile, LH is at work on a different set of cells within the follicle, encouraging increased production of androgen. The balance between the relative amounts of estradiol and androgen produced within each follicle determines its survival.

One follicle—the one that produces the most estradiol—eventually predominates. The more estradiol this follicle produces, the more FSH it attracts. But the estradiol it makes simultaneously signals the pituitary gland to cut back on its secretion of additional FSH. This, in effect, starves the other follicles for FSH and they begin to disappear, as the dominant follicle attracts more and more of the available FSH and makes more and more estradiol.

Eventually, the egg within this follicle develops the gelatinous coat described earlier and gets ready to leave the ovary and enter the fallopian tube. Meanwhile, the increasing levels of estradiol, along with a rise in progesterone and declining levels of FSH, prompt the pituitary to release a surge of LH.

When the egg is ready for release, roughly the 14th day of the normal menstrual cycle, LH levels peak. Release (ovulation) occurs, and the remnants of the dominant follicle remain behind, awaiting the next phase of the cycle, when they will be transformed into the corpus luteum, the "yellow body" that supports the developing baby, during the first three months of life.

The Second Phase: Preparing the Uterus

Now progesterone becomes the key hormonal player. The ruptured follicle, the first portion of its reproductive role completed, develops its own blood supply. It then starts to produce progesterone that simultaneously halts any further follicular growth and governs the preparation of the endometrium which has already been thickened in the first phase of the cycle. The corpus luteum also produces estrogen to help prepare the endometrium for potential pregnancy.

COMPLEX CHOREOGRAPHY OF THE REPRODUCTIVE HORMONES

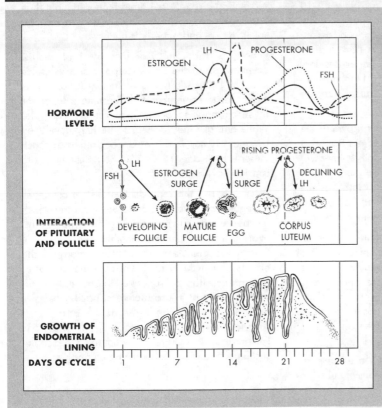

The monthly interplay of hormones begins with a surge of GnRH, or Gonadotropin Releasing Hormone (not shown). This triggers a burst of Follicle Stimulating Hormone (FSH) and a gradual increase in Luteinizing Hormone (LH). Responding to the FSH, a dominant follicle matures, releasing a surge of estrogen. This crescendo in estrogen levels prompts a burst of LH, which stimulates the remnants of the dominant follicle, now called the corpus luteum, to flood the system with progesterone. If conception doesn't occur, the system is self-limiting. Rising progesterone prompts a decline in LH; and less LH means less progesterone. When estrogen and progesterone levels hit bottom, it's the signal for a new surge of GnRH, starting the whole cycle anew.

About a week after you ovulate, your progesterone levels peak, then begin to decline along with your estrogen levels. If you have conceived a child, the developing placenta will produce yet another hormone called human chorionic gonadotropin (HCG). This hormone will maintain the corpus luteum, which will continue to produce progesterone to help maintain the pregnancy. On the other hand, if you are not pregnant, there will be no HCG, your LH levels will fall, and your corpus luteum will rapidly dry up and turn into a scar tissue. Low estrogen and progesterone levels will once again prompt the hypothalamus to speed production of GnRH, and your reproductive system will swing into action again.

Whether the goal is to increase your chances of conception or reduce the odds of pregnancy, many of the techniques described in the following chapters do their work by adjusting hormone levels at various points in this cycle. Birth control pills, shots, and implants all rely on this strategy, as do many fertility treatments. The understanding of this cycle by scientists has truly revolutionized our reproductive options. □

FROM MENARCHE TO MENOPAUSE

While we tend to think that the female reproductive system remains dormant until a girl is somewhere between 10 and 14, her sex hormones actually begin to function in the first few months after conception. In fact, GnRH, FSH and LH start to circulate in the fetus shortly after the ovaries develop. Surprisingly, the levels of FSH and LH in the developing baby are very similar to those found in postmenopausal women!

After a rather turbulent first year during which the newborn baby's system makes the final transition from reliance on her mother's hormones to her own, the reproductive system enters a dormant phase. FSH and LH levels fall to their lowest levels by the time girls are about two years old and then start to rise slowly again between the ages of four and ten.

Starting as early as age six, circulating levels of the male hormone, androgen, start to increase. This rise in androgen eventually causes the development of hair under the arms and in the pubic area. Meanwhile, estrogen stimulates breast development, and the sex hormones and glands begin to gear up for menarche, the onset of menses.

Even in an era when so many of the body's secrets are being unlocked, scientists still are not sure exactly what sets off the transformations of puberty.

However, at some point between the ages of 8 and 14 something causes pulses of LH to be secreted at a rate 2 to 4 times higher at night than during the day. This prompts estrogen and FSH levels to rise, and puberty is underway.

Puberty is traditionally defined by three events: development of the breasts, appearance of pubic hair, and the beginning of menstruation. It is important to remember that the time it takes for these changes to occur is extremely variable. While one girl may appear to be fully developed by age 11, her friend next door may not reach puberty until age 14 or 15. Both schedules are considered "normal."

After puberty, the reproductive system continues its regular cycles until around age 40, after which the perimenopausal years begin. At this point, ovarian function and the monthly menstrual cycle tend to become less regular, and many of the effects of estrogen in the body start to wane. Menopause (the cessation of the monthly cycle and the end of reproductive capacity) usually occurs between the ages of 45 and 55 in American women; the average age is about 51. For more on this stage in a woman's life, see the section on menopause beginning on page 351.

CHAPTER 18   **FERTILITY AND FAMILY PLANNING**

Overcoming Infertility: Tactics and Techniques

Elusive, unpredictable, demoralizing...the quest for fertility can be frustrating beyond words. Not only must both of you have smoothly operating reproductive systems, your timing must be impeccable as well. Intercourse has to take place when an egg is ripe for fertilization—and the window of opportunity is remarkably small.

In fact, after ovulation when an egg lies ready in the fallopian tube, it can be fertilized for only about 12 hours! This is why couples with no fertility problems whatsoever may still have difficulty conceiving quickly. Only 20 percent or so will succeed in the first month. For about half of the couples who've stopped contraception in order to conceive, it will take up to 3 months.

If you're having difficulty conceiving, you have plenty of company. Roughly 10 to 15 percent of American couples are having fertility problems at any given time. About 1 in every 5 married women in the U.S. seeks medical help to conceive at some point in her childbearing years.

Infertility, of course, can involve either or both partners. This chapter focuses on the difficulties you as a woman may face; but don't forget that it's essential for your partner to get a thorough check as well.

What Is "Infertility?"

Infertility is hard to pin down. A couple with no known reproductive problems might try for years to have a baby but fail simply because their timing was off. Are they infertile? Not physically, but they would be classified as such because infertility is usually defined as the inability to conceive after 1 year of unprotected sex.

Types of Infertility

Hypofertile couples have trouble conceiving quickly. Their fertility may be less than ideal or they may be having problems with timing, but they can eventually conceive without special treatment. For example, the man might have a low sperm count, or the woman might have endometriosis—roadblocks, but not brick walls.

Sterile couples won't be able to conceive without medical or surgical treatment. For example, the man might not create enough sperm to fertilize an egg, or the woman might have blocked fallopian tubes.

Infertility's Many Causes

A poorly functioning male reproductive system is the problem for 30 to 40 percent of couples seeking help for infertility. The man may have a low sperm count, sperm that move too slowly through the female reproductive system (low motility), semen that is too thick, or not enough of it.

Another 30 to 40 percent of fertility problems are caused by a malfunction in the female system. The most common, accounting for between 10 and 15 percent of all infertility, is the inability to release a healthy egg into the fallopian tube. Other problems include endometriosis, infection, or blocked tubes. In a significant percentage of couples (10 to 15 percent), sperm are unable to penetrate the mucus that lines the cervical canal leading to the uterus. About 10 percent of couples who seek help for infertility never learn the cause of their problem. Most turn out to be hypofertile and eventually do have children.

One important factor responsible for infertility in women is simply aging. Women tend to be most fertile in their early 20s. From then on, fertility declines rather slowly until about age 35, after which it becomes harder and harder to become pregnant. One in 7 couples is infertile if the woman is 30 to 34 years old; 1 in 5 is infertile if she is 35 to 40; and 1 in 4 can't conceive if she's 40 to 44.

Improving Your Chances

The remainder of this chapter will discuss the methods that physicians use to help couples who are having trouble conceiving. But before spending your time and money on specialists, consider these basic facts:

- Ovulation—prime time for fertilization—occurs in mid- to late morning, usually 12 to 16 days *before* your next menstrual period begins.
- The best time to have intercourse is on the day or evening before ovulation, so that sperm will already be waiting in the fallopian tube when the egg arrives.
- The missionary position (woman on her back, man on top) usually puts the uterus in the best position for receiving sperm. (For some women lying on the stomach is better. Your doctor can tell you which position is best for you.)
- You should lie still for about 10 minutes after intercourse to give the sperm that have entered the vagina enough time to proceed through the cervix.
- Since sperm can live in the fallopian tubes for 2 or 3 days longer, it is possible to have intercourse one day, ovulate the next day, and conceive on the third day—2 days after intercourse actually took place.
- Having intercourse at least 3 times during the week you expect to ovulate raises the odds that sperm will be present in the fallopian tubes when ovulation occurs.
- Fertility may be slightly impaired for a few months after you stop taking oral contraceptives or injectable or implanted hormones, but the effect will wear off.

SIGNS OF SUCCESSFUL OVULATION

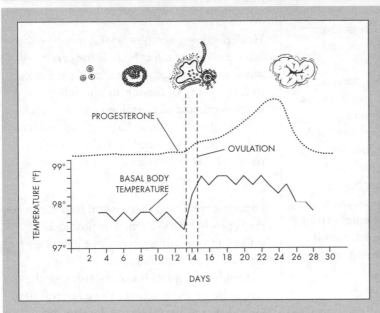

Since failure to ovulate is the most common cause of infertility in women, it's one of the first possibilities that your doctor will check. A change in your basal body temperature is one tell-tale sign of normal ovulation. If the temperature drops briefly, then jumps to a higher plateau, chances are that an egg has been successfully released. An increase in progesterone, produced by the remnants of the follicle after ovulation occurs, is also promising. If tests show higher levels during the second half of your cycle, any problem you may have probably lies elsewhere.

Tests For Infertility

If you have been trying to become pregnant unsuccessfully for a year, consider consulting a fertility specialist. Within 3 months of your first visit, you'll probably go through the following agenda.

Physical Workup

First, the doctor will perform a physical exam and take a thorough health history. You'll be asked many questions about your reproductive history, including how regular your periods are and whether you have ever had a sexually transmitted disease (STD). Some STDs, if untreated, can lead to pelvic inflam-matory disease (PID), impairing fertility even years later. Many other seemingly unrelated conditions, such as recurrent urinary tract infections and hypothyroidism, can cause infertility as well.

You will be asked to measure your basal body temperature (BBT) every day. The BBT is your lowest body temperature during waking hours. A measurable drop in temperature may *precede* ovulation by 12 to 24 hours. *After* ovulation, the sex hormone progesterone usually causes the body temperature to rise. Your doctor may measure your progesterone levels at various times since an increase during the second half of the monthly cycle suggests that ovulation has taken place.

One simple test that's usually part of the initial workup is an analysis of your partner's semen, which will be checked for the number and quality of sperm. Semen problems are frequently due to substances that can be eliminated, such as alcohol or illicit drugs (especially marijuana), caffeine, cigarettes, and certain prescription medications.

You'll probably also be given a postcoital test, performed after intercourse to assess the characteristics of your cervical mucus at the time of presumed ovulation, as well as the liveliness of the sperm that have just been deposited. Ideally, the test is performed 2 to 8 hours after intercourse on the day before ovulation. In this painless procedure, the physician collects a few drops of mucus from the cervix and examines it to see whether it can be stretched easily and to determine how slippery it is. Both qualities are needed by sperm attempting to enter the uterus.

Other Procedures and Tests

If results of the tests described above are normal, more complex procedures can be tried:

Hysterosalpingography (HSG) involves the insertion of a small tube into the cervix. A physician or radiologic specialist then injects dye. An x–ray of the uterus and fallopian tubes is taken and examined for any blockages or abnormalities. Although somewhat uncomfortable, an HSG usually doesn't require local anesthesia or require an overnight hospital stay.

Laparoscopy is another way of looking inside the reproductive system. The physician inserts an operating microscope called a laparoscope through a small incision made just under the navel. Looking through the scope, he or she examines the ovaries, fallopian tubes, uterus, and other internal structures. Laparoscopy is a surgical procedure

IF OBSTRUCTION IS THE SUSPECT

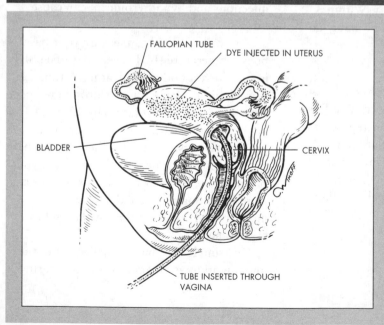

FALLOPIAN TUBE

DYE INJECTED IN UTERUS

BLADDER

CERVIX

TUBE INSERTED THROUGH VAGINA

To rule out the possibility of a physical barrier to conception, your doctor may recommend hysterosalpingography. This is nothing more than an x-ray of the uterus and fallopian tubes. A dye that blocks radiation is infused by a narrow tube inserted through the vagina and cervix. The resulting pictures show the exact position and dimensions of the crucial pathways the egg must travel on its way to successful implantation in the uterus.

that usually requires general anesthesia and sometimes a night in the hospital.

If a problem still hasn't surfaced, there are several laboratory tests that can help determine whether an infection, allergic reaction, or hormonal problem may be responsible for a couple's infertility. For example, sometimes a woman's immune system treats semen like germs, attacking and killing the sperm with antibodies. Or an infection with no symptoms in either partner may interfere with their reproductive systems, blocking the fallopian tubes or the passages through which sperm flow.

When the results of all tests are negative or normal, it's probably good news. The great majority of couples in whom no cause can be determined conceive a baby within 2 years of undergoing fertility testing.

Drug Therapy

A number of fertility drugs are available today. The choice depends on the specific cause or causes of a couple's problem. Drugs used to stimulate ovulation in women who don't ovulate naturally include clomiphene (Clomid, Serophene), bromocriptine (Parlodel), human menopausal gonadotropin (HMG), follicle–stimulating hormone (FSH), and gonadotropin–releasing hormone (GnRH).

Clomiphene is used most often. The drug can induce ovulation in 80 to 85 percent of women who take it; the resulting pregnancy rate is 40 to 50 percent, with slightly increased chance of multiple births (twins, triplets, or more).

Bromocriptine is reserved for women whose bodies generate too much of the hormone prolactin. Excessive levels of prolactin can disrupt the reproductive hormonal cycle by blocking FSH and LH, the two key hormones that promote growth and release of an egg (for more information, see chapter 17, "How the Reproductive System Works"). By restoring a normal hormonal balance, bromocriptine can induce ovulation in 80 percent of infertile women who take it.

Treatment with other hormones such as HMG and GnRH is still being explored, but they might be tried if the other drugs aren't working.

Surgery

If HSG or laparoscopy reveals an abnormality that can be repaired mechanically, your doctor may recommend surgery. This approach is usually best if you have adhesions (scar tissue), endometriosis, uterine fibroid tumors, or a physically abnormal uterus. Operations to correct these problems usually require hospitalization for several days and recovery at home for several weeks.

Assisted Reproductive Techniques

Modern technology has made pregnancies possible that would never have happened a few decades ago. Here's an overview of available techniques.

Artificial Insemination

Artificial insemination can be performed with your partner's sperm (Husband Insemination) or an unknown donor's sperm (Donor Insemination). The physician inserts a syringe containing a prepared sperm sample into the vagina and releases the solution into the cervical opening. The technique is used mostly for sperm problems but is also helpful when intercourse can't take place often enough to conceive.

WHEN THE PROBLEM IS FAILURE TO OVULATE

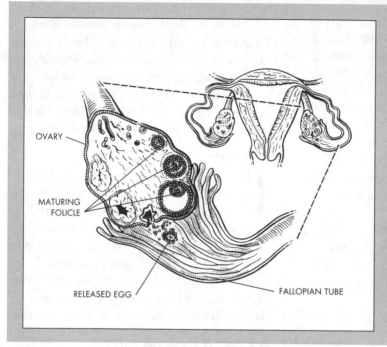

OVARY

MATURING
FOLICLE

RELEASED EGG

FALLOPIAN TUBE

The growth and release of a mature egg from the ovary depends on a precisely orchestrated—and easily interrupted—series of hormonal signals. For most infertile women, drugs that boost or supplement these signals are sufficient to trigger ovulation. Clomiphene citrate (Clomid, Serophene) works by coaxing an increased output of reproductive hormones from the pituitary gland. A more direct approach supplies the necessary hormones by injection. First a follicle stimulating hormone such as Metrodin or Pergonal is administered for 7 to 12 days. Then a single shot of the hormonal medication Profasi jump-starts release of the egg.

Intrauterine Insemination

If the cause of infertility is suspected to be the quality of the cervical mucus or an inability of the sperm to move toward the egg fast enough, intrauterine insemination can be tried. Bypassing the cervix, sperm are deposited directly into the uterus, from which they swim into the fallopian tubes. Conception rates for this technique range from 30 to 42 percent when cervical mucus is the problem and 14 to 43 percent when inadequate sperm are responsible. As in artificial insemination, sperm can be taken from your partner or a donor.

In Vitro Fertilization

July 25, 1978, marked the birth of the first "test–tube" baby. That landmark child was conceived outside the human body and implanted in her mother's uterus with a technique called in vitro fertilization (IVF). Today thousands of children conceived in vitro are leading healthy lives.

IVF, which requires a team of experts and takes several days, consists of four basic steps.

(1) The woman takes drugs that stimulate ovulation. A day and a half later, the doctor removes the eggs from her body. The eggs, which used to be "harvested" with laparoscopy in the hospital, can now be removed in the doctor's office.

(2) Meanwhile sperm are obtained form the partner or donor, usually on the same day the eggs are harvested.

(3) In a laboratory, eggs and sperm are combined in a special solution (culture medium) and the egg is fertilized.

(4) A solution containing the fertilized egg (embryo) is inserted through the cervical canal into the uterus. This transfer procedure usually takes place at least 48 hours after fertilization. The woman rests for at least 3 hours before going home.

While the success of IVF varies widely among doctors and institutions, the pregnancy rate is about 20 percent. Approximately three–fourths of these pregnancies continue to a successful delivery.

Gamete intrafallopian transfer (GIFT), another in vitro technique, is identical to IVF except that fertilization occurs in the woman's fallopian tube rather than in a test tube. The harvested eggs and prepared sperm are inserted into the fallopian tube at the same time. From there, the fertilized egg travels to the uterus, as it would under ordinary circumstances. Success rates for GIFT are slightly higher than for IVF. Because IVF is less costly, it's worth trying before the more expensive GIFT techniques. Researchers continue to explore new methods.

Key Points

Remember: *timing* and *time* are both critical factors in successful conception. Because the window of opportunity closes just 12 hours after ovulation, even the most fertile of couples has only a 20 percent chance of conceiving a child each month.

However, you have another 1 in 5 chance the following month—and the month after that—steadily increasing your cumulative odds of success. That's why *time* is so important. The majority of couples whose fertility evaluations turn up no identifiable problems will conceive a child unassisted within 2 years.

Patience, indeed, is among the most important of infertility therapies. Still, when you've been waiting 1 year, or 2 years, or more, hope founded on statistical odds can be little consolation. If you find your patience running out, remember that there are support groups to turn to across the nation. Ask your doctor or the nursing department of a local hospital for the organizations in your area, or consult the directory at the end of this book. □

CHAPTER 19   **FERTILITY AND FAMILY PLANNING**

Barrier Contraceptives: A Growing Array of Options

Women have been using barrier contraceptives for more than 3,000 years. Ancient Egyptians, Greeks, and Romans inserted a mixture of herbs, tree resins, and honey or oil into their vaginas. Some African women used hollowed–out okra pods as a vaginal pouch, somewhat like the modern female condom. Roman women used goat bladders in a similar manner while their partners used various forms of animal membrane as sheaths for the penis.

Today, millions of women and men rely on modern forms of barrier contraception both to prevent pregnancy and—more and more—to protect themselves against sexually transmitted diseases such as gonorrhea and especially HIV. Many women also choose barrier contraceptives to avoid the potential side effects and risks associated with the Pill, the IUD, and other forms of birth control.

Most barrier contraceptives are simple to use and are available without a prescription.

This chapter outlines the advantages and drawbacks of each of your options, from the familiar condom and diaphragm to new alternatives like the vaginal sponge and female condom.

Ensuring Success

Barrier contraceptives won't prevent pregnancy unless you and your partner remember to use them *every time you have sex*. That means planning ahead. Unlike methods such as the IUD or the Pill, barrier contraceptives need to be applied within a specific time before intercourse occurs. In addition, the barrier method you choose must be used correctly and consistently. Carelessness significantly increases the failure (pregnancy) rates for each method.

Failure rates for contraceptive methods are usually given as a percentage: the number of pregnancies expected to occur in a group of 100 women using the method for one year. The official rates vary. A "perfect" or ideal rate assumes that the couple uses the method absolutely correctly and without fail every time they have sex. In the real world, however, few couples manage to maintain a "perfect" record. Mistakes do happen: women forget the sponge or cap, insert the diaphragm incorrectly, or run out of spermicide.

The failure rates given in this chapter (see nearby table) are based on typical use—that is, allowing for a certain margin of error on the user's part. The effectiveness of a particular method may be higher when it is invariably used correctly and consistently.

Your Options

Couples today no longer have to rely on okra pods, herbs, tree resins, and goat bladders to prevent unwanted pregnancy. Now they can choose from a wide variety of devices and chemical formulations. Some work well alone. Others are even more effective when used in combination. For example, more unplanned pregnancies occur when couples rely solely on the male condom than when the woman also uses a barrier. But no matter which type you select, or combination you choose, remember that you must follow the guidelines given below for maximum protection.

The Condom

A long, thin, flexible sheath that fits over the erect penis, the condom has been in use for centuries. The first rubber condom was developed in the mid–1800s. Most modern condoms are made of latex.

Today, you can buy condoms in drug stores, supermarkets, and vending machines, usually rolled up in individual wrappers. They are often lubricated, and may be textured, colored, or treated with a spermicide. Using a latex condom in combination with a spermicide (see "Spermicides" later in this chapter) is one of the most effective ways to prevent sexually transmitted disease.

How it works. The condom keeps semen from entering the vagina. Whether made of latex or of a natural animal membrane, it will prevent pregnancy. However, because membrane condoms have microscopic pores (like the pores of your skin), *you cannot rely on them to prevent sexually transmitted diseases such as HIV.* Though the pores are small enough to block sperm cells, they are no obstacle to tinier microorganisms such as viruses. Many brands of condoms come treated with a spermicide that increases their effectiveness. Used alone, the condom has a failure rate of about 12 percent.

How to use it. Be sure to use a brand new condom with each act of intercourse. After your partner has an erection, but before it comes in any contact with your genital area, he should place a rolled–up condom on the tip of his penis. To leave room at the end of the condom for ejaculated semen, he must first pinch and hold the small receptacle at the tip, then unroll the rest of the condom all the way down to the base of the penis.

After ejaculation, your partner should grasp the condom at the base of his penis as he withdraws. Remember, too, that semen can leak out of the condom into the vagina if the penis is no longer erect. Used condoms should be thrown away—never reuse them.

If the condom is not already lubricated, you can add lubricant—but *never* use mineral oil, baby oil, or petroleum jelly with a latex condom. They will dissolve the latex, causing the condom to break. If you need extra lubricant, choose a water–soluble product such as K–Y Lubricating Jelly.

Pros and cons. Condoms are relatively inexpensive and readily available. They can be bought without a doctor's prescription,

SPERMICIDES—FOR AN EXTRA MEASURE OF SAFETY

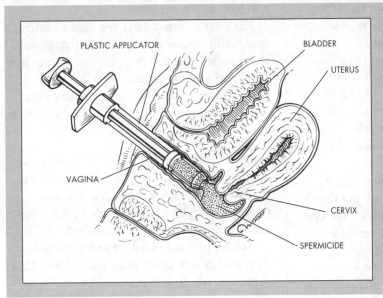

When applying a spermicide, make sure the applicator is filled to the top, then deposit the contents as close to the cervix as possible. It's best to use a diaphragm or cervical cap to hold the spermicide in place.

By themselves, spermicides are effective 4 times out of 5. When used as a backup for other barrier methods, the rate is even higher. Spermicides containing nonoxynol-9 have the important added advantage of providing a degree of protection against some sexually transmitted diseases.

and—if made from latex— offer protection against sexually transmitted disease.

However, use of a condom requires the cooperation of your partner, and some men dislike them. You may have to try several different brands before you find one that suits you both.

Some couples don't like interrupting sex to put on a condom. If you feel that donning one destroys sexual spontaneity, try to make it a ritual part of your mutual lovemaking.

You or your partner might be allergic to latex condoms. Signs of latex allergy include burning, itching, or irritation in the genital area. If your partner is allergic to latex, but you want the disease protection of a latex condom, he can wear an animal–membrane condom under the latex one. If you are allergic to latex, try the reverse: a latex condom under the natural–membrane variety.

Spermicides

Like condoms, spermicides are widely available. They come in foam, suppositories, cream, or jelly. For best effectiveness, all of these forms must be used with a condom, diaphragm, or cervical cap.

How they work. Spermicides contain a chemical that kills sperm. When you insert spermicidal foam or suppositories into the upper part of your vagina, the medication kills most sperm and helps prevent those that survive from entering your cervix. A diaphragm or cervical cap will hold spermicidal creams or jellies in place over the cervix. You can also use them to coat a condom.

Many brands of spermicide now contain nonoxynol–9, a chemical that helps protect against some types of STDs. Spermicidal foams and suppositories have a failure rate of about 21 percent.

How to use them. Spermicidal foams, creams, and jellies come with a plastic applicator threaded at one end to fit the mouth of the container. The creams and jellies come in tubes, the foam in an aerosol can.

To fill an applicator with cream or jelly, thread it onto the end of the tube with the plunger pushed all the way in. Holding the tube straight up with the applicator on top, gently squeeze until the cream or jelly fills the applicator and the plunger is pushed all the way out.

To load an applicator with spermicidal foam, first shake the can well, then put the applicator on top of it and bend it to one side (or, with some products, push it down) to trigger the valve and fill the applicator.

To apply the spermicide, lie down, insert the applicator into your vagina, and push in the plunger. The goal is to deposit the spermicide as close to the opening of your cervix as possible. Do not pull on the plunger to remove the applicator—this can remove some of the spermicide from the vagina.

You can insert spermicidal suppositories with your fingers or with the applicator that comes with the product. Place the suppository high up in your vagina, as close as possible to the cervix. Once it is in place, the natural secretions of the vagina will dissolve the suppository and make it foamy.

As with other barrier contraceptives, timing is important when using a spermicide. Follow the instructions on the package. Insert jelly and cream as shortly before intercourse as possible—no more than 15 minutes beforehand. You can apply foam up to 30 minutes in advance. You need to insert a vaginal suppository at least 10 minutes before intercourse to allow it to dissolve, but no more than 30 minutes in advance, or it will lose its effectiveness.

Each act of intercourse requires additional spermicide. Never douche right after using spermicide—this can push any remaining live sperm up into the cervix. Wait at least 6 hours before douching. Using a panty liner will keep you more comfortable if the spermicide leaks out of your vagina.

Pros and cons. Spermicides are readily available without a doctor's prescription and are easy to use. Look for those that contain nonoxynol–9, which gives added protection against sexually transmitted disease.

The biggest drawback of spermicides is their low effectiveness when used alone. This is particularly true of jelly and cream, but even foam and suppositories prevent pregnancy only about 79 percent of the time. For this reason, couples who need highly effective contraception should combine spermicide with another method, such as a condom, diaphragm, or cervical cap.

Some people are allergic to spermicides. If you experience burning or irritation in the genital area after using one, consult your doctor. You may need to switch brands or use another form of birth control.

The Diaphragm

Diaphragms have been around since the 1830s. They were the first major breakthrough for women seeking personal control over their fertility. Since then, improvements in design and effectiveness have maintained their popularity.

How it works. A flexible rubber device shaped like a shallow cup, the diaphragm is held in place over the cervix by the vaginal muscles. It serves to keep contraceptive cream or foam close against the cervix. Any sperm that find their way over the rim of the diaphragm will die when they encounter the spermicide. The diaphragm has a failure rate of about 18 percent.

Diaphragms are available in two types of rim: a flat ring, that can be squeezed into a flat oval; or an arcing or coil spring, that forms a bent circle when squeezed. The flat–ring type comes with an applicator to make insertion easier. You can insert an arcing or coil spring diaphragm with your fingers.

You can't get a diaphragm without a doctor's prescription. The devices come in various sizes and must be fitted by a doctor or other health professional. First, you'll need an examination to determine the size that's best for you. You'll then be shown how to insert the device, how to make sure it is in place, and how to remove it. Some clinics and doctor's offices dispense diaphragms themselves, while others will give you a prescription that can be filled at a pharmacy.

How to use it. It takes experience to place a diaphragm correctly. Your doctor or nurse should let you practice putting it in and should check to see whether you've placed it correctly. At the least, be sure to practice a little on your own before you use a diaphragm for the first time.

■ *Inserting an arcing or coil–spring diaphragm.* Before inserting the diaphragm, squeeze out a small amount—about a tea-spoonful—of spermicide into the rubber dome. Also spread a little around the inside of the rim. Take care not to put too much on

INSERTING A COIL-SPRING DIAPHRAGM

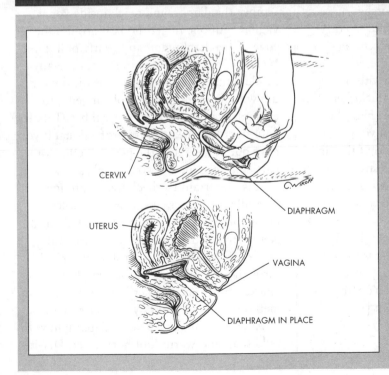

It takes a little practice, but placing a diaphragm correctly is basically a matter of making sure the cervix is completely covered. With the rim squeezed together, slide the diaphragm up and back into the vagina. Make sure the front edge is seated as shown; then feel your cervix with a finger to double-check for full protection. For best results, prior to insertion always spread a little spermicide inside the rim and on the dome.

CERVIX

DIAPHRAGM

UTERUS

VAGINA

DIAPHRAGM IN PLACE

the rim; this could cause the diaphragm to slip out of place.

Find a comfortable position—lying on your back, standing with one leg raised on a chair, or squatting with your knees apart. Squeeze the sides of the rim together between two fingers. Angling it toward the small of your back, insert it into your vagina, pushing it up and back with one finger as far as it will go. Push the front edge of the rim up behind your pubic bone.

When properly in place, the diaphragm should completely cover your cervix, with the back edge tucked between the cervix and the rear vaginal wall, and the front edge wedged behind your pubic bone. After inserting the diaphragm, feel your cervix with one finger to make sure it is completely covered. If it isn't, take out the diaphragm, apply a little more spermicide to the inside, and try again.

■ *Inserting a flat–spring diaphragm.* This type of diaphragm comes with a plastic applicator that has a series of small notches on one side. The notches are numbered to correspond to the size (the diameter in centimeters) of your diaphragm. To use the applicator, hold your diaphragm with the dome up and hook the rim onto the larger notch at the end of the applicator. Find the notch corresponding to the size of your diaphragm and hook the other end of the rim onto it. The diaphragm should be stretched into a flat oval, with the dome puckered into folds. Squeeze the spermicide into these folds and rub a little around the rim.

With the spermicide facing up, insert the applicator into the vagina. Angle it toward the small of your back, pushing it gently along the rear wall of the vagina. You are aiming for the small space between your cervix and the rear wall. When you have pushed it as far as it will go, twist the applicator to release the diaphragm, then remove the applicator. With one finger, push the front edge of the rim up behind your pubic bone. Check to make sure that the diaphragm covers your cervix.

■ *Timing is important.* Insert the diaphragm no more than 6 hours before you have intercourse. Any longer and the spermicide will weaken. If sex is delayed more than 6 hours, don't remove the diaphragm, but do insert additional spermicide just before intercourse. If you have sex again within 6 hours, apply more spermicide beforehand, without removing the diaphragm.

Wait at least 6 hours after intercourse before removing the diaphragm, but do not leave it in for more than 24 hours, as this increases your risk of a vaginal infection. Do not douche while the diaphragm is still in place; this can dilute the spermicide. To remove the diaphragm, reach inside your vagina with one finger, hook it around the edge of the diaphragm, and gently pull it out.

■ *Care of your diaphragm.* Do not use any product that is not intended specifically for use with a diaphragm. Petroleum jelly, for example, can disintegrate the rubber. Talk to your doctor or health care professional if you have questions about the possible effect of a particular product on your diaphragm.

It is important to check the diaphragm carefully for tiny cracks, tears and holes before inserting it. Hold it up to a light and *gently* stretch the rubber apart with your fingers. Take care not to push a fingernail through the rubber. If you see any holes or cracks, substitute another birth control method until you can buy a replacement.

After each use, wash your diaphragm with mild soap and warm (not hot) water. Dry it with a towel, dust it slightly with cornstarch (not powder), and store it in its case.

Although a diaphragm should last 2 years, have your doctor recheck the size at least once a year. If you have gained or lost 10 pounds or more, delivered a baby, or had an abortion, you'll need to be measured sooner.

Pros and cons. When used correctly, the diaphragm can be a fairly effective method of birth control. Many women rely on it for all or most of their childbearing years. Not only does it offer protection against unwanted pregnancy, it also appears to lower the risk of certain sexually transmitted diseases and of some types of precancerous changes in the cervix.

Unlike condoms and spermicides, a diaphragm can be inserted hours in advance of intercourse, permitting uninterrupted love-making. However, it does require some fore-thought, and you must have it in place every time you have sex. Leaking of spermicide and semen during the 6 hours after intercourse may prove to be uncomfortable, though wearing a panty liner can help.

Some women get repeated urinary tract infections while using the diaphragm. If your diaphragm is too large, the rim can press against the front wall of the vagina and irritate the urethra (the tube that carries urine from your bladder). Symptoms of a urinary tract infection include burning and pain during urination and a frequent urge to urinate. Call your doctor if you experience any of these problems. It may be a good idea to use another birth control method while you are undergoing treatment. After the infection has cleared up, make an appointment to get your diaphragm size rechecked.

The Cervical Cap

The cervical cap was originally developed in the 1800s, although it was not approved for use in the United States until 1988. To buy it, you'll need a doctor's prescription, and you must be fitted by a trained practitioner.

How it works. Somewhat similar to the diaphragm, the cervical cap is a small rubber dome that covers the cervix and holds spermicide against the cervical opening. The difference is that, instead of being anchored by the vaginal muscles and pubic bone, the snugly fitting cap is held in place by surface tension or suction.

The failure rate of the cervical cap for women who have never given birth is similar to that of the diaphragm—about 18 percent. In women who have delivered a baby, however, the rate rises to about 26 percent. Pregnancy and childbirth cause the cervix to become softer and more pliable, and hence less capable of staying in place.

How to use it. Most women find that it's a little harder to insert and remove a cervical cap than a diaphragm. It may take a little practice and patience until you get it right. After your doctor fits you for a cap, be sure you understand the steps for insertion and removal, as well as how to check for proper fit.

■ *Inserting the cap.* To use the cap, place a small amount of spermicide in the dome, filling it about a third of the way. Don't use too much, and don't put any on the rim of the cap. This could break the suction and cause the cap to slip out of place.

Find a comfortable position—you may want to lie down, stand with one leg raised on a chair, or squat with your knees apart. Squeeze the rim of the cap between your thumb and forefinger and insert it into your

PLACING A CERVICAL CAP

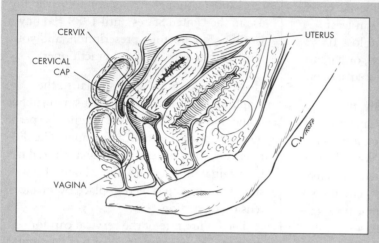

Cervical caps are held in place by suction, so it's important that you have a good fit. When maneuvering the cap into place, slide the upper rim along the rear wall of your vagina until it lodges behind the cervix with the cap pointing downward, then flip the lower edge of the rim up over the front of the cervix. As with a diaphragm, always apply a bit of spermicide to the dome—but with a cervical cap, avoid getting any on the rim.

vagina as far as you can. Then, with one finger, push it along the rear wall of your vagina and up to your cervix. Make sure that the dome of the cap is pointing down toward the opening of your vagina. Then push it up firmly onto your cervix.

Make sure that the cap fits snugly by running a finger all the way around the rim. If you have inserted the cap correctly, you should be able to feel your cervix through the cap, though it should not completely fill the dome. (This extra space allows room for the spermicide and cervical secretions.) During the first few months of use, check often to make sure the cap is in place.

Ask your doctor or pharmacist about obtaining an "introducer" for your cervical cap. This device may make insertion easier.

■ *Timing.* You can insert the cervical cap up to 48 hours in advance. Wearing it longer can cause a vaginal infection and is not recommended. You don't need to use more spermicide with repeated intercourse, but you must leave the device in place for at least eight hours after sex, and should not douche before taking it out. Use a method other than the cap during your period; the flow of menstrual blood could break the suction.

■ *Care of the cervical cap.* To remove the cap, reach into your vagina with one finger and tilt the cap to one side, breaking the suction. Then slip your finger under the rim and pull the cap out. After each use, wash the cap with mild soap and warm water. Clean the groove inside the rim with a cotton swab. Dry the cap and, if you wish, dust it lightly with cornstarch before storing it in its case.

Petroleum jelly and some other oils and lubricants can cause the rubber of the cervical cap to deteriorate. Do not use any of these products without first consulting your physician.

Some doctors recommend that you get a Pap smear before being fitted for a cervical cap, and another smear 3 months after you begin using it. You'll need another fitting if you have a miscarriage or deliver a baby. Cervical caps should be replaced every 1 to 2 years, depending on your doctor's advice.

Pros and cons. The cervical cap may be a good alternative for women who have had repeated urinary tract infections with use of the diaphragm. It's also more convenient (you can insert it up to 48 hours in advance), and less messy (you won't need as much spermicide). Like the diaphragm, it may also provide some protection against certain types of sexually transmitted diseases.

The cervical cap is not a good choice for all women. Some have difficulty inserting and removing it. Others cannot find a size to fit the shape of their cervix. In addition, the device is not available everywhere in the United States, and some doctors have not been trained to fit it.

The Vaginal Sponge

The vaginal sponge has provided women with an additional contraceptive alternative for over a decade. You can buy it in most drug stores and even in some supermarkets.

How it works. The vaginal sponge is made of a soft, synthetic, absorbent material saturated with spermicide. It has a dimple in the middle of one side and a loop attached to the other, and measures a little over two inches in diameter by three–quarters of an inch thick. It works by holding spermicide against the cervix while blocking the cervical opening.

For women who have had children, the sponge has a failure rate of about 28 percent; for childless women, it is comparable to the cervical cap and the diaphragm—about 18 percent. This difference is probably due to the changes in the cervix that result from pregnancy and childbirth.

USING THE VAGINAL SPONGE

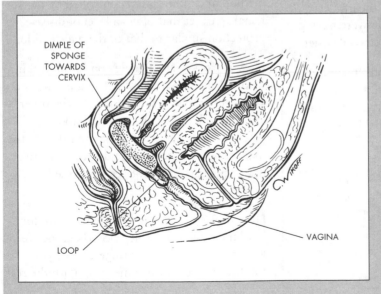

DIMPLE OF SPONGE TOWARDS CERVIX

LOOP

VAGINA

Unlike other barrier methods, the vaginal sponge need not be coated with spermicide, for it carries its own supply. Use a little warm water to wet the sponge and activate the spermicide. Remember to insert the sponge dimple-side up, with the loop facing downwards. You can put in the sponge up to a day before having sex—a significant advantage. The failure rate for women who haven't had children is the same as a diaphragm's—about 18 percent. However, if you've already had a child, chances of failure rise to a much higher 28 percent.

How to use it. Unwrap the sponge and wet it with warm water, then squeeze it until it becomes very foamy. This activates the spermicide. Take care not to wash out too much of the spermicide.

Hold the sponge between two fingers. With the dimpled side facing up, insert it into your vagina and push it up to your cervix. The dimple in the sponge should fit snugly over your cervix with the loop facing downward toward the opening of your vagina. Make sure the sponge completely covers your cervix.

You can insert the sponge up to 24 hours before having sex. Some women use more spermicide with additional intercourse, for added protection, but it is not mandatory. Do not leave a sponge in for more than 24 hours. The spermicide will lose its effectiveness, and you also run the risk of getting a vaginal infection.

Leave the sponge in place for at least 6 hours after sex. To remove it, reach inside your vagina, hook a finger through the loop attached to the sponge, pull it out, and throw it away. The sponge should never be reused.

You may find that the sponge has slipped away from your cervix during intercourse, making it hard to reach. Sitting on a toilet and bearing down as though you were having a bowel movement may make removal easier.

Pros and cons. The sponge is convenient and, because it can be inserted a full 24 hours in advance, allows more spontaneity than some other methods. It is readily available and does not require a doctor's prescription. For women without children, it can be as effective as the diaphragm and cervical cap.

If you are not used to inserting tampons or a diaphragm, it may take a little practice to master the sponge. On the whole, however, most women find the sponge easier to place than the cervical cap.

Some women experience vaginal dryness while using the sponge. A vaginal lubricant will alleviate this problem. Others may have an allergic reaction to the spermicide in the sponge. Consult your doctor if you experience burning, irritation, or itching in or around the vaginal area.

The Female Condom

The female condom, or vaginal pouch, is an important new contraceptive option. Approved for use in 1993, it will soon be available throughout the United States.

Like the male condom, but unlike other barrier devices, the female condom offers good protection against sexually transmitted disease as well as pregnancy. Although the diaphragm and cervical cap help shield the cervix against some types of infectious organisms, the vaginal walls remain exposed and vulnerable to viruses such as HIV. The female condom, however, completely covers the inside of the vagina as well as the cervix. It is the only method of contraception controlled by the female partner that offers a level of disease protection similar to that of the male condom.

How it works. The female condom is a thin, flexible sheath with a closed ring at one end and a slightly larger, open ring at the other. It appears to have a failure rate of about 13 percent—only slightly higher than that of the male condom. Because the device is relatively new, scientists have not yet confirmed this figure.

How to use it. To insert the female condom, hold the ring at the inner closed end between your thumb and middle finger. Place your forefinger against this inner ring with the rest

LATEST OPTION: THE FEMALE CONDOM

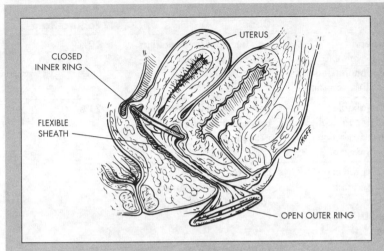

CLOSED INNER RING

UTERUS

FLEXIBLE SHEATH

OPEN OUTER RING

The closed inner ring of this tubular device should be seated just like a diaphragm. The open outer ring remains outside the vagina. Unlike the diaphragm, cap, and sponge, the female condom provides as much protection against STDs as its male counterpart, yet gives a woman full control. Another bonus: unlike the male condom, this version can be applied hours in advance of sex.

of the pouch hanging down. Then squeeze the sides of the ring together and insert it into your vagina as far as it will go. Push the front edge up behind your pubic bone. It should cover your cervix and be held in place between the cervix and the rear wall of the vagina—like a diaphragm.

The outer, open ring of the pouch hangs down outside your vagina. During sex, the vagina expands, taking up the slack in the pouch, and stretching the outer ring flat against the labia. Make sure the inner ring completely covers your cervix, and be careful not to twist the pouch. For added protection, you can use a spermicide.

The female condom is already prelubricated, and comes with extra lubricant in case you want to add more during sex. Add a few more drops if the pouch makes noise during

sex, if the penis dislodges it, or if the outer ring is pushed inside the vagina.

You can insert a female condom from several hours to a few minutes before sex. If you are menstruating, remove your tampon before inserting the condom. Your partner should avoid using a male condom at the same time.

Although you can leave the female condom in place after sex, you should replace it with a new one before each act of intercourse. Remove the pouch before standing up. Grasp the outer ring and squeeze it between your fingers to prevent spillage, then twist it and gently pull it out. Discard the pouch in the trash; never reuse it.

Pros and cons. The female condom is the first contraceptive that protects women against both pregnancy and sexually transmitted diseases such as HIV as effectively as the male condom. Since it requires no cooperation from a male partner, it gives a woman full control, and unlike the male condom, it can

BARRIER OPTIONS AT A GLANCE

Method	Pros	Cons	Failure Rate
Male condom (used alone)	Inexpensive, readily available No prescription needed STD and HIV protection	Can interrupt love–making Less effective when used alone	12%
Spermicides (used alone)	Readily available No prescription needed Some STD protection with nonoxynol-9	Can interrupt love–making Less effective when used alone	21%
Diaphragm (with spermicide)	Some STD protection Can be inserted in advance Recurrent UTI in some women	Exam and doctor's prescription required Takes practice to use	18%
Cervical cap (with spermicide)	Some STD protection Can be inserted in advance Can be left in place longer than diaphragm May be more convienient Avoids risk of UTI	Exam and doctor's prescription required Can be difficult to learn to use Less effective in women who have given birth	Women with children: 26% Women without children: 18%
Vaginal sponge	Readily available No prescription needed Used alone	Takes practice to use correctly May cause vaginal dryness Less effective in women who have given birth	Women with children: 28% Women without children: 18%
Female condom (used alone)	STD and HIV protection Can be inserted in advance	Not readily available Takes practice to use correctly	13%

be inserted hours in advance, eliminating the need for interruption. In addition, because the female condom does not have to be removed immediately after intercourse, like the male condom does, it can be less intrusive in the intimate moments after sex.

The female condom is made of polyurethane, a material that is thinner and more flexible than latex. Some couples who have used the female condom report that it is more comfortable for both partners than its male counterpart.

On the down side, inserting the female condom correctly may take some practice, and you may feel awkward until you get used to it. The condoms are also hard to find. At the moment, they are available only at certain clinics and women's health centers. However, once mass distribution gets underway, you should be able to find them in any pharmacy.

Making Your Choice

Is a barrier contraceptive the best type of birth control for you? Which kind should you use? The answers will depend on your health, life–style, and personal preferences.

Health Factors

If your health prevents you from using other forms of birth control, a barrier contraceptive may be a good alternative. Heart disease or high blood pressure, for example, rules out the Pill for some women, and a history of pelvic inflammatory disease can make an IUD risky. (For other contraindications, turn to chapters 20 and 21 which discuss these methods.)

Life–Style Issues

Anyone who has more than one sexual partner is at increased risk of contracting HIV and other sexually transmitted diseases. And even if *you* have only one sexual partner, your risk increases if *he* has more than one. In either situation, a barrier method—particlarly the male or the female condom—may be a wise choice—even if you are using another birth control method such as the Pill. (See chapters 11 and 13 on STDs and AIDS for more on your risk of these diseases.)

All of the barrier contraceptives require some degree of planning. Although some methods, such as the diaphragm and the cervical cap, can be inserted hours in advance, you must still have them and spermicide with you when the need arises. If you prefer spontaneity to planning every encounter, a barrier method may not be for you.

Personal Preferences

Some barrier methods require a certain amount of willingness and cooperation on the part of *both* partners. Applying condoms and spermicides in a moment of intimacy puts many people off. If either you or your partner feels this way, you'll be tempted to neglect the barrier device and should probably consider another method.

Here are some questions to ask yourself when considering a barrier method:

- How easy is it to use?
- Am I likely to use it every time I have sex?
- Does it require cooperation from my partner all or some of the time? What are his feelings?
- Does it provide enough protection from pregnancy on its own, or do I need to use a second contraceptive as well?
- Is it readily available? Do I need an exam and/or a doctor's prescription?
- How much does it cost?

Whatever method of contraception you choose, it's important that both you and your partner feel comfortable with it. If you're not sure you'll like a particular device, try it out. You can always switch to another method. Many couples rely on more than one barrier method, using a diaphragm, for example, some of the time, and condoms and spermicide at other times.

The availability, effectiveness, and disease–fighting properties of many barrier contraceptives have made them the choice of many women looking for alternatives to hormonal birth control and IUDs. Weigh the pros and cons. Talk with your partner. In this wide array of choices, there's bound to be one that's right for you. ☐

CHAPTER 20

FERTILITY AND FAMILY PLANNING

IUDs: Still Worth Considering

f intrauterine devices were automobiles, the Dalkon Shield would have been a Pinto," according to a 1992 news article in *USA Today*. The faulty design of both products warranted a massive recall and served to smudge the reputation of their manufacturers. Unlike the big–three Pinto manufacturer Ford Motor Company, IUD makers didn't fare so well; Dalkon's A.H. Robins Company declared bankruptcy due to lawsuits costing the company over $480 million, and other IUD manufacturers pulled out of the business because they could no longer afford liability insurance.

But IUDs didn't just fade into the sunset. Scientists improved them, making a second generation of the devices safer and more appealing. Now, American women are once again turning to IUDs for effective long–term birth control.

As you can imagine, researchers conducted numerous studies once women started experiencing problems with the Dalkon Shield. There were two kinds of problem: miscarriages and pelvic inflammatory disease (PID), an infection that can cause infertility. Earlier clinical studies indicated no association with either of these problems, but once the court battles started, researchers found astonishingly high rates of complications with the Dalkon Shield and an unexpected link between all types of intrauterine devices and PID.

Modern researchers have criticized both the conclusions of these older studies and the way they were conducted. After re–examining the data, they feel that other factors, such as life-style, may play a crucial role in the development of complications among women using an IUD.

Although there is no general consensus on the research findings, most experts agree that IUDs are an excellent contraceptive choice for most women as long as the devices are inserted under sterile conditions. Women at risk for sexually transmitted disease, however, should probably select another form of birth control.

What Was the Dalkon Shield?

Throughout this century, IUDs have been manufactured in many different shapes and sizes. The first devices came on the market in 1909. These simple nickel, bronze, and catgut rings later gave way to FDA–approved plastic devices that looked like squiggly S's (Lippes Loop, 1964–1985), ram's horns (Saf–T–Coil, 1967–1983), the number 7 (Copper–7, 1973–1986), and the letter T (Copper–T 380A, 1984– , Progestasert, 1976–, Copper–T, 1976–1986). A string (tail) attached to the bottom of each device protruded from the cervical opening. If you could feel the string with your finger, you could be sure your IUD was still in place. This tail also made removal easier.

The Dalkon Shield, introduced in 1970 and recalled in 1975, was a plastic device which looked like a round bug with one large eye and five legs on each side. It had a unique tail: not a single filament, but many fibers wound together and enclosed in a sheath. It was this string that led to its demise.

Some scientists now believe that the string had nothing to do with the increased rates of infection seen with the Dalkon Shield. It had been suggested that the string was a breeding ground for bacteria, and that it acted as a wick for bacteria, drawing them from the vagina up into the uterus and on into the fallopian tubes, thus causing dangerous infections. However, the theory did not hold up in subsequent testing, and another factor cast additional doubt: Although the Dalkon Shield came in two sizes—a large one for women who had given birth, and a smaller one for those who had never had children—

THE NOTORIOUS DALKON SHIELD

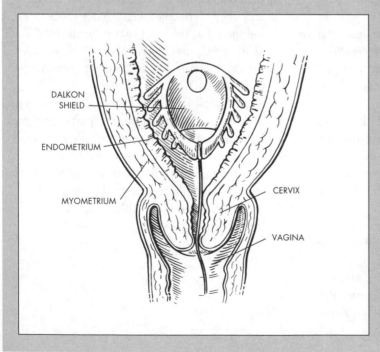

DALKON SHIELD

ENDOMETRIUM

MYOMETRIUM

CERVIX

VAGINA

A series of 12 deaths due to miscarriage-related infections in the early 1970s drove the popular IUD called the Dalkon Shield off the market, sent its manufacturer into bankruptcy, and tarnished the image of all IUDs for decades to come. No matter that some 2.8 million women had used the Shield, making the risk of death infinitesimally low, or that only one oversized version of the device was linked to the deaths: In little more than a decade, sales of all IUDs plummeted by more than two-thirds. Ironically, the fear of IUDs appears to be baseless. The rate of pelvic infection among IUD users is actually lower than among women using no contraceptive at all.

and both sizes had a multifilament string, only the larger size was associated with pregnancy–related deaths.

How IUDs Got a Bad Name

During the 1960s and 1970s, IUDs thrived. All of them were made of plastic (polyethylene), with some barium sulfate added so that they would show up on x–rays. The first American IUD, a large device called the Margulies Coil, caused a lot of bleeding and cramping and had a hard plastic tail that male sexual partners often found uncomfortable. The softer Lippes Loop replaced it. Later, the Saf–T–Coil and the short–lived Majzlin Spring came along.

Dalkon Shield became available at the same time as the U.S. Senate was holding inquiries into the safety of oral contraceptives. It was an immediate hit, especially among young women who had doubts about the pill. The year that A.H. Robins began marketing the Shield, the devices accounted for 66 percent of all IUDs sold, and by mid–1973, about 40 percent of all IUDs in use were Shields. By June 1974, when the FDA requested suspension of further sales, 2.8 million women had purchased the device.

Several months earlier, the FDA had urged physicians to remove IUDs immediately from any woman who became pregnant. Their recommendation was based on the fact that 12 IUD users had died after miscarriages left them with severe infections. Ten had the Dalkon Shield in place at the time, and two the Lippes Loop. After physicians began following the FDA's advice, IUD–related death from miscarriages ceased to be a problem.

However, these events led to further scrutiny of the Shield, and sparked an explosion of fear and distrust of all IUDs.

The data connecting the Dalkon Shield to miscarriage and even to death seemed overwhelming. Doctors reported that Dalkon Shield users were twice as likely to be hospitalized as other women, and that those who became pregnant while wearing an IUD—especially the Shield—increased their chance of dying by up to 50 times that of women with no IUD in place. Although some scientists pointed out weaknesses in the studies, women still avoided the device.

In the wake of the Dalkon Shield scandal, some researchers began charging that IUDs were also responsible for an increased risk of pelvic inflammatory disease. Initial studies showed that women using other forms of birth control did indeed have a lower rate of PID than did IUD users. Barrier methods blocked bacteria; and the Pill, by thickening the mucus in the cervix, made bacterial entry difficult.

However, when compared with women using no form of contraception at all, IUD users actually have a *lower* risk of PID. And researchers during the Dalkon Shield period were unaware of what we now know: The greatest risk factor for PID is frequent sex with multiple partners. Since use of IUDs peaked during the sexual revolution of the 1960s and 70s, IUDs mistakenly got the blame that increased sexual freedom deserved.

The Dalkon Shield disaster continued to cast a pall over all forms of intrauterine devices. IUDs containing copper—introduced during and shortly after the Shield publicity—never became popular in the United States. Total IUD sales declined from 2.2 million to 0.7 million between 1981 and 1988, and manufacturers found that the costs of defending lawsuits were prohibitive.

Although copper IUDs were never proved dangerous, most disappeared from the market by the late 1980s. Only two—the Copper–T 380A (the ParaGard) and the Progestasert—remain available in the United States today.

In other parts of the world, where the negative press about IUDs was never extensive, close to 100 million women now use these devices. In fact, they are the most popular form of birth control in such countries as China, Norway, Finland, and Egypt.

Recent worldwide studies suggest that:

- IUDs increase a monogamous woman's chances of getting PID only in the first 3 weeks to 3 months after insertion
- IUDs don't affect a woman's chances of having children in the future
- No women have died after an IUD–related miscarriage since 1977
- IUDs have the lowest failure rate of all reversible contraceptives (less than 1 percent)
- IUD users are more satisfied with their method than are women using any other type of birth control; 98 percent of IUD users report satisfaction, while 92 percent of Pill users and 87 percent of condom users say they are satisfied

Are Today's IUDs Right For You?

In order to decide whether you are a good candidate for an IUD, you need to know:

- How IUDs work
- How effective they are
- Who should avoid them
- What their advantages are
- Whether you can tolerate possible side effects and complications

How do IUDs Work?

Scientists aren't sure why the IUD is such an effective method of birth control. It was once thought that, as foreign objects, they produced an inflammatory response in the uterus that disrupted the implantation of a fertilized egg, but researchers haven't been able to prove this theory. In fact, when they look for fertilized eggs in the fallopian tubes of IUD users, they rarely find them. These studies should help ease the minds of women who are opposed to methods which prevent pregnancy by aborting a fertilized egg.

Now more researchers are fairly certain that IUDs are spermicidal. The inflammatory response may be enough to kill sperm before they ever get into the fallopian tubes to fertilize an egg.

There are two types of IUDs currently available in the United States, both of which have added pregnancy–preventing characteristics. The Copper T–380A, or ParaGard, is a T–shaped device with copper wire wound around the stem and copper tubing on the arms of the T. The frame also contains barium sulfate so that the IUD will show up on x–rays. The copper, besides intensifying the inflammatory response, has a chemical impact on the uterine lining, changing the normal levels of several enzymes. The environment copper creates throughout the reproductive tract is not friendly to eggs and sperm, making it unlikely that they will ever come together and form an embryo. The ParaGard remains effective for up to 8 years.

The Progestasert IUD is also T–shaped, but the vertical stem is actually a reservoir for 38 milligrams of progesterone, the naturally occurring hormone that helps bring about menstruation. Like Norplant implants or Depo–Provera (see chapter 21, "Hormonal Options: Pills, Shots, and Implants") the

THE OPTIONS TODAY

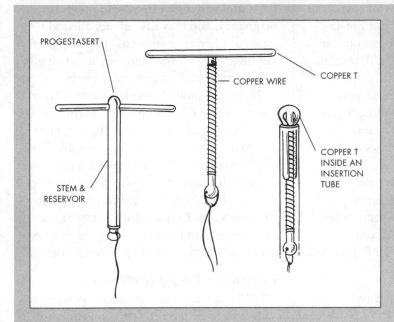

PROGESTASERT

COPPER WIRE

COPPER T

COPPER T INSIDE AN INSERTION TUBE

STEM & RESERVOIR

Only two IUDs have survived into the nineties: the Copper-T (or ParaGard) and the Progestasert. The Copper-T has the best track record of any contraceptive product: Your odds of becoming pregnant are only 1 in 500 during its first year of use. Odds with the Progestasert are not quite as favorable—over 1 in 100 in a given year—but it offers the added benefit of reduced cramping and bleeding for women with heavy periods.

device releases progesterone daily. This thickens cervical mucus, making it difficult for sperm to pass through the cervix. This IUD also diminishes cramping and blood loss, so it is an excellent choice for women who have heavy, uncomfortable periods. The Progestasert remains effective as long as it contains a sufficient amount of hormone; doctors usually replace it every year.

A similar device called the LevoNova—which is not available in the U.S.—contains a hormone known as levonorgestrel. It seems to be as effective as copper IUDs, and can be left in place for 7 years.

How Effective are IUDs?

Like the famous battery, the IUD "keeps working, and working, and working." Depending on the brand, it will protect you from pregnancy for up to 8 years. And, best of all, you don't have to do anything: There's no pill to remember or device to insert before sex. Some factors, however, including your age, your childbirth history, and your doctor's experience with IUD insertion, can reduce its effectiveness.

Failure rates for IUDs are the highest during the first two years. Still, in the first year of use for copper–releasing IUDs, only 2 women in every 1,000 will become pregnant. After eight years, the pregnancy rate for the ParaGard is still only 1.5 per 100 users—the lowest long–term rate of any copper IUD. For Progestasert, the pregnancy rate ranges from 1 to 3 women per 100 each year.

Who Should Avoid the IUD?

If you have a sexually transmitted disease—or risk getting one from a variety of sexual partners—you definitely should not use an IUD. In addition, if you're monogamous but aren't sure about your partner, an IUD might not be the best choice.

IUD manufacturers suggest that a good IUD candidate is a woman who already has had her children. Their concern arises, perhaps, from the potential for lawsuits over infertility, rather than from any medical data.

Known or suspected pregnancy precludes use of an IUD, as does active, recurrent, or recent pelvic infection. Here are some other problems you should discuss with your doctor before deciding whether an IUD is the right choice for you:

- Unexplained, irregular, or abnormal uterine bleeding
- Severe menstrual cramps or heavy periods
- Known or suspected cervical or uterine cancer, including a Pap smear whose results are inconclusive
- A history of endocarditis (heart inflammation), rheumatic heart disease, or the presence of artificial heart valves
- Problems with blood–clotting
- Reduced immune response (sometimes brought on by steroid treatment)
- Previous pregnancies while using an IUD
- A history of IUD expulsion from the uterus
- Abnormal uterine anatomy, such as a wall (septum) down the middle of the uterus, noncancerous tumors underneath the muscle surface which may increase bleeding, or a very thin cervical opening
- A copper allergy or Wilson's disease (excess copper in the body)
- Anemia
- A history of fainting

What Are the Advantages and Disadvantages?

IUDs are extremely effective in preventing pregnancy, and they are safe for the right women. They are easy to use because there's nothing to remember, and they don't change your normal cyclic hormonal pattern.

However, unlike some methods of birth control, IUDs offer no protection from STDs. The devices can also cause cramping, pain and extra bleeding when first inserted. They can be expensive: The Progestasert costs about $100, and the ParaGard is approximately $160. Insertion fees can add another $160 to $400. And if the doctor has little experience with inserting IUDs, the effectiveness of the device could be compromised.

Potential Complications

The most serious problems you might have with an IUD are infection, tubal pregnancy, and perforation of the uterine wall. These and other complications cause 1 in about every 100 to 300 IUD users to be hospitalized for intensive antibiotic treatment or surgery every year.

Infections

Insertion of an IUD can introduce bacteria into your uterus. Experts believe that most infections occurring from 3 weeks to 3 months after placement of an IUD are caused by unsterile insertion. Infections after that time are thought to be STDs.

The World Health Organization conducted a study recently which put to rest the nagging suspicion that IUDs cause pelvic inflammatory disease. In almost 23,000 IUD users studied, researchers found only 81 cases of PID. They also determined that PID risk was 6 times higher during the 20 days after insertion; and that the risk remained low for the next 8 years.

This study showed that PID occurred infrequently in women at low risk of sexually transmitted disease. It also found that PID was extremely rare in China, where more than half of all women of childbearing age use IUDs and where there are few cases of STDs. The researchers suggest that IUDs be left in place for as long as they are effective, and that physicians refrain from removing them periodically to combat potential infections, as some now do. Ironically, this routine removal followed by reinsertion can lead to even more infections.

Scientists are also investigating the benefits of using antibiotics, such as doxycycline, at the time of insertion to prevent infection. While some doctors don't recommend this yet, studies with small numbers of women have shown that preventative antibiotics can reduce the chance of infection by about 31 percent.

Still, if you get an infection for whatever reason while using an IUD, it can cause serious problems, including tubal infertility, peritonitis (infection of the entire abdomen), and liver damage. If bacteria get into your bloodstream, it can prove fatal.

Doctors can treat early infections successfully with antibiotics. If the infection isn't severe, your physician may opt to leave your IUD in place for a few days to see if the infection goes away. You will probably get a shot of Cefoxitin (Mefoxin) plus an oral dose of probenecid (1 gram), or a shot of Ceftriaxone (Rocephin) and a 2–week prescription for oral doxycycline (Doryx).

If your infection is severe, your doctor will almost certainly remove the IUD. If you require hospitalization, you may need intra-venous injections of Cefoxitin or Ceftriaxone, plus oral doxycycline over a two–week period.

Abdominal pain, a high temperature, bleeding, and discharge could be a sign of infection. If you experience any of these symptoms, contact your physician immediately.

Vaginitis and cervicitis (infections of the vagina and the passage to the uterus) are also more common among IUD users. It's possible that the strings irritate the cervix and predispose the user to this type of infection. Although vaginitis and cervicitis can easily be treated with antibiotics, their characteristic, strong–smelling discharge could signal a more serious uterine infection, such as PID. If your discharge has a peculiar odor, make sure your doctor checks you carefully to ensure your condition isn't serious.

DANGER SIGNS IN EARLY PREGNANCY

Contact your doctor immediately or go to the hospital emergency room if you develop any of these signs:

Warnings of Possible Miscarriage:
- Your last period was late, and now your bleeding is heavy—possibly with clots or clumps of tissue—and cramping is more severe than usual.
- Your period is prolonged and heavy—5 to 7 days of heavy flow.
- You have abdominal pain and fever.

Warnings of Possible Ectopic Pregnancy:
- You experience sudden intense pain, persistent pain, or cramping in the lower abdomen, usually on one side or the other.
- Your last period was late, and now you are having irregular bleeding and spotting with abdominal pain.
- You faint or feel dizzy, possibly a sign of internal bleeding.

Pregnancy

If pregnancy does occur, partial or complete—but undetected—expulsion of the IUD is at fault about one–third of the time. However, pregnancies can and will occur even when the IUD is properly placed.

IUD users have twice as many miscarriages as do nonusers; and ectopic pregnancy (a pregnancy developing outside the uterus) occurs more often among IUD users than among those who use the Pill, diaphragms, condoms, or spermicides.

If you do become pregnant, your doctor should remove your IUD immediately if the strings are still visible. After removal of an IUD with visible strings, the miscarriage rate is about 30 percent.

Removal is more difficult if the string can't be seen. If you want the pregnancy to continue, your doctor should not try to remove the IUD without the aid of sonographic guidance. This technique will help him or her avoid rupturing the membranes of the uterus.

Leaving the IUD in place during a pregnancy is not recommended. The chance of a miscarriage—and a life–threatening infection—increases 20–fold by the second trimester.

An ectopic pregnancy can cause a rupture and massive internal bleeding. Researchers believe that 1 in every 5 Progestasert users has an ectopic pregnancy each year, while 1 in 60 women using a copper IUD such as the ParaGard will have one. While women who use ParaGard have far fewer ectopic pregnancies than those who don't use any type of contraception, women using Progestasert have double the risk.

Learn to recognize the signs of possible miscarriage or ectopic pregnancy. (See the box about "Danger Signs In Early Pregnancy" nearby.)

Perforations

An IUD can puncture the wall of your uterus or your cervix, or can embed itself in the uterine wall. A puncture to the cervix can happen at any time, but a puncture to the uterus usually happens during insertion. Therefore, it is important to find a doctor experienced in placing IUDs. Your chance of perforation ranges from less than 1 in 1,000 to no more than 9 in 1,000.

You might not know that your IUD has slipped outside your uterus because there may not be any bleeding or pain. Other than pregnancy, disappearance of your IUD's strings may be the only sign you'll get that the IUD is no longer in place. X–rays can show lost IUDs, as can ultrasound; but ultrasound is not effective if fibrous tissue has built up in the abdomen or if the IUD is freely floating in the pelvic area.

A migrating IUD may or may not cause infection. An all–plastic device may not be a problem, even if you leave it in its new location. Copper IUDs usually get encased in fibrous adhesions and rarely produce serious symptoms. Talk with your doctor about the need to remove the IUD. Many health care professionals recommend leaving an out–of–place IUD in the abdomen. Removal requires laparoscopic surgery, in which a lighted tube is inserted through a one–inch incision in the abdomen.

Bleeding and Cramping

When you first get your IUD, it's not unusual to experience bleeding or spotting between periods, as well as heavier periods. This condition usually lasts for only a short time;

most IUD users report that by their third period, the bleeding has become more regular. In some cases, increased bleeding can lead to anemia if you're prone to that condition. That's why doctors often recommend iron supplements for IUD users. Vitamin C (200 milligrams 3 times daily) can improve spotting problems.

You might notice cramps, backache, and pelvic pain within 24 hours after you start wearing your IUD. You may also notice cramps or pelvic pain accompanying intercourse or breastfeeding, both of which cause the uterus to contract. Ovulation may be slightly more painful than usual, and you may also experience spotting at that time.

Since bleeding and cramping are common side effects of IUD use, but also can be indicative of PID, how do you know when you are in danger? It is often difficult to distinguish between a harmless side effect and a warning of possible infection. In general, you should call your doctor if you have pain and cramps that last longer than 12 to 24 hours and do not respond to pain relievers such as ibuprofen (Advil, Motrin).

Expulsion From the Uterus

Uterine contractions can push an IUD out of your uterus. Although it may seem hard to believe, many women don't even feel it happening.

During the first year of use, between 5 percent and 20 percent of IUD users experience a spontaneous expulsion of the device. Like infections, this is most likely to happen in the first few months, when the body is getting used to something foreign inside the uterus. It's more common in women who have a small uterus (2 and three–quarter inches or less) and in those who've never been pregnant. The more skilled the person

inserting the device, the less the possibility of expulsion. Other risk factors include childbirth at an early age, abnormal menstrual flow, and painful periods. Signs that could be a warning of expulsion are:

- Unusual vaginal discharge
- Bleeding or spotting
- Cramps and abdominal pain
- Strings that seem longer than normal or disappear
- An IUD tip that sticks out of the cervix
- An IUD that your partner can feel
- Signs of pregnancy

Expulsions are most likely to happen when you're menstruating, so always check sanitary pads and tampons, and don't forget to look into the toilet after you've used it. If you expel the device, you need to use another contraceptive until it's replaced.

Lost strings

Sometimes the string of an IUD can pull up into the uterus, giving you no way to know if the device is in its proper position. Your physician can use special instruments to find the strings. If they can't be found, he or she may have to remove the IUD and replace it with another one.

Reactions to copper

Allergies to copper are extremely rare, and it is even more unusual to retain high amounts of copper in body tissues (Wilson's disease). Copper IUDs release only about one-thirtieth of an adult's daily dietary requirement for copper.

If you are allergic to copper, you may notice a reaction resembling a skin rash after you start using the ParaGard.

THE INSERTION PROCEDURE

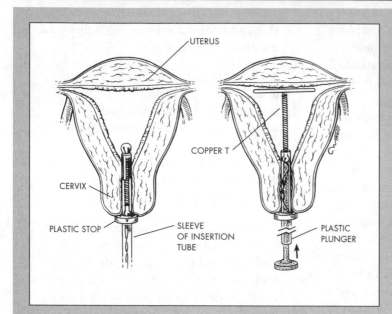

UTERUS

COPPER T

CERVIX

PLASTIC STOP

SLEEVE OF INSERTION TUBE

PLASTIC PLUNGER

Though a copper IUD can be left in place for up to 8 years with minimal attention, the initial insertion can be a minor ordeal. Done in the doctor's office or clinic, the procedure can be painful; and cramping can continue for up to a day. To insert the device, the doctor will pass a special applicator through the cervix into the lower end of the uterus. As it is pushed upwards with a plunger, the device unfolds to form a "T." A string is left protruding from the cervix to permit later removal.

What's Involved In Getting an IUD

If you've decided to use an IUD, you'll need to find a qualified physician to insert and eventually to remove the device. He or she should have completed at least 5 supervised insertions before trying it independently.

You may have to go to the clinic a few days before your scheduled insertion to be checked for infections. In any case, you will need a routine physical exam and a Pap test to check for the signs of infection right before the insertion.

To reduce the pain and cramping that usually occurs during the first 12 to 24 hours after an IUD insertion, take aspirin or ibuprofen an hour before your appointment. You may also want to have someone go with you to the clinic and drive you home, in case you feel queasy, shaky, or weak.

Insertion

The insertion procedure is simple and takes only 5 minutes. Many women feel pain, but some don't. To help you deal with the pain, your doctor may give you a "paracervical block," which consists of injections of lidocaine into your cervix. It will take effect in 2 to 5 minutes.

After the pelvic exam, your physician will determine the size and position of your uterus by using a procedure known as "sounding." He or she will open your vagina with an instrument called a speculum, and wash your cervix with a disinfectant. A long clamp called a tenaculum grasps your cervix and helps steady your uterus, minimizing the likelihood of perforation. Your doctor will push a uterine sound, a blunt rod–shaped instrument, through your cervical canal and into the uterus to determine whether your uterus is big enough to accommodate an IUD (it should be at least 2 and one–quarter inches) and if so, how deep he or she will need to insert the IUD to reach the top of the uterus (the fundus).

At this point, you're ready for the IUD. The doctor folds down the arms of the T–shaped device and loads it into a long tube. He or she inserts the tube into the uterus and releases the IUD by slowly and gently withdrawing the tube. This part of the procedure may cause cramping due to uterine contractions.

After insertion, you'll need to put one or two fingers into your vagina to check for your strings. Once you've located your cervix—it will feel smooth and round—you can touch the strings, which feel like nylon fishing line. Every month after your period you should check in this manner to ensure that you haven't expelled the device. You'll also want to make sure you can't feel the hard tip of the IUD coming out of your cervix.

You may have some bleeding and spotting during the first few days after insertion. This is normal, so don't worry. If the bleeding is heavy and constant, contact your doctor to rule out the possibility of infection.

Your first period will probably be a little heavier than normal; it also may come a few days early. You should schedule a follow–up appointment after your first period, sometime within 4 to 6 weeks of insertion. Don't wait longer than 3 months to have a checkup.

Unless you've just had a baby, you can have sex as soon as you like after an IUD insertion. Some doctors recommend using a backup method such as a condom during the first month to reduce your risk of infection. You don't need a backup method to protect you from pregnancy because an IUD is effective immediately.

Adverse Reactions After an Insertion

When the nerves of your cervix are stimulated, your blood pressure sometimes drops, or your heart rate may slow down. This could make you feel dizzy, nauseous, faint, and weak. Although most such reactions are mild and last only 15 to 30 minutes, convulsions and even heart arrest is possible. If your reaction is severe, your doctor may give you a drug called atropine.

WHAT'S THE BEST TIME FOR IUD INSERTION?

Because it's dangerous to insert an IUD into a pregnant woman, your doctor may suggest you schedule the procedure during your monthly period. Not only does that eliminate the possibility of pregnancy, but since your cervix is slightly dilated during your period, insertion will be easier.

If you are not pregnant you can have an IUD inserted ...

- Any time during your menstrual cycle, provided you are using another effective birth control method consistently, or have had a negative pregnancy test
- Any time during your menstrual cycle, if you haven't had sex since your last period
- Within six days of unprotected sex, if you want a post–intercourse (emergency) contraceptive.

If you have just been pregnant, you can have an IUD inserted...

- Immediately after or within 3 weeks of an uncomplicated first trimester miscarriage
- Immediately (within 10 minutes) following childbirth—by either vaginal or cesarean delivery
- Six weeks after giving birth if you are breast-feeding
- Six weeks postpartum, if you haven't had a period return, are not breast feeding, and have had a negative pregnancy test

Removal

There are several reasons to have an IUD removed. You may find you don't like it. You may wish to become pregnant. You may develop an infection or persistent side effects you can't tolerate. And, of course, at the end of an IUD's effective life—one year for the Progestasert and eight years for the ParaGard— you must have it removed and, if you wish, replaced.

Removal is usually easier and less painful than insertion. Your physician will take some of the same preliminary steps done for insertion, such as determining the position of the uterus. Once the strings are located, he or she will use a clamp to grab them and slowly pull the IUD out. The flexible arms of the T will fold up again as the device comes through the cervical canal.

If the strings can't be found, they may be just inside the cervical canal. The doctor may try to coax them out of your cervix with cotton–tipped swabs. If that fails, he or she will need to use a uterine sound again. Once the device is located, the physician will extract it with a pair of tweezer–like clamps. If this too fails, sonography may be necessary to locate the IUD.

The Next Generation of IUDs

Scientists are working on intrauterine devices that could cut down on expulsion rates and bleeding. One promising new IUD is called the FlexiGard or Cu–Fix. It is frameless, consisting of six copper sleeves strung on a surgical nylon thread that is knotted at one end. This string of copper is then "harpooned" into the lining at the top of the uterus, using a notched needle. So far, insertion has proved difficult for doctors taking part in the studies because the needle must be pushed hard–but not too hard– to attach the device.

Other modified and improved devices, including the French Ombrelle–250, the Cu–Safe (designed to be more flexible), and the TCu–380 Slimline (designed to make insertion easier), may also reach the market in the near future. □

CHAPTER 21   **FERTILITY AND FAMILY PLANNING**

Hormonal Options: Pills, Shots, and Implants

Women were preventing pregnancy long before there were any books about it—in fact, even before there was paper for printing the books. The first prescription for a contraceptive was written on papyrus around 1550 B.C. It seems to have called for crocodile dung to be inserted into the vagina, as the ancient Egyptians preferred. For ancient Arabians, elephant dung mixed with honey was the method of choice. And women in Northern Canada drank a potion of dried beaver testicles mixed with alcohol to avoid pregnancy.

Fortunately, technology has advanced to a point where we no longer have to rely on such methods of contraception. Modern science allows us to convert natural substances, such as the Mexican yam, into remarkably simple delivery systems, like tablets, subdermal implants, and shots.

Hormonal birth control methods—including oral contraceptives (the Pill), the Norplant implant, and Depo–Provera Contraceptive Injection—have several things in common. They are all highly effective and safe for most women; they all reduce cramp-

ing and pain related to the menstrual cycle; and they all require a doctor's prescription. Unfortunately, these forms of birth control offer little protection from sexually transmitted diseases; and all may be accompanied by health risks and side effects.

How Hormonal Methods Work

Pills, implants, and injections all have one goal: to prevent your reproductive system from producing a mature egg. They do this by tricking the system into skipping a key step in the interlocking cycle of hormone production that triggers the egg's release from the ovary. The deception works like this:

Under ordinary circumstances, the brain's **hypothalamus** produces **GnRH** (gonadotropin–releasing hormone). This prompts the **pituitary gland** to release **FSH** (follicle stimulating hormone) which travels to the ovaries through the bloodstream and causes a follicle to grow. The development of the follicle produces **estrogen,** which after about 10 days reaches high enough levels to trip off a surge of **LH** (luteinizing hormone) from the pituitary gland. The ovarian follicle releases a mature egg into the fallopian tube about 24 hours after this surge of LH, and the empty follicle becomes known as the **corpus luteum.** The cells of the corpus luteum produce **progesterone** and estrogen, which together stimulate the uterine lining to thicken with blood in preparation for nurturing a fertilized egg. Once the corpus luteum wanes and the lining is left with no hormonal support, it sloughs off during your monthly period. The low levels of estrogen and progesterone also signal the hypothalamus to start the process over again.

Since oral contraceptives (OCs) provide a steady level of both progestin (a substitute for progesterone) and estrogen every day, and

HOW HORMONAL METHODS SHORT-CIRCUIT THE REPRODUCTIVE CYCLE

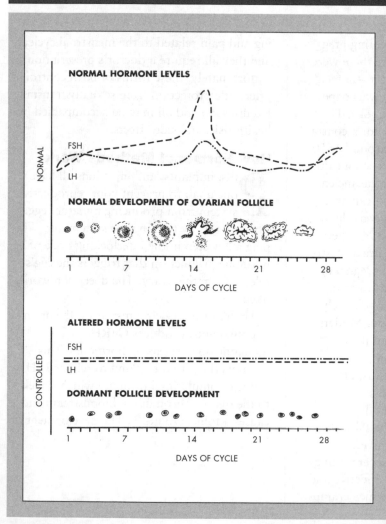

NORMAL HORMONE LEVELS

FSH

LH

NORMAL DEVELOPMENT OF OVARIAN FOLLICLE

NORMAL

1   7   14   21   28

DAYS OF CYCLE

ALTERED HORMONE LEVELS

FSH

LH

DORMANT FOLLICLE DEVELOPMENT

CONTROLLED

1   7   14   21   28

DAYS OF CYCLE

Hormonal contraceptives work by damping down the two key hormones that trigger ovulation. Follicle stimulating hormone (FSH), the substance that coaxes an egg towards maturity, is the first to be suppressed. Luteinizing hormone (LH), which ordinarily triggers release of the egg at mid-cycle, is also held down. Production of both these substances usually starts when the body senses a shortage of two other hormones: progesterone and estrogen, both produced in the ovaries. Hormonal contraceptives supply just enough of these substances to prevent start-up of the FSH/LH production cycle. Constant levels of estrogen and progesterone thus produce constant levels of FSH and LH, and the eggs remain dormant.

Norplant implants and Depo–Provera provide steady daily levels of progestin, there is no signal to the hypothalamus to release GnRH and therefore no signal to the pituitary gland to produce FSH and LH. Because FSH stimulates the ovaries to grow egg follicles, and LH triggers ovulation, their absence causes the ovary to be relatively dormant, and no egg is produced to a point where it could be released. Hormonal contraception locks the system into the same late phase of the cycle on a continuous basis, perpetually skipping the all–important release of GnRH.

Suppression of ovulation is the main mode by which OCs and Depo–Provera prevent pregnancy; the implant system causes ovulation suppression about 50 percent of the time. However, throughout each pill cycle, and continuously with Norplant implants and Depo–Provera, the mucous covering the cervix—the site where sperm enters the uterus—stays thick and sticky, making it very difficult for sperm to get through. This gooey impediment also acts on the sperm cell itself. It prevents fertilization by interfering with chemical changes inside the sperm that allow it to penetrate an egg's outer coating.

Even if ovulation and fertilization do take place, hormonal methods provide another measure of protection: changes to the uterine lining. Normally, estrogen initiates the thickening of the lining of the uterus in the first part of the cycle, while progesterone kicks in later to help the lining mature. Since both hormones are present throughout the pill cycle, and progestin is supplied continuously by implants and the shot, the usual hormonal variations are masked and the lining rarely has a chance to develop enough to nurture a fertilized egg.

All the hormonal methods currently available to us offer many benefits, including protection from cancer. However, they aren't 100 percent effective, and they aren't right for all women. To correct this, scientists are busy developing new forms of hormonal contraception which may be easier to use and may suit more women. These methods include biodegradable implants, pellets the size of a grain of rice, and a new product called the vaginal ring. Like a diaphragm, this device is removable. But unlike barrier contraceptives, it releases steady levels of progestins to prevent pregnancy.

Even without these new approaches, the array of choices at your disposal is varied and wide. Before you decide on a method take time to weigh the benefits and risks of all the forms of hormonal contraception available today. The following overview provides the basic information you'll need, but be sure to discuss any questions with your physician. Together you can find the approach that's optimal for you personally.

Oral Contraceptives

Birth control pills have been popular since the 1960s, and today they are relied upon by more than half of all women using a reversible method of birth control. Over the years, a tremendous amount of research has been done on their effects, but despite the large body of knowledge available, scientists are still at work investigating such things as the association between OCs and breast cancer.

Even if you think you're well informed about oral contraceptives, take this quick true/false quiz to determine your "Pill I.Q.":

- The Pill works by destroying the egg once it is released from the ovary.
- Taking the Pill too long makes it difficult for most women to conceive; it may even cause them to become sterile.
- A woman should take a short break from the Pill after she has used it for five years.
- Women over 35 years old should not take the Pill.
- Taking the Pill can lead to many types of cancer, including ovarian and endometrial cancer.

If you answered false to all these statements, you know more about the Pill than a great many people. A recent Gallup poll of over

THE PILL: PROS AND CONS

To help you decide whether oral contraception is for you, here's a brief overview of its pluses and minuses:

Advantages:
- Highly effective
- Does not interrupt sex
- Safe for most women
- Protects against ovarian and endometrial cancer
- Decreases menstrual cramps and pain
- Reduces menstrual blood flow, thereby reducing anemia
- Is easily reversible
- Is easy to use and discontinue
- Has been well researched

Disadvantages:
- Offers no protection from sexually transmitted diseases
- Can be expensive
- Produces rare but dangerous complications
- May cause mood changes
- May give rise to nuisance side effects such as headaches, weight gain, and breakthrough bleeding
- Must be taken every day

1,000 American women aged 18 to 44 found that knowledge is sorely lacking about this widespread method of birth control. For example, one–quarter of the survey's respondents believed that the Pill works by killing the egg, when in fact it inhibits egg production altogether.

Taking OCs for many years poses no increased risk of infertility, as was believed by 45 percent of the respondents. Experts say women don't need to take a break from the Pill, even after using it for long periods of time.

Forty–three percent of those interviewed said that women over age 35 shouldn't take OCs. However, the truth is that healthy nonsmoking women can use OCs all the way through menopause without any detriment to health.

More importantly, very few women interviewed for this poll knew that the Pill can actually protect women from certain health problems, including some types of cancer. Although it is clearly stated on the Pill package insert, less than 20 percent of women polled knew that the Pill helps reduce the incidence of ovarian and endometrial cancer, ovarian cysts, and benign cysts of the breast.

The Pill is not right for all women because, despite its beneficial effects, it is also associated with some risks. Doctors usually advise women likely to suffer from heart attacks, strokes, or blood clots—especially those who smoke—to choose some other type of contraception. Several other conditions, such as hypertension, diabetes, or sickle cell disease, also make Pill–taking risky.

The following information should help you improve your "Pill I.Q."

Your OC Options

Birth control pills come in packs of either 21 "active" pills (containing hormones), or packs of 28 pills, 21 of which are active and seven of which are inactive placebos. The placebo pills are simply a way of staying in the habit of taking a daily pill, even while having your period.

Either package, 21 days or 28 days, can be "monophasic" or "triphasic." Monophasic pills provide the same dosage level of hormones all through the active cycle, whereas triphasic pills give different dosage levels during each week of active pills. Triphasics were designed to more closely follow a woman's natural hormonal pattern. However, most experts say the fluctuations don't really matter and may even cause extra problems, such as increased "breakthrough" bleeding (sporadic menstruation) while on the Pill, or an increase in Pill-related headaches.

Birth control pills are either called "combined" OCs or "progestin–only" OCs. Combined pills are a combination of the hormones estrogen and progesterone. Progestin–only pills, also called minipills, lack the estrogen component. Since women shouldn't use estrogen–containing products when they are breastfeeding, minipills are often prescribed for women who want protection from pregnancy six weeks after they give birth. Minipills also have lower doses of progestin than combination forms, making them a good choice for women worried about metabolic effects of the hormones (but a bad choice for women who want highly effective birth control). They also require a woman to take them on a rigidly regular schedule.

How Effective Is the Pill?

Given all the ways the Pill discourages fertilization it's hard to believe that anyone can

ARE YOU A GOOD CANDIDATE FOR OCS?

You and your doctor should discuss the pros and cons of birth control pills. In general, pills might not be right for you if you:

- Are pregnant
- Are over 35 and a heavy smoker (more than 15 cigarettes a day)
- Are over 50 years of age
- Begin getting migraine headaches after you start using the Pill
- Are about to have major surgery which would immobilize you
- Are breastfeeding
- Have had a child in the last two weeks

Additionally, OCs might not be right for you if you have or have had in the past:

- Problems with blood clots (thrombophlebitis or cerebrovascular accidents)
- Heart disease
- Cancer of the breast or reproductive tract
- Liver problems or cancer
- Kidney disease
- High blood pressure
- Diabetes
- Active gallbladder disease
- Congenital hyperbilirubinemia (Gilbert's disease)
- Conditions which would make it difficult to take a pill every day (mental retardation, psychiatric illness, substance abuse)

get pregnant while using it. And in fact, the Pill does have an effectiveness rate of over 99 percent when used correctly, (taking an active tablet every day during the 21–day cycle). However, because women do forget to take a pill now and then, actual effectiveness in real–world use is about 97 percent.

That may sound pretty good, but remember that it does fall short of total certainty.

For example, even assuming the Pill is 99.5 percent effective, 84,000 of the 16.8 million women currently using OCs will have an unintended pregnancy, even if they take their pills correctly every day! If you are concerned about accidental pregnancy while using OCs, you should use a backup method—like a condom or spermicide—each time you have sex. In addition to allaying your fears about getting pregnant, a latex condom, unlike the Pill, will help protect you from the viral types of sexually transmitted disease.

The Benefits and Risks

OCs are among the most thoroughly studied drugs in the world. The vast body of data collected on them indicates that although they do have certain side effects, few women are likely to experience them. Moreover, most of the information on side effects was collected from studies of higher dose pills than those generally in use today. And research done in the Pill's early years involved women who had not been screened to see if they were good candidates. Today, women with a personal or family history of heart disease or other illnesses linked to the Pill are usually steered towards another method of birth control. If you are healthy, you don't smoke more than 15 cigarettes a day, and no one in your family has suffered from cancer, a heart attack, or very high cholesterol, you may never experience any of the more serious side effects.

The Pill can produce both "nuisance" side effects and more serious health problems. Included among the more serious potential effects are increased risk of cervical and liver cancer (and possibly breast cancer—studies so far are inconclusive), heart and blood vessel disorders (clots and high cholesterol), high blood pressure, increased blood sugar

levels, complications with the liver and gallbladder, cervical changes (increasing your risk for sexually transmitted diseases), eye problems, and delays in fertility once pills are discontinued. Some women at risk for these complications can continue taking OCs if they use them cautiously. Your doctor should be able to help you determine whether or not you should avoid the Pill.

Cancer: Women who have used OCs sometime in their lives are less likely to develop cancer by age 55 than women who have never taken the Pill. Oral contraceptives really do protect against certain kinds of cancer. If you use OCs for at least a year, your risk of developing endometrial cancer diminishes by 50 percent and it drops even more after three years of Pill use. The protection lasts up to 15 years after you stop using OCs.

Ovarian cancer, the most lethal of all female reproductive tract cancers, is also 40 percent less likely to develop in a woman who has used OCs. Even if you use OCs for as little as three months, you get some protection, but to get the full effect you need to take them for 5 to 10 years. If you use them for 10 years, your risk is reduced by 80 percent. The protection lasts for at least 10 to 15 years after discontinuation.

Endometrial and ovarian cancer are not the most common female cancers. Still, an estimated 2,000 cases of endometrial cancer and 1,700 cases of ovarian cancer were averted by Pill use in the 1980s.

OCs do not protect women from cervical cancer. In fact, the opposite may be true. Women who take the Pill for over a year appear to run an increased risk of developing this disease, the risk doubles when the medication is taken for 10 years. However, the most important risk factors for cervical cancer are not OCs, but rather the number of sexual partners a woman has had and how old she was when she first had sex. Exposure to human papillomavirus (HPV) and smoking also increase a woman's risk, while the use of barrier contraceptives, such as a diaphragm, condoms or spermicides protects against cervical cancer. It is difficult to determine the impact of these factors in women with cervical cancer who also used OCs, so research results have not been definitive. One study conducted by the Centers for Disease Control and Prevention (CDC) showed that women who used OCs didn't get cervical cancer more often than non–users. Instead, the higher rate of cancer diagnosed among these women was simply due to more careful screening, including more frequent Pap smears.

One woman in 9 will develop breast cancer during her lifetime, so it's not surprising that breast cancer is the main concern of anyone considering use of OCs. Unfortunately, despite a large body of scientific evidence showing no association between the two, a few studies have seemed to uncover an increased risk of breast cancer among those using OCs. Researchers aren't sure if these studies are important or if they are merely aberrations. It will probably take a decade or more before they reach a definitive conclusion. Many experts do agree that OC use is not associated with breast cancer after age 45. Some younger women, however, may be at higher risk. Several studies have shown that women who use OCs early in life, use them for longer than four years, and/or don't have a full term pregnancy early in life have a slightly increased risk for breast

SEE YOUR DOCTOR IF...

Here is an easy–to–remember acronym to help you determine whether to consult your doctor about what could be pill–related complications. Seek help if you experience jaundice, a breast lump, or any of the following warning signals:

A	Abdominal pain (severe)
C	Chest pain (severe), cough, shortness of breath
H	Headache (severe), dizziness, weakness, or numbness
E	Eye problems (vision loss or blurring), speech problems
S	Severe leg pain (calf or thigh)

Source: *Contraceptive Technology.* Irvington Publishers Inc., New York, NY, 1994.

cancer. (However, other research concludes the opposite.)

OC use has been implicated in a rare form of liver cancer known as hepatocellular carcinoma. However, since so few people ever develop this cancer, it has been difficult for researchers to determine with accuracy whether OCs were actually the cause. The largest study to include data about hepatocellular carcinoma found no association with OC use. In addition, death rates from liver cancer in the United States haven't changed since the introduction of OCs to the marketplace in the 1960s.

Despite a suggestion that OC use might lead to skin cancer, follow–up studies indicate no difference in the risk for Pill users versus nonusers. There is also no proven relationship between OCs and kidney cancer, colon cancer, gallbladder cancer, or pituitary tumors.

Heart and blood vessel disorders: Although concerns about cancer are usually foremost in the minds of women using OCs, the Pill's effects on blood chemistry are actually a greater cause for worry. Both the hormones in combined OCs are responsible for these problems, but in different ways.

The progestin component of OCs can alter the level of lipids (such as cholesterol) in the blood. Although estrogen works against this effect by increasing beneficial high–density lipoproteins (HDL) and lowering harmful low–density lipoproteins (LDL), progestin opposes the estrogen and does the opposite. Because high levels of LDL and depressed levels of HDL can cause fatty plaque to build up in the arteries, progestins have been implicated as a risk factor for coronary heart disease.

The estrogen component has been linked to a different problem: an increase in abnormal blood clotting, which can block circulation. A blood clot can appear in any blood vessel, but it is especially serious if it occurs in the brain, heart, or lungs.

Clots or blockages to blood flow can lead to serious and sometimes fatal complications that are usually associated with the following risk factors:

- Family history of heart attack or diabetes
- Previous heart or blood vessel disease
- Smoking
- High blood pressure
- Overweight
- Inactivity (either from too little exercise or from being immobilized)

If you have any of these risk factors, you should ask your physician whether the benefits from taking the Pill outweigh the possible dangers. Doctors and private clinics usually make this decision on a case-by-case basis. Public clinics may have stricter rules against giving OCs to women with certain risk factors.

Here is a description of the symptoms you might experience if you are suffering from a blood clot or blockage, and the technical name your doctor might use to describe it. If you think you have one of these problems, seek medical attention as soon as possible.

- Headache, impairment of the intellect, visual problems, weakness or numbness— *Cerebral infarction (stroke)*
- Chest pain, difficulty breathing, left arm and shoulder pain, weakness—*Myocardial infarction (heart attack)*
- Calf pain or swelling, heat or redness in the thigh, heat or tenderness in the lower leg, pain—*Thrombophlebitis*
- Chest pain, cough, shortness of breath— *Pulmonary embolism*
- Abdominal pain, vomiting, weakness— *Mesenteric vein thrombosis*
- Headache, loss of vision—*Retinal vein thrombosis*
- Cramps, lower abdominal pain—*Pelvic vein thrombosis*

High Blood Pressure: Although in itself not a life threatening condition, Pill–related high blood pressure—experienced by up to 5 percent of women taking high–dose pills—can lead to heart disease and stroke. If your blood pressure is over 140/90, you should stop taking OCs until it is under control. All women using the Pill should have their blood pressure checked once a year; for women with a history of blood pressure problems, a check once every six months is probably in order.

Increased Blood Sugar Levels: Estrogen and progestin not only can affect blood clotting and blood lipids, they can also raise blood sugar levels. Most experts believe these changes are so minimal, they have no clinical significance. For women with diabetes, however, the situation isn't so straightforward. Some doctors believe that diabetic women with no other risk factors can use OCs with minimal trouble, but others believe prescribing OCs to diabetics exposes them to unnecessary risks.

Liver and gallbladder complications: OCs can cause jaundice—a liver condition that makes the skin and eyes look yellow—but only 1 in 10,000 Pill users experience Pill related jaundice. OCs can also cause another rare liver condition known as hepatocellular adenoma. The risk of developing this condition is about 3 or 4 per 100,000 Pill users. Liver cancer is another rare complication. Gallbladder disease, which is fairly common among users—and non-users—of the Pill, is not life threatening but could require surgery.

Cervical changes: The thickness and strength of the cervical lining varies with the ebb and flow of reproductive hormones; and OCs can lead to an increase in the area of thin, vulnerable cervical tissue susceptible to sexually transmitted diseases (STDs). Most doctors recommend you use condoms for STD prevention while taking the Pill to prevent pregnancy, especially if you have more than one sexual partner and if you are less than 25 years old.

Eye problems: Use of older, high–dose OCs occasionally caused an inflammation of the optic nerve, resulting in blurred or double vision, swelling, pain, or even loss of sight. This almost never happens with today's OCs. However, any loss of vision warrants an immediate discontinuation of the Pill and a visit to an ophthalmologist or neurologist. You should also stop taking the Pill if a vision problem accompanies a migraine headache.

Returning to fertility: For most women, fertility comes back quickly after discontinuing OCs. However, 1 percent to 2 percent experience some delay in the return of normal reproductive cycles. In rare instances, hormones can stay suppressed for months or even years, though for the majority, menstrual cycles normalize within three months. Cycle suppression is more likely to cause infertility in older women, so if having a child is a high priority, you might consider switching to another reliable contraceptive method as you approach 30.

Nuisance Side Effects

Some women experience minor "nuisance" side effects while using the Pill. Of course, depending on your level of discomfort, a nuisance can become serious enough to warrant switching to a different OC or discontinuing the Pill altogether. Additionally, some minor side effects could actually be masking a condition that needs medical attention. Never hesitate to mention a side effect to your physician. Among the minor side effects the Pill sometimes produces are acne, breakthrough bleeding or spotting, breast tenderness, depression, headaches, nausea and weight gain.

Acne: Pill users may notice an improvement, a worsening, or no change in their acne. In some women, the progestin component of the Pill improves the acne; in others it works like the male sex hormone, androgen, and makes it worse. (Women produce androgen in small amounts.) Dietary, allergic, hygienic, or familial factors can also increase acne. A bad case could be a sign of an ovarian or adrenal tumor, although chances of this are minimal.

You have several options if you break out with acne while on the Pill. Recently, new lower dose pills containing so–called "new progestins," were introduced to the American market. These pills have been used in Europe and other parts of the world for over 30 years with great success. Although many claims are made about them, so far their only real benefit appears to be their lower androgenic properties. Ask your doctor about these pills containing progestins called norgestimate (Ortho–Cyclen, Ortho–Tricyclen) and desogestrel (Ortho–Cept, Ortho–Tricept, Desogen). A third new progestin called gestodene, which could actually be the best of the three because it can be used at the lowest dose, could become available in the U.S. sometime in the future.

The new pills are more expensive than the older high-dose pills, so you'll have to decide if improving your acne is worth the added expense. You might choose to switch to another of the older pills instead. You can also consider taking antibiotics, changing your diet, or using a special cleanser.

Breakthrough bleeding or spotting: Intermittent minor menstrual bleeding could mean that your pill isn't strong enough, or it could signal a pelvic infection, endometriosis, or ectopic pregnancy. Once your doctor has ruled out these more serious possibilities, he

or she will either switch you to a different pill (probably one with a higher dose of progestin or one of the new progestin pills) or counsel you to try to tolerate the bleeding and spotting for a little while longer, especially if you just started on the Pill. Breakthrough bleeding and spotting diminish rapidly over the first four months of pill use.

Most physicians do not recommend stopping the Pill because of this side effect. If you have any doubts, however, call your doctor.

Breast tenderness: If your breasts hurt, your doctor will first rule out pregnancy and breast cancer. He or she may then prescribe a different, lower dose pill.

You may also want to try wearing a different bra with better support. Also try to avoid vigorous exercise when you have the most discomfort.

Depression: It's difficult to prove a direct link between depression and the Pill. A woman who's chosen the Pill may still have strong moral or medical concerns about it. Starting on the Pill may also coincide with increased sexual activity, which may cause deep psychological conflicts for the user. This inner turmoil can easily seem like depression. It is important to decide whether there could be other reasons for your feelings, and to note whether your depression started or became worse when you began taking the Pill.

If you rule out depression from sources other than the Pill, there are several Pill–related remedies your doctor can try. Most likely the culprit is the progestin in the Pill, so your physician might try prescribing a pill with less of that hormone. Pill–related depression can be the result of fluid retention or a lack of vitamin B$_6$, among other causes. Talk with your doctor about the best plan of action. If your depression seems severe, he or she may suggest you discontinue the Pill and talk with a specialist.

Headaches: Although OCs sometimes initiate headaches or make them more severe, headaches can also be a warning of impending strokes or other circulatory disorders. Pay close attention to headaches that are different or more severe than those you had before starting on the Pill.

Estrogen seems to be the culprit in Pill–related headaches, so you might find relief by changing to a lower dose pill, or switching to a progestin–only method like Norplant implants or Depo–Provera. If you usually get headaches only during the week you're not taking pills—the placebo week—you might have what's called an estrogen withdrawal headache. To determine whether this is the case, consider using an estrogen supplement. For example, during your withdrawal week, you can try wearing a transdermal patch that releases estrogen through the skin.

Another approach to estrogen withdrawal headaches is simply to put off withdrawal from the Pill. Essentially, you postpone the headache by extending the amount of time you take active pills. A recent year–long study of 300 women showed that those who opted for an extended regimen—taking active pills for 9 weeks instead of 3 and then taking a withdrawal week—had fewer headaches. Continuing the active pills for the extra time caused no serious side effects and no decline in effectiveness.

It may seem unnatural to take pills for longer than the standard 3 weeks, but remember that the entire pill cycle is essen-

DRUGS THAT DEFEAT THE PILL

Have you ever known someone who became pregnant while taking the Pill, but who swore she took a tablet every day? The culprit could have been a drug interaction.

Certain drugs, notably anticonvulsant medications and some antibiotics, stimulate enzymes which absorb estrogen and progestins. This means less of the hormones from your OCs are available to prevent pregnancy. These drugs can also act on the Norplant system.

If you need to take these medications for only a few weeks, your doctor will probably advise you to use a backup contraceptive, such as condoms or spermicides. Long–term therapy may require you to switch from hormones. Here are some of the medications which can reduce the effectiveness of OCs and implants:

- Antibiotics: rifampin, chloramphenicol, cephalosporins, possibly metronidazole, nitrofurantoin.

- Anticonvulsants: phenobarbital, primidone, carbamazepine, ethosuximide, phenytoin.

- Antifungals: griseofulvin (does not affect Norplant implants).

Source: Outlook, Volume 9, Number 1, April 1991. Program for Appropriate Technology in Health (PATH), Seattle, WA.

tially unnatural. As one family planning expert puts it, "The day was made by God, the week was made by man."

Nausea: Although it could signal pregnancy, early miscarriage, or some nonreproductive disorder, when nausea is related to the Pill, it's the estrogen component that's at fault.

For a new Pill user, nausea usually subsides after the first few cycles or remains a nuisance only on the first day of each new cycle.

In addition to switching to a pill with a lower estrogen dose or to a progestin–only method, another possible remedy is taking your pill after a meal. Swallowing a pill before going to sleep has also helped some women.

If the nausea is so bad that you vomit within 1 hour of taking a pill, take another pill from an extra pack. Also, if you missed a pill and are trying to catch up, take the next 2 pills at least 12 hours apart. (For more information see the nearby box on "What To Do When You Miss a Pill.")

Weight gain: Some doctors refuse to acknowledge that the Pill can cause excessive weight gain. Although your doctor might switch you to a different pill, it could be because *you* believe it will help rather than because he or she thinks it will.

Weight gain that occurs after you start using the Pill may be caused by fluid retention or estrogen–induced fat deposits in the thighs, hips, and breasts. It may also be the result of reduced physical activity or increased intake of food. (The androgenic effects from the progestins in the Pill can cause an increase in appetite.)

Switching to lower dose pills or to pills with less progestin content can help, but increasing exercise and reducing caloric intake is often the best solution.

Emergency contraception

Contraception is usually thought of as a measure to be taken in advance of or during sex. But even though many women don't realize it, something still can be done after the fact —after unprotected sex; after a condom breaks; after a diaphragm, cap, or sponge becomes dislodged; or after a rape. Called by several names—such as the morning–after pill, postcoital contraception, emergency contraception, or interception—the regimen involves ingesting higher–than–normal doses of contraceptive hormones within 72 hours of intercourse, and then ingesting even more of the same hormones 12 hours later.

The drug companies that sell OCs don't have approval from the Food and Drug Administration to market their pills for emergency contraception, mainly because they haven't applied for it. However, physicians are allowed to prescribe an approved drug for any purpose they deem reasonable; so normal birth control pills—maybe ones similar to those in your drawer or purse—have been used after the fact since the early 1980s to prevent possible pregnancies.

There are several different postcoital treatment options available in the United States. The regimen of choice involves the use of an OC called Ovral, a high–dose pill containing the progestin norgestrel.

Here's how the regimen works: Two Ovral tablets are taken within 72 hours of unprotected sex; then 2 more Ovral tablets are taken 12 hours after the first dose. Because this much hormone can upset your system, always talk with your doctor before attempting emergency contraception of this type.

Depending on where you are in your menstrual cycle, postcoital pills work by either stopping release of an egg from the ovary, disrupting fertilization by the sperm, or pre-

NORPLANT: THE "NO HASSLE" APPROACH TO HORMONAL CONTRACEPTION

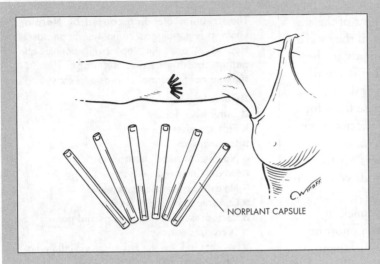

NORPLANT CAPSULE

The Norplant system requires just one trip to the doctor every 5 years—and nothing else! There's no daily pill to remember and nothing to fuss with before sex. The only major drawback to the system is the insertion procedure. Because the 6 levonorgestrel-filled capsules that make up the system must be placed under the skin, you can expect tenderness and swelling of your upper inner arm for a couple of days while the insertion site heals.

venting a fertilized egg from implanting in the lining of the uterus.

The most significant side effect is severe nausea, which affects about one–third of women using this regimen. However, this should stop a day or so after treatment. If the nausea is so severe that you have to vomit within an hour of taking the dose, you may need to take extra pills. You can also get anti–nausea medication from your doctor. Other side effects you might experience include headache, breast tenderness, dizziness, and fluid retention.

You should have your period in 2 or 3 weeks. If it hasn't started in 3 weeks, consider taking a pregnancy test. And don't forget to watch out for the Pill warning signs (turn to the "See Your Doctor…" box, page 267).

There are several other brands of pills containing norgestrel, including Lo/Ovral, Nordette, Levlen, Triphasil, and Tri–Levlen. If you are currently taking any of these pills, you can use them in an emergency, but you'll have to take twice the amount because they aren't as strong as Ovral. This means you will need to take four tablets within 72 hours, and then another four tablets 12 hours later. If you use the triphasic pills (Triphasil or Tri–Levlen), make sure you take only the pills designated for the last week. These are the ones with the right dose. Again, be sure to consult your physician before using OCs in this way.

Other progestin–based brands would probably work the same way, but they haven't been studied, so experts can't reliably make any recommendations.

Reported effectiveness rates for this treatment option vary, but a recent study found that emergency contraception of this type can be up to 75 percent effective, depending on where a woman was in her cycle when she had unprotected sex.

Norplant Implants

Oral contraceptives are the most widespread method of birth control, and they are well liked by most of the women who use them. However, if they were asked to name just one complaint about the Pill, most would probably say that it's hard to remember to take a tablet every day. To combat the problems that can arise from forgetting to take the Pill regularly (or not using a condom every time, or leaving the diaphragm at home...), researchers began searching for birth control methods you don't need to remember.

Scientists at the Population Council in New York City, an international, nonprofit contraceptive research organization, spent more than 20 years and over $20 million developing and introducing Norplant implants. This new system is effective for up to 5 years without replacement. Women around the world have been using the implants since the early 1980s. The Food and Drug Administration approved them for use in the United States at the end of 1990.

What the Implants Do

The Norplant implant system is a set of 6 matchstick sized, hormone-containing capsules made of flexible tubing. The tubing is a blend of silicone and plastic called Silastic. The capsules are inserted by a trained professional just below the skin of a woman's upper inner arm (the part of the arm that lies against the side of the rib cage when the arms are at rest). The doctor uses a device that looks like a syringe (called a "trocar") to place the capsules in a fan-like shape. Thin women will probably be able to see the cap

NORPLANT: PROS AND CONS

The irregular bleeding caused by Norplant implants is the biggest complaint among users. However, those who stop having periods altogether cite this as an advantage. Here's a summary of the implant's pros and cons:

Advantages
- Extremely effective
- Safe for most women
- Long-lasting
- No need to remember to use
- Doesn't interrupt sex
- No estrogen-related side effects
- Can stop the menstrual cycle
- Decreases menstrual cramps and pain
- Decreases anemia
- Possibly reduces the risk of pelvic inflammatory disease (PID)
- Possibly reduces the risk of endometrial cancer

Disadvantages
- Offers no protection against sexually transmitted diseases (STDs)
- Can be somewhat visible in thin women
- Costs more than other types of birth control at the outset
- Requires doctor's assistance and a surgical procedure for removal
- Can produce nuisance side effects, especially irregular bleeding

sules under the skin once they are inserted, but for most others they aren't noticeable.

Starting 24 hours after the capsules are placed under her skin, the user is protected from pregnancy by the progestin called levonorgestrel, which slowly leaks out of the capsules and enters the bloodstream. The implants contain no estrogen. They will continue to release progestin for up to 5 years. Because they are not biodegradable, they must then be removed. Your doctor can insert another set of implants at the same time the old set is removed, if you want to continue using the method.

The implants should be inserted within 7 days of the start of your menstrual cycle, just to make sure you aren't already pregnant. Although there is no evidence that the Norplant system will hurt a developing baby, most experts believe it's best not to expose it to hormones.

The insertion procedure is done on an out-patient basis. Your doctor will give you a local anesthetic to numb the area, then make a small incision. It takes about 15 or 20 minutes to place all 6 capsules. The area will probably be tender, bruised, or slightly swollen for a day or two.

If you want the implants removed—when the five–year effectiveness begins to wear off, you want to get pregnant, or you simply don't like the method—you will again need a minor outpatient surgical procedure. Removal is often more difficult than inser-tion, sometimes requiring 2 sessions before all 6 capsules are removed. Two visits are necessary when swelling of the surrounding tissue becomes an impediment to the doctor and a discomfort to you.

Removals often present a problem for doctors because your skin tissue forms an envelope around the implants, making them difficult to grab with the tweezer–like instru-ment often used to take them out. The tissue envelope, which gets thicker and harder to remove as time goes on, must first be dis-rupted before the capsules inside can be pulled out. Many clinicians can remove a set of six capsules in 30 minutes. Some take

longer, while others complete the procedure in as little as 10 minutes.

Twenty–four hours after the capsules have been removed, your protection from preg-nancy ends.

Many women and their doctors were dubious about the system's eventual success when it was first introduced in the United States. They wondered why women would want to have these tiny sticks buried beneath their skin. To their surprise, the odd new method became almost an instant hit. In just over 2 years, 750,000 American women have chosen the implant system.

Most of these women received the implants with the help of the Medicaid system or private insurers. Norplant implants do have high up–front costs; the kit itself is about $365, insertion costs can start at $100, and removal costs average $400 to $500. However, depending on where you live, the implants may cost less than or about the same as 5 years' worth of birth control pills.

How Effective Are the Implants?

The Norplant implant system is one of the most effective birth control methods in use today. During the first year after insertion, there is only one pregnancy per 500 users. The system becomes less effective towards the

DON'T USE NORPLANT IMPLANTS IF YOU

- Suspect you are pregnant
- Have abnormal, unexplained vaginal bleeding
- Take antiseizure medication or the antibiotic rifampin
- Have active thromboembolic disease (blood clots)
- Know or suspect you have breast cancer
- Have acute liver dysfunction

WHEN GROWTH WON'T STOP

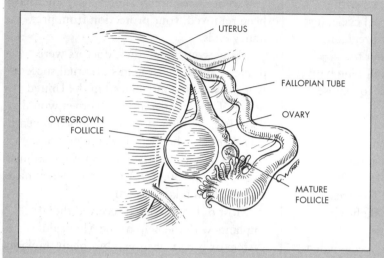

UTERUS

FALLOPIAN TUBE

OVARY

OVERGROWN
FOLLICLE

MATURE
FOLLICLE

Although the Norplant system prevents release of an egg, it will sometimes allow a follicle to begin developing. Lacking the usual hormonal cues that cause all but a dominant follicle to disappear at the end of a cycle, the out-of-control newcomer will continue to grow until it resembles a large ovarian cyst. In time, such enlarged follicles usually disappear. However, there is a slight danger of twisting or rupture, which could require surgery.

end of its useful life, so it is extremely important to have the capsules replaced at the 5 year mark.

The Benefits and Risks

Scientists have noted few if any serious complications with Norplant implants, probably because they don't contain estrogen, and release their contents slowly, thereby avoiding hormonal surges. To be on the safe side, the manufacturer relays warnings based on experience with the Pill, which contains estrogen. (For risks and complications of OCs, see preceding section of this chapter.) Other possible complications include bleeding irregularities, follicular abnormalities, tubal pregnancies, harm to the infant during breastfeeding, and thromboembolic disorders. Insertion site infections can also prove troublesome.

Bleeding irregularities: Since many women have irregular periods while using Norplant implants, it's possible that more serious conditions marked by vaginal bleeding could be overlooked. These conditions include cervical and endometrial cancer.

If you're like many other women, your period may gradually stop while you're using this method, a condition known as "amenorrhea." But if you use Norplant implants and you *suddenly* stop having periods after being regular, it could mean you're pregnant. If you have 6 weeks or more of amenorrhea following normal periods, take a pregnancy test.

Follicular abnormalities: In the normal reproductive cycle, many ovarian follicles compete to become the one dominant enough to produce an egg. Those follicles not quite making the grade degenerate in a process known as "atresia." Although Norplant implants suppress the ovulatory system in about 50 percent of users, sometimes follicles do start growing. Researchers have noted that in Norplant users, follicular atresia is sometimes delayed, causing follicles to grow beyond their normal size. These growths can't easily be distinguished from ovarian cysts. Although the enlarged follicles disappear on their own most of the time, if they twist or rupture, surgery may be required.

Tubal pregnancies: Tubal, or ectopic, pregnancies do occur among women using Norplant implants, but less often than among women using no method of birth control. If you begin to feel abdominal pain, especially after your implants have been in place for a long time, seek medical care to rule out ectopic pregnancy.

Breastfeeding: Progestin–only methods like Norplant implants and Depo–Provera have no impact on breast milk production; on the contrary, some studies show that milk production increases in the presence of progestins.

When studies were conducted on the Norplant system in the United States, some of the subjects were women who had the implants placed while they were breastfeeding. Six weeks after delivery, these women were given Norplant implants, and their breastfed children were then monitored for 3 years. Small amounts of the system's hormone could be found in the infants, but it did not affect their growth or health.

Unfortunately, no American women were studied earlier than 6 weeks after giving birth, making it impossible for the Food and Drug Administration to recommend the use of Norplant implants for women right after delivery. This lack of support from the FDA makes it difficult for doctors to recommend immediate postpartum insertion, even though studies outside the U.S. have documented its safety.

The issue is probably moot, because the act of breastfeeding can provide pregnancy protection for at least 6 weeks postpartum. Women in many developing countries (and even a small number of American women) actually use breastfeeding as a means of contraception. The method, which requires breast milk to be the infant's only source of nutrition, is known as the lactational amenorrhea method, or "LAM."

Thromboembolic disorders: Progestins are not known to cause the clots or blockages of blood vessels found in thromboembolic disease, but if you have an active case, your physician may suggest another method. If you develop any such disorder while using the implants, you should probably have them removed. If you had thromboembolic disease in the past, you are probably not a good candidate for Norplant implants.

Insertion site complications: With proper antiseptics, the insertion site seldom becomes infected. The skin can become irritated even several months after insertion, but this, too, is rare.

NEWER IMPLANTS MORE EFFECTIVE

Many women interested in receiving Norplant implants—especially when the method was first introduced—were told that they would be less effective in women weighing over 154 pounds. This is no longer the case.

Initially, the capsules were made of a dense material that somewhat reduced their effectiveness. All implants manufactured now contain softer, less dense tubing that allows for greater flow of hormones out of the tubes and into the bloodstream.

DEPO-PROVERA PROS AND CONS

Depo-Provera is becoming a popular option with women of all ages. To help you decide if you'd like to try the contraceptive injection, here's a quick list of advantages and disadvantages:

Advantages
- Extremely effective
- Safe for most women
- Long-lasting but easy to discontinue
- No need to remember to use
- No interruption of sex
- No estrogen-related side effects
- Possible cessation of the menstrual cycle
- Decreased menstrual cramps and pain
- Decreased anemia
- Possible reduction in risk of pelvic inflammatory disease and endometriosis
- Possible reduction in risk of endometrial cancer

Disadvantages
- Offers no protection against sexually transmitted diseases (STDs)
- Can delay return to fertility up to 2 years
- Lasts for 3 months with no option to discontinue during that time
- May produce nuisance side effects, especially irregular bleeding and weight gain

Nuisance Side Effects

Norplant implants can cause some of the same nuisance side effects as the Pill, including acne, breast tenderness, depression, headaches, nausea and weight gain. Other side effects that have been noted include nervousness and dizziness, skin rash, breast discharge, changes in appetite, and hair loss or growth. But by far the most common side effect of the implants is irregular bleeding.

In the many studies of the system, 60 to 100 percent of users experienced some kind of menstrual change, especially in the first few months. These changes can include bleeding for a longer time than usual per cycle (27.6 percent), spotting between periods (17.1 percent), frequent bleeding onsets (7.0 percent), infrequent or light bleeding (5.2 percent), or no bleeding at all (9.4 percent).

It is important to note that even with these irregular patterns of increased bleeding, women using Norplant implants lose less blood than women with normal menstrual cycles. Studies show that Norplant implant users have higher hemoglobin levels than nonusers do. This could prove beneficial for women prone to anemia.

Here is a list showing the rate of side effects seen during two multinational studies:

Condition	Study 1	Study 2
	(percentage)	*(percentage)*
Headache	16.7	18.5
Ovarian enlargement	11.6	3.1
Dizziness	8.1	5.6
Breast tenderness	6.8	6.2
Nervousness	6.8	6.2
Nausea	5.1	7.7
Acne	4.5	7.2
Rash	3.8	8.2
Breast discharge	3.5	5.1
Appetite changes	3.5	6.2
Weight gain	3.3	6.2
Hair loss or growth	1.8	2.6

If you are concerned about potential side effects, it might be a good idea to take the implant system for a kind of "test drive" before you pay a lot of money to have the capsules inserted. You can do this by taking a progestin-only OC called Ovrette for a cycle or two. It contains the same progestin as Norplant implants, and should give you some idea of how you will react once the implants are in place.

Depo–Provera Contraceptive Injection

If a woman has trouble remembering to take oral contraceptives or can't use them because of certain medical problems, and she doesn't want to use an implant because of its long–term effects, there is now a third option: Depo–Provera Contraceptive Injection.

Depo–Provera was approved by the U.S. Food and Drug Administration as a treatment for endometrial and kidney cancer in the early 1970s, but it took nearly 20 years of research to convince the agency to approve it as a contraceptive. Officials at the FDA were concerned about studies linking the drug to breast cancer, low birth–weight babies, and osteoporosis (brittle bones).

Four Shots a Year

Depo–Provera is a shot administered in the arm or buttocks every 90 days. It contains the synthetic hormone depot–medroxypro-gesterone acetate (DMPA). This hormone is similar to a woman's naturally occurring progesterone. Although not available in America until the end of 1992, DMPA has been used for contraception by almost 9 million women in over 90 countries.

The hormone in the shot is absorbed into the bloodstream from the muscle where it was given. It provides protection from preg-nancy within 2 weeks of the initial injection. Blood levels of DMPA remain high for about 4 weeks, then stabilize at a lower level.

You will probably be given a pregnancy test before your first injection because one study showed that DMPA users who were either pregnant at the time of their first shot or who got pregnant while using the drug were more likely to have low birth weight babies.

It's important that you get your shots reg-ularly. However, if you are going on an extended vacation and need one before 3 months are up, it will do no harm. You also have a grace period of about 4 weeks after the next shot is due. It is inadvisable to push the limit though, because some women have gotten pregnant by extending their three–month intervals. Shots cost about $30 to $40 or more, depending on where you live.

If you want to stop using Depo–Provera, there's good news and bad news. The good news is that, unlike Norplant implants which require a doctor's assistance to remove, you can discontinue Depo–Provera simply by not getting your next shot. The bad news is, once you've gotten a shot, you're committed for a full 90 days.

How Effective Are the Shots?

Depo–Provera is highly effective. Only 1 out of every 300 to 400 women on Depo–Provera will get pregnant.

The Benefits and Risks

Like Norplant implants, Depo–Provera con-tains no estrogen and is therefore free of estrogen–related side effects. It is, however, associated with its own set of complications: bleeding irregularities, cancer risks, bone mineral density changes, low birth weight babies, tubal pregnancies, drug interaction, and problems reestablishing fertility. Although breastfeeding while taking Depo–Provera poses no problem for the infant, some experts advise women to wait 6 weeks after childbirth before getting a shot.

Bleeding irregularities: You might have irreg-ular periods while using Depo–Provera. Since vaginal bleeding might also be a symptom of a more serious medical problem such as an infection or cancer, see your doctor if the bleeding is severe or persistent.

Cancer: Suspicion that Depo–Provera could cause breast cancer was based on high–dose animal studies later discredited by the FDA. Still, the stigma persisted. To resolve the issue, researchers in several different countries conducted studies involving thousands of women. Some of these studies found no increased risk for breast cancer, while others found a slightly higher risk among women who had taken Depo–Provera within the last 4 years and who were under 35 years of age. In June 1993, a panel of experts convened by the World Health Organization in Geneva, Switzerland, reviewed all the available data, and announced that Depo–Provera does not increase the overall risk of breast cancer. They also found no link between the drug and cervical cancer, the second most common cancer among women. Moreover, the panel stated that Depo–Provera can provide some protection from endometrial cancer.

Bone mineral density changes: During the FDA's evaluation of Depo–Provera, a study of 30 New Zealand women who had been using the drug for at least 5 years raised questions about a possible link with brittle bones. However, experts contend that the study was flawed because it involved too few women, failed to measure the women's prestudy bone density, and didn't consider such life-style factors as smoking.

The drug's suppression of a woman's naturally occurring estrogen could theoretically lead to a reduction in bone density. However, studies of women using Depo–Provera for noncontraceptive purposes have not shown this to be true. Scientists feel the results of the New Zealand study are inconclusive and that further research is needed to settle the issue.

Low birth weight babies: Women who are pregnant at the time of their first shot of Depo–Provera or who accidentally become pregnant a month or two after starting the drug are more likely to deliver babies with low birth weights. Although low-birth-weight babies are twice as likely to die as babies of normal weight, children exposed to Depo–Provera before birth and followed through adolescence show no signs of adverse health effects.

Tubal pregnancies: Tubal pregnancies can occur among Depo–Provera users, but less often than among women using an intrauterine device (IUD) or no birth control at all. If you begin to feel abdominal pain, see a doctor to rule out tubal pregnancy.

Drug interaction: The drug aminoglutethimide (Cytadren) can reduce the effectiveness of Depo–Provera. Cytadren is used to suppress adrenal gland function in patients with Cushing's syndrome and adrenal cancer.

Returning to fertility: Sixteen weeks after your last shot you should be able to conceive, but it could take 1 to 2 years for your periods to fully return to normal. In one study, more than half of the women who wanted to become pregnant conceived after 1 year; by the end of 2 years, 90 percent of women had conceived.

Breastfeeding: There is no evidence that Depo–Provera is harmful to nursing infants. However, the manufacturer takes a conservative approach by suggesting that a breastfeeding woman wait 6 weeks after giving birth before taking the medication.

Nuisance Side Effects

Depo–Provera can cause some of the same nuisance side effects as the Pill and Norplant implants: depression, headaches, weight gain, nervousness, and dizziness. As with the implant system, irregular bleeding is by far the most common side effect.

As you continue to use Depo–Provera, you'll notice less and less spotting or break-through bleeding, and finally will have no period at all. At the end of one year, 57 percent of women using Depo–Provera have no period, and by the end of two years, 68 percent have stopped menstruating.

Another significant side effect—probably the most undesirable one—is weight gain. Here is an example of the amount of weight gained by the average Depo–Provera user:

- After 1 year: 5.4 pounds gained
- After 2 years: 8.1 pounds gained
- After 4 years: 13.8 pounds gained
- After 6 years: 16.5 pounds gained

It seems that the weight gained by Depo–Provera users is related more to an increase in appetite than fluid retention. Reducing your fat and calorie intake and exercising regularly can help you prevent weight gain while using this method.

Whether you use Depo–Provera, Norplant, or the Pill, hormonal birth control takes the guesswork out of family planning and returns spontaneity to sex. It is the most effective method of contraception, and the risks it poses are minimal. As with any medication, it's important to watch for side effects and report them to your doctor. But, if you're like the majority of women, your problems most likely will be few. □

CHAPTER 22   **FERTILITY AND FAMILY PLANNING**

Those Other Approaches to Family Planning

Every "standard" birth control method has risks—vanishingly small, perhaps, but risks nonetheless. For some women, these methods are also burdened with unacceptable side effects. For many others, they pose a difficult moral dilemma.

For whatever reason, alternative approaches to family planning remain popular. Fertility awareness methods are gaining new adherents, while voluntary sterilization presents a safe and extremely effective option for all women who have completed their families. And, when all methods fail, termination of pregnancy remains a legal and widely used alternative.

Fertility Awareness

Fertility awareness, also known as natural family planning and the rhythm method, has enjoyed a recent resurgence in popularity because it encourages women to become more aware of their bodies and their monthly menstrual cycles while avoiding the use of chemical or mechanical forms of contraception.

To practice this technique, you must first determine your fertile days—the part of your menstrual cycle in which you are most likely to become pregnant. During these days, you then either abstain from sexual intercourse or use another form of birth control, such as a barrier method. Between 5 and 7 percent of American women use this family planning strategy, not only because it is completely safe and inexpensive, but also because it is the only method acceptable to all religions. Some researchers have theorized that using fertility awareness for family planning also builds self–esteem, since intercourse must be planned around the rhythms of a woman's body instead of relying on the protection of barriers or pills.

Nevertheless, fertility awareness is not as reliable as other contraceptive methods. Although its theoretical effectiveness is as high as 98 percent if used correctly *all the time*, its average effectiveness is much lower—anywhere from 30 to 70 percent for women who frequently forget their timing.

Fertility awareness also is difficult to use if you have very irregular menstrual cycles; and the daily record keeping that's required can be cumbersome.

As a result, some family planning experts advocate fertility awareness only for women who would not be unduly upset by an unintended pregnancy or for those who are motivated to follow the rules carefully. Fertility awareness can provide more reliable protection if you use two or more methods at the same time or add a backup form of contraception on your most fertile days.

No health risks are associated with fertility awareness. However, some researchers have linked this approach with higher rates of birth defects and miscarriages, since accidental pregnancies are more likely to occur very late in a woman's fertile period. Couples who delay intercourse until they believe the woman's fertile period has ended may inadvertently fertilize an "old" egg or fertilize an egg with "old" sperm. Either form of conception may lead to chromosome and other fetal abnormalities.

How Fertility Awareness Works

Although the average menstrual cycle lasts 28 days, the length of a cycle varies from woman to woman and even from one cycle to the next. Nevertheless, the number of days between ovulation and the beginning of the next menstrual period is fairly consistent—about 14 days.

You are most likely to become pregnant if fresh sperm are present in your reproductive tract at the time of ovulation. Since sperm are fertile for 2 to 4 days and a woman's egg is fertile for 12 to 24 hours, you are most apt to conceive if you have intercourse during the 4 days prior to or within 1 day after ovulation.

Certain reliable body signs indicate your most fertile period each month. They include specific changes in the color, amount, and texture of your cervical mucus as well as changes in your basal body temperature. To pinpoint your window of fertility, you can watch these signs, or calculate the most likely time of ovulation based on the average length of your menstrual cycle.

The Mucus Method

The cervical mucus discharged through your vagina changes throughout your menstrual cycle in response to normal hormonal variations. By noting these changes in color and consistency, you can detect ovulation. This technique involves checking your vagina and your cervical mucus daily with your fingers. If you're not comfortable with that, the mucus method is not a good choice for you.

To use the mucus method, also called the "Billings method" after the physician who developed it, place a finger inside your vagina at least once each day and notice how wet it feels. If you can collect any mucus on your finger, check it for stickiness and elasticity. Following menstruation, a woman typically experiences a few days when her vagina feels moist but not exactly wet, days when she has no cervical mucus. These are known as "dry" days.

Next you may notice thick, cloudy, sticky mucus with a white or yellowish tint, though your vagina may not actually feel wet. This mucus is a sign that you may be fertile, so you should avoid intercourse once it appears.

As ovulation approaches, the mucus becomes more abundant, clear, thin, slippery, and elastic—like raw egg white—and your vagina feels increasingly wet. These are signs that you're very fertile. The peak, or last, day of wetness and abundant mucus generally occurs at about the time of ovulation. To avoid pregnancy, refrain from intercourse for 4 days after this peak. By that time, you should notice that your vagina has reverted to the characteristics of the "dry" days.

Because blood masks other sensations of wetness during menstruation, the mucus technique alone may not give you enough advance notice of ovulation to prevent pregnancy—especially if you have very short menstrual cycles. The safest way to follow this method is to abstain from intercourse or use another method of birth control from Day 1 of your cycle until 4 days after your peak mucus day.

Before relying on the mucus method as a form of birth control, observe the changes for

KEEPING IN TIME WITH YOUR NATURAL RHYTHM

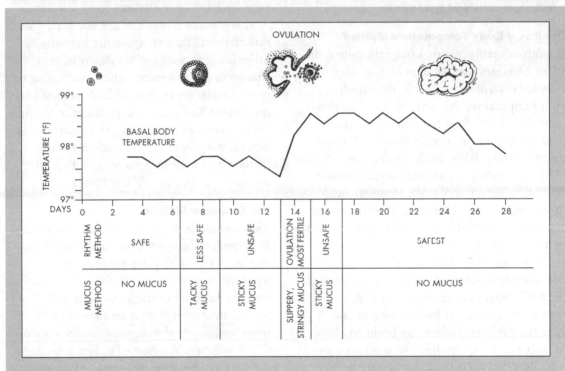

If you can accurately pinpoint the day when ovulation occurs, avoiding conception is easy. The egg remains fertile for a maximum of 24 hours; so if you refrain from sex for 4 days before ovulation (the longest that sperm can survive) and 1 day after, there's no way you'll get pregnant.

The catch word here is "accurately." The three ways of estimating the time of ovulation all have flaws. Body temperature drops briefly before ovulation, then rises. But other factors, such as fever, stress, or an interruption of regular sleeping habits, can nudge your temperature upward, sending a false "all clear." Peak production of cervical mucus occurs just as you ovulate. But menstrual flow, douches, and lubricants can all confuse the issue, making the true situation hard to judge. Going strictly by the calendar should work if your cycle is absolutely regular. Unfortunately, in many women it's not.

The bottom line: Rely totally on the rhythm method only if you wouldn't mind an unexpected pregnancy all that much.

at least 3 menstrual cycles so you can discern your individual pattern with some degree of confidence. Record your findings on a sheet of graph or notebook paper or on a special chart that you can obtain from your physician or a family planning clinic.

You should also be aware that variables such as vaginal infections, the use of vaginal spermicides, douching, the use of artificial lubricants, certain medications, and even the semen and secretions produced during intercourse can affect the accuracy of your mucus "readings."

The Basal Body Temperature Method

A woman's temperature often falls during the 12 to 24 hours preceding ovulation, then rises for several days after it. By recording your temperature fluctuations, you can determine the "safe" days for intercourse after ovulation. You can obtain these readings by using a special Basal Body Temperature (BBT) thermometer, an instrument sensitive enough to detect very small changes. Basal thermometers and blank charts to record the changes are available in many drugstores and family planning clinics.

To use the BBT method, take a five-minute reading of your temperature with the BBT thermometer every morning, just before you get out of bed. Be sure to take your temperature before you begin any kind of activity, drink anything, or smoke a cigarette. You may use the thermometer either orally or rectally, but be sure you always use the same technique at the same time.

Record your temperature every day on the special graph and connect the dots, so you can chart a line from one day to the next. When ovulation occurs, your temperature will rise by one-half to one degree Fahrenheit and you should stop having sex. When the temperature has been elevated for 3 days, you

can resume intercourse for the remainder of your menstrual cycle.

Before relying solely on BBT charting, you should record at least three menstrual cycles to make sure of your temperature pattern. Because your BBT rises only *after* ovulation, the safest way to use this technique is to avoid intercourse or use a backup method of birth control until you're certain ovulation has passed—in other words, from the beginning of menstruation—Day 1 of your cycle—until your BBT has been elevated for 3 full days.

A few other difficulties are associated with this method. Your temperature may rise for other reasons, such as illness, stress, or a change in your sleeping habits. According to one research study, one-fifth of women have no regular BBT pattern even when ovulating. Factors such as jet lag, dietary changes, irregular sleeping hours, the use of an electric blanket and even nightmares can also affect the accuracy of your BBT readings.

The Calendar Method

This method is the least reliable of the fertility awareness techniques. Since ovulation generally occurs 14 days prior to the onset of a woman's menstrual period, this technique uses the calendar to track the cycle and predict ovulation. You must then abstain from intercourse during the ovulatory period, which is generally assumed to last at least 7 days. The calendar technique is, of course, more reliable if you have regular menstrual cycles. If they vary widely, you should not expect this technique, alone, to provide adequate contraceptive protection.

Before using the calendar method, you should track at least 8 menstrual cycles. Note the shortest and longest cycles, then calculate the length of your fertile period by subtracting 18 from the total length of your *shortest* cycle to pinpoint your first fertile, or unsafe day, and subtracting 11 from the total length of your *longest* cycle to determine your last fertile, or unsafe day.

The first day of your period is called Day 1 of your menstrual cycle. Thus, if your cycle always lasts 28 days, you should abstain from intercourse from Day 10 (28–18=10) through Day 17 (28–11=17) of your menstrual cycle. If, however, your cycle varies from 26 days to 30 days, you should refrain from intercourse from Day 8 (26–18=8) until Day 19 (30–11=19) of your cycle.

Minimizing the Risks of Failure

The cardinal rule of fertility awareness is that self–discipline is essential to prevent pregnancy. When used perfectly and consistently, fertility awareness is a highly effective form of contraception. But if you're inclined to take risks and have intercourse on days when you are likely to be fertile, you would be wiser to choose another form of birth control.

Careful and routine recordkeeping is also essential to these techniques. You can increase your chances of success by attending a fertility awareness class or working with a physician, family planning clinic, or women's health center experienced in these methods. You can also increase the effectiveness of this form of contraception and pinpoint your fertility more accurately by using all three methods together.

Be sure to record several cycles before using any fertility awareness technique for birth control. If you later become confused about changes related to your menstrual cycle, don't take chances. Assume you're fertile and abstain from intercourse or use a backup method. If you miss a menstrual period or suspect for any other reason that you might be pregnant, or if your patterns are not clear, be sure to check with your doctor and get a pregnancy test.

Surgical Sterilization

Voluntary sterilization is the most popular contraceptive method in the world. Tubal ligation, the favored form of female sterilization, is more than 99 percent effective—the highest success rate of any form of contraception.

Numerous studies suggest that tubal sterilization is also remarkably safe. The fatality rate in the United States is reported to be as low as 4 per 100,000—much lower than that associated with many long–term contraceptives as well as with pregnancy itself. Pregnancy can cause serious, even life–threatening problems for women with such conditions as a blood clotting disorder or heart disease. For them, and for others who must avoid pregnancy to maintain their health, voluntary sterilization can be considered the contraceptive method of choice.

Surgical sterilization poses very few risks. In rare cases, a woman may suffer complications from the anesthesia, internal bleeding, or injury to surrounding structures such as the intestines. The risks are slightly higher for those who smoke, are overweight, have diabetes or pelvic inflammatory disease (PID), and for those who have had previous abdominal surgery. In an estimated 4 out of 10,000 operations, the procedure is unsuccessful or the tubes manage to reconnect, opening the way to an unexpected pregnancy, often occuring in the fallopian tubes. If this dangerous situation arises, the embryo must be surgically removed.

Very few women suffer any of these complications. Overall, voluntary sterilization is one of the safest, most economical and most effective methods of birth control available to women who've completed their families.

Male sterilization, or vasectomy, also is safe, simpler than female sterilization, and nearly as effective. The risk of death from a vasectomy is extremely low, and research studies have not identified any long–term health problems associated with the procedure.

Due to the *irreversible* nature of surgical sterilization, however, it is essential that you consider this choice carefully. Sterilization certainly frees a woman from the fear of an unwanted pregnancy and can actually enhance spontaneity and openness in a sexual relationship. Nevertheless, it will not solve emotional, marital, or sexual problems and

should *never* be chosen if any circumstance—a remarriage, the death of a child, or a change in financial status—might lead you to want another child.

Many women undergo sterilization after childbirth because it is convenient and economical, but you should consider this option with special care. The physical and emotional pressures of pregnancy could prompt you to make a choice you might later regret. In the unlikely case that your newborn develops medical problems or even dies, your decision could magnify your emotional pain. For these reasons, medical professionals often recommend that you take a few months after a pregnancy to make sure you want to proceed with the operation.

Although your partner's consent is not legally required, it's wise to make this decision together since it will have a permanent effect on your relationship. Remember, too, that you have a right to change your mind

THE ULTIMATE IN CERTAINTY

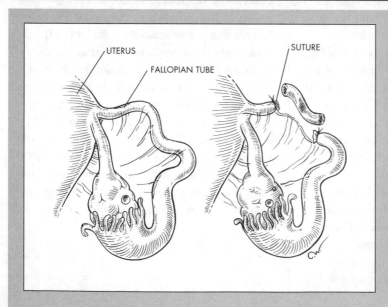

UTERUS

FALLOPIAN TUBE

SUTURE

Surgical sterilization in a procedure called "tubal ligation" is a just about 100 percent effective means of contraception. But be very cautious: Once it's done, there's no going back.

The operation itself is relatively minor. An incision of no more than 2 inches is required—less if the surgeon does a laparoscopy. The object—to block the route from ovary to uterus via the fallopian tubes—can be accomplished in a variety of ways. Here, the surgeon has removed a section of the tube and sutured closed the remaining ends.

about surgical sterilization at any time prior to the operation, even if you have already signed a consent form.

How Sterilization is Done

For women, sterilization means blocking or cutting the fallopian tubes so that eggs can no longer descend from the ovaries to encounter the sperm. This can be achieved through several different surgical procedures referred to jointly as tubal ligation. The actual method you undergo will depend upon your physical condition, the interval since your last pregnancy and, to some extent, your doctor's training and experience.

During a minilaparotomy, or "minilap," the physician makes an incision less than two inches long in your lower abdomen, near the pubic bone, bringing the fallopian tubes into direct view. The doctor then pulls the tubes through the opening, ties them off with bands or surgical clips, and stitches the incision closed. If this procedure is performed after childbirth, your physician will make the incision in the upper abdomen because pregnancy pushes the fallopian tubes higher in the body.

An alternative method, laparoscopy, is sometimes referred to as "Band–Aid®" surgery. The physician makes a small incision near the navel and, possibly, a second lower in the abdomen. Carbon dioxide or nitrous oxide gas is injected through the incision to expand the abdomen. The doctor then inserts a laparoscope—a tube that resembles a telescope equipped with a light—to view the abdominal cavity. The woman is tilted backwards slightly, with her head down, so that the intestines more readily move away from the fallopian tubes.

Once the fallopian tubes are in view, the physician inserts an instrument through either the laparoscope or a second incision and seals them with an electric current or ties them off. Once the tubes have been disconnected, the tiny incision(s) are stitched closed.

Tubal ligations also can be performed through the vagina during procedures known as colpotomy or culdoscopy. Long–term success rates and the risk of complications have not been firmly established for these techniques.

In rare cases, a physician may suggest a hysterectomy, or removal of the uterus, but this more complicated surgery should be considered only if other medical conditions are present and *never* strictly for the purpose of sterilization.

Getting Ready for the Operation

To prepare for your operation, do not eat or drink anything for 8 hours prior to the procedure. Arrange for someone to accompany you to the hospital or clinic, since you should not drive yourself home afterwards. Before leaving for the hospital, shower or bathe, carefully cleaning the area around your navel and pubic area.

Before the surgery, be sure that you are completely comfortable with your decision. Remember that you are entitled to change your mind at any time before the procedure. If you have any last–minute questions or misgivings, talk with your physician and consider canceling or rescheduling the operation.

The actual procedure is quick and relatively painless. In most cases, you will receive an injection of local anesthesia to numb the skin and surrounding tissue before the surgeon makes the incision. This allows you to remain awake and alert, yet feel no pain.

You may also receive medication to help you relax. Sometimes sterilization surgery is performed under general anesthesia; once in a while, spinal anesthesia is administered, numbing the lower half of your body.

Most tubal sterilizations—especially those done under local anesthesia—are performed on an outpatient basis. In these cases, the procedure takes less than an hour, and most women can resume their normal activities in 2 to 4 days. When performed after childbirth, tubal sterilization does not increase the length of your hospital stay beyond that required for regular postpartum recovery.

Minimizing Your Postoperative Problems

Female surgical sterilization is effective immediately. No backup form of birth control is needed after the procedure.

Tubal ligation does not trigger early menopause or alter your sexual functions. Your ovaries will continue to release an egg each month, and you will continue to menstruate. Because the tubes are blocked, however, the egg will dissolve and be absorbed by your body. Since your ovaries and uterus remain intact, your body will also continue to produce normal female hormones.

Though inconclusive, some research has suggested that tubal sterilization may be associated with heavier or more irregular menstrual bleeding and cramps, which may necessitate hysterectomy. On the other hand, a recent study of 78,000 premenopausal women found that tubal sterilization reduces the odds of developing ovarian cancer, the fourth leading cause of death in American women. Researchers theorize that severing the fallopian tubes may reduce the blood supply to the ovaries or cause undetected hormonal changes that inhibit cancer. In any event, women in the study who had received a tubal sterilization were only a third as likely to develop ovarian cancer as women with their tubes intact.

After your tubal ligation, plan to rest for at least 48 hours. Most women can then resume normal activities, though to allow the incision to heal, you should avoid lifting heavy objects for another week. You may bathe 48 hours after surgery, but avoid rubbing or pressing on the incision for at least 1 week, and be certain to dry the incision site carefully after bathing. You should also refrain from having intercourse for 1 week, then resume when it feels comfortable.

For the first few days, you may have some discomfort at the site of the incision, but an over–the–counter pain medicine should make you feel better. You may also feel some mild pain around your shoulders from the anesthesia and gas.

You should contact your doctor immediately if you develop a fever greater than 100.4 degrees Fahrenheit, fainting spells, persistent or steadily increasing abdominal pain, or any bleeding or pus at the incision site.

In addition, you should contact your doctor promptly if, at any time in the future, you suspect you might be pregnant. Though this is very rare after female sterilization, should it occur, the pregnancy is 20 times more likely to develop in the fallopian tubes. This is a dangerous situation that requires immediate medical intervention, since the rupture of a fallopian tube is a potentially life–threatening medical emergency.

Terminating Pregnancy

Abortion, or the termination of pregnancy, can be spontaneous or induced. The medical term for a spontaneous abortion is miscarriage. Termination of an unwanted pregnancy, or induced abortion, has been legal in the United States since 1973.

Abortion is not a method of contraception, since it is performed only after conception has occurred. Nevertheless, according to estimates by the U.S. government's National Institutes of Health, roughly half of the induced abortions in the United States each year follow a contraceptive failure. Some unplanned pregnancies are the aftermath of rape, incest or other forms of sexual abuse, while others are simply a result of inadequate sex education. Some women choose abortion when prenatal testing detects fetal abnormalities, or when personal circumstances change after a planned pregnancy occurs.

Whatever the reason, you should make a voluntary, carefully thought-out choice before having an abortion. Counseling is available from many sources, including your physician, your pastor, family planning clinics, social workers, and nurse practitioners. Although you'll probably want to discuss the situation with your partner and other loved ones, you should not feel forced into making a decision that you feel is irresponsible or immoral. Take time to explore your feelings about all the alternatives—raising the child, seeking an adoption, or having an abortion—before making your decision.

Abortion is safest for you when performed early in pregnancy—within the first 12 weeks after conception. After that time, the risks rise dramatically. An abortion performed before 9 weeks poses a 1 in 400,000 chance of death. But by the time 16 weeks have passed, the risk is 40 times greater, or 1 in 10,000. Although even this higher risk is merely comparable to that of continuing a pregnancy, physicians and family planning experts strongly urge a woman seeking an abortion to undergo the procedure as early in the pregnancy as possible.

A number of different surgical and drug-based techniques are available. During the first trimester, vacuum suction or aspiration is often used to draw the contents of the uterus through a narrow tube (cannula) attached to an electric or mechanical pump. This has become the most common technique, and results in the fewest complications. The procedure can be completed in a physician's office or clinic in less than 30 minutes, using local anesthesia. The size of the cannula is dependent on the length of the pregnancy.

RU-486 (mifepristone), often referred to as the "abortion pill" or "French pill" because of its widespread use in France, is a relatively safe, effective, nonsurgical early abortion measure. This steroid, which blocks the action of the female hormone progesterone, prevents the implantation of a fertilized egg in the uterus and can initiate menstruation even after implantation. Common side effects include abdominal cramps, dizziness, diarrhea, vomiting, and occasional heavy bleeding. The drug is most effective when used within 8 weeks of a woman's last menstrual period and followed by a dose of the hormone prostaglandin, which increases uterine contractions. Although RU-486 is not yet available in the United States, the U.S. Food and Drug Administration has indicated it would consider an application to market the medication.

From the later part of the first trimester on into the second trimester, other techniques come into use. During a vacuum curettage, the doctor stretches (dilates) the cervical opening so that a larger cannula can be used, then scrapes the uterus with a metal loop called a curette. This technique can be performed in a physician's office, clinic or hospital, usually under local anesthesia.

Dilation and curettage (D&C), a common gynecological procedure for diagnostic and therapeutic purposes, is also an option. Doctors sometimes recommend a D&C to ensure complete evacuation of the contents of the uterus. The procedure is usually performed in a hospital under general anesthesia.

Dilation and evacuation (D&E) is a newer method that combines dilation, suction, curettage and, possibly, forceps to terminate pregnancies after 12 weeks. In fact, this has become the most common procedure used for second trimester abortions. Because fetal tissue is larger and a woman's uterus is softer and more susceptible to perforation at this stage, only a skilled medical professional should perform a D&E. This procedure is typically completed in a hospital under general anesthesia.

During a medically induced or labor–induction abortion, the doctor injects saline, a natural body chemical called prostaglandin, or another solution into the amniotic fluid surrounding the fetus. This provokes uterine contractions, or labor, and expels the fetus and placenta from the woman's uterus. The procedure is typically done after detection of fetal abnormalities, and is used only after 16 weeks of pregnancy. It takes place in a hospital using local anesthesia to ease the discomfort of labor and delivery. An ultrasound may be performed prior to the procedure, and a D&C may be performed afterwards to remove any remaining tissue. Doctors often recommend a hospital stay of 1 to 2 days.

During the second trimester—and even later if a woman's life is in danger—a physician may also perform a hysterectomy. During this major surgical procedure, the fetus and placenta are removed through an incision in the abdomen and uterus, much the way a Cesarean section is performed. The operation is considerably riskier than other abortion procedures and is generally used only if other methods have failed.

In rare cases that involve other medical complications, the entire uterus is removed, preventing any future pregnancies.

During surgical abortion procedures, if you are Rh–negative, your doctor will give you immune anti–D globulin (RhoGAM) to prevent blood compatibility complications in future pregnancies. Women who undergo abortions may also be given antibiotics to prevent or treat infection, and blood transfusions if excessive bleeding occurs.

Complications can occur after any type of pregnancy termination, including miscarriage, but are more likely following improperly performed abortions and those performed after 16 weeks gestation. The problems, which range from mild to severe, include infection, bleeding, retained pregnancy tissue, perforation or tearing of the cervix or uterus, or allergic reaction to drugs or anesthesia used during the procedure. Some procedures—especially a vacuum aspiration performed very early in the pregnancy—can fail, and the pregnancy may continue. Some studies have suggested that chronic pelvic infection, which can increase a woman's risk for an tubal pregnancy or infertility, can be a delayed effect of abortion.

After most abortion procedures, you can resume your normal diet and activities. If possible, keep your schedule flexible for the first week following the abortion and avoid any strenuous activities during that time.

It's normal to experience some bleeding and cramps during the first 2 weeks following an abortion, but these should be no heavier than your normal menstrual period. To minimize the risk of infection, do not use tampons, do not douche and refrain from intercourse during the first week following the procedure. You should also check your temperature each day and call your doctor if it exceeds 100 degrees Fahrenheit. Your normal menstrual periods should resume 4 to 6 weeks after the procedure.

Watch for common danger signs that can indicate the presence of an infection, an incomplete abortion, or other complications. These include fever, chills, muscle aches, unusual fatigue, abdominal pain or cramping, tenderness in your abdomen, a bad-smelling vaginal discharge, or bleeding that is heavier than your menstrual period or lasts longer than 3 to 4 weeks. If any of these occur, contact your doctor immediately. And even if you don't experience any complications, schedule a return checkup with your doctor within a few weeks of the procedure. □

CHAPTER 23   **TOWARD SUCCESSFUL PREGNANCIES**

Strategies for a Healthy Pregnancy

It's one of the most exciting times in any couple's life: the planning, the preparation, and—finally—the reality of having a baby. Yet it's a worry–filled time too. You want to be certain you've done everything right, that you've given the little one every possible break along the way. In this chapter, you'll find the basic measures you need to take to make your pregnancy as trouble–free as possible, and your baby as healthy as can be.

Preparing for Pregnancy

Your body is the baby's home for its first 9 months. Ideally, you want to do everything possible to make that home as healthy as possible. Proper care of your body during pregnancy is crucial, but there are limits to what you can do once the baby is on the way. If you are planning a pregnancy, the best thing you can do is prepare your body *before* you conceive.

That's why most doctors recommend that you see a doctor (preferably the obstetrician/ gynecologist, or ob/gyn, you will see during your pregnancy) for what is known as a pre-conception checkup.

This visit enables your doctor to uncover any potential health problems before you get pregnant. These problems can then be prevented or treated. At the very least, you and your doctor will be aware of them so you can manage your pregnancy appropriately. It also gives you time to change your lifestyle to maximize your health before pregnancy, improve your chances of conceiving, and remove any potential dangers to the baby.

A preconception checkup is somewhat similar to the first visit after you know you are pregnant. If you see a doctor before you conceive, then your first prenatal visit will be more routine.

Here are some of the topics that may be discussed and tests that may be performed at a preconception visit. To be ready for the doctor's questions, you may need to obtain some information from your partner before seeing the doctor or ask your partner to go with you.

Topics You Should Discuss

Family history of genetic diseases and multiple births can be an important factor in your pregnancy and in the health of your baby. Since multiples run in the family, it will help your doctor to know whether you are more likely than the average woman to have them. If you or your partner know of a family history of a genetic disease, your doctor may want to test you both to see if either of you carries the genes for that disease. A blood test is sufficient in most cases. For example, Jews of central and eastern European ancestry are more likely to be carriers for Tay–Sachs disease; if both parents are carriers, chances are one in four that the child will have this fatal disease. Tay–Sachs' results can be difficult to interpret when the test is performed on a pregnant woman, so this test needs to be performed before pregnancy occurs. (If you're already pregnant, the father can still be tested. If he's negative, there's no danger the baby will inherit the disease.)

Your menstrual periods. The doctor will ask you about the pattern of your menstrual periods to check for any abnormalities that should be treated before you become pregnant or that might affect your ability to conceive. Keeping a diary of your periods can be helpful at this point.

Exposure to poisons at work or at home should be avoided before conception and during pregnancy. Radiation found in x–rays, known as ionizing radiation, also can harm a developing baby. If you are exposed to x–rays at work, you should ask for monthly readings of the amount of radiation before attempting to conceive. A pregnant woman should not be exposed to more than 0.5 rad total dose for the entire pregnancy, or 0.05 rad in any 1 month. It's best to avoid x–rays for medical purposes if possible. If you get a chest x–ray, for instance, it exposes your baby to about 0.008 rad. However, according to an April 1993 publication of the American College of Obstetricians and Gynecologists, radiation from video display terminals, color televisions, and microwave ovens is not dangerous during pregnancy. This is called non–ionizing radiation. Other health hazards at work include lead poisoning and, if you're a health-care worker, chemotherapeutic agents.

General health. Your doctor needs to know about any serious disease or chronic illness you may have. Diabetes, high blood pressure, heart disease, the connective tissue disease called systemic lupus erythematosus, and epilepsy and other seizure disorders can all affect pregnancy. Women with diabetes, for example, may need to change their medications before conceiving.

You and your partner may be asked about any history of sexually transmitted diseases because some STDs can make conception difficult, harm a developing baby, or affect management of pregnancy. For example, pelvic inflammatory disease brought on by a sexually transmitted infection can damage reproductive organs.

Medications. Even some over–the–counter drugs can affect a developing baby, so you should tell your doctor about every medicine you are taking. Some drugs can impair your ability to conceive; others could damage a fetus in the first few weeks before you know you are pregnant. If you take any medication regularly, you may need to stop taking it before trying to conceive, and you might need time to change your medication regimen.

High doses of vitamin and mineral supplements can also harm a fetus. If you are taking megadoses of supplements, tell your doctor about them so he or she can determine whether you need to stop them before attempting to conceive.

Birth control. If you've ever used an IUD, conception may be more difficult and your chances of a miscarriage are somewhat higher. If you have been using birth control pills, it will take from a few weeks to 3 months for your body to return to its normal hormonal cycles so that you can become pregnant. Conceiving immediately after stopping the pill, does not however, increase your chances of miscarriage or birth defects.

Prior pregnancies. Any problems with previous pregnancies can affect future pregnancies. Tell your doctor about any complications you experienced such as miscarriages, induced abortion, or premature or multiple births.

Examinations and Tests

A pelvic exam and a Pap smear will help identify any problem with the pelvic region and birth canal before pregnancy. If your doctor finds a condition requiring treatment, he or she may recommend further tests. Therapy will be much easier before you get pregnant.

Your weight. When you conceive, your pre–pregnancy weight, along with your weight gain during pregnancy, have an important bearing on your baby's health and will be monitored carefully. It's important to

IN THE BEGINNING

Well before you learn you're pregnant, amazing developments are already underway. Leaving the fallopian tube behind, the fertilized egg finds a resting place in the rich tissue of the endometrial lining, implants itself, and begins growing the placenta that will nourish the developing baby in the months ahead. Already, your intake of alcohol, tobacco, and drugs is a cause for concern. If you're even trying to conceive, it's time to cut out these potentially damaging substances. Remember, too, that certain prescription medications can be as just as damaging as an illegal drug. For more information see the table on Drug Risks in Pregnancy near the end of the book.

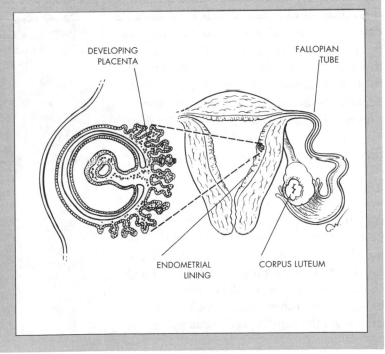

DEVELOPING PLACENTA

FALLOPIAN TUBE

ENDOMETRIAL LINING

CORPUS LUTEUM

do everything possible to reach your ideal weight before becoming pregnant.

Blood and urine tests. Your doctor will do a blood test for anemia, or insufficient iron in the blood. Because women lose blood through their periods every month, many begin pregnancy without enough iron. You can start to remedy this problem with an iron supplement or dietary changes if it is uncovered before conception. Another blood test determines the Rh factor. If you are Rh negative and your partner is Rh positive, there is potential for problems for the baby, particularly if this is not your first pregnancy. If your doctor knows both partners' Rh status, any difficulty usually can be prevented by administering a drug called Rho(D) Immuno Globulin (Human) (Rhogam), if necessary, at certain points before or after delivery. Urine will be analyzed for signs of kidney disease or diabetes.

Possible infection. You will be tested for hepatitis B, syphilis, and gonorrhea because these diseases can cause serious harm to the developing baby. Gonorrhea and syphilis can be cured prior to pregnancy. If you have hepatitis B the doctor will be prepared to give the baby hepatitis B immune globulin and the hepatitis B vaccine. Because the virus that causes AIDS can be passed to the baby, if you are at risk for AIDS, an HIV test will also be done at this visit.

Vaccinations. Your doctor will ask you if you have an immunity to German measles (rubella). Fifteen percent of women of childbearing age are not immune to German measles and if you become infected with it in the first 8 weeks of pregnancy, there is a high chance that your baby will be born deaf, blind, or with other serious problems. You cannot get the rubella vaccination while you are pregnant because the vaccine contains a weakened form of the virus. If you are not sure if you have the immunity, your doctor can do a blood test to confirm it. In addition, you should also update your tetanus and diphtheria boosters as needed and get a polio vaccine if you did not receive one as a child.

Getting Yourself in Shape

The nine months of pregnancy put a lot of stress on the body, but there are a number of things you can do before you conceive to make your pregnancy easier and healthier.

Weight

If you are under or overweight, try to get as close as possible to your optimal weight before conception. Underweight mothers are more likely to give birth to underweight and premature babies, even when they gain

YOUR OPTIMAL WEIGHT

These ranges are based on a Metropolitan Life Insurance table that allows for 3 pounds of clothes and 1 inch heels.

Height	Small Frame	Medium Frame	Large Frame
4'10"	102–111	109–121	118–131
4'11"	103–113	111–123	120–134
5'0"	104–115	113–126	122–137
5'1"	106–118	115–129	125–140
5'2"	108–121	118–132	128–143
5'3"	111–124	121–135	131–147
5'4"	114–127	124–138	134–151
5'5"	117–130	127–141	137–155
5'6"	120–133	130–144	140–159
5'7"	123–136	133–147	143–163
5'8"	126–139	136–150	146–167
5'9"	129–142	139–153	149–170
5'10"	132–145	142–158	152–173
5'11"	135–148	145–159	155–176
6'0"	138–151	148–162	158–179

weight normally during pregnancy. In addition, underweight women may not be able to gain enough during pregnancy to offset their low preconception weight. Women who are overweight before conceiving are more likely to develop diabetes during pregnancy and, due to increased weight of their babies, more likely to need Cesarean section. Weight loss is not advisable for any woman during pregnancy, so act before conceiving!

Exercise

If you do not have a regular exercise program, this is the time to start one, preferably one that you can maintain while you are pregnant. Carrying and nourishing a baby is hard work, and a fit woman is likely to feel better and be less fatigued during pregnancy than one who has avoided exercise most of her life. Some evidence suggests that women who are physically fit tolerate pregnancy and delivery better.

It's best to start an exercise program 1 year before becoming pregnant, but at the very least you should begin at least 3 months before conception to give your body a chance to adjust to the additional physical activity before facing the added challenge of carrying a child.

If you haven't exercised before, start slowly. Within 3 to 4 weeks, you should be able to perform aerobic (fitness) exercise for 30 minutes. If you have any medical problems, consult your physician before starting the program. Likewise, see a doctor if you experience any symptoms during exercise.

Resistance exercises, in which you lift weights so that your muscles are working against something, are also important and should be done 2 or 3 times a week on alternate days. Strengthening your muscles will help you recover more quickly from labor and delivery and give you more strength to carry the baby after birth. Because back pain can be a problem during pregnancy, exercises to strengthen the back can be helpful, too.

Alcohol, Tobacco, Caffeine, and Illegal Drugs

Alcoholic beverages have been proven to harm the developing baby. In particular, because the first 2 months after conception are so critical for healthy development, and because it is not known whether there is a "safe" level of alcohol consumption for a fetus, women should stop drinking before attempting to conceive. No form of alcohol is safer than any other; beer and wine are just as bad for the baby as hard liquor. Some studies suggest that women who drink before pregnancy tend to have smaller babies. Persistent and significant drinking during pregnancy can cause fetal alcohol syndrome, as a result of which infants may be born with brain, heart, and nervous system problems, distinctive facial abnormalities, and mental retardation.

Smoking increases your chances of a miscarrying during the first trimester. Mothers who smoke are also more likely to go into premature labor; have a premature rupture of membranes; experience third–trimester bleeding; have slower fetal growth, and deliver underweight babies. Prospective fathers who smoke should also quit. Studies indicate that a mother exposed to "passive smoking" during pregnancy is more likely to give birth to an underweight baby. You can't count on quitting smoking overnight, so it's best to start trying to withdraw from cigarettes well before attempting to conceive. Additionally, some evidence suggests that smoking impairs a woman's fertility. One study showed that 10.7 percent of smokers (women who smoked more than 20 cigarettes per day), compared with 5.4 percent of nonsmokers, failed to have a successful pregnancy within 5 years of stopping contraception. Smoking also affects sperm and may impair male fertility, too.

Caffeine. Many obstetricians recommend that pregnant women limit themselves to the equivalent of one cup of coffee daily. If you consume more than that—especially if you drink a lot of caffeine—withdrawal may take time, so start weaning yourself before you try to conceive. Some evidence suggests that in women who take in 400 milligrams of caffeine daily, the equivalent of four cups of coffee, the baby grows more slowly. Caffeine may also increase the risk of late first or second trimester miscarriage. Most studies find no association between caffeine consumption and low birth weight or birth defects but moderation is still best.

A few researchers have suggested that high caffeine consumption may also affect fertility. One study found that women who consumed more than 300 milligrams of caffeine daily (the equivalent of three cups of coffee) had a 27 percent lower chance of conceiving each cycle compared to women who consumed no caffeine. Women who consumed some caffeine but less than 300 milligrams daily were 10 percent less likely to conceive.

Illegal drugs are bad for your health, whether or not you are pregnant and they can only harm a baby. If you use them, it's imperative to stop before trying to conceive.

Folic acid

Women who have had a baby with a neural tube defect are at higher risk of having another baby with similar defects. Examples of neural tube defects are spina bifida, in which the spinal cord does not close completely, and anencephalopathy, in which part of the baby's brain and skull do not develop completely.

Most authorities recommend that anyone trying to conceive—and especially someone who's already had a baby with a neural tube defect—take 0.4 milligrams of folic acid daily starting 1 month before she plans to become pregnant and continuing at least for the first 3 months of pregnancy. In fact, the US Centers for Disease Control and Prevention now recommend that *all* women of child–bearing age consume 0.4 milligram of folic acid daily through diet or supplements. Your doctor can recommend a multivitamin that contains the right amount.

Prenatal care

Proper care of your body is crucial to a healthy pregnancy and baby. It's important to see your doctor as soon as you think you might be pregnant. Missing a period, or being a week or two late, is one possible sign of pregnancy, though it's not conclusive. Other indicators include nausea and vomiting, dizziness, and fatigue. A home pregnancy test is also an excellent indicator, but you should still see your doctor for confirmation.

Prenatal care enables your doctor to identify signs of any problems early. Your first visit to the doctor to confirm pregnancy will be similar to the preconception checkup. If you have had one of these checkups, then only a few tests will be repeated when your pregnancy is confirmed. Thereafter, if you are between 18 and 35 with no known medical problems you will probably see your doctor

WHERE THE WEIGHT GAIN GOES

Maternal	
Uterus	2 lbs
Breasts	1 lb
Blood	2.75 lbs
Water	3.7 lbs
Fat	7.4 lbs
Subtotal	16.85 lbs
Fetal	
Fetus	7.5 lbs
Placenta	1.4 lbs
Amniotic fluid	1.75 lbs
Subtotal	10.65 lbs
Total	**27.5 lbs**

Adapted from Hytten, FE, Leitch, I (eds.):
The Physiology of Human Pregnancy,
ed 2. Oxford, England, Blackwell Scientific
Publications, 1971.

once a month until week 28 of pregnancy, every 2 or 3 weeks until week 36, then every week until the baby is born. The age of the baby is dated from the first day of your last menstrual period.

Visits after the first one are brief and involve measuring the fetal heart rate, the size of the baby, fetal activity, your blood pressure, your weight, and the length of your abdomen (to measure uterus size—another way of measuring the baby). The doctor will also ask for a urine specimen to check for protein and sugar. At times during the pregnancy, urine will also be checked for signs of infection. The doctor will also ask you if you are experiencing any symptoms.

Other tests that may be performed at some point during pregnancy include blood tests, glucose tolerance tests to check for gestational diabetes, and ultrasound. Some women will have an amniocentesis or chorionic villus sampling to detect abnormalities in the baby. These tests are discussed further in the next chapter. A pelvic exam is part of the initial visit and generally is not repeated until the 36th week of pregnancy, or later, unless there is a complication.

Nutrition During Pregnancy

What you eat and how much weight you gain while pregnant has a major impact on your baby's health. This is one time when even the most body-conscious woman can feel that it's all right to gain weight!

How Much Weight to Gain

How much you should gain varies with your weight before pregnancy. Underweight women should gain 28 to 40 pounds, normal weight women should gain 25 to 35 pounds, and overweight women should gain 15 to 25 pounds (if very overweight, even less.) If you are of normal weight you should gain about 2 to 4 pounds in the first trimester and three-quarters to 1 pound per week thereafter. Underweight women should gain about one and a quarter pounds per week in the second and third trimester and overweight women should gain a half to three-quarters of a pound each week during that time.

Don't worry too much about retaining your pregnancy weight; most women lose about two-thirds of it by the time they leave the hospital, and much of the rest is lost within 6 months. The reason for this becomes apparent when you see that in most women, only about a quarter of the weight is fat. The average amount of weight retained 6 months after delivery is 3 pounds.

CORRECT MENU FOR A HEALTHY PREGNANCY

Food	Daily Servings
Dark–green and dark–yellow vegetables	1
Vitamin C fruits and vegetables	2
Other fruits and vegetables	1 (or more)
Breads and cereals	4 (or more)
Milk and milk products	4
Protein foods (Poultry, fish, eggs, meat)	2
Beans, nuts	2

Food and Drink

Pregnant women should consume 2,500 calories per day, 300 more than women who are not pregnant. Almost any diet with sufficient calories supplies enough of all the minerals you need except iron. Recommended Daily Allowances of vitamins and minerals during pregnancy and a daily menu for pregnant women can be found in the boxes nearby.

You will need to eat about 27 percent more protein than what's recommended for women who are not pregnant—a total of 60 grams a day. Meat, fish, poultry, eggs, milk, and other dairy products are excellent sources. Milk and dairy products have the added advantage of providing calcium.

Drink at least eight 8–ounce glasses of water or other fluids a day. Coffee and tea don't count as they cause you to lose fluid but if you do drink them, make sure they're decaffeinated. Avoid diet soda, and other artificially sweetened foods and drinks, as aspartame may harm your baby.

Vitamins and Minerals

You will need more iron, calcium, folic acid, and zinc. With the exception of iron, these substances can generally be obtained through diet. When you do use salt, make sure it is iodized to ensure that you get enough iodine. Don't take supplements without consulting your doctor. Too much vitamin A, B_6, C, D, E, or K, or too much zinc, iron, or selenium, can be harmful during pregnancy.

Women whose diets are deficient in some nutrients or who have other special needs may have to take supplements. However, even the recommended amounts of certain prenatal vitamin and mineral supplements can lead to total ingestion of far more of certain substances than is required, so it's important to ask your doctor what you should take. Many physicians recommend that women take supplemental iron in their second and third trimesters, and the amount that most healthy women need is contained in many prenatal vitamins. Ask your doctor if he or she thinks you need a supplement. Take iron at bedtime or between meals with water or citrus juice—never with milk, because calcium makes it harder for the body to absorb iron.

What's Safe During Pregnancy?

You may feel that your regular lifestyle has become severely restricted due to your pregnancy, and it may be difficult to give up certain habits. It is important to remember, however, that you are doing what is necessary to ensure your health and the health of your baby.

Exercise

Most women can continue their exercise routine after becoming pregnant. But don't start or intensify an aerobic exercise regimen while pregnant. The American College of Obstetricians and Gynecologists recommends brisk walking, swimming, and stationary cycling as the safest exercises during this period. Tennis and jogging in moderation are acceptable if you start before becoming pregnant. If you were not getting enough exercise before conceiving, stick to brisk walking. You should discuss your exercise program with your doctor, both at the start and as you progress through your pregnancy.

The American College of Obstetricians and Gynecologists recently revised its recommendation regarding exercise in pregnant women to remove limits on intensity and heart rate. However, the guidelines say that there is no need to exercise strenuously because mild to moderate exertion can maintain cardiovascular fitness. One definition of moderate exercise is a 30-minute aerobic workout, twice or three times weekly at 50 percent to 85 percent of maximum capacity. The College recommends letting your own body be your guide; do not exercise to the point of exhaustion.

Less oxygen is available for aerobic activity during pregnancy, so even well-conditioned pregnant women may not be able to continue their prepregnancy regimens at the same level. Aerobic exercise does raise body temperature, and high body temperatures early in pregnancy can increase the risk of certain birth defects. The ideal way to monitor this is to check your rectal temperature after completing your typical exercise regimen. Since this is not a realistic option at the gym, most doctors recommend checking your pulse instead, with a goal of keeping it below 140. If you do get overheated (a temperature exceeding 101 degrees Fahrenheit), try to keep cooler by drinking more water, wearing lighter clothing, or exercising for a shorter time. *Do not use hot tubs or saunas while pregnant.*

After the third month of pregnancy, do not exercise while lying on your back, since this can reduce your heart rate, lower your blood pressure, cause dizziness, and reduce blood flow to the baby.

Even women who got no exercise before pregnancy can benefit from a mild weight training program to strengthen their back, leg, and other muscles needed to carry the baby. You should build up gradually to avoid injury. Always check with your doctor before starting such a regimen.

Strengthening the muscles in the pelvic region can help support the uterus, ease deliv-

VITAMINS AND MINERALS: YOUR NEEDS IN PREGNANCY

	Daily Allowance
Calcium	1,200 (milligrams)
Phosphorous	1,200 (milligrams)
Magnesium	300 (milligrams)
Iron	30 (milligrams)
Zinc	15 (milligrams)
Vitamin A	800 (milligrams)
Vitamin D	10 (milligrams)
Vitamin E	10 (milligrams)
Vitamin C	70 (milligrams)
Thiamin	1.5 (milligrams)
Riboflavin	1.6 (milligrams)
Niacin	17 (milligrams)
Vitamin B-6	2.2 (milligrams)
Folic acid	400 (micrograms)
Vitamin B-12	2.2 (micrograms)

Nutrition During Pregnancy, American College of Obstetrics and Gynecologists Technical Bulletin, April 1993.

ery, and speed the return of normal muscle tone after delivery. You can locate the pelvic muscles by spreading your legs apart while urinating, then stopping and starting the flow of urine several times. Once you have found these muscles, you can exercise them anywhere. Contract them hard for 5 seconds, then gently release them. Ideally, this should be done 20 to 30 times a day. These movements are known as Kegel exercises.

Avoid contact sports or other activities during which you risk colliding with someone or falling on your abdomen, since your baby could be injured. Examples include downhill skiing and horseback riding. If you have had complications in previous pregnancies, your doctor may advise you to avoid exercising altogether.

Work

Healthy women with uncomplicated pregnancies whose jobs pose no more risk than that of other everyday activities can stay at work right up to labor, and resume working several weeks after giving birth. Any job that requires severe physical strain should be avoided, however. As pregnancy progresses, strenuous work will become more tiring. On the other hand, activity such as heavy housework or child care is actually associated with a less than average rate of miscarriage.

As with exercise, it's important to rest during the day as you become tired. Women who have had complications during other pregnancies should minimize physical work. It's also wise to avoid working with toxic substances that could harm the baby, just as you would avoid them while trying to conceive.

Travel

Travel is acceptable except within a month or so of your due date. The main risk is not in the journey itself but in the chance that a complication may develop or labor may begin while you are far from medical services. If you must be away late in pregnancy or for a prolonged period, ask your doctor to recommend a local physician you can contact in an emergency. If you are traveling abroad, be sure to take whatever dietary precautions are needed at your destination.

When traveling by car, fasten the seat belt with the lap portion under your abdomen and across the upper thighs. Stop the car, get out and walk every hour and a half or so to prevent swelling and reduce discomfort. You should also do this on a plane or train. As with any drugs, do not take motion sickness medications without consulting your doctor.

Sexual intercourse

Some physicians suggest that you refrain from intercourse during the last 4 weeks of pregnancy. Aside from this possible restriction, intercourse is safe unless you are at risk for miscarriage or early labor. Women experiencing vaginal bleeding are at risk for miscarriage and should avoid intercourse.

Some data show that 1 woman in 4 is less interested in sex during the first trimester of pregnancy. Some women also lose interest during the last trimester.

Light bleeding may occur after intercourse, possibly due to minor injury to the cervix, which is engorged with blood during pregnancy. If this is the reason, you and your partner may merely need to avoid deep penetration. Still, you should call your doctor to be sure there is no problem.

Abdominal cramps after intercourse are common, but if they continue and worsen over an hour, notify your doctor. It could mean contractions are starting. Some pregnant women may leak fluid from their breasts during sexual activity but this does not present a medical problem.

Avoiding Infection

Raw meat and cat litter both can contain an organism called *Toxoplasma* that can cause miscarriage, stillbirth, or an infection in the baby or mother. Wash your hands immediately after handling raw meat and make sure the meat is well cooked, also avoid cleaning litter boxes or gardening in soil frequented by cats.

Poisons

It's best to avoid contact with hazardous materials such as harsh cleaning solutions, paint fumes, paint removers, etc. Some other materials you might not think of are garden fertilizers, herbicides, and pesticides; arts and crafts glues, solvents, and photographic chemicals; and chemical hair dyes. If you absolutely must use these types of products, wear gloves and make sure you have adequate ventilation (both of which are a good idea anyway). Lead is also highly toxic. The two most common ways you can be exposed to lead are through inhaling particles of flaking lead–based paint and drinking lead–tainted water. You can have your drinking water tested if you think it might contain dangerous levels of lead or you can simply drink bottled water. Your doctor can do a blood test to detect lead levels in your system.

Other Concerns

Douching can cause complications that can kill the developing baby.

Tub baths in the last trimester of pregnancy should be avoided, as your balance may be off and you may be more likely to slip and fall.

Dress in whatever is comfortable. Avoid constricting garters and tummy–control pantyhose because they can interfere with blood flow. Many women find maternity pantyhose to be very supportive, particularly towards the end of the pregnancy. Shoes with heels are fine if you are comfortable and can balance yourself although many women feel better in low heels or flats. You probably will need new bras since breasts increase by about two cup sizes during pregnancy. You may also need larger shoes, as your feet may swell in the last 2 months.

Sleep on your side instead of your back after the third month. The weight of the enlarged uterus can constrict some of your major blood vessels if you lie flat on your back.

Treating Common Problems

Most women encounter some of the problems and discomforts discussed here. Generally, they are not serious, but if you have any questions, or your symptoms seem out of the ordinary, contact your doctor.

Digestive

Nausea and vomiting are very common in early pregnancy. Eat several small meals throughout the day, rather than three larger ones, and drink plenty of liquids. Avoid any foods that cause nausea. Although it's called morning sickness and usually passes after the

WHY ALL THE PROBLEMS?

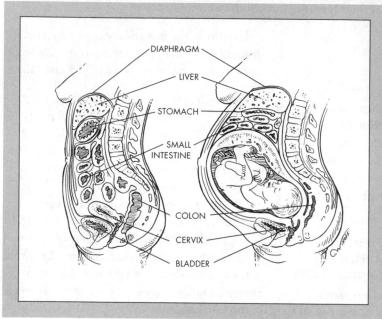

It's easy to see. As the baby grows, it exerts increasing pressure on virtually all your internal organs. Upward pressure on the stomach can lead to heartburn; downward pressure on the bladder can keep you heading for the bathroom. Hemorrhoids develop as the uterus presses on the rectum. And all the extra bulk up front means backaches for many women nearing term.

first trimester, many women experience nausea and vomiting throughout the day and, sometimes, throughout their pregnancy.

Constipation is also a common problem. Getting enough fiber from bran, fruits, and raw vegetables is important. Proper diet, along with enough fluids, engaging in reasonable amounts of daily exercise, and, sometimes, using mild laxatives such as prune juice or milk of magnesia should prevent constipation if you did not have this problem before you were pregnant.

Heartburn is a third common digestive problem. It occurs as the uterus pushes on the stomach, forcing acid up into the esophagus. Again, eating smaller, more frequent meals rather than three larger meals can help. Avoid bending over or lying flat. Antacids may relieve discomfort.

Cravings are not harmful as long as you eat the substances in moderation and also consume healthy foods. Rarely, some pregnant women crave, and eat, items such as laundry starch, clay, dirt, or chopped ice. See your doctor if you have any really unusual cravings. Some may indicate that you are not getting enough iron, and a supplement may be in order.

Fatigue and Headache

Most women complain of being tired early in pregnancy. This feeling usually goes away by the fourth month and is considered to be normal. Fatigue can also be due to anemia, or insufficient iron in the blood. A simple blood test can reveal anemia and your doctor may recommend an iron supplement. Don't start taking supplements on your own. Too much iron can be dangerous.

Headaches are also common in early pregnancy and usually go away by the fourth or fifth month. It's safe to take Tylenol for headache relief. Headaches in later pregnancy can be a sign of serious complications, such as high blood pressure, and should be reported to your doctor immediately.

Vaginal and Urinary Symptoms

Increased vaginal discharge. Many women develop thicker, more plentiful, more odorous discharge for no apparent reason. The discharge can, however, be caused by infection—yeast infections are more common during pregnancy. Any infection needs to be treated so if you think you have one, don't wait until your next scheduled appointment to call your doctor.

Frequent urination is a problem for many women as their large uterus presses on the bladder and their hormone balances are altered. Some women lose urine when they move or cough. The pelvic exercises described earlier in this chapter may help.

Urinary tract infections are more common during pregnancy. Most doctors will test your urine at each visit but call your doctor immediately if you experience burning during urination. Untreated urinary infections can trigger premature labor. Your doctor will know which antibiotics are safe to take during pregnancy.

Other Physical Discomforts

Breast swelling is common and, for many women, uncomfortable. There really is no solution except to wear a very supportive bra, 24 hours a day, if necessary.

Hemorrhoids occur as the uterus presses on the veins of the rectum. They sometimes develop for the first time during pregnancy but are more likely to occur if you've been troubled by them earlier. Pain–relieving creams, warm soaks, and drugs that soften stool can help. As always, check with your doctor before using any over–the–counter medication while you are pregnant.

Backache develops late in pregnancy in many women, especially those with poor posture. A fitted maternity girdle can alleviate backache due to your new shape. Rest, supportive shoes, and massage also help. Exercises that strengthen the back muscles can make you less vulnerable to back problems.

Varicose veins often can develop in the legs, external genitals, or abdominal wall, especially when there is a family history of this complication. Wearing elastic support stockings and raising your legs when possible can help prevent and alleviate varicose veins.

Fluid retention is a common occurrence in late pregnancy, and is rarely serious. If you see swelling in your hands and face, however, it can be a sign of a serious complication called preeclampsia (pregnancy–induced high blood pressure) and should be reported to the doctor immediately. Preeclampsia should be treated to ensure that blood flow (and thus oxygen and nourishment) to the baby remains unrestricted, and to prevent an even more serious condition called eclampsia (pregnancy-related convulsions) that can be fatal to both mother and baby.

Leg cramps can be caused by a deficiency of calcium in a form that your body can use, or by getting too much phosphorus. Your doctor may tell you to drink less milk, and stop taking supplements containing calcium phosphate. Instead, the doctor may prescribe calcium carbonate or calcium lactate tablets. Leg massage, flexing the feet, and applying heat can relieve the pain. Avoid pointing your toes when you stretch your legs in the morning since this can cause cramps. Also, lead with the heel when you walk.

If Complications Get Serious

This chapter dealt with the kind of pregnancy we all hope for—full of little discomforts, but basically trouble–free. However, if you've had problems in previous pregnancies, are under 18 or over 35, have a medical condition, or believe that you are at risk for a difficult pregnancy for other reasons, you'll probably also want to read chapter 25, "Potential Complications You Should Keep in Mind" later in this section. □

CHAPTER 24   **TOWARD SUCCESSFUL PREGNANCIES**

Prenatal Tests to Consider

Pregnancy is incredibly exciting, but it's also a bit scary. As the reality of having a baby sets in, it's hard not to worry about whether your baby will be healthy. In the old days, doctors simply told women not to think about it.

Modern women think a lot about such things. Today's expectant mothers are much better informed than were their own mothers, and have heard about many of the more than 3,000 congenital disorders parents can pass along to their babies. Fortunately, there are now several prenatal tests that can help reassure the majority of expectant parents that their babies are just fine. And when there is a possible problem, these tests give the couple time to go through counseling and make an informed decision about continuing the pregnancy.

In addition to all the high-technology techniques generally available to pregnant women in the 1990s, there are many routine prenatal procedures that have been keeping babies safe for decades. Certain common laboratory tests are repeated every time you see your doctor; others are done periodically throughout the pregnancy.

Routine Tests

During your first prenatal appointment your doctor will determine your blood type and test for anemia, exposure to such sexually transmitted diseases as syphilis and AIDS, and perhaps for signs of drug abuse. He or she will also examine your vaginal secretions for the presence of gonorrhea, which can cause potentially serious eye infections if transmitted to a baby during birth.

You will also have a Pap smear to rule out possible cancer of the cervix and a urine test to detect the presence of bacteria that could indicate a current or potential infection. Your doctor also needs to know whether you have ever been exposed to rubella (German measles). This childhood disease can produce severe birth defects if contracted during pregnancy. This initial battery of tests gives the physician a fairly good idea of your overall health.

Certain tests must be repeated at every prenatal visit to make sure you—and your baby—stay healthy. Your blood pressure will be checked regularly. Your doctor will also examine your urine. Too much sugar in the urine could mean you are developing gestational diabetes; too much protein could indicate the danger of toxemia.

In the fourth month of pregnancy, the doctor will probably check your blood again for anemia. In the sixth month of pregnancy, he or she will take a specimen from the cervix to test for the presence of group B streptococcus. If these bacteria are present, you may be treated as soon as labor starts in order to keep the baby from becoming infected during birth.

Later at 28 weeks, you will probably have a glucose tolerance test to check for diabetes. Women who are already diabetic will need this test earlier and will probably have it done more than once.

At the beginning of a glucose tolerance test, a small amount of your blood is drawn and examined to determine how much sugar is present. Following this you will drink a fruit-flavored preparation with a high concentration of glucose. Then blood will be drawn at various intervals and tested to determine how well your body is able to handle—and get rid of—all this extra sugar.

Any further testing depends on your medical and family history and that of the father, as well as the course of your pregnancy. Despite the fears common to all parents that something could be wrong with their baby, the incidence of chromosomal and other congenital defects has been greatly reduced by the common use of such procedures as amniocentesis, ultrasound, chorionic villi sampling, and alpha-fetoprotein screens.

Ultrasound

The advent of ultrasonography gave physicians a safe way of examining a developing baby without the risk of invading the womb or disturbing the pregnancy. Ultrasound uses sound waves bouncing off the baby—and anything else in the womb—to create a picture of the pregnancy without the potentially harmful effects often associated with x-rays.

The procedure is now used routinely to date a pregnancy, since it allows the doctor to see whether the size of the baby corresponds with the reported length of time since conception. Ultrasound also helps physicians monitor the baby's growth during the pregnancy if there is any concern that the baby is too small or too large.

Ultrasound is helpful in confirming or ruling out pregnancy; determining the presence of more than one baby; assessing the development, health, and location of the placenta; and checking the volume of amniotic fluid in the uterus.

These sound-wave pictures also help physicians look for suspected congenital abnormalities. With ultrasound, doctors are actually able to see the baby's organs and central nervous system and look at the baby's bones to make sure the skull, arms and legs are the right size for its prenatal age.

Your doctor will order an ultrasound if he or she cannot hear a heartbeat, if the baby isn't moving or there is a change in the pattern of movement. The doctor will also want to take a look at the placenta when there is any bleeding—especially if the bleeding occurs early or late in the pregnancy.

As the time of delivery nears, ultrasound helps physicians determine the baby's position (presentation) and identify any potential problems that might interfere with birth. If a baby has to be delivered early, ultrasound helps ensure that it is mature enough to survive. If the infant seems to be overdue, the doctor can use ultrasound to check on its size.

Ultrasound has greatly improved the safety of other diagnostic procedures such as amniocentesis and chorionic villi sampling. Indeed, without the road map the ultrasound picture provides, many physicians and parents would probably consider the risk of such testing far too great.

Ultrasound is a simple, quick procedure. The physician either inserts a probe into the vagina or moves what is called a transducer back and forth across the abdomen. Either way, the instrument records the echoes of sound waves bouncing off anything encountered in the uterus. These echoes make pictures that are shown on a sort of television screen attached to the unit.

The single biggest drawback is that women who are having an abdominal ultrasound must drink a lot of water beforehand and aren't allowed to go to the bathroom until after the examination. Any woman who has ever been pregnant knows just how uncomfortable a really full bladder can be.

Apart from all the medical benefits of ultrasound, prospective parents also have the thrill of actually seeing their baby months before he or she arrives. Those grainy pictures do much to make up for all the aches and pains of the first few months of pregnancy. The pictures also kick-start the parent-child bonding that, in the old days, didn't begin until well after delivery.

Amniocentesis

Amniocentesis is the granddaddy of modern prenatal testing. This procedure has been available to expectant mothers for some 30 years and has now become routine for the increasing number of pregnant women over 35, when the chance of problems with the baby goes up.

Doctors recommend amniocentesis when either parent or a previous child has a chromosome abnormality, when either parent is a carrier for certain disorders, when an earlier child was born with a neural tube defect such as spina bifida (a partially open spinal column), or when there is a family history of such chromosomal disorders as Down syndrome.

Physicians also suggest amniocentesis if the mother has a history of miscarriage. Another potential reason is the presence of too much alpha-fetoprotein in the mother's blood. This substance is produced by the baby, and an excessive amount could indicate a potentially serious problem with the pregnancy.

During the pregnancy, the baby floats in a liquid called amniotic fluid. As the baby matures, cells from his or her body are discarded into the fluid. Amniocentesis enables physicians to retrieve these cells and study the genetic information they contain. The presence—or absence—of certain chemicals in the fluid also helps doctors determine how well the baby is doing.

Amniocentesis is generally performed during the 16th or 17th week of pregnancy. The procedure can be done any time from week 14 through week 20. Before week 12, it's unlikely that the body has produced enough amniotic fluid for a good specimen. The problem with waiting until the 19th or 20th week is that the mother will be in her

AMNIOCENTESIS: WEIGHING THE RISKS

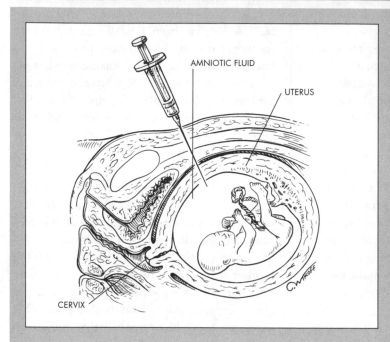

AMNIOTIC FLUID

UTERUS

CERVIX

If there's a danger that the baby will be born with a congenital defect, your doctor will probably recommend amniocentesis to rule the problem out. This test requires a sample of the baby's cells, which are always present in the surrounding amniotic fluid. Collecting the sample is not without risk, since the doctor must insert a needle directly into the uterus. However, the odds of a mishap are extremely low. When done in the 16th week of pregnancy, only 1 in 200 procedures results in loss of the baby.

fifth month by the time the test results are available, and the longer you wait, the more difficult it is to perform a therapeutic abortion should the couple decide to terminate the pregnancy. Amniocentesis is sometimes done toward the end of the pregnancy to see whether the baby's lungs are mature enough to allow him or her to breathe independently in case of premature labor or the need for an early delivery due to a medical problem.

During amniocentesis, you recline on a table and are hooked up to an ultrasound machine. First the position of the baby and placenta are located by ultrasound. The doctor will then swab your abdomen with an antiseptic and insert a long thin needle into your uterus. There is a burning or stinging sensation and a feeling of pressure as the physician maneuvers the needle to obtain a

small amount of amniotic fluid. (Some physicians give their patients a local anesthetic; others do not, since the anesthetic needle causes about the same amount of discomfort as the other one.)

Ultrasound is a very important part of the amniocentesis procedure. It helps the doctor locate the placenta and keep the needle far away from the baby when taking the specimen, thus avoiding potential complications.

There is a slight risk that amniocentesis will trigger premature labor or that the mother could develop an infection. In rare cases, there may be a little bit of vaginal bleeding or some loss of amniotic fluid. Most women, however, merely have some mild cramping—if anything—and are able to resume their normal routine soon after the procedure.

The amniotic fluid specimen is sent to a special laboratory that performs genetic studies. The fluid is cultured in a laboratory dish, and the cells are allowed to grow. The cells are then examined for any chromosomal abnormalities.

Test results are generally available within 1 to 2 weeks. Most prospective parents learn that all is well and are then able to enjoy the final months of the pregnancy. When the studies indicate a possible problem with the baby, the couple still has enough time to carefully consider the difficult choice that confronts them.

Although amniocentesis cannot diagnose such sex-linked disorders as hemophilia or muscular dystrophy—which occur only in males—the test can determine the sex of the baby. If the baby is a girl, the parents need not worry. If the baby is a boy, there is a 50-50 chance that the child will be affected if the mother carries the gene for the disease.

Chorionic Villus Sampling

The chorionic villi are slender projections attached to the chorion, a membrane which eventually becomes the part of the placenta closest to the baby. Since this membrane begins to develop as the result of fertilization, the material contained within the chorion—and the chorionic villi—accurately reflects the baby's genetic recipe. Physicians can test a sample of this material for a wide range of congenital conditions.

Chorionic villi sampling offers a big advantage over amniocentesis because it can be done as early as the eighth week of the pregnancy. Test results are generally completed within two weeks. Therefore, the preg-

nancy can be terminated if necessary, early in the second trimester—or even within the first trimester—when a therapeutic abortion is most safely performed. The relatively early diagnosis also allows couples to make this difficult decision in private, before the pregnancy is apparent to family and friends.

The procedure is currently performed in a hospital, generally between weeks 9 and 12 of the pregnancy. The sample is obtained by snipping or suctioning the tiny, finger-like villi.

As with amniocentesis, ultrasound monitoring establishes the whereabouts of the fetus and the placenta. The area of entry is swabbed with an antiseptic agent to prevent infection. The physician then inserts a needle either through the vagina and the cervix, or through a small incision in the abdomen. The needle is maneuvered into place following the map provided by the ultrasound. The doctor will pump the needle several times to obtain a sufficient sampling of chorionic villi.

Results for tests that do not require the cells to be grown in a culture are usually ready in a day or two. Tests that do require a cell culture may take up to two weeks to complete.

Many women experience emotional and physical fatigue following this procedure. There also may be some bleeding. The bleeding is not a cause for concern unless it lasts longer than two days. The risk of miscarriage is about the same as that associated with amniocentesis. However, many couples having this test believe that the benefit of a much earlier diagnosis far outweighs the still-slight risk of a miscarriage. (There is still some debate over the possibility that this test may sometimes cause deformities.)

FOR EARLIER TEST RESULTS: CHORIONIC VILLUS SAMPLING

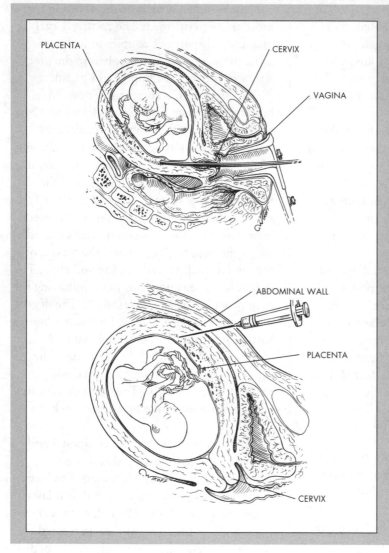

This relatively new test allows your doctor to detect a congenital defect in the baby as early as 8 weeks into the pregnancy. The genetic content of the chorion, a membrane in the placenta, parallels that of the baby itself. To obtain as sample, some of the tiny villi that line the chorion are sucked out through a narrow tube advanced into the uterus through the cervix and vagina, or directly into a needle inserted through the abdomen. Risks involved in this procedure are comparable to those of amniocentesis: in approximately 1 in 200 cases, the baby is lost.

Alpha-Fetoprotein

Alpha-fetoprotein (AFP) is a type of protein produced only by a fetus or the fetal yolk sac. The mother-to-be does not produce this substance on her own. Screening for AFP involves analyzing the level of the protein in the mother's blood. The test is generally performed between the 16th and 18th weeks of pregnancy.

An excessive amount of AFP in your blood could indicate that the baby has a neural tube defect such as the spinal deformity known as spina bifida. There could also be a high AFP reading if more than one fetus is producing the alpha-fetoprotein. An elevated level may also indicate that the pregnancy is more advanced than the initial estimate. An abnormally low amount of AFP may point to the possibility of Down syndrome or another chromosomal problem.

It is important to remember that this is only a screening test. It is not a diagnostic procedure. AFP testing will not tell you for sure that something is wrong, but rather that the matter should be pursued further. For example, if a second AFP test also showed low AFP levels, you would be advised to have amniocentesis to rule out the possibility of Down syndrome.

The AFP test itself is safe. However, if the test falsely indicates that there may be a problem when everything is really fine, mother and baby could then be exposed to the unnecessary risk of a more invasive procedure.

The statistics associated with this screening test are overwhelmingly on the side of a normal baby. Before subjecting that baby to any unnecessary risk, it's essential to obtain a second test—and perhaps a second opinion—from physicians experienced in genetic testing. There are still other studies to expect late in the pregnancy. Your doctor may ask you to lie quietly for an hour and count the number of times your baby moves to make sure the child is active enough. A sluggish baby may already be a baby in trouble. If there is concern about the baby's heart rate, you will be hooked up to a special fetal monitor that traces each heartbeat.

If there is any reason to believe that the baby is at risk during the last month of the pregnancy—or if the baby is overdue—you will have what is called a "non-stress" test. Your doctor will have you lie on a table while a fetal monitor records the baby's heartbeat in relation to its activity. This record allows physicians to see exactly how well the baby is doing.

If a baby's performance is worrisome, the doctor may order a stress test. In this procedure, you are given a small amount of oxytocin, the drug used to induce labor when the contractions don't start on their own. The doctor will then use ultrasound to see how well the baby will be able to handle the demands of labor and delivery. The major drawback is that the oxytocin could start actual labor. That's why such testing is performed in a hospital near the labor and delivery suites.

Many other prenatal tests are currently being studied and will no doubt be commonplace someday. Indeed, it really hasn't been that long since AFP screens and chorionic villi sampling were brand new procedures. As each new test becomes available, your odds of having a healthy baby should continue to improve. □

　　　　　　　　　　　　　　　　　　　TOWARD SUCCESSFUL PREGNANCIES

Potential Complications You Should Keep in Mind

Every woman who is about to have a baby hopes the entire 9 months will be healthy and trouble–free. For 10 to 20 percent of pregnancies, however—about 875,000 a year in the United States alone—one or more conditions arise to complicate matters. Obtaining good medical care, preferably starting before the pregnancy even begins, is the best way to ensure a safe journey through pregnancy. After identifying any potentially dangerous conditions, the doctor will take every step possible to protect both mother and baby.

What constitutes a "complication"? Simply put, it's any condition that might endanger the health and safety of mother, baby, or both. Being considered at "high risk" merely alerts you (and your doctor) to watch carefully for danger signs and do all you can to prevent trouble. Pregnancy, labor, and delivery can still proceed normally, and the baby is likely to be just fine.

Why is the outlook so much better now than it once was? First, doctors know what to look for. Second, many tests are available to assess suspected problems. (See chapter 24,

"Prenatal Tests to Consider.") Third, if the mother–to–be follows her doctor's instructions, many of the complications of pregnancy will not affect the baby and will disappear after delivery.

Physicians and midwives have been trained to recognize danger signs early in pregnancy. They can even take some preventive measures beforehand. Since overweight causes difficulties in pregnancy, for example, doctors often advise heavy women to shed pounds before they conceive. Women suspected of carrying the gene for a hereditary disease may choose to undergo genetic testing and counseling while they are still considering pregnancy.

Your obstetrician can also tap the expertise of a specialist, such as a perinatologist, who routinely handles medical problems during late pregnancy and immediately after birth. A neonatologist, a pediatrician who works exclusively with newborns, can be called in to advise about problems that occur (or are expected to occur) shortly after delivery. Women who develop gestational diabetes, a blood sugar condition that begins during pregnancy, may need to see both a diabetologist and an obstetrician regularly throughout pregnancy.

If you are told that your pregnancy is "complicated" or "high risk," don't panic. Keep in mind that even an "uncomplicated" pregnancy isn't necessarily problem–free. In fact, most so–called normal pregnancies involve physical discomfort. Your body undergoes many changes to create a small but cozy space in which the baby can flourish until it's out on its own.

When you (and your partner) first learn that pregnancy is going to be "complicated," you'll naturally feel frightened and depressed. The best way to allay those feelings is to learn as much as you can about your particular problem.

Ask your doctor for pamphlets or a list of suggested books. Call a professional association or self–help group such as those listed at the end of this book. Ask your hospital's medical librarian for recent articles on the subject. Perhaps your doctor or a nurse in the obstetrics department of your hospital can put you in touch with a woman who has gone through the same difficulties.

Think through your pregnancy realistically. When choosing an obstetrician, remember that the distance from your home to the doctor's office and the hospital could become important in case of an emergency. Since you'll rely on your doctor for continued reassurance, education, and support, make sure you're on the same wavelength. If he or she recommends bed rest for days, weeks, or even months, don't hesitate to look for assistance with your everyday responsibilities. One not–for–profit organization that specializes in advising women who need extended bed rest

is Sidelines. (See "Directory of Support Groups" at the end of this book.)

Be alert for any condition that might cause the baby to be born early. Prematurity is the cause of 85 percent of neonatal injury and death in the United States. That helps explain why your doctor wants your pregnancy to last as close to the full 40 weeks as possible. The "magic number" is 36 weeks. At that point the baby's lungs have matured enough to allow it to breathe on its own. Babies born before 33 to 34 weeks usually must rely on a respirator or other assisted breathing for a while.

Symptoms such as bleeding are important warning signs that something may be wrong. They provide an opportunity to seek medical care and make things right. Think of your high–risk pregnancy as a *high–awareness* pregnancy.

When the Baby is Lost

Some circumstances make an end of the pregnancy inevitable. They include:

Ectopic ("Out–of–Place") Pregnancy

In this situation, the embryo becomes implanted outside its rightful place—the uterus—most often in the fallopian tubes. The usual symptoms are lower abdominal pain and bleeding. Since such an embryo could endanger your life if allowed to grow, your doctor must remove it surgically as soon as possible after diagnosis. You are more likely to have an ectopic pregnancy if you have had a pelvic inflammatory disease or other sexually transmitted disease, have had an ectopic pregnancy previously, or have undergone previous tubal surgery. You are also at greater risk if your mother took the anti–miscarriage drug DES.

Miscarriage

At least 10 to 30 percent of pregnancies end in miscarriage (loss of the fetus before the 20th week of gestation). It usually happens even sooner—by the tenth week—when you may not even realize you're pregnant. In most miscarriages (85 percent), a genetic disorder in the egg has made it impossible for the fetus to develop normally. Other causes include congenital abnormalities; infection; and exposure to drugs or chemicals. Because any woman who has had 3 or more miscarriages in a row is said to be prone to "recurrent miscarriage," all her subsequent pregnancies are classified as high risk and must be monitored closely.

Risk factors for a miscarriage include early or late pregnancy (age under 18 or over 35); endometriosis; placental abruption (see below); uterine infection from a sexually transmitted disease or another cause; fibroid tumors or uterine scar tissue; malnutrition; exposure of either parent to radiation or toxic chemicals; smoking; excessive alcohol intake; previous miscarriages; and hormone problems. For more information see chapter 27, "What To Do When Miscarriage Strikes."

Extreme Prematurity

This is usually defined as birth at less than 24 weeks. High–tech neonatal intensive–care units are saving increasingly smaller infants, but they can't save the tiniest ones.

Molar Pregnancy

In this rare condition, clinically called a hydatidiform mole, the fertilized egg degenerates and the placenta deteriorates into a mass of tissue that a doctor must remove by surgery, vacuum extraction, or other means. Risk factors include a maternal age of less than 20 or more than 40, chromosomal abnormalities, hormone imbalance, and possibly nutritional deficiencies. A woman who thinks her pregnancy is progressing normally may realize she has a problem because of nausea or bleeding. The doctor may notice that her uterus seems too large for the length of her pregnancy; that she has high blood pressure, fluid buildup, and too much protein in her urine—all signs of a dangerous condition called preeclampsia; and that there are no fetal heart sounds. Molar pregnancy is usually diagnosed in the second, third, or fourth month, usually by ultrasound.

Troublemakers Part I: Maternal Health Problems

Any woman who has had problems with a previous pregnancy, whether it resulted in a healthy child or not, is considered at risk in subsequent pregnancies. If a close blood relation, especially her mother, had a problem pregnancy, the doctor may judge that a risk factor as well, though it is highly unlikely that exactly the same problem would occur.

Even if you've had no previous problems, there are numerous medical conditions you might have that could affect the unborn baby.

Common diseases, infections, chemical imbalances, and other health factors pose special dangers for the fetus unless they are carefully controlled. That's why you need close medical attention throughout your pregnancy.

Diabetes Mellitus

This condition, in which your body lacks sufficient insulin to process the sugars it relies on, can cause numerous complications. Without adequate medical treatment, it poses an increased risk of birth defects, very large babies (more than 9 or 10 pounds at birth), too much amniotic fluid (hydramnios), pregnancy-induced high blood pressure (preeclampsia), respiratory distress syndrome in the baby, miscarriage, premature birth, and stillbirth. About 1 to 2 percent of pregnant women have diabetes mellitus before becoming pregnant; some develop it during pregnancy (gestational diabetes). Routine testing of all pregnant women is usually done at 24 to 28 weeks of gestation.

Part of the usual treatment for diabetes, whether chronic or gestational, is a diet carefully regulated to remain low in sugar. Many women learn how to monitor their own blood sugar levels at home every day with a blood glucose meter or strips (available at many pharmacies and home health supply stores). One small drop of blood is enough for such tests. If necessary, a woman can control her blood sugar level with diet (frequent small meals), exercise, and self–injected insulin. She can also perform simple urine tests with dipsticks (specially treated paper strips) at home. Other tests sometimes given to women with chronic or gestational diabetes to assess the health of the baby include fetal nonstress tests and alpha–fetoprotein tests (see chapter 24, "Prenatal Tests to Consider").

If you have diabetes mellitus, you may need brief hospitalization to stabilize blood glucose levels, especially immediately after the condition has been diagnosed. The doctor may decide to perform a cesarean section or induce labor before 40 weeks of gestation if your condition or the baby's condition warrants that step. You can take insulin safely during pregnancy, although you should not use the oral diabetes medications tolbutamide (Orinase) and chlorpropamide (Diabinese), which increase the risk of fetal defects.

High Blood Pressure

High blood pressure during pregnancy is a leading cause of fetal loss in midterm and late pregnancy. If untreated, high blood pressure can cause the baby to grow inadequately, to be born prematurely, and to undergo fetal distress during labor. It also can seriously threaten the mother's health.

About 7 percent of pregnant women have high blood pressure. Your chances of developing it are greatest during your first pregnancy,

COMMON SOURCES OF DISCOMFORT IN AN "UNCOMPLICATED" PREGNANCY

- Digestive problems, such as heartburn
- Dizziness
- Emotional upset
- Excessive body warmth
- Fatigue
- Gas, constipation
- General aches
- Headaches
- Hemorrhoids
- Increased or decreased desire for sex
- Increased urination
- Nausea and vomiting
- Pelvic pressure
- Sleeping problems
- Sore nipples and breasts
- Stuffy nose
- Swollen ankles and feet
- Swollen or bleeding gums
- Varicose veins
- Especially in late pregnancy:
    Back pain
    Leg cramps
    Shortness of breath
    Unsteady balance

especially if you're a teenager or over 30, are overweight, or have a history of hypertension. Other risk factors include diabetes, multiple births (such as twins or triplets), too much water in the amniotic sac surrounding the fetus and lack of prenatal care.

An early tipoff to high blood pressure is any sign of fluid retention, such as a puffy face or swollen fingers, blurred vision, or severe headaches. Other symptoms are pain in the upper abdomen and a weight gain of more than 2 or 3 pounds in 1 week during the last month of pregnancy.

All pregnant women should have a routine blood pressure reading at each visit to the doctor. If you seem to be developing problems your doctor may ask you to return to the office for more frequent readings or may teach you to take your blood pressure at home. Treatment may include blood pressure medications, such as methyldopa (Aldomet) and hydralazine (Apresoline); but you should not take Reserpine (Diupres, Hydropres, others) and propranolol (Inderal, Inderide) during pregnancy, unless absolutely necessary. Lying in bed, especially on your left side, promotes blood supply to the kidneys and uterus. Doctors recommend a high–protein, low–salt diet and forbid all smoking.

If you already have high blood pressure, it raises your chances of developing the condition known as preeclampsia. In addition to hypertension, the symptoms of this serious condition include water retention and protein in the urine, indicating a kidney problem. As a result, the baby may be premature, underweight, and weak due to poor nutrition and a shortage of oxygen. The doctor may prescribe dietary changes and bed rest, as well as medications such as magnesium sulfate and phenotoin (Dilantin) to prevent possible seizures. Delivery may be scheduled as soon as it's safe for the baby.

Untreated preeclampsia is a life–threatening condition that can damage the mother's kidneys, liver, eyes, and brain and may lead to coma or convulsions (eclampsia). Between 3 and 5 percent of pregnant women with eclampsia die; 20 percent of their babies suffer the same fate. Fortunately, women who receive close medical attention throughout their pregnancies rarely develop the problem. Typically, eclampsia is discovered when a woman who has had uncontrolled high blood pressure throughout pregnancy arrives at the emergency room to give birth without the benefit of any prenatal care.

Kidney Disease

Diseases of the kidney—relatively rare in pregnancy—may be caused by lupus, diabetes, or an untreated bladder infection. The mother may develop high blood pressure, and other dangerous conditions, and the baby may be born prematurely. Fever, flank pain, or blood in the urine—the chief symptoms of kidney infection—require immediate medical care.

Heart Disease

Extra weight and water retention—common during pregnancy—make the heart pump harder. A pregnant woman with heart disease should call the doctor immediately if she experiences any dizziness, discomfort, or pain. She should be sure to include adequate iron and folic acid in her diet and restrict her salt intake. The obstetrician will exercise special caution when prescribing medications and may ask a heart specialist (cardiologist) to help oversee the pregnancy.

Sickle–Cell Anemia

Advances in the treatment of this disease, which almost exclusively attacks blacks, has greatly improved the chances of a successful pregnancy. Pregnant women may need blood transfusions every 1 to 3 weeks, starting in the first trimester. Urinary tract infections are twice as common in women with the sickle–cell gene, and these infections must receive prompt treatment.

Lupus

Systemic lupus erythematosus (SLE) is called an autoimmune disorder because the body attacks its own connective tissue. The rate of miscarriage and fetal loss in women with SLE is much higher than average. Flareups are common both during pregnancy and after childbirth, although remission is possible. Sometimes diagnosis only comes after repeated miscarriages.

Thyroid Imbalance

About 1 in 200 pregnant women have hyper-thyroidism; their thyroid glands produce too much hormone. Those with too little hormone (hypothyroidism) are sometimes infertile; but when pregnancy occurs, they can receive medical treatment to help prevent miscarriage and any problems with the baby. Children born to women with thyroid imbal-ance typically have low birth weight.

PKU

Phenylketonuria is a congenital condition that can lead to mental retardation and seizures when left untreated. If a mother–to–be has this condition it can leave the baby with birth defects—small brain, mental retardation, and heart problems—or miscarriage. Any woman who was born in a U.S. hospital since the 1960s should have had a PKU test at birth. To reduce the danger to a developing baby,

who may inherit the disorder in any case, doctors prescribe a low–phenylalanine diet prior to conception. Among other things, the mother should be especially careful to avoid aspartame (Nutrasweet), which releases phenylalanine after being digested.

Epilepsy and Other Seizure Disorders

Pregnancy changes the metabolism and balance of hormones in the body, altering the response to medication and increasing the probability of seizures in women with epilepsy. According to the Epilepsy Foundation of America, women taking epilepsy medications also have a 2 to 3 times greater risk of bearing a child with a birth defect. If the doctor thinks it's advisable, a woman who has had no seizures for a long time and wants to become pregnant can stop taking her medication briefly to see what happens. Sometimes however, there is no choice but to continue the drugs, whether she's pregnant or not. In any event, genetic counsel-ing and prenatal testing are advisable. Close monitoring throughout the pregnancy is vital.

Age

Age is considered a risk factor because many problems are more likely to occur before age 20 or after age 35. For example, the chance that the baby will have Down syndrome is 9 times greater at 40 than at 30—although even at the increased rate, it's still less than 1 percent. At age 45, however, the incidence of Down syndrome increases to 3 percent. Diabetes and high blood pressure strike 1.3 percent of pregnant women under 35 but 6 percent of those over 35. Labor tends to last longer after age 35, and the chances of having twins or triplets increases. First births between ages 30 and 39 have doubled in the past 15 years, and those in women over age 40 have increased by 50 percent; so more and more pregnant women find themselves in the high risk category.

Viral Infections

Infections caused by viruses are hard to treat and threaten potentially serious problems to the baby.

Rubella (German measles). A fairly innocuous illness in itself, rubella during pregnancy can cause serious harm to a developing baby. If rubella occurs during the first 8 to 12 weeks of pregnancy, there's a 50 to 80 percent chance that the baby will have such serious birth defects as mental retardation, blindness, hearing loss, and heart disease. Miscarriage or stillbirth are other possibilities. Almost a third of those babies whose mothers had rubella during pregnancy die within 4 months after birth. Termination of the pregnancy is often considered by expectant mothers who develop rubella. Vaccinations prompted by widespread awareness of this serious danger have dramatically lowered the number of babies affected by the disease while still in the uterus.

If you have a rash, low fever, swollen glands, and symptoms of the common cold, you could be suffering from rubella. A blood test will tell you whether you have had the disease—and whether the infection was recent. Immune globulin will lessen the effects of the virus if you decide to continue the pregnancy. Any woman who has never had rubella or been immunized against it—a group that includes about 10 to 15 percent of women of childbearing age in the United States—should receive the vaccine at least a few months before she tries to become pregnant.

Chickenpox. Chickenpox may play a role in preterm labor and birth defects. If you are pregnant and have never had chicken pox, you should get an injection of chickenpox immune globulin. If you contract the disease during late pregnancy and have it during labor, when it can be fatal to your baby, the doctor can give an injection of the globulin to the fetus through the placenta.

WHEN TO CALL THE DOCTOR

If the typical discomforts of pregnancy progress to severe and troubling symptoms such as those listed below, it's a sign that something could well be wrong. Don't hesitate to call your doctor is you have any of these signs.

Blurred vision
Chills; fever greater than 100° Fahrenheit
Clots or pieces of tissue in your vaginal discharge
Cramping or abdominal pain
Extreme nausea and vomiting
Fainting
Frequent or severe headaches
Leakage or flow of clear liquid from your vagina
Pain in your side or back
Pain or burning when you urinate
Spotting or bleeding
Swollen face or fingers
Unusual thirst

In late pregnancy:
Frequent regular contractions before 36 weeks
No movement of the fetus for 8 to 10 hours

Mother's Use of DES

From about 1941 to 1971, many women with a history of miscarriage, premature delivery, moderate bleeding during pregnancy, or diabetes took a drug called diethlystilbestrol (DES). Years later, evidence showed that these women had increased their own risk for breast cancer and their daughters' risk for miscarriage, ectopic pregnancy, and premature delivery—among other problems. If your mother took DES when she was pregnant with you—and you should check all available medical records if you're not sure—be sure to discuss the situation with your gynecologist, preferably before becoming pregnant.

Sexually Transmitted Diseases

If you develop a sexually transmitted disease (STD) during pregnancy, you must get treatment immediately. Should you notice even the slightest evidence of an STD *before* conception, see your doctor right away, to prevent any risk to a future baby.

Syphilis. An untreated mother can pass syphilis on to a developing baby for up to 4 years after she contracted it. The baby may develop serious deformities and irreversible brain damage, and may even die from the disease. Fortunately syphilis responds well to penicillin and other antibiotics.

Chlamydia. Vaginal infection, pain during intercourse, and a general run–down feeling suggest infection with chlamydia. When present during pregnancy, chlamydia makes premature birth, miscarriage, or stillbirth 10 times more likely to occur. A baby delivered vaginally may contract the virus and develop eye disease (conjunctivitis) a few days later; doctors successfully treat this infection with antibiotic eye ointment. Erythromycin is the safest antibiotic treatment for chlamydia during pregnancy.

Gonorrhea. A woman with gonorrhea during pregnancy may go into labor before her due date; her baby may not grow properly and may develop conjunctivitis 2 to 7 days after birth. Penicillin or antibiotics will help prevent these problems.

Cytomegalovirus (CMV). In the United States, CMV is the most common viral infection of the uterus. Symptoms are similar to those of mononucleosis: sluggishness and general exhaustion. If contracted early in pregnancy, CMV can cause bleeding and liver disease in the mother, and may be a reason to opt for termination of the pregnancy. Symptoms of the virus in the baby may not appear immediately. A child with CMV might have hearing difficulties, learning disabilities, and a tendency to contract infections during the first 2 years of life.

Genital herpes. Babies born to mothers with active herpes lesions around the vagina can contract the disease directly from the sores. If laboratory tests confirm the infection, the mother can use acyclovir (Zovirax) to reduce the chance of fetal infection. Infection with herpes during pregnancy increases the risk of miscarriage and premature delivery. A child born to an infected mother may grow slowly or may even die. Doctors sometimes recommend cesarean section to keep the baby away from the sores. While there is no known cure for herpes, it can disappear for long periods of time. If you know you have had herpes, or think you might have, be sure to tell your doctor so that he or she can test you, especially toward the end of your pregnancy.

HIV infection and AIDS. Babies of women who are positive for human immunodeficiency virus (HIV), which causes AIDS, have a 25 to 30 percent chance of acquiring the infection during pregnancy. Extreme illness and early death are usually inevitable, although azidothymidine (AZT) has recently shown promise for protecting newborns against their mothers' HIV infection.

Nonviral Infections

Bacterial infections are easier to treat than viral infections.

Urinary tract infections. Two to 10 percent of pregnant women have urinary tract infections (UTIs). Most don't even realize it until the laboratory report comes in. One reason doctors routinely ask pregnant patients for urine specimens starting with the first appointment is their interest in treating a UTI as soon as possible.

Bladder infections (cystitis), the most common type of UTI, occur in a great many women (and in some men and children, too). The likelihood of developing cystitis increases during pregnancy and is especially strong in women who have had UTIs before. Changes in the immune system during pregnancy may be one reason for this increased risk. Also, the growing baby can cause the uterus to press against the bladder, preventing it from emptying completely and creating a breeding ground for bacteria (see chapter 10, "Putting an End to Urinary Tract Infections" for more information).

Infection can spread from the bladder up through the ureters to the kidney. Dangerous and painful in themselves, kidney infections can lead to premature birth. Doctors treat pregnant women with penicillin—usually ampicillin or amoxicillin—and the cephalosporins. Although the baby can't "catch" a UTI from its mother, a tendency for such infections may be hereditary.

Toxoplasmosis. Babies who contract this parasitic disease between conception and the twenty–fourth week tend to be born small and run the risk of developing liver disease, convulsions, blindness, brain abnormalities, and mental retardation. Since toxoplasmosis organisms live in raw or incompletely cooked meat and are carried in cat feces, pregnant women should eat only well–done meat and should avoid changing cat litter.

Hepatitis (inflammation of the liver). The risk to the baby is serious when the mother has chronic hepatitis B or C. Hepatitis A, which also requires treatment, has fewer dangerous side effects during pregnancy. To prevent neonatal hepatitis the doctor will give the baby hepatitis B immune globulin and vaccine immediately after birth. All male and female healthcare workers should get a vaccination before starting a child. The mother is also tested for hepatitis B during her pregnancy.

Troublemakers Part 2: Conditions That Result from Pregnancy

Gestational diabetes

About 5 percent of pregnant women develop diabetes for the first time during pregnancy. Gestational diabetes poses the same risks to the baby as chronic diabetes, but usually disappears after the baby is born. The mother's risk of having diabetes in a future pregnancy or later in life, however, may go up.

You're more likely to get gestational diabetes if you had the condition before; if an earlier pregnancy ended in stillbirth; if a family member has diabetes; if you suffer from recurrent vaginal or urinary tract infections; or if you're overweight or over 25 years of age. When risk factors are present, your doctor will give you oral glucose tolerance tests earlier than the usual 24 to 28 weeks of gestation.

Chronic vomiting

Nausea and vomiting, especially during the first 3 months, are probably the most universally known signs of pregnancy. In some cases, the vomiting is frequent enough to produce weakness, dehydration, and eventual damage to the kidneys and liver. Stress and fear worsen the situation. If vomiting is serious, a woman may need hospitalization so that she can receive nutrients intravenously.

How much vomiting is too much? If you throw up more than 3 or 4 times a day, are unable to hold any food down, lose weight, faint, run a fever, or urinate less than usual, call your doctor immediately. Since vomiting can destroy tooth enamel, it's important to keep your teeth and gums very clean and see a dentist for frequent cleaning.

Bleeding

Although between 25 and 50 percent of pregnant women experience some spotting, especially at the beginning, any bleeding during pregnancy is cause for concern. The doctor may tell you to go to bed and stay there until 48 hours after the bleeding has stopped. Very heavy bleeding (hemorrhaging) requires an emergency trip to the hospital. During the second and third trimesters, any bleeding is usually caused by the placenta (see the following pages). If you experience vaginal bleeding, call your doctor right away. Describe the color and amount of blood, any associated symptoms, the type of pain (if any), and what you were doing when you started to bleed.

Excess—or Too Little—Amniotic Fluid

When there is too much fluid in the amniotic sac that surrounds the baby inside the uterus, the mother has hydramnios. The condition can develop suddenly or gradually. The extra fluid can prevent normal chest expansion, thus causing shortness of breath. Premature labor and delivery may result as well. The doctor may perform amniocentesis (withdrawing amniotic fluid with a long needle) one or more times to remove some of the excess fluid. Hospitalization may be necessary.

Oligohydramnios, an equally serious situation, occurs when there is too little amniotic fluid. To prevent compression of the umbilical cord and other problems, the doctor may deliver the baby early.

Intrauterine Growth Retardation (IUGR)

When a newborn measures less than 18 inches or weighs less than 5 pounds, it has IUGR. Small babies are weaker than larger ones and require more medical help. If your baby doesn't seem to be growing enough, the physician may prescribe bed rest to increase its oxygen supply and nutrition. Remember, though, that smaller mothers tend to have smaller babies.

Premature Rupture of Membranes (PROM)

Many conditions of pregnancy can cause the membranes to break too early, sometimes necessitating a quick trip to the hospital, followed by delivery. (For more information, see chapter 26, "What to Expect during Labor and Delivery.")

Rh Incompatibility

If the father's and the baby's blood contains a component called Rh factor, but the mother's does not, the baby can develop Rh disease. (In the United States, only 15 percent of whites and 5 percent of blacks are Rh negative.) Problems occur, usually in a second pregnancy or later, if a few cells of fetal blood leak into the mother's, typically at the time of delivery. The mother's Rh–negative system treats these cells as foreign objects, producing antibodies against them. If the baby is still in the uterus—and in future pregnancies—antibodies can enter and destroy some of the baby's red blood cells, leading to anemia, heart failure, and death.

The doctor may decide to deliver early if amniocentesis—evaluation of a sample of the amniotic fluid—reveals too much bilirubin, an orange–yellow pigment formed when blood cells break down. A substantial amount of bilirubin suggests that Rh antibodies from the mother have destroyed the fetal cells, and that there is an Rh incompatibility problem.

A drug called $RH_O(D)$ immune globulin (Gamulin Rh, RhoGAM, others) prevents Rh antibodies from forming. It is given to Rh–negative women within 72 hours of delivering an Rh–positive baby (or having a miscarriage, abortion or amniocentesis), to protect future pregnancies from Rh incompatibility. Some doctors also inject $RH_O(D)$ immune globulin at 28 to 32 weeks of gestation. The fetus or newborn can also receive blood transfusions directly, if necessary.

Placenta Previa

In about 1 out of 200 pregnancies, the placenta develops abnormally low in the uterus. Because the walls of the lower third of the uterus are thinner than those of the upper uterus, the mother's blood supply is smaller

PLACENTA PREVIA ("PLACENTA FIRST")

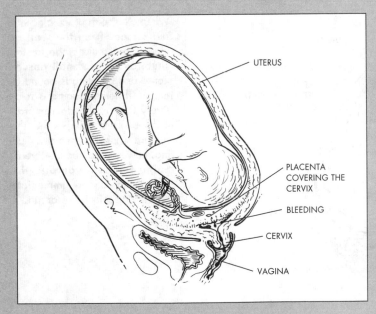

UTERUS

PLACENTA COVERING THE CERVIX

BLEEDING

CERVIX

VAGINA

When the placenta blocks normal access to the birth canal at the end of a pregnancy, cesarean delivery is usually a must. However, placenta previa discovered early in the pregnancy (during the first 20 weeks) usually corrects itself. If your doctor discovers this problem, the most likely prescription will be bed rest.

there. If this situation develops you may notice spotting during the last trimester, usually after 30 weeks. In addition, the lower uterine walls may cover some or all of the cervix. Since this location would make a vaginal birth difficult or impossible, and the fetus needs a healthy blood supply, the doctor usually orders bed rest to prevent excessive bleeding. If the condition is discovered during the first 20 weeks, the placenta may migrate out of the way. Sexual intercourse is inadvisable. Ninety percent of the time, in early cases, the situation corrects itself; and the vast majority of women who develop this condition deliver perfectly normal babies with few complications.

Placenta previa can be total, partial, or marginal. Risk factors include previous placenta previa, a previous cesarean section, scar tissue in the uterus, 5 or more pregnancies, and being more than 35 years old. Possible causes range from unusual fetal position or a multiple pregnancy to previous uterine surgery, advanced age, or congenital abnormalities.

The mother may suspect something is wrong when she experiences severe bleeding, which can lead to anemia and low blood volume. Or she may see a discharge of bright–red blood but have no pain or cramping. Even if placenta previa occurs without symptoms, the doctor may find it on a routine ultrasound scan or one performed for other reasons.

After delivery of the baby in placenta previa, the uterus may be unable to contract tightly enough to shut off the blood vessels shorn away when the placenta detached from the uterine wall. To prevent hemorrhage and the possibility of subsequent shock, the mother may need intravenous fluids and blood infusions as well as medication that will encourage the uterus to contract. Even if

IF THE PLACENTA TEARS AWAY

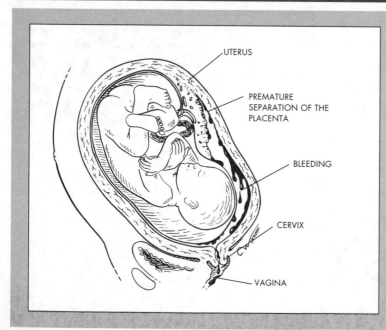

UTERUS

PREMATURE SEPARATION OF THE PLACENTA

BLEEDING

CERVIX

VAGINA

When all or part of the placenta tears loose from the wall of uterus, the medical term for the situation is "placental abruption" and bleeding is bound to occur. If hemorrhaging is relatively minor, the doctor may order bed rest in hopes that the rupture will heal. Heavy bleeding, however, can be life-threatening for both you and the baby, and calls for immediate delivery, usually by cesarean.

she does not hemorrhage, she may have to take oral or intravenous antibiotics after delivery of a placenta previa to prevent uterine infection.

Placental Abruption

In this rare emergency, the placenta shears partly or entirely loose from the uterus before delivery. About half the time, this occurs after the 36th week, when immediate cesarean section is safe. Symptoms include vaginal bleeding after the 20th week, nausea and vomiting, and severe abdominal pain. Abruption occurs more often in women who have had many previous pregnancies, particularly those with high blood pressure and preeclampsia.

Multiple Births

Twins, triplets, and more are considered a "complication" of pregnancy because multiple fetuses have greater nutritional needs than a single baby and place additional strain on the mother's body. Sleeping, eating, and remaining physically comfortable may pose challenges sooner than in a one-baby pregnancy. The risks of high blood pressure, hydramnios, and postpartum hemorrhage are also higher. About half of multiple births are premature.

Doctors often advise bed rest or a drastic reduction of activity and stress, sometimes for most of the pregnancy. Cesarean section is usually recommended for triplets and quadruplets. Preeclampsia is 3 to 5 times more common with twins than with solo babies; it occurs in 20 to 30 percent of all twin pregnancies. If you are having more than one baby, contact one of the advocacy groups for parents of "multiples," such as the International Twins Association in Denver and the Triplet Connection in Stockton, California.

Postmaturity

About 10 percent of pregnancies extend beyond their projected due dates. Any pregnancy that's still going strong 2 or more weeks after that date is considered "postmature," especially if the mother's or baby's health seems in jeopardy. After 40 weeks' gestation, the amount of oxygen and nutrients reaching the baby begins to decline. Furthermore, if a baby grows too large, there's less chance of a normal vaginal birth. An overterm baby is also more likely to undergo fetal distress during labor, especially if the mother is 35 or older and this is her first child.

Many doctors prefer to induce labor 2 weeks beyond the due date; others wait. Ultrasound scans and electronic fetal monitoring help determine whether the fetus is healthy and can wait for delivery. The tests may be done biweekly.

Tests and Procedures

If you have a complicated pregnancy, your doctor is likely to recommend quite a few of the tests and procedures described in chapter 24, "Prenatal Tests to Consider." Amniocentesis is often performed at 34 to 39 weeks to evaluate fetal maturity (and the feasibility of early delivery) in cases of high blood pressure, Rh incompatibility, diabetes, and postmaturity.

Other tests commonly given to women with high risk pregnancies are biophysical profiles (to evaluate fetal heart rate and activity) and sonography (ultrasound). Women with diabetes are taught to test themselves. Home uterine monitoring for conditions such as high blood pressure and premature labor allows many women to remain safely at home despite difficulties during pregnancy.

Medications During Pregnancy

The U.S. Food and Drug Administration has categorized all federally approved medications according to their known or suspected safety—or lack of safety—during pregnancy. We still don't know much about the effects of many drugs on the pregnant woman and her baby, partly because doctors have been extremely reluctant to prescribe almost any medication since the thalidomide scare of the 1960s and the DES discoveries of the 1980s. Your doctor will insist on overseeing any and all drugs you take during pregnancy—including aspirin, which may seem harmless, but can, in fact, affect the baby.

Antibiotics

Some infections, such as sexually transmitted diseases and urinary tract infections, are serious enough to require medication during pregnancy, despite the potential risks. Don't take anything without your doctor's permission and supervision, and be sure to tell him or her about any illness or symptoms you may have.

Drugs to Delay Labor

These drugs are given either orally or intravenously to postpone labor that starts too soon—usually at 20 weeks or later. The goal is to keep the pregnancy on course long enough to allow the baby's lungs to mature to the point that it can breathe on its own.

Tocolytic medications, such as indomethacin (Indocin), ritrodine (Yutopar), terbutaline (Brethaire, Bricanyl), and magnesium sulfate, act in different ways but can have similar effect on labor. All of them have potential side effects, such as palpitations, nausea, and nasal congestion.

Drugs to Induce Labor

When labor has begun but then stalls, the physician may give you an injection to "jump–start" the uterine muscles. The drugs used include Pitocin and Syntocinon. Doctors sometimes prescribe Prostaglandin gel to encourage softening and thinning of the cervical opening in preparation for delivery.

Reassurance

Despite complications, most "high–risk" pregnancies end with the birth of a healthy baby. Doctors already have the means to control most threats, and they're learning more all the time.

Unfortunately, newspapers and popular magazines often report new treatments before they've really been proven. The reports are usually brief and sound conclusive. In fact, research may be flawed or need to be repeated many times before its results will be accepted by most physicians. Still, whenever you read about a condition or treatment that could affect your pregnancy, don't hesitate to discuss your concerns with your doctor. Visit often, call when you have questions, and follow his or her advice, even if it's hard. Remember, the best way to protect your baby is to take good care of yourself. □

CHAPTER 26

What to Expect During Labor and Delivery

Childbirth is one of the most memorable and rewarding events of a couple's life. No matter how often a woman gives birth, each experience is an intimate and unique celebration of life. Though labor and delivery are not without pain and some degree of anxiety, if you remain confident, well-informed and fully supported by your partner and your doctor, you're likely to have no problem handling the awesome task of bringing a child into the world

Because the unexpected can happen at any time, you may not always be able to control every aspect of your labor and delivery, but don't let this bother you. You can maintain a sense of emotional control by asking questions, challenging assumptions about routine procedures, and openly sharing your hopes and fears with your partner and your physician. Whether you deliver vaginally or by cesarean section, receive anesthesia or experience "natural" childbirth, use a hospital delivery room or birthing center, the experience is yours alone, and every decision will be made in your best interest and that of your child.

Toward the end of your pregnancy, you eagerly await the arrival of your child as the culmination of nine months of careful planning and preparation. If this is your first child, you may feel a mixture of excitement and nervousness when you think about the delivery. And to be perfectly honest, you may also feel restless and irritable as the growing baby exerts greater demands on your body.

This jumble of emotions is completely normal and natural. As your due date draws near, you'll want to know exactly when labor will start and when your baby will be born. But although the process of labor is well understood, no one knows exactly why it starts, and your doctor won't be able to predict either the start of labor or how long it will last. Your due date is a best estimate, but only about 5 percent of women who carry their babies to term actually deliver on that day. The rest deliver from several days to several weeks before or after their due dates.

Nevertheless, you may begin to notice changes in your body that are commonly recognized as signs of impending labor. During a first pregnancy, the baby may "drop," or engage in the birth canal 2 to 3 weeks before labor begins. You may suddenly feel as though you can breathe more easily, though the increased pressure on your bladder may also cause you to urinate more frequently. In subsequent pregnancies, this "lightening" may occur only a few hours before labor.

The irregular contractions you may have experienced throughout your pregnancy or the third trimester may increase in frequency and intensity. You may have a sudden burst of energy, often referred to as the "nesting instinct," and feel compelled to take on a major domestic project, such as waxing a floor, baking bread, or reorganizing a closet. Hours to days before labor, the small mucus "plug" that has sealed your cervix throughout pregnancy may begin to stretch, then break apart as the cervix shortens and thins out in a process called "effacing." Once this occurs, pink-tinged mucus, or "bloody show," may be discharged from your vagina.

When you notice these signals, you should begin to finalize plans for the care of other children, arrange your transportation to the hospital, and call your doctor for last-minute instructions. Pack a small suitcase, placing any items you will need during labor in a separate bag. Continue to practice any breathing techniques you may have learned during childbirth preparation or Lamaze classes. They can help to distract you from pain and relax you during labor. (See the box "Breathing Techniques Help Bring Relief.")

One additional sign often indicates that labor is imminent. The downward pressure of the baby's head against the amniotic sac may cause these membranes to rupture. The breaking of your "water" can occur as a trickle or a gush of odorless, colorless amniotic fluid. Alert your medical attendants as soon as this happens. Once the sac has broken, labor is imminent, often beginning spontaneously within 12 to 24 hours. In fact, in many women, the membranes don't rupture until labor is already underway.

Once your water breaks, keep your vagina clean to minimize the risk of infection. Don't take a bath, douche, or engage in sexual intercourse. Be prepared to describe when and how the membranes ruptured, and also be alert to any discoloration of the fluid—from yellow or tan to brown or green. This indicates the presence of meconium, a waste product discharged by your baby's bowels, which can be an indicator of fetal distress.

When Labor Begins

Your uterus is a powerful muscle that tightens and relaxes rhythmically during labor, allowing the cervix to stretch open and help to push your baby through the birth canal. Although every woman's labor is different, at the outset, you may begin to feel a pattern of dull cramps similar to menstrual cramps in your lower back or pelvis. If these remain regular for an hour or more, last at least 30 seconds, and gradually increase in intensity—even if you change position or move around—your labor has begun.

Your physician will probably have given you some guidelines about when to contact him or her once labor begins. If this is your first pregnancy, stay home awhile, so you can relax and remain unencumbered by the hospital routine and environment. Take a walk, catch a nap, enjoy a long shower, sip liquids (clear liquids only), read a book, or engage in any activity that will entertain and distract you and allow you to preserve your energy. Most physicians recommend that during a first labor, a woman wait until contractions are five minutes apart for an hour before coming to the hospital or birth center. In subsequent pregnancies, you may be advised to come sooner, since your labor can progress much more quickly.

You should contact your physician immediately if you notice any vaginal bleeding other than the pinkish "show," if the baby doesn't move for an unusually long time, or if you have constant, severe pain rather than intermittent contractions. These signs can indicate such potentially serious conditions as placenta previa, in which the placenta may be blocking the exit from the uterus, or placental abruption, in which the placenta begins to prematurely separate from the uterus and limit the baby's oxygen supply. If your physician suspects any complications, you'll be asked to come to the birth center as quickly as possible so your condition can be checked and your baby can be monitored throughout the remainder of your labor.

After you are admitted to the hospital, your physician, nurse or birth attendant will

LABOR FROM BEGINNING TO END

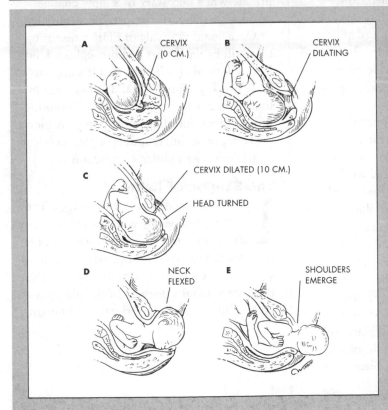

A CERVIX (0 CM.)

B CERVIX DILATING

C CERVIX DILATED (10 CM.)
HEAD TURNED

D NECK FLEXED

E SHOULDERS EMERGE

As the first contractions of labor begin, the baby's head lies waiting on the inner side of the still-closed cervix (A). During the early and active phases of the first stage of labor, the cervix begins to open (dilate), finally reaching a diameter of 8 centimeters (B). In the transition phase that follows (C), the cervix dilates an additional 2 centimeters and the baby's head advances towards the birth canal.

During the second stage of labor (D and E), the baby's head emerges from the birth canal, followed almost immediately by the rest of the body. In the third stage, which quickly follows delivery, the placenta and membranes are expelled by a few final, weak contractions. From start to finish, the process averages 12 hours for a first baby, less for later children.

want to discuss the events leading to labor. Your vital signs will be checked and recorded, and special attention will be paid to your baby's fetal heart tones and fetal heart rate (FHR), both important indicators of the baby's response to the stress of childbirth. You will be asked when you last ate and how much you consumed. Be sure to tell your physician if you want your partner or older children to be present at the delivery, or if you have made any other special arrangements.

Unless there's concern about complications such as placenta previa or the risk of infection, your doctor will perform a vaginal examination to check the baby's position, the dimensions of your pelvis, and the effacement and dilation of your cervix. A blood sample may be taken and a urine specimen may be tested for protein. You should challenge any hospital procedures that seem medically unnecessary, such as extensive shaving of your pubic area or administration of an enema. There is rarely any need for these outdated rituals, but though they have been eliminated in many birth centers, they persist in some institutions.

Depending on the status of your labor, your baby's position and heart rate, and additional factors such as a previous cesarean delivery or a post-term pregnancy, your physician may recommend electronic fetal monitoring now or at some point during your labor. Many hospitals routinely use external electronic FHR monitoring for 20 to 30 minutes after admission to establish the baby's baseline heart rate and check variations, such as beating slower during uterine contractions. If you need fetal monitoring, the doctor or birth attendant will place two belts around your abdomen to hold two small monitoring instruments in place.

Once your membranes have ruptured, the baby can be monitored internally with a small electrode threaded through your vagina. At the same time, if there's any question about the force of labor, your doctor may place a small plastic tube, or catheter, in your uterus to measure the strength of your contractions.

Numerous studies comparing continuous FHR monitoring and listening to the baby's heart rate with a stethoscope or other device have shown little difference in detecting fetal distress during labor in an otherwise uneventful pregnancy. If your baby's heart rate is normal and your labor is progressing steadily, continuous monitoring is probably unnecessary—and unduly restrictive. Instead, your birth attendant should encourage you to walk around, lean against your partner, urinate when necessary or simply change positions to stay as comfortable as possible.

Occasional intervals of FHR monitoring may still be recommended throughout labor. You will need continuous monitoring only if there are any signs of fetal distress, such as the presence of meconium-stained amniotic fluid, vaginal bleeding, a drop in your blood pressure, or an interruption in your cervical dilation despite regular contractions.

The Stages of Labor

Labor is divided into three stages. The first stage begins with the onset of contractions and ends when the cervix is fully dilated (to 10 centimeters). The second stage involves delivery of the baby, and the third stage entails delivery of the placenta and membranes, or "afterbirth." Although

DECIDING WHERE TO DELIVER

Today, women have more options about how and where to deliver their babies than ever before. A hospital remains the choice of many, since it provides the security of extensive medical technology in the event of a complication for the mother or child. Many hospitals offer single rooms that allow you and your partner the privacy to participate more fully in childbirth and care of the newborn. Be sure the staff understands and respects the role your partner wants to play in the birth of your baby well before you check in.

Some medical centers now have separate birthing centers in place of their old labor and delivery wards. These centers are more homelike than the maternity section of the hospital, though a woman still has access to medical help, should it become necessary. Home delivery is another alternative advocated by some women who want childbirth to be as natural as possible, but because emergencies, though rare, can be catastrophic when they do occur, most physicians advise against this. Many obstetrical practices now include one or more midwives. Midwifery is one of the world's oldest and most respected professions. Some midwives only work in medical centers, while others also offer assistance with home deliveries. In one study, women who were assisted by midwives in hospital birth centers reported significantly higher satisfaction than those under the care of physicians in traditional hospital settings. There were no differences in Apgar scores in either group, despite the fact that the midwife-assisted mothers were not monitored electronically, and the rate of cesarean deliveries in both groups was similar. The study concluded that women should be offered choices in obstetrical care, including the selection of a birth attendant.

Women who receive competent and compassionate care throughout labor and delivery are much more likely to remain calm and self-controlled during childbirth and experience the greatest satisfaction. Because of the complications that can arise, a hospital birthing center, combining a warm environment for routine deliveries with access to intensive medical care if necessary, appears to offer women, their babies, and their partners with the best of both worlds.

---

the length of labor varies considerably, women experiencing their first full-term childbirth usually have the longest labors. About half will exceed 12 hours, and 2 in 10 will last longer than 24 hours. After the first baby, labor is usually shorter. Three-quarters of women deliver within 12 hours, and only one in 50 labor for more than 24 hours.

The first and longest stage of labor has three distinct phases: the *early*, or latent, phase; the *active* phase; and the *transition*. During the early phase of labor, contractions are often widely spaced—perhaps 10 minutes or more apart—and feel like a tightening or pulling in your back or groin. They can vary considerably in frequency and intensity. At this point you may feel excited, sociable and talkative, or you may be a bit nervous. Most women remain at home during this phase, during which the cervix dilates from 0 to 4 centimeters, and later arrive at the birth center in active labor.

The Active Phase

As you progress from the early to the active phase, your attention focuses completely on labor. Your contractions occur about 3 minutes apart, last about 45 to 60 seconds, and become more centered in your abdomen. They also become stronger and more rhythmic, peaking and receding like waves.

Your determination may waver during this phase of labor. Extra reassurance from your partner and birth attendant can help you stay focused. Breathing exercises and other relaxation techniques also become more important as your cervix dilates to 8 centimeters—nearly wide enough to allow for your baby's birth.

During the active phase, you may begin to long for relief from the pain and tension of labor. Though medication is an obvious solution for your discomfort, you must consider the safety of the baby. Many drugs cross the placenta and affect the baby, making its heartbeat and breathing more sluggish throughout the remainder of labor and after delivery. For this reason, many doctors recommend concentrating on one contraction at a time and relying on your partner, rather than medication, to help maintain your focus.

If your pain is so intense that it actually impedes your progress, however, medication may help you to relax so that contractions can remain steady and vigorous. Two basic kinds of pain medication—analgesics and anesthetics—are used during childbirth.

Analgesics will relieve most of the pain. Drugs used include Demerol, Sublimaze, Nubain, Stadol, morphine, and fentanyl injected into a muscle or vein. These medications are not designed to provide a pain-free labor, but, in appropriate dosages, they can make you more comfortable.

Potential side effects of these drugs include nausea, vomiting and an abnormally fast heartbeat. They present some additional risk to the baby, but if handled properly pose no significant threat. Large doses, however, can interrupt your labor pattern, and if this happens, additional medications such as oxytocin (Pitocin, Syntocinon) may be needed to reestablish strong contractions.

Regional anesthetics completely eliminate the pain. The most common types used during labor include:

Paracervical block. Medication is injected into your cervix, usually during the first stage of labor, to provide you with pain relief from contractions and dilation without interfering with the urge or ability to push. This drug may not work properly in up to one-third of women, and it must be repeated every hour to maintain numbness. It is no longer used frequently.

Pudendal block. The anesthetic is injected through the vaginal wall during the second stage of labor to relieve pain in the perineum (the area between the vagina and the rectum). It may be used in an otherwise unmedicated childbirth. The medication does not interfere with the urge or ability to push and generally masks the effects and repair of an episiotomy—the incision made to enlarge the vaginal opening.

Spinal or saddle block. A single injection of regional anesthetic is made into your spinal canal, numbing the complete lower abdominal and perineal area. This type of anesthetic is rarely used during labor but may be suggested if a forceps or cesarean delivery is required. Administration of a spinal block completely removes the urge to push and may lower your blood pressure. In rare cases, it causes a severe headache when it wears off.

Epidural or caudal block. A needle holding a thin, flexible tube is threaded into the space between your spinal cord and your vertebrae. When the needle is removed, the anesthetic can flow continuously through the tube. Like a spinal block, this procedure provides full pain relief in the perineal area. Dosages can easily be changed or discontinued. Most physicians consider the epidural block to be the optimal method of pain relief for uncomplicated labor or non-emergency cesarean births because it allows a woman to remain fully alert. Nevertheless, the anesthetic requires up to 20 minutes to take full effect and may leave a painful "hot spot". In addition, it may diminish uterine contractions, bringing on the need for oxytocin. The risk of a forceps delivery is also increased.

Transition

Transition is the time when the cervix dilates the final two centimeters. This is the most difficult phase of labor, and produces the hardest, longest, and most frequent contractions. Fortunately, transition is relatively short, sometimes lasting for only two or three contractions. Even in a first labor, transition rarely takes longer than one hour.

During transition, contractions occur every two to three minutes and last 60 to 90 seconds. You have little relief between them, and their intensity may cause you to feel frightened and overwhelmed. While you may have enjoyed your partner's presence and physical touch throughout the early part of labor, transition may suddenly make you feel withdrawn, irritable, and short-tempered. You may develop chills, become nauseous, or feel the urge to have a bowel movement. These physical sensations reflect the descent of your baby into the birth canal and can become more intense as you enter the second stage of labor.

Though you may feel overwhelmed by the power of your own body, transition is not the time to begin analgesics. The best strategy for withstanding transition is to cooperate with your contractions instead of fighting them. Heating pads, hot water compresses, changes in position, breathing exercises, music, meditation, and visualization techniques all can serve as effective alternatives for pain relief. Even women who have received a regional anesthesia may want to consider withdrawing their medication as their cervix nears full dilation so they can begin to feel their contractions and push more effectively.

BREATHING TECHNIQUES HELP BRING RELIEF

During active labor, your goal is to remain as relaxed as possible so your cervix can continue to dilate, and you can provide your baby with a generous oxygen supply in preparation for birth. The following breathing techniques, used alone or in combination, can be effective throughout labor. If you master these techniques during your pregnancy, you may find you can vary the patterns during labor to provide the most effective relief.

- **Deep, cleansing breaths.** Take these long, deep breaths at the beginning and end of each contraction.
- **Slow, chest breathing.** Take these slow, focused breaths 8 to 10 times per minute during the early, milder contractions of the first stage of labor.
- **Rapid chest breathing.** Using the same technique as you employed in early labor, double the speed of these more focused chest breaths as the first stage of labor continues and contractions increase in frequency and intensity.
- **Shallow chest breathing.** Use this shallow, panting technique at the peak of your most intense contractions.

Common Complications of Labor

The rate of cesarean births in the United States has skyrocketed from 5 percent in the 1960s to nearly 25 percent since the 1980s. Many factors have contributed to this increase, including the frequency of repeat cesarean delivery, the use of electronic fetal monitoring, the declining use of vaginal breech and forceps deliveries, and the drift toward surgical intervention for "failure to progress" in labor. While cesarean delivery is certainly safer today than during the 1960s and obviously indicated in extremely high-risk situations or emergencies, it still causes a higher rate of maternal injuries than vaginal delivery.

Cesarean delivery is often accepted as the inevitable outcome to a complication arising during labor. Based on the experience of the past two decades, however, most experts agree that surgical intervention is not always in the best interests of the woman or baby. In order to make an informed decision, it's important to understand some of the common complications that can occur during labor.

Premature Rupture

Most women begin labor spontaneously when their membranes rupture and their pregnancies have reached full term. When labor does not begin within 12 to 24 hours, the situation is described as "premature rupture of the membranes" (PROM). Because PROM certainly plays a role in high cesarean rates, more doctors are proceeding with a quick induction of labor after a PROM at full-term. Although the "wait-and-see" approach has been associated with fewer cesarean deliveries than the use of oxytocin to stimulate contractions, one large study has concluded that induction of labor using vaginal suppositories containing prostaglandin E2 is a viable option for han-

dling PROM—especially in women experiencing a first labor. In the study, the rate of cesarean section in the women who received prostaglandin was half that of those who either received oxytocin or waited for the onset of labor.

Failure to Progress

Physicians generally agree that once active labor has begun, a woman's cervix should dilate 1.2 cm to 1.5 cm per hour. Sometimes dilation falters during the active phase despite regular contractions. This condition is known as "failure to progress." Because labor can be interrupted for a variety of reasons, the immediate cause is not always clear to the woman or her physician. Should this occur, your doctor will perform a pelvic exam, check your vital signs, and monitor the baby for a short period of time. If all appears well, he or she can take a hands-off approach or consider the possibility of "actively managing" your labor.

A number of procedures are effective in reestablishing labor. If your amniotic sac has not yet broken, your doctor may suggest breaking it manually, a procedure known as amniotomy. Because rupturing the membranes commits a woman to delivery, this can be a risky strategy during the latent phase, when false labor is always a possibility. Several research studies have concluded, however, that amniotomy performed during active labor actually shortens its duration by up to 2 hours. Moreover, the rate of vaginal delivery increases, and there is no added risk of injury to the woman or baby.

Physicians disagree on how to handle the 10 percent of pregnancies that extend beyond

40 weeks. The main goal is to avoid injury or death to the baby due to lack of oxygen or intake of meconium in the lungs—established risks in post-term pregnancies. Some doctors advocate inducing labor at 41 to 42 weeks, while others recommend fetal monitoring until labor begins spontaneously. In one large study of women with post-term but otherwise uncomplicated pregnancies, the induction of labor resulted in a lower rate of cesarean delivery, mainly because there was less fetal distress. In any event, few clinicians allow a pregnancy to continue past 42 weeks. In these rare instances, labor is often induced with prostaglandin gel or oxytocin.

Pelvic Size

Certain variations in a woman's anatomy also can lead to complications during labor. During vaginal delivery, the baby must be propelled through your pelvic area by the contractions of your uterus and your own "bearing down." In general, a woman's

pelvis is large enough and shaped properly to allow for the baby's passage. In fact, unless you have a history of pelvic fracture or bone or neuromuscular disease, your physician should not discourage you from trying a natural delivery strictly on the basis of your pelvic dimensions. Even if your pelvic area is smaller than average, it may still be big enough for your baby if the rest of your labor progresses normally.

Nevertheless, in some cases, the size of the baby's head does exceed the dimensions of the birth canal. If this happens, labor will almost certainly fail to progress during the second stage; and the first stage of labor may be irregular as well. If the size of the baby is the cause of a woman's "failure to progress," she will need a cesarean.

Position of the Baby

In more than 95 percent of full-term labors, the baby's head is "presenting" —pointed toward— the cervix. Typically, the baby's

DANGERS OF A BREECH PRESENTATION

When the baby passes head-first through the birth canal—as it does 95 percent of the time—the rounded top of the cranium has a chance to mold to the contours of the passage and slide through without incident. But when the baby is delivered buttocks or feet-first, the chances that the head will be caught in the narrow canal increase dramatically. Deaths following breech deliveries are 4 times more likely than normal, usually as a result of nerve damage or suffocation. A breech presentation is now generally considered a signal for cesarean delivery.

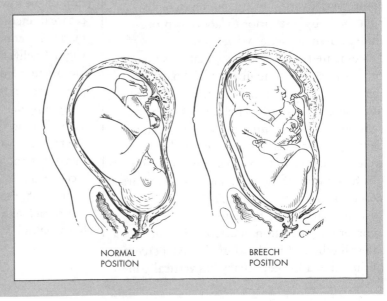

NORMAL POSITION

BREECH POSITION

head is tucked against its chest, with the crown of the head facing the birth canal in preparation for delivery. In some unusual situations, a baby's face, forehead, or top of the head is presenting. If the baby remains in either of the latter two positions throughout labor, a cesarean delivery may be necessary since the broadest part of the baby's head may be too wide to clear your pelvis. A full-face presentation is very rare. Unless you've already had several children, your physician will almost certainly insist on cesarean delivery should this occur. Vaginal delivery increases the risk of injury to the baby's neck or spinal cord.

When the baby's buttocks or feet are presenting at labor, the position is commonly called "breech." Prior to the 1960s, when cesarean delivery carried much higher risks for the mother, these infants were nearly always delivered vaginally, even though they faced a greater risk of injury or death during childbirth. Safer cesarean procedures have all but eliminated the rigors of labor for breech babies. Nevertheless, some physicians are attempting to reduce the incidence of breech cesarean deliveries by attempting to reposition the baby just prior to labor—a procedure known as "external version." Documented reports indicate that version is often successful, though 1 out of 3 babies may revert to breech presentation afterwards, and there is a risk of complications such as a twisted umbilical cord. An attempt at vaginal delivery in a breech presentation under well-managed conditions, including continuous fetal monitoring, is gaining some support within the medical community.

The position—or attitude—of the baby is another consideration in determining the safest method of birth. More than 99 percent of the time, a full-term baby lies vertically in the uterus. In the remaining cases, known as a transverse lie, the baby's back faces the birth canal. A baby in this position when labor begins almost always must be delivered by cesarean.

A Past Cesarean

More and more women are being encouraged to attempt a vaginal birth, after a previous cesarean delivery (VBAC). If you are considering VBAC, you and your doctor need to discuss several factors, including the type of incision made in your uterus during your previous cesarean delivery, the size of your pelvis, whether you are carrying twins or have a breech presentation, and certain medical conditions you may have, such as diabetes or high blood pressure. Despite the slightly higher risk, none of these factors necessarily eliminates the VBAC option.

Fear of uterine rupture has been the reason most often cited for the outdated medical dictum, "Once a cesarean, always a cesarean." Rupture of a uterine scar can result in the baby's death and severe injury to the mother. Nevertheless, widespread adoption of the low transverse, or horizontal, cesarean incision in the uterine wall has dramatically reduced the risks faced in future vaginal deliveries. Moreover, many of the factors that led to an initial cesarean—breech presentation, fetal distress, failure to progress—may not be present during a second labor. Counterbalancing the risks is the fact that vaginal delivery has fewer complications and a shorter recovery period than a cesarean.

In 1988, the American College of Obstetricians and Gynecologists issued guidelines making VBAC a preferred, rather than

MEASURING LABOR IN CENTIMETERS

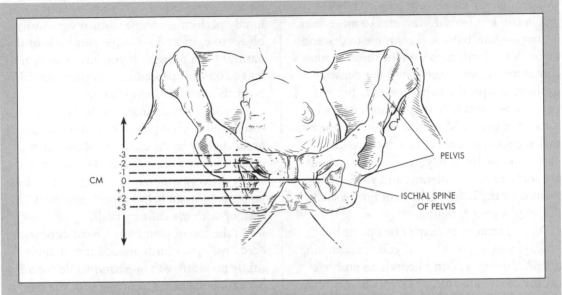

The second stage of labor officially begins when the baby's head settles into the upper end of the birth canal, 3 centimeters from the center of the pelvis. When the top of the head reaches the center point, the baby has achieved "0" station. Three centimeters later, the baby has reached the lower end of the birth canal, and delivery is underway. This centimeter-by-centimeter advance can last more than 2 hours—or be over in 15 minutes!

optional, procedure under most circumstances. Specifically, the College recommends that women with one previous low transverse cesarean should be encouraged to attempt labor in a later pregnancy, and women with two or more low transverse incisions should not be discouraged from trying vaginal birth. However, the group cautions that women with a classic vertical incision should not risk labor, and it advises physicians offering the VBAC option to have the staff and equipment available to perform an emergency cesarean if necessary.

Vaginal Delivery

When the widest part of the baby's head has settled into the birth canal, it is said to be engaged, or positioned for the second stage of labor. At this point, your contractions may slow to four or five minutes apart and become less intense. Your birth attendant will encourage you to push when each contraction begins and will monitor the baby's "descent" on a regular basis. When the baby's head is even with the lower bones of your pelvis, its position will be recorded as "0" station. As the baby's head continues to move through the birth canal, the stations will be identified as

+1, +2, +3, etc., in reference to the baby's progress in centimeters.

Throughout the second stage of labor—which can last from 15 minutes to more than 2 hours—your baby will continue to descend through the birth canal. As the force of your contractions, combined with your conscious pushing, propel the baby, you may become very tired—especially if your labor has been long or rigorous. Most women find, however, that the second stage of labor is physically and emotionally satisfying. The contractions are often easier to tolerate, and your excitement over the baby's imminent birth usually outweighs your fatigue.

Your partner can help at this point by bracing you as you push. If you're attempting a VBAC delivery, don't hesitate to push vigorously. The nine months of pregnancy and the rigors of your labor have provided a reliable test of your incision's strength.

As the second stage of labor progresses, the perineal area between the vagina and rectum will begin to stretch. Your doctor may make a small incision or episiotomy, in this region, to prevent the perineal skin from tearing during childbirth. Though fewer physicians advocate episiotomies as a routine part of every delivery, they are still commonly performed. Some women vigorously object to episiotomies as the antithesis of the natural birth process. If you have strong feelings about this procedure, tell your physician or birth attendant beforehand.

As your baby approaches the bones and soft tissue of your pelvis, its pliable head will mold slightly to the contours of the birth canal. Once its head slips under your pubic bone, delivery is imminent. At this juncture, your partner can help support your back or legs, or with the delivery itself.

As the top of your baby's head appears, or "crowns," your birth attendant will apply subtle pressure with one hand while reaching beneath your pelvis to prepare for the baby's birth. In rare cases, forceps or vacuum extraction may be necessary to help guide the baby's head through the birth canal.

At this point, you may be told to pant, rather than continuing to push, so the baby's head can be delivered gently rather than bursting out. You may want to watch the

THE EPISIOTOMY ISSUE

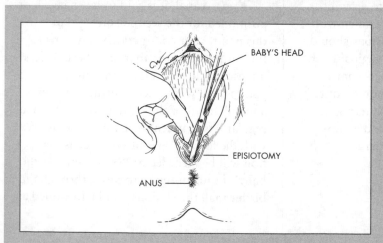

BABY'S HEAD

EPISIOTOMY

ANUS

As the baby emerges, there's a chance that skin between the vagina and anus will be stretched to the breaking point. To prevent uncontrolled tearing, many physicians routinely make the minor incision called an episiotomy. Because the procedure is considered routine, if you don't want it done you should be sure to let your doctor know in advance.

birth in a mirror. When the head is through, your birth attendant will check to ensure that the umbilical cord remains free of the baby's neck. He or she will then immediately clear the baby's mouth and nostrils of mucus. With your next contraction, the attendant will deliver the baby's body, then clamp and cut the cord. As soon as the infant's general condition has been assessed—usually using Apgar scores—you will be able to cuddle and enjoy your baby.

Within a few minutes of birth, your rapidly diminishing uterine contractions will cause the placenta to separate from the uterine wall. Generally, you can expect the placenta to be expelled rapidly. You may be given oxytocin to stimulate contractions while your uterus is massaged to reduce bleeding. If you delivered by VBAC, your birth attendant will carefully check your old incision for any evidence of injury.

The doctor will examine the placenta, and inspect your cervix and vagina for any tears or bruises. If you have had an episiotomy, the doctor will stitch it closed. In the meantime, you and your partner will probably be oblivious to these final details as you share the joy of your new child.

Cesarean Delivery

Despite its detractors, cesarean delivery continues to be one of medicine's most important and—often lifesaving—operations. Physicians continue to recommend cesarean delivery when they consider labor unsafe for either mother or baby, when delivery is necessary but labor cannot be induced, when the baby's size or presentation precludes vaginal birth, and when a medical emergency occurs.

A cesarean may be called for if the placenta is blocking the exit of the uterus (placenta previa), if you have had a classic cesarean incision, or if you have a history of uterine surgery or abnormalities. If such medical conditions as diabetes mellitus or hypertension threaten the baby's welfare, you may need preterm cesarean delivery if labor induction fails. Cesarean birth also is a safe alternative when anatomical problems of the uterus or birth canal prevent successful vaginal delivery.

Maternal or fetal emergencies necessitate immediate delivery. These include untimely separation of the placenta from the uterus, bleeding from placenta previa, protrusion of the umbilical cord, or an active vaginal infection such as herpes. Roughly one-fifth of all cesarean deliveries are prompted by an emergency condition.

Although repeat cesarean delivery is no longer mandatory, approximately 40 percent of women attempting VBAC ultimately require another cesarean. If this occurs, you should be proud of your efforts and never feel that you have failed yourself or your baby.

Cesarean deliveries are classified by the type and location of uterine incision. The two most common incisions in the United States are vertical cut in the upper portion of the uterus—often called a "classic" incision—and the transverse, or "Kerr" incision in the lower portion of the uterus. The transverse incision is a safer procedure than the classic.

Although a variety of anesthetic techniques are used, an epidural block is often the anesthesia of choice for a cesarean delivery. During a particularly difficult or emergency cesarean, when there's no time to wait for an epidural anesthetic to take effect, the doctor may use general anesthesia. Though it can slightly increase such additional risks to the mother as the chance of inhaling gastric backflow (aspiration) and the danger of cardiac or respiratory arrest, the value of the surgery usually outweighs the risks of anesthesia. The baby usually suffers no harm because delivery often takes place before the anesthesia has time to cross the placenta.

Prior to surgery, a nurse or attendant may wash and shave your abdomen and cleanse the area with a special antiseptic lotion. You will probably need a catheter to remove urine from your bladder during the operation and will likely be given an intravenous (IV) line to provide you with additional fluid.

As the cesarean delivery begins, the physician will cut open your abdomen and uterus in quick succession, rupture the membranes, and carefully guide the baby's head through the incision. You may feel a tugging sensation around your abdomen. The baby's mouth and nostrils will be suctioned, then the body gently delivered. The entire process can take less than five minutes.

Once the doctor has checked the baby, you or your partner may be able to hold the infant while the doctor manually removes your placenta, checks your uterus, and begins to stitch the incisions closed. The doctor will gently massage your uterus to expel any blood clots. You will be carefully watched for any signs of bleeding or infection during the period immediately following the birth.

Possible complications of cesarean delivery include fever, wound infection, bleeding, aspiration during general anesthesia, urinary tract infections, inflammation of the endometrium and blood clots. Complications are estimated to occur in 25 percent of all cesarean operations; the mother dies in roughly one out of every 1,000 cesarean deliveries. As many as one-fourth of these deaths are related to anesthesia.

Most women should begin walking within a day of their cesarean delivery, when a urinary catheter is no longer necessary. You can usually start eating a soft diet on the day after the operation, and you'll probably leave the hospital approximately 3 days after delivery. During your recovery, you may have to use a stool softener and a mild pain reliever. You will probably need to visit your doctor 2 to 3 weeks after leaving the hospital so he or she can examine your incision and remove any sutures or staples. □

CHAPTER 27   **TOWARD SUCCESSFUL PREGNANCIES**

What To Do When Miscarriage Strikes

Miscarriage can leave a couple severely shaken as the anticipation of having a baby suddenly turns to grief over a loss. Many feel devastated and guilty even if the miscarriage occurs during the early weeks or months of the pregnancy. However, while it's normal to blame some specific act or situation, miscarriages are rarely triggered by factors under the partners' control.

Exercising, a minor fall, or sexual intercourse does not typically cause a miscarriage. The fetus is well protected by the mother's bones and muscle as well as by the amniotic fluid in which it floats. There is also no evidence that conceiving while taking birth control pills increases the risk of miscarriage. Becoming pregnant while using an IUD, however, does make you more likely to miscarry or develop an infection.

As many as 30 percent of all pregnancies end in miscarriage, half of them before the woman even realizes she is pregnant. Fortunately, most women who miscarry, even more than once, can become pregnant again and give birth to a healthy baby. If you have had a miscarriage and want to try again, work with your doctor to learn the reason for the loss and to plan future pregnancies. Closely monitored pregnancies are especially important for women who have miscarried.

Your doctor may refer to a miscarriage as a "spontaneous abortion," since "abortion" is the medical term for any interrupted pregnancy. A miscarriage, or spontaneous abortion, is the loss of a pregnancy before the fetus can survive outside the womb, usually within the first 20 weeks.

Warning Signs

Any bleeding from the vagina during pregnancy suggests the possibility of miscarriage. Call your doctor about any abnormal vaginal bleeding, even if you do not think you are pregnant. Bleeding or spotting may be the first sign that you are pregnant and that the pregnancy is at risk. Staining or bleeding does not necessarily mean that you will miscarry, however. About 20 to 25 percent of pregnant women have some spotting or bleeding early in pregnancy, and about half of these pregnancies continue successfully.

Bleeding that signals possible miscarriage is usually light. It can be brown or bright red and may occur repeatedly over many days. If the bleeding persists or increases, the chances of losing the baby are higher. Mild pain, such as cramping or low backache, usually develops at some point after the bleeding has started. Some women experience severe abdominal pain and dizziness.

If you have been bleeding and an ultrasound scan (sonogram) indicates that the fetus is alive, your doctor probably will ask you to rest in bed as much as possible. Avoid sexual activity. The doctor will monitor you to be sure that bleeding and cramping remain mild, that the cervical canal from the uterus stays closed in order to retain the baby in the uterus, that sonograms continue to show fetal heart movements, and that the fetus is growing. More than 90 percent of first–trimester pregnancies continue when ultrasound scans indicate that the baby is alive.

Rarely, early in pregnancy, fluid is suddenly released from the vagina without bleeding or pain. If you experience this, call your doctor immediately. You will probably be instructed to stay in bed and watch for further leakage, bleeding, cramping, or fever. If, after a few days, you have none of these things, your doctor may tell you that it is safe to go back to daily activities. Avoid intercourse and any other vaginal penetration. If you do develop bleeding, pain, or fever, however, miscarriage may be inevitable.

Types of Miscarriage

Miscarriages differ according to 2 main factors: how far the pregnancy has progressed and how much of the fetus and other elements of preg-

nancy, such as the placenta, have been expelled from the body. To prevent infection, it's important to ensure that all material related to pregnancy has been either expelled naturally or removed from the uterus.

Inevitable Miscarriage

When bleeding and pain are accompanied by the breaking of membranes (the amniotic sac surrounding the fetus) and the widening of the cervix, the pregnancy is viewed as lost (inevitable miscarriage). Uterine contractions to expel the fetus usually begin soon after these symptoms develop.

Incomplete and Missed Miscarriages

In some miscarriages, the body does not expel all the elements of pregnancy. This is called an *incomplete* miscarriage. At other times—in about 1 percent of pregnancies—the body does not discharge the fetus, the placenta, or any other elements of the pregnancy for several weeks, even though the fetus has died. This is known as a *missed* miscarriage. It is a possibility when a woman has neither menstrual periods nor any signs of pregnancy. Breasts may return to their prepregnancy state, for example, or the woman may lose a few pounds. Not all missed miscarriages are preceded by warning signs.

An incomplete or missed miscarriage that takes place early in pregnancy is usually removed with either suction or dilation and curettage (D&C), "opening" the uterus and scraping out its contents, through the vagina, with an instrument called a curette. These procedures not only clear the uterus but also prevent infection. When incomplete miscarriage occurs later in pregnancy, the doctor may have to induce labor to remove the fetus.

Minimizing the Risk of Miscarriage

Most miscarriages are caused by chromosomal (genetic) abnormalities and other physical factors that are beyond your control. There are, however, steps you can take to reduce the risk of losing a pregnancy.

Don't smoke. Smoking increases the risk of losing a genetically normal baby. One study showed that women who smoked more than 14 cigarettes a day were about twice as likely to miscarry, regardless of their age or use of alcoholic beverages. The risk of losing a pregnancy increases with the number of cigarettes a woman smokes. On the other hand, giving up smoking at any time during the pregnancy will benefit the baby. Since passive smoke is also dangerous, it's wisest if no one in your household smokes during the pregnancy.

Don't drink alcoholic beverages or much caffeine. Having an alcoholic drink twice weekly doubled the risk of losing normal babies in one study; drinking alcohol every day tripled the risk of such miscarriages. Similarly, consuming large amounts of caffeine—more than 4 cups of coffee per day (or the equivalent in other substances that contain caffeine) slightly increases the chance of miscarriage. The risk appears to rise with the amount of caffeine consumed; and doctors generally recommend limiting intake to one cup of coffee per day.

Avoid radiation and poisons. Exposure to high levels of radiation or toxic substances increases the risk of miscarriage. The dangers of various levels of radiation are discussed in the chapter on "Strategies for a Healthy Pregnancy." Arsenic, lead, formaldehyde, benzene, and ethylene oxide can cause miscarriage. Make sure you are not exposed to these substances at work or anywhere else while pregnant or trying to conceive.

Prevent trauma to the abdomen. Don't participate in sports such a skiing that might involve serious falls. Stab wounds or injuries from the steering wheel or seat belt in a car, especially during the second trimester, sometimes cause miscarriage. See the nearby box for the right way to wear a seat belt when you are visibly pregnant.

Check out all medications with your doctor. Certain prescription and over–the–counter drugs are associated with fetal abnormalities and miscarriages. Consult your doctor before taking any medication when you are pregnant or trying to conceive. Some drugs can damage the fetus and cause miscarriage before you even know you are pregnant.

Causes of Miscarriage

In general, miscarriage is more common in women over 35 years old and in pregnancies involving more than one fetus. In some multiple pregnancies (twins, triplets, or more), one or more of the fetuses survives even after another one dies. The dead fetus leaves the mother's body when the surviving baby is born.

Some of the factors discussed in this section are more common after repeated—that is, 3 or more—miscarriages. About 1 in 200 women has repeated miscarriages, which physicians call recurrent spontaneous abortion. In many cases—perhaps most—even these miscarriages happen by chance and do not signal a problem in either or both partners. Often no cause is found.

Chromosomal abnormalities.

Problems in the chromosomes of the embryo, by far the most common reason for loss of pregnancy, are found in more than half of miscarriages occurring in the first 13 weeks. Miscarriages apparently eliminate about 95 percent of fertilized eggs or embryos with genetic problems—perhaps nature's way of ending a pregnancy in which the child would be unable to survive. Spontaneous abortions of this type usually occur before the woman knows that she is pregnant. Most chromosomal problems happen by chance, have nothing to do with the parents, and are unlikely to recur.

Sometimes, however, chromosomal abnormalities are caused by the parents' genes. This is more likely if the woman has had repeated miscarriages or if either parent has relatives or a child with birth defects. Genetic testing and analysis of fetal material from the miscarriage can help the doctor identify the problem.

Illness

Miscarriages are much less common in the third trimester. Those that occur are more likely to be due to maternal factors, such as an illness in the mother, than to genetic abnormalities in the baby.

Women with poorly controlled diabetes are at great risk for miscarriage. Those whose diabetes is controlled, however, whether it existed before the pregnancy or developed after conception (gestational diabetes), are no more likely to lose a pregnancy than other women. A woman may not know that she has diabetes, however, until it is discovered during a search for the cause of repeated miscarriages. The routine blood and urine tests given

during pregnancy are an effort to identify this problem while it still can be remedied.

Other diseases and conditions linked to increased risk of miscarriage include systemic lupus erythematosus (SLE, or lupus), high blood pressure, and certain infections, such as rubella (German measles), herpes simplex, and chlamydia. Experts disagree about the role of hypothyroidism, or an underactive thyroid gland, in miscarriage, but it's likely that a severe case increases the risk.

With conditions such as diabetes, treating or controlling the problem can improve the odds of a successful pregnancy. Special monitoring may also be required.

Hormone Imbalance

Some women do not make enough progesterone, the hormone that prepares the lining of the uterus to nourish a fertilized egg; and if the uterine lining cannot sustain an egg, miscarriage will occur. Progesterone supplements, given by injection or in vaginal or rectal suppositories, can correct this problem. The medication also can make it more difficult for a dead fetus to be expelled. A blood test and a biopsy of a small amount of tissue taken from the uterine lining can determine whether you are producing enough progesterone naturally. Hormone imbalance also can be caused by diabetes mellitus or thyroid disease.

Abnormalities of the Uterus and Cervix

Anything physically wrong with the uterus or cervix can lead to a miscarriage. Some defects may be present from birth. Fibroids—noncancerous growths made of uterine muscle tissue—can also be at fault. So can a weak cervix that widens too early in pregnancy without any warning signs of labor, releasing the fetus from the uterus.

These physical problems account for up to 15 percent of repeated miscarriages. To diagnose such problems, the doctor may inject the cavity of the uterus with some fluid, then take an x–ray of your uterus and fallopian tubes. Another technique is to examine the inside of your uterus through a long, thin instrument (hysteroscope) inserted through the vagina and cervix. In another procedure, the doctor may make a small incision in the lower abdomen and insert a laparoscope, through which he or she can inspect the pelvic organs. Surgery can correct many abnormalities in the uterus but your doctor probably won't recommend it until all other causes of miscarriage have been ruled out. After surgery, 70 to 90 percent of pregnancies are successful.

Though a weak cervix is a relatively rare condition, it's almost impossible to detect before it becomes apparent during pregnancy, usually after the 15th week. Once discovered, it is likely to disrupt every pregnancy. To remedy the problem, after the first trimester, but before the cervix has dilated (widened) to a certain point, your doctor can reinforce the cervix with sutures, which will be removed when the baby reaches term. Women with bleeding, uterine contractions, or ruptured membranes should not undergo this procedure.

Immune System Problems

A developing baby is half made up of foreign genetic material from the father. Some women have repeated miscarriages because their bodies see each baby as an invading organism and attack it with antibodies. Ordinarily, many elements of the immune system work together to ensure that the mother's body does not reject the baby. But when this coordination fails, a miscarriage follows. Treatments for such problems in the immune system are experimental and should not be tried until other causes for repeated miscarriage have been ruled out. Some research centers have tried to "immunize" the mother with the father's white blood cells, but so far without good results.

Certain autoimmune diseases and abnormalities also increase the risk of miscarriage. Women whose blood contains certain types of antibodies are at particularly high risk. These women may have no symptoms other than trouble retaining a pregnancy, but a blood test can determine whether the antibodies are present. If so, heparin, prednisone, and aspirin during pregnancy can help prevent miscarriage. About 70 to 75 percent of women with lupus-associated antibodies who are treated with these drugs are able to deliver. In any case, if you have these blood abnormalities, you should have your doctor watch you closely. The baby may grow too slowly or develop other complications.

After Miscarriage

Miscarriages due to random natural factors are so common that they are not considered medically significant until you've had 3 in a row. At that point, the problem is officially classified as "recurrent miscarriage," and your doctor will recommend a complete diagnostic workup.

The investigation will probably start with a detailed interview. Which tests are performed will depend on your own personal and medical history, the father's history, and how many miscarriages you have had. You will be tested for infections of various kinds, possibly including sexually transmitted diseases. Blood tests may be done for hormonal problems or a malfunction in the immune system. You and your partner may be tested for chromosomal abnormalities and genetic diseases as well. The lining of your uterus may be analyzed from a small sample. The doctor may order x–rays of your uterus and fallopian tubes to look for a blockage, fibroid, or scar tissue.

Knowing as much as possible about why the miscarriages are happening can increase the chances of having a normal pregnancy in the future. It's best to postpone trying to conceive again until your medical evaluation is complete. More than likely, you *can* carry a baby to term. Unless the problem involves autoimmune antibodies, chromosomal abnormalities, or a weak cervix, there's a 70 to 85 percent chance of success, even after 3 miscarriages.

Recovering Emotionally

Allow yourselves to grieve after losing a pregnancy. Many couples feel a renewed sense of emptiness and loss at the time the baby would have been born. Consider joining a self–help group such as one of those listed at the end of this book. Your obstetrician or local hospital may be able to suggest others. Try not to blame yourself. Instead, concentrate on finding out what went wrong—and how you can make it right.

Some couples want to conceive again quickly. While such a step may be physically possible, it is psychologically unwise. Nevertheless, sex can be resumed safely within 2 to 4 weeks after miscarriage. A woman's body usually is prepared for another pregnancy after 1 or 2 normal menstrual periods. Ovulation can occur as little as 2 weeks after a miscarriage.

Give yourselves enough time to recover emotionally from your loss before facing the challenges of another pregnancy. As with any major life event, it's important to balance the need to grieve with the need to move on. And remember, most couples who experience a miscarriage can go on to have a healthy baby. □

CHAPTER 28

Understanding the Change

In a phenomenon some sociologists have dubbed "youth creep," the meaning of middle age in America today is different than what it was just a generation ago. Doctors now consider 55, rather than 40, as the turning point into middle age. Women reaching their 40s and 50s today can look forward to a vigorous, active, and healthy middle and old age — particularly if they take responsibility for the preventive health care that can help keep them in good physical and mental condition.

Changes At Midlife

Women may notice the first signs of bodily changes in their menstrual patterns, skin, and shape as early as their late 30s. Menopause — the cessation of the menstrual cycle — is certainly the most notable sign of advancing age for women. The hormonal changes that spur the end of menstruation affect our entire bodies, from the texture of our skin to the condition of our heart and bones.

The medical definition of menopause is the end of menstruation, so menopause can only be diagnosed after the fact. But the bodily changes leading up to menopause may take place over a decade. Most women reach menopause between the ages of 45 and 55. At age 52, 80 percent will no longer be menstruating. There does not appear to be any consistent relationship between a woman's age at the onset of menopause and her age at her first menstruation, nor does marriage, childbearing, height, weight, or use of oral contraceptives appear to make a difference. However, women who smoke do tend to reach menopause a year or two earlier than nonsmokers.

Menopause Without Mystery

Until quite recently, menopause was something of a "taboo" topic, and often not discussed even between mothers and daughters or among close friends. Now that the huge "baby boom" generation (known for its openness and take-charge attitude toward medical care) is entering its middle years, discussion of menopause appears more frequently in the media and in private conversations. A recent survey indicates that menopause is now also discussed more openly among women and men at work. By taking some of the mystery out of this natural process, women and men are learning how to cope with everyday changes.

Most of today's women will live 25 to 30 years—one-third of their lives—after menopause. An understanding of the body's physiological changes during this phase of life can ease the transition, and equally important, better prepare you to safeguard your health during your later years.

Is Menopause A Deficiency Disease?

Within the medical community, there's a debate about whether menopause should be viewed as a natural process or as a health threat. Some physicians see menopause as a hormone deficiency syndrome associated with dysfunction of the ovaries, requiring diagnosis and treatment. Their argument is based on the fact that menopausal women are at increased risk for developing health disorders. For example, for every 2,000 postmenopausal women, 20 will develop heart disease; 11 will develop severe bone loss (osteoporosis); six will develop breast cancer; and three will develop endometrial cancer. The risk of some of these diseases can be reduced by treating menopause with hormonal replacement therapy (HRT), and some physicians strongly believe that this treatment should be used by all women who have no medical reason to avoid it.

Other professionals object to the "medicalization" of menopause, believing that it perpetuates negative cultural perceptions of aging as a time of decay that should be feared, rather than as a normal developmen-

tal stage in a woman's life. They, too, acknowledge that the risk of certain diseases rises after menopause and encourage various preventive strategies.

Premature and Induced Menopause

There are certain situations that bring about menopause earlier than usual. About one percent of women cease menstruating before age 40. This is called premature menopause or premature ovarian failure. The reasons for it are largely unknown. In some cases, severe infections or tumors in the reproductive tract damage the ovaries and precipitate menopause. Other possible causes are exposure to radiation, chemotherapy drugs, and surgery that impairs blood flow to the ovaries.

When a woman has her ovaries surgically removed or rendered nonfunctional through radiation therapy, induced or artificial menopause occurs. Because this results in an abrupt and almost total loss of estogen in the body, symptoms of induced menopause can be particularly severe. The condition is usually a side effect of treatment for abdominal disease, such as ovarian cancer. Elective removal of the ovaries is sometimes used to prevent ovarian cancer particularly where there is a family history of the disease. The practice is highly controversial in premenopausal women, though less so in postmenopausal women. In the past, it was also common to remove the ovaries during a hysterectomy (surgical removal of the uterus), but today in premenopausal women the ovaries are left in place whenever possible.

The Menstrual Cycle

A brief overview of the menstrual cycle is essential to understanding what happens to the body during menopause. Taking a close look at how your body functions will help increase your sense of comfort and familiarity, and place the sometimes puzzling symptoms of menopause into perspective.

Monthly Ovarian Cycle

While men manufacture sperm each day, often into advanced age, women are born with a single lifetime supply of egg cells that are released from the ovaries gradually throughout the menstrual years. The entire structure of an egg, with its surrounding flat sheet of cells, is called a follicle. The ovarian cycle begins when the follicular cells swell, absorbing a cholesterol-rich fluid that is then converted into steroid hormones — predominantly estrogen, a woman's most important sex hormone. These hormones act as chemical messengers that orchestrate the menstrual cycle, which lasts an average of 28 days. Some of these hormones escape the follicle into the bloodstream and travel throughout the body. Not only do the sex organs need estrogen to function, but almost every part of

WHAT'S MISSING IN MENOPAUSE

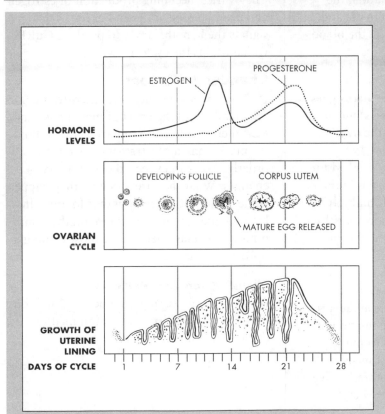

HORMONE LEVELS

ESTROGEN

PROGESTERONE

DEVELOPING FOLLICLE

CORPUS LUTEM

MATURE EGG RELEASED

OVARIAN CYCLE

GROWTH OF UTERINE LINING

DAYS OF CYCLE   1   7   14   21   28

Menopause occurs when the ovaries shut down and menstruation ends. But, as the diagram at left shows, more than menstruation is at stake. During the regular monthly cycle, the egg-bearing follicles within the ovaries produce first a burst of estrogen, then a follow-up surge of both estrogen and progesterone. When ovulation stops, so does virtually all production of these hormones.

Because estrogen plays many roles in the female body—including maintenance of bone density, stimulation of breast tissue, and nurture of the vaginal membranes—its loss has numerous ramifications, collectively known as the "Change."

your body is affected by the hormones produced by the ovaries.

The ovary raises many follicles each month but usually only one follicle matures to reach ovulation. Ovulation occurs when the egg is released from its follicle — leaving the ovary, entering the fallopian tube, and journeying toward the uterus. If the egg is fertilized by a sperm, pregnancy occurs.

The cycle continues after ovulation with the reconnection and multiplication of the cells of the ruptured follicle in the ovary. The former follicle grows and takes on a yellow color, thus its name, corpus luteum ("yellow body"). As the corpus luteum grows, it secretes increasing amounts of estrogen and progesterone, raising the levels of these hormones in the blood. If the egg is not fertilized by the fourteenth day after ovulation, the cells of the corpus luteum begin to die and, simultaneously, hormone levels in the blood decline sharply.

Monthly Uterine Cycle

Along with ovarian changes, the uterus goes through a cycle of its own. When stimulated by the estrogen secreted during the ovarian cycle, the lining of the uterus (the endometrium) develops to serve as a bed for the fertilized egg. As hormone levels in the blood rise, the endometrial cells multiply, and blood vessels grow to provide nourishing oxygen, causing an increase in the thickness of the endometrial tissue.

When hormone levels drop at the end of the ovarian cycle, the blood vessels in the endometrium begin to deteriorate and deprive the cells of nourishment. The elimination of blood, mucus and the dead cells from the endometrial tissue, in the form of menstrual blood flow, generally occurs for three to five days. This signals the start of a new cycle.

The Control Center

The entire monthly cycle is controlled by certain centers in the brain. The hypothalamus, located in the base of the brain, releases several hormones directly into the bloodstream.

One of these, gonadotropin releasing hormone (GnRH), prompts the pituitary gland to secrete two hormones called the gonadotropins: follicle stimulating hormone (FSH) and luteinizing hormone (LH). These hormones control the ovaries. FSH stimulates the development of follicles in the ovaries. LH causes ovulation and changes the ruptured follicle into the corpus luteum. In turn, the progesterone produced by the corpus luteum prevents the pituitary from releasing additional FSH and LH, thus preventing the growth of new follicles until the next cycle. The ovaries' declining production of estrogen and progesterone at the end of the cycle signals the hypothalamus to produce GnRH, which begins the cycle anew.

Changes to Expect

Some women continue to menstruate normally until the onset of menopause and then simply cease to have periods. But for most women, the transition is not so orderly. You can expect to see a variety of changes. What they are and why they happen is the subject of the section that follows. In later chapters, you'll find more on the symptoms and management of the most troubling of these problems.

Changing Hormonal Patterns

A woman's egg supply, as much as 2 million in the ovaries at birth, is programmed for depletion. When the supply is almost

MENOPAUSE AT A GLANCE

The wide array of problems shown in this diagram may seem daunting; but fortunately, few women experience every one of them. Hot flashes are the most common complaint. However, these annoying sensations pass in due course, while other symptoms may pose a much greater long-term threat. Be particularly alert for lower back pain, which may signal the onset of osteoporosis, the bone-weakening disorder that leaves older women prey to fractures. Remember, too, that menopause robs you of estrogen's protective effect on the heart, and that heart disease is the Number One killer of women. (For more information, turn to chapter 12, "Heart Disease: The Greatest Threat of All.")

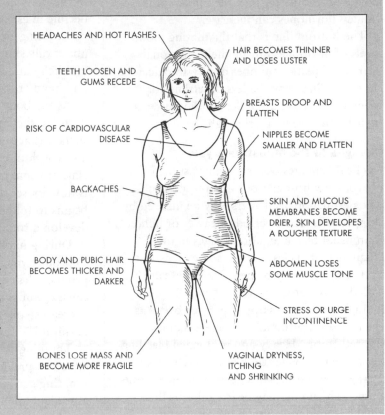

HEADACHES AND HOT FLASHES

TEETH LOOSEN AND GUMS RECEDE

RISK OF CARDIOVASCULAR DISEASE

BACKACHES

BODY AND PUBIC HAIR BECOMES THICKER AND DARKER

BONES LOSE MASS AND BECOME MORE FRAGILE

HAIR BECOMES THINNER AND LOSES LUSTER

BREASTS DROOP AND FLATTEN

NIPPLES BECOME SMALLER AND FLATTEN

SKIN AND MUCOUS MEMBRANES BECOME DRIER, SKIN DEVELOPES A ROUGHER TEXTURE

ABDOMEN LOSES SOME MUSCLE TONE

STRESS OR URGE INCONTINENCE

VAGINAL DRYNESS, ITCHING AND SHRINKING

exhausted because of the aging process, or the ovaries are surgically removed, the menstrual cycle comes to an end. In fact, the reproductive cycle begins to change several years before menopause, a period referred to as perimenopause.

During this time, typically starting in the late 40's, the ovaries' response to the various stimulating hormones produced by the brain becomes unsynchronized, until eventually the aging ovaries fail to respond at all. They start to produce less progesterone, losing their ability to ovulate and develop the subsequent

corpus luteum. When ovulation stops, estrogen levels decline and menstruation ceases.

As ovulatory cycles become more irregular throughout perimenopause, the body's sensitive hormonal rhythm is thrown off and menstruation may vary more from month to month. In addition, two hormones known as androgens begin to play a bigger role. Though referred to as male sex hormones, they are in fact produced in small amounts by the female body as well. As levels of the female hormones decline, the impact of these "male" hormones can increase.

The bottom line is that fluctuating blood levels of hormones during the transitional years can create a number of physiological changes. These may be less unsettling for women who have an understanding of what their bodies are going through.

Changes In The Menstrual Cycle

Cyclical Changes occur for the vast majority of women whose periods do not just stop. The perimenopausal years may be marked by skipped menstrual periods, heavier or lighter than usual bleeding, and changes in the frequency of cycles. During some menstrual cycles, no egg may be produced; these are called anovulatory cycles.

Light, short, or skipped periods occur as the ovaries' hormonal response becomes unpredictable. Heavy and prolonged bleeding arise when a longer than normal release of estrogen overstimulates growth of the uterine lining. The lining may be irregular or thickened and may not slough off completely or evenly, causing menstruation to stop and start again. Clotting may be noticeable in menstrual bleeding.

The physical changes that accompany the menstrual cycle may also become less predictable and regular. Such signs as breast tenderness, fluid retention and headache may occur at unpredictable times.

Fertility declines as a woman enters her 40s, but it does not disappear entirely until menopause is complete. To avoid unplanned pregnancies, doctors recommend using birth control until a full year has passed since the last menstrual cycle.

Muscle Tone and Elasticity

Skin and mucous membranes in various parts of the body become drier because of the decline in estrogen levels and the aging process in general. Women who once worried about oily skin may now find their skin dry and itchy and may need to apply moisturizers and hand creams.

As the body ages and the estrogen level declines, the fatty layer beneath the skin surface that makes the skin appear supple and youthful begins to shrink from a loss of elasticity and moisture. The outer skin layer is now looser than the deeper layers, and begins to fold and wrinkle. The skin may also develop a rougher texture.

During midlife, it is especially important to protect your skin from the sun. Aging skin produces less melanin, the pigment that causes your skin to tan instead of burn. This decreases your natural protection from harmful UV rays.

Thinning skin also reveals any harmful effects of previous years of sun exposure. Limiting sun exposure and using sunscreen is a prudent and effective way to delay aging of the skin.

Vaginal changes are the first sign of approaching menopause for some women, while many do not notice changes until five to ten years after menopause. As estrogen levels drop, the vulva and vagina lose elasticity, resulting in vaginal dryness, itching and a shrinking process known as vaginal atrophy in which the vagina becomes shorter and narrower at the opening. Vaginal membranes also become thinner, hold less moisture, and lubricate more slowly. The thinner vaginal lining becomes more susceptible to tears. Reduced secretion of cervical mucus can add to the problem. The result of all these changes can be discomfort, vaginal infections, and painful intercourse.

Breast Changes are also apparent as estrogen's stimulation of the breast tissue is reduced, causing glandular tissue to shrink. Loss of elasticity causes the breasts to droop and flatten, losing their earlier fullness. Nipples become smaller and flatter and may lose their erectile properties.

Women who have been bothered by breast tenderness and cysts related to the menstrual cycle are often relieved to find that these symptoms disappear after menopause.

Abdominal wall tone may lessen gradually as we age, resulting in a protruding stomach. Regular exercise to strengthen the abdominal muscles can help maintain muscle tone.

A sudden increase in the size of the abdomen may be the first warning sign of ovarian tumors. Stomach enlargement may also be caused by inadequate nutrition or exercise, but should be seen promptly by your gynecologist.

Hair, Bones, and Teeth

Hair all over the body can change in texture and quantity during menopause. For some women, the increased effects of the body's androgens can result in darker, thicker and wiry body hair on the pubis, underarms, face, chest, lower abdomen, and back. This sprouting of excess, coarse hair, known as hirsutism, is usually related to hormonal changes. However, not all cases of hirsutism are menopause-related, so check with your physician for proper diagnosis.

The softer hair on your head also begins to change in texture as you reach your forties. A loss of luster occurs because individual hair shafts begin to thin and dry as a result of hormonal changes. The replacement process for normal daily hair loss becomes slower, and new replacement hair is generally dryer, with less shine. Many women also note a thinning of pubic and underarm hair after menopause. Female baldness, a rare problem, may begin about age forty. See a dermatologist if hair loss persists.

Changes in hair texture and thickness can be minimized by avoiding over-styling. Good nutrition can also slow the brittleness of hair that comes with normal aging.

Bone strength is critical at all ages but particularly during and after menopause. As estrogen and progesterone levels fall drastically, the bones begin to lose mass. This causes them to become progressively more fragile. Backaches, common in midlife, may indicate the beginning of bone loss as a result of declining estrogen levels. These pains are localized, beginning in the lower back. Severe loss of bone becomes a condition called osteoporosis, which strikes at least half of all women age 50 and older. In fact, by the time a woman is 80, she may have lost 40 percent of her bone mass. Osteoporosis leaves a woman vulnerable to bone fractures, especially in the hip, spine, and wrist.

Teeth and the mouth are similarly affected. Dental problems that can occur around midlife, such as receding gums or loose teeth, may be related to declining levels of estrogen and a loss of bone mass. Gingivectomy, a procedure to repair the gums after periodontal disease, is a common oral surgery proce

MENOPAUSE: MYTHS AND REALITIES

Myth: *Menopausal women are unhappy and depressed.*

Reality: Most women cope very well with the physical challenges of menopause. Serious mental health problems do not increase. While some women may experience emotional distress, this is often related to sleep disturbance and deprivation due to hot flashes.

Myth: *All women going through menopause are plagued by hot flashes.*

Reality: About 80 percent of American women experience only mild symptoms, or none at all, during menopause. When hot flashes do occur, in most cases they are mild and disappear after a few months, rarely persisting for more than 2 or 3 years.

Myth: *Menopause is the end of your sex life.*

Reality: Libido, or sexual desire, does decline with aging, but many women continue to enjoy a satisfying sex life deep into old age. Some women find sex more enjoyable after menopause when concerns about pregnancy are past.

dure for women in midlife, especially for those prone to osteoporosis. Maintenance of your teeth and gums, including daily cleaning, and flossing, professional cleaning and regular checkups, will help reduce your risk of these dental problems.

"Classic" Menopausal Changes

Hot flashes, flushes, or night sweats are the most common characteristics of menopause. Some women experience a simple warming sensation throughout the body. Others feel acute flushes that begin with a sensation of pressure in the head similar to a headache, which then leads to a feeling of heat or burning in the face, neck, and chest, followed immediately by an outbreak of sweating. In most cases, hot flashes are mild and disappear after a year or two. But the frequency can vary from 1 or 2 a week to 1 or 2 per hour, and a few women experience them acutely for as long as 2 or 3 years.

The exact physiological cause of this upset in body temperature control is not yet known. Low estrogen levels alone are not responsible; it appears that estrogen must be present, and then withdrawn, for hot flashes to occur. The feeling may be precipitated by a hormonally induced imbalance in the body's temperature-control center, resulting in a drop in core body temperature and a subsequent attempt by the body to activate heat centers to re-adjust the body's "thermostat." (See the next chapter for a discussion of remedies.)

Short term memory loss has been cited as a problem by women in midlife, although this phenomenon has not been carefully documented and memory lapses have not as yet been linked to changing hormone levels during menopause. Forgetfulness may be related to stress or lack of sleep. Anecdotal reports suggest that memory problems in the perimenopausal period tend to disappear after menopause. If the problem persists, you should see your doctor.

Emotional issues loom large for many women during menopause, but contrary to previous conventional wisdom, studies now show that there is no increase in serious psychiatric disorders in women experiencing menopause. Minor emotional distress, however, may be a natural response to the changes a woman faces during this period.

Two changes in physical function that occur around the time of menopause may take a particularly heavy toll on a woman's psychological state. Hot flashes may keep you up at night, leading to chronic sleep deprivation which can reduce your mental and coping abilities. Vaginal changes that result in painful intercourse may interfere with your sexual pleasure and psychological health. There may also be other factors, currently unknown, that create coping challenges for women in the years immediately surrounding menopause.

Weight gain, while a common occurence around menopause, has not been shown to be directly related to hormonal changes. There is a natural redistribution of fat over the abdomen and hips. That may be due in part to changes in the endocrine system; but weight gain most likely results from reduced muscle tone, reduced physical activity, increased appetite and calorie intake, and other effects of the aging process. Increased physical activity and a nutritious, balanced diet, can minimize weight gain.

Heart Health

Women rarely die of heart disease before menopause because estrogen provides protection against it—partially by helping to keep cholesterol levels in check. For reasons not completely understood, there is a relationship between hormone levels and the development of the plaque-like substances inside the blood vessels that can cause blockage and lead to heart disease.

A women's risk of cardiovascular disease rises dramatically after menopause. Surgical menopause likewise increases the risk for heart disease, even in young women. In fact, the younger a woman is when her ovaries stop functioning, the greater her risk for heart attack and although women tend to worry more about breast cancer, heart disease is considerably more lethal — it is the number one killer of American women. One in seven women, ages 45 to 64, has some form of heart disease. This number increases to one in three over the age of 65.

Thus menopause itself is a risk factor for cardiovascular disease, along with high blood pressure, smoking, family history, poor diet, high blood cholesterol, diabetes, and obesity. Hormone replacement therapy (HRT) may help to promote cardiovascular health; but reducing the risk factors that are within your control can be equally important. Proper nutrition, regular exercise, maintaining your proper weight, and quitting smoking are key strategies for ensuring your cardiovascular health during midlife and beyond.

Bladder Control

Women in peri- and postmenopause may experience mild stress incontinence, defined as the loss of a little urine in response to sudden muscular stress, such as jogging, sneezing, coughing, laughing, or emotional distress. Many women also experience urge incontinence, the sensation that they need to urinate with great urgency, even though the bladder may be empty. These problems occur when declining estrogen levels cause cell deterioration and diminished muscle control in the urethra, bladder, and vagina.

Severe incontinence problems are rare and are not related to menopause. If incontinence goes beyond the mild form usually associated with menopause, you should see your doctor for proper diagnosis and treatment. (See the next chapter for exercises that help prevent or treat incontinence.)

Repeated urinary tract infections (UTIs), are also common in menopausal women. The deterioration of cells in the urinary tract produces an easily torn and bruised surface, creating an hospitable environment for the bacteria that cause UTI.

Mid-Life Medical Checkup

Most women will live many vital, useful, and enjoyable years after menopause. To stay healthy during this phase of life, preventive health measures and medical care are needed. When the signs of mid-life changes begin to appear, it's a good reminder to set up an appointment for a thorough medical checkup. A good relationship with a doctor who is aware of your health history and personality can give you an excellent resource to turn to when questions about menopausal signs and symptoms arise. □

CHAPTER 29

COPING WITH MENOPAUSE

Five Common Problems and Their Remedies

The effects of hormonal gyrations during the years surrounding menopause can be extremely powerful and disconcerting. This is especially true if a woman interprets the changes as signaling the "end of life" rather than a "change of life." Three or four generations ago menopause did signal the beginning of the end. In 1900, the average age of menopause was 46, and the life expectancy of women was 51. But today, most women can expect to live one-third of their lives after menopause. According to medical expert Dr. Leon Speroff, "the menopause should and can mark the beginning of a new and promising period of life, relatively free from previous obligations, ready for new career choices, more education, and new ventures."

Many of the upsets of the menopausal period can be regarded as temporary inconveniences that most women find they can manage quite well on their own. A good understanding of what is happening to your body and how other women cope with these changes can help with the adjustment. So

can an understanding doctor who can make recommendations tailored to your particular problems, health history, and life-style.

There is no totally "normal" menopause; each woman experiences this transition somewhat differently. A woman's final menstrual period commonly occurs between ages 45 and 55, but the process that leads up to menopause occurs gradually, easing the body's adjustment to shifting hormonal patterns. Women are affected in varying degrees by the uncomfortable symptoms that can accompany menopause, such as irregular menstrual cycles, hot flashes, disturbed sleep patterns, vaginal discomfort, and the emotional difficulties these problems can cause.

Some women barely notice the changes and experience no interruption in their daily routines, but about 60 percent of women approaching the age of menopause experience some symptoms due to biochemical changes taking place within. Symptoms often subside naturally as the menopausal years progress. Other women experience symptoms suddenly or very intensely, and seek medical relief for their debilitating effect.

This chapter focuses on the most common symptoms of the menopausal period and the non-pharmaceutical strategies that can relieve them. A discussion of pharmaceutical remedies can be found in the chapter on hormone replacement therapy.

Irregular Menstrual Cycles

A change in your menstrual pattern is usually the first sign of menopause. During the time referred to as perimenopause, which for some women can last as long as 5 or even 10 years, the menstrual cycle is likely to become less predictable. Some women notice changes as early as their late 30s.

Because the decline of ovarian function occurs gradually, only 10 to 15 percent of women experience an abrupt cessation of menstruation. During this time, women whose periods do stop abruptly are apt to get a pregnancy test. It's important to note that pregnancy can occur, even amidst irregular cycles, so to ensure greatest accuracy, a blood test is recommended over standard urine tests.

For most women the change is more gradual, with a steady decrease in both the amount and duration of menstrual flow, until it eventually ceases to occur. Typically, the transition takes about four years. During this time, it may become difficult to keep track of your menstrual cycles, with periods occurring late or early, cycles being skipped, and the flow becoming heavier or lighter than previously experienced. This unpredictability is usually the biggest inconvenience of irregular cycles.

Irregular and longer cycles occur as hormonal regulators become less reliable. As menopause nears, the periods become further apart and the flow becomes lighter. If menstruation doesn't occur for 6 months to a year, menopause probably has occurred. If you have vaginal bleeding after a prolonged lack of menses you should see your doctor; it could be a sign of disease.

More frequent or heavier bleeding may also be experienced during the menopausal years. This occurs when estrogen continues to stimulate the uterine lining, while production of the progesterone needed to counteract its growth declines. Thus, when the lining is shed, the flow is much heavier than usual. Cigarette smoking and excessive alcohol intake can make a woman more susceptible to heavy irregular bleeding.

Declining ovulation may also shorten the menstrual cycle, so that periods come so close together that you bleed throughout the month. A 7 to 10 day menstrual period is not uncommon and bleeding between periods may also occur. Any unusual menstrual patterns should be evaluated by your doctor, to make sure they are truly due to changing hormone levels, rather than such conditions as fibroid tumors, polyps, uterine cancer, or cervical cancer.

To Stay In Control

Once medical problems are ruled out, the challenge for a woman with unpredictable menstrual patterns is to find ways of decreasing the inconvenience.

One method is to keep track of your cycles with an ongoing written record. This allows you to notice overall patterns in a system that seems to have gone completely awry. It also provides you with a record to bring to your doctor for evaluation. Making quick notes on your calendar may make the process less tedious.

To keep a log, note the beginning and end of your cycle, the type of flow, and when any accompanying symptoms, such as cramps, sore breasts, or bloating, occur. Also note bleeding that occurs at any time other than the end of your monthly cycle.

Even women who keep a chart, however, may still be taken by surprise by unexpected menstruation. Many women in this predicament find it helpful to continue to keep some form of sanitary protection handy at home, and in their purse.

If heavy bleeding becomes an ongoing problem, discuss the condition with your doctor. Depending on your individual case and where you are in the menopausal process, possible medical remedies include low dose birth control pills to regularize the menstrual cycle and reduce bleeding; progesterone therapy to cause regular monthly shedding of the uterine lining; and hormone replacement therapy. If the bleeding is associated with uterine fibroids (benign tumors), your doctor may recommend surgical removal of either the fibroids or the entire uterus (hysterectomy).

Body Temperature: Hot Flashes, Hot Flushes

The most common symptom of the perimenopausal period is an upset in the body's thermostat that results in episodes of warmth and flushing. Although the hot flash or flush can cause discomfort, it does not in and of itself, present a health hazard and does not indicate disease.

Your first hot flash can be a startling experience. It may begin like a headache, with a pressure in the head, or as a sudden sensation of intense warmth. The "flash" increases in intensity until a feeling of heat or burning occurs in the face, neck, and chest. Your skin may redden and increase in temperature by as much as seven degrees. You may feel an urgent need to remove a sweater, jacket, or nightgown, and cool yourself by grabbing for a fan, throwing off covers, or standing by an open window. An outbreak of sweating, particularly affecting the upper body, may immediately follow the hot flash. Sweating cools down the skin temperature, causing the shivers. Less common symptoms which may accompany a hot flash include palpitations, weakness, fatigue, faintness and vertigo.

Hot flashes vary in frequency, intensity and duration. The average length of a hot flash is 4 minutes, though it can last from a moment to as long as 10 minutes. Frequency varies from 1 to 2 an hour to 1 to 2 a week.

Hot flashes trouble three-fourths of women experiencing natural or surgical menopause. However, only 10 to 15 percent of women find them debilitating. Eight out of 10 women who experience hot flashes get them for more than a year, but only 25 percent get them for more than 5 years. Hot flashes can occur as early as age 42. Heavier women tend to experience hot flashes less often, perhaps due to the estrogen produced in fatty tissue.

For some women, a hot flash is not unbearable and they easily go on with their daily routine. For others, it can be an intolerable disruption to their lives. The greatest problem the hot flash brings about is disturbed sleep patterns. A women experiencing regular hot flashes may wake several times, or even hourly, during the night. Some women wake up sweating profusely, in a phenomenon known as night sweats, and need to change the sheets or their night clothes.

Sleep deprivation affects people differently. A profound sleep disturbance may cause memory disorders or make concentration difficult. Some women feel anxiety, or suffer from fatigue or muscle aches. Lack of sleep can also cause a woman to cry easily and feel mentally and physically exhausted.

Coping With Hot Flashes

For the majority of women, hot-flash symptoms begin to subside within four to six years after their last menstrual period. Studies have shown that women who exercise are less likely to experience hot flashes. Among smokers, however, the incidence rises, probably due to the effect smoking has on the hormonal output of the ovaries.

Though there is no way to eliminate hot flashes short of drug therapy, many women develop ways to cope that help them get through the experience gracefully. For example, they learn not to wear turtlenecks or they switch from wool to cotton sweaters. Dressing in layers that can be quickly removed when feeling warm is also a good idea.

Embarrassment and concerns about what others are thinking is a common reaction. To allay your worries, you might ask a friend, or your spouse, to give you an accurate picture of how you look when experiencing a hot flash. As intense as it feels to you, close observers may not even realize that you appear slightly flushed and moist. If this is the case, ignoring the experience during a business meeting or other public event may be the best course.

On the other hand, if you perspire so profusely that it is obvious to others, you may want to plan what you will do if a hot flash strikes at an inconvenient time. It may be best to excuse yourself and head for the ladies' room, or to be prepared with a brief joke or explanation to ease yourself through the moment. With over 40 million American women set to experience menopause in the next 2 decades, public understanding of hot flashes is likely to expand. Though you may not be able to predict when the next one will occur, you can be prepared to react. Confidence, patience, self-assurance and a sense of humor will help ease the frustration.

Hot flashes lead more women to seek professional medical assistance than any other symptom of menopause. Estrogen therapy is the principal treatment eliminating hot flashes quickly and completely. Beneficial results include an end to the symptoms and thus relief from the constant awakening that can end in chronic sleep deprivation. Restored sleep patterns bring measurable improvements to memory, as well as decreased anxiety and irritability.

Other medications are also somewhat effective in reducing hot flashes. These include clonidine (Catapres TTS), and naloxone (Talwin NX, Narcan). If you cannot or do not wish to take hormone replacement therapy, ask your doctor about alternative medications. But be aware, that like all drugs, these can cause side-effects about which you should be informed.

Mood Swings

There is no increase in severe psychiatric illness in women during or after menopause. Indeed, depression is less —not more—common among middle-aged women.

Some psychological symptoms, however, do tend to occur around menopause. Emotional problems may arise in the period just preceding menopause, and decline one to two years into the postmenopausal period. It is unlikely that these symptoms are indeed related to changing hormonal levels. Fatigue, nervousness, headaches, insomnia, depression, irritability, joint and muscle pain, dizziness, and heart palpitations are among the symptoms women frequently report to their doctors.

Some emotional disturbances can be associated with the sleep deprivation that occurs as a result of hot flashes. Changing sexual patterns due to untreated vaginal atrophy can also be psychologically distressing for some women. Other changes at this point in life, such as children leaving home, career disappointments, or fear of aging, can also induce bouts of emotional turmoil.

The value of estrogen therapy for psychological complaints is not established, but a woman's outlook can often be improved simply by relief from hot flashes, insomnia, and vaginal atrophy.

Coping with Emotional Changes

Anticipating the physical and emotional changes likely to occur during menopause can help you get through this time with a minimum of friction and despair. Many women find that simply identifying the fact that they are in a bad mood or feeling irritable helps them and those around them adjust to a temporarily difficult situation. It also helps to distinguish trivial annoyances that get blown out of proportion because of moodiness from the real sources of anger and frustration. Some women call a "time out" when they are feeling out of sorts and delay any discussion of serious issues for another time. A chance to discuss emotional and physical symptoms with other women also undergoing menopause can provide support and comfort. Reading books and magazine articles about other women's menopausal reactions can also help.

After menopause, many women report what anthropologist Margaret Mead identified as "postmenopausal zest." This sense of well-being, hard-won individuality, and positive attitude toward life propels women into an especially rewarding period of their lives. So it can be comforting for women undergoing unpredictable mood swings to realize that there's something to look forward to a little further down the road.

Vaginal Discomfort

Because estrogen plays such a significant role in a woman's reproductive system, the decline in estrogen that accompanies menopause brings significant changes in all the reproductive organs. Some women begin to experience vaginal problems during perimenopause, but for most, it does not become a problem until five to ten years after menopause.

As a woman ages, lubrication of the vagina in response to sexual arousal, occurs more slowly. With the drop in estrogen the vaginal lining becomes thinner, drier and less elastic, and over time, the vagina shrinks. Burning and itching sensations may signal vaginal dryness which can be aggravated by reduced secretion of cervical mucus. All of these factors can cause pain or bleeding during intercourse, known medically as dyspareunia.

In addition, these changes make the vagina more vulnerable to injury because the tissues are more easily traumatized. This, in turn can increase the likelihood of local bacterial infection.

These difficulties can lead to a steep decline in sexual desire because of discomfort, embarrassment, or misinformation. However, for couples who adjust to the situation by using slower, gentler sexual techniques and vaginal lubricants, it need not be a problem. In fact, an active sexual life can help maintain vaginal health, as well as having a positive impact on a couple's self-esteem.

Coping with Vaginal Changes

The best way to combat vaginal dryness is to remain sexually active throughout life. Regular sex increases blood flow to the vagina, stimulating the mucous membrane and exercising the surrounding muscle. A study of postmenopausal women found that women who achieved orgasm by any means 3 or more times a month were less likely to suffer vaginal atrophy than those who had intercourse less then 10 times a year.

Using over-the-counter vaginal lubricants can make intercourse more comfortable. Water soluble lubricants such as K-Y Lubricating Jelly, or vaginal moisturizers such as Replens are recommended. Avoid oil-based lubricants, such as petroleum jelly or baby oil; because they are not easily cleaned away, they are a breeding ground for bacterial infection.

Hormone replacement therapy is also an effective cure for vaginal dryness. Estrogen cream applied locally also restores the lubricating capacity of the vagina. However, estrogen cream carries the same risks as oral or transdermal estrogen. (See chapter 31, "Hormone Replacement Therapy: Weighing the Pros and Cons.")

Treating vaginal dryness can keep it from devastating a woman's sex life. Sexual responsiveness reaches a peak for women in the late 30s and remains on a high plateau into the 60s. Some women even discover an increase in desire after menopause. They find sex more enjoyable without the fear of unwanted pregnancy and the interruptions caused by contraception and menstruation.

Preventing Bladder Problems

Lower estrogen levels also cause a loss of muscle tone and control in the bladder and urethra. When stress is put on the bladder—due to sneezing, coughing, laughing or jogging—a momentary loss of control can occur resulting in a small amount of leakage. Called urinary stress incontinence, this problem is more likely to occur in women who have had one or more children.

Urge incontinence can also be a problem for some women. It takes the form of a sudden overwhelming feeling of having to go to the bathroom even when the bladder contains very little urine. Whichever the type, urinary incontinence usually does not go beyond the mild condition associated with perimenopause. Nevertheless, it's important to see your doctor for an accurate diagnosis.

Kegel Exercises

Mild urinary stress incontinence is a temporary problem that can be controlled. Kegel exercises, named after the doctor who invented them, help to strengthen the pelvic floor, and are usually effective for those who do them diligently. This easy-to-do exercise can be done anywhere, without anyone being aware of it.

Locate your pelvic muscles by contracting the vaginal opening as if trying to stop the flow of urine. Hold the contraction for a count of three, relax and repeat. You may

AN END TO INCONTINENCE

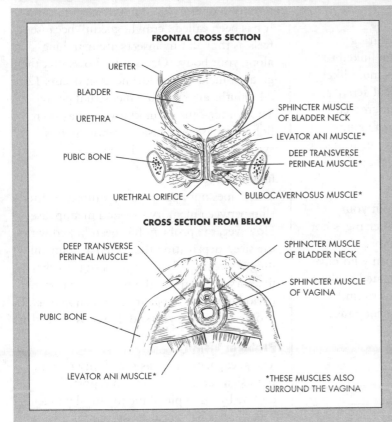

FRONTAL CROSS SECTION

URETER
BLADDER
URETHRA
PUBIC BONE
URETHRAL ORIFICE

SPHINCTER MUSCLE OF BLADDER NECK
LEVATOR ANI MUSCLE*
DEEP TRANSVERSE PERINEAL MUSCLE*
BULBOCAVERNOSUS MUSCLE*

CROSS SECTION FROM BELOW

DEEP TRANSVERSE PERINEAL MUSCLE*
PUBIC BONE
LEVATOR ANI MUSCLE*

SPHINCTER MUSCLE OF BLADDER NECK
SPHINCTER MUSCLE OF VAGINA

*THESE MUSCLES ALSO SURROUND THE VAGINA

The mild incontinence that sometimes comes with menopause is easily remedied—provided you're willing to stick to a daily routine of Kegel exercises. All you need do is clench the muscles surrounding your vagina for a count of three, relax, and repeat 10 times. You should do between 5 and 10 sets of this exercise each day.

not be able to maintain this squeeze, but with practice the muscles will get much stronger. Another method is to alternately contract and relax the muscles quickly. Repeat a series of 10 muscle contractions several times each day, for a total of 50 to 100 contractions.

Making these exercises part of your daily routine is probably all you need to restore bladder control. To help alleviate urge incontinence, delay trips to the bathroom as much as possible. This will aid in restraining reflex responses. Urge incontinence and mild stress incontinence are frequently eliminated by hormone replacement therapy.

Other Menopausal Symptoms

More than 50 symptoms have been blamed on the hormonal changes of the menopause. Because a proven link between these symptoms and declining estrogen levels has not been established, some believe that they have other origins. Symptoms that are thought to be clearly not a result of menopause are: weakness, fatigue, anorexia, nausea, vomiting, gas, constipation, and diarrhea.

Unexplained symptoms are often attributed to anxiety or other emotional imbalances, but much research is yet to be done. What follows summarizes the current thinking on symptoms women commonly ask about.

Weight Gain

Women do tend to gain weight during menopause, but this has not been linked to hormonal changes. The cause is more likely a combination of reduced physical activity, declining muscle tone, possibly increased caloric intake, and other effects of aging. Increased physical activity and a nutritious, balanced diet can minimize weight gain.

Breast Changes

If your breasts are sore throughout your cycle, it may be due to hormonal changes not unlike those in pregnancy, when breast tenderness is also a problem. Women who have experienced breast tenderness related to their menstrual cycle are often relieved to find that symptom disappears after menopause.

Itchy Skin

Some women experience a prickling, itching sensation on the skin, known as formication. It has been called "crawling skin" because it feels as though tiny insects are marching along your body. One study shows that the greatest incidence of formication occurs 12 to 24 months after the last menstrual period. Though the cause is unknown, it has been linked with menopause. Eventually this symptom disappears on its own.

Memory Loss

There does not appear to be a direct relationship between memory loss and menopause. However, the problem has been linked with the sleep deprivation that often accompanies "night sweats." Some reports suggest that memory problems in the perimenopausal period tend to disappear after menopause. If problems persist, you should see your doctor.

Problem Vision

Visual capacity, such as the ability to read road signs at night, has been reported to decline by a sample of menopausal women. This change has not been systematically studied, and can not as yet be directly linked to hormonal changes during menopause. □

CHAPTER 30

Holding Back Osteoporosis

People tend to think of their bones as an unshakable foundation—a strong and solid support system for the muscles and inner organs. However, our skeletal structure isn't solid at all, but composed of living, growing cells. Our bones depend on a dynamic balance of available minerals (such as calcium) and the hormones that control mineral absorption, to stay strong and healthy well into old age.

Osteoporosis, the condition that turns so many elderly women into smaller, shrunken, weakened versions of their former selves, is not inevitable. It is possible to grow older and still stand tall, walk confidently, retain strong bones, and enjoy a great deal of physical strength. Today, women can benefit from increasing medical knowledge about how to ward off this disease that weakens bone.

In fact, osteoporosis, the "silent thief" that robs us of bone strength, can often be prevented, or at least minimized, by simple improvements in nutrition and exercise before bone loss begins, generally around age 35. And even those already affected by severe bone loss, can take preventive measures to minimize the risk of disabilities.

Though 25 million Americans, mostly women, are affected by osteoporosis, surveys show that most (3 out of 4) women from ages 45 to 75 have never spoken to their doctor about the disease. This is a missed opportunity, because there is much you can do during and after menopause to protect yourself from this disease. This chapter outlines steps you can take to strengthen your bones and contribute to your better overall health and well–being as you get older.

The Framework: Understanding Bones

Bone cells, which store 99 percent of the calcium in our bodies, are continuously breaking down and building up, in a process called remodeling. The cells, which are interlaced with nerves and blood vessels, both collect calcium molecules from the bloodstream and release calcium back into

INSIDE A BRITTLE BONE

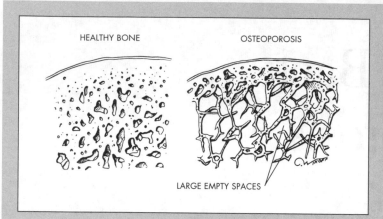

HEALTHY BONE   OSTEOPOROSIS

LARGE EMPTY SPACES

When the life-long process called bone remodeling slows, calcium leaches out faster than bone cells can restore it. The result is an increasingly porous skeletal structure given to tiny fractures you may never notice. As the disease progresses and bone density declines, major fractures of the hip, spine, or wrist become ever more likely.

circulation. The retained calcium adds to bone mass and keeps the skeleton strong.

As we age, the balance of retained versus lost calcium tends to tip in the wrong direction, with more calcium leaching out of our cells than is taken in. Losing a certain amount of bone mass is therefore a natural result of the aging process. However, after menopause, lower estrogen levels cause an accelerated rate of bone loss in most women, making them vulnerable to osteoporosis.

In osteoporosis, the bones become progressively more porous, making them more likely to break. Imagine osteoporatic bone as a honeycomb or Swiss cheese, and you can understand how the slightest trauma can cause debilitating bone fractures—typically occurring in the hip, spine, and wrist.

Since the loss of crucial bone mass usually occurs without symptoms or pain, osteoporosis can go undetected for years—until a fracture occurs. In young people, a broken bone usually heals itself in a month or two, but in old age, the process is slower and some fractures never fully heal.

A woman's lifetime risk of developing a hip fracture is equal to her combined risk of developing breast, uterine, and ovarian cancer. Hip fractures leave many women permanently disabled; and within 6 months following the injury, between 15 and 20 percent of patients will die because of a hip fracture and its complications. One in 3 women over 50 suffer vertebral fractures, which can lead to height loss and a stooped posture.

Hormones and Bone Strength

Our body balances the two processes of building new bone and removing old bone through the actions of a variety of hormones, including estrogen. Estrogen plays a dual role in bone metabolism: It facilitates the absorption of calcium from the blood into the bone and inhibits the loss of calcium from the bone. Bone density peaks in women about age 35. After this time, and especially when estrogen levels drop after menopause, bone loss exceeds new bone formation.

Normal estrogen levels help to ensure an adequate level of calcium in the blood, which, in turn, influences muscle and nervous-system functions. As estrogen levels decline, calcium blood levels can drop excessively, stimulating the production of another hormone called PTH. This hormone, which is secreted by the parathyroid gland, then triggers the leaching of calcium from the reservoir in the bones to correct the deficit in the blood, at the expense of bone health.

Bone loss accelerates after menopause, but varies considerably among individuals, for there is a wide variation in blood hormone levels among postmenopausal women. A woman can lose from one-half to 6 percent of her bone mass per year. This percentage may be even higher for women who experience surgical or chemically-induced menopause, in which the estrogen supply is abruptly cut down. By the time a woman is 80, she can easily have lost 40 percent of her bone mass. Once bone is lost it cannot be restored with tissue of equal strength or, as yet, be replaced.

Are You At Risk?

The risk of developing osteoporosis varies according to a number of factors, including sex, race, weight, and family history. People who enter midlife with light, thin bones have a smaller margin of bone mass that they can safely lose, and are therefore more vulnerable to bone disease.

Risk Factors You Cannot Control

Gender. Women generally have lighter, thinner bones than men. At age 35, men have 30 percent more bone mass than women, and they lose bone more slowly as they age. Because of the decrease in estrogen produc-

tion that occurs during menopause, just being a woman puts you in the high-risk group for developing osteoporosis.

Race. Caucasian and Asian women have lower bone density than blacks by as much as 5 to 10 percent. The lighter your complexion, the greater the risk for developing osteoporosis. Women with very fair skin, freckles, and blond or reddish hair are at the highest risk of all. Osteoporosis is less of a problem for African-Americans.

Build. Having a delicate frame or weaker bones predisposes you to a higher fracture risk. Overall muscle tone also plays a role in the likelihood of sustaining an injury.

Onset of Menopause. Undergoing early menopause, naturally or surgically, increases your risk, because you will have reduced levels of estrogen for a longer period of time than you would with normal menopause. Because of the abrupt cessation of estrogen production that accompanies surgical menopause, women whose ovaries are removed (69 percent in one study) tend to show signs of osteoporosis within 2 years after surgery if no hormone replacement therapy is instituted. When medically possible, doctors recommend keeping your ovaries intact in order to maintain estrogen production, even if a hysterectomy (removal of the uterus) is necessary.

Heredity. Having a mother, grandmother, or sister with a diagnosis of osteoporosis or its symptoms ("dowager's hump" or multiple fractures) increases your risk. Body type, as well as a possible genetic predisposition to osteoporosis, can be passed from one generation to the next.

Controllable Factors

Exercise. The amount of exercise you get has a major impact on bone strength and growth. Bones tend to lose mass from inactivity; on the other hand, the mechanical stress of exercise—especially weight–bearing exercise—such as jogging, walking, and tennis—has been shown to stimulate bone growth and improve strength.

Weight. Heavier women are at a smaller risk for osteoporosis since bone mass is positively affected by a slight excess of fat. Fat tissue converts other hormones to estrogen, even after menopause, and estrogen, as we know, aids with the absorption of calcium.

Childlessness. Never having children puts you at higher risk of bone loss because you won't experience the temporary surges of estrogen that accompany each pregnancy. These surges help to protect against osteoporosis later in life.

Calcium. Calcium is critical for building bones. You may have less bone mass than you should if you haven't been getting the recommended daily allowance of 1,200 milligrams per day throughout your life. Studies have shown that over 75 percent of American women get less than 800 milligrams of calcium a day; one out of four ingests less than 300 milligrams a day. For post-menopausal women, a high daily intake of 1,000 to 1,500 milligrams is recommended.

Smoking. Women who smoke generally experience menopause up to a year and a half earlier than nonsmokers, and thus face a longer period of estrogen deficiency and accompanying bone loss. Smoking also hampers efficient processing of calcium.

REMODELING IN PROGRESS

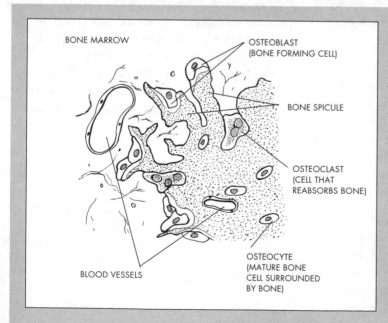

BONE MARROW

OSTEOBLAST
(BONE FORMING CELL)

BONE SPICULE

OSTEOCLAST
(CELL THAT
REABSORBS BONE)

BLOOD VESSELS

OSTEOCYTE
(MATURE BONE
CELL SURROUNDED
BY BONE)

Deep within the bones, an army of cells constantly tears down aging bone mass and builds it anew. Since estrogen fosters new growth, the reduced levels found in menopause can quickly lead to a reduction in bone density. Adequate supplies of calcium *throughout life* can alleviate the problem. After menopause, hormone replacement therapy can boost the bones' calcium absorption, preventing osteoporosis in three-quarters of the women at risk.

HIDDEN FRACTURES PLAGUE ONE WOMAN IN THREE

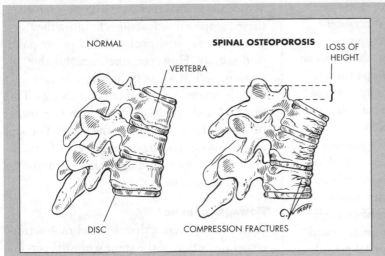

NORMAL   **SPINAL OSTEOPOROSIS**   LOSS OF HEIGHT

VERTEBRA

DISC   COMPRESSION FRACTURES

A persistent low backache, or sudden localized pain, could be a warning sign of compression fractures in the vertebrae of the spine. But for many, these breaks cause little pain, and may go undetected for years. For some, the only tip-off is a noticeable loss of height, which can reach as much as 8 inches.

Smokers have a higher rate of vertebral fractures than nonsmokers.

Alcohol. Consuming more than two alcoholic drinks daily can decrease calcium absorption. It also interferes with the vitamin D synthesis that helps the bones absorb calcium.

Medical Factors

Lactose Intolerance. This problem is caused by the deficiency of the enzyme, lactase, which aids in the digestion of milk products. Less milk means less calcium. Sixty percent of women with osteoporosis (but only 15 percent of the general population) are lactose intolerant.

Medications. Commonly prescribed steroids like cortisone and prednisone, thyroid for hypothyroidism, and phenobarbital or phenytoin (Dilantin) for seizures all interfere with the body's ability to absorb calcium from food or calcium supplements.

Medical Conditions. Women with anorexia, Celiac disease, (an intolerance of certain grain products), diabetes, chronic diarrhea, kidney, or liver disease are all more likely to develop osteoporosis.

Warning Signs of Osteoporosis

Loss of bone mass produces minimal symptoms, while it quietly eats away skeletal strength, making bones more susceptible to fracture. For some women, a fracture may therefore be the first outward sign of osteoporosis. A broken bone as the result of a minor jolt, such as a wrist fracture following a simple fall, is a good reason to suspect the development of osteoporosis. An x-ray of the fracture can confirm the extent to which the break was caused by deterioration of the bone. Fortunately, for many women there are other, less dramatic signs to watch for.

Backache

Because the vertebrae are the most common site of fracture in osteoporotic women, an early symptom of the disease is a persistent backache in the lower part of the spine. Sudden muscle spasms or pain in the back can occur while you are resting or doing routine daily tasks. This sudden pain is often caused by the spontaneous collapse of small sections of the spine that have been severely thinned or weakened over time. Unlike back pain due to other causes, this pain is localized and seldom spreads. Seeking treatment from an orthopedic specialist or gynecologist is important. Those who develop osteoporosis often begin to notice more severe backaches about 9 and a half years after their last menstrual period or 13 years after surgical menopause.

Height Loss

Spinal osteoporosis is rarely diagnosed until spinal bones have broken. These breaks occur at the weakest points of the spinal column—places where the spine naturally curves. Women are often unaware that they have these compression fractures because they don't always cause prolonged or severe pain, or disability. However, one unmistakable warning sign is a loss of height, which is directly related to spinal crush fractures. This loss of 2-and-a-half up to as much as 8 inches occurs in the upper half of the body. You can and should watch for development of spinal osteoporosis by routinely measuring and recording your height.

"Dowager's Hump"

With a loss of height due to vertebral fractures comes distortion of the spine's normal curves. This can lead to the development of a "dowager's hump"—a protrusion in the upper back and a shortening of the chest area, that leaves the ribs practically sitting on the pelvic region. One consequence is more difficulty in

NO NEED FOR "DOWAGER'S HUMP"

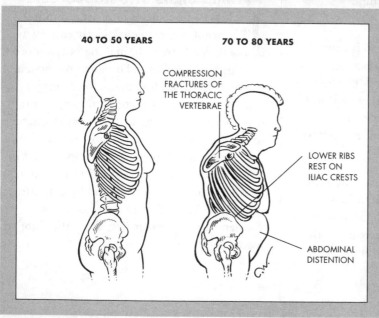

40 TO 50 YEARS

70 TO 80 YEARS

COMPRESSION FRACTURES OF THE THORACIC VERTEBRAE

LOWER RIBS REST ON ILIAC CRESTS

ABDOMINAL DISTENTION

This unbecoming distortion of the spine is a direct result of osteoporosis and the spinal fractures that accompany it. Take measures to prevent osteoporosis now and you'll avoid this development in your later years.

digesting food. Another is the impact on your appearance and self–esteem. This hunchback–like appearance is not a natural part of growing older or the result of poor posture; it is a clear indication of osteoporosis.

Tooth Loss

Tooth loss during midlife and the thinning of bones supporting the teeth is another indication of osteoporosis. The loss of tooth–bearing bone, called periodontal disease, is common among osteoporotic women. This bone thinning may be detected early by dental x–rays. To prevent periodontal disease, menopausal women should take extra care with their dental hygiene. This includes regular checkups and cleanings, brushing, and daily cleaning with dental floss or a Water Pik to retrieve food particles below the gum line.

Detecting Osteoporosis: Bone Density Screening

If you are at high risk for developing osteoporosis, or if you have already seen the early warning signs, discuss an evaluation of your skeletal health with your doctor. Ordinary x–rays do not detect osteoporosis until at least 30 percent of the bone is already lost and the disease has progressed much further than is healthy. But sophisticated technology is now available for earlier detection of bone loss, when it can still be stopped or perhaps reversed.

Several different methods of bone screening exist, all of which are painless, involve low–dose x–ray procedures, and range in cost from $75 to $250. Make sure you use a facil-

ity that does bone density testing on a regular basis. Most large hospitals have the necessary equipment, and some even have special osteoporosis centers.

The most popular and accurate test to date is dual–photon absorptiometry (DPA), which scans the entire body. The test takes about 20 to 40 minutes, with a 5 mrem dose of radiation (a full dental x–ray is 300 mrem). Single–photon absorptiometry (SPA) scans are quicker and less expensive—taking less than 15 minutes and costing less than 100 dollars—but they only measure bone density in the arm and heel, which is not particularly helpful in predicting vertebral or hip fractures. Be sure to discuss your test results with a qualified medical professional.

If you already have osteoporosis, bone density screenings can help you monitor your condition. Another approach to bone density screenings is to establish a baseline DPA bone mass measurement just before you reach menopause, and then get periodic tests to see how your bones are changing. The medical community is not in agreement with baseline DPAs, and most insurance carriers will only cover the cost of SPA testing. However, with the possibility that increasingly sophisticated methods of bone testing will be developed, screening for menopausal women may become more routine.

Preventing Osteoporosis

While the effects of osteoporosis are most often seen in later life, your risk is determined by your level of bone mass at age 35. For this reason, it is important to build bone to its peak density prior to menopause. It is essential for young women to be aware of risk factors and to take steps to slow bone loss and improve bone remodeling. However, women in their

CALCIUM RICH FOODS: A SAMPLER

Food	Portion	Calories	Calcium (mg.)
Cream of Wheat, Instant	1 cup, cooked	130	185
Cheese			
American	1 ounce	107	195
Cottage	1 cup	239	211
Swiss	1 ounce	104	259
Milk			
Skim	1 cup	89	303
Whole, fat 3.5%	1 cup	159	288
Yogurt from skim milk	1 cup	127	452
Fish			
Flounder	3 ounces	61	55
Sardines, canned	8 medium	311	354
Scallops, cooked	3 1/2 ounces	112	115
Fruit			
Orange	1 medium	73	62
Figs, dried	5 medium	274	126
Vegetables			
Broccoli, raw	1 stalk	32	103
Broccoli, cooked	2/3 cup	26	88
Collards, cooked	1/2 cup	29	152
Parsley, raw	3 1/2 ounces	44	203
Watercress, raw	3 1/2 ounces	19	151

50s and 60s can also benefit by taking immediate anti–osteoporosis action. These steps focus on diet and exercise.

Calcium

Calcium, the primary component of bone tissue, is the key factor in maintaining bone strength. But if you diet, fast, or habitually eat little, your daily calcium requirements are probably not being met. In addition, excess consumption of protein, sodium, sugar, alcohol, and caffeine has been shown to decrease absorption of calcium from your diet. And a certain amount of calcium is lost naturally each day through excretion. Since your body needs calcium to function, it tries to compensate for all of these deficits by taking calcium from your bones.

This situation is further complicated as a woman reaches menopause. Since estrogen increases the absorption of calcium into your system, lower estrogen levels generally mean you need to take in more calcium. Your body *will absorb calcium without estrogen—but only at a lower rate.*

Calcium needs vary according to unique requirements, but the bottom line is: To build bone mass, you need calcium. Studies have shown that women consume less than half of the calcium they need, pre-, peri-, and post-menopause. For a woman in her twenties, 650 milligrams of calcium may be adequate. But by menopause, most women need to ingest about 1,000 milligrams of calcium a day in order to prevent a loss of bone mass. Women in their 40s should consume 1,000 to 1,500 milligrams of calcium every day. After menopause, 1,500 milligrams daily is suggested for women who are not on hormone replacement therapy. Because your body can absorb only about 600 milligrams of calcium at a time, it is advisable to consume calcium–rich foods at separate sittings.

Ideally, calcium should come from a natural diet. Devising a plan to promote adequate calcium levels includes making calcium–rich foods—such as dairy products, nuts, leafy greens, broccoli, rhubarb, salmon, sardines—a regular part of your diet. Skim milk is just as valuable to your bones as high–fat whole milk.

Women who are lactose intolerant should consider using LactAid, which supplies the enzyme needed for proper digestion of milk products. Calcium–rich yogurt is another alternative because it is easier to digest than other dairy products.

Analyze your diet to learn how much calcium you are actually getting each day. Using the nearby chart can help you become more aware of calcium content in food, and aid you in shifting slowly to a new nutritional program.

Calcium supplements are recommended if you or your doctor feel your calcium needs are not being met through your diet. The recommended amounts are the same for dietary calcium: 1,000 to 1,500 milligrams of elemental calcium daily for women in their 40s, and 1,500 milligrams. for postmenopausal women not on hormone replacement therapy. Don't overdo it. Excessive calcium can create other problems in the body, such as promoting kidney stones and hardening of the arteries.

The most important point about supplements is absorption. To be properly absorbed calcium supplements must dissolve quickly in the stomach. Yet in recent studies about half of the pills on the market failed to dissolve fast enough. You can test your brand of choice at home. Drop a tablet into a container with 2 to 4 ounces of vinegar, stirring twice. After 30 minutes the pill should have completely dissolved or disintegrated into fine particles. If not, change brands.

Calcium citrate is the preferred formulation of many doctors because it is easily absorbed (especially by older women who make less gastric hydrochloric acid), and does not need to be taken with meals. To ensure best absorption, calcium should be taken in two daily doses, preferably at breakfast and dinner. Also, for some women calcium needs to be accompanied by daily doses of vitamin D (see below) or it is likely to go unabsorbed.

Antacids have become a newly touted source of calcium. However, with alternatives like calcium–rich food and pure calcium supplements, there's reason to wonder why anyone would choose antacid tablets as a major source of calcium. Though antacids may be less expensive than supplements, many contain aluminum, which can actually cause your body to lose calcium. (Two popular brands, Tums and Titralac, are aluminum–free, however.)

If you need to take an antacid for its intended purpose, there's nothing wrong with taking one that contains calcium. However, taking antacids solely for their calcium content is not recommended. Taken five to six times a week, they may be harmless; but in excessive amounts they can cause constipation and may lead to the formation of kidney stones and other urinary problems. In addition, certain pre–existing medical conditions can be aggravated by antacids, including colitis, stomach or intestinal bleeding, irregular heartbeat, and kidney disease.

Other Vitamins and Minerals

Vitamin D is essential to ensure adequate supplies of calcium in your body because it not only helps the body absorb calcium but also promotes its uptake into the bone. But very few foods in our diet are rich in vitamin D so you may be at risk of a deficiency. It's important to monitor your intake of this crucial vitamin, or the efforts you make to get adequate supplies of calcium may be futile.

The recommended daily dose of Vitamin D is 400 international units (IU). If you do opt to get your daily dose from supplements, be aware that amounts *over* 1,000 IU a day can interfere with calcium absorption. Also, because vitamin D is stored in the body for long periods of time, megadoses can be toxic.

Most women need supplements of no more than 400 IU daily—and only during winter in cloudy regions at that. For women over 65 years of age, supplements of 800 IU per day are usually the most that's recommended.

Vitamin D is present in such foods as egg yolk, certain fish, fish liver, and butter. Fortunately, it is also added to milk, bread, cereals, and other foods. An 8 ounce glass of milk contains 100 IU of vitamin D. Exposure to sunshine for about 15 minutes a day can also trigger the body's formation of needed vitamin D.

Magnesium is an important mineral for strong teeth and bones because it helps your body utilize calcium and vitamin D. Physicians agree that your daily magnesium dosage should be at least half the amount of calcium you consume on a daily basis—for example, 600 milligrams of magnesium to 1,200 milligrams of calcium. Provided you eat a balanced diet, however, your chances of having a magnesium deficiency are very low.

Phosphorus is a mineral necessary to metabolize calcium, and should be consumed in amounts equal to your calcium intake. However, most Americans get too much phosphorus by eating excessive quantities of red meat, white bread, processed cheese, and soft drinks. Excess phosphorus, like excess vitamin D, actually accelerates bone demineralization and increases urinary calcium levels. To keep your phosphorous level in line, avoid consuming large quantities of foods labeled as containing sodium phosphate, potassium phosphate, phosphoric acid, pyrophosphate, or polyphosphate.

Exercise and Posture

Physical activity affects bone strength because bone mass increases or decreases in response to the demands placed on it. Developing and maintaining good exercise habits can significantly reduce your risk of age–related bone fracture. Women who work out regularly have a bone density that is often 10 percent higher than that of women who do not. Research also shows that just 3 hours a week of weight–bearing exercise can decrease bone loss by as much as 75 percent. In addition, exercise increases muscle tone and mass, which serves to cushion and support bones and makes falls due to unsteadiness less likely.

Weight bearing exercises, which work the muscles against gravity, are the key to creating positive stress on your bones. These exercises includes jogging, aerobics, dancing, and tennis. Walking is also an excellent way to strengthen the back, legs, and stomach muscles. Though swimming and biking provide less positive bone stress, these exercises do help to increase muscle tone.

Just as exercise has profound effects on the strength of bone, the way you sit and stand everyday affects the way your bones shape themselves. If you slouch, your bones will grow to conform to that curvature. If you sit and stand with an erect posture, your bones will have a tendency to grow straight.

Hormone Replacement Therapy

Long term Hormone Replacement Therapy (HRT) after the onset of menopause improves calcium absorption and has been shown to prevent osteoporosis in 75 to 80 percent of women. It is especially effective in women with chemically or surgically induced menopause. HRT is usually continued for 8 to 10 years or more after menopause, the time when women experience bone loss at an accelerated rate. In order for HRT to be fully effective, a woman's calcium, vitamin D, and magnesium intake should be at recommended levels.

The medical community is still debating the best dosage and length of time for HRT. To make an informed decision about whether you should consider this therapy, see the next chapter.

Coping with Osteoporosis

Once osteoporosis has been diagnosed, treatment usually consists of vitamin D, adequate calcium intake, and perhaps estrogen supplements. Current scientific research is evaluating other approaches such as calcitonin injections and sodium–fluoride treatments.

If you already have osteoporosis, your doctor is also likely to advise appropriate exercise regimens that strengthen, but do not fracture, the bones. Exercise will not cure osteoporosis, but it can help you preserve the bone mass you do have, strengthen your back and hips, maintain flexibility, and steady your gait. Within only 6 months, a regular exercise program can reduce your risk of bone fractures. The best program is one you can continue on a regular basis.

In addition to specific treatment programs, you may need to make other adjustments in your daily life to reduce your risk of sustaining an injury. The following recommendations are made by the National Osteoporosis Foundation:

- Wear sturdy, low–heeled, soft–soled shoes; avoid floppy slippers and sandals.
- Ask your doctor whether any medications you are taking can cause dizziness, light–headedness, or loss of balance. If so, is there anything you can do to minimize these side effects.
- Minimize clutter throughout the house.
- Secure all rugs; avoid using small throw rugs that can slip and slide.
- Remove all loose wires and electrical cords that can cause tripping.
- Make sure treads and handrails are installed on staircases and remain secure.
- Keep halls, stairs and entries well lighted.
- Use nightlights in the bedroom and bath.
- In the bathroom, use grab bars and nonskid tape in the shower or tub.
- In the kitchen, use nonskid rubber mats near the sink and stove.
- Avoid using slippery waxes; watch out for wet floors; clean up spills immediately.
- When driving, wear seat belts and adjust seat properly. □

CHAPTER 31

Hormone Replacement Therapy: Weighing the Pros and Cons

Whether or not to undergo hormone replacement therapy (HRT) may be one of the most difficult decisions facing a woman at mid–life. The medical community itself is divided on the issue. Some experts recommend hormone treatments for all menopausal women who have no outright reason to avoid it; others are opposed to the treatment for most women. Many doctors cautiously recommended hormone therapy for some, but not all, women.

The question of whether hormone therapy is right for you cannot be answered with a simple yes or no. The decision should be influenced by a number of factors, including:

- The severity of the immediate physical symptoms caused by declining hormonal levels.
- Your individual risk for osteoporosis and heart disease.
- Your individual risk for cancers of the breast and reproductive system.

The attempt to balance short– and long–term health concerns against HRT's potential risks has been a source of great uncertainty for many women. In fact, one survey found that one–third of the women who are given prescriptions for hormones don't bother to fill them. Rather than avoiding the issue, or staying in the dark about hormone replacement therapy, each woman needs to know the full range of both the benefits and risks. The goal of this chapter is to help you make an informed decision based on your individual needs.

The Controversy

In the 1950s and 1960s, doctors enthusiastically prescribed estrogen to relieve menopausal symptoms. The drug was promoted by many doctors and the popular media as a "fountain of youth" that would slow the aging process and make women feel more attractive. By 1975, estrogen was one of the top five prescription drugs in the United States.

Then, in the mid–seventies, the darker side of estrogen replacement therapy came to view. Estrogen use was linked to a four– to

WHO SHOULD CONSIDER HRT?

Hormone therapy maybe helpful to you if you:

- Have non–functioning ovaries
- Have had both ovaries surgically removed
- Begin to experience symptoms of early menopause before you are 45
- Experience extreme menopausal discomfort
- Are at a high risk of osteoporosis
- Are at a high risk of cardiovascular disease

Hormone therapy should be avoided if you:

- Are pregnant
- Have a family history of or have had uterine, or ovarian cancer (perhaps breast cancer, too)
- Have large fibroids, or benign uterine tumors
- Have venous thrombosis, or blood clotting problems
- Have gall bladder or liver disease

ten–fold increase in the risk of endometrial cancer (cancer of the uterine lining). A panic spread among many users, and after 1976 the use of estrogen declined. In response, doctors cut the standard dose of estrogen in half. Soon they learned that the risk of uterine cancer could be dramatically cut or even eliminated by combining estrogen with progestin, a synthetic form of the female hormone progesterone.

Today, lower dosages and combination therapy have become the norm. However, despite these modifications, HRT remains controversial, with opposing views on menopause fueling the dispute. Some scientists view the changes that occur in a woman's body in midlife as the onset of a "hormone deficiency disease." Noting the many ways that a lack of estrogen has a negative, aging effect on the body, they encourage women to replenish their body's supply of reproductive hormones for the rest of their lives, if possible. Thus, hormone therapy is urged not only as treatment for symptoms in the short–term, such as hot flashes or vaginal dryness, but recommended as a long–term preventive measure against heart disease and osteoporosis.

And, indeed, the evidence is piling up that, for a significant percentage of women, the hormonal changes brought by menopause do contribute to chronic disease and early death. In 1991, a Food and Drug Administration committee recommended that hormone therapy be made available to "virtually all" postmenopausal women, except those for whom it is clearly a danger.

Those who oppose hormone replacement therapy criticize the "medicalization" of menopause—that is, the tendency to view the changes at mid–life as a disease that automatically requires medication, rather than a natural life process. They question whether hormone therapy—especially the use of progestin in combination with estrogen—should be prescribed as a long–term preventive measure before there are enough long–term clinical trials to fully guarantee its safety and effectiveness. In addition, some object to the routine prescribing of hormones for healthy women because of the known risks associated with the treatment.

Women's health groups also fear that the marketing of long–term hormone therapy to doctors by pharmaceutical companies, combined with these companies' financial domination of hormone research, has restricted the scope of public discussion. Still, currently ongoing studies, discussed later in this chapter, should yield definitive findings on the benefits and risks of hormone therapy. Some women have also accused the male medical establishment of promoting the use of hormones to keep women "younger." However, HRT advocates aren't necessarily men. A 1989 study from Massachusetts General Hospital in Boston found that female doctors are 19 times more likely than their male counterparts to prescribe HRT (though the ratio dropped to 50/50 among male and female *gynecologists.*)

Although HRT usage is on the increase, the majority of postmenopausal women still do not take hormones. Hormonal changes are a normal part of mid–life, and many women experience menopause with few discomforts. For those who do experience intense, unpleasant symptoms during menopause, however, hormone replacement therapy can bring effective relief.

The Basics

The main role of estrogen is to control the functioning of the reproductive organs, though researchers have found estrogen receptors—which are taken as evidence of estrogen sensitivity—in the brain, liver, skin, bone, fat, muscle, and blood vessels. At menopause, a woman's estrogen levels decline dramatically.

Estrogen replacement therapy (ERT) is a medical treatment in which a woman's estrogen level is artificially increased, restoring premenopausal levels on a short– or long–term basis. HRT refers to a treatment that combines both estrogen and a progestin, a form of the hormone progesterone. Developed to sever the link between ERT and endometrial cancer, HRT is not needed if you have had your uterus removed by a hysterectomy.

No one form of estrogen is better than another. The method, dose, and presence or absence of a progestin are the main variables in hormone therapy, rather than which type of estrogen is administered.

Available Methods

Hormone Pills are the most often prescribed and easiest way of taking HRT. The benefit of this method is that when estrogen in pill form is processed by the liver (where cholesterol is produced), it more readily increases the level of high–density lipoproteins (HDL), the "good" cholesterol, than do some other methods. However, the hormone can be changed when processed in the liver, resulting in unwanted side effects if the dose proves too high.

Injections are one way of bypassing the liver. With this method, you receive hormone shots directly into the muscle. The drawback is that injections fail to maintain steady blood levels of the hormone; initially high levels decrease over time. Because shots can be spaced no more than a month apart, this method imposes the cost and inconvenience of frequent visits to the doctor, plus the need for regular monitoring of hormone levels in the blood.

An estrogen–filled patch, usually placed on the buttocks or upper arm, feeds hormones directly into the bloodstream, again bypassing the liver. Each patch lasts several days. Unfortunately, this method does not seem to have the same beneficial effects on HDL levels as estrogen taken orally.

Implants—pellets surgically placed under the skin twice a year—were popular in the 1960s and 1970s. But because of a cumulative effect, after several years, estrogen levels in the blood were shown to rise as much as 2 to 3 times higher than those obtained from the standard oral dose. Because hormone levels delivered by implants cannot be easily adjusted, most doctors now view them as outdated. In addition, insertion can be uncomfortable and result in infection. If you do choose implants, your estrogen blood levels should be monitored regularly.

Creams containing estrogen and progestin can be applied directly to the skin—usually over the abdomen, arms or thighs. This method also bypasses the liver, eliminating the possibility of high–dose side effects generated by liver metabolism. Creams allow for balanced treatment because a specific dose is administered daily; but applications can be messy, and you can inadvertently apply an improper amount. Like implants, creams can produce higher blood levels of estrogen than standard oral regimens so your blood estrogen levels should be monitored if you opt for this method.

Vaginal creams containing estrogen can be helpful for women who have only vaginal menopausal symptoms, such as dryness, itching, or painful intercourse. Contrary to common belief, estrogen *does* enter the bloodstream when applied vaginally, so the same risks and benefits apply to this method as for other forms of estrogen.

Dosage

The most common prescription for menopause is an oral dose of 0.625 milligram of conjugated estrogens—a combination of naturally occurring estrogens—taken with 5 milligrams of the progestin medroxyprogesterone acetate. This usual prescription contains about one–sixth the amount of estrogen and progestin found in birth control pills.

Discuss with your physician whether lower or higher doses of hormones may be right for you. Some women use low dose HRT, such as 0.3 milligram of estrogen rather than the standard 0.625, and 2.5 milligrams of progestin instead of 5 milligrams. Doses as low as 0.3 milligram of estrogen may relieve symptoms, but may also offer little or no protection against osteoporosis or heart disease. Thus, lower doses may be appropriate for a woman who is not at high risk for heart disease or osteoporosis, but who does suffer from menopausal symptoms such as hot flashes.

Regimen

Combined therapy. A common sequential regimen for oral administration is a daily dose of estrogen with a daily dose of progestin added for the first 14 days of the month. Another sequential regimen is a dose of estrogen for the first 25 days of each month with progestin taken during days 15 to 25. (This regimen is losing favor, however, because it's difficult to keep track of the doses.)

These regimens can result in side effects such as breast tenderness, bloating, fluid retention, and depression. In addition, menstrual bleeding occurs in 80 to 90 percent of women on a sequential regimen when the progestin is withdrawn. Lowering the dose of progestin usually remedies these symptoms, but the lowest effective progestin dose required to offset the risk of uterine cancer in sequential regimens has not been established.

A continuous, daily regimen, as opposed to traditional sequential treatment, allows the use of lower doses of progestin. Thus, progestin–induced side effects, such as bleeding, tend to improve with continuous therapy. However, even in a continuous regimen, 40 to

60 percent of patients still experience some bleeding during the first six months of treatment. Since no method of drug alteration has been found to prevent this bleeding, the only approach is to wait it out. Though the bleeding will usually cease over time, some women find its irregularity difficult to manage. Some opt to return to a sequential program, where withdrawal bleeding occurs predictably each month.

Estrogen–only treatment. A woman can safely take estrogen "unopposed," that is, without the addition of progestin, if she has had her uterus removed. However, many women who cannot tolerate treatment with progestin because of adverse side effects such as menstrual–like bleeding, mood swings, and bloating also opt for unopposed estrogen. When there is no progestin to offset the uterine cancer risk of estrogen alone, doctors recommend an annual endometrial biopsy.

The Benefits of HRT

Despite the ongoing controversy, HRT is still widely prescribed because there do appear to be clinically proven benefits: protection against osteoporosis and heart disease, and relief of menopausal symptoms.

Preventing Osteoporosis

Bone loss, which begins naturally around age 35, accelerates dramatically at menopause. The prevention of osteoporosis, the progressive thinning of bone, is one major reason why women are advised to take long–term hormone or estrogen therapy (see the preceding chapter). Hormone therapy's effectiveness in preventing bone loss is firmly established. In numerous studies, postmenopausal women who have undergone some form of hormone therapy—either estrogen alone or estrogen with progestin—for at least a decade, show significantly less bone loss than women who have not. For women with a high risk of osteoporosis, hormone replacement therapy provides a clear benefit and could be lifesaving.

Contrary to popular belief, hormone or estrogen therapy is not useless if you have already developed osteoporosis. Although calcium supplements, proper nutrition, and exercise can help preserve bone mass, estrogen can effectively halt and even reverse the degenerative process of osteoporosis. The treatment can be started at almost any point after menopause. Continued hormone treatment is needed in order to sustain its preventive effects against bone deterioration. Once the therapy is stopped, postmenopausal bone loss resumes. Since osteoporosis–induced fractures are most likely in women aged 75 to 80, this can translate into decades of preventative hormone therapy.

Preventing Heart Disease

The mechanisms by which estrogen protects the heart are not fully understood, but one significant contribution is its capacity for improving a woman's metabolism of fats and cholesterol. Estrogen's protective effect comes from its ability to raise the "good" high–density (HDL) cholesterol associated with a reduced risk of heart disease, while also decreasing low–density (LDL) cholesterol or "bad" cholesterol. For this reason, a woman's risk of heart disease is lower than that of men the same age until shortly after she passes menopause. Eventually risk levels even out, but nonetheless, 40 percent of a woman's greater life expectancy can be attributed to early protection from heart disease.

With the declining estrogen levels that accompany menopause, the risk of heart disease doubles for women as HDL cholesterol declines and LDL cholesterol increases. While very few premenopausal women are affected by cardiovascular disease, it has now become the number–one killer of women over the age of 50 in the United States. (See chapter 12, "Heart Disease: The Greatest Threat of All.")

Within the last few years, doctors have begun advising long–term hormone replacement therapy as a heart disease preventive, especially for those women at high risk of the disease. The ongoing Nurses' Health Study, coordinated by Harvard University, has followed 48,470 postmenopausal women with no previous heart disease and found that those who take estrogen have 50 percent fewer heart attacks than those who do not, and the death rate from cardiovascular disease is about 50 percent less. Although these results are impressive, other variables may be involved. Women who take estrogen therapy tend to be healthier, and therefore at a lower risk of heart disease, anyway. Better diet and health care among women on hormone replacement therapy also may contribute, to some extent, to the lower death rate.

Though an overwhelming majority of studies have now shown that estrogen therapy significantly reduces a post-menopausal woman's risk of heart disease, it's still not clear how heart disease risk is affected when a woman takes progestin as part of her treatment. Short–term studies indicate that by increasing the levels of the "bad" LDL cholesterol, the progestins blunt—but do not negate—estrogen's beneficial effect on the heart. But because the impact of progestin is influenced by dose and duration of the hormonal therapy, long–term studies are needed.

As a preventative measure, long–term hormone therapy has proven its value against heart disease and osteoporosis. However it's misleading to suggest that taking HRT works as a quick fix for such voluntary risk–taking as cigarette smoking, heavy drinking, poor diet, or lack of exercise, all of which contribute to both heart disease and osteoporosis. In fact, 60 to 70 percent of the decrease in mortality from heart disease that has occurred over the last three decades in the United States can be directly attributed to preventative health strategies, such as giving up smoking, reducing blood pressure, and lowering cholesterol.

Relief of Menopausal Symptoms

Temporary hormone replacement therapy can reduce or eliminate many of the uncomfortable symptoms of menopause. Some women find relief by taking HRT for a year or two, and have no menopausal symptoms when the hormones are stopped. If your symptoms do recur, as they do for some women, your doctor may then recommend long–term treatment.

Hot flashes. About 75 percent of women entering menopause experience hot flashes—a sudden reddening of the skin on the upper body and face accompanied by a feeling of intense heat and often by profuse perspiration. These frequent and unpredictable episodes may awaken you at night, causing sleep deprivation. In most women, hot flashes occur for a year or two after the onset of menopause; but in 25 to 50 percent of women, they continue for more than 5 years. Although the physiology of the hot flash is still not understood, its correlation with lower levels of estrogen following menopause has been clearly established. Most women find relief from hot flashes with hormone therapy.

Alternative treatments, such as drug therapy with the clonidine patch (Catapres–TTS), are designed to target hot flashes specifically, though they offer less effective relief than hormone therapy. Their advantage is that, unlike hormone therapy, they do not affect your entire body chemistry. If controlling hot flashes is your main concern, discuss treatment options with your physician.

Vaginal atrophy. Because low estrogen production brings a loss of elasticity in the skin, many postmenopausal women experience atrophic changes of the vagina—a loss of muscle tone and strength in the vaginal wall. Vaginal dryness, which can result in burning, itching, and painful intercourse, can be remedied with postmenopausal hormone therapy. Recurrent urinary tract infections that result from abrasions due to vaginal dryness are also effectively prevented with hormone treatment.

Some women get significant relief in a month, but therapy can take 6 to 12 months, so don't be discouraged if you do not see immediate results. To maintain relief, you will most likely have to continue taking estrogen. Stopping treatment usually brings a recurrence of the problem.

Nonhormonal, water–soluble, over–the–counter lubricants (such as Replens or Astroglide) can be an effective alternative to hormonal treatment.

Urinary incontinence. The postmenopausal loss of pelvic tone that causes urinary stress incontinence in some women can be improved with hormone therapy. However, the Kegel exercises described in Chapter 29 are a more effective way of restoring muscle tone, and you don't need a prescription. Most doctors recommend diligently performing these exercises rather than using HRT solely to cure incontinence.

Emotional distress. Women do not experience a greater rate of mental illness with the onset of menopause. However, if you are plagued by debilitating menopausal symptoms such as hot flashes, you may succumb to other problems such as fatigue, nervousness, irritability, and depression. Hormonal therapy can restore your sense of well–being by alleviating such symptoms. However, emotional distress that goes beyond the normal sadness that accompanies serious life events, such as the death of a loved one, is probably better treated by a psychiatrist or psychologist than by hormonal treatment.

Other symptoms. Hormone therapy may improve short–term memory and slow overall body deterioration. It also improves skin collagen, bringing smoother and thicker skin, firmer breasts, and improved muscle tone.

The Major Risks of HRT

As most women who are familiar with HRT know, the major drawback of hormone replacement therapy is an increased risk of certain types of cancer. For many women, cancer strikes greater fear than do uncomfortable menopausal symptoms, osteoporosis, or even heart disease, despite the fact that heart disease is a far greater killer. The best way to make a decision on HRT is to learn as much as you can, consider your own health, and discuss your situation with your doctor.

Uterine Cancer

Estrogen therapy, unopposed by progestin, increases a postmenopausal woman's chances of developing uterine cancer from an average of 1 in 1,000 to as much as 1 in 100. The risk increases with the duration of exposure and the dose of estrogen. For example, women taking estrogen for 8 years show an eight–fold increase in the rate of uterine cancer at 8 years, a ten–fold increase at 10 years, and so forth.

Estrogen's ability to cause cell growth, indispensable when it thickens the uterine lining during your monthly cycle, helps explain its notorious connection to uterine cancer. It has been suggested that the more cells made in a particular organ, the greater the likelihood that a few of those new cells will be abnormal and turn cancerous.

Uterine cancer is the most serious risk of estrogen therapy. However, adding progestin, which inhibits the growth of the uterine lining, to the hormonal regimen dramatically reduces that risk. The appropriate dose of progestin continues to be an important issue, because of its tendency to undermine estrogen's cardiovascular benefits. In addition, progestin–induced side effects cause problems for many women, forcing them to opt for estrogen–only treatment or to abandon hormone therapy altogether. Only women who have had their uterus removed may safely take estrogen alone. If you do take estrogen alone and you have not had a hysterectomy, yearly examination of the uterine lining is crucial. Even if you are on combination therapy, monitoring for uterine cancer is advisable if you experience any abnormal bleeding.

Breast Cancer

Sufficient evidence exists to indicate the *possibility* of a slightly increased risk of developing breast cancer with prolonged postmenopausal estrogen use. Most studies show that the increase in the incidence of breast cancer occurs after 10 to 15 years of estrogen use. Aside from duration, it's thought that high doses may be at fault. The type of estrogen may also affect your level of risk.

Because of estrogen's possible link with breast cancer, many doctors advise women to take the therapy for 5 years or less following menopause. Though this strategy can remedy the short–term symptoms of menopause, discontinuation of the therapy allows bone loss to resume at its postmenopausal, pre–HRT rate. If you are at greater risk of developing osteoporosis than breast cancer, you may want to consider continued hormone treatment.

The evidence on the impact of combined estrogen–progestin treatment on a woman's risk of breast cancer is still limited. Future studies, along with more experience should provide better answers to the outstanding questions about using both estrogen and progestin.

Though the possibility of a link between hormone replacement therapy and breast cancer is controversial, you should keep it in mind as a part of making an informed decision. As a preventive measure, you should be checked thoroughly for any tumors with a careful physical examination and a mammogram before you start hormone or estrogen therapy. Once you are on hormone therapy, you should examine your own breasts monthly and have yearly mammograms and physical exams. (See chapter 37, "Your Best Insurance Against Breast Cancer.")

Because there is evidence that breast cancer is a hormone responsive tumor, hormone therapy is not recommended for women who have had breast cancer. The interplay between a family history of breast cancer and HRT is less certain, but still something to take into account. So, if you are suffering from severe hot flashes, vaginal dryness, or other menopausal symptoms, and you have a family history of breast cancer, you need to weigh the risks and benefits with your doctor.

Gallbladder Disease

As with oral contraception, taking hormone or estrogen therapy can double your risk of developing gallstones. For women at high risk of gallstone attacks, oral hormone therapy should be avoided because it contributes to the formation of cholesterol crystals in the bile duct, which in turn supports the growth of gallstones. If you do decide to take hormone therapy, consider taking it via patch or vaginal cream.

Side-Effects of HRT

Although most women respond well to hormone replacement therapy, you may notice one or more of the following side effects.

Vaginal Bleeding

Uterine bleeding is the most common reason for stopping hormone therapy. This menstrual–like bleeding is called withdrawal bleeding, because it occurs when progestin is withdrawn from the treatment. While bleeding diminishes and ceases within a year for about two–thirds of women on progestin, some women will continue to bleed periodically as long as they take the therapy.

Breakthrough bleeding, which is spotting at other than the expected time, may also occur. Whether you are troubled with bleeding depends on the dose, regimen, hormone chosen and your individual response.

One way to reduce or eliminate this side effect is to alter the way progestin is given. Research is currently underway for new ways to take the hormone that will eliminate bleeding. If this side effect is unmanageable for you, discuss treatment alternatives with your doctor.

Breast Pain

Hormone therapy may cause swollen or tender breasts, especially if progestin is added to your treatment. It's unpleasant, but rarely is the pain so severe that the medication needs to be changed or stopped. If you do experience severe ongoing pain, hormone therapy may have to be discontinued and started at a lower dose.

Other Side Effects

A 2- to 3-month adjustment period is often necessary for women beginning hormone replacement therapy. Other reported side effects include: nausea, cramping, headaches, fluid retention, vaginal discharge, depression, irritability, weight gain, and bloating.

Estrogen may also have adverse effects on some patients with seizure disorders and migraine headaches. In rare cases, it can also interfere with liver function, raise blood pressure, or promote the growth of benign uterine fibroids. The amount of hormone that can cause side effects, as well as the amount needed to remedy menopausal symptoms, varies from woman to woman, so tell your physician about any problems you may have. Changes can be made in the method, dosage, or schedule of your treatment.

Making the Decision

The decision to use or not to use HRT ultimately belongs to you. It can be a tough decision informed by competing influences.

Trying to decide whether to take medication now to prevent disease that may occur in 20 years is a daunting prospect. Most women base their decision on matters much closer to home. For example, a woman with a family history of breast cancer may resist taking hormones until she can no longer tolerate her severe menopausal symptoms. But after being on estrogen and progestin, she may become reconciled to the therapy as it eliminates her hot flashes, restoring her normal sleep patterns and improving her mood. She worries about cancer, but believes with her doctor that she can monitor her situation through monthly self–exams, an annual checkup and an annual mammogram. Given the uncertainty of the statistics on heart disease and cancer, another woman may choose to avoid hormone therapy altogether. Though the risk of heart disease is greater than that of breast cancer, many women tend to be more worried about breast cancer because of the disease's physical and emotional toll. A woman may reason that there are other ways to prevent heart disease but no known ways to prevent breast cancer, and so resolve to eat a low–fat diet and exercise regularly instead of taking hormones.

Every woman entering menopause should have a physical examination and then talk with her doctor about her overall health, her family history and her physical and psychological concerns. Working with your doctor to assess your risk factors accurately should help you determine whether the benefits of hormone replacement therapy outweigh the risks for you personally. If you are concerned about HRT, consider other effective nonmedical therapies for addressing your needs, and seek a second opinion before initiating a course of treatment. Plan on yearly visits with your doctor for a complete physical exam.

The Future of HRT

Doctors are hopeful that the first large–scale clinical trial of hormone replacement therapy will provide a more definitive basis for decision–making. The three–year study by the National Institutes of Health (NIH), called PEPI (Postmenopausal Estrogen/Progestin Interventions), is following 875 women randomly placed in five groups, each with a different treatment: estrogen alone, estrogen and progestin in three combinations or doses, and a placebo. The study is measuring the effects of the drugs on cholesterol, blood pressure, and bone density, as well as on the incidence of breast and uterine cancer. Hormone use is also being correlated with personal matters, such as sexual satisfaction, mood, and general outlook on life.

Another NIH effort is the Women's Health Initiative, a 14–year clinical trial that will track, among other things, the incidence of heart disease, osteoporosis, and breast and uterine cancer in 25,000 postmenopausal women taking either estrogen or a combination therapy. Together, these two studies should provide answers to the many questions both doctors and patients are asking today. □

CHAPTER 32   **CONQUERING EMOTIONAL PROBLEMS**

Coming to Grips with Stress

Stress: It's the buzzword of the 90s, especially among women who do too much. Few human conditions receive so much credit...and so much blame. "I work better under stress," is the refrain of many successful professional women. Yet for a harried single mother trying to juggle a career and two small children stress can add up to a severely debilitating problem.

What exactly is this universal challenge called stress? In broad, general terms, it's any event that forces us to adapt to a new set of circumstances. For practical purposes, however, it's broken down into specific situations called stressors.

Stressors range from minor to major, and can include daily annoyances, pressures at home or on the job, marital discord, emergencies, accidents, illness and injury—even hostile weather conditions. It's important to remember that joyous occasions as well as difficult ones can be stressful. Without stress, our existence would lack the ups and downs that give life its substance and meaning. Too little of it leads to boredom; too much can undermine your health.

When confronted with a stressful situation, your body responds with a chain of biochemical reactions that can affect your entire system. Any real or imagined emergency sets in motion a series of changes designed to enable you to "fight or flee" the "danger." Responding to complex triggers from the brain, the adrenal glands release adrenaline and other hormones. Immediately, your heart rate and blood pressure increase, your pupils dilate, and you feel a heightened sense of alertness.

There are three stages in this stress response: alarm, resistance, and exhaustion. During the alarm phase, when you first notice a stressor, you may perspire and feel flushed. Muscles in your stomach and limbs may tighten. During emergencies, some people feel a surge of extraordinary strength that allows them to do things they never could before.

In the resistance phase, the release of other hormones works to bring the body back to normal. Then, as you recover from the stressful episode, you'll probably feel exhausted.

The stress response we experience during an emergency is a normal reaction to an abnormal incident: The body has safely and naturally protected itself from danger. But unrelieved, unremitting stress keeps your body in a constant state of alert and can seriously affect your health.

How Much Stress Is Too Much?

There's no clear–cut answer. The same type of stress may cause problems for one woman and have no effect on another. Richard Rahe, a pioneering stress researcher, estimated the degree of difficulty people have in adjusting to certain stressful changes in their lives. He rated these experiences in "Life Change Units" (LCUs), with scores ranging from 25 for a change in political beliefs or a minor illness to 105 for the death of a spouse or child. The higher your total LCUs during a given period, the more careful you should be to handle your stress appropriately. (See table nearby.)

Keep in mind, though, that the LCU of a stressful event varies from one woman to the next. Recent studies have shown that while pleasant events certainly cause stress, unpleasant ones take on an even greater toll. Some people can handle major stressors successfully while life's constant little hassles find them unable to cope. What looms as a challenge for one person strikes another as a mild annoyance.

It's Not All in Your Head

The changes your body undergoes in reaction to stressors may produce symptoms that can literally make you sick. When unrelenting or frequently repeated stressors overwhelm your personal coping skills, you can

"LIFE CHANGE UNIT" RATINGS OF COMMON STRESSORS

Exactly how much stress are you under? Any change means stress; and the more profound the change, the greater its impact. Use the ratings below to gauge the cumulative effect of the readjustments you're currently experiencing in your life. Note that a sudden burst of relatively minor events can easily cause as much stress as a major loss or disaster.

Stressful event	LCU
Child leaving for college	28
Major change in eating habits	29
Vacation	29
Job promotion	31
Major change in sleeping habits	31
New romantic relationship	32
Breaking up	35
Troubles with co–workers	35
Changing jobs	38
Major change in living conditions	39
Major purchase	39
Troubles with boss	39
Major dental work	40
Injury or illness that hospitalized you or kept you in bed a week or more	42
Marital reconciliation	42
Accident	44
Marriage	50
Major change in health or behavior of family member	52
Miscarriage or abortion	53
Marital separation	56
Job demotion	57
Loan or mortgage foreclosure	57
Decreased income	60
Pregnancy	60
Divorce	62
Death of brother or sister	64
Getting fired	64
Death of parent	66
Death of spouse or child	105

develop symptoms of illness or experience a worsening of pre–existing symptoms.

Stress can affect your body's immune response, and make you more vulnerable to illness. Clinical studies show a relationship between stress and resistance to infection: For example, there is evidence that people under stress are more prone to contract common colds. But physical reactions to stress are highly individual. Medical experts aren't certain why one woman under stress gets stomachaches, while another has headaches. Many doctors and researchers now believe that environmental factors combined with a woman's genetic make–up and her innate coping skills determine her personal reaction to stress.

Therefore, it's important to understand the way your body reacts to stress. If you experience any of these symptoms frequently, it's quite possible that stress is the culprit.

- Cardiovascular irregularities
- Digestive disorders
- Sleep difficulties
- Menstrual problems
- Migraines and headaches
- Neck aches and back spasms
- Skin disorders—
  hives, acne, and other rashes

Stress can also cause or aggravate such potentially destructive or unhealthy behavior as smoking, drinking, nail–biting, forgetfulness, an increased or decreased desire to eat, and nervousness.

Cardiovascular Irregularities

According to a recent study, stress plays a role in the development of heart disease, especially in postmenopausal women. Older women who took stressful mental tests had higher blood pressures and heart rates than did men or younger women. Researchers who monitored all three groups as they went about their daily activities noted that post-menopausal women were three times as likely to respond to stress with episodes of abnormal heart function. This finding is especially important for middle–aged or elderly women whose arteries are already clogged.

■ *How to help yourself:* Employ the stress–reduction techniques and follow the dietary suggestions outlined at the end of this chapter. Ask your doctor whether you are a candidate for estrogen–replacement therapy, since the estrogen loss that follows menopause may make the heart more vulnerable to the effects of stress.

Digestive Disorders

The chemical reactions unleashed by stress have a direct effect on the digestive tract, and women are far more likely than men to seek medical help for stomach and bowel complaints. There are a number of digestive ailments that have close links to stress.

Nonulcer dyspepsia (NUD), a catchall term for stomach cramps and discomfort that can't be linked to a specific cause, is a common digestive disorder in women. Not a true disease, NUD is difficult to diagnose because neither blood tests, nor physical exams or X–rays can confirm its existence. When gastrointestinal tests fail to indicate a more serious condition, your doctor may say you have NUD.

■ *How to help yourself:* Try over–the–counter remedies such as Mylanta or Maalox. During times of stress, resist the impulse to change your eating habits, but make certain your diet is well–balanced. See your doctor if symptoms persist or worsen.

Irritable Bowel Syndrome (IBS), or "spastic colon," is thought to affect up to 19 percent of Americans; 85 percent of IBS–sufferers are women. Symptoms include moderate to severe cramping, bloating, and bouts of constipation and diarrhea. IBS may be stress–triggered.

■ *How to help yourself:* If you experience chronic stomach discomfort, see your doctor or a specialist in gastroenterology. He or she will most likely conduct a series of tests to rule out other disorders, including lactose sensitivity, parasitic diseases, allergic reactions, ulcerative colitis, and Crohn's disease. Physicians sometimes prescribe antispasmodic drugs such as Donnatal and Bentyl, or low doses of antidepressants, to ease spasms. A high–fiber diet can relieve constipation.

Ulcers are diagnosed through endoscopy and barium x–rays. For years doctors thought stress produced ulcers and made them worse. Now, however, medical experts agree that a bacterium is the initial cause of most ulcers.

■ *How to help yourself:* Your doctor may prescribe a medication such as Zantac, Tagamet or Pepcid to reduce the amount of hydrochloric acid your stomach produces. He or she may also advise you to cut down on alcohol; caffeine; carbonated beverages; and rich, fried, or fatty foods. The recommended cure, however, is a course of antibiotics. One new therapy combines two antibiotics and Pepto–Bismol. Ninety percent of women treated this way experience relief, and after treatment, their ulcers rarely recur.

Sleep Disorders

Insomnia, the inability to fall or stay asleep easily, is one of the most common signs of stress, and perhaps one of the most difficult to avoid. It is a double threat for the already stressed–out woman who especially needs the restorative energy that comes with a good night's sleep.

■ *How to help yourself:* Most women experience an occasional sleepless night, and this is no cause for alarm. But if sleeplessness persists for more than a few days, follow these helpful do's and don'ts:

DO:
■ Eat dinner early; make it light on fat and heavy on complex carbohydrates.
■ Check with your doctor to see if your medications are a problem. Over–the–counter cold remedies and diet pills can cause wakefulness.
■ Try a glass of warm milk.
■ Set yourself a regular sleep schedule: Go to bed and arise at the same time every day.
■ Take a warm, relaxing bath a couple of hours before bedtime.
■ Employ the relaxation exercises described later in this chapter.
■ Exercise in the afternoon.
■ Aim for a peaceful evening; save conflicts with family members for the daylight hours.
■ Leave yourself some "wind–down" time for an hour or two before you go to bed.

DON'T:
■ Drink alcoholic beverages in an attempt to get sleepy. You'll only disrupt your sleep pattern.
■ Read, work, or watch television in bed. If you can't sleep, get up and go to another room.
■ Have a heavy meal close to bedtime.
■ Let a night or two of insomnia upset you. Worrying about sleep only makes it harder.

Fatigue

Fatigue is often a way of life for busy working women and mothers. It can come from chronic, unrelieved stress; sleep–deprivation; or a variety of illnesses.

If you feel constant fatigue, first determine whether you are getting all the sleep your body needs. Sleep restores the body, allowing it to repair damage caused by stress and other factors. Women who lead stressful lives actually need more sleep than do other women because their bodies demand more sleep recovery time. Sleep–deprived women show diminished mental alertness and performance; over time, unchecked fatigue can lead to depression and illness.

Are you getting enough sleep? "Yes" answers to the following questions are a sign that you're not.

- Do you need an alarm to wake up?
- Do you hit the snooze button regularly?
- Do you fall asleep quickly? (Women who get enough sleep take about 15 minutes to fall asleep; sleep–deprived women fall asleep within about five minutes.)
- Do you find yourself falling asleep during the day?

A vacation is a good time to determine how much sleep you need. After three or four days, note how long you sleep naturally. This is the amount of sleep your body needs to get consistently, whether it's 4, 8 or 10 hours.

FIGHT OR FLIGHT

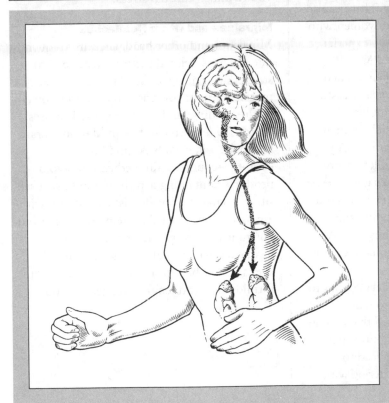

Faced by a threat, your body responds with a complex cascade of chemicals. The hypothalamus, alerted by the brain, pumps out a specialized hormone that ultimately prompts the two adrenal glands (perched atop the kidneys) to release the energizing hormone known as adrenaline. The result — faster pulse, higher blood pressure, sharpened awareness — is the "fight or flight" response we call stress.

■ *How to help yourself:* Determine how much sleep you need, then make a point of getting it regularly. Follow the suggestions for insomnia if you have trouble falling or staying asleep. Take short naps if at all possible. Eat a well–balanced diet with plenty of fresh fruits and vegetables and schedule at least three brisk 20 to 30–minute walks each week.

Menstruation, Infertility, and Pregnancy

When a woman undergoes prolonged stress, her levels of estrogen and progesterone can decrease. This can sometimes lead to decreased sex drive and menstrual irregularities such as delayed periods or none at all.

The menstrual cycle is also subject to physical stressors: The menses of women athletes are often irregular and sometimes cease during times of excessive training, as do those of women who suffer from two serious eating disorders: anorexia and bulimia. There is also evidence to support the fact that women who suffer stress may be more likely to experience the uncomfortable symptoms of PMS.

Can stress affect fertility? When women have trouble conceiving, it can be a stressful time—especially for those undergoing high–tech fertility treatments. Such women get little comfort from well–meaning people who suggest they "just relax and let nature take its course." For them, there's good news: 80 to 90 percent of the time, infertility has a physiological cause. Stress does enter the picture, however, for women whose severe stress causes a decrease in hormonal levels or irregular menstrual cycles.

Stress during pregnancy can be dangerous to both mother and baby. A study conducted at the University of Texas indicated that certain chemicals released during times of stress (epinephrine and norepinephrine) can lead to uterine and cervical changes, interfering with

oxygen and blood flow to the developing child. Women who had an especially difficult time coping with stress during their pregnancies were more likely to have babies that were born prematurely or at a low birth weight.

■ *How to help yourself:* Moderate, regular exercise (a brisk, 20– to 30–minute walk three times a week is ideal) has been found to relieve many menstrual and PMS discomforts, including cramps and bloating. Some medical experts also suggest that certain vitamins, E, for example, can be useful in lessening symptoms of PMS. Avoid or lessen your intake of salt, sugar, alcohol, caffeine, and fat. If symptoms persist, see your doctor. During pregnancy, make certain to get the best prenatal care available and follow your obstetrician's advice about rest, exercise, and diet. Make certain to tell your doctor if you're under unusual stress.

Migraines and Other Headaches

Migraines and other headaches are frequently due to stress–related factors. Reactions to stress that can trigger headaches include: muscle tension, constriction of blood flow, teeth–grinding, and even congested sinuses.

■ *How to help yourself:* A mild to moderate headache will usually respond to over–the–counter pain medication; avoid products containing aspirin if you have a sensitive stomach. Your dentist can fit you with a plastic mouth guard to help you stop grinding your teeth at night. True migraine headaches—pain that causes nausea and keeps you in bed for hours—present a more formidable treatment challenge. See your doctor. He or she may prescribe special migraine medications or refer you to a pain clinic for sophisticated treatment. (See chapter 14, "Taking Control of Headache" for additional details.)

Back and Neck Aches

When stress produces muscle tension, painful spasms in the neck and back can result. Some 80 percent of us will experience neck or back pain at some point during our lives. Your posture, the chair you use, the type of work you do, and your muscle tone can all effect your susceptibility to back and neck pain.

■ *How to help yourself:* Hot showers, massages, heating pads, and over–the–counter analgesics are usually enough to relieve simple, temporary back and neck pain. Take preventative measures: Include stretching exercises in your daily routine and use a well designed chair. Learn how to lift and carry heavy objects properly; remember to always bend your knees, not your back. It's better to get help carrying a heavy object than to seek help for an injury. When back pain is persistent, severe, or incapacitating, it's time to see your doctor. He or she may prescribe muscle relaxants or other medication, or may refer you to specialist.

Skin Disorders

Stress can cause or exacerbate a broad variety of skin conditions, including acne, hives, lichen planus (itchy, flat purplish bumps on your wrists, forearms, abdomen, and back), neurodermatitis, and psoriasis. Since so many other factors—including allergies, prescription and over–the–counter medications, and overexposure to the sun—can also affect the skin, the best first step is to seek the advice of a good dermatologist whenever you are troubled with a persistent, uncomfortable skin rash, eruption, or inflammation.

Coping With Stress

To alleviate your stress–related problems you must first understand your personal reaction to stress. Each woman has her individual stress threshold. What pushes one woman to distraction may be ignored—or even welcomed—by another. For example, a high powered woman executive might find a vacation away from the office extremely stressful. Even the absence of stress can be stressful. Many middle–aged women have a particularly hard time coping with the "empty nest" syndrome that hits when children grow up and leave home.

Stress can be, if not a silent killer, at least, a silent challenge to peaceful, healthy living. Still, it's worth remembering that stress has its good points too. It can work as an alarm system to protect you against serious damage. Highly stressful situations can even add spice, dimension, and excitement to your life. Most important, keep in mind that life's most joyous occasions—the birth of a baby, college entrance, a wedding, a new job or a promotion—can all create stress that strains your psyche, yet still be well worth the strain.

To cope with stress you must first recognize your own limits. Know what stressors disturb you. Be aware of times in your life that are particularly stressful. If you experience a few major stressful events within a short period of time, be extra–gentle with yourself. Acknowledge that you're going through a difficult time. Try to gain control of the situation by asking yourself, "How can I change this?" Make time to rest and relax. Adopt a program of healthy eating and exercising. Choose the coping strategies that suit you best.

Diet

There's no substitute for a well–balanced diet to help your body handle the ravages of stress. While researchers have yet to prove a connection between psychological stress and the need for vitamin supplements, nutritionists often recommend a diet high in vitamins C, E, and B.

Whether you take these supplements or not, follow these tips for a healthy, stress–fighting diet.

Include...
- Raw fruits and vegetables
- Complex carbohydrates (new dietary guidelines suggest 6 to 11 servings a day)
- More fish and poultry
- A good breakfast every day
- Low–fat foods

Be sparing with...
- Refined sugar
- Salt
- Alcoholic and caffeinated beverages
- Fatty and fried foods

Coping Strategies

The best way to manage severe or chronic stress is to treat yourself tenderly. Acknowledge that you're going through a difficult time, then reward yourself. Self–indulgence isn't selfish, it's essential to your well–being. Choose from this list of personal rewards—or add your own—when you're stressed–out:

Take a...
- Walk
- Vacation
- Break
- Nap
- Course (in something not job–related)

Make time to...
- Play
- Garden
- Go shopping (the window variety will do)
- Read
- Laugh
- Cry
- Make love
- Watch a movie, a play, TV—or the sunset
- Exercise

Biofeedback

Biofeedback is an ideal way to learn how to manage moderate to severe stress. It is a painless, electronic process that takes in and processes information about your body's involuntary response to stressors, then relays it back to you so you can learn to modify these previously unwitting reactions. Though it sounds complicated, biofeedback is a simple way to help you learn how to relax.

Biofeedback has been found to be particularly helpful for dealing with migraines, muscle tension and spasms, teeth grinding, and stress–related effects on the circulatory system.

Relaxation Exercises

When you feel caught in a particularly stressful situation, try this special breathing exercise:

1. Sit as comfortably as possible in a chair or on the floor. Dim the lights if you can.
2. Inhale deeply, through your nose. Expand your lungs with air as fully as possible. Visualize the air coming through the top of your head, down all the way to the bottom of your lungs.
3. Breathe out slowly through your nose. Visualize the air rising slowly up through your body and out through the top of your head.
4. Repeat until calm.

Meditation

Meditation is a way of relaxing and emptying the mind of all outside stimuli. It has been practiced for centuries, and is frequently recommended today as an excellent way to ease stress. There are many techniques. One approach you might want to try is called the Benson Relaxation Response.

Before you begin:

■ Plan to make meditation a regular part of your daily routine. Set aside 10 to 20 minutes each day at the same time, if possible. Before breakfast is a good time.

While you meditate:

■ Sit quietly in a comfortable position.
■ Eliminate distractions and interruptions during the period you'll be meditating.
■ Commit yourself to a specific length of time and try to stick to it.
■ Pick a focus word or short phrase that's firmly rooted in your personal belief system. A nonreligious person might choose a neutral word like *one, peace,* or *love.* Others might use the opening words of a favorite prayer from their religion.
■ Close your eyes.
■ Relax your muscles.
■ Breathe slowly and naturally, repeating your focus word or phrase silently as you exhale.
■ Assume a passive attitude. Don't worry about how well you're doing. When other thoughts come to mind, simply say, "Oh, well," and gently return to the repetition.
■ Continue for 10 to 20 minutes. You may open your eyes to check the time, but do not use an alarm. After you finish: Sit quietly for a minute or so, at first with your eyes closed and later with your eyes open. Do not stand for one or two minutes.
■ Plan for a session once or twice a day.

You may try some of the other stress–reducing techniques and therapies that many find effective. They include visualization, yoga, dance and art therapy, and massage.

Listening to Yourself

Many people under stress make matters worse by telling themselves things like "I'll never make it," and "it always happens to me." Take time to sort out what you're really thinking. If your reactions are self–defeating or causing additional stress, make a deliberate effort to change them. Tell yourself "I've gotten through tough situations before, and I'll get through this one." Though it may seem unlikely that this will make a difference, some people find that it really does help them cope.

If All Else Fails

There is no rule that says you must deal with stress single–handedly. If a major problem like a chronic disease is causing you stress, seek out a support group or a workshop. And if you feel overwhelmed by multiple stressors, remember that there's nothing wrong with seeing a good doctor or therapist. □

CHAPTER 33

CONQUERING EMOTIONAL PROBLEMS

Dealing With Anxiety, Depression and Chronic Fatigue Syndrome

You don't have to be a woman to suffer from anxiety, depression, or chronic fatigue syndrome, but it certainly helps. Women are about twice as likely as men to seek treatment for these disorders.

Some studies show that women actually do suffer certain types of these disorders more than men, while for other conditions, men and women appear to be stricken at the same rate, with women more likely to seek treatment. Either way, the bottom line is: don't be surprised if you or someone you know has one of these illnesses. Just look at the numbers: an estimated 18 million Americans have severe anxiety, more than 15 percent have had or will have a serious depression at some time in their lives and chronic fatigue syndrome has been estimated to affect as many as 5 million people.

But Don't We All Feel That Way?

Imagine you're keyed up planning a wedding, feeling restless, and not sleeping as well as usual. Or you're sad for a few weeks following the death of a friend. Or one Monday after a busy weekend, you feel more tired than usual.

Sound familiar? These are all normal feelings and normal responses to the events of life. Everyone feels anxious, depressed or fatigued for short periods of time, and the feelings usually pass on their own. A job change, marriage or divorce, financial problems, a new baby, illness of a loved one, or even an argument with a friend or colleague are all good reasons for some of these feelings.

In fact, even positive events can produce these reactions. The anxiety and fatigue that can accompany a whirlwind two–week vacation tour or a cross–country move to a great new job can be real and significant.

But—if you have feelings of anxiety, depression, or fatigue that severely disrupt your daily life or persist for more than a few weeks, or if your feelings seem out of proportion to the event that caused them—or if there is no specific cause—then it's time to see your doctor. Anxiety and depression are treatable mental illnesses, and incapacitating fatigue can be an important symptom of disease, including chronic fatigue syndrome.

What Kind of Doctor?

The first step is to get an initial diagnosis from your regular internist or family practitioner. Your family doctor can screen you for underlying medical conditions or medications that could be causing or contributing to the way you feel. Usually, the doctor will ask you about your medical history, perform blood and urine tests, and, if appropriate, take x–rays. Your doctor may then refer you to a specialist for treatment. Severe anxiety and depression are real illnesses—not signs of "weakness"—and should be treated by a psychiatrist, psychologist or social worker. Chronic fatigue syndrome is a medical condition that can be treated by your regular doctor, a specialist in the syndrome, or an immunologist. In some cases, you may be referred to a neurologist for an assessment.

Anxiety

Anxiety is a feeling of being keyed up and extra alert. Your heart may race or you may get "butterflies" in your stomach. You may feel short of breath or generally jittery. You're likely to have a feeling of impending danger.

These reactions are the way our bodies prepare to cope with stress. All the senses become tuned up and on alert in the presence of a threat. These reactions derive from the primitive "fight or flight" response that enabled early humans to deal quickly with dangerous situations.

Everyone is likely to have that kind of anxiety response in urgent situations, such as a fire or other emergency. But we also get these feelings in the course of our daily routines. Time pressures, traffic tie–ups, social jitters, a new job, or waiting for test results can all produce anxious feelings; and these feelings are normal and healthy.

But anxiety ceases to be positive when it is painful or prolonged, or when the response is out of proportion to the cause. When anxiety interferes with your daily life or when it becomes incapacitating fear, it becomes an illness called an anxiety disorder.

Causes of Anxiety Disorder

The causes of anxiety disorder are not clear. Researchers are currently investigating a number of factors including chemical imbalances, enzyme deficiencies, hormones, the role of emotional traumas, and the interaction between emotions and brain chemistry.

Diagnosing Anxiety Disorder

There is no specific test for anxiety, but after ruling out medical causes, your doctor will compare the symptoms you are having with the definitions of anxiety disorders in the American Psychiatric Association Diagnostic and Statistical Manual (DSM). Anxiety disorders are divided into seven (sometimes overlapping) categories: generalized anxiety disorder; simple phobias; social phobias; agoraphobia; panic disorder; obsessive–compulsive disorder; and posttraumatic stress disorder.

Generalized Anxiety Disorder can typically leave you feeling constantly edgy or jumpy, and worrying excessively. You may suffer from shortness of breath, palpitations, dizziness, or nausea. For a diagnosis of generalized anxiety disorder, you must have the symptoms for more than six months, and in relation to at least two areas of your life (such as overwhelming concern about your health and your finances). The disorder can cause both psychological and physical complaints, ranging from edgy feelings to stomach trouble, sexual problems, and insomnia.

Phobias are involuntary fear reactions that are inappropriate to the situation. They produce a strong sense of dread, and those with the illness do everything possible to avoid the source of their fear. There are three (often overlapping) categories.

Simple phobias are based on a fear of a specific object or situation, such as heights, driving, or flying, even when the object of the fear poses no real threat or danger. Almost anything can become the object of a simple phobia.

Extreme anxiety about being judged by others or fears about behaving in a way that will lead to public embarrassment are signs of a social phobia. People with this disorder often dread speaking, eating or writing in public, or using public restrooms.

Agoraphobia is a complex set of fears about being alone or feeling trapped in a public place. It is often accompanied by panic disorder. Agoraphobia can be debilitating, even to the extent that some people with this disorder become completely housebound.

Panic Disorder. A panic attack is a period of intense fear or discomfort, when you feel confronted with immediate, mortal danger. It has been described as a feeling of life or death in a situation that is not truly dangerous. During a panic attack, you may have shortness of breath, dizziness, palpitations, feelings of unreality, hot flashes or chills. Some

people believe they are losing control or even dying. People who have four or more panic attacks in a month, or one or more panic attacks followed by persistent fear of another attack are diagnosed with panic disorder.

Obsessive–Compulsive Disorder. Unpleasant and unwanted thoughts that preoccupy and intrude on one's daily life are a sign of obsessive–compulsive disorder. For example, a woman may have the thought that she could harm her children. These thoughts, while disturbing, are almost never acted upon. They are usually accompanied by repetitive routines and rituals that serve to make the person feel a bit more comfortable. For instance, some people with this disorder feel compelled to wash their hands repeatedly. Others check and re–check that the stove is off or a door is locked. Some hoard things or count things.

Posttraumatic Stress Disorder is a condition brought on by the experience of surviving a severe or unusual physical or mental trauma (such as war, rape, or kidnap), or disasters such as fire, flood, or plane crash. Symptoms range from reliving the traumatic event over and over to feeling emotionally numb. Victims of this disease often have trouble sleeping and suffer recurrent nightmares.

Treating Anxiety Disorders

Everyday anxiety responds to simple measures that you can take yourself, such as regular aerobic exercise, time management, learning to let your feelings out with a trusted friend, or relaxation training. But when anxiety is severe, professional treatment is necessary. The good news is that anxiety disorders are among the most treatable emotional illnesses, and while they are certainly distressing, they are rarely dangerous.

Treatment is usually two–pronged, combining drug therapy and psychotherapy. Drugs are useful for short–term relief, while long–term improvement usually requires some behavioral and life–style changes.

Psychotherapy, including cognitive and behavioral therapies, can be helpful in reducing anxiety. Behavioral therapy involves gradually exposing you to the object or situation that causes your anxiety. Cognitive therapy helps you learn to control unrealistic or negative thinking patterns that may be contributing to your anxiety.

Drugs are available to help treat and manage the symptoms of various anxiety disorders. Benzodiazepines such as diazepam (Valium), lorazepam (Ativan) and alprazolam (Xanax) are commonly used to treat generalized anxiety disorders.

Panic attacks are treated with drugs containing tricyclic antidepressants, such as Etrafon, Triavil, and Limbitrol. Also used for panic are certain benzodiazepines such as alprazolam (Xanax).

For obsessive–compulsive disorders, doctors can prescribe clomipramine (Anafranil). To control the physical symptoms of phobias such as severe stage–fright, beta–blocking drugs such as propanolol (Inderol) are sometimes prescribed.

Outlook

People with anxiety disorders do get better. With proper management, most people with an anxiety disorder can expect to live normal, fulfilling lives.

Depression?

Like anxiety, depressed feelings strike almost everyone at some time. And like anxiety, depression is an appropriate response to some situations. But depression that is overwhelming and persistent is a serious illness. An estimated 15 percent of people with severe depression commit suicide and many more make a suicide attempt. Depression is the most common emotional disorder in women, about one–fourth of all women suffer from depression at some time in their lives.

Since we all tend to use the term depression to describe the "blues", people often think a serious depression is simply more of the same, a problem that will pass in time. But serious depression is more than the ordinary feelings of grief, disappointment, or burnout that are normal, short–lived responses to real disappointment or loss. People suffering from depression are suffering from an illness, just like a physical illness such as appendicitis or diabetes. And just like a physical illness, serious depression doesn't respond to common sense, you cannot just snap out of it, and it doesn't improve when things get better. Most important, despite some commonly held views, it is not a sign of a weak character, or lack of will power. Certainly it's not a disorder that implies failure in your life: Ludwig van Beethoven, Winston Churchill, Charles Dickens, Abraham Lincoln, and Virginia Woolf, among many other famous historical figures, all suffered from depression at one time or another.

Causes of Depression

There are many theories about the cause of depression. Recent research suggests that some people are biologically inclined to react with depression when they experience a stress overload. Another suspected culprit is an imbalance of certain chemical messengers in the brain, particularly a substance called serotonin. Other theories suggest that depression is a result of anger turned inward towards oneself, an ingrained sense of helplessness, or patterns of negative thinking.

Depression can also be caused by illnesses (such as thyroid or adrenal gland problems, infections, and multiple sclerosis), by drug or alcohol abuse, and by prescription medications. For example, among the drugs that can cause depression are some of those prescribed for high blood pressure, heart disease, pain relief, stomach and intestinal problems, and Parkinson's disease. Anticonvulsants, sedatives, sleeping pills, oral contraceptives, antibiotics, and cancer chemotherapy drugs can also be at fault.

Diagnosing Depression

Depression is not always easily diagnosed and many women go from doctor to doctor with vague complaints of fatigue, difficulty sleeping, irritability, poor concentration, or stomach and intestinal distress until someone finally realizes they are seriously depressed. (This is often referred to by physicians as "masked depression.") You should suspect depression if you find that in addition to all of your symptoms, you are simply not able to enjoy yourself.

There is no specific diagnostic test for every type of depression but a thorough medical examination and interview with a psychiatrist, psychologist or neurologist can help make a diagnosis. Since specific medical

PRIME SUSPECTS IN DEPRESSION: THE CHEMICAL MESSENGERS OF THE BRAIN

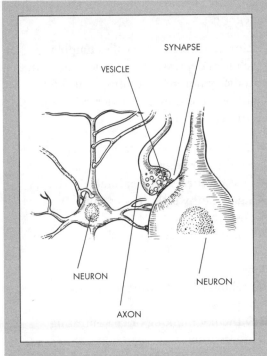

To pass messages among themselves, nerve cells in the brain release bursts of chemicals that briefly stimulate receptors on a neighboring cell, then quickly disappear. These chemicals, called neurotransmitters, are manufactured within the cell and stored in tiny bubbles (vesicles) at the end of the cell's tentacle-like axons. They travel to the receiving cell across a tiny gap called the synapse.

To eliminate one burst of a neurotransmitter and prepare for the next, the chemical is either destroyed by the receiving cell or taken back by the sending cell in a process called "reuptake." Serotonin, a neurotransmitter that plays a central role in the brain, appears to be in short supply among the depressed; and a number of antidepressant drugs are thought to work by preventing serotonin's destruction or reuptake. The celebrated drug Prozac, for instance, is classified as a "serotonin uptake inhibitor."

conditions can cause depression, if indicated, your doctor will do diagnostic tests to make sure that a physical illness is not the underlying cause. Depression disorders fall into three categories:

Major depression, also called unipolar or clinical depression, is a syndrome with specific symptoms that affect your body, emotions and thoughts. Criteria for a diagnosis of depression include:

- Depressed mood most of the day, nearly every day
- Loss of interest in pleasurable activities
- Significant weight loss or gain
- Disturbed sleep
- Constant fidgeting or a slowdown in movement
- Fatigue, loss of energy
- Feelings of guilt, worthlessness, hopelessness
- Difficulty thinking or concentrating
- Indecisiveness
- Recurrent thoughts of suicide

If you have at least five of these symptoms and they interfere with your daily life, the condition is called major depression. If you have fewer than five or if the symptoms are mild and do not interfere with daily life, the condition is called mild depression.

Bipolar depression, which used to be called manic depression, causes not only the "lows" of major depression, but also a mood swing to a wild euphoric state. These "highs," or manic episodes, can be extremely disruptive.

Most people with bipolar depression go for many months between episodes of depression or mania. Women are more likely than men to have more frequent episodes, called rapid cycling.

Criteria for a diagnosis of the manic phase of bipolar depression include:

- Less need for sleep
- Talkativeness
- Distractibility
- Flight of ideas
- Increase in goal–directed activities—either socially, at work, in school or sexually—or restlessness and agitation
- Inflated self–esteem
- Excessive involvement in pleasurable activities that have high potential for negative consequences, such as buying sprees, sexual indiscretions, or foolish business investments

If you have these symptoms in a milder form insufficient to disrupt your daily life, the condition is called hypomania.

Postpartum Depression. Many new mothers suffer from some degree of "baby blues," after childbirth. They find themselves crying or laughing easily and often. They feel anxious and have trouble concentrating. Typically, this situation lasts a few weeks.

For some new mothers, however, the blues become a serious postpartum depression that can, without treatment, last more than a year. Anxiety, fatigue, phobias, an inability to enjoy life, sleep disturbance, lack of appetite, and guilt are common. If you suffer from postpartum depression, you may be overly anxious about the care and health of your baby or doubt your ability to be a good mother. If you are a first–time mother, you are more likely to have mild baby blues rather than serious postpartum depression.

Postpartum depression may be caused by a number of physical, psychological and social factors that accompany childbirth. Two important contributors may be postpartum hormone levels and the inevitable sleep deprivation that comes with a new baby. Your expectations, family situation, and the baby's personality and condition may all also contribute.

Related Disorders

Depression and Premenstrual Syndrome (PMS). PMS is not depression, although if you have PMS you may have some of the same symptoms (see chapter 3, "PMS: Sorting Fact from Fiction.") PMS is considered a recurring mood disorder, caused by hormonal changes related to menstruation. Researchers are investigating the relationship of PMS to depression.

Seasonal Affective Disorder (SAD) is a cyclical mood disturbance that affects mostly women. It is often related to a lack of light, and usually occurs in the fall and winter. Most people with SAD become depressed when the days are short and get better as the days lengthen in the spring. (Paradoxically, a few feel better in the winter, worse in the spring, and summer.) Researchers are investigating a link between SAD and the hormonal changes that accompany menstruation.

Treating Depression

A combination of psychotherapy and medication is usually helpful in treating major and bipolar depression. Psychological approaches, including cognitive (learning), behavioral, and interpersonal therapies, can help you understand patterns of negative thinking and can help you develop a more positive outlook.

Treatment for postpartum depression may include counseling, cognitive therapy, and medication. Most doctors suggest that new mothers also seek out social support systems such as new mothers groups. Some women find relaxation training to be helpful. About two–thirds of women with postpartum depression recover in one year.

Seasonal Affective Disorder (SAD) is treated with both antidepressants and exposure to bright sun or special treatment lights.

Drugs used in treating depression can take several weeks to become effective. They require close medical follow–up to monitor potential side effects.

There are three common types of antidepressant medication. Drugs in one category may work very well for a particular individual, while another type has little effect. There is no way to predict which type is best for a specific patient, so don't be surprised if your doctor has to try several different prescriptions before finding the medication that works best for you.

The newest type of antidepressant, called serotonin uptake inhibitors, includes the widely publicized drug fluoxetine (Prozac). Other drugs in this category are paroxetine (Paxil), sertraline (Zoloft), and the new drug venlafaxine (Effexor), which affects several of the brain's chemical messengers. These drugs claim to have fewer side effects than some of the others.

A second major type, called tricyclic antidepressants, is thought to work by increasing the availability of another brain chemical called norepinephrine. Included in this category are amitriptyline (Elavil, Endep), imipramine (Tofranil), nortriptyline (Aventyl, Pamelor), desipramine (Norpramin, Pertofrane), and amoxapine (Asendin).

A third category, known as MAO inhibitors, is often tried when other antidepressants fail. Included in this group are phenelzine (Nardil), tranylcypromine (Parnate), and isocarboxazid (Marplan). MAO inhibitors cause dangerous interactions with a number of foods and need to be taken with care.

Falling outside these three categories are medications such as buproprion (Wellbutrin), trazodone (Desyrel), and maprotiline (Ludiomil). Lithium (Lithonate) is prescribed for treatment of the manic phase of bipolar depression, and is now also being used for recurrent depressive episodes.

For a small group of people, psychotherapy and drug therapy are not effective. Electroconvulsive therapy (ECT), also known as shock therapy, can be helpful to these people. New methods of ECT are painless and pose little risk of harm. The most common side effect is a limited, temporary loss of memory.

Outook

Depression usually has a beginning and end, but many people who have major depression once will have it again. Major depressions generally last six months to two years; the average duration is nine months.

Bipolar depression tends to be a lifelong condition, requiring close medical supervision. If you learn to manage this condition effectively, as most people do, you can lead a fully–functioning life.

Chronic Fatigue Syndrome

While debilitating fatigue is the hallmark of chronic fatigue syndrome (CFS), a feeling of weariness is not, by itself, a sure sign of this illness. People with CFS have a combination of symptoms, including sore throat, swollen glands, low–grade fever, muscle pain, and confusion. The symptoms may come and go, vary in intensity from mild to incapacitating, and last for months or years. Exercise often makes CFS worse.

People with CFS describe it as feeling like a terrible case of flu that never gets better. A typical victim, previously well and active, suddenly comes down with a flu–like condition. Then, instead of getting better, she develops a chronic illness that includes a severe, prolonged fatigue.

CFS is not well understood: it was only officially described by the Centers for Disease Control and Prevention in 1988. Research into its causes and treatments is just beginning and no clear answers have emerged. The condition goes by several names: you may hear it called chronic fatigue immune dysfunction syndrome (CFIDS), chronic Epstein–Barr, or myalgic encephalomyelitis.

Most disturbingly, you may still find doctors who do not believe the syndrome exists, or doctors who believe CFS patients are actually suffering from depression, or even faking it.

It is not even certain how many people have the illness: estimates in the United States range from 100,000 to five million. Although most people diagnosed with CFS are young adult women, the condition occurs in people of all ages and races and of both sexes. CFS is not contagious.

Causes of CFS

Current thinking is that CFS probably has more than one cause; research generally falls into two areas: immune dysfunction or a viral cause. Experts pursuing the viral theory say it is not clear whether there are several viruses that each happen to cause the same syndrome, or whether the disease results from a combination of viruses working together. Some research shows that people with CFS may have an abnormal response to viruses in general. Some viruses, such as Epstein–Barr and human herpes virus 6, have been considered as possible causes, but there is no conclusive evidence for any single virus.

Recent research into the immune dysfunction theory has found that cytokines, an immune system component normally active in fighting infections, may be involved in CFS.

Two other areas under investigation are a link between CFS and allergies and the relationship of CFS to inflammation of the central nervous system.

Diagnosing CFS

Since there is no one conclusive lab test for CFS, diagnosing the syndrome means ruling out all the things it isn't—a very difficult task. For example, CFS shares symptoms with medical disorders such as lupus, multiple sclerosis, and Lyme disease, as well as with depression, so these conditions must all be ruled out before CFS can be seriously considered.

CFS is defined by a menu of factors, including two major criteria, ten symptoms and three physical signs. The general diagnostic rule is that you must fulfill both major criteria, have six or more of the ten symptoms and at least two of the three physical signs, or have eight or more symptoms in the absence of physical signs.

The two major criteria are:
- New onset of persistent fatigue that reduces activity 50 percent, and does not get better with bedrest
- Fatigue not explained by other medical or psychiatric illness

The ten symptoms are:
- Mild fever or chills
- Sore throat
- Painful lymph nodes
- General muscle weakness
- General muscle pain
- Prolonged fatigue after physical activity
- Generalized headaches
- Pain that moves from one joint to another without swelling or redness
- Forgetfulness, excessive irritability, confusion, or inability to concentrate
- Sleep disturbance

The three physical signs are:
- Low–grade fever
- Dry inflamed throat
- Swollen or tender lymph nodes in neck or armpits

Treatments for CFS

There is no proven cure for CFS. Treatments in current use only help relieve symptoms. Most doctors recommend improving general health and physical condition. If you have CFS, you should eat a balanced diet, get adequate rest, and exercise as much as your condition allows—walking is most frequently recommended.

You must also learn to set limits and pace yourself, since stress can often make the symptoms worse. For many people, lifestyle changes may be necessary. For example, you may need to take a job closer to home, or switch to a less stressful occupation. Many people with CFS cannot work full time while they are ill.

Pain management programs may help with severe muscle pain or headache, while sleep disorders can often be treated at a specialized sleep disorder center; relaxation training may help reduce stress; some alternative therapies, such as acupuncture, have helped some patients. Support groups and counseling may also be helpful.

Drug Treatment for CFS has met with mixed results. There are reports of success in treating symptoms of CFS with a number of products, including antiviral drugs, antidepressants and medications that boost the immune system. But few drugs for CFS have gone through formal clinical testing, and none have shown clear benefits. Recent tests of antiviral agents such as acyclovir (Zovirax), and immunoglobulin (Gamimune, Gammagard, others) have been inconclusive, working no better than dummy pills in some tests.

Some doctors use pain relievers, non-steroidal anti–inflammatory drugs, and injections of gamma globulin (Gammar), vitamin B_{12} and magnesium for relief of general symptoms.

Support groups. Because chronic fatigue syndrome is not well understood, you may want to be in touch with the national organizations that offer the latest information on the illness. There are also patient organizations that can help you find a support group. Many people with CFS find these groups helpful in dealing with the effects of the disease on their lives. For information, check the directory at the end of this book.

Outlook

The good news is that CFS does not seem to get worse over time. Often the first episode is the worst, with relapses becoming fewer and milder over time. Typically, symptoms come and go, and worsening symptoms are rare.

People with CFS generally tend to improve, even if they do not recover completely. Most people with CFS make significant changes in their lifestyles while they have the disease, and learn to accept new limits. Some people recover spontaneously in a few weeks or months.

There are no reports of death from CFS. □

CHAPTER 34　　　　　　　　　　　**CONQUERING EMOTIONAL PROBLEMS**

Battling Anorexia, Bulimia…and Obesity

You see their photos everywhere: gaunt models strutting the latest in fashion, skinny socialites dining in trendy restaurants, svelte young actresses partying till dawn at the newest club. No wonder American women seem obsessed with their weight.

But when is thin too thin? And when does dieting turn into a life–threatening eating disorder?

Over the past few years, the media have been filled with the tragic stories of famous women whose abnormal eating behavior led to serious health problems and even death. For the most part, these women suffered from anorexia nervosa or bulimia nervosa. Together these eating disorders affect approximately 8 million Americans—mostly young women and teenaged girls. At the opposite extreme, excessive overweight (obesity), while rarely deadly in itself, increases your risk of life–threatening medical conditions ranging from breast cancer to heart disease.

All three of these problems represent normal diet gone awry. Anorectic women relentlessly pursue thinness by literally starving themselves for varying periods of time. Victims of bulimia suffer repeated binges of eating followed by purging through self–induced vomiting, laxatives, and similar measures. Seriously overweight women— defined medically as those who are more than 20 percent over their ideal weight—are often plagued by compulsions to eat.

It's important to remember that these disorders are not merely the normal variations in eating we all go through. Dieting is not automatically a sign of anorexia any more than an occasional eating binge such as consuming an entire package of cookies in one sitting means you are suffering from bulimia. If you're 5 or 10 pounds overweight, you may feel "fat," but that doesn't make you medically obese.

Anorexia Nervosa

The word anorexia means "loss of appetite," but this name is misleading. Anorectics—95 percent of whom are women—often have a normal appetite but because of an abnormal fear of being fat and a distorted body image, they're convinced that they're obese and refuse to eat. In most cases their weight is within—or below—acceptable limits. Anorexia is considered a psychological disorder because there is no known physical cause for the extreme weight loss associated with the condition.

Tipoffs of Anorexia

You may be anorectic if you:

- Lose at least 25 percent of your original weight.
- Have not had a physical or mental illness that could have caused the weight loss.
- Think of yourself as fat even if you're not.
- Fear being overweight and losing control over your eating behavior.
- Refuse to eat enough to maintain or return to a normal weight.
- Fail to menstruate for at least three consecutive months.
- Feel that all of your energy is going into controlling your weight.
- Feel that staying hungry is the only way you can avoid becoming fat.

Other signs that you may have anorexia include growth of a fine covering of hair all over your body, sensitivity to cold, and constipation. You may also feel depressed or anxious.

Weight loss is the most visible symptom of anorexia. Most anorectics drastically reduce the amount of food they eat. Some cut back mainly on certain types of "fattening" foods such as bread and sweets, while others eat less of everything. Sometimes anorectics lose control and go on an eating binge. Like bulimics, they usually follow this binge with laxatives or self–induced vomiting, to prevent food from being absorbed into the body.

Many anorectics are compulsive exercisers, and their typical program is far more strenuous than normal. Women with anorexia often devote a major portion of their waking hours to aerobics, weight training, calisthenics, or running.

While most women worry about their weight and diet at some point in their lives, the anorectic organizes her life around food. If a social occasion involves eating, she'll decline the invitation. The dieter, on the other hand, will generally put in an appearance and try not to eat too much.

Who's at Risk?

Anorexia is most likely to begin sometime between adolescence and the early 20s, but it can appear in children under the age of 10 or in women as old as 70. Although the disorder receives a great deal of publicity, it's relatively rare. For example, among teenage girls—the group at highest risk—the rate of anorexia is under 1 percent. While the disorder is most common among the middle and upper classes, it occurs in all social classes and ethnic groups.

Certain personality traits increase the risk of developing anorexia. Anorectic girls are often described as "model children" or perfectionists. Many have overcontrolling parents who are themselves fascinated by fitness and appearance. Faced with the impossible task of always being perfect, these girls discover that they can take charge of at least one aspect of their lives by exerting control over their eating and their weight.

Family background may also predispose a woman to anorexia. If you have a mother or sister with anorexia, you are more likely to have the problem than if there were no history of the disorder in your family. However, in a number of cases, there is no familial link.

Why It Happens

Anorexia and eating disorders are unhealthy responses to stress, painful feelings, and other problems. While the specific cause is unknown, the condition seems to stem from a combination of psychological, biological, familial, and cultural factors.

The teens and early twenties are tumultuous years for a woman. Moods and emotions can swing wildly from one day to the next. The dutiful daughter turns into the rebel, eager to assert her independence—sometimes in self-destructive ways.

Some researchers see anorexia as a power struggle between a strong-willed girl and her dominating parents. Starving herself, she unconsciously shows that she is in control of her own body and affirms that her parents are powerless to stop her.

Since anorexia usually causes menstrual periods to stop and breasts to flatten, other experts theorize that girls who refuse to eat may be expressing a desire to remain children, free of adult bodies, adult sexual relationships, and adult responsibilities.

Stress can play a major role in anorexia. Taking an exam, moving to a new home, starting college or a new job, becoming pregnant, and beginning or ending a relationship may sometimes push a woman into beginning the heavy dieting that ends with anorexia.

Our equation of thinness with beauty, social success, and even desirability is also at fault. In America, the pressure to be thin is intense. Most young women can handle it successfully, but a few respond in extreme ways, such as anorexia.

For some adolescents, ordinary biology poses a problem. As their bodies mature, many girls discover that they can no longer eat as they used to without gaining weight. Most can cut back as needed; a few lose control. Sensible dieting is fine, but when *low* calories become *no* calories, it's time to admit there's a problem.

Consequences of Anorexia

Ironically, most anorectics develop an intense interest in food and a fascination with recipes and cookbooks. They spend many hours planning menus, buying groceries, and preparing meals for others, yet eat next to nothing themselves. This preoccupation may grow stronger as the pounds continue to drop off.

Stringent dieting leads to muscle and fat loss. The body begins to look like a skeleton, bones protrude, legs resemble matchsticks, and breasts disappear. Facial muscles tighten because there is no layer of fat beneath the skin to cushion them.

Anorexia can last for many years and cause severe health problems. Besides weight loss and absence of menstrual periods, the physical consequences of anorexia may include:

- Anemia
- Constipation, digestive discomfort, and abdominal bloating
- Dehydration, muscle cramps, and tremors
- Dental problems
- Downy body hair on the face, back or arms
- Dry skin
- Dull and brittle hair
- Excessively low blood pressure
- Icy hands and feet
- Irregular heartbeat

If anorexia remains untreated, it can be fatal. Some victims literally starve themselves to death or die of conditions related to their malnourished state. Others commit suicide.

How Doctors Decide It's Anorexia

Doctors look for such common signs of anorexia as a patient's conviction that she needs to lose weight, a weight loss of at least 25 percent, and absence of at least 3 consecutive menstrual periods. The physician must also rule out other medical problems that could be responsible for the weight loss.

There is no laboratory test for anorexia, although your doctor may draw blood to check for physical problems such as anemia. Since several other physical diseases and mental disorders cause many of the same physical problems, your physician will rely mainly on your attitude toward eating and information about your behavior in making a diagnosis.

Getting Treatment

Self–help doesn't work for anorexia because the victims do not consider themselves sick. Most believe they are doing the right thing and are convinced that their attitude toward food and weight is reasonable. They are quite happy to go on starving themselves and rarely seek medical care on their own—at least not for the anorexia itself. They may see a doctor because they are concerned about missing their periods or are worried about other physical symptoms. Sometimes concerned parents take their daughter to a physician because her extreme weight loss makes them suspect she is anorectic.

If you think you have anorexia or are worried about a family member, ask your physician for an evaluation and a referral to someone who can help. If the situation seems life–threatening, go immediately to a hospital emergency room or call a crisis hotline (listed in the Yellow Pages under Crisis Intervention Service).

Anorectics need more than orders to "eat more." The first step is to restore a normal or near–normal body weight. In extreme cases, when the anorectic has lost so much weight that her life is in danger, the priority is to save her from starvation. After stabilizing her weight, the anorectic must relearn normal eating behavior and abandon drastic weight loss strategies, such as excessive exercise and vomiting or purging. This can't be achieved without coming to grips with the personality or family problems that have helped cause the illness.

The best way to conquer anorexia is to catch and treat it early. If you have this dangerous eating disorder, your doctor may hospitalize you until you have gained weight. If you decide to stay home, you'll need regular medical checkups and counseling.

Some anorectics undergoing hospital in-patient treatment programs try to continue controlling their weight by flushing food down the toilet, making themselves vomit, or taking laxatives. They also find ways to make their weight seem higher during examinations. Experienced doctors and nurses know how to handle such deceptions.

Because they understand the anorectic's fear of being fat, physicians, nurses, or others treating her usually encourage her to gain only the minimum weight necessary for her height to maintain normal, healthy body functions, such as menstruation and temperature control.

Stopping such dangerous weight–loss tactics as self–induced vomiting and the frequent use of laxatives can produce some side effects. You may temporarily gain weight as your body becomes rehydrated. Cramps, abdominal fullness, and constipation may continue for some time during this readjustment period. If you experience any of these symptoms, don't panic and revert to the habits that made you sick. Your body must go through these changes on its way back to health.

If you've suffered extreme weight loss, treatment may include forced nutrition through intravenous infusions and tube feeding. However, many anorectics resent these measures which they regard as an attempt to control their behavior and weight, and this, in turn, makes recovery even more difficult.

Counseling and therapy are essential to recovery from anorexia. Individual psychotherapy will help the anorectic face her problem, while family therapy helps those close to her change patterns of behavior that may have contributed to the disorder. Many patients also benefit from group therapy or support groups where they can share their feelings and gain strength from others who have the same problems. Nutritional counseling can be a practical help.

Occasionally, physicians prescribe medications such as tranquilizers, antidepressants, and lithium carbonate. Unfortunately, no drug now on the market has proven successful in treating anorexia, though some of the new antidepressants have been helpful. A combination of individual and family therapy is usually the best route to recovery.

Is Recovery Possible?

An estimated 50 to 70 percent of anorectics in treatment return to their normal or near–normal weight. Reaching this goal takes at least 6 months. About 15 to 20 percent will have an occasional relapse. Women who force themselves to vomit, and purge with laxatives are at highest risk for failure. They may binge intermittently during or after treatment. If you fit this description, you need to continue seeing your doctor or therapist for help and encouragement. Fifteen to 20 percent of anorectics need treatment for many years.

For those who don't try to beat the disease, the prognosis is guarded. An estimated 10 to 20 percent of anorectics die from related problems. The cause of death ranges from starvation and suicide to heart problems brought on by imbalances in the body due to excessive vomiting. Some women succumb to infections and diseases that overcome their weakened immune systems.

Treatment substantially improves the odds of survival. Among those who seek therapy, the mortality rate is only 5 percent. Recovery rates may grow even higher in coming years as researchers find better ways of fighting this very dangerous disorder.

Bulimia Nervosa

The hallmark of bulimia is a repeated uncontrollable urge to eat large amounts of food in a short time. After this binge, the bulimic often induces vomiting or uses laxatives, enemas, or diuretics to prevent weight gain. Some bulimics never purge themselves, but most go on strict diets between binges.

Until 15 or 20 years ago, doctors considered bulimia and anorexia two aspects of the same disorder. The conditions do have some characteristics in common. Both mainly affect women—particularly teens and young adults—and both are marked by binges of eating. However, while women with anorexia are obsessed by the urge to become ever thinner, those with bulimia usually maintain a normal weight and start a binge/purge cycle to avoid getting fat.

Profile of a Bulimic

All victims of bulimia are plagued by irresistible urges to binge on food. During a binge, bulimics often choose foods—such as ice cream, candy bars, puddings and cookies—that are high–fat, high–sugar, easy–to–swallow, and easy–to–vomit afterward. Bulimics usually gorge in secret. A binge typically lasts about 2 hours—although some are shorter or longer—and only stops when the bulimic gets a stomachache, feels sleepy, or is interrupted.

After a binge, self–induced purging is the norm. Bulimics usually make themselves vomit or use laxatives, diuretics, or diet pills to get rid of all the excess food. Some then follow a strict diet or exercise compulsively to undo the damage until the cycle begins all over again.

Women with this eating disorder often feel depressed, ashamed, and guilty after a binge. They realize that their behavior is abnormal, and that they are out of control.

The pattern of binge eating varies. Some bulimics binge several times a day for a few days, then not at all for a long time. Others follow a predictable pattern, such as binging and purging 3 times a week. Some binge only in response to certain stressful situations. The behavior may go on for years, although many bulimics often eat normally between phases of binging and purging. A few bulimics are totally given over to the binge and purge pattern and never maintain a normal diet. The amount of food consumed during a binge also varies considerably, but is always much more than the bulimic would ordinarily eat in a day.

Who's at Risk?

While young and middle or upper class women are particularly susceptible to bulimia, the disorder strikes people of all economic backgrounds and is found among all ethnic groups. The illness usually begins between the ages of 15 and 24, but it can occur in younger or older women and in men. If you are a young woman, your odds of developing bulimia are estimated to be between 1 in 10 and 1 in 20.

Studies have shown that bulimics frequently have obese parents or siblings, which may explain their exceptional fear of becoming fat themselves. Studies have also found that close family members of bulimics suffer from depression more often than would be expected.

Some bulimics adopt this abnormal eating pattern for professional reasons. Dancers, actors, models, and athletes whose careers depend on low body weight often stay thin by purging themselves with laxatives or inducing vomiting. They do not, however, always indulge in binge eating.

Why It Happens

To date there is no conclusive evidence linking bulimia to such biological factors as chemical imbalance in the brain. According to one theory, after you have eaten a usual amount of food, your brain sends a message to turn off the desire to eat more. But if you have starved yourself or followed a strict diet between binges, you are in a food–deprived state. When you resume eating during a binge, the turnoff message may fail to work. You then continue eating well beyond the point where you ordinarily would stop.

A few researchers have suggested that physical, psychological, or especially sexual abuse in childhood may cause bulimia later in life. These findings are controversial, and the role child abuse plays in causing bulimia is unclear.

Social pressures could also play a part. Society's emphasis on thinness as the ideal form of feminine beauty may be what causes some young women to become so afraid of the idea of becoming fat that they fall into the binge/purge pattern of bulimia. One thing is certain: If you are susceptible to bulimia, your first episode may be triggered by a stressful situation such as school problems, death in the family, career changes, divorce, or pregnancy.

Consequences of Bulimia

Unlike anorectics, most bulimics know that their behavior is abnormal and that their eating binges are not merely ordinary overeating. They also know that anxiety and depression sometimes trigger their episodes. However, they are usually unable to break the binge and purge cycle without professional help.

If you have bulimia, you're probably fascinated with food. You enjoy reading articles about food, buying cookbooks, and talking about food and cooking. Food and eating become ways to escape from life's many stresses.

You probably plan well for your binges, hoarding food, buying special treats, and preparing elaborate dishes. The foods you choose may be those you do not let yourself have at other times because you think they are "bad" and will make you gain weight. Sweets fit into this category.

You are also careful to conceal your illness. You may go to a number of different stores so that your purchases do not cause attention. Perhaps you tell the checkout clerks that you have a large family or are planning a party as a way to explain your overflowing shopping cart.

During the binge, you may abandon normal table manners and stuff yourself, gulping food as fast as you can. If you are sure you will not be discovered, you may eat at a more normal pace. By the time you're finished, you may have consumed 3 to 30 times more than you would normally eat in a day.

You probably have a secret place to binge—perhaps a closet. You have also found ways to vomit without being discovered; locked bathrooms are a popular choice. Because of your secrecy, you may have been able to hide your binge and purge episodes from your parents, husband, siblings, or roommates for years.

This destructive behavior eventually takes a toll on your body. Physical consequences of bulimia include:

■ Broken blood vessels in the face and bags under the eyes

■ Dehydration, fainting spells, tremors, and blurred vision

■ Indigestion, cramps, abdominal discomfort, bloating, gas and constipation

■ Internal bleeding and infections

■ Laxative dependency and damage to the bowels

■ Liver and kidney damage

■ Loss of tooth enamel from repeated vomiting

■ Suicidal depression

■ Swollen glands in the neck under the jaw.

■ Upset of the body's fluid/mineral balance, possibly causing rapid or irregular heartbeats or even a heart attack

■ Weight fluctuations from alternating diets and binges

■ Rupture of the esophagus (upper gastric tract)

Though bulimia is not as deadly as anorexia, fatalities do occur.

How Doctors Decide It's Bulimia

A physician who suspects bulimia looks for signs and symptoms established by the American Psychiatric Association:

■ Recurrent episodes of binge eating

■ A feeling of a lack of control over eating behavior during the binges

■ Regular self–induced vomiting, use of laxatives or diuretics, strict dieting or fasting, or vigorous exercise in order to prevent weight gain

■ A minimum average of two binge eating episodes a week for at least three months

■ Persistent excessive concern with body shape and weight

Getting Treatment

Bulimics may not develop the life–threatening medical problems that anorectics are prey to. Bulimics are generally treated with psychotherapy rather than the hospitalization and constant supervision required for some anorectics. There are exceptions to this guideline. If you feel suicidal or severely depressed, you may have to be hospitalized briefly for examination and preparation of a treatment plan. You may also need a short stay in the hospital if your bulimia has caused physical problems that require medical attention.

Unlike anorectics, who deny their illness and resist treatment, some bulimics want help and are willing to try to change their behavior. If you do begin treatment, you should realize, however, that you may experience some initial side effects. Temporary weight gain may occur as your body begins to retain fluid again; and symptoms such as constipation, abdominal fullness, and cramps may continue for some time.

The goal of treatment is to change your eating patterns while maintaining your normal weight. Your therapist will help you to uncover and deal with unconscious motives for your compulsion to binge and work with you to change your attitude toward food and weight. You will also be taught ways to overcome bad habits that keep you focused on food, such as maintaining records of how much food you eat, counting calories, weighing yourself frequently, and constantly reading recipes and cookbooks. You will have to stop labeling foods as "good" and "bad" and accept the fact that it is all right to eat high–calorie or sweet foods in moderation.

While antidepressants and other medications are sometimes tried during treatment of anorexia, they do not seem to break the binge/purge cycle of the typical bulimic. Research also shows that after initial improvement, many bulimics receiving drug therapy regress to their former behavior. Because these powerful medications may produce undesirable side effects, doctors usually reserve them for cases in which severe depression accompanies the bulimia.

Neither medication or individual therapy are always the answer to bulimia. If you're having trouble the doctor may recommend family therapy and group sessions with other bulimics. Other options include daytime care in a clinic or hospital and supervised use of a self–help manual.

Is Recovery Possible?

Although bulimia is not as dangerous as anorexia, doctors have found that it's more difficult to treat, and the recovery rate is lower. By one estimate, about 40 percent of bulimics respond well to treatment, 40 percent have moderate success, and 20 percent show no improvement. Relapses are common and can be triggered by any stressful event such as school exams, career change, illness, marriage, or divorce.

Your chances of returning to a normal life may be better if you can establish a good relationship with your therapist or physician. If you feel comfortable during treatment, you may return for more help if you have a relapse. It is also important to avoid taking a job associated with food preparation or serving. Bulimics who become cooks or wait-resses often resume their former dangerous eating patterns.

Obesity

Although simply being overweight is not a disorder of the same caliber as anorexia and bulimia, it's still a major health problem and a cause of concern and frustration for millions of Americans. If you have trouble keeping your weight down, you're far from alone. About a quarter of the population is technically classified as "obese."

The Official Definition

Medically speaking, obesity is not just another word for "fat." To be considered obese, you must weigh at least 20 percent more than the norm for a woman of your height and bone structure. What's more, there are four grades of obesity. If you are 20 percent heavier than your ideal weight, you are slightly obese. At 40 percent above normal you are moderately obese; at 50 percent, morbidly obese; and at 100 pounds or more over the weight you should be, you are hyperobese.

Doctors worry about obesity because it is a contributing factor in a variety of danger-ous medical conditions including diabetes, high blood pressure, and heart disease.

Who's at Risk?

Obesity often runs in families, although the exact nature of this apparent genetic influence on body weight is still unknown. Since you can't pick your parents, you can't control your predisposition to developing this disorder.

Obesity is also related to your economic background. Being overweight is more common in working–class groups than in the wealthy, possibly because less affluent people cannot afford the expensive diet and exercise programs favored by the rich. In addition, among the well–off, it is unacceptable to be obese or even moderately heavy, while working–class people are more tolerant of weight problems.

Gender and age also influence your weight. About twice as many women as men qualify as obese; and in both women and men, weight often increases with age.

Your ethnic background also makes a difference. Eskimos, for instance, tend to have slower metabolisms, burning energy more slowly than others and generally tending to be heavier. In this country, obesity is a greater problem for blacks than for whites.

Why It Happens

If you think the answer is "too much food," you're not entirely wrong. However, there are a couple of factors that determine what's too much. Inactivity reduces your calorie requirement, making more of what you eat unnecessary. A slow metabolism that burns fewer calories does the same. Psychological factors can also contribute to the problem. If you turn to food for comfort in times of stress, chances are greater that you'll wind up overeating.

Consequences of Obesity

Medical consequences aside, severe over-weight can lead to numerous other problems, including real psychological difficulties. Subtle put–downs, outright criticism, and even insults all take their toll. Years of discrimination can batter self–esteem to the point that psychotherapy is needed along with an attack on the excess weight.

How Doctors Gauge Obesity

A doctor generally decides that you are obese simply by looking at you. Most doctors form mental images of the various categories of obesity, from moderate to hyperobese. After judging your appearance, the doctor will then confirm his or her impression by more objective means.

The most common method is by comparing your weight to the figures on standard height and weight charts. These charts are based on life insurance company statistics. They list a range of *ideal* weights for various heights and body frames. At each height, the ideal weight-range for people with a particular type of frame can vary more than 20 pounds; and for a given height, the range from the lowest weight in the small–frame category to the heaviest in the large–frame category can be as high as 40 pounds.

Some experts argue that these height and weight charts are inaccurate for one reason or another. They are widely used, however, and provide a standard baseline for making decisions about weight.

Another common way of measuring obesity is called the skinfold "pinch test." To test you in this way, a doctor measures folds of skin at various parts of your body.

When you see a doctor for treatment of obesity, your examination is likely to include questions about obesity in your family. You will also be asked about your eating and exercise habits, use of cigarettes and alcohol, your occupation, and your experiences with gaining and losing weight in the past. During your physical examination, the doctor will check for signs of other medical conditions that might be responsible for your excess weight. Lower than normal activity of the thyroid or adrenal glands are two possibilities. However, these and other medical conditions are to blame in only about 1 percent of obesity cases.

Attacking the Problem

There's no way around it: to rid yourself of obesity you need to diet rigorously, though regular exercise is also helpful in shedding pounds and keeping them off. Although both over–the–counter and prescription medications help take off pounds temporarily, there is little evidence that they are effective in helping you maintain weight loss over the years.

The best diet includes nutritious foods served in smaller portions than you're in the habit of eating. Be sure to check with your doctor before undertaking low carbohydrate diets, liquid protein fasts, and other "fad diets." Some can be dangerous. Liquid diets of the past, for example, caused several deaths and hospitalizations; the dieters apparently starved to death because the liquids provided only a few hundred calories per day.

Losing weight can be a struggle, particularly if your problem is severe enough to classify you as obese. You may find help and support from local chapters of such organizations as Weight Watchers and Overeaters Anonymous. These groups can offer both advice on weight loss and a chance to ease your feelings of isolation by talking with people who understand what you're going through. (For more information, see the directory of support groups at the end of the book.)

Medical treatment ranges from dieting under a doctor's supervision to outpatient or residential programs. These treatment programs are usually run by private doctors; some are associated with hospitals.

In an outpatient program, you will have regular consultations with the physician or other professionals. You will probably eat prepackaged diet foods for several months before gradually reverting to other foods. To prevent you from reverting to your old eating habits, the treatment may include behavior modification counseling.

Residential programs are more comprehensive; many include various forms of psychotherapy designed to treat obesity as an addiction. A residential program may charge thousands of dollars; outpatient therapy can cost you several hundred dollars or more per month.

Surgery is reserved only for people who are massively obese or whose health is at risk. The two most common surgical techniques are liposuction and intestinal bypass. In liposuction, a tool is inserted under the skin to suck fat from the body. In bypass surgery, the digestive flow is routed past the large and small intestines to reduce the amount of food absorbed. Both surgical techniques can be dangerous and should only be used as a last resort.

How To Increase the Odds of Success

Unfortunately, success rates for long–term weight loss are low. It is estimated that only 20 percent of patients lose 20 pounds and keep them off for more than 2 years. An even smaller percentage maintain higher rates of weight loss.

Your best chance for success is a multi–pronged attack, employing a variety of strategies and emphasizing maintenance of weight loss more than the initial loss of excess fat. A well–rounded treatment program that includes a low calorie diet, counseling to help change eating behavior, regular exercise, and social support is the approach most likely to work. It also helps to have a close, supportive relationship with your therapist or physician. Above all, you must be motivated to attain your goal and keep the pounds off. □

CHAPTER 35

CONQUERING EMOTIONAL PROBLEMS

Coping After A Sexual Assault

The word rape evokes images of being accosted by a strange man carrying a weapon, attacked by an intruder in your home, or kidnapped and forced at knife–point to perform degrading sexual acts against your will. The reality, however, is that in many cases the rapist is someone the victim knows— most likely a family member or a date. One researcher found that in more than 40 percent of rape cases, the victim identified her husband or friend as her attacker. Another study found that 84 percent knew the attacker. Many rapes occur at the place where the victim and the attacker meet—often one or the other's home—instead of a secluded parking lot or dark alley.

The odds are that one of every four women you know has been the victim of a sexual assault at some time in her life. If you've been raped yourself, you know that the pain doesn't end with the attack. You face the possibility of medical complications and of continuing emotional trauma. You also face decisions about whether to tell your family and friends, and whether you want to report the attack to the police.

Should You Tell?

Despite volumes of scientific evidence proving that rape is an act of assault, many people—jurors, professionals, and even attackers themselves—hold on to a false belief that the victim is somehow at fault. For these people, rape is a purely sexual act. They believe the woman, through her dress and behavior, must surely have provoked the assault, and that she merely got what she asked for. Of course, that's not true. One study found that more than 50 percent of rape survivors did not physically try to resist their victims, not because they were enjoying the attack, but out of fear of being more seriously injured or even killed. Less than 20 percent had dared to fight back.

Rape is not just an act of sex. It is an act of violence and aggression in which one person attempts to exert absolute control and domination over another. Women who flirt are not asking to be attacked. Rape victims are not "bad girls." They're pretty and unattractive, thin and overweight, healthy and disabled, very young and very old.

The fact that you did not fight back during a rape does not mean that you encouraged or enjoyed it. Even a spontaneous orgasm is not a sign of consent, it's simply a biological response.

At a time like this you need the support of your family and friends. But even though they mean well, they may not be there for you. Those closest to you may be so enraged over the mere fact that the assault could have happened that they lash out in all directions. They may even turn their anger on you. Some may say you "got what you deserved." Others may suspect you of lying about your role in the attack.

Only about 1 in 10 rapes is reported to the police. If the attacker was someone you know, making a report can be especially troubling. Fortunately, many police officers are especially trained to help you through this difficult time, so don't be afraid to tell them your story.

Your First Priority: Medical Treatment

Even if you think you're all right, see your own doctor or go to the hospital emergency room as soon as possible after the rape. The assault may have left you with undetected injuries that need prompt treatment. After examining you thoroughly, the physician will perform tests for sexually transmitted diseases and pregnancy and will collect evidence you'll need if you decide to prosecute the attacker. Since some of this

evidence is lost after 36 hours, it's especially important to get immediate medical attention.

Do not shower, douche, change clothes, or otherwise try to clean up before going to the emergency room. Bring along a change of clothes; the ones you were wearing during the attack will be kept for evidence. You may want to take a trusted friend, a family member, or a rape crisis worker with you for support.

What to Expect in the Emergency Room
You will probably speak to a nurse or other emergency room personnel before the doctor sees you. First they will ask routine questions about your vital statistics, medical insurance, allergies, and the type of birth control you use. They also need to know whether you're in pain, when you last had sex before the rape, and the date of your last period. By finding out how recently you menstruated, they can determine how likely it is that the attacker made you pregnant.

They will also ask questions about the assault; for example, whether the rapist used a condom, whether he bled or had an ejaculation, and whether you scratched him. Tell the doctor or nurses everything you recall. If you're not sure of the details, simply say you don't remember. The answers you give to their questions may become part of the record if you go to court.

A nurse may also take pictures of your visible injuries. (Sometimes it takes several days for bruises and other injuries to appear, so you will want to ask a friend to take instant photographs of anything that shows up after your hospital visit.)

The Examination
Next, a doctor will examine your vagina and treat anything that needs attention. He or she will also look for semen or other signs of

sexual intercourse and take samples of secretions from all areas involved in the attack.

A doctor, nurse, or technician will trim and comb your pubic hair to check for foreign tissue or fluids. You may be asked for a blood sample to test for the presence of alcohol or other drugs and a urine sample to find out if you were pregnant before the assault.

The Danger of
Sexually Transmitted Disease

You'll also be tested for sexually transmitted diseases (STDs), including gonorrhea, chlamydia, genital herpes, syphilis, and AIDS. If the rapist has an STD, there's a reasonable chance that he has passed it on to you through his semen or blood.

It takes 3 to 5 days to get the results back from initial STD testing. You'll also need follow–up tests 90 days later. Because of the chance that you were exposed to gonorrhea or chlamydia, the doctor will probably start treatment without waiting for the test results.

Symptoms of gonorrhea, if left untreated may be very mild, and you might not even notice them. You may have some abdominal pain, burning during urination, and a vaginal discharge. It is possible to get a gonorrhea infection in your mouth or anus, as well as in your vagina.

With chlamydia, you may notice a thin discharge from your vagina, as well as stomach pain and a burning sensation when you urinate some time after the exposure.

Trichomoniasis and vaginosis are forms of vaginal inflammation that can be caused by sexually transmitted organisms. They produce burning and itching sensations, odor, and a discharge.

In women, STD symptoms are not as noticeable as they are in men, and some types show no early warning signs at all. You

---

DOS AND DON'TS AFTER AN ASSAULT

DO...
- Seek medical help as soon as possible
- Bring a change of clothes to the emergency room
- Get tested for sexually transmitted disease
- Inquire about emergency contraception
- Remember that what you say to medical personnel could be used in court

DON'T...
- Shower...
- Douche, or...
- Change clothes until after the exam
- Hesitate to call the police

---

should report anything unusual—discomfort or discharge, for example—to your doctor.

Syphilis begins with genital sores—which may go unnoticed—and progresses into flu–like symptoms. This disease is so contagious that it can be passed on just by kissing, and, if left untreated, it will eventually attack other organs, causing heart trouble, blindness, and severe mental illness. For more on this and other STDs, turn to chapter 11, "Coming to Terms with Sexually Transmitted Disease."

AIDS—acquired immune deficiency syndrome—leads to the total destruction of the immune system, but unless you get tested, you can carry the HIV virus that causes it for years without knowing it. You may be tested for the virus at the emergency room, but because this infection is slow to show up in tests, you will have to be retested again 6 months later and again after a year. Finding out that you have this terminal illness could be devastating, but it's still better to know. Doctors do have drugs that can improve and prolong your life. For more information, see chapter 13, "The Growing Danger of AIDS."

If there is even a remote chance that you have gotten HIV or another STD, it's best to abstain completely from sex until you're sure you don't have it. If you do have sex, be sure to use a condom to help avoid the possibility of passing on HIV or other serious STDs to your partner.

Avoiding Unwanted Pregnancy

Unless you were using birth control at the time of the rape, there is a risk of pregnancy. If you choose not to carry an unwanted fetus to term, you have several options. For example, your doctor can give you emergency, or "morning after," hormonal treatment or insert an intrauterine device (IUD) to prevent a fertilized egg from developing in your uterus. Fortunately your chance of pregnancy is extremely low—between 2 and 4 percent—unless the attack took place in the middle of your menstrual cycle.

The Emotional Toll

Most if not all women experience some sort of emotional trauma after a sexual assault. These disturbances may not show up for months—or even years—but they can be a very real disruption in your life.

For half of all rape victims, emotional symptoms persist for months or years; so it is never too late to seek medical or emotional support if you feel you need it. In fact, some childhood victims continue to experience problems well into their adulthood.

Sexual assault victims are at higher risk than other women of developing a serious depression, substance abuse, and emotional problems. Indeed, survivors of sexual assault are 2 to 4 times more likely to have serious emotional problems as a result of the attack.

Two of the most common reactions are depression and what has come to be called posttraumatic stress disorder, or PTSD. How the rape affects you depends in part on the type of attack, the level of violence, how long it has been since the attack, whether you have a history of emotional problems, and the type of person you are.

First Reactions

Immediately after the attack, you'll probably feel confused and extremely afraid. A few hours later, these feelings will give way to depression, exhaustion, and restlessness. In about two weeks, you'll begin to feel better emotionally; but three weeks later, your symptoms may worsen again.

You may experience severe bouts of fear and depression and have problems with self–esteem, social adjustment, and sexual dysfunction for up to 18 months after the assault. These symptoms will probably last at least 6 years. Women who were raped as children may repress the memory, only to have it resurface full force years later.

It's important to talk with a professional about your assault and your reactions to it. A psychiatrist, therapist, or counselor specially trained to work with rape victims can help you understand that you really are the victim and not to blame for what happened. Vent your anger, fear, desperation, even guilt—and discuss how you feel about the attack at the present time. In that way you can learn how to deal with your emotions and get on with your life.

Posttraumatic Stress Disorder

First recognized in soldiers returning from battle, PTSD is also known as shell–shock and battle fatigue. This anxiety disorder is a common response of people who have been exposed to extreme violence, such as assault and rape.

Posttraumatic stress disorder can take several forms:

Posttraumatic stress response, an early form of PTSD, may go almost unnoticed. Rape victims sometimes develop generalized fears associated with the rape. Fear of being alone or going out after dark can keep you from participating in your normal activities. You may become afraid of all men or find it hard to trust or be intimate with anyone.

Posttraumatic stress disorder develops when these systems persist. If left untreated, anxiety can turn into full–blown depression.

Two of the most common signs of PTSD are insomnia and severe nightmares. You might relive the assault over and over; flash-backs and nightmares may be so strong that you actually seem to be experiencing the event. You may become obsessed with the encounter and what could happen if you see the rapist again.

Panic attacks can accompany PTSD. They usually occur in response to a specific stimu-lus, such as a frightening environment. Your fear may make you hyperventilate and may even convince you that you are dying. Relaxation exercises and other coping tech-niques, such as deep breathing, can help you control the panic attacks.

Depression

Many cases of depression are thought to be the result of chemical imbalances in the brain. However, people can also develop a crippling depression in response to an outside event such as rape.

If you are a rape victim, fear that no one will believe you, problems with a relation-ship, or feelings of self–blame are all reason enough for profound depression. You may feel helplessness, hopelessness, and worthless-ness. The very act of rape is dehumanizing. In all probability, the person who assaulted you said demeaning things to convince you that you deserved the attack.

Clinical depression is not the same as "the blues." It is often so debilitating that its suf-ferers cannot manage to get out of bed or feed themselves, much less participate in the routine of work, family and school. Unfortunately, it can lead to self–destructive behavior, substance abuse, even suicide. If you find yourself sliding into a deep depres-sion, you owe it to yourself to fight back. See a specialist and get the treatment you need.

Sexual Dysfunction

Rape victims often have sexual problems after an attack. Reactions range from wild promiscuity to a complete lack of desire and a total inability to respond. Even the thought of having sex may be disgusting. However, most women regain their normal sex drive within a few months after the rape.

Treatment for Emotional Problems

If you don't talk with a counselor or therapist in the emergency room, you will probably want to contact one later as you sort through your emotions following the attack. Ask your doctor, religious advisor, friends, or rape crisis center for a referral; call one of the mental health associations listed in your telephone book.

Some people still believe you have to be "crazy" to need or want therapy, or that seeking help is a sign of weakness. Don't be led astray by such misconceptions; some problems are too serious to handle alone.

Like everyone else, doctors and therapists have their own beliefs about sexual assault, rapists, and their victims. Look for a counselor with experience treating women like you, and ask up front how he or she feels about rape perpetrators and victims.

It is also appropriate to ask about how much therapy will cost, when payments are due, and whether treatment is covered by insurance. Counseling can be expensive, particularly if you must continue for a long time; but low cost or free services are available if you cannot afford the usual fees. You are under no obligation to continue treatment if the therapist makes you feel uncomfortable.

Both psychotherapy and medical therapy can help you deal with emotional problems. The most common medical treatment employs prescription drugs, such as antidepressants, to relieve your symptoms. Antidepressants work by changing the level of chemicals in the brain that are believed to be responsible for moods. If you are prescribed an antidepressant, be prepared to wait. Most of these drugs take time to work, and it may be weeks before you feel any improvement. Anxiety disorders, such as PTSD or panic attacks, respond to tranquilizers, psychotherapy, or a combination of the two.

Only a doctor can prescribe these drugs for you. He or she needs to monitor your response to make sure they are helping you and not causing unpleasant or dangerous side effects.

Discuss all medications and your reactions to them with your doctor, and be sure to call the office if you have questions or concerns.

Physicians, psychologists, social workers, and licensed counselors all can provide psychotherapy. You may choose one–on–one, family, or group counseling. (Some women's centers have groups for survivors of rape or incest.) "Behavior Therapy" is often helpful in treating conditions such as fears and phobias.

In therapy, you will have a chance to talk about what has happened to you and to vent your anger. You may also learn coping skills, relaxation techniques, communication skills, and techniques for controlling your rage.

Therapy doesn't have to be formal. Some women find that reading, self–help programs, volunteer work, and social activities help them recover. Others need to confront their rapists. Sometimes writing about the attack and your feelings during and after it can be therapeutic. If you decide to prosecute your attacker, keeping a journal can also help you sort out what to tell the police or your lawyer.

Will therapy cure your problems? There are no guarantees. It helps to know that you're not alone, that someone understands what you're going through and knows how to deal with it. Chances are you'll begin to feel better after a few sessions, although most rape victims find that time in itself is also a great healer. Give therapy a try and see if it enables you to regain control over your body and your life.

The Police and the Courts

The judicial system sometimes appears unsympathetic and even hostile to a victim of sexual assault, especially when the rapist is her husband or lover. The legal definition of rape varies from state to state; and in some places a man cannot legally rape his wife. Though the law may not always have a definition for marital rape, it most certainly does occur—often together with other types of violence and emotional abuse. Regardless of your relationship to the attacker, you always have the right to say no to sex.

Many advocates for rape victims believe that everyone who is sexually assaulted should report the incident to the authorities. You've probably heard of women who have followed that advice and feel as if they were raped all over again by the judicial system. Others say they just want to get on with their lives, and telling and re–telling their story to investigators, attorneys and jurors keeps them from putting the experience behind them. Nevertheless, making a police report may be the best course for the sake of both your personal safety and your emotional well–being.

If you decide to report the crime, it's best to do it soon after the attack. The police may even come to the emergency room to talk to you and collect evidence. They will ask you to give information about yourself, the person or people who assaulted you and the place where the rape occurred. Be sure to tell them whether you think your assailant will attack you again, so they can set up a plan to protect you. The police will also ask you for an exact description of the assailant and will have you sign a statement. They should also explain about your state's procedures for pressing charges. (You probably will not have to do so if you choose not to.)

The fact that you press charges does not mean the case will ever be prosecuted or that you will have to appear on the witness stand. If the case does go to court, it may be months or even years before it is heard; and your attacker's attorney probably will do everything possible to postpone the trial.

When you press charges, the attacker will be jailed, then in all probability released on bond. He'll be given a couple of hearings in which a judge will formally tell him the charge, assign him a lawyer if he can't afford one, and determine whether there is enough evidence for the case to go to a grand jury.

If the case goes forward, the grand jury will decide whether the evidence warrants an indictment. At several points in this process, the accused will have an opportunity to enter a plea; he may opt to plead guilty, perhaps to a lesser offense, in exchange for a lighter sentence.

If the case does go to trial, you will probably have to testify in open court. However, it isn't as degrading as it once was. Most states now have laws that prevent the defense attorney from bringing up the victim's sexual history in an attempt to discredit her, and the law in general seems to be growing more sensitive to victims' rights.

That is definitely not to say that you'll have an easy time. It is the defense attorney's job to try to convince the jury that his client—your attacker—is innocent and should be released without punishment. In doing so, he may insist that you consented to have sex; that you were at fault because you did something "wrong," such as going back to the man's apartment or having too much to drink; that you are blaming his client for something someone else did; or that no sexual activity occurred.

Rape can be hard to prove. You should understand that if the district attorney declines to prosecute, if the case is thrown out of court, or if your attacker is found not guilty, it doesn't mean you weren't raped or that you did something wrong. A "not guilty" verdict doesn't prove the rapist's innocence; it simply means the prosecution didn't have enough evidence to meet the level of proof required for a conviction.

You may also be able to sue your attacker in civil court for damages (mental and physical) that he has caused you. Talk to an attorney about your options. Many states and counties have referral services that can put you in touch with a lawyer if you need one.

Moving On

Though the road ahead may be long and difficult, you *can* recover from sexual assault. You can't expect things to ever be exactly the same as they were before, but you still can be certain that your life will return to normal. Do give yourself a few days to start sorting things out before going back to your routine activities. Don't dwell on the attack to the exclusion of all else. Always remember that you are not the guilty one, and that it's okay to feel anger and grief. Remember, too, that a strong support network of family, friends, and professionals can help you regain the most important component for your recovery—your sense of control. □

CHAPTER 36   **DEALING WITH CANCER**

Breast Cancer: Great Odds of a Cure

Rightly or wrongly, breast cancer is the disease that women dread most. A woman's chances of developing heart disease are actually much higher. Other forms of cancer are equally devastating and harder to cure. But somehow it's still breast cancer that grips our attention.

Maybe it's because almost everyone knows someone who's had it. Or because it strikes many women in the prime of their lives. Whatever the reason, the raw statistics are frightening in themselves:

■ Breast cancer hits 1 out of every 9 American women.
■ There are 100,000 new cases each year; the majority are women between 40 and 70 years old.
■ It is the leading cause of death in women aged 40 to 55 and causes more deaths than any other form of cancer from age 15 onward.

Now for the good news: Breast cancer has a very high cure rate—over 95 percent—when diagnosed early. Unfortunately, some women are so frightened of the "big C" that they don't call their physician even when they find a lump. Doctors can do much to fight this killer, but only if you give them the opportunity. It is impossible to overemphasize the importance of performing regular breast self–exams and getting regular mammograms during the high–risk years that surround menopause.

Whose Chances are Worst?

No one understands exactly why breast cancer seems to run in some families and not others, but physicians are getting better at predicting which of us is more likely to be stricken. Whatever the underlying reason may be, family history definitely does play a significant role. If your mother or sister—or both—have had breast cancer, your estimated risk is 10 to 15 times higher than that of a woman whose close female relatives are breast cancer–free. Breast cancer in a more distant relative, such as a cousin, is not currently considered to be a risk factor.

The older you are, the greater your chance of developing this frightening disease. Breast cancer rarely occurs before the age of 20. The odds of developing it gradually increase after that, leveling off for a bit after menopause, then starting to rise again at age 65. Many doctors now believe that age becomes a serious consideration after 40—particularly between ages 40 and 44—and again after 60.

The longer a woman remains fertile, the greater her chances of developing breast cancer. If you started having periods early (before the age of 12), stop having them late (after the age of 55), or have them for more than 30 years, you're in the high–risk group. Some doctors and medical researchers speculate that the factors that eventually trigger the development of breast cancer begin to work as soon as a girl enters puberty. The process continues until she reaches her early 40s.

Pregnancy seems to short–circuit the process under certain circumstances. The earlier a woman completes her first full–term pregnancy, the less likelihood she has of contracting the disease. For example, a woman's lifetime risk of developing breast cancer drops by as much as 70 percent when she has a baby before her eighteenth birthday. This beneficial effect steadily tapers off during her 20s and seems to vanish entirely by the time she reaches the age of 30.

Women who have their first baby after the age of 35 are twice as likely to develop breast cancer as those who give birth while still in their teens. As a matter of fact, postponing childbirth until your 30s seems to be more risky than never having a baby.

Although some reports seem to indicate that women with only one or two children are at a somewhat higher risk, having a large family will not reduce your odds of getting breast cancer. Nor does abortion play a significant role. And what of the widespread belief that breastfeeding naturally protects a nursing mother from breast cancer? At present, it's still under scientific debate.

Like early motherhood, the removal of the ovaries seems to offer some protection against breast cancer. If a woman's ovaries are surgically removed while she is still in her mid–to–late thirties, her chances of getting breast cancer can fall by as much as 75 percent. The risk–reducing benefits of this operation decline steadily as a woman nears the age of 40, then disappear entirely.

Other probable risk factors are harder to pinpoint. For example, breast cancer is most common among Caucasians and occurs much less often among Asians. But despite a very low rate of breast cancer among Japanese women who stay at home, the risk rises sharply among those who have moved to the United States—a phenomenon that has convinced some scientists of a link between environment and development of the disease.

Breast cancer also occurs more frequently among overweight women; city dwellers; and those who have previously had cancer of the (other) breast, ovary, or endometrium (the lining of the uterus). Women from high–income families are also at greater risk, perhaps because they can afford to eat rich, fatty foods that can raise estrogen levels in the body. This female hormone is thought to promote the growth of a breast cancer once it gets started.

Because the breast is extremely vulnerable to the effects of radiation, previous exposure to radiation increases the odds of breast cancer, especially for women exposed before the age of 30. Exposure as a young girl is a particular cause for worry.

Your chances of getting breast cancer probably increase further with each additional risk factor you sustain, but experts are not sure by how much. If you have even one, the safest course is to have regular breast exams every 3 to 6 months, so that if a cancer does develop it can be stopped in time.

The Estrogen Connection

Researchers have spent decades investigating the role of the natural female hormone estrogen—and the oral contraceptive pills that contain it—in the development of breast cancer. After all these years, however, there's still no clear answer.

At present, the experts have no evidence that oral contraceptives trigger breast cancer (although estrogen has caused tumors in lab animals). A study conducted by the federal Centers for Disease Control and Prevention found that even high-risk women who had used oral contraceptives for long periods of time ran no greater risk of breast cancer than those who do not take the Pill. Indeed, some studies have found that oral contraceptives that combine estrogen with another hormone may actually offer some protection against breast cancer.

One clinician has noted that if the Pill did in fact promote breast cancer, we certainly should have seen an increase in the disease by now. There are, however, a couple of provisos. Doctors still advise caution for women over the age of 35, who are typically warned against using oral contraceptives anyway for a variety of other reasons, including the increased possibility of stroke. It's also believed that estrogen may hasten the development of an existing breast cancer in genetically susceptible women. And it has been found that, once breast cancer occurs, the hormone stimulates its growth in a significant percentage of women, particularly those who develop benign breast lesions after they begin taking estrogen supplements.

Surgical removal of the ovaries, which creates an artificial menopause and ends a woman's natural production of estrogen, markedly reduces her risk of developing breast cancer, especially if she is in her mid–thirties. About half of women with advanced breast cancer will go into remission after this procedure. (On the other hand, some other women have had a remission while *taking* estrogen.)

Warning Signs to Watch For

For nearly 80 percent of women with breast cancer, the discovery of a mass or lump in the breast is the first sign that something is amiss. Fortunately, 3 out of every 4 lumps discovered turn out to be noncancerous, but if you do find a suspicious lump, it's still best to call your doctor right away.

Most women discover breast lumps themselves, either by accident or while performing a monthly self–examination. Because early detection is crucial for a cure, you need to learn the right way to examine your breasts each month. The next chapter "Your Best Insurance Against Brest Cancer," provides you with detailed instructions. Once you know the feel of a "normal" breast, you'll quickly recognize any little change.

Nearly half of all lumps appear at the top of the breast on the side nearest the armpit. For some reason the lumps occur in the left breast slightly more often than in the right. It is important to remember, though, that lumps can turn up anywhere within the breast, and that more than 20 percent of the time breast cancer is found when there's no lump at all.

If you do find a lump, your breast may be tender, or it may feel normal. There could be some discomfort or a "pulling sensation." Cysts, which are benign, tend to move freely within the breast, so when a lump appears to be immobile, or the skin is dimpled or puckered, doctors tend to suspect that the growth is malignant. However, this is not a certainty.

A discharge from the nipple is the second most common sign of a potential problem. The discharge may be clear, bloody, or colored. It is important to understand that a discharge can be perfectly normal in women who are not breastfeeding. In this case, a small amount of discharge usually comes out of several openings in *both* breasts.

A spontaneous discharge that occurs without squeezing the breast is a far greater cause for concern. A discharge coming from the same general location in one breast may well indicate the presence of an underlying mass. Although a bloody discharge occasionally may occur during pregnancy, it can also be a significant warning sign of cancer. The older the woman, the greater the possibility that the discharge is caused by cancer. The odds are even higher if she also has a lump.

Other signs of cancer include a change in the shape or size of the breast or swelling of the skin that covers it. The breast tissue may feel thicker, even though there is no lump. There may be pain or redness of the skin. The nipple may be sore or retract inside the breast. You should have a doctor examine any sores on the nipples or breast that do not clear up after two weeks of treatment with a prescribed cream or lotion. In most cases, the doctor will

need to take a sample for microscopic examination (a biopsy) to check for cancer.

As breast cancer progresses, signs and symptoms become unmistakable, including skin ulcers and extensive swelling and redness of the breast and swelling of the arm. The nipple may retract into the breast, and the breast may retract into the chest.

Next Steps If You Find a Lump

If you notice a lump or anything else that seems suspicious, the next step will be an examination, followed by a mammogram and a biopsy.

Mammography

This well–known procedure is essentially an x–ray of the breast. It is an important weapon in the fight against breast cancer. Mammograms are invaluable not only for examining a known lump, but also for detecting lumps too small to feel. A tumor can keep growing for as long as 7 years before you or your doctor can feel it; and some masses buried deep within the breast or under the arm can be detected only by a mammogram. Without this procedure, such cancers can reach the dangerous stage before you even know about them. For more on mammography and its importance in regular cancer screening, turn to the next chapter.

Once a lump is discovered, by mammography or otherwise, your doctor can make a reasonable guess about the likelihood of malignancy based on the physical signs he or she finds during the examination. However, several other diseases have similar signs and symptoms, and a mammogram can only show the size and location of a mass. To be certain about a lump, only a biopsy will do.

Biopsy

All lumps are presumed guilty until proven innocent, even though nearly 4 out of 5 lumps are noncancerous. Any lump—and anything suspicious on a mammogram—is automatically a signal for a biopsy. Your physician will also recommend a biopsy if a nipple is inflamed, encrusted, or has scaly lesions that don't go away, *or* if it is leaking a bloody fluid.

If you haven't yet gone through menopause and you don't have any signs or symptoms that point to the possibility of cancer, your doctor may decide to wait through one complete menstrual cycle before proceeding. During this time he or she will check to see whether the lump goes away or is in any way affected by the hormonal changes that occur before, during, and after menstruation. On the other hand, if you have a history of cysts, or if the physician strongly suspects the mass is a relatively harmless cyst, he or she may do a needle biopsy right in the office.

This procedure, also known as fine needle aspiration, is fast, relatively painless and can help ease your anxiety *if* the lump is only a cyst and not a tumor. The doctor simply swabs the area with an antiseptic solution, then inserts a thin needle into the lump and draws off the fluid. The procedure can be done under local anesthesia.

A cyst is little more than a fluid–filled sac; a mass has more substance. The needle should have no trouble penetrating a cyst, but may encounter resistance if the lump is a solid mass and potentially malignant.

If the lump is really a cyst, the sac will collapse as soon as the fluid is removed, and the lump will suddenly disappear. In this case you will need a mammogram just to be sure, as well as another examination in 2 or 3 weeks. If the lump has not returned, there generally is no further cause for concern. However, a follow–up biopsy *is* needed if the doctor isn't able to get any fluid; if the fluid is bloody; if the mass does not completely

FINE NEEDLE ASPIRATION

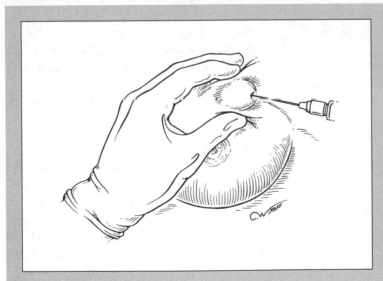

This minor office procedure can quickly reveal whether a breast lump is a benign cyst or something more worrisome. To find out, the doctor inserts a thin needle into the lump and draws out the liquid contents. If the fluid is greenish or straw-colored, you're dealing with a harmless cyst. If it contains blood, further tests are needed: The doctor will smear a sample on a glass slide and send it to be examined for abnormal cells. The whole procedure takes only a few minutes, and requires no advance preparation.

disappear after the fluid is drawn; if the "cyst" returns after two "successful" aspirations; or if the mammogram is suspicious.

Another possible procedure is a core needle biopsy, which uses a larger needle to take a sample of the mass. This approach, which does require local anesthesia, can be helpful for large tumors that might be difficult to remove in the office. However, a negative result could be misleading. In other words, even though the small sample contains no cancer cells, there's no guarantee that the entire mass is cancer–free.

If there is any doubt about the results of a needle biopsy, your doctor will order a surgical biopsy. This is necessary because the only way to be sure of the diagnosis is to look at the abnormal tissue under a microscope. If the lump is small—and your doctor feels it's not malignant—the surgeon will probably do an excisional biopsy, removing the entire mass. If the lump is larger, an incisional biopsy can be done instead. This procedure removes a small specimen from the mass, usually providing enough tissue for a diagnosis without having to make a large incision. However, if a diagnosis cannot be made without more tissue, the surgeon may decide to do an excisional biopsy and take the rest of the lump.

Biopsies are often performed on an outpatient basis. In the old days, the woman remained in the operating room while the pathologist examined the specimen. If the diagnosis was cancer, her breast was removed immediately. Clinical studies eventually showed that there was no need to do the biopsy and surgery in a single step. In the increasingly popular two–step approach, the biopsy is done at an outpatient clinic and surgery, if necessary, is performed in a hospital a week or so later.

A short delay between biopsy and surgery doesn't harm a woman's chance of survival, but does allow her time to discuss the proposed treatment and possible breast reconstruction with her physician. The doctor, in turn, has time to order a chest x-ray, blood tests, and other laboratory procedures that help determine whether the cancer has spread from the breast to the bones, lungs, liver or brain. If the cancer is localized, these test results can establish a baseline against which the doctor will compare follow–up tests done every three months after surgery.

The movement towards the two–step outpatient approach to biopsies has removed much of the fear that once kept women from seeking help when they felt a lump. In fact, as women take increased responsibility for their health care decisions, more and more of them are likely to request a biopsy. These women are no longer content with well–intended reassurances that the doctor is "almost 100 percent sure that there is nothing to worry about." These women want answers that only a biopsy can provide.

Biopsy of a non–cancerous mass may also reveal the first signs of an early cancer in the surrounding "healthy" tissue. Without a doubt, biopsy remains the best–possible way to identify malignancies while the cancer is still highly curable.

Ultrasound

Ultrasound, another diagnostic tool, forms a picture by bouncing sound waves off the mass. Ultrasound takes longer to perform than a needle biopsy, and the results are generally not as good. However, it can be helpful in locating masses in younger women whose breasts are more dense and harder to see on a mammogram. Ultrasound is most useful in evaluating masses that lie deep within the breast and thus cannot be felt or reached with a needle.

Staging the Spread

With the diagnosis firmly established, the doctor is free to focus on determining whether the cancer has spread, and, if so, how far. This evaluation, or "staging," involves ranking the cancer from Stage I (early cases) to Stage IV (advanced cases). For the precise description of each stage, see the box nearby. There is no single "best" operation or treatment for breast cancer. Much depends on whether the disease is localized (only in the breast) or disseminated (in other parts of the body as well). Unfortunately, it is often difficult to tell whether the cancer has spread. There is no definitive laboratory test for this, and many women don't have any symptoms at all.

Treatment: Assessing the Options

Prompt treatment is essential. Without surgery, radiation, or chemotherapy, a woman who has breast cancer will almost surely die. Fortunately, the chances for long–term survival—and cure—are excellent if the cancer is caught early enough.

Once the physician has determined the type of breast cancer, the size and location of the primary tumor, and the extent of the disease, it's time to discuss the various treatment options. The doctor will recommend the course of treatment that he or she believes will provide the best results with the fewest disabling side effects.

THE FOUR STAGES OF BREAST CANCER

Staging the breast cancer provides some general guidelines to help the doctor decide what type of treatment has the best chance of curing the disease. The National Cancer Institute has developed the following criteria for classifying the extent of breast cancer:

Stage	Extent
I	The tumor is no larger than 2 centimeters (about 1 inch), and the cancer has not spread beyond the breast.
II	The tumor is 2 to 5 centimeters (about 1 to 2 inches), and/or the cancer has spread to the lymph nodes under the arm.
III	The tumor is larger than 5 centimeters (two inches), the cancer involves more of the underarm lymph nodes, and/or the cancer has spread to other tissues near the breast.
IV	The cancer has spread to other organs in the body, most often to the bones, liver, lungs, or brain.

The goal of the therapy is to prevent the spread of cancer if the disease is confined to the breast and to minimize the possibility of a recurrence of cancer in the future. For women whose cancer has already spread, the physician will develop a treatment plan that eases any pain or other symptoms. This is called palliative therapy.

Mastectomy—surgical removal of the breast—offers a good chance of a cure for Stage I and II breast cancers. Surgery may also be successful for some Stage III cancers *if* they have not invaded other parts of the body. Women with Stage IV breast cancer receive palliative treatment.

Surgery

There are many different types of surgery for breast cancer—from removing just the lump to removing the entire breast and the muscles in the chest. The surgeon may also remove some—and possibly all—of the lymph nodes under the arm.

The lymph nodes are part of the body's lymphatic system, which filters waste from the tissues and carries fluids that help the body fight infection. The lymphatic system transports fluids very efficiently and, if invaded by cancer cells, can carry them throughout the body. Surgeons remove at least a sampling of the lymph nodes near the breast to check whether the cancer has reached the nodes. The extent of "nodal involvement"—the number of lymph nodes with cancer—helps the physician determine how much radiation or chemotherapy a woman needs after surgery.

For many years, women went into the hospital for a biopsy not even knowing whether they even had cancer and often woke up several hours later to find that their breast was gone. Advocates of this one–step approach to biopsy and treatment believed that a simple surgical procedure involved less risk than waiting between biopsy and surgery. Treatment began immediately and the woman had less stress and anxiety because the ordeal was over much sooner. The one–step approach was also cheaper and involved only one hospitalization.

Times have changed. Many women and physicians now favor the two–step approach. This not only allows the doctor time to better evaluate the disease, but also gives the patient a chance to consider the different treatment possibilities, obtain a second opinion if she wants, make any necessary arrangements at work or at home, and get herself mentally and emotionally ready to fight the disease.

Whatever treatment a woman chooses, she needs to have her physician's support. It's very important for doctor and patient to discuss the situation thoroughly and make sure they agree on what's best. The bottom line for most women is to go with the approach that offers them the best chance for survival. There are many choices:

Radical Mastectomy

In a radical mastectomy, the surgeon removes the entire breast, both chest muscles, and all of the lymph nodes under the arm. Also known as the Halsted radical mastectomy, after the surgeon who developed the procedure in the 1890s, this operation was the standard breast cancer treatment until just a few years ago.

Surgeons believed that removing the entire breast was the best way to get rid of all of the cancer—assuming that the disease hadn't yet spread beyond the breast. Taking out all the lymph nodes made it possible to better determine the extent of any spread.

There were many drawbacks to such extensive surgery. Women sometimes lost movement in the arm and shoulder and experienced numbness, discomfort, and swelling of the arm. The surgery was very disfiguring—some called it mutilation. After the operation, the chest looked hollow and the scar unsightly. Breast reconstruction was possible, but very difficult.

Over the years, scientific studies have shown that removing the chest muscles doesn't improve a woman's prognosis and isn't necessary if the cancer is found early. Today, doctors seldom perform radical mastectomies.

FROM RADICAL TO MODIFIED RADICAL

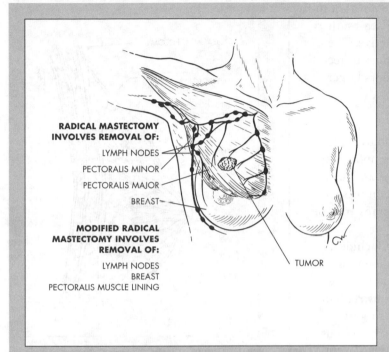

RADICAL MASTECTOMY INVOLVES REMOVAL OF:

LYMPH NODES
PECTORALIS MINOR
PECTORALIS MAJOR
BREAST

MODIFIED RADICAL MASTECTOMY INVOLVES REMOVAL OF:

LYMPH NODES
BREAST
PECTORALIS MUSCLE LINING

TUMOR

Radical mastectomy, which removes both pectoral muscles along with the breast and lymph nodes, has been discredited in all but severe cases. A modified radical mastectomy, which leaves one or both muscles intact, is now considered just as effective in stopping the cancer's spread. With less muscle and nerve damage to contend with, women suffer fewer complications after the operation and find subsequent breast reconstruction to be less of a problem.

Modified Radical Mastectomy

The modified radical mastectomy is an updated version of the standard radical and is the procedure of choice for most women with early–stage breast cancer. The operation involves removing the breast, the lymph nodes, and the lining that covers the two chest muscles. The muscles themselves are usually left in place, although the smaller muscle is sometimes removed.

This operation delivers survival rates for women with early breast cancer that are just as good as those achieved with a radical mastectomy. The surgery effectively removes local cancer without causing muscle and nerve damage. Women experience fewer complications and have more muscle strength in the arm.

The chest also looks a lot better, and this can be a great morale booster. In addition, breast reconstruction is much easier to perform after a modified radical.

Although many women don't decide to have reconstruction until several months or even years after their cancer surgery, it is important to discuss the possibility beforehand so that the surgeon can help prepare the area for eventual operation. The type of incision used in the mastectomy, for example, can make a big difference in subsequent reconstructive surgery.

If reconstruction seems likely, the plastic surgeon will probably advise having a modified radical mastectomy because this operation allows the best cosmetic result possible.

Some women still view any removal of the breast as mutilation, but in some cases, there is little choice if they want to survive. The National Cancer Institute continues to recommend breast removal for tumors larger than three–quarters of an inch.

Total or Simple Mastectomy

In this operation, the surgeon removes the breast and maybe a few of the lymph nodes closest to the breast. Presumably, any invasion of cancer cells will show up in these lymph nodes first. Radiation therapy may or may not follow the surgery.

The benefits of this approach include a great reduction in swelling, because most (or all) of the lymph nodes are left alone. The operation also makes breast reconstruction easier than does more extensive surgery.

The drawbacks, however, can be serious. The breast, of course, is still removed, and there is always the possibility that the cancer has already spread to some of the lymph nodes that have not been examined. In that case, the cancer will remain undiscovered until the disease has progressed much farther.

Partial or Segmental Mastectomy

With this procedure, the surgeon removes the tumor along with a portion of the tissue around it. This wedge also includes some skin and the lining of the chest muscle just below the tumor. The surgeon may also remove some or all of the lymph nodes. Women who have this type of surgery also receive radiation therapy.

If the breast is large, this approach leaves most of it intact. However, a woman with smaller breasts will definitely see a change in breast shape after the surgery. The amount of

OTHER OPTIONS

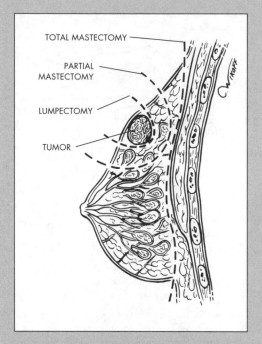

Three alternatives to modified radical mastectomy leave more of the breast area intact:

Simple mastectomy stops with removal of the breast and, at most, a few nearby lymph nodes. There's less postoperative swelling, and reconstruction is easier.

Partial mastectomy takes only a portion of the breast, as the name implies. However, the surgeon may also remove lymph nodes and a portion of the chest muscle's lining.

Lumpectomy, the least damaging of all the options, focuses on the tumor, but may include lymph nodes as well. The operation leaves a scar, but can render reconstruction unnecessary.

Doctors are still debating the effectiveness of these operations. Because a potentially cancerous lymph node may be left behind, radiation therapy is used as a backup precaution after a partial mastectomy or lumpectomy, and after some simple mastectomies as well.

postoperative swelling generally depends on the number of lymph nodes removed. Loss of muscle strength in the arm is not a problem.

Lumpectomy

The popular name for this operation, which involves removing only the tumor, is somewhat misleading. Many surgeons also take out the lymph nodes through a second incision in the armpit. Radiation therapy follows the surgery.

There is much debate about a lumpectomy's effectiveness in comparison with more extensive surgery. Some physicians want to see more research on survival rates before they perform the procedure; others believe it can be a safe alternative to mastectomy. The National Cancer Institute does not advise a lumpectomy when the tumor is larger than three-quarters of an inch.

Lumpectomy is not without some drawbacks. The resulting scar tissue in the breast can make follow-up breast examinations difficult. Swelling in the arm is a possibility whenever lymph nodes are removed.

Women who have a large lump removed from a small breast are likely to notice a significant change in the shape of the breast. Since the procedure itself can make it more difficult to correct any resulting "deformities," many plastic surgeons do not recommend a lumpectomy for small-breasted women or those whose tumor is located under the nipple.

On the other hand, many women do not need reconstruction after a lumpectomy. To make a decision, you really need to discuss the prospects with both a general surgeon and a plastic surgeon.

After Surgery: Reconstruction

It took a while, but physicians have come to realize that treating breast cancer involves more than just getting rid of the tumor. The psychological impact of losing a breast varies, but for many women it means some very real grieving. Doctors are learning to ask women whether they've considered reconstructive surgery, and women are learning to speak up.

Obviously, the medical team is most concerned with saving the woman's life. But if the surgeon knows that she eventually plans to have reconstruction, he can tailor the operation to help ensure a natural-looking result from future plastic surgery.

Many women prefer to have reconstruction immediately; others put it off for years. The decision to perform immediate reconstruction depends on many factors, including age, the size and location of the tumor, and the stage of the disease.

The benefits of having reconstructive surgery at the time of breast removal are obvious, and there is little evidence that the cosmetic surgery impedes successful treatment of the cancer. Doing the procedures back to back, however, does mean an additional two to seven hours of surgery and anesthesia.

Inserting a saline or silicone prosthesis into a pocket created in the breast takes much less time than transplanting tissue from the stomach. The plastic surgeon can also craft a new nipple and areola (the red area surrounding the nipple) if necessary. This latter procedure, which is done after the initial healing is completed, entails grafting tissue from the inner thigh or vagina.

If it is necessary to delay reconstruction during chemotherapy or radiation therapy, the surgeon can implant a small prosthesis at the time of breast removal. This temporary prosthesis helps stretch the skin and eliminates the need for excessive skin grafts when the full–sized prosthesis is eventually inserted.

Some women prefer to wear a breast prosthesis, that fits into a pocket in a custom–designed brassiere. Many others, however, feel that surgical reconstruction makes them feel more attractive and normal.

Radiation's Role

Radiation therapy involves beaming x–rays at the site of the tumor to kill the growing cancer cells. X–rays may sterilize the tissue around the tumor site— and possibly under the arm—and keep the cancer from spreading or returning.

Although researchers are still studying the long–term success rate of radiation therapy, this treatment appears to be a promising option for early–stage cancer. Radiation is also used to shrink an especially large tumor prior to surgery or to slow the growth of inoperable tumors.

Radiation appears to be as effective as a mastectomy in treating early–stage cancer and unlike surgery, it lets a woman keep her breast; tissue surrounding the tumor generally remains undeformed. However, radiation is more often used following a lumpectomy than as a sole primary treatment.

There are two types of radiation. The doctor may beam a concentrated booster dose at the original tumor site or implant radioactive materials within the breast. The five–day–a–week treatment usually lasts for five weeks.

Some women undergoing radiation develop a skin reaction similar to a sunburn and complain of itchy or peeling skin. However, the skin usually regains its normal appearance as soon as treatment ends. Radiation therapy may also cause a temporary decrease in the blood's disease–fighting white cells and increase the risk of developing an infection.

Follow–Up Treatment

In the past few years, physicians have recognized that adjutant (additional) treatment may improve the survival rate in early–stage breast cancer. A decade ago, it was assumed that women with no evidence of cancer in their lymph nodes went home after surgery and had a relatively good chance of remaining cancer–free with no further treatment.

Yet experience has shown that cancer does return in up to 30 percent of cases. And research over the past 75 years has consistently found that half of the women undergoing treatment for "curable" tumors never reach the 10–year survival milestone.

Since there is no way to be sure who is likely to have a recurrence, the National Cancer Institute now strongly recommends follow–up treatment with drugs (chemotherapy) or hormones to improve the odds of beating breast cancer. Doctors regard this "extra treatment" as an insurance policy, hopefully ridding the system of any hidden cancer that may remain and preventing or at least delaying any return of the disease.

Chemotherapy

If you have breast cancer, your doctor may prescribe a combination of drugs most likely to destroy remaining cancer cells. This anticancer "cocktail" is usually administered intravenously, generally every 3 to 4 weeks for anywhere from 4 to 24 months. Some drugs may be swallowed or injected into a muscle. At one time physicians used a single drug, but studies have shown that the various combinations are more effective.

Chemotherapy is generally recommended if there is any spread of the cancer—even to a single lymph node—because of the chance that surgery or radiation therapy will fail to eliminate all "residual" disease.

Radiation targets a specific part of the body. Chemotherapy, on the other hand, is a systemic treatment: The drugs reach every part of body. The strategy is to attack any remaining cancer cells no matter where the drugs are found.

The problem with this strategy is that the drugs are very strong. They attack many types of cells and, as a result, can produce debilitating side effects such as nausea, vomiting, fatigue, and hair loss. Because they can damage healthy cells, the body is less able to fight infections and other diseases.

Despite the drawbacks, chemotherapy works. Anticancer drug treatment can increase a woman's chance of reaching the 10–year survival mark by as much as 35 percent. If the disease has already spread, chemotherapy will generally shrink up to 60 percent of the tumors. About 20 percent of the women under treatment will have no sign of cancer after completing chemotherapy.

The even better news is that some of the newer drugs cause fewer and less severe side effects. Some women are lucky and don't have any side effects at all. Administering certain drugs before chemotherapy can help reduce nausea and vomiting, too. Regular laboratory tests can alert the doctor to any damaging effects on the body's ability to fight infection and other diseases.

Hormonal Therapy

It is not uncommon for cancer to return. It eventually recurs in up to half of the women who have surgery or radiation to treat the original tumor. Additional treatment with radiation or chemotherapy greatly improves a woman's odds against having a recurrence, but there are still no guarantees.

The possibility of a recurrence weighs heavily on anyone who has had breast cancer. Fortunately, there are some very promising new treatments. Hormonal therapy, for example, is proving to be particularly effective.

Studies indicate that some cancers need the female hormone estrogen (or sometimes progesterone) to grow. Pathologists now test the tissue removed at biopsy for the presence of estrogen receptors. If the tumor has these receptors, it means that the cancer is "receptive" to estrogen and probably will not grow as well or as quickly if deprived of the hormone.

This is pretty much how hormonal treatments work: They either block or eliminate a woman's natural supply of estrogen.

About two–thirds of women with breast cancer have estrogen–receptive tumors and can benefit from hormonal therapy. According to the National Cancer Institute, when a tumor has both estrogen and progesterone receptors, there is an 80 percent chance that the cancer will respond to hormone treatment.

Anti–estrogen treatment may involve removing the ovaries in women younger than 40 years of age. This operation effectively halts the body's estrogen production and produces a high rate of remission in younger women.

A drug called tamoxifen has also proved to be very effective, particularly in older women who have already completed menopause. Tamoxifen works by attaching itself to the estrogen receptors and blocking the estrogen from doing its cancer–promoting work. The drug is taken twice a day for up to 5 years.

Pregnancy and Breast Cancer

One out of every 35 women with breast cancer is also pregnant. Although the incidence of breast cancer found during pregnancy is lower (1 in 3,000), the implications are very serious— both for the mother and for her baby.

The overall breast cancer survival rate of 50 percent drops to 15 to 20 percent if the woman is pregnant. And although the generally poor prognosis improves greatly—climbing to a survival rate of 70 to 80 percent—if the cancer is caught early, unfortunately it rarely is. By the time the cancer is diagnosed, it has usually progressed to a stage that carries a much less favorable prognosis.

According to one theory, breast changes that occur naturally during pregnancy may obscure Stage 1 tumors. Another possibility is that increased hormonal activity during pregnancy may accelerate the natural progression of the disease. It's also thought that the increased blood supply to the breasts that occurs during pregnancy may help spread the cancer.

Although there currently is no hard evidence for the theory that pregnancy speeds the growth of tumors in the breast, and no proof that a therapeutic abortion improves a patient's prognosis, many physicians still suspect that pregnancy does play a role.

Treating breast cancer in a pregnant woman is problematic. Many of the drugs used in chemotherapy are known to harm a developing fetus; radiation therapy is similarly unwise because of the potential risk to

the baby. The decision as to how best to treat the cancer can only be made after careful consideration of such variables as the length of the pregnancy, the extent of the cancer, the probable prognosis, and the wishes of the mother–to–be.

Women who develop breast cancer while pregnant should not breastfeed their babies. It is possible that both breasts could contain cancer and that the increased blood supply in a nursing mother's breast could help feed a growing tumor.

Although pregnancy before the age of 18 markedly reduces a woman's likelihood of developing breast cancer in the first place, there is no evidence that having a baby will protect a woman against a *recurrence* of breast cancer. On the other hand, there's also no evidence that a woman who has undergone breast cancer treatment before conceiving should terminate her pregnancy if there is no sign that the cancer has recurred.

Since breast cancer usually occurs in women over 35, it rarely affects expectant mothers. However, if you have had the disease and are considering becoming pregnant, talk to your family doctor or cancer specialist before making your final decision. He or she will help you determine if it is safe for you to have a child.

The Need for Follow–up Care

Follow–up care is crucial, especially during the first 5 years after the initial diagnosis. According to the National Cancer Institute, 60 percent of the recurrences of breast cancer appear in the first 3 years; another 20 percent happen in years 4 and 5. The remainder can show up from 5 to 20 years later.

If you've had breast cancer, your physician will schedule regular office visits to examine your breasts, scars, chest, underarms, and neck. From time to time, the doctor will perform a complete physical examination and order a mammogram. Every 3 months or so, there will be a battery of blood and urine tests to make sure there is no sign of cancer in other parts of the body. Because breast cancer is most likely to travel to the lungs, bones, and liver, periodic chest x–rays and bone and liver scans will also be necessary.

The physical healing after breast cancer treatment takes a few weeks. The psychological scars take much longer. Many women find that it helps to meet with other cancer survivors who truly understand the fear and anger that can follow a diagnosis of breast cancer. They cope by learning to live in the present and not dwell on the unknown. And, like all women, they can take comfort in the steadily growing number of women who have fought the disease and survived. □

CHAPTER 37   **DEALING WITH CANCER**

Your Best Insurance Against Breast Cancer

The best way to beat breast cancer is to catch it early. Detecting and treating a malignant tumor in its earliest stages gives you a better than 9 out of 10 chance of surviving the disease for at least 5 years. Although breast cancer usually hits older women—two–thirds are over age 50—you're never too young to be on the lookout for this dangerous killer. The American Cancer Society and other health organizations have developed guidelines to help you and your doctor find the disease before it causes irreparable damage:

- Examine your breasts every month.
- Make sure a physician or other health care professional examines your breasts every year, beginning at age 20.
- Have a baseline mammogram by the time you reach 40, a screening mammogram every one or two years between 40 and 49, and a yearly mammogram beginning at age 50.

Unfortunately, studies indicate that fewer than one–third of American women give themselves monthly breast self–examinations (BSEs), even though more than 75 percent of all breast cancers are found by women themselves— usually by accident. Too often, women hesitate to perform a BSE because they are "too busy" or "don't know what to look for." Some are simply afraid of finding the very thing they dread: a lump in their breast.

Likewise, fewer than half of the women who should receive routine mammograms actually do. Although the National Cancer Institute recently revised its guidelines, declaring that mammograms before age 50 save no additional lives, the move was extremely controversial, and the American Cancer Society continues to recommend mammograms for women in their 40s. Whichever guidelines you choose to believe, it's still clear that too many women neglect this potentially life–saving test. They may feel they do not need an annual mammogram because there is no family history of breast disease. If their first mammogram is normal, they may decide there's no need for another.

IS IT A LUMP...OR A GLAND?

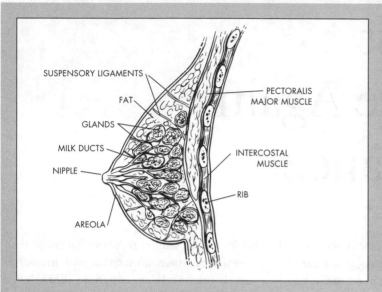

SUSPENSORY LIGAMENTS

FAT

GLANDS

MILK DUCTS

NIPPLE

AREOLA

PECTORALIS MAJOR MUSCLE

INTERCOSTAL MUSCLE

RIB

Distinguishing a lump from a normal milk gland during your breast self-exam may be difficult at first. There's always a possibility, too, of overlooking a lump amid all the glandular tissue of the breast. Your doctor can help you learn to feel the difference; and regular monthly self-exams will quickly make you familiar with your breasts' own unique textures.

They also avoid testing due to lack of insurance reimbursement, concern about radiation exposure, discomfort during the procedure, and failure to understand the benefits of mammography.

Nevertheless, this three–step approach to early breast cancer detection is just as important to a woman's overall physical health as proper diet, regular exercise, and the avoidance of tobacco and other harmful substances. BSE, clinical breast examinations, and mammography are a woman's best insurance against breast cancer.

The Breast Self–Exam

Every woman should perform a BSE once a month. Because breasts can be more tender, swollen, and lumpy prior to your period, the best time to do the exam is day 5 to day 7 of your menstrual cycle (5 to 7 days after your period starts). If you take oral contraceptives or hormones, check your breasts before starting a new pack of pills. Continue to examine your breasts during pregnancy, even though your breasts might feel lumpier and more swollen than usual; although rare, breast cancer can appear while you are pregnant. If you've had a hysterectomy or have passed menopause, you should schedule a BSE for the first day of each month.

You may feel embarrassed about examining your breasts—especially if you haven't done so in the past. Remember that you should know your body better than anyone else, and a BSE allows you to become better acquainted with the unique appearance and texture of your own breasts. Noncancerous breast conditions are common in many women, and regular BSEs can help you to distinguish between "normal" and "suspicious" tissue. In fact, some experts recommend that, initially, women conduct a BSE every day for a month until they learn the "geography" of their breasts.

If you don't know how to get started, your doctor can provide you with additional information that describes the structure of the breast and the composition of its tissue. Your doctor may also have a model that allows you to feel the differences between breast lumps and the normal glandular tissue involved in milk production, as well as underlying fatty tissue.

The Visual Inspection

Breast self–examination is not difficult to master and requires only a few minutes each month. To begin, stand in a comfortable, private, well–lighted room, where you can view your breasts in a large mirror. First inspect them visually to check for anything unusual, such as discharge from your nipples, or puckering, dimpling, or scaling of the skin. Then, clasp your hands behind your head and press your hands forward while watching your breasts closely in the mirror. Finally, press your hands firmly on your hips and bow slightly toward the mirror, pulling your shoulders and elbows forward.

During this inspection, check for the following characteristics:

Size and Symmetry: Breasts vary greatly in size based on age, heredity, childbirth, breast-feeding, weight changes, and birth control pills or other hormones. In any event, they should be fairly symmetrical and point slightly to the outside. Your physician should examine any deviation.

Texture and shape: Most breasts are firm and rounded, though your breasts may become more flaccid after pregnancy, breastfeeding, or menopause.

Skin color: The color of your breasts depends on your own individual pigmentation. Although your breasts may be lighter than other areas not usually exposed to the sun, the color should be uniform throughout. Unusual coloration may indicate underlying problems. Redness suggests an infection, such as mastitis, a common inflammation of the mammary glands during breastfeeding. A blue hue might be caused by an increased blood supply to the area. Because this may indicate an abnormality, be sure to discuss it with your doctor.

Surface appearance: Breast skin normally looks smooth, although during pregnancy, breastfeeding, or a sudden weight gain, you may develop stretch marks that are reddish when they first appear and whiten with age. When these occur on both breasts, there is no cause for concern. Skin that develops an "orange peel" texture or dimpling, however, may be a sign of cancer.

Moles, growths, and sores: Watch for the appearance of any unusual growth on the skin, and be alert for a change in any existing growth.

Nipples and areola: Inspect the nipples and areola (the pigmented skin surrounding the nipple) for size, symmetry, color, direction, rashes, lesions, or discharge. Both nipples should be about the same size, as should the areola. Pregnancy and breastfeeding cause the size of these breast structures to increase and become more prominent.

Like the surrounding skin, pigmentation of the nipples varies in hue; but the color should be the same on both breasts. Any abnormal coloration—redness or a bluish hue—may indicate infection or an increased blood supply to the area and should be evaluated by a physician.

Most nipples point outward, though some women have nipples that are retracted, or pointed inward. If a nipple normally points outward but suddenly pulls in either spontaneously or when you move your arms, there may be a growth nearby. If you notice any rashes, growths, or ulcerations on the nipples, bring them to your doctor's attention.

Spontaneous nipple discharge is another warning sign, though many women can squeeze a tiny amount of clear, yellowish or milky discharge from their nipples—especially toward the end of pregnancy and throughout breastfeeding. Be sure to discuss any pinkish, bloody, or foul–smelling discharge with your physician.

The Manual Examination

The second half of your breast self–exam may be easier to complete in the shower, where your fingers can glide over soapy skin and make it easier for your to concentrate on the texture of your breasts. Raise your left arm and use the sensitive pads—not the tips—of the first three fingers of your right hand to begin pressing, or exploring, your left breast. Make small, circular motions. Begin at the outermost part of your breast and move slowly clockwise around the breast toward the nipple and areola. Vary the pressure in each spot from light to heavy, checking changes in skin texture, changes below the surface, and changes closer to your ribs. Complete this portion of the exam without lifting your hand, then squeeze your nipple to check for a discharge. Finally, repeat the entire process with the other breast.

Feeling the lymph nodes is the next step in your exam. The first sign of many breast cancers is a hardened, enlarged or fixed

THREE THINGS TO CHECK IN YOUR MANUAL EXAM

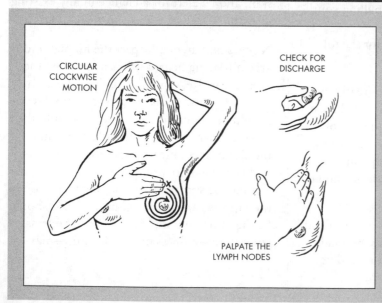

CIRCULAR CLOCKWISE MOTION

CHECK FOR DISCHARGE

PALPATE THE LYMPH NODES

Although thoroughly exploring your breast tissue is the longest part of the self-exam, other elements are just as important. A hard or swollen lymph node in the armpit area near your breast may be the first tip-off that cancer is developing. A pinkish discharge from the nipple could also be a warning sign.

Note the circumference-to-tip pattern you should follow as you feel each breast. Remember, too, that you should vary the pressure so that you feel both the superficial texture and the tissue deep within.

lymph node. Raise your left arm and again use the pads of your first three fingers to explore the area in and around your armpits for any unusual lump or mass under the skin; then repeat under the opposite arm.

After towel drying, repeat the inspection while lying flat on your back. Place a pillow or your folded towel under your left shoulder to flatten your left breast, then raise your left arm over your head. If you're large–breasted, roll slightly away from your left side to make it easier to examine your breast tissue. Palpate the left breast using the circular technique described earlier. Check the nipple and palpate the lymph nodes, then repeat on your right side.

Women with breast implants should perform a BSE every month and get a doctor's examination every 6 months to a year. Contact your physician if you notice any change in the texture, size, shape, color, or appearance of either breast; a discharge or unusual sensation around the nipple; burning or pain in the chest area; stiffness in the chest, shoulder, or upper arm; or lumps in the breast or underarm area.

What Else A Lump Could Be

Even if you discover something unusual during your BSE, don't panic. Many women have harmless breast conditions, and four–fifths of the lumps found during a self–exam turn out to be noncancerous, or benign.

One thing you may detect is a thickening in the breasts. This is often the result of a **fibrocystic condition** marked by localized solid or fluid–filled lumps that form and swell somewhat during the premenstrual period. The condition is benign; and it's estimated that up to half of all women between the ages of 35 and 50 develop it. After menopause, it gradually diminishes. Though fibrocystic lumps pose no threat to your health and most researchers believe the condition is too widespread to be considered a risk for cancer, the lumps are often difficult to distinguish from malignancies and should be evaluated by a doctor.

Benign lumps also come in other shapes and sizes:

Cysts are smooth, fluid–filled sacs that can be soft or firm. They are often sensitive to the touch during the premenstrual period. Cysts are typically found in both breasts and appear most often when a woman is 35 to 50 years of age.

Fibroadenomas are composed of fibrous and glandular tissue. They feel solid, round, and rubbery. They often move freely and are painless to the touch. These lumps appear most often in women under the age of 30 and are twice as common in black women. Although they are benign, most doctors recommend that they be removed since they will not clear up on their own and may continue to grow—especially during pregnancy and breastfeeding.

Lipomas are single, painless lumps that most often appear in older women. Varying in size from a dime to a quarter, they are composed of fatty tissue. They are slow–growing, soft, and movable. Doctors often recommend laboratory examination of a sample of the tissue (a biopsy), or complete removal, to confirm a diagnosis.

Intraductal papillomas are small, wart–like growths in the milk ducts near the nipple. Usually occurring in women during their 40s, these nodules develop near the edge of the nipple and can cause it to bleed.

NONCANCEROUS LUMPS

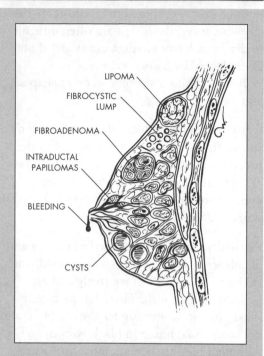

LIPOMA
FIBROCYSTIC LUMP
FIBROADENOMA
INTRADUCTAL PAPILLOMAS
BLEEDING
CYSTS

If you do feel a lump, chances are it's a false alarm. Four out of five lumps are the harmless growths illustrated here:

- Fibrocystic lumps, which tend to swell in rhythm with the menstrual cycle, and diminish after menopause
- Cysts, which generally are found in both breasts and appear most often between the ages of 35 and 50
- Fibroadenomas, solid, round, and rubbery, which are found more often in younger women
- Lipomas—painless lumps the size of a coin—which develop slowly, primarily in older women
- Intraductal papillomas, small nodules underneath the edge of the nipple, which typically appear during your 40s

Even if you feel certain that a lump is just one of these growths, you should still see your doctor. Diagnostic tests are needed to conclusively rule out cancer.

Though these conditions are no cause for alarm, only your doctor can make an accurate diagnosis. Be sure that he or she knows about any change in your breasts—no matter how small or seemingly insignificant. If you are still menstruating, the doctor may advise you to monitor the lump for one or two cycles to see if it varies with your normal hormonal fluctuations. If you are past menopause, immediate evaluation may be necessary, since older women are at higher risk for breast cancer. A woman of 70 is twice as likely to develop the disease as a woman aged 50.

A monthly BSE is a woman's first line of defense. It is especially important for younger women and is crucial for detecting changes that may develop between annual medical checkups. Nevertheless, BSE is not a substitute for clinical examinations and regular screening mammograms. All women should have a doctor examine their breasts every year as part of their annual checkup. If your physician skips your breast exam, ask for one.

Your annual checkup is also an ideal time to learn how to perform a BSE. Ask your doctor to demonstrate the technique, then repeat it so he or she can see whether you're doing it correctly. BSE training also may be available through health education classes at your local hospital, women's center, or corporate wellness program.

Mammograms

For detecting breast cancer in its earliest stages, screening mammography is the single most effective method of all. Mammograms are vital because they can locate a lump too small to be found during a self–exam.

Mammography is simply a breast x–ray. It allows the x–ray specialist, or radiologist, to see the internal structures of your breasts without the need for injection of dyes or contrast materials. Screening mammography can uncover unexpected problems in women with no other symptoms. Diagnostic mammograms—which are conducted in virtually the same manner—help identify a lump or other change found during a BSE or clinical breast examination. Overall, the accuracy of mammography in combination with BSE is greater than 90 percent, though mammography can fail to show some tumors—even some large enough to be felt—especially in dense breasts of younger women.

In addition to following the general American Cancer Society mammography screening guidelines, your physician may recommend the use of mammograms earlier or more frequently if he or she thinks you may be at higher risk for breast cancer. About 1 in every 5 women is at greater risk due to a family history of the disease (a mother, sister or aunt with breast cancer). You are also at greater risk if you have never been pregnant or had your first child after age 30, began menstruating early, or had a late menopause. In addition, some research studies have indicated that women over 40 whose mammograms reveal especially prominent milk ducts or dense breast tissue have a greater chance of developing breast cancer.

Radiation exposure from a mammogram is minimal. There is much evidence to support the belief that the benefits of detecting and successfully treating early breast cancer far outweigh any hypothetical risks from the x-ray—especially for women over age 50. Other imaging technologies, such as magnetic resonance imaging (MRI), are under investi-

gation as alternatives to mammography, but their development may take years.

An estimated 12,000 U.S. medical facilities perform and interpret mammography tests. Recent federal regulations required all of them to meet national quality control standards and receive federal certification by October 1, 1994. The new standards are similar to but stronger than voluntary guidelines in effect since the late 1980s. When scheduling a mammogram, double-check to be sure the facility observes these new standards.

What To Expect

Mammography requires no special dietary or physical restrictions, though your doctor may advise you not to use deodorant, talcum powder, or skin lotions on your breast or underarms on the day of the test. You should also wear a two-piece outfit, since you'll have to undress from the waist up. You may feel nervous, frightened or embarrassed by the idea of disrobing to the waist and having your breasts manipulated for various x-ray views. Don't hesitate to voice your concerns to your physician and the mammography technologist prior to the procedure. Ask the technologist to explain beforehand what to expect. Many of these professionals are sensitive to a woman's desire for modesty and a sense of self-control.

During a mammogram, each breast will be gently flattened between two plastic plates so all of the tissue can be viewed. The x-ray machine will send a tiny amount of radiation through your breast to create an image. Generally, screening mammograms include two views of each breast—from the top and from the side—and take only 10 to 15 minutes to complete.

Although mammography is relatively painless, some women feel uncomfortable because the breast is compressed during the procedure. This pressure is necessary to obtain good detail of the breast on the x–ray film and only lasts a few seconds. Though mammography is effective at any time during the menstrual cycle, women who are still having periods may want to schedule the procedure during the first two weeks of their cycle, when their breasts are less swollen and tender.

Be sure to ask your doctor when the test results will be available. A long delay causes many women intense anxiety; so, many hospitals and women's health centers have responded with full–service screening programs that offer results within 30 minutes of the test. Your doctor or the radiologist who reads the x–ray films should be on hand to talk with you about the results. If any additional views are necessary, you can often have more x–rays taken on the spot. Your doctor can also schedule procedures such as a biopsy within 24 hours.

Women with breast implants should also follow regular screening guidelines for mammography. Tumor detection is more difficult after breast enlargement, especially in women who have developed scar tissue around the implants, have their implants in front of muscle, or have little breast tissue to begin with—which is often the case after implant surgery. The Food and Drug Administration (FDA) recommends that you choose a radiologist who has experience with breast implants. The mammogram should be taken with a more thorough technique called a "modified compression view," since both saline and silicone implants can obscure x– rays.

It's important to tell your mammography technologist that you have breast implants so that he or she can exercise special care during the test. The radiologist will take 4 to 6 low–dose x–rays of each augmented breast,

pushing the implant away from your breast tissue to get the best possible views. The technique requires more time—about 20 to 30 minutes—and generally costs slightly more than a basic screening mammogram.

Some groups have suggested that women with breast implants have more frequent mammograms in order to detect implant rupture or silicone that has leaked into breast tissue. However, an FDA advisory panel has recommended against this because of the danger posed by increased radiation exposure. In addition, the FDA warns that compression of the breast during mammography may rupture the implant, particularly if it's the type filled with saline. If you have breast implants, talk to your doctor about the advisability of having more frequent mammography. He or she will help you decide whether the benefits outweigh the possible risks.

Next Steps
When There's A Problem

If any lumps are found during an examination and screening, your doctor will need to do additional tests. At this point, you should remember that only about 20 percent of biopsied breast lumps are cancerous. Even malignant masses, when diagnosed early, respond very favorably to treatment. If surgery is required, often removal of the lump and a small amount of surrounding tissue is all that's necessary. And, most women treated for early breast cancer do not experience a recurrence.

The first step will probably be a diagnostic mammogram to assess the mass. If this raises any suspicion of breast cancer, your physician may recommend one or more of these additional diagnostic tests:

Ultrasound sends high–frequency sound waves into the breast, then converts the echoes from those waves into an image of the breast's interior. Ultrasound is an accurate way of distinguishing between solid and fluid–filled lumps; but it cannot detect small calcium deposits that may indicate cancer, and it does not identify small tumors. If your doctor discovers a suspicious lump during pregnancy, ultrasound may be preferable to a mammogram for the sake of the baby.

Thermography measures heat patterns given off by the skin. "Hot spots" may suggest an abnormality. Although thermography has no known risks, doctors do not consider it as reliable as mammography. However, it is sometimes used as a supplement to the x–ray procedure.

Diaphanography, or transillumination, shines a bright light through the breast. This experimental technology can indicate the difference between a solid mass and a cyst but does not detect the small cancers that a mammography can reveal.

Needle aspiration determines whether a lump is solid or fluid–filled. If the lump is a cyst, the doctor drains the fluid and sends it to a laboratory to check for the presence of cancer cells. The procedure is generally done in a physician's office or clinic using a local anesthetic, and further treatment is rarely needed.

Needle core biopsy (also called stereotactic breast biopsy and mammo–test) is used to remove a core of tissue from a solid lump. Using a computerized x–ray technique, your doctor will guide a needle into the suspicious breast area to obtain a sample for microscopic examination. The procedure uses a local anesthetic, leaves no scar and is consid-

ered highly accurate. More and more physicians are choosing this technique to confirm a diagnosis and develop a treatment plan.

Surgical biopsy is still the predominant method of confirming a suspicion of cancer. After removing the breast lump surgically, your doctor will have the tissue examined under a microscope. You can usually have this procedure done in a walk–in care center under local or general anesthesia and go home the same day.

If you are uncertain about the need for any of these tests, don't hesitate to discuss your concerns frankly with your physician, and feel free to get a second opinion, perhaps from a breast specialist or breast health clinic. The American Cancer Society has chapters in every major U.S. city that can provide you with additional information.

The National Cancer Institute hotline at (800) 4–CANCER can send you publications or a refer you to a specialist if you want a consultation.

Above all, remember that self–exams and mammograms can truly be life–savers. Though they seem a nuisance, they are a critical safeguard you should never pass up. Every year, 46,000 American families lose a mother, sister, wife, or daughter to breast cancer. Don't allow yourself to become a part of the statistic. □

CHAPTER 38   **DEALING WITH CANCER**

Cervical Cancer: The One That's Preventable

I f you're one of the millions of women who regularly visit their obstetricians and gynecologists for routine pelvic examinations and Pap tests, then you are part of the good news about cervical cancer. This disease is almost 100 percent curable when it is diagnosed in its early stages and treated promptly. Pap tests are the single most effective method for identifying irregularities in cervical cells that could develop into cancer. Since the 1940s, when the Pap test was first introduced, the death rate for cervical cancer has declined by nearly 75 percent.

The battle against cervical cancer is far from won, however. Approximately 13,500 women are diagnosed with cervical cancer each year. As many as 4,500 of these women will die from the disease because it was diagnosed too late for effective treatment. Sadly, many of these deaths could be prevented with regular screening and early treatment.

Cervical cancer is not as common as other cancers that affect women. Breast cancer is far more prevalent, striking approximately 180,000 women in 1992. In the same year, more than 20,000 women developed ovarian cancer, and nearly 12,000 women died from it.

Early Warning; Gradual Progression

B arely more than an inch long, the cervix is the narrow end of the uterus that opens into the upper part of the vagina. Lined with mucous membrane similar to that found inside the mouth, the cervix is made up of connective tissue. This tiny passage is laced with a network of nerves that respond to pressure by sending electrical messages to the brain and spinal cord. Several weeks prior to labor and childbirth, as pressure from the uterus grows, the cervix thins and begins to expand—or dilate—to accommodate the movement of the baby through the birth canal.

Cervical cancer usually develops over a long period of time. At the outset, formerly healthy cells in the cervix begin to develop abnormally for some reason. Here are the stages of progression.

THREE STAGES OF ABNORMAL GROWTH

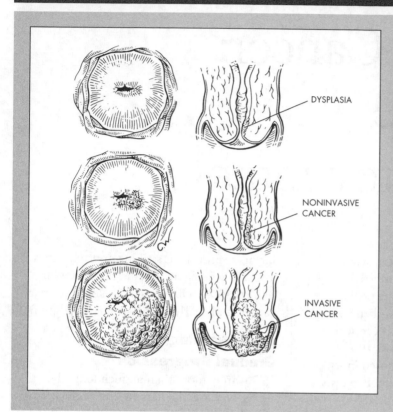

DYSPLASIA

NONINVASIVE CANCER

INVASIVE CANCER

Nearly half the time, the slightly abnormal cell growth called cervical *dysplasia* will go away on its own. But the abnormal cells can become frankly cancerous; and if they do, decisive treatment is called for immediately. Eliminating the cancer while it is *noninvasive*—still confined to the surface of the cervix—makes a complete cure almost a certainty. However, if the cancer is allowed to continue and become *invasive*—attacking deeper layers of tissue—the odds of stopping it decline rapidly.

Cervical intraepithelial neoplasia (CIN). Also called cervical dysplasia, CIN is not cancer but the first of the cellular changes that may develop into cancer *in some women.* A Pap test detects these abnormal changes. However, no test can predict whether CIN will develop into cancer, which is why early detection and treatment of any abnormality is so important.

Cervical dysplasia is a fairly common condition; more than 55,000 women are diagnosed with it each year. Increasingly, women are developing cervical dysplasia at younger and younger ages—during their late teens to early 20s.

Noninvasive Carcinoma. A very early form of cervical cancer is known as carcinoma *in situ.* It also may be called noninvasive carcinoma. This abnormality involves only the top layer of cervical cells, not deeper layers of tissue in the cervix or elsewhere in the reproductive tract. Without treatment, carcinoma *in situ* usually will develop into invasive cervical cancer. Carcinoma *in situ* occurs most often in women between 30 and 40 years of age.

Invasive Cervical Cancer. At this stage, cancer has penetrated deep into the cervix and possibly into neighboring tissues and organs. Invasive cervical cancer is nearly 100 percent curable when diagnosed early and treated promptly. However, when the disease has spread outside the reproductive tract, it can be effectively treated in only 5 percent of cases. Invasive cervical cancer occurs most frequently in women between the ages of 40 and 60.

Who's at Risk?

All women are at risk for cervical dysplasia and cervical cancer. As with many other forms of cancer, researchers are unsure of the exact cause. Several factors have been identified, however, that could increase your chances of developing cervical dysplasia and cervical cancer. These risk factors include:

Cigarette smoking. Chemicals from cigarettes and cigarette smoke have been found in the cervical tissue of women who smoke. These chemicals may damage cervical cells and weaken their ability to fight off infection, as well as make them more vulnerable to abnormal development. The exact mechanism linking cigarette smoking and cervical cancer has not been established, however.

Early sexual activity. Women who have sex at an early age may be more susceptible to cervical cancer than other women. One reason for this risk is that the developing cells in the cervix of a young woman are more fragile than the mature cervical cells of older women, and more likely to be damaged from the slight abrasions caused by frequent intercourse. Teenagers who smoke *and* have frequent sex double their risk.

Sexually transmitted diseases (STDs). Cervical dysplasia may develop after a sexually transmitted infection. Herpes simplex virus type II, a common STD, was once suspected as a cause of cervical dysplasia. However, research has shown that this virus cannot change normal cells into abnormal ones. Although the link between a specific STD and cervical cancer has yet to be identified, these diseases are believed to increase overall risk. Indeed, the connection between HIV (the AIDS virus) and cervical cancer is so strong that women with the virus are now advised to get a Pap test every 6 months.

Women with multiple partners have a greater chance of contracting sexually transmitted diseases. Teenagers are especially at risk for STDs, including human papilloma virus (HPV) and herpes. Even a woman with only one partner can still be at risk for STDs if her partner has had many others. Several STDs, including syphilis, gonorrhea, *chlamydia*, and HIV are increasing at alarming rates in the U.S. teen population.

Human papilloma virus (HPV). There are 60 known types of this sexually transmitted virus, but only a few can cause cells to become cancerous. One form of HPV produces genital warts and also is suspected of causing the cellular changes that may lead to cervical cancer. Up to 90 percent of cervical cancers show evidence of HPV infection. On the other hand, many women are diagnosed with HPV but never develop dysplasia or cervical cancer. The symptoms caused by HPV can be treated, but the virus itself cannot be "cured." Symptoms often recur after treatment. If your doctor diagnoses HPV but finds no dysplasia, aggressive treatment is not necessary.

Age. The risk of cervical cancer rises with age and, when first diagnosed, cervical cancer in older women tends to be more advanced. Ironically, few women over age 65 have Pap smears regularly. Furthermore, one research study reports that after age 44, women no longer listed the Pap smear as the major reason for visiting a physician's office. You, too, may mistakenly believe that once you r̩ch menopause, you no longer need routine gynecological exams. In fact, nothing is further from the truth.

Income. Women in low income groups develop CIN and cervical cancer 5 times as often as women in higher economic brackets. One explanation for this discrepancy in cancer rates is that poor women are less likely to have regular access to cancer screenings and follow-up care.

Race. African-American women are twice as likely to develop cervical cancer, and to have a more advanced cancer when first diagnosed than are Caucasian women. Cervical cancer rates are also higher for Hispanic and Native American women. However, a predisposition for developing cervical cancer is not passed from mother to daughter, as with breast cancer.

Symptoms of CIN and Cervical Cancer

Cervical dysplasia and early stages of cervical cancer have no visible symptoms. An abnormal Pap test is the first indication that something may be wrong. The test itself does not confirm CIN or cervical cancer; however, it does indicate that some cervical cells are abnormal.

In more advanced cervical cancer, the most common symptom is irregular bleeding. Two-thirds of women with advanced cervical cancer experience bleeding between periods, with heavier or lighter amounts than normal menstrual flow, or are troubled by bleeding following intercourse. Eventually the bleeding becomes constant. In some women, however, cervical cancer can spread dramatically to other areas in the body before it causes any bleeding.

Pain in the pelvic area, legs, and back, and discomfort while urinating (caused by pressure from a tumor), or blood in the urine, may also indicate advanced disease.

Detecting and Treating Abnormal Cells

Because early detection greatly increases the chances that treatment for CIN or cervical cancer will be successful, it's crucial that women be screened for signs of cervical disease. The main screening method is the Pap smear. If the results of the Pap are abnormal, a series of tests can determine the reason for the problem. Here are the procedures for detecting and evaluating abnormal cervical cells.

Pap Test

This simple procedure involves scraping some cells with a cotton swab or small "cyto" brush from the mucous membranes where the cervix and vagina meet. It is in this area that cell changes begin which could lead to cervical cancer.

The cells are deposited on a glass slide and sent to a laboratory where it is examined by a cytopathologist—an expert in the study of diseased cells. The lab report will describe the type and severity of any cell changes found. Cell appearance from the Pap test will be rated as normal, or as showing mild (CIN I), moderate (CIN II), or severe dysplasia (CIN III); carcinoma *in situ*; or invasive cancer.

What an Abnormal Pap Test Can Mean

If your physician tells you that the results of your Pap test are abnormal, it's a good idea to ask how your results were described by the laboratory. A basic understanding of your Pap test can help explain the additional diagnostic procedures your doctor will probably recommend.

If the abnormal results are due to an infection, other diagnostic tests probably won't be needed. Infections actually are the most common cause of abnormal Pap tests. Yeast infection (or candidiasis) as well as viral infections like herpes and HPV (genital warts) can cause inflammation of cervical cells. The treatment for yeast and bacterial infections is usually antibiotics. Your doctor may recommend a follow–up Pap test within 1 to 2 months to make sure the treatment was effective.

As many as 20 percent of all Pap tests may be inaccurate—reporting abnormal results when nothing irregular is present. A second Pap test can help validate suspicious findings. It's important not to have a second Pap test too quickly because the cervical cells need time to repair themselves after an exam.

What's Next After an Abnormal Pap

If infection is not the cause of your abnormal Pap results, your doctor most likely will recommend further diagnostic tests for cancer. These may include **colposcopy, endocervical curettage (ECC), loop electrocautery excision procedure (LEEP),** or **conization.** Each of these diagnostic procedures will involve a **biopsy** (removal for microscopic evaluation) of cervical tissue. A pelvic examination is also part of the diagnostic evaluation to determine whether there are any serious abnormalities in the pelvic region.

Most primary care physicians will perform the basic diagnostic and treatment procedures for mild to moderate dysplasia. When conization is necessary, you should see a gynecolo-

THE CERVIX: STRONG, DELICATE, VULNERABLE

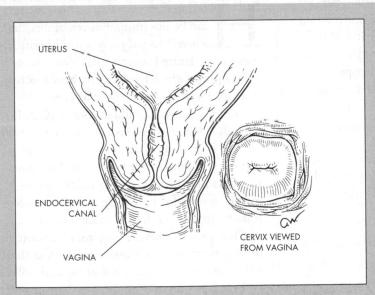

UTERUS

ENDOCERVICAL CANAL

VAGINA

CERVIX VIEWED FROM VAGINA

This tiny corridor between the uterus and the vagina must be strong enough to keep a developing baby securely in place during pregnancy, yet elastic enough to allow delivery at term. Lined with delicate mucous membrane, it is prey to infection by the human papilloma virus (HPV), a sexually transmitted disease linked to the development of cervical cancer in ways yet to be explained. If you've been diagnosed with HPV—or any other STD—you should schedule regular Pap tests to check for early signs of cancer.

gist—especially if the biopsy will be performed for treatment of invasive cancer.

Doctors generally agree that a step–by–step approach to diagnosis usually is preferable to immediate aggressive treatment. This limits the impact on the cervix as much as possible, especially before a complete biopsy has been performed. Continued or prolonged invasive treatments can erode and weaken the cervix.

Colposcopy. During this procedure, your physician inserts a viewing scope (colposcope) into the vagina to magnify the region for inspection. For this procedure, a Schiller test, a rinse of acetic acid solution applied with a cotton swab, is administered to turn abnormal areas yellow or white. Small portions of these abnormal areas can then be removed for biopsy with a special punch instrument.

A colposcopy takes about 15 minutes and is performed in your doctor's office. Although the procedure may be uncomfortable, it is not painful. You may feel some discomfort—similar to menstrual cramps—when cervical tissue is removed for biopsy.

Endocervical curretage (ECC). Often performed during a colposcopy, ECC involves scraping cells from the inner portion of the cervix. Even when the outside of the cervix appears normal through a colposcope, the inner cervix, which can't be viewed, could pose a problem. Adenocarcinoma, for example, is a form of cancer that grows in the upper portion of the cervix and is difficult to detect without an ECC. It is common in young women and spreads quickly. Together, colposcopy and ECC can reliably identify most cervical cancers.

Loop electrocautery excision procedure (LEEP) and conization. These two more extensive methods of diagnosing abnormal tissue may also be used as treatments for CIN and early invasive cervical cancer.

With LEEP, abnormal or suspicious cervical tissue is removed with a sharp wire loop and the site is cauterized—burned to eliminate any remaining abnormal tissue. With conization, a cone–shaped section of the cervix is cut with a scalpel or a laser and removed for biopsy. This procedure requires general anesthesia and usually is performed as outpatient surgery in the hospital. Most doctors suggest conization only when other diagnostic tests have revealed cancerous abnormalities. Conization helps to assess how much tissue is diseased. Because it requires removal of part of the cervix, it should be recommended only when invasive cervical cancer is suspected and a comprehensive diagnosis is necessary, and only after biopsies from other tests have indicated severe abnormalities.

Treating CIN

Hearing that your Pap test is abnormal can be upsetting. But remember that, when detected early, most abnormalities can be treated successfully. Your treatment options are determined by how much diseased tissue is present in your cervix.

One alternative in mild dysplasia (CIN I) is a "watch and wait" approach. As many as 40 percent of mild dysplasia cases will return to normal without further treatment. Frequent Pap tests may be all your physician recommends to monitor mild dysplasia. Be sure to follow through on this recommendation.

Moderate and severe dysplasia (carcinoma *in situ*) need more aggressive treatments that either destroy or remove the abnormal cells.

These treatments include: **hysterectomy** (surgically removing the uterus and the cervix), **cryosurgery** (freezing the site with carbon dioxide or nitrous oxide), **electrocautery** (burning away the abnormal cells with an electric rod), **laser vaporization** (destroying the cells with a laser beam), **excising** (cutting out the diseased area), and **conization.**

Hysterectomy

This operation is sometimes recommended to treat CIN III (preinvasive cancer). But with other treatment options available, hysterectomy may not be the first choice for most women, especially if they are still interested in having children. This operation is major surgery with unique risks and benefits. It should be discussed carefully with your physician.

Long-term effects. Hysterectomy has significant consequences. When the uterus is removed, a woman no longer menstruates. If the ovaries are left intact, they continue to produce hormones until natural menopause occurs. But if they are removed during hysterectomy, menopausal symptoms such as hot flashes, vaginal dryness, and night sweats will suddenly begin. Hormone replacement therapy can prevent or minimize these symptoms. Although sexual function should not be impaired beyond the effects of vaginal dryness, some women describe changes in sexual sensation following a hysterectomy. In some cases, the vagina is slightly shortened.

For many women, a hysterectomy is an emotional issue. Regardless of whether a woman still wants to, or is able to, have children, removal of the uterus can affect her identity as a female. This is a legitimate issue to consider and to come to terms with when deciding whether to have the operation.

Recovery from hysterectomy takes between 4 and 6 weeks, although many women feel fatigued for longer periods. Actual hospitalization is normally several days to a week.

Electrocautery, Cryosurgery, and Laser Vaporization

These treatments destroy the abnormal cells on the surface of the cervix, allowing eventual growth of new healthy cells. The procedures can be performed in the physician's office, usually with no anesthesia.

Electrocautery often causes more pain during and after the procedure than newer methods, and it leaves more scar tissue on the cervix. For these reasons, it is used less frequently now than in the past. Still, it is effective in treating CIN I and II.

Cryosurgery and laser surgery cause cramp-like pain during the procedures and some vaginal discharge for several weeks afterwards. Bleeding may follow laser treatment. After either procedure, some women will need a second treatment to ensure all the abnormal tissue has been destroyed.

Advantages and Disadvantages. The area affected by cryosurgery in particular can be difficult to control. This can result in the destruction of either too much or not enough tissue, depending on the size of the probe. Laser surgery is slightly more likely than cryosurgery to destroy the diseased tissue the first time, but often is more expensive. Other benefits of laser treatment include its precision—it destroys only diseased tissue—and its reach—it can be directed at abnormalities farther inside in the cervix that are inaccessible to cryosurgery and electrocautery.

Follow–up. After electrocautery, cryosurgery, or laser treatment, nothing should be inserted into the vagina for several weeks. This means no tampons, douching, or intercourse. Pap smear and colposcopy should be performed in 4 months to determine whether the treatments were successful. Pap smears may not return to normal for some time following these treatments because of the trauma to the cervical cells. To be certain, Pap testing should continue at 6–month intervals until you and your physician are comfortable with the status of your lab reports.

Excision

This is both a treatment method (it removes damaged tissue) and a diagnostic tool. Excised tissue can be biopsied. The edges of the diseased area also can be evaluated to ensure that all the abnormal cells have been removed. This type of assessment is more difficult with methods such as cautery and vaporization that completely destroy the tissue.

If It's Cervical Cancer

If a biopsy confirms that abnormal cells are either preinvasive (CIN III or carcinoma *in situ*) or invasive cancer, your physician will want to move quickly to determine the extent and location of the disease. You may be referred—or want to consider referral—to a gynecologist who specializes in the treatment of cancer of the reproductive system.

Frequently, when advanced disease is suspected, larger portions of tissue must be removed for an accurate biopsy to help determine treatment. Dilation and curretage (D & C), a procedure in which the cervix is dilated and the sides of the cervical canal and uterus

are scraped with a small spoon-shaped instrument, is another diagnostic procedure the doctor may use.

Other tests are used to determine if the disease has spread from the cervix to other parts of the body. This process of assessment is called staging and includes a comprehensive pelvic exam, performed under anesthesia, blood and urine tests, and a chest x–ray. Computed tomography scans (CT or CAT scans), ultrasound, and magnetic resonance imaging (MRI scans) of the bones, liver, and spleen are other diagnostic tests used to identify diseased areas.

Treating Cervical Cancer

Preinvasive cancer (carcinoma *in situ*) can be treated with the same procedures described for cervical dysplasia. However, conization or hysterectomy are more frequently recommended to prevent the disease from spreading. Without treatment, carcinoma *in situ* usually develops into invasive cancer. Untreated, invasive cervical cancer will travel to other pelvic structures, then invade the lymph nodes located in the groin, then finally spread into the lungs, liver, and bones. Your doctor may refer to cancer that has spread beyond the pelvis and groin as metastasis.

Surgery and radiation therapy are equally successful treatment options for invasive cervical cancer. Chemotherapy does not work as well against cervical cancer as it does against other forms of the disease, but doctors do prescribe it to treat recurrent cervical cancer.

Surgery

Surgery is used to treat cancer when the disease is confined to the cervix. Options include total hysterectomy (removal of the cervix and uterus); radical hysterectomy (removal of the cervix, uterus, upper vagina, and the lymph nodes in the area); surgical removal of the tumor; or, if a woman wants to preserve her ability to carry a child, merely conization. The choice of procedure depends on a woman's age and overall health as well as the size of the tumor.

The consequences of hysterectomy have already been touched on. But, as serious as this surgery is, both medically and emotionally, it may be the best option for treating cervical cancer. It's important to discuss the risks and benefits of the procedure, as well as the long-term consequences, with your doctor.

Radiation Therapy

Radiation therapy, which destroys the ability of cells to grow and divide, can be used alone or in combination with surgery to treat large tumors and cancers that have grown beyond the cervix. Two forms of radiation therapy are employed: internal radiation, in which radioactive implants are placed directly into the cancerous site, and external radiation, in

which a machine directs high doses of radiation into the diseased tissue.

Internal radiation, called brachytherapy, destroys less of the healthy tissue around the cancer and causes fewer side effects than external radiation. Radioactive implants are inserted through the vagina, into the cervix and the uterus. Internal radiation is not always possible if the disease or earlier surgery has dramatically altered the region.

External radiation can be administered on an outpatient basis and is normally given 5 days a week for several weeks. Internal radiation usually requires a short hospital stay; the implant is left in place for 2 to 3 days.

Side Effects. The side effects of radiation therapy are uncomfortable and can be emotionally distressing. Radiation kills normal tissue, and the body reacts negatively to this aggressive treatment. Radiation for cervical cancer destroys the ovaries. Side effects may also include diarrhea, nausea, vomiting,

DEFINING CANCER

The decision about how to treat any invasive cancer is based on how much tissue the cancer has penetrated. A classification system, also called **staging,** is used to describe how far cancer has spread. For cervical cancer, these 5 stages and the rates of survival after treatment for each stage, are:

Stage	Areas Reached	Survival Rate
Stage 0	carcinoma in situ	100% 5-year survival
Stage I	Cancer is confined to the cervix	85% 5-year survival
Stage II	Cancer extends to the upper third of the vagina, or the tissue around the uterus, but not the pelvic wall	50 to 60% 5-year survival
Stage III	The lower third of the vagina and/or the pelvic side-wall and possibly the kidneys are diseased	30% 5-year survival
Stage IV	Cancer has spread beyond the reproductive tract involving the bladder or rectum, and has invaded distant organs (most often the lungs or liver), the bones, or other systems in the body	5% 5-year survival

bladder irritation and painful urination, weight loss and loss of appetite, fatigue, loss of vaginal sensation (when the vagina is included in the radiation field), and skin reactions. These side effects vary among women undergoing this treatment and those symptoms directly related to radiation usually disappear after treatment. Because the ovaries are destroyed, radiation also brings on the symptoms of menopause such as hot flashes, vaginal dryness, and night sweats.

Follow-up care. After treatment for cervical cancer, Pap tests are recommended every 2 months for the first year, every 4 months during the second year, every 6 months in the third and fourth year after surgery, and once a year thereafter. Pap tests can be inconclusive or inaccurate if a woman has received radiation therapy because radiation causes changes in cellular structure. For these women, biopsies are a better test. Three months after the tissue damage from treatment has healed, a biopsy should reveal only normal cells.

The Odds of a Cure

Not all cervical cancer responds to radiation therapy. In addition, disease returns in approximately one-third of all women treated for advanced cancer, usually within 2 years after therapy. Recurring cancer after treatment with radiation is most commonly found in the cervix, the uterus, upper vagina, and the pelvic wall. Cancer that returns after hysterectomy usually is found in the upper part of the vagina, where the cervix used to be located.

These symptoms indicate possible recurrence: weight loss, unexplained swelling in one or both legs, bloody vaginal discharge, pain in the thigh or buttock. When advanced cancer recurs in the pelvic area, prognosis is generally favorable. If the cancer has spread to locations beyond the pelvic area, however, the chances for recovery are less favorable.

Good Reasons For Optimism

A discussion of cervical cancer should not end on a pessimistic note. There is overwhelming evidence that when the disease is diagnosed early and treated effectively, a woman has every reason to expect complete recovery.

The key word here is "early." That's why every woman needs to make a commitment to have regular Pap tests and take other steps to prevent CIN and cervical cancer. Yearly Pap tests should begin at age 18, or whenever a woman becomes sexually active.

Using condoms during sex can help prevent sexually transmitted diseases such as AIDS, as well as other infections that may contribute to the development of cervical cancer. Quitting smoking not only improves overall health but also reduces risk of CIN and cervical cancer.

Most important, be an informed consumer. Know your options when considering treatment for dysplasia or cervical cancer. Open a dialogue with your doctor. Find out exactly why he or she is recommending certain treatments or tests. When reviewing the consequences of major surgery or radiation, don't lose sight of the risk inherent in inaction. Stay well-informed and you'll make the choice that's best for you and your family. □

CHAPTER 39

Making Sense of Your Pap Test

There it is: the little postcard reminding you that it's time to schedule a physical exam...and your Pap test. It's an easy reminder to cast aside. After all, didn't you have a Pap test just a little while ago? Why have one so often? What exactly does it mean, anyway?

Actually, this little test is one of the most important developments in women's health in decades. It's a screening test for cancer of the cervix; and since its introduction there has been a dramatic decline in deaths from the disease.

A study in British Columbia showed that, for every 100,000 people, there were 13 to 14 deaths per year from cervical cancer in 1958; in 1966, this number decreased to 11 to 12 and in 1974 it was down to 5 to 6, a 50 percent decrease. The most recent statistics show that the mortality from cervical cancer in the United States in 1988 was only 3 per 100,000.

In addition to detecting cancer and precancer, the Pap test may also show evidence of vaginal infections, such as yeast, Trichomonas, or viral infections. If your Pap test suggests inflammation, your doctor may do further tests to identify infections of the uterus, fallopian tubes, or vagina, which sometimes take hold without any warning symptoms. Rarely, the Pap test detects cells being shed from within the uterus (endometrial cells), which could signify excessive growth of this tissue.

When to Have a Pap Test

How often you need a Pap test has been somewhat controversial: the American Cancer Society and the American College of Obstetrics and Gynecology, along with several other health organizations, currently recommend the following: if you are sexually active, or are 18 years of age or more, you should have a Pap test and pelvic exam every year for 3 consecutive years. After 3 normal reports the test can be repeated less often, every 2 to 3 years, depending on your risk for cervical cancer. If you have had a hysterectomy, and as a result do not have a cervix, you may still be advised to have a Pap test from your vaginal walls to detect cancer there.

Reasons for an Annual Test

You are considered to be at increased risk of cervical cancer, and should therefore have a Pap test every year, if you:

- Have HPV (Human Papilloma Virus, the virus that causes genital warts—often detected *only* by a Pap test since many who carry the virus actually have no warts)
- Smoke
- Began having sex at an early age
- Have had many sexual partners
- Use birth control pills
- Have an impaired immune system (for example, have HIV or AIDS)
- Are being treated with drugs that suppress your immune system
- Have had radiation therapy
- Were born after your mother took DES while carrying you (DES, given years ago to prevent miscarriage, was subsequently discovered to increase the child's risk of cervical or vaginal cancer in later life.)
- Have a sexual partner who is "high–risk" (has genital warts, for instance)

You may be surprised to learn that you are at increased risk. In fact, some of these factors have only recently been discovered, and are still unfamiliar to most women. Doctors are also aware that a few of these factors offer benefits that far outweigh their role in cervical cancer. For example, it would be unwise to discontinue birth control pills given the protection they afford not only against pregnancy, but also against endometrial and ovarian cancer.

How the Test is Done

The Pap test relies on minute samples of tissue from the lining of the cervix; and these samples must be taken from very specific points.

The cervix is actually the lowermost part of the uterus. A cylinder projecting into the vagina, it surrounds a tiny canal leading out from the uterus. The interior of the canal is lined with tissue filled with glands that produce mucus. This is called glandular or "columnar" tissue. The end of the cervix is lined with tissue that is flat and smooth like the lining of the vagina and is, in fact, continuous with the vagina. This is called flat or "squamous" tissue. These 2 types of tissue meet at the squamo–columnar junction, which is the area where precancer and cancer are most likely to arise and therefore the area of greatest importance in a Pap test. (A sample from further inside the cervical canal is also needed.)

The squamo–columnar junction is not fixed but rather undergoes continuous changes during puberty and the childbearing years, as squamous or flat tissue slowly covers over the glandular tissue that grows out of the cervical canal. This process is called the squamous metaplasia. The squamo–columnar junction is usually found at the opening of the cervical canal (the "os") or on the outside part of the cervix (the "portio") during a woman's reproductive years, but often recedes up into the canal after menopause, making an accurate Pap smear difficult. For this reason, postmenopausal women are more likely to have Pap tests reported as "inadequate sample" or "unsatisfactory."

Women whose mothers took DES while pregnant with them may have a very large area of glandular or columnar tissue on the

CANCER-PRONE ZONE WHERE VAGINA AND CERVIX MEET

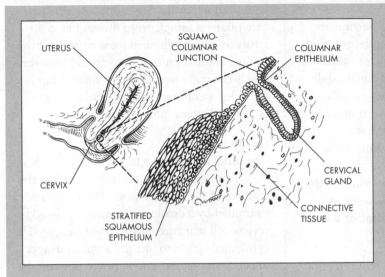

UTERUS
SQUAMO-COLUMNAR JUNCTION
COLUMNAR EPITHELIUM
CERVIX
CERVICAL GLAND
STRATIFIED SQUAMOUS EPITHELIUM
CONNECTIVE TISSUE

The mucus-producing lining of the cervical canal (called "columnar" tissue after the shape of its outer cells) meets the surface covering of the vagina (made up of squamous epithelial cells) at a line of demarcation called the "squamo-columnar junction." It is in this shifting zone of disparate cells that abnormal growth is most likely to arise. Central to the Pap test is an adequate sample from this important point.

outside of the cervix, even extending into the vagina. Some experts believe that this is the reason for the increased risk of cancer among women exposed to DES, although there is currently no definitive proof.

A good Pap test requires more than just knowing the right tissue to sample. Your preparation and the doctor's instruments are also important, and accurate interpretation is a necessity.

Preparation

You should not douche, or use any medications or creams in your vagina or have intercourse for 24 to 48 hours prior to having a Pap test. This is because douching may remove cells, and vaginal creams and fluids from intercourse can obscure or hide cells shed from the cervix. Blood can also obscure cervical cells, so if you are menstruating and

your flow is heavy, you should schedule your exam for after your period. In fact, some pathologists (doctors who specialize in analyzing tissue) recommend that a Pap test should be delayed until 14 days after your period.

Tools of the Test

A wooden spatula and Q–tip have been the usual means for collecting cells for a Pap test for many years. Recently, doctors have begun using new tools such as the cytobrush, cervix brush, and plastic spatulas because they collect more cells, providing a better sample. The major drawback is that tools with a brush–like surface are more abrasive and more likely to cause bleeding. For this reason, they are usually not used for pregnant women.

Taking the Sample

1) Your doctor will insert a tool called a speculum into your vagina using water as a lubricant if necessary; K-Y Jelly and other commercial lubricants can obscure the cells in the sample. If there is a large amount of discharge on the cervix, the doctor will gently wipe it off.

2) The next step is to scrape the outside of the cervix carefully with the spatula, rotating it 360 degrees to ensure a sample of the entire area. This sample is smeared on a glass slide in as thin a layer as possible, then quickly "fixed" by spraying or immersing it in a fixative. This preserves the cells in the state which they were found and prevents drying.

3) Next, the endocervical canal is sampled with a Q–tip or cytobrush, again rotating the tool 360 degrees to sample the entire canal. This sample is smeared on the same or a new slide, and fixed.

If you were exposed to DES before birth, your doctor may take an additional sample from the upper two–thirds of the vagina to check for vaginal cancer that could possibly result from that exposure. Some doctors also advocate taking a sample from the vagina in an effort to detect cells shed from cancers of the uterus, fallopian tubes, or ovaries. However, this is generally not necessary since it rarely provides useful information, and there are tests that better evaluate these problems.

Getting Results

The slides are sent to a laboratory for evaluation. First, the samples are stained so that the features of the cells are clear. Then they are examined by a cytologist (someone trained to review cell structure under a microscope). The cytologist's job is to identify abnormal–appearing cells among the many normal ones on the slides; every cell must be evaluated.

HOW A PAP SMEAR IS TAKEN

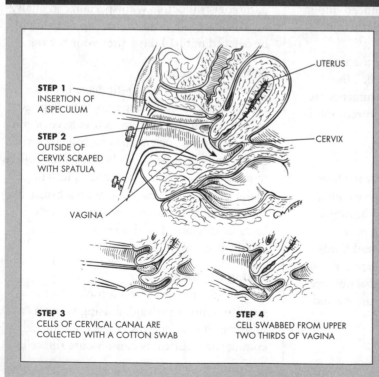

STEP 1
INSERTION OF
A SPECULUM

STEP 2
OUTSIDE OF
CERVIX SCRAPED
WITH SPATULA

VAGINA

UTERUS

CERVIX

STEP 3
CELLS OF CERVICAL CANAL ARE
COLLECTED WITH A COTTON SWAB

STEP 4
CELL SWABBED FROM UPPER
TWO THIRDS OF VAGINA

To gain free access to the cervix, the doctor first inserts into the vagina a device called a speculum (Step 1). With a tiny wooden or plastic spatula, the doctor then takes a scraping from the entire outer circumference of the cervix (Step 2). The cells inside the cervix must also be sampled, so the next part of the procedure calls for insertion of a Q-tip or brush into the cervical canal itself (Step 3). Finally, some doctors follow up by swabbing a cell sample from the upper two-thirds of the vagina (Step 4).

How Reliable are the Results?

The accuracy rate of the Pap test is estimated to be 80 to 90 percent. Thus, you have as much as a 1 in 5 chance that any given test will be wrong. The most likely kind of error is called a false–negative. This means that the test fails to detect a cell abnormality that is present on the cervix. Another kind of error is a false–positive, which means that the test results indicate a cell abnormality that is not actually there. The error rate seems high but there are a number of points where error may occur.

Types of Error

Patient preparation. Douching can remove abnormal cells from the cervix. Using vaginal creams or medications, or having intercourse prior to the Pap test, can introduce substances that obscure abnormal cells. Menstrual blood can also obscure the cells.

Sampling error. It is always possible, when collecting the sample, to miss an area of abnormal cells. This can occur even though your doctor is well–trained and experienced. It is called an inherent error, which means that there is no way to completely eliminate the possibility of its happening. In addition, if the sample dries before fixation (this can happen in seconds, as it is a very thin layer), or is not properly fixed, it may defeat interpretation.

Errors of interpretation. When cervical cells shed, they begin to degenerate as part of their normal life cycle. This degeneration is liable to misinterpretation during laboratory examination, resulting in a false–positive report of abnormalities. This is another source of inherent error. Also, errors can easily arise if the cytologist is not well–trained, uses poor judgment, or has inadequate time to thoroughly inspect the slide. For this reason, quality–control in cytology labs is currently a hot topic; standards for the number of slides screened per cytologist per day and unannounced tests of judgment are being reviewed and may be revised. Who should pay for the quality–control programs in this era of cutting medical costs is an equally hot topic of debate.

What To Do About Reliability

The 10 to 20 percent error rate has resulted in two important recommendations: First, if you are at increased risk for cervical cancer, you should have an annual Pap test. The likelihood of a false–negative test 2 years in a row is low. Second, if you receive an abnormal Pap test report, you should talk to your doctor about a further evaluation. A single abnormal report is not a diagnosis.

What the Report Tells You

In 1991, a new system to report Pap test results was introduced. This system, called Bethesda, gives results in a more descriptive way than previously. First, the adequacy of the sample is described and if the cytologist or pathologist notes an infection, it is described as well. If there are abnormalities in the squamous cells from the end of the cervix, they are described and attributed (if possible) to infection, inflammation, or precancerous changes. Sometimes it is not possible to classify the abnormality, so the cells are described as atypical, of undetermined significance.

Cells that appear to be undergoing a transformation to cancer are classified as either low–grade or high–grade "squamous intraepithelial lesions" (SIL). Low–grade SIL includes mildly precancerous cells and those showing signs of infection with HPV. They are grouped together because cytologists and pathologists cannot consistently distinguish between them, and because the recommendations for treatment and follow–up are usually similar. High–grade SIL includes moderately or severely precancerous cells and the condition in which the full thickness of the cervical lining contains abnormal cells (carcinoma in situ). Treatment and follow–up is the same for all of these types of lesions.

The cytologist will also describe any abnormalities in the glandular cells. With these cells, even the description of atypical is worrisome, because cancer of the glandular tissue is believed to start deep in the gland, may not shed for a long time, and may not be detected until well established. As a result, abnormal glandular cells always warrant further evaluation. Sometimes glandular cells from within the uterus (endometrial cells) are found; these may or may not warrant further evaluation, depending on where you are in your menstrual cycle, whether you've passed menopause, and whether or not the cells are described as atypical.

Interpreting the Report

If your Pap test results are anything other than normal, you should discuss them with your doctor and be prepared to take the next steps. Remember that the test does not yield a diagnosis; rather, it is a screen that suggests what the appropriate next steps should be.

Unsatisfactory or Inadequate Sample

If your results come back as unsatisfactory or inadequate, it means that the cytologist did not find enough cells on the slide to evaluate, or that no glandular cells were found. In some cases, you'll want to have a repeat test, especially if you have previously had an abnormal test or have risk factors for the abnormal cell growth called dysplasia. In other cases, your doctor may believe that he or she obtained as good a sample as possible, and that repeat testing is not necessary. This may very well be the case if you are post-menopausal and your squamo–columnar junction is high in the cervical canal. In any case, you should discuss the significance with your doctor. You should feel free to request a repeat test if you desire, even if your doctor does not feel it is necessary.

Infection

The Pap test may report Trichomonas (a sexually–transmitted vaginal infection), Candida (yeast) or large amounts of bacteria, usually Gardnerella (the most common bacteria normally found in the vagina). You can have these infections without any symptoms. Your doctor may want to do further testing which usually involves taking a sample of vaginal discharge and inspecting it under a microscope for the presence of these organisms.

Rarely, a Pap test may indicate the presence of cells that appear to be infected with the Herpes virus. Pap tests are not reliable as a test for Herpes and the results should never be offered as a definitive diagnosis. Instead, your doctor should take a culture that tests specifically for Herpes.

Reactive or Repair–related Changes

These changes are sometimes seen if you've had an infection or a recent cervical procedure, such as a biopsy. They may also be found in Pap tests from women who are post-menopausal, because the lack of estrogen that was previously produced by the ovaries can cause the vaginal and cervical lining to become very thin and inflamed (atrophic vaginitis). In addition, women who use an

WHAT "PAP" STANDS FOR

Pap is not an acronym. It's short for Papanicolaou, the name of the doctor who invented the test. His description of the procedure was first published in 1941. After years of research and verification, the test came into general use in the 1950s.

IUD (intrauterine device) for contraception often have reactive changes on their cervix, due to slight irritation from the IUD string. And you can get a similar irritation leading to a reactive change if you frequently use a diaphragm or cervical cap. Finally, women who have radiation treatment of the pelvis may also show reactive changes. Generally, if the cause of a reactive change is known, no further evaluation or treatment is advised. If the cause is not known, a repeat exam may be suggested.

Squamous Cell Abnormalities

Atypical squamous cells of undetermined significance means that the cytologist found cells that appear abnormal, but that the exact cause of the abnormality is not clear. If the cytologist can make this determination, the report should suggest whether the cause is more likely to be inflammation or precancer. Generally your doctor will recommend a repeat Pap test or further evaluation.

Low–grade squamous intraepithelial lesion means that cells have been found which appear to be undergoing a transformation to a state of uncontrolled growth. If the cell growth is described as low–grade, the abnormality is considered mild. In about half of these cases, the cells spontaneously revert to normal. However, there is a 25 percent chance that the abnormality may persist and

another 25 percent chance that it will progress to a higher degree of abnormality, and thus to cancer. In these situations, further evaluation is always recommended.

High–grade squamous intraepithelial lesion is a discovery of cells that are moderately or severely abnormal and are undergoing a transformation to a state of uncontrolled growth. The likelihood that these cells will progress to cancer is 50 to 75 percent. If the report finds that these cells are present, the next step is a biopsy to see if the cells are, in fact, cancerous.

Cancer. If the cells readily appear to be cancer, your doctor will do a biopsy to confirm the Pap test report.

Glandular Cell Abnormalities

Endometrial cells are shed from the lining of the uterus and they can sometimes show up on a Pap test. If you were in the middle of your period during the Pap smear, this is a normal finding; even if you were not actively menstruating, endometrial cells could have been seen. There are 2 situations where endometrial cells in a Pap test may indicate a state of rapid or uncontrolled growth in the uterine lining. First, if repeated Pap tests show endometrial cells when you are not actively menstruating, and second, *anytime* these cells are seen on a Pap test when you are post-menopausal. In either of these cases, your doctor should suggest further evaluation with a biopsy of the lining of the uterus. Also, if the endometrial cells are described as appearing abnormal, further evaluation is warranted even if you have not reached menopause.

Atypical glandular cells of undetermined significance are glandular cells that are abnormal in appearance without an obvious cause. This is more worrisome than the same finding applied to squamous cells, because cancer arising in glandular cells can develop undetected for a long time. The cells also may have descended from high in the cervical canal, above the area normally sampled by the endocervical brush. The test report should state whether the abnormality is more likely due to inflammation or a precancerous process. Regardless, this finding should always be evaluated further with colposcopy (a visual inspection of the cervix) and endocervical curettage (scraping the cervical canal with a sharp instrument to obtain a large sample of cells).

Cancer of glandular cells. If cancer is seen in the glandular cells, your doctor will want to confirm the Pap test results.

Next Steps

If you've received an abnormal Pap test result, your doctor may recommend any one of a number of further diagnostic tests. These are covered in greater detail in chapter 38, "Cervical Cancer: The One That's Preventable."

Colposcopy

A colposcopy is generally the first test done after an abnormal Pap test result. It is a visual inspection of the cervix using a low-power microscope.

In a colposcopy, your doctor is looking for rapidly growing areas of tissue, abnormal blood vessel patterns, or abnormal surface contour. If any of these abnormalities are seen, your doctor will take a biopsy (small pieces of tissue) and send it to a pathology laboratory for a definitive diagnosis. A diagnosis by biopsy is considered 100 percent accurate, unlike a Pap test report.

A cervical biopsy is usually painless, although some cramping may occur afterward. If you find cervical manipulation painful, ask your doctor for a local anesthetic (similar to that used in dental procedures). Endocervical curettage, or scraping the endocervical canal with a sharp instrument to obtain a large sample of glandular cells, is also often done during a colposcopy. After the biopsy, your doctor may apply medication to the cervix to stop or prevent bleeding; this may result in a dark vaginal discharge resembling coffee grounds that can last up to a week. You will be told not to use tampons, douche, or have intercourse for several days, until the biopsy sites have healed and the risk of infection has passed.

If colposcopy does not provide a view of the entire squamo–columnar junction, or show an abnormal area that extends high into the cervical canal, your gynecologist may recommend conization of the cervix. This is a minor operation in which a part of the cervix surrounding the canal, including the squamo–columnar junction, is surgically removed. It is performed in an operating room, with anesthesia and is usually done on an outpatient basis (no overnight hospitalization). A pathologist will evaluate the tissue and determine whether precancerous growth is present; if so, it has often been entirely removed, and no further treatment is necessary.

Endometrial Biopsy

If endometrial cells are reported on a Pap test in a postmenopausal woman, or on repeated Pap tests in a premenopausal woman who is not menstruating at the time of the Pap test, doctors usually recommend a biopsy of the tissue that lines the uterus. The presence of these cells in a Pap test, even if they are normal in appearance, may mean that the endometrium is growing at an abnormally rapid rate, undergoing a transformation to a state of uncontrolled growth. This transformation is called endometrial hyperplasia and is considered a precancerous state. It is important to detect and treat this condition before it becomes cancer.

If the Diagnosis Is Dysplasia

If precancerous or uncontrolled cell growth (dysplasia) is diagnosed on a cervical biopsy, your doctor will discuss the next steps with you. Mild dysplasia may be managed with observation, repeating cervical evaluation by Pap test, colposcopy, and biopsy at intervals of 3 to 6 months. Over time, mild dysplasia will either resolve on its own or progress to moderate/severe dysplasia. These forms of dysplasia should always be treated, and you and your doctor may also decide to treat a mild dysplasia right away. Methods of treatment include laser vaporization, excision with electrical loop, freezing, or conization as described above. All of these methods are considered 90 percent curative when performed properly. The 10 percent failure or recurrence rate is considered unavoidable. For this reason, follow–up is especially important. Cervical evaluation by colposcopy, Pap, or both should be carried out at 3 to 6 month intervals for 1 to 2 years after treatment.

More Good Reasons to Get Your Test

The Pap test is not perfect but it is one of the few tests available to detect pre-cancer and therefore prevent cancer from developing. It is easy, relatively inexpensive, and can be done during a visit for contraception or other health care.

Women who avoid having a Pap for reasons of discomfort should be aware that doctors can be gentle; if yours is not, you should ask for a softer touch. If your request is disregarded, don't be afraid to find another doctor, getting a referral from a friend or local hospital.

And remember that although the Pap test has a significant error rate, the greatest error of all is to avoid having it; prevention is still the best medical care! □

CHAPTER 40

Ovarian Cancer: Facing the Facts

O f all the cancers to which women are prey, this is the deadliest. By the time it's discovered in the majority of cases, odds of a cure have already dropped to little more than 1 in 10.

Fortunately, this kind of cancer is also quite rare. Your overall chances of developing it are 1 in 100—in contrast to a breast cancer rate of 1 in 9. Even if you're in the group at greatest risk—women in their 50s and 60s—the odds against you are still only 1 in 70. In a typical year, some 20,000 American women find out they have ovarian cancer, and more than 12,000 die from it.

Like all cancers, this one is most dangerous when discovered late. Hope of a cure in the most advanced stage is only 5 percent. On the other hand, there's much more reason for optimism if your doctor finds the disease early, when chances of a cure are 2 to 1 in your favor. The catch, however, is in finding it.

The Symptoms

O ne of the reasons ovarian cancer is so deadly is that it frequently doesn't have any symptoms in its earlier stages. To compound the problem, because the ovaries are located deep within the abdomen there's no way to do a self–examination on a regular basis, as you can with your breasts. And when the disease does produce symptoms, they can often be confusing, possible signaling many other conditions, or meaning nothing at all.

The most frequent symptoms are vague stomach discomfort, an expanded abdomen, or abnormal bleeding. But many women have these types of nonspecific symptoms throughout their lives and therefore don't bother telling their doctor. By the time you are troubled enough to see your doctor, or your doctor feels (palpates) an ovarian tumor during the course of a normal examination, the disease may have spread too far to stop.

Happily, even when your doctor does find an ovarian mass, it does not always mean cancer. In fact, the great majority of ovarian masses detected in premenopausal patients are benign and eventually disappear on their own. If you are over 50, an enlargement is considered potentially more serious—since the ovary shrinks during menopause, and ovarian cancer occurs more frequently in women in their 50s and 60s. Still, even masses found in postmenopausal women are often just benign cysts.

Who's at Greatest Risk

As with many cancers, doctors just don't know what exactly causes the growth of cancerous ovarian cells. Current theory is that a number of factors—some controllable, many not—may influence the development of ovarian cancer. One proposal suggests a link between the number of times a woman ovulates during her life and her risk of developing ovarian cancer: The more she has ovulated, the greater the risk.

Some researchers have noted that for 99.9 percent of the human history, women ovulated much less frequently than they do today, since so much time was spent in pregnancy and breast feeding. One expert has estimated that our remote ancestors might have had only about 50 menstrual cycles in an entire lifetime compared to more than 400 that the average American woman has today.

Whether this theory is true or not remains to be proven, but it may help explain why the following factors tend to increase the risk of ovarian cancer:

- Ovulation for more than 40 years
- Never being pregnant or having your first pregnancy after age 30
- Late menopause

The theory might also help explain why oral contraceptives, pregnancy, and breastfeeding appear to protect against ovarian cancer, since you don't ovulate when you are on the Pill, pregnant, or breastfeeding. In fact, one study showed that using oral contraceptives, even for just a few months, can markedly reduce the risk of ovarian cancer, with the protection lasting for years.

Other factors—unrelated to ovulation—that are thought to increase the risk of ovarian cancer include:

- A family history of ovarian or uterine cancer (especially mother or sister)
- Having had breast cancer or benign breast disease
- Having had colon or rectal cancer or polyps

A history of mumps infection before the start of menstruation and a diet high in animal fat may also play a role. Researchers have speculated that the use of talcum powder in the vaginal and anal area might increase the risk of ovarian cancer, perhaps because the powder can enter the reproductive tract and settle on the ovary, possibly causing irritation.

How the Disease is Diagnosed

If your doctor feels a mass that might indicate an enlarged ovary, he or she will usually send you for an ultrasound (sonogram) of the pelvic area. This is a painless diagnostic test that allows your doctor to see your internal reproductive organs by bouncing sound waves off of them. It is usually performed in the doctor's office. Generally, if a mass is small, and only one ovary is involved, the chances are very good that it is benign (non–cancerous). It may still require treatment (see chapter 9, "What You Need to Know About Ovarian Cysts"), but at least you will know it's not cancer.

A blood test called the CA–125 assay can also provide useful diagnostic information, especially in postmenopausal women. This test also measures a substance that can be associated with ovarian tumors. A higher level of this substance than is normal, coupled with an ultrasound that shows a significant mass, can lead your doctor to suggest that further exploration is needed. However, like many tests, the CA–125 assay can produce a false positive result, predicting that a cancer is present, when, in fact, the mass is benign.

If the ultrasound and blood tests suggest that a mass might be cancerous, your doctor will recommend a laparotomy (surgery done through the abdomen), in order to make a clear diagnosis.

Stages of Ovarian Cancer

If your doctor makes a diagnosis of ovarian cancer, he or she will categorize it as one of 4 stages of the disease. Stage I is the earliest stage in which only the ovaries are involved. About two–thirds of Stage I patients can look forward to a cure. In Stage II, the cancer will have spread from an ovary to other parts of the pelvis. As with most cancers, as the disease begins to spread, survival rates decrease. About half of those diagnosed with Stage II ovarian cancer will survive after treatment. The majority of cases are diagnosed at Stage III, at which point the disease involves the lymph nodes and/or other parts of the abdomen. About 13 percent of patients diagnosed with Stage III cancer are cured. The most advanced form is Stage IV which has a very low survival rate—only about 5 percent of those diagnosed with Stage IV ovarian cancer will survive for five years. The overall five–year survival of all patients with ovarian cancer, regardless of stage, is about 30 percent.

CANCER'S INSIDIOUS ATTACK ON THE OVARIES

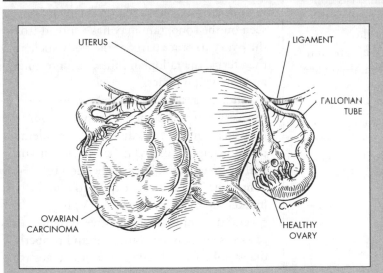

UTERUS

LIGAMENT

FALLOPIAN TUBE

OVARIAN CARCINOMA

HEALTHY OVARY

Because ovarian cancer often develops without any troubling symptoms, your only warning could be discovery of an enlarged ovary during your annual physical exam. If your doctor does encounter a mass while checking your pelvic area, he or she will probably follow up with an ultrasound look at the internal organs, followed by a blood test for a tumor-related substance. Surgery may be needed if both tests suggest the possibility of cancer.

Kinds of Ovarian Tumors

Ovarian tumors tend to arise from three different kinds of ovarian tissue: About 85 percent grow from epithelial tissue, the kind of tissue that covers most internal and external surfaces of the body and its organs; about 10 percent from stromal cells, the cells that make up the connective tissue framework of an organ; and the remaining 5 percent come from germ cells (the egg cells and their precursors).

Tumors that grow from these kinds of cells can be benign, on the borderline between benign and malignant, or purely malignant. The ones that are malignant vary in their severity: Some spread quickly; others are easier to control.

Treatment Strategies

If you are diagnosed with ovarian cancer, your treatment will depend on the malignancy and stage of the tumor; in other words, what kind of tumor it is and how far it has spread.

Surgery

Surgery is almost always the first step in treating ovarian cancer because the cancerous tissue must be removed. If the cancer is confined to the ovary and has not spread to the lymph nodes or to other parts of the abdomen, your doctor will try to ensure that you'll still be able to have children, if you are of childbearing age. However, since ovarian cancer can spread rapidly, this is not always possible; your doctor's primary goal is to do what needs to be done to eradicate the cancer and prolong life. Even when an early stage cancer is confined to a single ovary, it is occasionally necessary to remove the other ovary and the uterus, if your doctor is concerned that the cancer will spread.

The primary operation for ovarian cancer is a laparotomy. This is considered major surgery in ovarian cancer patients, since the surgeon usually must make a vertical incision between the belly button and the pubic area in order to reach the cancerous tissue in the abdominal or pelvic area. A laparotomy should not be confused with a laparoscopy. The latter procedure requires only a small incision below the belly button, through which an instrument called a laparoscope is inserted. (For more on laparoscopy, see chapter 9.)

Since surgery for ovarian cancer is usually relatively extensive, you can expect to go under general anesthesia, in which you are completely unconscious, rather than get a regional or local anesthetic that would numb only the abdominal and pelvic areas.

The surgery is considered both diagnostic and therapeutic. In other words, your doctor will be looking to see how far the cancer has spread, and then will remove all signs of it. This is very important because the tumor that your doctor may have felt on the ovary or seen on the sonogram may have spread from the ovary to other parts of the body such as the uterus, the fallopian tubes, the intestines, and the lymph nodes.

After surgery, you will be brought to a recovery room, and then a hospital room. Not surprisingly, you can expect considerable pain during the following few days, but you will be given painkilling medication to control it. You can also expect to remain hooked up to an intravenous (IV) line for several days until your digestive system recovers enough for you to eat and properly digest solid food. If any part of the digestive system was removed, you will probably be on IV feeding for a longer period.

As with all surgery, the first few days afterward are the most critical. You will probably be monitored carefully for infection, blood clots, and internal bleeding, all of which tend to occur earlier rather than later in the postoperative period. You should expect to be in the hospital for about a week, if there are no complications, and to convalesce at home for several weeks. Once you are home, be sure to call your doctor if you have fever, persistent bleeding, pain that is not relieved by medication, or any other unexpected symptoms.

Chemotherapy and Radiation

Whether you receive chemotherapy and radiation depends on the stage and malignancy of the cancer and how your individual case is being managed. These forms of treatment are generally used after surgery to destroy any cancerous tissue that was too small to have been detected during the operation.

You are less likely to get chemotherapy or radiation if you have a Stage I cancer (limited to one or both ovaries). More advanced cancers are often treated by chemotherapy, radiotherapy, or both, after the initial surgery is finished.

Radiation treatment can be administered either by an external machine or by putting a solution containing a radioactive substance into the abdomen.

Chemotherapy—the use of potent anti–cancer drugs that are selectively toxic to malignant cells and tissue—is usually started 2 to 4 weeks after surgery. There are many different kinds of drugs, and they can be given individually or in various combinations. How you get chemotherapy will depend on which drugs your doctor decides to use, but usually treatment is given for 1 to 3 days at a time and repeated every 3 to 4 weeks. The entire treatment period may last several months.

Chemotherapy is usually given intravenously, but the medications are sometimes instilled (poured drop by drop) directly into the abdomen. This method of administration is thought to maximize contact between the drug and the cancerous tissue, although intravenous drugs seem to work just as well. Also, because drugs delivered directly to the abdomen don't enter your circulation first, which would affect the entire body, they may have fewer side effects than they do when they are taken orally or intravenously.

The most effective medications studied so far include cisplatin (Platinol), carboplatin (Paraplatin), doxorubicin (Adriamycin, Rubex), cyclophosphamide (Cytoxan, Neosar), melphalan (Alkeran), chlorambucil (Leukeran), and hexamethylmelamine. Chemotherapy drugs are very powerful and can have side effects ranging from severe nausea and fatigue to actually causing other kinds of cancer such as leukemia. If you need to undergo chemotherapy (for ovarian or any other type of cancer), talk with your doctor and be sure to obtain comprehensive counseling about what to expect and how to deal with it.

Second–Look Procedures

Although you will be monitored constantly during both chemotherapy and radiation, sometimes it is very difficult to tell if the surgery and follow–up treatment have eradicated all the cancer. As a result, you may undergo what is known as a "second–look laparotomy so that your doctor can see first–hand whether any cancer has slipped past the treatments. A negative (no apparent cancer) second–look operation is a good sign. Unfortunately, it is not a guarantee. The best judge of cure in ovarian cancer is time.

Beating the Odds

Because ovarian cancer gives so few warning signs, and because there's no way you can check for it yourself, your annual checkup is your best—and possibly your *only*—hope of discovering the disease while it's still easily curable. Make sure you get a thorough pelvic exam every year, complete with palpation of the ovaries. If you feel you have any reason for concern, don't hesitate to ask your doctor about a sonogram and the CA–125 assay. If you're lucky, you'll find they weren't needed at all. □

CHAPTER 41   **DEALING WITH CANCER**

Stopping Endometrial Cancer in Time

There's no way around it: Endometrial cancer is a dreaded, potentially lethal disease. Still, there is plenty of reason for optimism. If the cancer is caught soon enough—before it's had a chance to spread beyond the uterus—the odds of a cure are excellent. Eight out of 10 women treated at this stage of the disease can expect to go on with their lives for a minimum of 5 years. And happily, 3 out of 4 cases are discovered at this early, curable stage.

But make no mistake about it: The key word here is "early." Keeping alert for the first signs of a problem is your best guarantee of successful treatment and long–term survival.

The telltale sign to watch for, as with so many other diseases of the reproductive system, is abnormal bleeding from the vagina. But what, exactly, does "abnormal" bleeding mean?

In this instance, what we're talking about is a relatively unalarming watery discharge that begins with some streaks of blood and may contain more blood later on. This symptom may seem somewhat vague, but

that's no reason to dismiss it. When a woman encounters this problem, she should see a physician promptly, especially if she is entering or past menopause, when her menstrual periods end.

After menopause, when normal bleeding has stopped, any bleeding is considered "abnormal." And cancer of the endometrium—the lining of the uterus—appears most often around or after menopause. So any irregular bleeding in a woman entering, or about to enter, menopause is not a routine matter. Approximately 25 percent of postmenopausal bleeding is due to some form of cancer of the uterus.

Endometrial cancer, however, can begin with no symptoms. If the disease progresses unnoticed to a more advanced stage, the first warning sign could be pelvic pain or pressure as fluid accumulates in the abdomen. Fortunately, it is usually discovered before reaching this point.

What is Endometrial Cancer?

Cancer is abnormal tissue growth brought about by uncontrolled division of the cells that make it up. In endometrial cancer the tissue involved is the inner lining of the uterus. When communication and interdependence break down among the cells of this lining, new cells develop faster than existing ones die. The excess cells continue trying to create tissue and perform their normal tasks, but have neither the room nor the regulation to do it properly.

Without order, they multiply, pile up, and eventually form excess tissue that has no function except to grow. As the tissue increases, it forms tissue masses, known as tumors. Some are benign (noncancerous), some malignant (cancerous). Cancerous tumors can destroy normal uterine tissue and break away to spread from one organ to

another, invading other parts of the body. This spreading is called metastasis.

Endometrial cancer is one of two major cancers that occur in the uterus. In 3 out of 4 cases, it first develops in the glandular cells of the lining. Later, it may affect their supporting structure known as the stroma. If it spreads, it usually moves into the wall of the uterus, the myometrium. Further growth can project it into the cervix at the mouth of the uterus, and the bladder, bowel, and lower abdominal cavity. The lymph and blood systems may also circulate it to more distant areas of the body, such as the lung or the liver.

An entirely different form of uterine cancer called *sarcoma* begins in the smooth muscle of the uterine wall. It grows rapidly and may eventually reach the endometrium to involve the surface cells of the uterine lining. While sarcoma presently accounts for only about 5 percent of uterine cancer, its diagnosis is

WHERE UTERINE CANCER BEGINS

In nearly three-quarters of all cases, uterine cancer establishes its initial foothold in the glandular cells that line the surface of the endometrium. Uncontrolled multiplication of these cells leads first to *hyperplasia*—an excessive number of cells—then to *tumors* formed by a large mass of abnormal cells. If an endometrial tumor is cancerous, it will penetrate deep into the uterine wall, destroying normal tissue as it goes and eventually spreading to nearby organs.

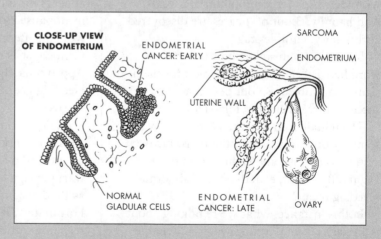

A totally unrelated type of tumor arises deep within the muscular wall of the uterus, reaching the endometrium at the surface only in its later stages. Called a *sarcoma,* this tumor spreads more quickly than endometrial cancer and is therefore more dangerous. Fortunately, it is also quite rare, accounting for only 1 uterine cancer in 20.

becoming more frequent. (See the nearby box on "Other Cancers of the Uterus.")

Distinct from endometrial cancer are the benign tumors known as fibroids. These abnormal growths seldom cause pain, but can become large enough to be uncomfortable as they press on organs around the uterus and eventually produce bleeding. They do not usually invade nearby tissues or organs, however, and can be removed surgically. (For more information, see Chapter 7, "Your Treatment Options for Fibroids.")

Benign or Malignant?

Endometrial hyperplasia—an abnormal increase in the cells of the endometrium—is common among women who are nearing menopause and who seldom ovulate. It is not in itself cancerous, but can change progressively to become malignant.

Since it can be a forerunner of endometrial cancer, your doctor will investigate it carefully once it's discovered. Treatment—or lack of it—depends on which of three classes of hyperplasia is identified:

- *Cystic hyperplasia* is generally considered unlikely to become malignant, but will be monitored regularly.
- *Adenomatous hyperplasia* is likely to progress to cancer in 25 percent of women who develop it, and generally requires some type of treatment.
- *Atypical hyperplasia* is more serious yet, and may call for surgical removal of the uterus.

Endometrial cancer itself is broken down into four classifications: *adenocarcinoma, adenosquamous carcinoma, papillary serous carcinoma,* and *clear cell carcinoma.* Adenocarcinoma accounts for 3 of 4 cases of endometrial cancer. Fortunately, it is the easiest to treat, with the best chance of success.

Risks, Large and Small

As with most other cancers, how and why endometrial cancer develops is still an unsolved mystery. Because the most common variety, adenocarcinoma, appears far more frequently at and after menopause, usually in women in their 60s and 70s, it is considered a slow–growing cancer. The chances of developing it are greater for women who:

- Began to menstruate at an early age
- Went through menopause late (after the age of 53)
- Are considerably overweight
- Never had a child

While endometrial disease is not inherited, there is a tendency for it to appear more often in relatives. Women who develop ovarian tumors, which stimulate estrogen production, are also at higher risk, as are women with endometrial hyperplasia.

The Role of Excess Weight

Diabetes and/or high blood pressure are also common in those who develop endometrial cancer, but the excess weight that accompanies these problems is probably the factor at work. Women who are 50 pounds overweight are 9 times as likely to develop the disease as women of normal weight. Excess fatty tissue turns certain hormones into a form of estrogen, and women with high levels of estrogen are twice as likely to develop endometrial cancer.

OTHER CANCERS OF THE UTERUS

The vast majority (perhaps 95 percent) of cancers of the uterus are endometrial cancers, 75 percent of which are adenocarcinomas. The remaining 25 percent are: adenosquamous (18 percent), papillary serous (6 percent), and clear cell carcinomas (1 percent). These three grow more rapidly and are deadlier than adenocarcinoma.

An entirely different type of cancer—uterine sarcoma—begins in the smooth muscle of the uterine wall or the connective tissue called the stroma, which supports the endometrium. The various types of uterine sarcomas include leiomyosarcoma, endometrial stromal sarcoma, and mixed Müllerian sarcoma. They, too, are deadlier and grow faster than adenocarcinoma.

Low-grade stromal sarcoma enlarges the uterus uniformly, while the high-grade stromal sarcoma protrudes into the endometrial cavity, invading the lymphatic channels and blood vessels of the myometrium, the muscular wall of the uterus. Both types spread readily. The low-grade type has come back as long as 20 years after removal of the primary tumor. While 80 percent of women with the low-grade tumors survive at least 5 years, only 15 to 25 percent who develop the high-grade type do.

Mixed Müllerian sarcoma grows rapidly and usually spreads. It typically appears around the age of 70. Pelvic pain and vaginal discharge often accompany bleeding. The tumor contains both stroma and epithelial cells, either of which may be benign or malignant. If the sarcoma has no stroma cells, it is called carcinosarcoma. Once it has spread outside the uterus or penetrated half the depth of the myometrium, it can be deadly. Müllerian adenosarcoma is, on the other hand, a less malignant cancer that develops both in older and younger women. It may recur, but survival at 5 years exceeds 50 percent.

Leiomyosarcoma represents only 1 percent of malignant uterine tumors. It usually arises from the wall of the uterus, causing pain and bleeding. The uterus is usually enlarged. Women who have it are in their 40s and 50s.

A few cancers found in the uterus are not really "uterine" at all. Because a number of organs—bladder, rectum, colon, lymph nodes—lie close to the uterus and some—ovaries and fallopian tubes—are actually connected to it, a cancer originating in any of these organs can spread to the uterus.

Estrogen and Increased Risk

Heavy use of estrogen replacement therapy (ERT) is clearly a factor in the development of endometrial cancer in some women. This is especially true if the estrogen is not combined with progesterone, or a similar compound called progestin. Estrogen and progesterone are important controls in the reproductive cycle. Until menopause, estrogen stimulates a build-up of the endometrium to accept a woman's egg, then prompts it to shed the excess tissue if conception does not take place. When estrogen levels decline after menopause, a woman faces problems ranging from depression and "hot flashes" to increased risk of coronary heart disease and osteoporosis (brittle and easily broken bones). ERT overcomes these effects, but it can also stimulate the endometrium to bleed and can increase the likelihood of endometrial hyperplasia, which in turn can progress to adenocarcinoma. To reduce this risk, doctors often supplement ERT with progestin treatment, which has been demonstrated to reverse endometrial hyperplasia.

Other Risk Factors

A history of certain other diseases also increases the chances of developing endometrial cancer. Polycystic ovarian disease, ovarian tumor, or colon or rectal cancer are among the culprits. Women who have had breast cancer are more prone to develop endometrial cancer; and the breast-cancer-drug tamoxifen has also been linked to an increased risk of endometrial disease. In fact, any history of cancer of a woman's reproductive organs increases the risk. Additionally, in the under 40 age group, this disease occurs 3 times as often in women with endometriosis, a disease of abnormal endometrial tissue development outside the uterus.

You can see that hormone levels affect many of these risk factors in some way. Nevertheless, it is unlikely that any single factor triggers the disease. In fact, 2 in 5 cases of endometrial cancer appear to have no connection to abnormal functioning of the system that produces the hormones.

When Does It Strike?

Endometrial cancer is diagnosed in nearly 40,000 women annually in the United States. It represents 6 percent of all cancers in women. It occurs more often than any other cancer of the reproductive tract, now exceeding cervical cancer, which for most of this century ranked number one.

Unlike endometriosis, which affects women almost entirely in their childbearing years, endometrial cancer occurs overwhelmingly in women who have reached or are reaching menopause. Three of 4 women with the disease are postmenopausal. Of these, the majority are between 61 and 75. Overall, it is most often diagnosed in women who are between 55 and 60 years of age.

As our population ages, the number of endometrial cancer cases is increasing. However, fatalities from endometrial cancer are not keeping pace. In 1990, when 40,000 cases were diagnosed, only 4,000 women succumbed to the disease. By comparison, cervical cancer was diagnosed in only 13,500 women that year, but took the lives of 6,000. Overall, the mortality rate from endometrial cancer is now about 3 women in 100,000.

Endometrial cancer's lower death rate—despite its higher incidence—is primarily a result of early detection. Because bleeding usually provides a clear warning early in the disease, the cancer can be caught while it is still confined to the uterus. At this early stage, it is the easiest cancer to treat outside of skin cancer.

Stages Of Development

Endometrial cancer can progress through five stages, from tissue abnormalities like hyperplasia to cancer extended to the bladder, bowel, or other parts of the body. Among its targets as the cancer spreads are the wall of the uterus (called the myometrium), the cervix and vagina, the nearby lymph nodes, the bladder, the bowel, the abdominal cavity, and even more distant organs and lymph nodes. The fact that cancer spreads to distant areas of the body by way of the lymphatic system has focused a lot of attention in recent years on carefully checking the lymph nodes near the uterus and cervix, since seemingly unaffected nodes can still spread the malignancy.

If endometrial cancer does recur, it is likely to happen quickly. In 8 out of 10 women who have a recurrence, the new cancer develops in the first 2 years after the

STAGES OF ENDOMETRIAL CANCER

Cancer Development	Treatments
O. Endometrial hyperplasia (abnormal cell growth)	Progestin to reverse hyperplasia. D&C to remove potentially cancerous tissue. Women treated for this stage should not take estrogen or, if they must, should have a hysterectomy to preclude estrogen-dependent cancer in the uterus.
I. Cancer found only in the body of the uterus	Hysterectomy and removal of the ovaries and fallopian tubes is recommended. Nearby lymph nodes will be removed and tested for cancerous cells. Radiation, to all or part of the pelvis, may be suggested if cancer has spread to the nodes.
II. Uterine body and cervix involved, but no cancer outside the uterus	Removal of uterus, ovaries and fallopian tubes, usually with external and/or internal radiation outside before or after surgery. Removal of para–aortic lymph nodes to examine for disease. Radical hysterectomy may be done in some cases, with removal of pelvic lymph nodes and the connective tissue that holds the uterus in place.
III. Cancer beyond the uterus but not outside the pelvis	Surgery, often with radiation therapy before or after the operation.
IV. Cancer beyond pelvis in bladder, bowel or other areas of the body	Treatment depends on the location of tumors and the symptoms. Possible hormonal therapy when other areas involved. Internal and external radiation when surgical removal is not possible.

first was found and treated. The recurrence is usually in some organ distant from the uterus, due to metastasis by a cancer cell that was not destroyed or removed in the original treatment.

What Can You Do?

Though there is nothing you can do to treat endometrial cancer yourself, if you are aware of the early warning signs and know your degree of risk, you can certainly help prevent, or at the least, detect the disease. Make a list of your family risk factors. Do you, for example, have a close rel-

ative who developed cancer of the reproductive organs or breast? This information can help a doctor evaluate your risk. Take a look at the other risk factors discussed above, and add any to your list that apply to you. If you have diabetes and/or high blood pressure or if you are seriously overweight, get these factors under control with medication and diet.

If you are using estrogen replacement therapy, be sure you know how much you are taking. Have regular checkups by a physician. If you are a premenopausal woman who has several cancer risk factors, your physician may prescribe oral contraceptives to reduce the danger.

Above all, do not believe any old wives' tales about endometrial cancer—that it is a benign disease or that its spread to lymph nodes is not important. This disease is *not* benign. It is true that the 5–year survival rate is 8 out of 10 for women treated before the cancer has had a chance to spread beyond the uterus. Nevertheless, 1 in 4 women who have endometrial cancer eventually die from it.

Diagnosis: Difficult but Crucial

Accurate diagnosis must (1) differentiate endometrial cancer from other possible illnesses; (2) locate the particular cancer type; and (3) judge how far the disease has progressed. When you consider that benign conditions—fibroid tumors, endometrial hyperplasia, and the start of normal menopause—all produce symptoms similar to early cancer, and also consider that several other cancers of the uterus progress more rapidly than endometrial cancer, it is obvious that diagnosis is not easy.

The Examination

To begin with, the doctor will take a woman's medical history and review her symptoms. Next is a complete physical exam of the pelvis—the uterus, ovaries, fallopian tubes, vagina, bladder, and rectum. This allows the physician to evaluate the source of the bleeding and the condition of nearby organs that could likely affect or be affected by the uterus. Later, if endometrial cancer is found, the information obtained will help determine whether it has progressed. The doctor will also order routine blood and urine tests. Occasionally, if a woman is too frail or too overweight for a routine examination, the doctor may use ultrasound to picture the inside of the uterus.

Taking a Biopsy

All other tests aside, the key to a definitive diagnosis is laboratory examination of a sample of endometrial tissue to check for abnormal cells. This procedure of removing and examining tissue is called *biopsy*. There are many ways of collecting the sample. Irrigation, suction, or brush techniques are all possibilities though they may not obtain enough tissue, and occasionally miss cancer cells or misidentify normal cells as cancerous. The *PAP smear,* used to detect cancer of the cervix, is accurate only half the time in identifying endometrial cancer, primarily because abnormal endometrial cells lose the features that clearly mark them by the time they reach the cervix, where the PAP smear is collected. Even the well–known *dilation and curettage* usually referred to as a D&C, in which the uterus is scraped or tissue snipped out while the woman is under anesthesia, can sometimes miss the diagnosis.

One newer alternative to a D&C is *diagnostic hysteroscopy*, in which a light–bearing telescope is inserted into the uterus so the physician can view the entire cavity and the surface of the endometrium. It is an outpatient procedure that requires a local anesthetic and lasts only a few minutes. Using this technique, the doctor is able to select specific tissue for removal and analysis.

Examining the Tissue

Once a biopsy is obtained, a pathologist examines the cellular make–up of the tissue to determine if it contains cancerous cells.

WHAT TO EXPECT FROM A "D&C"

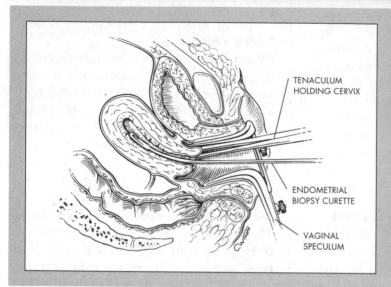

TENACULUM
HOLDING CERVIX

ENDOMETRIAL
BIOPSY CURETTE

VAGINAL
SPECULUM

The "D" portion of this procedure is *dilation*—opening up the cervix to permit access to the uterus. "C" stands for *curettage*, or scraping tissue samples from the surface of the endometrial lining of the uterus. To maintain a clear entry to the uterus, the doctor uses a speculum to brace open the walls of the vagina, and a tenaculum to hold back the lips of the cervix. A D&C helps in diagnosing endometrial cancer, but surgery is needed for a cure.

The pathologist decides what kind they are and what their stage of development is. The less–defined each cell and the more the cancer looks like a solid mass of cells instead of normal endometrial cells, the more severe the cancer is likely to be.

Other Tests

Prior to an operation, the biopsy is sometimes followed by more comprehensive testing. The doctor may decide to measure the size, location, and density of tumors with *computed axial tomography,* the so–called CAT scan. It can also show if the cancer has spread beyond the uterus into the pelvic lymph nodes. *Intravenous pyelography* (a type of x-ray) locates growths in the urinary tract. *Magnetic resonance imaging* or MRI supplies cross–sectional images of internal organs.

In addition, the tumor cells may be examined to determine their ability to accept progestin. If the cancer is due to overstimulation by estrogen, taking opposing progestin may

become part of the treatment. Overall, comprehensive diagnosis takes less time than it might seem since many tests are conducted at the same time. A basic yes or no can often be given after the first visit to the doctor. From these diagnostic procedures, he or she can tailor a treatment plan to suit the woman and her disease.

Treatment Choices

The stage of the cancer's development is the key consideration in selecting a treatment. The decision is affected by both the degree to which the cancer has penetrated the wall of the uterus and the extent to which it has spread beyond it.

If a younger woman with a 0 stage malignancy (see the box on "Stages of Endometrial Cancer") wants to keep her ability to have children, she may simply have a D&C combined with progestin treatment. However, a hysterectomy or removal of the uterus before cancer has spread beyond it is the treatment most likely to produce a cure. For a post-menopausal woman, it may be combined with removal of the ovaries and fallopian tubes. There may be more extensive surgery to remove various lymph nodes if the disease has spread or was not diagnosed until it reached an advanced stage. Radiation therapy is another possibility. It may be given both internally and externally. Sometimes it begins before surgery and is resumed afterwards. In other cases, it may not start until after the original surgery. Radiation is used more frequently for advanced stages of cancer.

Chemotherapy is primarily a palliative, a means of reducing the effects of endometrial cancer and prolonging survival. It does not cure the cancer, and is more likely to become part of the treatment in the more advanced stages.

Hysterectomy

A successful hysterectomy—which requires 2 to 3 hours under general anesthesia—removes all cancerous tissue without spreading cancer cells to other tissues and organs.

During the operation, the surgeon removes the uterus either through an incision in the lower abdomen or at the top of the vagina. Any suspicious tissue outside the uterus is also taken out and samples of tissue and fluid from the entire pelvic area are taken and analyzed for any cancerous cells. Both ovaries and fallopian tubes are also usually removed, so that the estrogen they produce can pose no further threat of stimulating new cancer.

Effects of Hysterectomy. The effects of a hysterectomy accompanied by removal of the ovaries include depression—even in women past menopause—as well as increased risk of coronary heart disease and osteoporosis. Getting out of bed and walking may be a little difficult the day after surgery, but it is important to try. Vaginal bleeding and discharge for a day or two is not unusual. While it will probably be possible to go home in 4 to 7 days, convalescence may last several weeks. Depending on the particular patient and the stage the cancer had reached, the physician may start her on estrogen replacement therapy within weeks or months with progestins prescribed to balance the estrogen.

HOW HYSTEROSCOPY WORKS

A relatively new device called the hysteroscope allows doctors to do a direct visual examination of the endometrium. The lighted tip of the instrument is inserted through the vagina and cervix into the uterine cavity. There the doctor can inspect any abnormal tissues and, using a tiny electrified loop, can even take samples for later lab analysis.

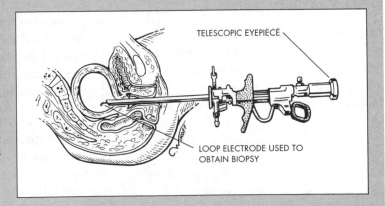

TELESCOPIC EYEPIECE

LOOP ELECTRODE USED TO OBTAIN BIOPSY

Follow-up visits to the doctor will be necessary every three to four months.

Radiation Therapy.

The need to avoid vital organs and systems while removing cancerous tissue limits the extent of any surgery. Radiation thus takes on a bigger role in treatment of more advanced cancer that has spread beyond the uterus. However, it may also be used in early stages to destroy cancerous cells that are difficult for the surgeon to see or reach, and has even been used alone in some early–stage patients. (Success rates, however, are not as good.) There are two ways of administering the radiation. When treatment is from the outside, an x–ray machine aims a radiation beam at the pelvis, reaching the uterus, cervix, and pelvic lymph nodes. The external treatment usually is given once a day for 4 to 5 weeks. In internal radiation, a number of tiny metal cylinders containing the radioactive elements radium or cesium are implanted in the uterus for a few days.

Radiation will also successfully treat cancer in the peritoneum (the covering of the pelvic organs) or in the ovaries or vagina. At higher stages of cancer development, the doctor may use both internal and external radiation. It is often combined with hormones and chemotherapy to reach the areas to which the cancer has spread.

Experimental Treatments

Immunotherapy is being investigated in a number of clinical trials although it is not yet an accepted form of treatment. Immunotherapy may fight cancer in a variety of ways:

- Strengthening the body's immune system to resist cancer
- Eliminating or suppressing body reactions that allow cancer to grow
- Sensitizing a cancer cell so it is more easily destroyed

Also under study are *biological response modifiers*, natural substances the body makes to fight cancer, that have now been manufactured in the laboratory. Currently, they are being tested only in endometrial cancer patients whose disease is severe or has recurred.

Chemotherapy

Many drugs used in breast cancer treatment are also used to fight endometrial cancer. They may slow progression of the disease, causing tumors to shrink, but rarely provide a cure. They are used to reach areas not accessible through surgery with more precision than radiation affords. If a woman's individual profile suggests she may respond to several of them, the doctor may prescribe a combination.

Doxorubicin (Adriamycin, Ribex) is an antibiotic that has been in use for some time to fight widespread cancer growth.

Cyclophosphamide (Cytoxan) and **cisplatin** (Platinol) are injected to break up cancer cell development. They act on new cancer growths in endometrial, ovarian, and bladder cancer, and are often given together. Several studies have shown that half the patients with widespread cancer will respond to a combination of these two drugs and doxorubicin.

Mesna (Mesnex) and **ifosfamide** (Ifex) are used in treatment of advanced endometrial cancer on a small scale. They are injected together because Mesnex prevents the urinary tract inflammation produced by Ifex.

Tamoxifen, which has been used for almost 20 years to treat advanced breast cancer, is now under study for prevention of breast cancer, as well as for use against some endometrial cancers. Unfortunately, in several trials women treated for advanced breast cancer at the usual tamoxifen dosage had double the risk of developing endometrial cancer. That risk is the same as a woman on estrogen. Although tamoxifen, taken by mouth, appears to work *against* estrogen's promotion of breast cancer cell growth, it acts *like* estrogen in other systems of the body.

Hormonal Treatments

Megesterol (Megace) is a progestin taken by mouth to treat severe, widespread endometrial cancer. It balances or reduces any estrogen buildup that promotes tumor growth. Progesterone–based medroxyprogesterone (Amen, Cycrin, Depo–Provera, others) and hydroxyprogesterone do the same. Depo–Provera is given by injection; the others can be taken orally. In the type of endometrial cancer related to estrogen overstimulation and endometrial hyperplasia, where the disease is at stages 0 or I (see the box on "Stages of Endometrial Cancer"), this progestin treatment has stopped or reversed tumor growth. It may even allow women past menopause to begin or continue estrogen therapy as long as they have regular checkups.

Disease and Treatment Damage

Since radiation and chemotherapy affect normal cells as well as cancer cells, side effects are often severe. Chemotherapy may suppress bone marrow, from which blood cells are formed, and thereby cause anemia. Nausea and vomiting, resulting in loss of fluids, can cause kidney problems. Another effect is inflammation of the inside of the mouth. In a few patients, urinary and rectal inflammation and fistulas (abnormal passages between organs) may show up months and even years after radiation. If the disease reaches a late stage, with cancerous growths in many areas of the body, the side effects of treatment added to the effects of the disease, can become nearly intolerable. However, doctors now have a number of strategies that help make therapy much more comfortable:

- Combining treatments
- Adding drugs that combat side effects
- Using lowest effective dosages
- Limiting radiation or drug therapy for certain patients

Any woman suffering from endometrial cancer and the effects of treatment needs a great deal of emotional and medical support. For sources of emotional and social assistance, see the "Directory of Support Groups" at the end of this book. For relief of physical pain and discomfort, the doctor can draw on a wide variety of medications and therapeutic techniques.

Pain Relief

Pain relievers—both narcotic and non-narcotic—are standard treatment for advanced endometrial cancer. Most frequently used are narcotic medications such as codeine, meperidine (Demerol), oxycodone (Percodan), and, particularly, morphine. If oral forms of these drugs cause nausea or vomiting, the doctor will prescribe injectable and suppository forms instead. For pain caused by pressure on nerves, transcutaneous (through the skin) electric nerve stimulation, called "TENS," often gives relief.

The woman under treatment and her medical team must be continually alert to the adverse effects, of the more powerful painkillers. Other medications that help are antidepressants, tranquilizers, anti–inflammatory drugs, sedatives, and antinausea medications. The choice of medicines depends on the individual patient's problems.

Prospect for Recovery?

As long as cancer has failed to spread beyond the uterus, the outlook is encouraging. And since this depends on early recognition, prompt diagnosis is crucial. If you have abnormal vaginal bleeding, your doctor must take great care to establish the cause. The biopsy stage of the process is especially important, since it's the step that determines whether there is a cancer, a benign tumor, or a forerunner of cancer.

Once you've been treated, the most important step you can take is getting regular follow–up care. The danger that some of the cancer was missed is, unfortunately, always a reality. As with any disease, thorough check-ups are your best insurance for complete, long–lasting recovery. □

PART TWO

A Woman's Handbook of Medicines

Brand name:

ACCUTANE

Pronounced: ACC-u-tane
Generic name: Isotretinoin

Why is this drug prescribed?

Accutane, a chemical cousin of vitamin A, is prescribed for the treatment of severe, disfiguring cystic acne that has not cleared up in response to milder medications such as antibiotics. It works on the oil glands within the skin, shrinking them and diminishing their output. You take Accutane by mouth every day for several months, then stop. The antiacne effect can last even after you have finished your course of medication.

Most important fact about this drug

Because Accutane can cause severe birth defects, including mental retardation and physical malformations, a woman *must not* become pregnant while taking it. If you are a woman of childbearing age, your doctor will ask you to sign a detailed consent form before you start taking Accutane. If you accidentally become pregnant while taking the medication, you should immediately consult your doctor.

How should you take this medication?

Take Accutane with food. Follow your doctor's instructions carefully.

Depending on your reaction to Accutane, your doctor may need to adjust the dosage upward or downward. If you respond quickly and very well, your doctor may take you off Accutane even before the 15 or 20 weeks are up.

After you finish taking Accutane, there should be at least a 2-month "rest period" during which you are off the drug. This is because your acne may continue to get better even though you are no longer taking the medication. Once the 2 months are up, if your acne is still severe, your doctor may want to give you a second course of Accutane.

Avoid consumption of alcoholic beverages.

Read the patient information leaflet available with the product.

Do not crush the capsules.

■ *If you miss a dose...*
Take the forgotten dose as soon as you remember. If it is almost time for your next dose, skip the one you missed and go back to your regular schedule. Do not take 2 doses at the same time.

■ *Storage instructions...*
Store at room temperature, away from light.

What side effects may occur?

Side effects cannot be anticipated. If any develop or change in intensity, inform your doctor as soon as possible. Only your doctor can determine if it is safe for you to continue taking Accutane.

■ *More common side effects may include:*
Conjunctivitis ("pinkeye")
Dry or fragile skin
Dry, cracked, inflamed lips
Dry mouth
Dry nose
Itching
Joint pains
Nosebleed

■ *Less common side effects may include:*
Bowel inflammation and pain, chest pain, decreased night vision, decreased tolerance to contact lenses, depression, fatigue, headache, nausea, peeling palms or soles, rash, skin infections, stomach and

intestinal discomfort, sunburn-sensitive skin, thinning hair, urinary discomfort, vision problems, vomiting

Why should this drug not be prescribed?

You should not take Accutane if you are sensitive to or have ever had an allergic reaction to parabens, the preservative used in the capsules.

If you are a woman of childbearing age, you should not take Accutane if you are pregnant, if you think there is a possibility you might get pregnant during the treatment, or if you are unable to keep coming back to the doctor for monthly checkups, including pregnancy testing.

Special warnings about this medication

When you first start taking Accutane, it is possible that your acne will get worse before it starts to get better.

If you are a woman of childbearing age and you are considering taking Accutane, you will be given both spoken and written warnings about the importance of avoiding pregnancy during the treatment. You will be asked to sign a consent form noting that:

- Accutane is a powerful, "last resort" medication for severe acne;
- You must not take Accutane if you are pregnant or may become pregnant during treatment;
- If you get pregnant while taking Accutane, your baby will be at high risk for birth defects;
- If you take Accutane, you must use effective birth control from 1 month before the start of treatment through 1 month after the end of treatment;
- You must test negative for pregnancy within 2 weeks before starting Accutane, and you must start Accutane on the

second or third day of your menstrual period;
- You may participate in a program that includes an initial free pregnancy test and birth control counseling session;
- If you become pregnant, you must immediately stop taking Accutane and see your doctor;
- You have read and understood the Accutane patient brochure and asked your doctor any questions you had;
- You are not currently pregnant and do not plan to become pregnant for at least 30 days after you finish taking Accutane;
- You have been invited to participate in a survey of women being treated with Accutane.

Some people taking Accutane, including some who simultaneously took tetracycline, have experienced headache, nausea, and visual disturbances caused by increased pressure within the skull. See a doctor immediately if you have these symptoms; if the doctor finds swelling of the optic nerve at the back of your eye, you must stop taking Accutane at once and see a neurologist for further care.

Be careful driving at night. Some people have experienced a sudden decrease in night vision.

Some people taking Accutane have had problems regulating their blood sugar level.

You may not be able to tolerate your contact lenses during and after your therapy with Accutane.

You should stop taking Accutane immediately if you have abdominal pain, bleeding from the rectum, or severe diarrhea. You may have an inflammatory disease of the bowel.

You should not donate blood during your therapy with Accutane and for at least a month after you stop taking it.

Possible food and drug interactions when taking this medication

While taking Accutane, do not take vitamin supplements containing vitamin A. Accutane and vitamin A are chemically related; taking them together is like taking an overdose of vitamin A.

Special information if you are pregnant or breastfeeding

Accutane causes birth defects; do not use it while pregnant. Nursing mothers should not take Accutane because of the possibility of passing the drug on to the baby via breast milk.

Recommended dosage

The recommended dosage range for Accutane is 0.5 to 2 milligrams per 2.2 pounds of body weight, divided into 2 doses daily, for 15 to 20 weeks. The usual starting dose is 0.5 to 1 milligram per 2.2 pounds per day.

People whose disease is very severe or is primarily on the body may have to take up to the maximum recommended dose.

If after a period of 2 months or more off therapy, severe cystic acne persists, your doctor may prescribe a second course of therapy.

Overdosage

Any medication taken in excess can have serious consequences. If you suspect an overdose of Accutane, seek medical attention immediately.

- *Overdosage of Accutane, like overdosage of vitamin A, can cause:*
  Abdominal pain
  Dizziness

Dry, cracked, inflamed lips
Facial flushing
Incoordination and clumsiness
Headache
Vomiting

Generic name:

ACETAMINOPHEN

See Tylenol, page 777.

Generic name:

ACETAMINOPHEN WITH CODEINE

See Tylenol with Codeine, page 779.

Generic name:

ACETIC ACID

See Aci-Jel, page 502.

Brand name:

ACHROMYCIN V CAPSULES

Pronounced: A-kro-MY-cin Vee
Generic name: Tetracycline hydrochloride
Other brand name: Sumycin

Why is this drug prescribed?

Achromycin V, a "broad-spectrum" antibiotic, is used to treat bacterial infections such as Rocky Mountain spotted fever, typhus fever, and tick fevers; upper respiratory infections; pneumonia; gonorrhea; amoebic infections; and urinary tract infections. It is also used to help treat severe acne and to treat trachoma (a chronic eye infection) and conjunctivitis ("pinkeye"). Tetracycline is often an alternative drug for people who are allergic to penicillin.

Most important fact about this drug
Tetracycline should not be used during the last half of pregnancy or in children under the age of 8. It may damage developing teeth and cause permanent discoloration.

How should you take this medication?
Achromycin V should be taken exactly as prescribed by your doctor. Be sure to use the entire prescription. If you are taking a liquid form of the drug, shake well before using.

Do not use outdated Achromycin V. Outdated tetracycline is highly toxic to the kidneys.

Do not take antacids containing aluminum, calcium, or magnesium (e.g., Mylanta, Maalox) while taking this medication. They will affect the absorption of the drug.

Take Achromycin V 1 hour before or 2 hours after meals. Foods, milk, and some other dairy products affect absorption of the drug.

Achromycin V should be continued for at least 24 to 48 hours after your symptoms have subsided.

■ *If you miss a dose...*
Take it as soon as you remember. If it is almost time for your next dose and you take Achromycin V once a day (e.g., for acne), take the dose you missed, and then take the next one 10 to 12 hours later; if you take it twice a day, take the dose you missed, and then take the next one 5 to 6 hours later; if you take 3 or more doses a day, take the one you missed, and then take the next one 2 to 4 hours later. Then go back to your regular schedule.

■ *Storage instructions...*
Store capsules at room temperature. Keep the liquid form of tetracycline in the refrigerator, but do not allow it to freeze.

What side effects may occur?
Side effects cannot be anticipated. If any occur or change in intensity, inform your doctor as soon as possible. Only your doctor can determine if it is safe for you to continue taking Achromycin V.

■ *More common side effects may include:*
Anemia, blood disorders, blurred vision and headache (in adults), bulging soft spot on the head (in infants), diarrhea, difficult or painful swallowing, dizziness, extreme allergic reactions, genital or anal sores or rash, hives, inflammation of large bowel, inflammation of the tongue, inflammation of the upper digestive tract, increased sensitivity to light, loss of appetite, nausea, rash, ringing in the ears, swelling due to fluid accumulation, vision disturbance, vomiting

■ *Less common or rare side effects may include:*
Inflamed skin, liver poisoning, muscle weakness, peeling, throat sores and inflammation

Why should this drug not be prescribed?
Do not take this medication if you are sensitive to or have ever had an allergic reaction to Achromycin V or any other tetracycline medication.

Special warnings about this medication
If you have kidney disease, make sure the doctor knows about it. A lower than usual dose of Achromycin V may be needed.

Tetracycline drugs can make you more prone to sunburn when you are in sunlight or ultraviolet light. Take appropriate precautions.

Some adults may develop a headache and blurred vision while taking tetracycline, and infants may develop a bulging soft spot on the head. Contact your doctor if you experience or notice these symptoms. They usually disappear soon after the medication is stopped.

As with other antibiotics, use of this medication may cause other infections to develop. Contact your doctor if this occurs.

If you are taking Achromycin V over an extended period of time, your doctor will perform blood, kidney, and liver tests periodically.

Possible food and drug interactions when taking this medication

If Achromycin V is taken with certain other drugs, the effects of either could be increased, decreased, or altered. It is especially important to check with your doctor before combining Achromycin V with the following:

Antacids containing aluminum, calcium, or magnesium, such as Mylanta and Maalox
Blood thinners such as Coumadin
Oral contraceptives
Penicillin (Amoxil, Pen Vee-K, others)

Special information if you are pregnant or breastfeeding

Achromycin V is not recommended for use during pregnancy. It can affect the development of the unborn child's bones and teeth. If you are pregnant or plan to become pregnant, inform your doctor immediately. Achromycin V appears in breast milk and may affect a nursing infant. If this medication is essential to your health, your doctor may recommend that you stop breastfeeding until your treatment is finished.

Recommended dosage

Your doctor will adjust your dose on the basis of the condition to be treated, your age, and risk factors such as kidney problems.

You should use this drug for at least 24 to 48 hours after symptoms and fever have subsided. For a streptococcal infection, doses should be taken for at least 10 days.

ADULTS

For most infections, the usual daily dose is 1 to 2 grams divided into 2 or 4 equal doses, depending on severity.

For treatment of brucellosis
The usual dose is 500 milligrams 4 times daily for 3 weeks; the drug should be accompanied by streptomycin.

For treatment of syphilis
You should take a total of 30 to 40 grams, divided into equal doses over a period of 10 to 15 days.

Gonorrhea patients sensitive to penicillin can take tetracycline, starting with 1.5 grams, followed by 0.5 gram every 6 hours for 4 days, to a total dosage of 9 grams.

For urethral, endocervical, or rectal infections in adults caused by Chlamydia trachomatis
The usual dose is 500 milligrams, 4 times a day, for at least 7 days.

CHILDREN 8 YEARS OF AGE AND ABOVE

The usual daily dose is 10 to 20 milligrams per pound of body weight divided into 2 or 4 equal doses.

Overdosage

Any medication taken in excess can have serious consequences. Seek medical attention immediately if you suspect an overdose of Achromycin V.

Brand name:

ACI-JEL

Pronounced: ASS-ee-jel
Generic ingredient: Acetic acid

Why is this drug prescribed?

In some cases of vaginitis, the level of acidity in the vagina becomes too low. Applying Aci-Jel internally restores the acidity and keeps it within the normal range.

Most important fact about this drug

Your doctor will test your vaginal acidity periodically to determine how long you will have to continue treatment.

How should you take this medication?

Aci-Jel comes with an applicator. Fill the applicator with the vaginal jelly, insert it into your vagina, and push the plunger to release the medication.

■ If you miss a dose...
Return to your regular schedule with the next dose.

■ Storage instructions...
Store Aci-Jel at room temperature.

What side effects may occur?

Although side effects are rare, a few women have experienced local stinging and burning when using Aci-Jel.

Why should this drug not be prescribed?

There are no reported reasons for avoiding this medication.

Special warnings about this medication

No safety hazards have been reported by women using Aci-Jel.

Possible food and drug interactions when taking this medication

There are no known food or drug interactions with Aci-Jel.

Special information if you are pregnant or breastfeeding

The effects of Aci-Jel during pregnancy have not been adequately studied. If you are pregnant or plan to become pregnant, inform your doctor immediately. It is not known whether this medication appears in breast milk and whether it could affect a nursing infant. If this drug is essential to your health, your doctor may advise you to discontinue breastfeeding until your treatment with Aci-Jel is finished.

Recommended dosage

The usual dose is 1 applicatorful in the vagina, morning and evening. Your doctor will decide how long you should continue using the medication, according to your response.

Overdosage

There are no reports of overdosage with this medication.

Generic name:

ACYCLOVIR

See Zovirax, page 804.

Brand name:

ADAPIN

See Sinequan, page 744.

Generic name:

ALPRAZOLAM

See Xanax, page 795.

Generic name:

AMITRIPTYLINE

See Elavil, page 580.

Generic name:

AMITRIPTYLINE WITH PERPHENAZINE

See Triavil, page 772.

Generic name:

AMOXAPINE

See Asendin, page 513.

Generic name:

AMOXICILLIN

See Amoxil, page 503.

Generic name:

AMOXICILLIN WITH CLAVULANATE

See Augmentin, page 519.

Brand name:

AMOXIL

Pronounced: a-MOX-il
Generic name: Amoxicillin
Other brand names: Trimox, Wymox

Why is this drug prescribed?

Amoxil, an antibiotic, is used to treat a wide variety of infections, including: gonorrhea, middle ear infections, skin infections, upper and lower respiratory tract infections, and infections of genital and urinary tract.

Most important fact about this drug

If you are allergic to either penicillin or cephalosporin antibiotics in any form, consult your doctor before taking Amoxil. There is a possibility that you are allergic to both types of medication; and if a reaction occurs, it could be extremely severe. If you take the drug and feel signs of a reaction, seek medical attention immediately.

How should you take this medication?

Amoxil can be taken with or without food. If you are using Amoxil suspension, shake it well before using.

■ *If you miss a dose...*
Take it as soon as you remember. If it is almost time for the next dose, and you take 2 doses a day, take the one you missed and the next dose 5 to 6 hours later. If you take 3 or more doses a day, take the one you missed and the next dose 2 to 4 hours later. Then go back to your regular schedule.

■ *Storage Instructions...*
Amoxil suspension and Pediatric drops should be stored in a tightly closed bottle. Discard any unused medication after 14 days. Refrigeration is preferable.

What side effects may occur?

Side effects cannot be anticipated. If any develop or change in intensity, inform your doctor as soon as possible. Only your doctor can determine if it is safe for you to continue taking Amoxil.

■ *Side effects may include:*
Agitation, anemia, anxiety, changes in behavior, confusion, diarrhea, dizziness, hives, hyperactivity, insomnia, nausea, rash, vomiting

Why should this drug not be prescribed?

You should not use Amoxil if you are allergic to penicillin or cephalosporin antibiotics (for example, Ceclor).

Special warnings about this medication

If you have ever had asthma, hives, hay fever, or other allergies, consult with your doctor before taking Amoxil.

You should stop using Amoxil if you experience reactions such as bruising, fever, skin rash, itching, joint pain, swollen lymph nodes, and/or sores on the genitals. If these reactions occur, stop taking Amoxil unless your doctor advises you to continue.

For infections such as strep throat, it is important to take Amoxil for the entire amount of time your doctor has prescribed. Even if you feel better, you need to continue taking Amoxil. If you stop taking Amoxil before your treatment time is complete, you may get other infections, such as glomerulonephritis (a kidney infection) or rheumatic fever.

If you are diabetic, be aware that Amoxil may cause a *false positive* Clinitest (urine glucose test) result to occur. You should consult with your doctor about using different tests while taking Amoxil.

Before taking Amoxil, tell your doctor if you have ever had asthma, colitis (inflammatory bowel disease), diabetes, or kidney or liver disease.

Possible food and drug interactions when taking this medication

If Amoxil is taken with certain other drugs, the effects of either could be increased, decreased, or altered. It is especially important to check with your doctor before combining Amoxil with the following:

Chloramphenicol (Chloromycetin)
Erythromycin (E.E.S., PCE, others)
Oral contraceptives
Probenecid (Benemid)
Tetracycline (Achromycin V, others)

Special information if you are pregnant or breastfeeding

Amoxil should be used during pregnancy only when clearly needed. If you are pregnant or plan to become pregnant, inform your doctor immediately. Since Amoxil may appear in breast milk, you should consult your doctor if you plan to breastfeed your baby.

Recommended dosage

Dosages will be determined by the type of infection being treated.

ADULTS

Ear, Nose, Throat, Skin, Genital, and Urinary Tract Infections
The usual dosage is 250 milligrams, taken every 8 hours.

Infections of the Lower Respiratory Tract
The usual dosage is 500 milligrams, taken every 8 hours.

Gonorrhea
The usual dosage is 3 grams in a single oral dose.

Gonococcal Infections Such as Acute, Uncomplicated Anogenital and Urethral Infections
3 grams as a single oral dose.

CHILDREN

Children weighing 44 pounds and over should follow the recommended adult dose schedule.

Children weighing under 44 pounds will have their dosage determined by their weight.

Dosage of Pediatric Drops:
Use the dropper provided with the medication to measure all doses.

All Infections Except Those of the Lower Respiratory Tract
   Under 13 pounds:
      0.75 milliliter every 8 hours.
   13 to 15 pounds:
      1 milliliter every 8 hours.
   16 to 18 pounds:
      1.25 milliliters every 8 hours.

Infections of the Lower Respiratory Tract
   Under 13 pounds:
      1.25 milliliters every 8 hours.
   13 to 15 pounds:
      1.75 milliliters every 8 hours.
   16 to 18 pounds:
      2.25 milliliters every 8 hours.

Children weighing more than 18 pounds should take the oral liquid. The required amount of suspension should be placed directly on the child's tongue for swallowing. It can also be added to formula, milk, fruit juice, water, ginger ale, or cold drinks. The preparation should be taken immediately. To be certain the child is getting the full dose of medication, make sure he or she drinks the entire preparation.

ELDERLY
The elderly should use Amoxil cautiously.

Overdosage
Any medication taken in excess can have serious consequences. If you suspect an overdose, seek medical attention immediately.

■ *Symptoms of Amoxil overdose may include:*
Diarrhea
Nausea
Stomach cramps
Vomiting

Generic name:

AMPICILLIN

See Omnipen, page 699.

Brand name:

ANAPROX

Pronounced: AN-uh-procks
Generic name: Naproxen sodium

Why is this drug prescribed?
Anaprox, a nonsteroidal anti-inflammatory drug, is used to relieve mild to moderate pain and menstrual cramps. It is also prescribed for relief of the inflammation, swelling, stiffness, and joint pain associated with rheumatoid arthritis, osteoarthritis (the most common form of arthritis), and for juvenile arthritis, ankylosing spondylitis (spinal arthritis), tendinitis, bursitis, acute gout, and other conditions.

Most important fact about this drug
You should have frequent checkups with your doctor if you take Anaprox regularly. Ulcers or internal bleeding can occur without warning.

How should you take this medication?
Your doctor may ask you to take Anaprox with food or an antacid to avoid stomach upset.

Take this medication exactly as prescribed by your doctor.

If you are using Anaprox for arthritis, it should be taken regularly.

■ *If you miss a dose...*
Take the forgotten dose as soon as you remember. If it is almost time for your next dose, skip the one you missed and go back to your regular schedule. Never take 2 doses at the same time.

■ *Storage instructions...*
Store at room temperature in a tightly closed container.

What side effects may occur?

Side effects cannot be anticipated. If any develop or change in intensity, inform your doctor as soon as possible. Only your doctor can determine if it is safe for you to continue taking Anaprox.

■ *More common side effects may include:*
Abdominal pain, bruising, constipation, diarrhea, difficult or labored breathing, dizziness, drowsiness, headache, hearing changes, heartburn, indigestion, inflammation of the mouth, itching, light-headedness, nausea, rapid, fluttery heartbeat, red or purple spots on the skin, ringing in the ears, skin eruptions, sweating, swelling due to fluid retention, thirst, vertigo, vision changes

■ *Less common or rare side effects may include:*
Abdominal bleeding, black stools, blood in the urine, change in dream patterns, changes in hearing, chills and fever, colitis (inflammation of the large intestine), congestive heart failure, depression, general feeling of illness, hair loss, inability to concentrate, inability to sleep, inflammation of the lungs, kidney disease or failure, menstrual problems, muscle weakness and/or pain, peptic ulcer, severe allergic reactions, skin inflammation due to sensitivity to light, skin rashes, vomiting, vomiting blood, yellow skin and eyes

Why should this drug not be prescribed?

If you are sensitive to or have ever had an allergic reaction to Anaprox, aspirin, or similar drugs such as Motrin, or if you have had asthma attacks caused by aspirin or other drugs of this type, you should not take this medication. Make sure your doctor is aware of any drug reactions you have experienced.

Special warnings about this medication

Remember that peptic ulcers and bleeding can occur without warning.

This drug should be used with caution if you have kidney or liver disease. It can cause liver inflammation in some people.

Do not take aspirin or any other anti-inflammatory medications while taking Anaprox, unless your doctor tells you to do so.

Anaprox contains sodium. If you are on a low sodium diet, discuss this with your doctor.

Use with caution if you have heart disease or high blood pressure. This drug can increase water retention.

Anaprox may cause vision problems. If you experience any changes in your vision, inform your doctor.

Anaprox may cause you to become drowsy or less alert; therefore, driving or operating dangerous machinery or participating in any hazardous activity that requires full mental alertness is not recommended.

Possible food and drug interactions when taking this medication

If Anaprox is taken with certain other drugs, the effects of either could be increased, decreased, or altered. It is especially important to check with your doctor before combining Anaprox with the following:

Antiseizure drugs such as Dilantin
Aspirin
Beta blockers, including blood pressure
    drugs such as Inderal
Blood thinners such as Coumadin
Lithium (Lithorate)
Loop diuretics such as Lasix
Methotrexate
Naproxen in other forms such as Naprosyn
Oral diabetes drugs such as Micronase
Probenecid (Benemid)

Special information
if you are pregnant or breastfeeding

The effects of Anaprox during pregnancy have not been adequately studied. If you are pregnant or plan to become pregnant, inform your doctor immediately. Anaprox appears in breast milk and could affect a nursing infant. If this medication is essential to your health, your doctor may advise you to discontinue breastfeeding until your treatment with this medication is finished.

Recommended dosage

ADULTS

Mild to Moderate Pain, Menstrual Cramps, Acute Tendinitis and Bursitis
The starting dose is 550 milligrams, followed by 275 milligrams every 6 to 8 hours. You should not take more than 1,375 milligrams a day.

Rheumatoid Arthritis, Osteoarthritis, and Ankylosing Spondylitis
The starting dose is 275 milligrams or 550 milligrams 2 times a day (morning and evening). Your physician can adjust the doses for maximum benefit. Symptoms should improve within 2 to 4 weeks.

Acute Gout
The starting dose is 825 milligrams, followed by 275 milligrams every 8 hours, until symptoms subside.

CHILDREN

Juvenile Arthritis
The usual daily dosage is a total of 10 milligrams per 2.2 pounds of body weight, divided into 2 doses. Dosage should not exceed 15 milligrams per 2.2 pounds per day.

The safety and effectiveness of Anaprox have not been established in children under 2 years of age.

ELDERLY

Your doctor will determine the dosage based on your particular needs. Adjustments in the normal adult dosage may be needed.

Overdosage

Any medication taken in excess can cause symptoms of overdose. If you suspect an overdose of Anaprox, seek medical attention immediately.

■ *The symptoms of Anaprox overdose may include:*
Drowsiness
Heartburn
Indigestion
Nausea
Vomiting

Brand name:

ANDROID

Pronounced: AN-droyd
Generic name: Methyltestosterone
Other brand names: Testred, Oreton Methyl

Why is this drug prescribed?

Android, a synthetic male sex hormone, is given to help develop and/or maintain male sex characteristics in boys and men who, for some reason, are not producing enough of the hormone on their own. A relatively short course of Android is sometimes used to try to trigger pubertal changes in boys whose puberty seems delayed. Android may also be given to women who have certain advanced, inoperable forms of breast cancer.

Most important fact about this drug

Because of potentially serious adverse health effects, Android is *not* recommended as a treatment for athletes who want to enhance their physique and/or improve their performance.

How should you take this medication?

Do not change from one brand to another without consulting your physician. The tablets may be either swallowed or dissolved in the cheek. Take them exactly as prescribed.

If you are taking methyltestosterone buccal tablets (those dissolved between the gum and the cheek) be careful not to swallow them. Avoid eating, drinking, or smoking while the tablet is in place.

■ *If you miss a dose...*
If you take 1 dose a day, take the forgotten dose as soon as you remember. If you do not remember it until the next day, skip the one you missed and go back to your regular schedule. Do not take 2 doses at the same time.

If you take 2 or more doses a day, take the missed dose as soon as you remember. If it is almost time for your next dose, skip the one you missed and go back to your regular schedule. Do not take 2 doses at the same time.

■ *Storage instructions...*
Store away from heat, light, and moisture.

What side effects may occur?

Side effects cannot be anticipated. If any develop or change in intensity, inform your doctor as soon as possible. Only your doctor can determine if it is safe for you to continue taking Android.

In men, possible adverse effects include breast development, annoyingly frequent and persistent erections, and (at high dosage) decreased sperm count.

In women, possible adverse effects include irregular or no menstrual periods, deepened voice, and enlarged clitoris.

Elderly males risk enlarged prostate or prostate cancer.

■ *Other possible side effects include:*
Acne, allergic reactions, anxiety, bloating, depression, excess body hair, headache, itching, burning, or tingling skin, jaundice, male-pattern baldness, nausea, sex-drive changes (increase or decrease)

Why should this drug not be prescribed?

Do not take Android if you are sensitive to or have ever had an allergic reaction to a synthetic male hormone.

Men with breast or prostate cancer should not take Android.

Women should not take Android during pregnancy, since the drug may masculinize the genitals of a female fetus.

Special warnings about this medication

Extreme caution is needed when giving Android to a child. If taken for too long by a boy who has not yet reached puberty, the drug may prematurely halt bone development so that the youngster never reaches full height. For safety's sake, any young boy being treated with Android should have X-rays of the wrist and hand every 6 months so the doctor can monitor his bone growth.

Women taking Android should be alert for signs of virilization: acne, deepened voice, enlarged clitoris, increased hairiness, and irregular menstrual periods. If the drug is not discontinued promptly while such changes are still mild, the masculinizing effects may be permanent.

An adult man taking Android should report too frequent or persistent erections to his doctor immediately.

An adult woman should report any hoarseness, acne, or changes in the menstrual cycle.

People who already have heart, kidney, or liver disease may risk fluid accumulation and congestive heart failure.

Possible food and drug interactions when taking this medication

If Android is taken with certain other drugs, the effects of either could be increased, decreased, or altered. It is especially important to check with your doctor before combining Android with the following:

Blood thinners such as Coumadin
Insulin
Oxyphenbutazone (antiarthritis and antigout medication)

With any of these, you may need a reduced dosage while taking Android.

Special information if you are pregnant or breastfeeding

If you become pregnant while taking Android, notify your doctor immediately. If the unborn baby is a girl, the drug may cause her to develop certain sexual abnormalities: enlargement of the clitoris, formation of a pseudo-scrotum, and malformation of the vagina. These fetal abnormalities are especially likely if Android is taken during the first 3 months of pregnancy. It is not known whether Android is excreted in breast milk. If this medication is essential to your health, your doctor may advise you to stop breastfeeding until your treatment with Android is finished.

Recommended dosage

The dosage prescribed by your doctor is determined by your age, sex, diagnosis, response to the drug, and other factors. The following are only general guidelines.

Androgen Replacement Therapy in Males
The suggested daily dosage is 10 to 50 milligrams in oral form. For delayed puberty, dosage is generally at the lower end of this range, and is prescribed for a limited time, usually 4 to 6 months

Androgen Therapy in Female Breast Cancer
The usual daily dose is 50 to 200 milligrams in oral form.

Overdosage

Although no specific overdosage information is available for Android, any medication taken in excess can have serious consequences. If you suspect an overdose, seek medical attention immediately. Watch for nausea and bloating or swelling.

Brand name:

ANSAID

Pronounced: AN-sed
Generic name: Flurbiprofen

Why is this drug prescribed?

Ansaid, a nonsteroidal anti-inflammatory drug, is used to relieve the inflammation, swelling, stiffness, and joint pain associated with rheumatoid arthritis and osteoarthritis (the most common form of arthritis).

Most important fact about this drug

You should have frequent checkups with your doctor if you take Ansaid regularly. Ulcers or internal bleeding can occur without warning.

How should you take this medication?

Your doctor may ask you to take Ansaid with food or an antacid.

Take this medication exactly as prescribed by your doctor.

If you are using Ansaid for arthritis, it should be taken regularly.

■ If you miss a dose...
Take the forgotten dose as soon as you remember. If it is almost time for your next dose, skip the one you missed and go back to your regular schedule. Never take 2 doses at the same time.

■ Storage instructions...
Store at room temperature.

What side effects may occur?

Side effects cannot be anticipated. If any develop or change in intensity, inform your doctor as soon as possible. Only your doctor can determine if it is safe for you to continue taking Ansaid.

■ More common side effects may include:
Abdominal bleeding, abdominal pain, anxiety, constipation, depression, diarrhea, dizziness, gas, general feeling of illness, headache, inflammation of the nose, indigestion, loss of memory, nausea, nervousness, rash, ringing in ears, sleepiness, swelling due to fluid retention, tremors, trouble sleeping, urinary tract infection, vision changes, vomiting, weakness, weight changes

■ Less common or rare side effects may include:
Altered sense of smell, anemia, asthma, blood in the urine, bloody diarrhea, bruising, chills and fever, confusion, conjunctivitis (pinkeye), heart failure, hepatitis, high blood pressure, hives, inflammation of the mouth and tongue, inflammation of the stomach, itching, kidney failure, lack of coordination, nosebleed, peptic ulcer, pins and needles, sensitivity of skin to light, severe allergic reaction, skin inflammation with or without sores and crusting, swelling of throat, twitching, vomiting blood, welts, yellow eyes and skin

Why should this drug not be prescribed?

If you are sensitive to or have ever had an allergic reaction to Ansaid, aspirin, or similar drugs such as Motrin, or if you have had asthma attacks caused by aspirin or other drugs of this type, you should not take this medication. Make sure your doctor is aware of any drug reactions you have experienced.

Special warnings about this medication

This drug should be used with caution if you have kidney or liver disease. Kidney problems are most likely to develop in such people, as well as in those with heart failure, those taking diuretics (water pills), and the elderly.

Do not take aspirin or similar drugs while taking Ansaid, unless your doctor tells you to do so.

Ansaid can cause vision problems. If you experience a change in your vision, inform your doctor. Blurred and/or decreased vision has occurred while taking this medication.

Ansaid prolongs bleeding time. If you are taking blood-thinning medication, this drug should be taken with caution.

This drug can increase water retention. If you have heart disease or high blood pressure, use with caution.

If you want to take Ansaid for pain less serious than that of arthritis, be sure to discuss the risks of using this drug with your doctor.

Possible food and drug interactions when taking this medication

If Ansaid is taken with certain other drugs, the effects of either could be increased, decreased, or altered. It is especially important to check with your doctor before combining Ansaid with the following:

Aspirin
Beta blockers such as Inderal and Tenormin
Blood thinners such as Coumadin
Cimetidine (Tagamet)
Diuretics such as Lasix and Bumex
Methotrexate
Oral diabetes drugs such as Micronase

Special information
if you are pregnant or breastfeeding

The effects of Ansaid during pregnancy have not been adequately studied. If you are pregnant or plan to become pregnant, inform your doctor immediately. Ansaid appears in breast milk and could affect a nursing infant. If this medication is essential to your health, your doctor may advise you to discontinue breastfeeding until your treatment is finished.

Recommended dosage

ADULTS

Rheumatoid Arthritis or Osteoarthritis:
The usual starting dosage is a total of 200 to 300 milligrams a day, divided into 2, 3, or 4 smaller doses (usually 3 or 4 for rheumatoid arthritis). Your doctor will tailor the dose to suit your needs, but you should not take more than 100 milligrams at any one time or more than 300 milligrams in a day.

CHILDREN

The safety and effectiveness of Ansaid have not been established in children.

ELDERLY

The elderly are among those most apt to develop kidney problems while taking this drug.

Your doctor will determine the dosage according to your needs.

Overdosage

Any medication taken in excess can cause symptoms of overdose. If you suspect an overdose of Ansaid, seek medical attention immediately.

■ *The symptoms of Ansaid overdose may include:*
Agitation, change in pupil size, coma, disorientation, dizziness, double vision, drowsiness, headache, nausea, semiconsciousness, shallow breathing, stomach pain

Brand name:

ANUSOL-HC

Pronounced: AN-yoo-sol AICH-SEE
Generic name: Hydrocortisone
Other brand name: Hytone

Why is this drug prescribed?

Anusol is a steroid cream for use on the skin. It is prescribed to treat certain itchy rashes and other inflammatory skin conditions.

Most important fact about this drug

When you use Anusol-HC, you inevitably absorb some of the medication through your skin and into the bloodstream. Too much absorption can lead to unwanted side effects elsewhere in the body. To keep this problem to a minimum, avoid using large amounts of Anusol-HC over extensive areas, and do not cover it with airtight dressings such as plastic wrap or adhesive bandages unless specifically told to by your doctor.

How should you use this medication?

Use Anusol-HC exactly as directed, and only to treat the condition for which your doctor prescribed it.

Anusol-HC is for use only on the skin. Be careful to keep it out of your eyes.

Apply the medication directly to the affected area.

If you are using Anusol-HC for psoriasis or a condition that has been difficult to cure, your doctor may advise you to use a bandage or covering over the affected area. If an infection develops, remove the bandage and contact your doctor.

■ *If you miss a dose...*
Apply it as soon as you remember. If it is almost time for the next dose, skip the one you missed and go back to your regular schedule.

■ *Storage instructions...*
Keep the container tightly closed, and store it at room temperature, away from heat. Protect from freezing.

What side effects may occur?

Side effects cannot be anticipated. If any develop or change in intensity, inform your doctor as soon as possible. Only your doctor can determine if it is safe for you to continue using Anusol-HC.

■ *Side effects may include:*
Acne-like skin eruptions, burning, dryness, growth of excessive hair, inflammation of the hair follicles, inflammation around the mouth, irritation, itching, peeling skin, prickly heat, secondary infection, skin inflammation, skin softening, stretch marks, unusual lack of skin color

Why should this drug not be prescribed?

Do not use Anusol-HC if you are sensitive to or have ever had an allergic reaction to any of its ingredients.

Special warnings about this medication

Avoid covering a treated area with waterproof diapers or plastic pants. They can increase unwanted absorption of Anusol-HC.

If you use this medication over large areas of skin for prolonged periods of time—or cover the treated area—the amount of the hormone absorbed into your bloodstream may eventually lead to Cushing's syndrome: a moon-faced appearance, fattened neck and trunk, and purplish streaks on the skin. You can also develop glandular problems or high blood sugar, or show sugar in your urine. Children, because of of their relatively larger ratio of skin surface area to body weight, are particularly susceptible to overabsorbtion of hormone from Anusol-HC.

Long-term treatment of children with steroids such as Anusol-HC may interfere with growth and development.

If an irritation develops, stop using the medication and contact your doctor.

Possible food and drug interactions when using this medication

No interactions have been reported.

Special information if you are pregnant or breastfeeding

The effects of Anusol-HC during pregnancy have not been adequately studied. If you are pregnant or plan to become pregnant, inform your doctor immediately. It is not known whether this medication appears in breast milk in sufficient amounts to affect a nursing baby. To avoid any possible harm to your baby, use Anusol-HC sparingly, and only with your doctor's permission, when breastfeeding.

Recommended dosage

ADULTS

Apply Anusol-HC to the affected area 2 to 4 times a day, depending on the severity of the condition.

CHILDREN

Limit use to the least amount necessary, as directed by your doctor.

Overdosage

Extensive or long-term use can cause Cushing's syndrome (see "Special warnings about this medication"), glandular problems, higher than normal amounts of sugar in the blood, and high amounts of sugar in the urine. If you suspect an overdose of Anusol-HC, seek medical treatment immediately.

Brand name:

ASENDIN

Pronounced: a-SEND-in
Generic name: Amoxapine

Why is this drug prescribed?

Asendin relieves the symptoms of depression. It is believed to work by readjusting the balance of certain natural chemicals in the brain.

Most important fact about this drug

Serious, sometimes fatal, reactions can occur when drugs such as Asendin are taken with another type of antidepressant called an MAO inhibitor. Drugs in this category include Nardil, Marplan, and Parnate. Do not take Asendin within two weeks of taking one of these drugs. Make sure your doctor and pharmacist know of all the medications you are taking.

How should you take this medication?

Take Asensin exactly as prescribed. Don't be discouraged if you feel no immediate effect. Relief of symptoms usually begins within 2 weeks, and sometimes in as few as 4 to 7 days.

Asendin can cause dry mouth. Sucking hard candy or chewing gum can help this problem.

■ *If you miss a dose...*
  If you take Asendin once a day at bedtime and don't remember until morning, skip the missed dose. If you take several doses per day, take the forgotten dose as soon as you remember. If it is almost time for your next dose, skip the one you missed and return to your regular schedule. Never try to "catch up" by doubling the dose.

■ *Storage instructions...*
Asendin can be stored at room temperature. Protect it from excessive heat.

What side effects may occur?
Side effects cannot be anticipated. If any develop or change in intensity, inform your doctor as soon as possible. Only your doctor can determine if it is safe for you to continue taking Asendin.

■ *More common side effects may include:*
Anxiety, blurred vision, confusion, constipation, difficulty sleeping, dizziness, drowsiness, dry mouth, excessive appetite, excitement, fatigue, fluid retention, headache, increased perspiration, lack of muscle coordination, nausea, nervousness, nightmares, rapid, fluttery heartbeat, restlessness, skin rash, tremors, weakness

■ *Less common side effects may include:*
Abdominal pain, blood disorders, breast enlargement and excessive or spontaneous flow of milk in women, diarrhea, difficulty urinating, dilation of the pupils of the eye, disorientation, disturbed concentration, extremely high body temperature, fainting, fever, gas, hepatitis, high blood pressure, hives, impotence, incoordination, increased or decreased sex drive, itching, low blood pressure, menstrual irregularity, numbness, painful ejaculation, peculiar taste, rapid heartbeat, ringing in the ears, seizures, sensitivity to light, stuffy nose, teary eyes, tingling or pins and needles in arms and legs, upset stomach, vomiting, weight gain or loss

Why should this drug not be prescribed?
Do not use Asendin while taking an MAO inhibitor. (See "Most important fact about this drug.") Also, do not take Asendin if you are recovering from a heart attack, or if you are sensitive to or have ever had an allergic reaction to amoxapine or dibenzoxazepine medications.

Special warnings about this medication
Asendin may cause facial and body twitching known as tardive dyskinesia.

Neuroleptic malignant syndrome (NMS) has also occurred in people using Asendin. NMS is characterized by extremely high body temperature, rigid muscles, excessive perspiration, altered mental state, and irregular pulse, blood pressure, and heartbeat. Report any of these symptoms to your doctor immediately.

Use Asendin with care if you have had difficulty urinating, angle-closure glaucoma, or increased pressure within the eye.

Be very careful in using Asendin if you have a seizure disorder or have had one in the past.

If you have a heart condition, use Asendin with caution. There have been reports of heart attack and stroke in patients taking this type of antidepressant.

Antidepressants can cause allergic reactions such as skin rashes or fever in some people. This usually occurs during the first few days of treatment. If these symptoms develop, stop taking the medication and consult your doctor.

Asendin may cause you to become drowsy or less alert. Be careful driving, operating machinery or appliances, or doing any activity that requires full mental alertness until you know how you react on Asendin.

Possible food and drug interactions when taking this medication
Asendin may increase the effects of alcohol. Do not drink alcohol while taking this medication.

If Asendin is taken with certain other drugs, the effects of either could be increased, decreased, or altered. It is especially important to check with your doctor before combining Asendin with the following:

Albuterol (Ventolin, Proventil)
Anticholinergics such as Bentyl
Barbiturates/sedatives such as phenobarbital
 (Donnatal) and Seconal
Cimetidine (Tagamet)
MAO inhibitors (antidepressant drugs such as
 Nardil and Marplan)
Other central nervous system depressants
 such as Percocet and Halcion

Special information
if you are pregnant or breastfeeding

Although the effects of Asendin during pregnancy have not been adequately studied, stillbirths and decreased birth weight have appeared in animal studies. Asendin should be used only if the potential benefits outweigh the potential risks. If you are pregnant or plan to become pregnant, inform your doctor immediately. Asendin appears in breast milk and could affect a nursing infant. If this medication is essential to your health, your doctor may advise you to stop breastfeeding until your treatment is finished.

Recommended dosage

Effective dosages of Asendin may vary from one person to another.

ADULTS

The usual starting dosage is 50 milligrams 2 or 3 times daily. If you tolerate the drug well, your doctor may increase the dosage to 100 milligrams 2 or 3 times daily by the end of the first week. If that dose is not effective after 2 weeks, your doctor may increase the dose even further.

When the effective dosage has been established, your doctor may have you take the drug in a single dose (not to exceed 300 milligrams) at bedtime.

CHILDREN

Safety and effectiveness have not been established in children under the age of 16.

ELDERLY

In general, lower dosages are recommended for the elderly. The recommended starting dosage of Asendin is 25 milligrams 2 or 3 times daily. If you tolerate it well, your doctor may increase the dosage by the end of the first week to 50 milligrams 2 or 3 times daily. A daily dosage of 100 to 150 milligrams may be enough for many elderly people, but some may need up to 300 milligrams.

Overdosage

Any medication taken in excess can have serious consequences. If you suspect an overdose of Asendin, seek medical treatment immediately.

■ *Symptoms of Asendin overdose may
 include:*
 Coma
 Convulsions
 Kidney failure
 Severe, protracted epileptic seizures
Generic name:

ASPIRIN

Pronounced: ASS-per-in
*Brand names: Empirin, Ecotrin, Genuine
 Bayer*

Why is this drug prescribed?

Aspirin is an anti-inflammatory pain medication (analgesic) that is used to relieve headaches, toothaches, and minor aches and pains, and to reduce fever. It also temporarily relieves the minor aches and pains of arthritis, muscle aches, colds, flu, and menstrual discomfort. In some patients, a small daily dose of aspirin may be used to ensure sufficient blood flow to the brain and prevent stroke. Aspirin may also be taken to decrease recurrence of a heart attack or other heart problems.

Most important fact about this drug

Aspirin should not be used during the last 3 months of pregnancy unless specifically prescribed by a doctor. It may cause problems in the unborn child or complications during delivery.

How should you take this medication?

Do not take more than the recommended dose.

Do not use aspirin if it has a strong, vinegar-like odor.

If aspirin upsets your stomach, use of a coated or buffered brand may reduce the problem.

Do not chew or crush sustained-release brands, such as Bayer time-release aspirin, or pills coated to delay breakdown of the drug, such as Ecotrin. To make them easier to swallow, take them with a full glass of water.

■ *If you miss a dose...*
Take it as soon as you remember. If it is almost time for your next dose, skip the one you missed and go back to your regular schedule. Never take 2 doses at the same time.

■ *Storage instructions...*
Store at room temperature.

What side effects may occur?

Side effects cannot be anticipated. If any develop or change in intensity, inform your doctor as soon as possible. Only your doctor can determine if it is safe for you to continue using aspirin.

■ *Side effects may include:*
Heartburn
Nausea and/or vomiting
Possible involvement in formation of stomach ulcers and bleeding
Small amounts of blood in stool
Stomach pain
Stomach upset

Why should this drug not be prescribed?

Do not take aspirin if you are allergic to it, if you have asthma, ulcers or ulcer symptoms, or if you are taking a medication that affects the clotting of your blood, unless specifically told to do so by your doctor.

Special warnings about this medication

Aspirin should not be given to children or teenagers for flu symptoms or chickenpox. Aspirin has been associated with the development of Reye's syndrome, a dangerous disorder characterized by disorientation, and lethargy leading to coma.

If you have a continuous or high fever, or a severe or persistent sore throat, especially with a high fever, vomiting and nausea, consult your doctor. It could indicate a more serious illness.

If pain persists for more than 10 days or if redness or swelling appears at the site of inflammation, consult your doctor.

If you experience ringing in the ears, hearing loss, upset stomach, or dizziness, consult your doctor before taking more aspirin.

Possible food and drug interactions when taking this medication

If aspirin is taken with certain other drugs, the effects of either could be increased, decreased, or altered. It is especially important to check with your doctor before combining aspirin with the following:

Acetazolamide (Diamox)
ACE-inhibitor-type blood pressure
    medications such as Capoten
Anti-gout medications such as Zyloprim
Arthritis medications such as Motrin and
    Indocin
Blood thinners such as Coumadin
Certain diuretics such as Lasix
Diabetes medications such as DiaBeta and
    Micronase
Diltiazem (Cardizem)
Dipyridamole (Persantine)
Insulin
Seizure medications such as Depakene
Steroids such as prednisone

Special information
if you are pregnant or breastfeeding
The use of aspirin during pregnancy should be discussed with your doctor. Aspirin should not be used during the last 3 months of pregnancy unless specifically indicated by your doctor. It may cause problems in the fetus and complications during delivery. Aspirin may appear in breast milk and could affect a nursing infant. Ask your doctor whether it is safe to take aspirin while you are breastfeeding.

Recommended dosage
ADULTS

Treatment of Minor Pain and Fever
The usual dose is 1 or 2 tablets every 3 to 4 hours up to 6 times a day.

Prevention of Stroke
The usual dose is 1 tablet 4 times daily or 2 tablets 2 times a day.

Prevention of Heart Attack
The usual dose is 1 tablet daily. Your physician may suggest that you take a larger dose, however.

CHILDREN

Consult your doctor.

Overdosage
Any medication used in excess can have serious consequences. If you suspect symptoms of an aspirin overdose, seek medical treatment immediately.

Brand name:

ASPIRIN FREE ANACIN

See Tylenol, page 777.

Brand name:

ATIVAN

Pronounced: AT-i-van
Generic name: Lorazepam

Why is this drug prescribed?
Ativan is used in the treatment of anxiety disorders and for short-term (up to 4 months) relief of the symptoms of anxiety. It belongs to a class of drugs known as benzodiazepines.

Most important fact about this drug
Tolerance and dependence can develop with the use of Ativan. You may experience withdrawal symptoms if you stop using it abruptly. Only your doctor should advise you to discontinue or change your dose.

How should you take this drug?
Take this medication exactly as prescribed by your doctor.

■ *If you miss a dose...*
If it is within an hour or so of the scheduled time, take the forgotten dose as soon as you remember. Otherwise, skip the dose and go back to your regular schedule. Do not take 2 doses at once.

■ *Storage instructions...*
Store at room temperature in a tightly closed container, away from light.

What side effects may occur?

Side effects cannot be anticipated. If any develop or change in intensity, inform your doctor as soon as possible. Only your doctor can determine if it is safe for you to continue taking Ativan.

If you experience any side effects, it will usually be at the beginning of your treatment; they will probably disappear as you continue to take the drug, or if your dosage is reduced.

■ *More common side effects may include:*
Dizziness
Sedation (excessive calm)
Unsteadiness
Weakness

■ *Less common or rare side effects may include:*
Agitation, change in appetite, depression, eye function disorders, headache, memory impairment, mental disorientation, nausea, skin problems, sleep disturbance, stomach and intestinal disorders

■ *Side effects due to rapid decrease or abrupt withdrawal of Ativan:*
Abdominal and muscle cramps, convulsions, depressed mood, inability to fall or stay asleep, sweating, tremors, vomiting

Why should this drug not be prescribed?

If you are sensitive to or have ever had an allergic reaction to Ativan or similar drugs such as Valium, you should not take this medication.

Also avoid Ativan if you have the eye disease, acute narrow-angle glaucoma.

Anxiety or tension related to everyday stress usually does not require treatment with Ativan. Discuss your symptoms thoroughly with your doctor.

Special warnings about this medication

Ativan may cause you to become drowsy or less alert; therefore, driving or operating dangerous machinery or participating in any hazardous activity that requires full mental alertness is not recommended.

If you are severely depressed or have suffered from severe depression, consult with your doctor before taking this medication.

If you have decreased kidney or liver function, use of this drug should be discussed with your doctor.

If you are elderly or if you have been using Ativan for a prolonged period of time, your doctor will watch you closely for stomach and upper intestinal problems.

Possible food and drug interactions when taking this medication

Ativan may intensify the effects of alcohol. Avoid alcohol while taking this medication.

If Ativan is taken with certain other drugs, the effects of either could be increased, decreased, or altered. It is especially important to check with your doctor before combining Ativan with barbiturates (phenobarbital, Seconal, Amytal) or sedative-type medications such as Valium and Halcion.

Special information
if you are pregnant or breastfeeding

Do not take Ativan if you are pregnant or planning to become pregnant. There is an increased risk of birth defects. It is not known whether Ativan appears in breast milk. If this medication is essential to your health, your doctor may advise you to discontinue breastfeeding until your treatment is finished.

Recommended dosage

ADULTS

The usual recommended dosage is a total of 2 to 6 milligrams per day divided into smaller doses. The largest dose should be taken at bedtime. The daily dose may vary from 1 to 10 milligrams.

Anxiety

The usual starting dose is a total of 2 to 3 milligrams per day taken in 2 or 3 smaller doses.

Insomnia Due to Anxiety

A single daily dose of 2 to 4 milligrams may be taken, usually at bedtime.

CHILDREN

The safety and effectiveness of Ativan have not been established in children under 12 years of age.

ELDERLY

The usual starting dosage for the elderly and those in a weakened condition should not exceed a total of 1 to 2 milligrams per day, divided into smaller doses, to avoid oversedation. This dose can be adjusted by your doctor as needed.

Overdosage

Any medication taken in excess can have serious consequences. If you suspect an overdose, seek medical attention immediately.

■ *The symptoms of Ativan overdose may include:*
Coma
Confusion
Low blood pressure
Sleepiness

Brand name:

A/T/S

See Erythromycin, Topical, page 587.

Brand name:

AUGMENTIN

Pronounced: awg-MENT-in
Generic ingredients: Amoxicillin, Clavulanate
potassium

Why is this drug prescribed?

Augmentin is used in the treatment of lower respiratory, middle ear, sinus, skin, and urinary tract infections that are caused by certain specific bacteria. These bacteria produce a chemical enzyme called beta lactamase that makes some infections particularly difficult to treat.

Most important fact about this drug

If you are allergic to either penicillin or cephalosporin antibiotics in any form, consult your doctor *before taking Augmentin.* There is a possibility that you are allergic to both types of medication and if a reaction occurs, it could be extremely severe. If you take the drug and feel signs of a reaction, seek medical attention immediately.

How should you take this medication?

Augmentin may be taken with or without food.

Shake the suspension well before using.

■ *If you miss a dose...*
Take it as soon as you remember. If it is almost time for the next dose, and you take 2 doses a day, take the one you missed and the next dose 5 to 6 hours later. If you take 3 or more doses a day, take the one you missed and the next dose 2 to 4 hours later. Then go back to your regular schedule.

■ *Storage instructions...*
Store the suspension under refrigeration and discard after 10 days. Store tablets away from heat, light, and moisture.

What side effects may occur?

Side effects cannot be anticipated. If any develop or change in intensity, inform your doctor as soon as possible. Only your doctor can determine if it is safe for you to continue taking Augmentin.

■ *More common side effects may include:*
Diarrhea/loose stools
Itching or burning of the vagina
Nausea or vomiting
Skin rashes and hives

■ *Less common side effects may include:*
Abdominal discomfort, anemia, arthritis, black "hairy" tongue, blood disorders, fever, gas, headache, indigestion, itching, joint pain, muscle pain, skin inflammation, skin peeling, sores and inflammation in the mouth and on the tongue and gums

■ *Rare side effects may include:*
Agitation, anxiety, behavioral changes, change in liver function, confusion, dizziness, hyperactivity, insomnia

Why should this drug not be prescribed?

If you are sensitive to or have ever had an allergic reaction to any penicillin medication or if you have an infectious disease such as mononucleosis, do not take this drug.

Special warnings about this medication

Augmentin and other penicillin-like medicines are generally safe; however, anyone with liver, kidney, or blood disorders is at increased risk when using this drug. Alternative choices may be available to your doctor.

If you have diabetes and test your urine for the presence of sugar, you should ask your doctor or pharmacist if this medication will interfere with the type of test you use.

Allergic reactions to this medication can be serious and possibly fatal. Let your doctor know about previous allergic reactions to medicines, food, or other substances before using Augmentin. If you experience a reaction, report it to your doctor immediately and seek medical treatment.

Possible food and drug interactions when taking this medication

Augmentin may react with the antigout medication Benemid, resulting in changes in blood levels. A reaction with another antigout drug, Zyloprim, may cause rashes. Notify your doctor if you are taking either of these drugs.

Do not take Augmentin when using Antabuse (disulfiram).

Special information if you are pregnant or breastfeeding

The effects of Augmentin during pregnancy have not been adequately studied. Because there may be risk to the developing baby, doctors usually recommend Augmentin to pregnant women only when the benefits of therapy outweigh any potential danger. Augmentin appears in breast milk and could affect a nursing infant. If Augmentin is essential to your health, your doctor may advise you to stop nursing your baby until your treatment with this drug is finished.

Recommended dosage

ADULTS

The usual adult dose is one 250-milligram tablet every 8 hours. For more severe infections and infections of the respiratory tract, the dose should be one 500-milligram tablet every 8 hours. It is essential that you take this medicine according to your doctor's directions.

CHILDREN

The usual total daily dosage is 20 milligrams per 2.2 pounds of body weight per day, divided into 4 doses and taken every 8 hours. For middle ear infections, sinus infections, and lower respiratory infections, the dose should be 40 milligrams per 2.2 pounds per day, divided into smaller doses and taken every 8 hours. Severe infections should be treated with the higher recommended dose. Children weighing 88 pounds or more will take the adult dosage.

Overdosage

Augmentin is generally safe; however, large amounts may cause overdose symptoms, including exaggerated side effects listed above. Suspected overdoses of Augmentin must be treated immediately; contact your physician or an emergency room.

Brand name:

AVC

Pronounced: A VEE CEE
Generic name: Sulfanilamide

Why is this drug prescribed?

AVC is used to treat yeast infections caused by *Candida albicans*, a type of fungus. AVC rapidly relieves vulvovaginitis—the itching, redness, and irritation of the external sex organs (vulva) and the thick, cottage cheese-like discharge that usually accompany yeast infections.

Most important fact about this drug

Although you should begin to feel better soon after you start using AVC, you must continue treatment for a full 30 days, including during your menstrual period, to prevent a relapse. If you still have symptoms after completing your treatment, see your doctor.

How should you take this medication?

Use this medication exactly as prescribed.

To administer, follow these steps:

1. Load the applicator to the fill line with cream, or unwrap a suppository, wet it with warm water, and place it in the applicator as shown in the instructions you received with the product.
2. Lie on your back with knees drawn up.
3. Gently insert the applicator high into the vagina and push the plunger.
4. Withdraw the applicator and discard it if disposable, or wash with soap and water.

To keep the medication from getting on your clothing, wear a sanitary napkin. Do not use a tampon because it will absorb the medicine. Wear cotton underwear; avoid synthetic fabrics such as rayon or nylon.

Dry the genital area thoroughly after a shower, bath, or swim. Change out of a wet bathing suit or damp workout clothes as soon as possible. Yeast is less likely to grow in a dry environment.

Do not scratch if you can help it. Scratching can cause more irritation and can spread the infection.

■ *If you miss a dose...*
Insert it as soon as you remember. If it is almost time for your next dose, skip the

one you missed and go back to your regular schedule.

■ *Storage instructions...*
Store AVC at room temperature and protect from cold. Keep the suppositories away from excessive moisture. The cream will darken with age.

What side effects may occur?

Side effects cannot be anticipated. If any develop or change in intensity, stop using the medication immediately and inform your doctor as soon as possible. Ony your doctor can determine if it is safe for you to continue using AVC Cream or Suppositories.

■ *Side effects may include:*
Increased discomfort
Vaginal and vulvar burning

Why should this drug not be prescribed?

If you are sensitive to sulfa drugs or if you have ever had an allergic reaction to them, you should not use AVC. Make sure your doctor is aware of any drug reactions you have experienced.

Special warnings about this medication

Sulfa drugs can be absorbed into your bloodstream and may produce serious, even life-threatening reactions in women who are especially sensitive to them.

Take special care when using vaginal applicators and suppositories after the seventh month of pregnancy.

If you have any itching or burning, or any other unusual symptoms, stop using the medication and contact your doctor.

Possible food and drug interactions when taking this medication

No interactions have been reported.

Special information if you are pregnant or breastfeeding

The effects of AVC during pregnancy have not been adequately studied. If you are pregnant or plan to become pregnant, inform you doctor immediately. Sulfa drugs may appear in breast milk and have caused jaundice in newborn infants. If this drug is essential to you health, your doctor may advise you to discontinue breastfeeding until your treatment with AVC is finished.

Recommended dosage

AVC CREAM

Insert 1 applicatorful (about 6 grams) of cream in your vagina once or twice daily for 30 days.

AVC SUPPOSITORIES

Insert 1 suppository in your vagina once or twice daily for the full 30-day period of therapy.

Overdosage

Although there have been no reports of overdosage with AVC, any medication taken in excess can have serious consequences. If you suspect an overdose, seek medical attention immediately.

Brand name:

AVENTYL

See Pamelor, page 708.

Generic name:

AZITHROMYCIN

See Zithromax, page 800.

Brand name:

BACTRIM

Pronounced: BAC-trim
Generic ingredients: Trimethoprim,
Sulfamethoxazole
Other brand names: Cotrim, Co-Trimoxazole,
Septra

Why is this drug prescribed?

Bactrim, an antibacterial combination drug, is prescribed for the treatment of certain urinary tract infections, severe middle ear infections in children, long-lasting or frequently recurring bronchitis in adults that has increased in seriousness, inflammation of the intestine due to a severe bacterial infection, pneumonia in patients who have a suppressed immune system (*Pneumocystis carinii* pneumonia) and for travelers' diarrhea in adults.

Most important fact about this drug

Sulfamethoxazole, an ingredient in Bactrim, is one of a group of drugs called sulfonamides, which prevent the growth of bacteria in the body. Rare but sometimes fatal reactions have occurred with use of sulfonamides. These reactions include Stevens-Johnson syndrome (severe eruptions around the mouth, anus, or eyes), progressive disintegration of the outer layer of the skin, sudden and severe liver damage, a severe blood disorder (agranulocytosis), and a lack of red and white blood cells because of a bone marrow disorder.

Notify your doctor at the first sign of an adverse reaction such as skin rash, sore throat, fever, joint pain, cough, shortness of breath, abnormal skin paleness, reddish or purplish skin spots, or yellowing of the skin or whites of the eyes.

Frequent blood counts by a doctor are recommended for patients taking sulfonamide drugs.

How should you take this medication?

It is important that you drink plenty of fluids while taking this medication in order to prevent sediment in the urine and the formation of stones.

Bactrim works best when there is a constant amount in the blood. Take Bactrim exactly as prescribed, try not to miss any doses. It is best to take doses at evenly spaced times day and night.

If you are taking Bactrim suspension, ask your pharmacist for a specially marked measuring spoon that delivers accurate doses.

■ *If you miss a dose...*
Take the forgotten dose as soon as you remember. If it is almost time for your next dose, skip the one you missed and go back to your regular schedule. Do not take 2 doses at once.

■ *Storage instructions...*
Store tablets and suspension at room temperature and protect from light. Keep tablets in a dry place. Protect the suspension from freezing.

What side effects may occur?

Side effects cannot be anticipated. If any develop or change in intensity, inform your doctor as soon as possible. Only your doctor can determine if it is safe for you to continue taking Bactrim.

■ *More common side effects may include:*
Hives
Lack or loss of appetite
Nausea
Skin rash
Vomiting

■ *Less common or rare side effects may include:*

Abdominal pain, allergic reactions, anemia, chills, convulsions, depression, diarrhea, eye irritation, fatigue, fever, hallucinations, headache, hepatitis, inability to fall or stay asleep, inability to urinate, increased urination, inflammation of heart muscle, inflammation of the mouth and/or tongue, itching, joint pain, kidney failure, lack of feeling or concern, lack of muscle coordination, loss of appetite, low blood sugar, meningitis (inflammation of the brain or spinal cord), muscle pain, nausea, nervousness, red, raised rash, redness and swelling of the tongue, ringing in the ears, scaling of dead skin due to inflammation, sensitivity to light, severe skin welts or swelling, skin eruptions, skin peeling, vertigo, weakness, yellowing of eyes and skin

Why should this drug not be prescribed?

If you are sensitive to or have ever had an allergic reaction to trimethoprim, sulfamethoxazole or other sulfa drugs such as Septra, you should not take this medication. Make sure that your doctor is aware of any drug reactions that you have experienced.

Unless you are directed to do so by your doctor, do not take this medication if you have been diagnosed as having megaloblastic anemia, which is a blood disorder due to a deficiency of folic acid.

This drug should not be prescribed for infants less than 2 months of age.

Bactrim is not recommended for preventative or prolonged use in middle ear infections and should not be used in the treatment of streptococcal pharyngitis (inflammation or infection of the pharynx due to streptococcus bacteria).

Special warnings about this medication

Make sure your doctor knows if you have impaired kidney or liver function, have a folic acid deficiency, are a chronic alcoholic, are taking anticonvulsants, have been diagnosed as having malabsorption syndrome (abnormal intestinal absorption), are in a state of poor nutrition, or have severe allergies or bronchial asthma. Bactrim should be used cautiously under these conditions.

If you have AIDS (acquired immunodeficiency syndrome) and are being treated for *Pneumocystis carinii* pneumonia, you will experience more side effects than will someone without AIDS.

Possible food and drug interactions when taking this medication

If Bactrim is taken with certain other drugs, the effects of either could be increased, decreased, or altered. It is especially important to check with your doctor before combining Bactrim with the following:

Amantadine (Symmetrel)
Anticonvulsants such as Dilantin
Blood thinners such as Coumadin
Diuretics (in the elderly) such as
   HydroDIURIL
Methotrexate (Rheumatrix)
Oral diabetes medications such as Micronase

Special information if you are pregnant or breastfeeding

The effects of Bactrim during pregnancy have not been adequately studied. If you are pregnant or plan to become pregnant, notify your doctor immediately. The drug should not be taken at term. Bactrim does appear in breast milk and could affect a nursing infant. It should not be taken while breastfeeding.

Recommended dosage

ADULTS

Urinary Tract Infections and Intestinal Inflammation
The usual adult dosage in the treatment of urinary tract infection is 1 Bactrim DS (double strength tablet) or 2 Bactrim tablets, or 4 teaspoonfuls (20 milliliters) of Bactrim Pediatric Suspension every 12 hours for 10 to 14 days. The dosage for inflammation of the intestine is the same but is taken for 5 days.

Worsening of Chronic Bronchitis
The usual recommended dosage is 1 Bactrim DS (double strength tablet), 2 Bactrim tablets, or 4 teaspoonfuls (20 milliliters) of Bactrim Pediatric Suspension every 12 hours for 14 days.

Pneumocystis Carinii Pneumonia
The recommended dosage is 20 milligrams of trimethoprim and 100 milligrams of sulfamethoxazole per 2.2 pounds of body weight per 24 hours divided into equal doses every 6 hours for 14 days.

Travelers' Diarrhea
The usual recommended dosage is 1 Bactrim DS (double strength tablet), 2 Bactrim tablets, or 4 teaspoonfuls (20 milliliters) of Bactrim Pediatric Suspension every 12 hours for 5 days.

CHILDREN

Urinary Tract Infections or Middle Ear Infections
The recommended dose for children 2 months of age or older, given every 12 hours for 10 days, is determined by weight. The following table is a guideline for this dosage:

22 pounds, 1 teaspoonful (5 milliliters)

44 pounds, 2 teaspoonfuls (10 milliliters) or 1 tablet

66 pounds, 3 teaspoonfuls (15 milliliters) or 1 and a half tablets

88 pounds, 4 teaspoonfuls (20 milliliters) or 2 tablets or 1 DS tablet

Intestinal Inflammation:
The recommended dose is identical to the dosage recommended for urinary tract and middle ear infections; however, it should be taken for 5 days.

Pneumocystis Carinii Pneumonia
The recommended dose, taken every 6 hours for 14 days, is determined by weight. The following table is a guideline for this dosage:

18 pounds, 1 teaspoonful (5 milliliters)

35 pounds, 2 teaspoonfuls (10 milliliters) or 1 tablet

53 pounds, 3 teaspoonfuls (15 milliliters) or 1 and a half tablets

70 pounds, 4 teaspoonfuls (20 milliliters) or 2 tablets or 1 DS tablet

The safety of repeated use of Bactrim in children under 2 years of age has not been established.

ELDERLY

There may be an increased risk of severe side effects when Bactrim is taken by the elderly, especially in those who have impaired kidney and/or liver function or who are taking other medication. Consult with your doctor before taking Bactrim.

Overdosage

If you suspect an overdose of Bactrim, seek emergency medical attention immediately.

■ *Symptoms of an overdose of Bactrim include:*
Blood or sediment in the urine, colic, confusion, dizziness, drowsiness, fever, headache, lack or loss of appetite, mental depression, nausea, unconsciousness, vomiting, yellowed eyes and skin

Brand name:

BENZAC W

See Desquam-E, page 565.

Brand name:

BENZAGEL

See Desquam-E, page 565.

Brand name:

BENZAMYCIN

Pronounced: BEN-za-MI-sin
Generic ingredients: Erythromycin, Benzoyl peroxide

Why is this drug prescribed?
A combination of the antibiotic erythromycin and the antibacterial agent benzoyl peroxide, Benzamycin is effective in stopping the bacteria that cause acne and in reducing acne infection.

Most important fact about this drug
If you experience excessive irritation or dryness, stop using Benzamycin and notify your doctor.

How should you use this medication?
Use Benzamycin 2 times per day, once in the morning and once in the evening, or as directed by your doctor. Apply to the affected areas after thoroughly washing, rinsing with warm water, and then gently patting dry.

■ *If you miss a dose...*
Apply it as soon as you remember. If it is almost time for your next dose, skip the one you missed and go back to your regular schedule.

■ *Storge instructions...*
This medication should be stored in your refrigerator in a tightly closed container and discarded after 3 months. Do not freeze.

What side effects may occur?
Very few side effects have been reported with the use of Benzamycin. However, those reported include:

Abnormal redness of the skin
Dryness
Itching

If any develop or change in intensity, inform your doctor as soon as possible. Only your doctor can determine if it is safe for you to continue taking Benzamycin.

Why should this drug not be prescribed?
If you are sensitive to or have ever had an allergic reaction to erythromycin or benzoyl peroxide, or any other ingredients in Benzamycin, you should not take this medication. Make sure your doctor is aware of any drug reactions you have experienced.

Special warnings about this medication
Benzamycin Topical Gel is for external use only. Avoid contact with your eyes and mucous membranes.

Benzamycin may bleach hair or colored fabric. Avoid contact with scalp and clothes.

As you use this antibiotic, organisms that are resistant to it may start to grow. Your doctor will have you stop taking

Benzamycin and will give you a medication to fight the new bacteria.

Possible food and drug interactions when using this medication

If Benzamycin is used with other acne medications, the effects of either could be increased, decreased, or altered. Always check with your doctor before combining any other prescription or over-the-counter acne remedy with Benzamycin.

Special information if you are pregnant or breastfeeding

The effects of Benzamycin during pregnancy have not been adequately studied. If you are pregnant or plan to become pregnant, inform your doctor immediately. It is not known whether Benzamycin appears in breast milk. If this medication is essential to your health, your doctor may advise you to discontinue breastfeeding your baby until your treatment with this medication is finished.

Recommended dosage

ADULTS

Apply to affected areas twice daily, once in the morning and once in the evening.

CHILDREN

The safety and effectiveness of Benzamycin have not been established in children under 12 years of age.

Overdosage

There is no information available on overdosage.

Brand name:

BENZASHAVE

See Desquam-E, page 565.

Generic name:

BENZOYL PEROXIDE

See Desquam-E, page 565.

Generic name:

BROMOCRIPTINE

See Parlodel, page 711.

Generic name:

BUPROPION

See Wellbutrin, page 793.

Brand name:

BUSPAR

Pronounced: BYOO-spar
Generic name: Buspirone hydrochloride

Why is this drug prescribed?

BuSpar is used in the treatment of anxiety disorders and for short-term relief of the symptoms of anxiety.

Most important fact about this drug

BuSpar should not be used with antidepressant drugs known as monoamine oxidase (MAO) inhibitors. Brands include Nardil and Parnate.

How should you take this medication?

Take BuSpar exactly as prescribed. Do not be discouraged if you feel no immediate effect. The full benefit of this drug may not be seen for 1 to 2 weeks after you start to take it.

■ *If you miss a dose...*
  Take the forgotten dose as soon as you remember. If it is almost time for your

next dose, skip the one you missed and go back to your regular schedule. Never take 2 doses at the same time.

■ *Storage instructions...*
Store at room temperature in a tightly closed container, away from light.

What side effects may occur?
Side effects cannot be anticipated. If any develop or change in intensity, inform your doctor as soon as possible. Only your doctor can determine if it is safe for you to continue taking BuSpar.

■ *More common side effects may include:*
Dizziness, dry mouth, fatigue, headache, light-headedness, nausea, nervousness, unusual excitement

■ *Less common or rare side effects may include:*
Anger/hostility, blurred vision, bone aches/pain, confusion, constipation, decreased concentration, depression, diarrhea, fast, fluttery heartbeat, incoordination, muscle pain/aches, numbness, pain or weakness in hands or feet, rapid heartbeat, rash, restlessness, stomach and abdominal upset, sweating/clamminess, tingling or pins and needles, tremor, urinary incontinence, vomiting, weakness

Why should this drug not be prescribed?
If you are sensitive to or have ever had an allergic reaction to BuSpar or similar mood-altering drugs, you should not take this medication. Make sure your doctor is aware of any drug reactions you have experienced.

Anxiety or tension related to everyday stress usually does not require treatment with BuSpar. Discuss your symptoms thoroughly with your doctor.

The use of BuSpar is not recommended if you have severe kidney or liver damage.

Special warnings about this medication
The effects of BuSpar on the central nervous system (brain and spinal cord) are unpredictable. Therefore, you should not drive or operate dangerous machinery or participate in any hazardous activity that requires full mental alertness while you are taking BuSpar.

Possible food and drug interactions when taking this medication
Although BuSpar does not intensify the effects of alcohol, it is best to avoid alcohol while taking this medication.

If BuSpar is taken with certain other drugs, the effects of either can be increased, decreased, or altered. It is especially important to check with your doctor before combining BuSpar with the following:

The blood-thinning drug Coumadin
Haloperidol (Haldol)
MAO inhibitors (antidepressant drugs such as Nardil and Parmate)
Trazodone (Desyrel)

Special information if you are pregnant or breastfeeding
The effects of BuSpar during pregnancy have not been adequately studied. If you are pregnant or plan to become pregnant, inform your doctor immediately. It is not known whether BuSpar appears in breast milk. If this medication is essential to your health, your doctor may advise you to discontinue breastfeeding until your treatment is finished.

Recommended dosage
ADULTS

The recommended starting dose is a total of 15 milligrams per day divided into smaller doses, usually 5 milligrams 3 times a day. Every 2 to 3 days, your doctor may increase the dosage 5 milligrams per day as needed. The daily dose should not exceed 60 milligrams.

CHILDREN

The safety and effectiveness of BuSpar have not been established in children under 18 years of age.

ELDERLY

The use of BuSpar in the elderly has not been thoroughly researched. However, no unusual age-related effects have been identified. The usual dose is 15 milligrams per day divided into smaller doses.

Overdosage

Any medication taken in excess can have serious consequences. If you suspect an overdose of BuSpar, seek medical attention immediately.

■ *The symptoms of BuSpar overdose may include:*
Dizziness
Drowsiness
Nausea or vomiting
Severe stomach upset
Unusually small pupils

Generic name:

BUSPIRONE HYDROCHLORIDE

See BuSpar, page 527.

Generic name:

BUTALBITAL, ACETEMINOPHEN, AND CAFFEINE

See Fioricet, page 598.

Generic name:

BUTALBITAL, ASPIRIN, AND CAFFEINE

See Fiorinal, page 600.

Generic name:

BUTALBITAL, CODEINE, ASPIRIN, AND CAFFEINE

See Fiorinal with Codeine, page 602.

Generic name:

BUTOCONAZOLE

See Femstat, page 596.

Brand name:

CAFERGOT

Pronounced: KAF-er-got
Generic ingredients: Ergotamine tartrate, Caffeine

Why is this drug prescribed?

Cafergot is prescribed for the relief or prevention of vascular headaches—for example, migraine, migraine variants, or cluster headaches.

Most important fact about this drug

The excessive use of Cafergot can lead to ergot poisoning resulting in symptoms such as headache, pain in the legs when walking, muscle pain, numbness, coldness, and abnormal paleness of the fingers and toes. If this condition is not treated, it can lead to gangrene (tissue death due to decreased blood supply).

How should you take this medication?

Cafergot is available in both tablet and suppository form. Be sure to take it exactly as prescribed, remaining within the limits of your recommended dosage.

Cafergot works best if you use it at the first sign of a migraine attack. If you get warning signals of a coming migraine, take the drug before the headache actually starts.

Lie down and relax in a quiet, dark room for at least a couple hours or until your feel better.

Avoid exposure to cold.

To use the suppositories, follow these steps:

1. If the suppository feels too soft, leave it in the refrigerator for about 30 minutes or put it, still wrapped, in ice water until it hardens.
2. Remove the foil wrapper and dip the tip of the suppository in water.
3. Lie down on your side and with a finger insert the suppository into the rectum. Hold it in place for a few moments.

■ *If you miss a dose...*
  Take this medication only when threatened with an attack.

■ *Storage instructions*
  Store at room temperature in a tightly closed container away from light. Keep suppositories away from heat.

What side effects may occur?

Side effects cannot be anticipated. If any develop or change in intensity, inform your doctor as soon as possible. Only your doctor can determine if it is safe for you to continue taking Cafergot.

■ *Side effects may include:*
  Fluid retention
  High blood pressure

Itching
Nausea
Numbness
Rapid heart rate
Slow heartbeat
Tingling or pins and needles
Vertigo
Vomiting
Weakness

■ *Complications caused by constriction of the blood vessels can be serious. They include:*
  Bluish tinge to the skin
  Chest pain
  Cold arms and legs
  Gangrene
  Muscle pains

Although these symptoms occur most commonly with long-term therapy at relatively high doses, they have been reported with short-term or normal doses.

Why should this drug not be prescribed?

If you are sensitive to or have ever had an allergic reaction to ergotamine tartrate, caffeine, or similar drugs, you should not take this medication. Make sure your doctor is aware of any drug reactions you have experienced.

Unless directed to do so by your doctor, do not take this medication if you have coronary heart disease, circulatory problems, high blood pressure, impaired liver or kidney function, or an infection, or if you are pregnant.

Special warnings about this medication

It is extremely important that you do not exceed your recommended dosage, especially when Cafergot is used over long periods. There have been reports of psychological dependence in people who have abused this drug over long periods of time. Discontinuance of the drug may produce withdrawal symptoms such as sudden, severe headaches.

If you experience excessive nausea and vomiting during attacks making it impossible for you to retain oral medication, your doctor will probably tell you to use rectal suppositories.

This drug is effective only for migraine and migraine-type headaches. Do not us it for any other kind of headache.

Possible food and drug interactions when taking this medication

If Cafergot is taken with certain other drugs, the effects of either could be increased, decreased, or altered. It is especially important to check with your doctor before combining Cafergot with the following:

Beta-blocker drugs (blood pressure medications such as Inderal and Tenormin)

Drugs that constrict the blood vessels, such as Epipen and the oral decongestant Sudafed

Macrolide antibiotics such as PCE, E.E.S., and Biaxin

Nicotine (Nicoderm, Habitrol, others)

Special information if you are pregnant or breastfeeding

Do not take Cafergot if you are pregnant. Cafergot appears in breast milk and may have serious effects in your baby. If this medication is essential for your health, your doctor may advise your to discontinue breastfeeding.

Recommended dosage

Dosage should start at the first sign of an attack.

ADULTS

Orally

The total dose for any single attack should not exceed 6 tablets.

Rectally

The maximum dose for an individual attack is 2 suppositories.

The total weekly dosage should not exceed 10 tablets or 5 suppositories.

A preventive, short-term dose may be given at bedtime to certain people, but only as prescribed by a doctor.

Overdosage

If you suspect an overdose of Cafergot, seek emergency medical treatment immediately.

■ *Symptoms of Cafergot overdose include:* Coma, convulsions, diminished or absent pulses, drowsiness, high or low blood pressure, numbness, shock, stupor, tingling, pain and bluish discoloration of the limbs, unresponsiveness, vomiting

Brand name:

CALCIMAR

Pronounced: KAL-si-mar
Generic name: Calcitonin-salmon

Why is this drug prescribed?

Calcimar is a synthetic form of calcitonin, a naturally occurring hormone produced by the thyroid gland. Calcimar reduces the rate of calcium loss from bones. Since less calcium passes from the bones to the blood, Calcimar also helps control blood calcium levels. Calcimar is used to treat:

Paget's disease (abnormal bone growth leading to deformities)

Hypercalcemia (abnormally high calcium

blood levels)
Postmenopausal osteoporosis (bone loss occurring after menopause)

Most important fact about this drug
Calcimar has been reported to cause serious allergic reactions (such as shock, difficulty breathing, wheezing, and swelling of the throat or tongue) in a few people.

How should you take this medication?
Calcimar is taken by injection, given by either you or your doctor. If you are injecting Calcimar yourself, it is important to follow your doctor's instructions carefully so that you inject Calcimar correctly. Calcimar is for injection under the skin or into a muscle; do not inject it into a vein.

You can minimize side effects such as nausea, vomiting, and skin flushing by taking the injection at bedtime.

Do not use Calcimar solution if it has changed color or has particles floating in it.

If you are taking Calcimar for postmenopausal bone loss, you should be sure your diet provides enough calcium and vitamin D. Foods that are good sources of calcium include dairy products (such as milk and cheese) and fish. Good sources of vitamin D include fish (such as salmon, sardines, and tuna), liver, and dairy products. Sunlight is an indirect source of vitamin D.

■ *If you miss a dose...*
If you take calcimar twice a day, take it as soon as you remember if it is within 2 hours of your scheduled time. Then go back to your regular schedule. If you do not remember until later, skip the dose you missed and go back to your regular schedule.

If you take Calcimar once a day, take it as soon as you remember, then go back to your regular schedule. If you do not remember until the next day, skip the dose you missed and go back to your regular schedule.

If you take Calcimar every other day, take it as soon as you remember if it is the day you are scheduled to take it. Then go back to your regular schedule. If you do not remember until the next day, take the dose you missed when you remember it, then skip a day and start your schedule again.

If you take a dose of Calcimar 3 times a week, take the dose you missed the next day, then set each injection back a day for the rest of the week. The following week, go back to your regular 3 days.

Whatever your schedule, never take 2 doses at once.

■ *Storage instructions...*
Store in the refrigerator.

What side effects may occur?
Side effects cannot be anticipated. If any develop or change in intensity, inform your doctor as soon as possible. Only your doctor can determine if it is safe for you to continue taking Calcimar.

■ *More common side effects may include:*
Inflamed skin where Calcimar has been injected
Nausea
Vomiting

■ *Less common side effects may include:*
Flushed face, flushed hands, severe allergic reaction, skin rashes

Why should this drug not be prescribed?
You should not be using Calcimar if you are allergic to it.

Special warnings about this medication

Calcimar may cause an abnormally low blood level of calcium, resulting in muscle cramps, spasms, and twitches in the face, feet, and hands.

Before taking Calcimar for the first time, you should consider having a skin test to determine whether you are allergic to the drug.

People who take Calcimar on a long-term basis should have periodic urine and blood tests to determine the ongoing effects of Calcimar.

It is important to let your doctor know how you respond to this drug; some people may develop an antibody to Calcimar, and it may become less effective.

Possible food and drug interactions when taking this medication

There are no interactions listed for this drug.

Special information if you are pregnant or breastfeeding

The effects of Calcimar in pregnancy have not been adequately studied.

Pregnant women should use Calcimar only if the potential benefits clearly outweigh any potential risks to the unborn child. It is not known whether Calcimar appears in breast milk. Women are usually advised not to take Calcimar while breastfeeding an infant.

Recommended dosage

Your doctor will tailor the dosage according to your individual requirements and the condition being treated. Do not change the dose without consulting your doctor.

If you are taking Calcimar for postmenopausal osteoporosis, ask your doctor about taking supplemental Vitamin D and calcium.

Overdosage

Any medication taken in excess can have serious consequences. If you suspect an overdose, seek medical help immediately.

- *Symptoms of Calcitonin overdose may include:*
  Nausea
  Vomiting

Generic name:

CALCITONIN-SALMON

See Calcimar, page 531.

Generic name:

CALCIUM CARBONATE

See Caltrate 600, page 533.

Brand name:

CALTRATE 600

Pronounced: CAL-trait
Generic name: Calcium carbonate
Other brand names: Os-Cal 500, Oystercal 500

Why is this supplement prescribed?

Caltrate is a supplement for women who do not get enough calcium in their diets or have a need for more calcium. Calcium supplements may reduce the rate of bone loss and help prevent osteoporosis (brittle bones). Calcium is also needed for the heart, muscles, and nervous system to work properly. The vitamin D in Caltrate + Vitamin D helps the body absorb calcium, while the extra iron in Caltrate + Iron &

Vitamin D supplements diets deficient in iron.

Most important fact about this supplement

If you do not get enough calcium in your diet, a calcium supplement may help prevent serious bone disease, especially later in life.

How should you take this supplement?

Follow the dosing instructions on the bottle. Do not take more than the recommended dose. Take calcium with meals, even if only a light snack. Drink a full glass of water or juice when taking a calcium supplement.

Certain foods, such as spinach, rhubarb, bran, whole cereals, and dairy products reduce absorption of calcium supplements. Allow 2 to 3 hours between taking calcium and eating any of these foods.

- *If you miss a dose...*
  If you are taking the calcium supplement on a regular schedule, take the dose you missed as soon as possible and then go back to your regular dosing schedule.

- *Storage instructions...*
  Store at room temperature.

What side effects may occur?

No side effects have been reported.

Why should this supplement not be used?

If you have any medical problems, check with your doctor before starting on a calcium supplement.

Special warnings about this supplement

Do not take more calcium than suggested on the packaging, as too much may cause excessive levels of calcium in the blood or increase the chance of kidney stones.

Possible food and drug interactions when taking this supplement

Be sure to tell your doctor if you are taking any medications, because dietary supplements and certain medications should not be used together. For example, if you are taking a tetracycline antibiotic, take your calcium supplement at least 1 hour before or 3 hours after you take the antibiotic.

Certain other drugs also may interact with calcium. Check with your doctor before combining calcium with the following:

Atenolol (Tenormin)
Iron preparations such as Feosol
Quinolone antibiotics such as Cipro and
  Floxin

Special information if you are pregnant or breastfeeding

Ask your doctor whether you should take a calcium supplement while you are pregnant or breastfeeding. Taking too much of any supplement may be harmful to you or your unborn child.

Recommended dosage

For Caltrate 600, Caltrate 600 + Iron & Vitamin D, and Caltrate 600 + Vitamin D tablets, use the following dosage recommendations:

ADULTS

The usual dose is 1 or 2 tablets daily or as directed by your doctor.

Overdosage

Mega doses of any dietary supplement can be harmful. If you have unexplained symptoms and suspect an overdose, check with your doctor.

Brand name:

CATAFLAM

See Voltaren, page 790.

Brand name:

CECLOR

Pronounced: SEE-klor
Generic name: Cefaclor

Why is this drug prescribed?

Ceclor, a cephalosporin antibiotic, is used in the treatment of ear, nose, throat, respiratory tract, urinary tract, and skin infections caused by specific bacteria, including staph, strep, and E. coli. Uses include treatment of sore or strep throat, pneumonia, and tonsillitis.

Most important fact about this drug

If you are allergic to either penicillin or cephalosporin antibiotics in any form, consult your doctor before taking Ceclor. There is a possibility that you are allergic to both types of medication; and if a reaction occurs, it could be extremely severe. If you take the drug and feel signs of a reaction, seek medical attention immediately.

How should you take this medication?

Take this medication exactly as prescribed. It is important that you finish taking all of this medication to obtain the maximum benefit.

This medication works fastest when taken on an empty stomach. However, your doctor may ask you to take this drug with food to avoid stomach upset.

Ceclor suspension should be shaken well before using.

■ *If you miss a dose...*
Take it as soon as you remember. If it is almost time for your next dose, skip the one you missed and go back to your regular schedule. Never take 2 doses at the same time.

■ *Storage instructions...*
Keep Ceclor capsules in the container they came in, tightly closed. Store at room temperature.

Regrigerate Ceclor Suspension. Discard any unused portion after 14 days.

What side effects may occur?

Side effects cannot be anticipated. If any develop or change in intensity, inform your doctor as soon as possible. Only your doctor can determine if it is safe for you to continue taking Ceclor.

■ *More common side effects may include:*
Diarrhea
Hives
Itching

■ *Less common or rare side effects may include:*
Blood disorders (an increase in certain types of white blood cells), liver disorders, nausea, skin rashes accompanied by joint pain, vaginal inflammation, vomiting

Other problems have been reported in patients taking Ceclor, although it is not known whether the drug was the cause. Check with your doctor if you suspect a side effect.

Why should this drug not be prescribed?

If you are sensitive to or have ever had an allergic reaction to Ceclor or similar drugs, you should not take this medication. Make sure your doctor is aware of any drug reactions you have experienced.

Unless you are directed to do so by your doctor, do not take this medication if you have a history of gastrointestinal problems, particularly bowel inflammation (colitis). You may be at increased risk for side effects.

Special warnings about this medication

Ceclor may cause a false positive result with some urine sugar tests for diabetics. Your doctor can advise you of any adjustments you may need to make in your medication or diet.

Ceclor occasionally causes diarrhea. Some diarrhea medications can make this diarrhea worse. Check with your doctor before taking any diarrhea remedy.

Oral contraceptives may not work properly while you are taking Ceclor. For greater certainty, use other measures while taking Ceclor.

Possible food and drug interactions when taking this medication

If Ceclor is taken with certain other drugs, the effects of either could be increased, decreased, or altered. It is especially important to check with your doctor before combining Ceclor with the following:

Certain antibiotics such as Amikin
Certain potent diuretics such as Edecrin and
   Lasix
Oral contraceptives
Probenecid (Benemid)

Special information
if you are pregnant or breastfeeding

The effects of Ceclor during pregnancy have not been adequately studied. If you are pregnant or plan to become pregnant, this drug should be used only when prescribed by your doctor. Ceclor appears in breast milk and could affect a nursing infant. If this medication is essential to your health, your doctor may advise you to stop nursing your baby until your treatment with Ceclor is finished.

Recommended dosage

ADULTS

The usual adult dose is 250 milligrams every 8 hours. For more severe infections (such as pneumonia), your doctor may increase the dosage.

CHILDREN

The usual daily dosage is 20 milligrams per 2.2 pounds of body weight per day divided into smaller doses and taken every 8 hours. In more serious infections, such as middle ear infection, the usual dose is 40 milligrams per 2.2 pounds of body weight per day divided into smaller doses. The total daily dose should not exceed 1 gram.

Overdosage

■ *Symptoms of Ceclor overdose may include:*
   Diarrhea
   Nausea
   Stomach upset
   Vomiting

If other symptoms are present, they may be related to an allergic reaction or other underlying disease. In any case, you should contact your doctor or an emergency room immediately.

Generic name:

CEFACLOR

See Ceclor, page 535.

Generic name:

CEFIXIME

See Suprax, page 749.

Brand name:

CEFTIN

Pronounced: SEF-tin
Generic name: Cefuroxime axetil

Why is this drug prescribed?
Ceftin, a cephalosporin antibiotic, is prescribed for mild to moderately severe bacterial infections of the throat, lungs, ears, skin, and urinary tract, and for gonorrhea.

Most important fact about this drug
If you are allergic to either penicillin or cephalosporin antibiotics in any form, consult your docter *before taking* Ceftin. There is a possibility that you are allergic to both types of medication; if a reaction occurs, it could be extremely severe. If you take the drug and feel signs of a reaction, seek medical attention immediately.

How should you take this medication?
Ceftin can be taken on a full or empty stomach. However, this drug enters the bloodstream and works faster when taken after meals.

Take this medication exactly as prescribed: It is important that you finish taking all of this medication to obtain the maximum benefit.

Ceftin for children is available only in tablet form. If your child cannot swallow the tablet whole, the tablet may be crushed and mixed with food such as applesauce or ice cream. However, the crushed tablet has a strong, bitter taste. If your child cannot swallow the tablet or won't take the medication due to the taste, check with your doctor so that an alternative therapy can be considered.

■ *If you miss a dose...*
Take it as soon as you remember. If it is almost time for your next dose and you take 1 dose a day, take the missed dose and the next dose 10 to 12 hours later. If you take 2 doses a day, take the missed dose and your next dose 5 to 6 hours later. Then go back to the regular schedule. Do not take 2 doses at once.

■ *Storage instructions...*
Store at room temperature in a tightly closed container.

What side effects may occur?
Side effects cannot be anticipated. If any develop or change in intensity, inform your doctor as soon as possible. Only your doctor can determine if it is safe for you to continue taking Ceftin.

■ *More common side effects may include:*
Colitis
Diarrhea
Nausea
Skin rashes, redness, or itching
Vomiting

■ *Less common or rare side effects may include:*
Dizziness, headache, seizures, vaginal inflammation, yeast infection

Why should this drug not be prescribed?
Ceftin should not be prescribed if you have a known allergy to penicillin, cephalosporins, or other drugs.

Special warnings about this medication
Inflammation of the bowel (colitis) has been reported with the use of Ceftin; therefore, if you develop diarrhea while taking this medication, notify your doctor.

Continued or prolonged use of Ceftin may result in an overgrowth of bacteria that do not respond to this medication and can cause a second infection. You should take this drug only when it is prescribed by your doctor, even if you have symptoms like those of a previous infection.

Possible food and drug interactions when taking this medication

It is important to consult with your doctor before taking this drug with probenecid, a gout medication.

If diarrhea occurs while taking Ceftin, consult with your doctor before taking an antidiarrhea medication. Certain drugs, such as Lomotil, may cause your diarrhea to become worse.

This medication may cause a false test result indicating sugar in your urine.

Special information if you are pregnant or breastfeeding

The effects of Ceftin during pregnancy have not been adequately studied. If you are pregnant or plan to become pregnant, inform your doctor immediately. Ceftin appears in breast milk and could affect a nursing infant. If this medication is essential to your health, your doctor may advise you to discontinue breastfeeding until your treatment with this medication is finished.

Recommended dosage

ADULTS

The usual dose for adults and children over 12 years of age is 250 milligrams, 2 times a day. For more severe infections the dose may be increased to 500 milligrams, 2 times a day. The usual dose for urinary tract infection is 125 milligrams, 2 times a day. This dose may be increased to 250 milligrams 2 times a day for severe infection.

The usual dosage for gonorrhea is a single dose of 1 gram.

CHILDREN

The usual dose for children up to 12 years of age is 125 milligrams, 2 times a day.

In middle ear infections, for children under 2 years of age the usual dosage is 125 milligrams, 2 times a day. For children 2 years of age and older it is 250 milligrams, 2 times a day.

ELDERLY

No adjustment of the usual adult dose is necessary.

Overdosage

Any medication taken in excess can have serious consequences. Overdosage with cephalosporin antibiotics can cause brain irritation leading to convulsions. If you suspect an overdose, seek medical attention immediately.

Generic name:

CEFUROXIME

See Ceftin, page 537.

Brand name:

CENTRAX

Pronounced: SEN-tracks
Generic name: Prazepam

Why is this drug prescribed?

Centrax is used in the treatment of anxiety disorders and for short-term relief of the symptoms of anxiety. In addition, doctors sometimes prescribe it to treat alcohol and narcotic withdrawal. It belongs to a class of drugs known as benzodiazepines.

Most important fact about this drug

Tolerance and dependence can occur with the use of Centrax. You may experience withdrawal symptoms if you stop using this drug abruptly. Discontinue or change your dose only in consultation with your doctor.

How should you take this medication?

Take this medication exactly as prescribed by your doctor.

■ *If you miss a dose...*
Take it as soon as you remember. If it is almost time for your next dose, skip the one you missed and go back to your regular schedule. Never take 2 doses at the same time.

■ *Storage instructions...*
Store Centrax at room temperature, protected from moisture.

What side effects may occur?

Side effects cannot be anticipated. If any develop or change in intensity, inform your doctor as soon as possible. Only your doctor can determine if it is safe for you to continue taking Centrax.

■ *More common side effects may include:*
Dizziness
Drowsiness
Fatigue
Lack of muscular coordination
Light-headedness
Weakness

■ *Less common or rare side effects may include:*
Blurred vision, confusion, dry mouth, excessive sweating, fainting, genital and urinary tract disorders, headache, itching, joint pain, palpitations, skin rashes, slurred speech, stomach and intestinal disorders, swelling of feet, tremors, vivid dreams

Why should this drug not be prescribed?

If you are sensitive to or have ever had an allergic reaction to Centrax or similar drugs, you should not take this medication.

Unless you are directed to do so by your doctor, do not take this medication if you have the eye condition known as acute narrow-angle glaucoma.

Centrax should not be prescribed if you are being treated for other emotional disorders more serious than anxiety.

Anxiety or tension related to everyday stress usually does not require treatment with Centrax. Discuss your symptoms thoroughly with your doctor.

Special warnings about this medication

Centrax may cause you to become drowsy or less alert; therefore, driving or operating dangerous machinery or participating in any hazardous activity that requires full mental alertness is not recommended.

If you are severely depressed or have suffered from severe depression, consult with your doctor before taking this medication.

If you take Centrax for a prolonged period of time, your doctor should perform periodic blood and liver tests.

If you have kidney or liver disease, this drug should be used with caution.

Possible food and drug interactions when taking this medication

Like alcohol, Centrax is a central nervous system depressant. Do not drink alcohol while taking this medication.

If Centrax is taken with certain other drugs, the effects of either could be increased, decreased, or altered. It is especially important to check with your doctor before combining Centrax with antidepressants and central nervous system depressants, including the following:

Barbiturates (Phenobarbital)
Cimatidine (Tagamet)
Guanabenz (Wytensin)
MAO inhibitors (antidepressant drugs such as Nardil, Marplan, and Parnate)
Major tranquilizers such as Mellavil and Thorazine
Narcotic pain medications such as Demerol and Percocet

Special information
if you are pregnant or breastfeeding

Do not take Centrax if you are pregnant or planning to become pregnant. There may be an increased risk of birth defects. This drug may appear in breast milk and could affect a nursing infant. If this medication is essential to your health, your doctor may advise you to discontinue breastfeeding until your treatment with this medication is finished.

Recommended dosage

ADULTS

The usual dosage is a total of 30 milligrams per day divided into small doses. Your doctor will adjust the dose gradually to between 20 and 60 milligrams per day, depending on what you need.

Centrax can also be taken as a single dose at bedtime. The recommended starting dose is 20 milligrams. To maximize the anti-anxiety effect with a minimum of daytime drowsiness, your doctor may increase the dose up to a total of 40 milligrams.

CHILDREN

Safety and effectiveness have not been established in children under 18 years of age.

ELDERLY

In the elderly, the usual daily dose is 10 to 15 milligrams, divided into smaller doses.

Overdosage

Any medication taken in excess can have serious consequences. If you suspect an overdose, seek medical attention immediately.

Generic name:

CEPHALEXIN

See Keflex, page 628.

Generic name:

CEPHRADINE

See Velosef, page 788.

Generic name:

CHLORDIAZEPOXIDE

See Librium, page 634.

Generic name:

CHLORDIAZEPOXIDE WITH AMITRIPTYLINE

See Limbitrol, page 636.

Generic name:

CHOLINE MAGNESIUM TRISALICYLATE

See Trilisate, page 775.

Brand name:

CHRONULAC SYRUP

Pronounced: KRON-yoo-lak
Generic name: Lactulose
Other brand name: Duphalac

Why is this drug prescribed?
Chronulac treats constipation. In people who are chronically constipated, Chronulac increases the number and frequency of bowel movements.

Most important fact about this drug
It may take 24 to 48 hours to produce a normal bowel movement.

How should you take this medication?
Take this medication exactly as prescribed. If you find the taste of Chronulac unpleasant, it can be taken with water, fruit juice, or milk.

■ *If you miss a dose...*
Take the forgotten dose as soon as you remember; but do not try to "catch up" by taking a double dose.

■ *Storage instructions...*
Store at room temperature. Avoid excessive heat or direct light. The liquid may darken in color, which is normal.

What side effects may occur?
Side effects cannot be anticipated. If any develop or change in intensity, inform your doctor as soon as possible. Only your doctor can determine if it is safe for you to continue taking Chronulac.

■ *Side effects may include:*
Diarrhea
Gas (temporary, at the beginning of use)
Intestinal cramps (temporary, at the beginning of use)
Nausea

Potassium and fluid loss
Vomiting

Why should this drug not be prescribed?
Chronulac contains galactose, a simple sugar. If you are on a low-galactose diet, do not take this medication.

Special warnings about this medication
Because of its sugar content, this medication should be used with caution if you have diabetes.

If unusual diarrhea occurs, contact your doctor.

Possible food and drug interactions when taking this medication
If Chronulac is taken with certain other drugs, the effects of either could be increased, decreased, or altered. It is especially important to check with your doctor before combining Chronulac with non-absorbable antacids such as Maalox and Mylanta.

Special information if you are pregnant or breastfeeding
The effects of Chronulac during pregnancy have not been adequately studied. If you are pregnant or plan to become pregnant, inform your doctor immediately. Chronulac may appear in breast milk and could affect a nursing infant. If this medication is essential to your health, your doctor may advise you to stop breastfeeding until your treatment is finished.

Recommended dosage
The usual dose is 1 to 2 tablespoonfuls (15 to 30 milliliters) daily. Your doctor may increase the dose to 60 milliliters a day, if necessary.

Overdosage
Any medication taken in excess can have serious consequences. If you suspect an

overdose, seek medical treatment immediately.

■ *Symptoms of Chronulac overdose may include:*
Abdominal cramps
Diarrhea

Brand name:

CIPRO

Pronounced: SIP-roh
Generic name: Ciprofloxacin hydrochloride

Why is this drug prescribed?

Cipro is used to treat infections of the lower respiratory tract, the skin, the bones and joints, and the urinary tract. It is also prescribed for infectious diarrhea; and some doctors also prescribe Cipro for certain serious ear infections, tuberculosis, and some of the infections common in AIDS patients.

Because Cipro is effective only for certain types of bacterial infections, before beginning treatment your doctor may perform tests to identify the specific organisms causing your infection.

Most important fact about this drug

Cipro kills a variety of bacteria, and is frequently used to treat infections in many parts of the body. However, be sure to notify your doctor immediately at the first sign of a skin rash or any other allergic reaction. Although quite rare, serious and occasionally fatal allergic reactions—some following the first dose—have been reported in patients receiving this type of antibacterial drug. Some reactions have been accompanied by collapse of the circulatory system, loss of consciousness, swelling of the face and throat, shortness of breath, tingling, itching, and hives.

How should you take this medication?

Cipro may be taken with or without meals but is best tolerated when taken 2 hours after a meal.

Drink plenty of fluids while taking this medication.

Cipro, like other antibiotics, works best when there is a constant amount in the blood and urine. To help keep the level constant, try not to miss any doses, and take them at evenly spaced intervals around the clock.

■ *If you miss a dose...*
Take it as soon as you remember. If it is almost time for your next dose, skip the one you missed and go back to your regular schedule. Never take 2 doses at the same time.

■ *Storage instructions...*
Cipro should be stored at room temperature.

What side effects may occur?

Side effects cannot be anticipated. If any develop or change in intensity, inform your doctor as soon as possible. Only your doctor can determine if it is safe for you to continue taking Cipro.

■ *More common side effects may include:*
Abdominal pain/discomfort
Diarrhea
Headache
Nausea
Rash
Restlessness
Vomiting

■ *Less common side effects may include:*
Abnormal dread or fear, achiness, bleeding in the stomach and/or intestines, blood clots in the lungs, blurred vision, change in color perception, chills, confusion,

constipation, convulsions, coughing up blood, decreased vision, depression, difficulty in swallowing, dizziness, double vision, drowsiness, eye pain, fainting, fever, flushing, gas, gout flare up, hallucinations, hearing loss, heart attack, hiccups, high blood pressure, hives, inability to fall or stay asleep, inability to urinate, indigestion, intestinal inflammation, involuntary eye movement, irregular heartbeat, irritability, itching, joint or back pain, joint stiffness, kidney failure, labored breathing, lack of muscle coordination, lack or loss of appetite, large volumes of urine, light-headedness, loss of sense of identity, loss of sense of smell, mouth sores, neck pain, nightmares, nosebleed, pounding heartbeat, ringing in the ears, seizures, sensitivity to light, severe allergic reaction, skin peeling, redness, sluggishness, speech difficulties, swelling of the face, neck, lips, eyes, or hands, swelling of the throat, tender, red bumps on skin, tingling sensation, tremors, unpleasant taste, unusual darkening of the skin, vaginal inflammation, vague feeling of illness, weakness, yellowed eyes and skin

Why should this drug not be prescribed?

If you are sensitive to or have ever had an allergic reaction to Cipro or certain other antibiotics of this type, you should not take this medication. Make sure that your doctor is aware of any drug reactions that you have experienced.

Special warnings about this medication

Cipro may cause you to become dizzy or light-headed; therefore, you should not drive a car, operate dangerous machinery, or participate in any hazardous activity that requires full mental alertness until you know how the drug affects you.

Continued or prolonged use of this drug may result in a growth of bacteria that do not respond to this medication and can cause a secondary infection. Therefore, it is important that your doctor monitor your condition on a regular basis.

Convulsions have been reported in people receiving Cipro. If you experience a seizure or convulsion, notify your doctor immediately.

This medication may stimulate the central nervous system, which may lead to tremors, restlessness, light-headedness, confusion, and hallucinations. If these reactions occur, consult your doctor at once.

If you have a known or suspected central nervous system disorder such as epilepsy or hardening of the arteries in the brain, make sure your doctor knows about it when prescribing Cipro.

You may become more sensitive to light while taking this drug. Try to stay out of the sun as much as possible.

If you must take Cipro for an extended period of time, your doctor will probably order blood tests and tests for urine, kidney, and liver function.

Possible food and drug interactions when taking this medication

Serious and fatal reactions have occurred when Cipro was taken in combination with theophylline (Theo-Dur). These reactions have included cardiac arrest, seizures, status epilepticus (continuous attacks of epilepsy with no periods of consciousness), and respiratory failure.

Products containing iron, multi-vitamins containing zinc, or antacids containing magnesium, aluminum, or calcium, when taken in combination with Cipro, may interfere with absorption of this medication.

Cipro may increase the effects of caffeine.

If Cipro is taken with certain other drugs, the effects of either also could be increased, decreased, or altered. These drugs include:

Cyclophosphamide (Cytoxan)
Cyclosporine (Sandimmune)
Metoprolol (Lopressor)
Phenytoin (Dilantin)
Probenecid (Benemid)
Sucralfate (Carafate)
Theophylline (Theo-Dur)
Warfarin (Coumadin)

Special information
if you are pregnant or breastfeeding

The effects of Cipro during pregnancy have not been adequately studied. If you are pregnant or plan to become pregnant, notify your doctor immediately. Cipro does appear in breast milk and could affect a nursing infant. If this medication is essential to your health, your doctor may advise you to discontinue breastfeeding your baby until your treatment is finished.

Recommended dosage

ADULTS

The length of treatment with Cipro depends upon the severity of infection. Generally, Cipro should be continued for at least 2 days after the signs and symptoms of infection have disappeared. The usual length of time is 7 to 14 days; however, for severe and complicated infections, treatment may be prolonged.

Bone and joint infections may require treatment for 4 to 6 weeks or longer.

Infectious diarrhea may be treated for 5 to 7 days.

Urinary Tract Infections
The usual adult dosage is 250 milligrams taken every 12 hours. Complicated infections, as determined by your doctor,

may require 500 milligrams taken every 12 hours.

Lower Respiratory Tract, Skin, Bone, and Joint Infections
The usual recommended dosage is 500 milligrams taken every 12 hours. Complicated infections, as determined by your doctor, may require a dosage of 750 milligrams taken every 12 hours.

Infectious Diarrhea
The recommended dosage is 500 milligrams taken every 12 hours.

CHILDREN

Safety and effectiveness have not been established in children and adolescents under 18 years of age.

Overdosage

Any medication taken in excess can have serious consequences. If you suspect an overdose, seek medical attention immediately.

Generic name:

CIPROFLOXACIN

See Cipro, page 542.

Brand name:

CLEOCIN T

Pronounced: KLEE-oh-sin
Generic name: Clindamycin phosphate

Why is this drug prescribed?
Cleocin T is an antibiotic used to treat acne.

Most important fact about this drug
Although applied only to the skin, some of this medication could be absorbed into the

bloodstream; and it has been known to cause severe—sometimes even fatal—colitis (an inflamation of the lower bowel) when taken internally. Symptoms, which can occur a few days, weeks, or months after beginning treatment with this drug, include severe diarrhea, severe abdominal cramps, and the possibility of the passage of blood.

How should you take this medication?
Use this medication exactly as prescribed. Excessive use of Cleocin T can cause your skin to become too dry or irritated.

- *If you miss a dose...*
  Apply it as soon as you remember. If it is almost time for your next dose, skip the one you missed and go back to your regular schedule.

- *Storage instructions...*
  Store at room temperature. Keep from freezing.

What side effects may occur?
Side effects cannot be anticipated. If any develop or change in intensity, inform your doctor as soon as possible. Only your doctor can determine if it is safe for you to continue taking Cleocin T.

The most common side effect is skin dryness.

- *Less common or rare side effects may include:*
  Abdominal pain, bloody diarrhea, burning or abnormal redness of skin, colitis, diarrhea, oily skin, peeling skin, skin inflammation and irritation, stomach and intestinal disturbances

Why should this drug not be prescribed?
If you are sensitive to or have ever had an allergic reaction to Cleocin T or similar drugs, you should not use this medication.

Make sure your doctor is aware of any drug reactions you have experienced.

Unless you are directed to do so by your doctor, do not take this medication if you have ever had an intestinal inflammation, ulcerative colitis, or antibiotic-associated colitis.

Special warnings about this medication
Cleocin T contains an alcohol base, which can cause burning and irritation of the eyes. It also has an unpleasant taste. Use caution when applying this medication so as not to get it in the eyes, nose, mouth, or skin abrasions. In the event of accidental contact, rinse the affected area with cool water.

Use with caution if you have hay fever, asthma, or eczema.

Possible food and drug interactions when taking this medication
If you have diarrhea while taking Cleocin T, check with your doctor before taking an antidiarrhea medication, as certain drugs may cause your diarrhea to become worse.

The diarrhea should not be treated with the commonly used drugs that slow movement through the intestinal tract, such as Lomotil or products containing paregoric.

Special information if you are pregnant or breastfeeding
The effects of Cleocin T during pregnancy have not been adequately studied. If you are pregnant or plan to become pregnant, inform your doctor immediately. Cleocin T may appear in breast milk and could affect a nursing infant. If this medication is essential to your health, your doctor may advise you to discontinue breastfeeding your baby until your treatment with this medication is finished.

Recommended dosage

ADULTS

Apply a thin film of gel, solution, or lotion to the affected area 2 times a day.

If you are using the lotion, shake it well immediately before using.

CHILDREN

The safety and effectiveness of Cleocin T have not been established in children under 12 years of age.

Overdosage

Although there is no information on Cleocin T overdose, any medication taken in excess can have serious consequences. If you suspect an overdose, seek medical attention immediately.

Brand name:

CLEOCIN VAGINAL CREAM

Pronounced: KLEE-oh-sin
Generic name: Clindamycin phosphate

Why is this drug prescribed?

Cleocin Vaginal Cream is used to treat bacterial vaginosis, an infection of the vagina. The infection, which is probably sexually transmitted, often produces a gray or yellow discharge with a fishy smell that increases after you wash your external genitals with alkaline soap.

Before prescribing Cleocin, your doctor will test the vaginal discharge in the laboratory and examine it under the microscope to make certain that you do not have a yeast infection or another sexually transmitted disease (STD) such as chlamydia, gonorrhea, or herpes simplex.

Most important fact about this drug

Keep using Cleocin Vaginal Cream for the full time of treatment, even if the infection seems to have disappeared. If you stop too soon, the infection could return. Continue the treatment even if you have a period.

How should you take this medication?

Use this medication exactly as prescribed by your doctor.

Each tube of Cleocin comes with seven disposable plastic applicators. Remove the cap from the tube and screw an applicator on the threaded end of the tube. Roll the tube from the bottom while squeezing it gently to force the medication into the applicator. Stop squeezing when the plunger reaches the top of the applicator and no longer moves. Unscrew the applicator from the tube and replace the cap.

While lying on your back, firmly grasp the applicator barrel and insert it into your vagina as far as possible without causing any discomfort. Slowly push the plunger until it stops.

Carefully withdraw the empty applicator from your vagina and discard it.

To keep the medication from soiling your clothing, wear a sanitary napkin. Do not use a tampon because it will absorb the medication. Wear cotton underwear; avoid synthetic fabrics such as rayon or nylon.

Do not scratch if you can help it. Scratching can cause more irritation and can spread the infection.

■ *If you miss a dose...*
   Take the forgotten dose as soon as you remember. If is almost time for the next dose, skip the one you missed and go back to your regular schedule.

■ *Storage instructions...*
Store Cleocin Vaginal Cream at room temperature and protect from freezing.

What side effects may occur?

Side effects cannot be anticipated. If any develop or change in intensity, stop using the medication immediately and inform your doctor as soon as possible. Only your doctor can determine if it is safe for you to continue using Cleocin Vaginal Cream.

■ *More common side effects may include:*
Inflammation of the cervix
Inflammation of the vagina
Irritation of the vulva
Yeast infection caused by *Candida albicans*

■ *Less common side effects may include:*
Frothy pale yellow or green smelly vaginal discharge with vaginal burning and itching

■ *Rare side effects may include:*
Abdominal pain, constipation, diarrhea, dizziness, headache, heartburn, hives, nausea, rash, vertigo, vomiting

When other clindamycin preparations are applied to the skin or taken by mouth or injection, side effects may develop. Although Cleocin Vaginal Cream has a lower concentration of clindamycin than these other medications, it is possible the following reactions will appear when you are using it.

■ *Side effects from clindamycin applied to the skin may include:*
Abdominal pain, burning sensation, inflammation of the hair follicles, oily skin, peeling skin, severe inflammation of the large intestine (bowel), skin redness, stomach and intestinal problems

■ *Side effects from clindamycin taken by mouth or injection may include:*
Abdominal pain, arthritis in more than one joint, diarrhea, hives, inflammation of the upper gastric tract, nausea, severe allergic reaction, skin rash, skin redness, vomiting, yellow skin and eyes

Why should this drug not be prescribed?

Do not use Cleocin Vaginal Cream if you are sensitive to clindamycin or lincomycin or if you have ever had an allergic reaction to these drugs.

If you have a history of Crohn's disease (a chronic inflammation of the large intestine), ulcerative colitis (repeated episodes of inflammation of the large intestine and rectum), or inflammation of the bowel caused by antibiotics, do not use Cleocin Vaginal Cream.

Special warnings about this medication

When taken orally or by injection, clindamycin can cause pseudomembranous colitis, a disease which produces diarrhea, fever, and stomach cramps. Even though Cleocin is only applied to the vagina, a small percentage of the medication is absorbed into your system and could cause colitis. If you have diarrhea while using Cleocin Vaginal Cream, call your doctor for advice. Regular diarrhea medications could be dangerous.

The mineral oil in Cleocin Vaginal Cream may weaken latex or rubber products such as condoms or diaphragms. Wait at least 72 hours after stopping treatment with Cleocin before using these contraceptive devices.

Do not have vaginal intercourse while using this medication.

If you accidentally get Cleocin Vaginal Cream in your eyes, it can cause burning and irritation. Rinse immediately with large amount of cool tap water.

This medication may promote a vaginal yeast infection. If you develop itching, redness, and irritation in your vagina or vulva, or a thick, cottage cheese-like discharge, inform your doctor.

Possible food and drug interactions when taking this medication
There are no reports of interactions with other drugs you would use at home. Cleocin does interact with certain drugs used prior to surgery.

Special information if you are pregnant or breastfeeding
The effects of Cleocin Vaginal Cream during pregnancy have not been adequately studied. If you are pregnant or plan to become pregnant, inform your doctor immediately. It is not known whether clindamycin appears in breast milk when the drug is applied to the vagina. However, when clindamycin is injected or taken by mouth, the medication does make its way into breast milk. If Cleocin Vaginal Cream is essential to your health, your doctor may advise you to discontinue breastfeeding until your treatment is finished.

Recommended dosage
Insert 1 applicatorful (about 5 grams) of Cleocin Vaginal Cream in your vagina each night, preferably at bedtime. Continue using the medication for 7 consecutive days or as prescribed by your doctor.

Overdosage
An overdose of Cleocin Vaginal Cream is unlikely. However, any medication taken in excess can have serious consequences. If you suspect an overdose, seek medical attention immediately.

Generic name:

CLINDAMYCIN
See Cleocin T, page 544, Cleocin Vaginal Cream, page 546.

Brand name:

CLINORIL
Pronounced: CLIN-or-il
Generic name: Sulindac

Why is this drug prescribed?
Clinoril, a nonsteroidal anti-inflammatory drug, is used to relieve the inflammation, swelling, stiffness and joint pain associated with rheumatoid arthritis, osteoarthritis (the most common form of arthritis), and ankylosing spondylitis (stiffness and progressive arthritis of the spine.) It is also used to treat bursitis, tendinitis, acute gouty arthritis, and other types of pain.

The safety and effectiveness of this medication in the treatment of people with rheumatoid arthritis who are incapacitated, almost or completely bedridden, in wheelchairs, or unable to care for themselves, have not been established.

Most important fact about this drug
You should have frequent checkups with your doctor if you take Clinoril regularly. Ulcers or internal bleeding can occur without warning.

How should you take this medication?
Take this medication exactly as prescribed by your doctor.

If you are using Clinoril for arthritis, it should be taken regularly.

■ *If you miss a dose...*
Take it as soon as you remember. If it is almost time for your next dose, skip the one you missed and go back to your regular schedule. Never take two doses at the same time.

■ *Storage instructions...*
Do not store in damp places like the bathroom.

What side effects may occur?

Side effects cannot be anticipated. If any develop or change in intensity, inform your doctor as soon as possible. Only your doctor can determine if it is safe for you to continue taking Clinoril.

■ *More common side effects may include:*
Abdominal pain, constipation, diarrhea, dizziness, gas, headache, indigestion, itching, loss of appetite, nausea, nervousness, rash, ringing in ears, stomach cramps, swelling due to fluid retention, vomiting

■ *Less common or rare side effects may include:*
Abdominal bleeding, abdominal inflammation, anemia, appetite change, bloody diarrhea, blurred vision, change in color of urine, chest pain, colitis, congestive heart failure, depression, fever, hair loss, hearing loss, hepatitis, high blood pressure, inability to sleep, inflammation of lips and tongue, kidney failure, liver failure, loss of sense of taste, low blood pressure, muscle and joint pain, nosebleed, painful urination, pancreatitis, peptic ulcer, sensitivity to light, shortness of breath, skin eruptions, sleepiness, Stevens-Johnson syndrome (blisters in the mouth and eyes), vaginal bleeding, weakness, yellow eyes and skin

Why should this drug not be prescribed?

If you are sensitive to or have ever had an allergic reaction to Clinoril, aspirin, or similar drugs, or if you have had asthma attacks caused by aspirin or other drugs of this type, you should not take this medication. Make sure that your doctor is aware of any drug reactions that you have experienced.

Special warnings about this medication

Peptic ulcers and bleeding can occur without warning.

This drug should be used with caution if you have kidney or liver disease; it can cause liver inflammation in some people.

Do not take aspirin or any other anti-inflammatory medications while taking Clinoril, unless your doctor tells you to do so.

Nonsteroidal anti-inflammatory drugs such as Clinoril can hide the signs and symptoms of an infection. Be sure your doctor knows about any infection you may have.

Clinoril can cause vision problems. If you experience a change in your vision, inform your doctor.

If you have heart disease or high blood pressure, this drug can increase water retention. Use with caution.

If you develop pancreatitis (inflammation of the pancreas), Clinoril should be stopped immediately and not restarted.

Clinoril may cause you to become drowsy or less alert. If this happens, driving or operating dangerous machinery or participating in any hazardous activity that requires full mental alertness is not recommended.

Possible food and drug interactions when taking this medication

If Clinoril is taken with certain other drugs, the effects of either could be increased, decreased, or altered. It is especially important to check with your doctor before combining Clinoril with the following:

Aspirin
Blood thinners such as Coumadin and
    Panwarfin
Cyclosporine (Sandimmune)
Diflunisal (Dolobid)
Dimethyl sulfoxide (dmso)
Lithium
Loop diuretics such as Lasix
Methotrexate
Oral diabetes medications
The anti-gout medication Benemid

Special information if you are pregnant or breastfeeding

The effects of Clinoril during pregnancy have not been adequately studied; drugs of this class are known to cause birth defects. If you are pregnant or plan to become pregnant, inform your doctor immediately. Clinoril may appear in breast milk and could affect a nursing infant. If this medication is essential to your health, your doctor may advise you to discontinue breastfeeding until your treatment with Clinoril is finished.

Recommended dosage

ADULTS

Osteoarthritis, Rheumatoid Arthritis, Ankylosing Spondylitis
Starting dosage is 150 milligrams 2 times a day. Take with food. Doses should not exceed 400 milligrams per day.

Acute Gouty Arthritis or Arthritic Shoulder and Joint Condition
400 milligrams daily taken in doses of 200 milligrams 2 times a day.

For acute painful shoulder, therapy lasting 7 to 14 days is usually adequate.

For acute gouty arthritis, therapy lasting 7 days is usually adequate.

The lowest dose that proves beneficial should be used.

CHILDREN

The safety and effectiveness of Clinoril have not been established in children.

Overdosage

Any medication taken in excess can cause symptoms of overdose. If you suspect an overdose, seek medical attention immediately.

■ *Symptoms of Clinoril overdose may include:*
Coma
Low blood pressure
Reduced output of urine
Stupor

Brand name:

CLOMID

See Clomiphene Citrate, page 550.

Generic name:

CLOMIPHENE CITRATE

Pronounced: KLAHM-if-een SIT-rate
Brand names: Clomid, Serophene

Why is this drug prescribed?

Clomiphene is prescribed for the treatment of ovulatory failure in women who wish to become pregnant and whose husbands are fertile and potent.

Most important fact about this drug

Properly timed sexual intercourse is very important to increase the chances of conception. The likelihood of conception diminishes with each succeeding course of treatment. Your doctor will determine the need for continuing therapy after the first course. If you do not become pregnant after 3 courses, your doctor will stop the therapy.

How should you take this medication?
Take this medication exactly as prescribed by your doctor.

■ *If you miss a dose...*
Take it as soon as you remember. If it is time for your next dose, take the 2 doses together and go back to your regular schedule. If you miss more than 1 dose, contact your doctor.

■ *Storage instructions...*
Store at room temperature in a tightly closed container, away from light, moisture, and excessive heat.

What side effects may occur?
Side effects occur infrequently and generally do not interfere with treatment at the recommended dosage of clomiphene. They tend to occur more frequently at higher doses and during long-term treatment.

■ *More common side effects include:*
Abdominal discomfort
Enlargement of the ovaries
Hot flushes

■ *Less common side effects include:*
Abnormal uterine bleeding, breast tenderness, depression, dizziness, fatigue, hair loss, headache, hives, inability to fall or stay asleep, increased urination, inflammation of the skin, light-headedness, nausea, nervousness, ovarian cysts, visual disturbances, vomiting, weight gain

Why should this drug not be prescribed?
If you are pregnant or think you may be, do not take this drug.

Unless directed to do so by your doctor, do not use this medication if you have an uncontrolled thyroid or adrenal gland disorder, an abnormality of the brain such as a pituitary gland tumor, a liver disease or a history of liver problems, abnormal uterine bleeding of undetermined origin, ovarian cysts, or enlargement of the ovaries not caused by polycystic ovarian syndrome (a hormonal disorder causing lack of ovulation).

Special warnings about this medication
Your doctor will evaluate you for normal liver function and normal estrogen levels before considering you for treatment with clomiphene.

Your doctor will also examine you for pregnancy, ovarian enlargement, or cyst formation prior to treatment with this drug and between each treatment cycle. He or she will do a complete pelvic examination before each course of this medication.

Clomiphene treatment increases the possibility of multiple births; also, birth defects have been reported following treatment to induce ovulation with clomiphene, although no direct effects of the drug on the unborn child have been established.

Because blurring and other visual symptoms may occur occasionally with clomiphene treatment, you should be cautious about driving a car or operating dangerous machinery, especially under conditions of variable lighting.

If you experience visual disturbances, notify your doctor immediately. Symptoms of visual disturbance may include blurring, spots or flashes, double vision, intolerance to light, decreased visual sharpness, loss of peripheral vision, and distortion of space.

Your doctor may recommend a complete evaluation by an eye specialist.

Ovarian hyperstimulation syndrome (or OHSS, enlargement of the ovary) has occurred in women receiving treatment with clomiphene. OHSS may progress rapidly and become serious. The early warning signs are severe pelvic pain, nausea, vomiting, and weight gain. Symptoms include abdominal pain, abdominal enlargement, nausea, vomiting, diarrhea, weight gain, difficult or labored breathing, and less urine production. If you experience any of these warning signs or symptoms, notify your doctor immediately.

To lessen the risks associated with abnormal ovarian enlargement during treatment with clomiphene, the lowest effective dose should be prescribed. Women with the hormonal disorder, polycystic ovarian syndrome, may be unusually sensitive to certain hormones and may respond abnormally to usual doses of this drug. If you experience pelvic pain, notify your doctor. He may discontinue your use of clomiphene until the ovaries return to pretreatment size.

Because the safety of long-term treatment with clomiphene has not been established, your doctor will not prescribe more than 3 courses of therapy.

Possible food and drug interactions when taking this medication
No food or drug interactions have been reported with clomiphene therapy.

Special information if you are pregnant or breastfeeding
If you become pregnant, notify your doctor immediately. You should not be taking this drug while you are pregnant.

Recommended dosage
The recommended dosage for the first course of treatment is 50 milligrams (1 tablet) daily for 5 days. If ovulation does not appear to have occurred, your doctor may prescribe up to 2 more courses of treatment.

Overdosage
Taking any medication in excess can have serious consequences. If you suspect an overdose of clomiphene, contact your doctor immediately.

Generic name:

CLORAZEPATE

See Tranxene, page 769.

Generic name:

CLOTRIMAZOLE

See Gyne-Lotrimin, page 612.

Brand name:

COGNEX

Pronounced: COG-necks
Generic name: Tacrine hydrochloride

Why is this drug prescribed?
Cognex is used for the treatment of mild to moderate Alzheimer's disease. This progressive, degenerative disorder causes physical changes in the brain that disrupt the flow of information and affect memory, thinking, and behavior. As someone caring for an Alzheimer's patient, you should be aware that Cognex is not a cure, but has helped some patients.

Most important fact about this drug

Do not abruptly stop Cognex treatment, or reduce the dosage, without consulting the doctor. A sudden reduction can cause the person you are caring for to become more disturbed and forgetful. Taking more Cognex than the doctor advises can also cause serious problems. Do not change the dosage of Cognex unless instructed by the doctor.

How should you take this medication?

This medication will work better if taken at regular intervals, usually 4 times a day. Cognex is best taken between meals; however, if it is irritating to the stomach, the doctor may advise taking it with meals. If Cognex is not taken regularly, as the doctor directs, the condition may get worse.

- *If you miss a dose...*
  Give the forgotten dose as soon as possible. If it is within 2 hours of the next dose, skip the missed dose and go back to the regular schedule. Do not double the doses.

- *Storage instructions...*
  Store at room temperature away from moisture.

What side effects may occur?

Side effects cannot be anticipated. If any develop or change in intensity, tell the doctor as soon as possible. Only the doctor can determine if it is safe to continue giving Cognex.

- *More common side effects may include:*
  Abdominal pain, abnormal thinking, agitation, anxiety, chest pain, clumsiness or unsteadiness, confusion, constipation, coughing, depression, diarrhea, dizziness, fatigue, flushing, frequent urination, gas, headache, inflamed nasal passages, insomnia, indigestion, liver function disorders, loss of appetite, muscle pain, nausea, rash, sleepiness, upper respiratory infection, urinary tract infection, vomiting, weight loss

- *Less common side effects may include:*
  Back pain, hallucinations, hostile attitude, purple or red spots on the skin, skin discoloration, tremor, weakness

Be sure to report any symptoms that develop while on Cognex therapy. You should alert the doctor if the person you are caring for develops nausea, vomiting, loose stools, or diarrhea at the start of therapy or when the dosage is increased. Later in therapy, be on the lookout for rash, yellowing of the eyes and skin, or changes in the color of the stool.

Why should this drug not be prescribed?

People who are sensitive to or have ever had an allergic reaction to Cognex should not take this medication. Before starting treatment with Cognex, it is important to discuss any medical problems with the doctor. If during previous Cognex therapy the person you are caring for developed jaundice (yellow skin and eyes), which signals that something is wrong with the liver, Cognex should not be used again.

Special warnings about this medication

Use Cognex with caution if the person you are caring for has a history of liver disease, certain heart disorders, stomach ulcers, or asthma.

Because of the risk of liver problems when taking Cognex, the doctor will schedule weekly blood tests to monitor liver function for the first 18 weeks on treatment. After 18 weeks, blood tests will be given every 3 months. When the doctor increases the dose of Cognex, he or she will resume weekly monitoring of the liver for at least 6 weeks. If the person you are caring for develops any liver problems, the doctor may temporarily discontinue Cognex treatment until further testing shows that the liver has returned to normal. If the doctor resumes Cognex treatment, he or she will reinstate weekly monitoring of the liver.

Before having any surgery, including dental surgery, tell the doctor that the person is being treated with Cognex.

Cognex can cause seizures, and may cause difficulty urinating.

Possible food and drug interactions when taking this medication

If Congex is taken with certain other drugs, the effects of either could be increased, decreased, or altered. It is especially important that you check with your doctor before combining Cognex with the following:

Antispasmodic drugs such as Bentyl and
   Cogentin
Bethanechol chloride (Urecholine)
Cimetidine (Tagamet)
Theophylline (Theo-Dur)

Special information if you are pregnant or breastfeeding

The effects of Cognex during pregnancy have not been studied; and it is not known whether Cognex appears in breast milk.

Recommended dosage

ADULTS

The usual starting dose is 10 milligrams 4 times a day, for at least 6 weeks. Do not increase the dose during this 6-week period unless directed by your doctor. The doctor may then increase the dosage to 20 milligrams 4 times a day.

Restarting Cognex Therapy
The recommended restarting dose if 10 milligrams 4 times a day for 6 weeks.

The doctor may adjust the dose at regular intervals.

CHILDREN

The safety and effectiveness of Cognex have not been established in children.

Overdosage

Any medication taken in excess can have serious consequences. If you suspect an overdose, seek medical attention immediately.

■ *Symptoms of Cognex overdose include:*
  Collapse
  Convulsions
  Extreme muscle weakness, possibly ending
    in death (if breathing muscles are
    affected)
  Low blood pressure
  Nausea
  Salivation
  Slowed heart rate
  Sweating
  Vomiting

Brand name:

COLACE

Pronounced: KOH-lace
Generic name: Docusate sodium

Why is this drug prescribed?

Colace, a stool softner, promotes easy bowel movements without straining. It softens the stool by mixing in fat and water. Colace is helpful for people who have had recent recent rectal surgery, people with heart problems or high blood pressure, patients with hernias, and women who have just had babies.

Most important fact about this drug

Colace is for short-term relief only, unless your doctor directs otherwise. It usually takes a day or two for the drug to achieve its laxative effect; some people may need to wait 4 or 5 days.

How should you take this medication?

To conceal the drug's bitter taste, take Colace liquid in half a glass of milk or fruit juice; it can be given in infant formula. The proper dosage of this medication may also be added to a retention or flushing enema.

- *If you miss a dose...*
  Take this medication only as needed.

- *Storage instructions...*
  Store at room temperature. Keep from freezing.

What side effects may occur?

Side effects are unlikely. The main ones reported are bitter taste, throat irritation, and nausea (mainly associated with use of the syrup and liquid). Rash has occurred.

Why should this drug not be prescribed?

There are no known reasons this drug should not be prescribed.

Possible food and drug interactions when taking this medication

No interactions have been reported with Colace.

Special information if you are pregnant or breastfeeding

If you are pregnant, plan to become pregnant, or are breastfeeding your baby, notify your doctor before using this medication.

Recommended dosage

Your doctor will adjust the dosage according to your needs.

You will be using higher doses at the start of treatment with Colace. You should see an effect on stools 1 to 3 days after the first dose.

ADULTS AND CHILDREN 12 AND OLDER

The suggested daily dosage is 50 to 200 milligrams.

In enemas, add 50 to 100 milligrams of Colace or 5 to 10 milliliters of Colace liquid to a retention or flushing enema, as prescribed by your doctor.

CHILDREN UNDER 12

The suggested daily dosage for children 6 to 12 years of age is 40 to 120 milligrams; for children 3 to 6 years of age, it is 20 to 60 milligrams; for children under 3 years of age, it is 10 to 40 milligrams.

Overdosage

Overdose is unlikely with the normal use of Colace.

Brand name:

CONDYLOX

Pronounced: CON-de-lox
Generic name: Podofilox

Why is this drug prescribed?

Condylox is used to treat external genital warts.

Most important fact about this drug

Use Condylox solution only on the surface of the skin. Do not use it for warts in the area between the vagina and rectum, or for warts on mucous membranes in the linings of various parts of the body, including the vagina, rectum, and urethra.

How should you take this medication?

Use this medication exactly as prescribed by your doctor.

To help you understand the right way to apply Condylox solution and to correctly identify the warts that need treatment, your doctor will demonstrate the proper technique for the first treatment. Your doctor may also give you an instruction sheet with a diagram of the female genital area to enable you to see exactly where to apply the medication. A patient information leaflet is also available with the product.

After you have a thorough understanding of how and where to apply Condylox, use the cotton-tipped applicator supplied with the product to treat your warts. Touch the wart with the drug-dampened applicator, applying only enough to cover the wart. Do not apply too much medication.

Be sure to limit treatment to less than one and a half square inches of wart tissue and to no more than 10 drops of Condylox solution per day. Let the solution dry before letting parts of your body touch the wart. When you have finished, dispose of the applicator and wash your hands.

If your condition does not completely clear up after 4 weeks of treatment, check with your doctor; he or she may want to consider using another medication.

■ *If you miss a dose...*
Resume your normal schedule with the next dose.

■ *Storage instructions...*
Store at room temperature. Avoid excessive heat. Do not freeze.

What side effects may occur?

Side effects cannot be anticipated. If any develop or change in intensity, tell your doctor as soon as possible. Only your doctor can determine if it is safe to continue using Condylox solution.

■ *More common side effects may include:*
Burning
Erosion (the wearing away of the skin surface)
Inflammation
Itching
Pain

■ *Less common side effects may include:*
Bleeding, blistering, blood in the urine, chafing, crusting, dizziness, dryness and peeling, edema (swelling with fluid), inability to retract the foreskin, inability to sleep, offensive or bad odor, pain with intercourse, scarring, skin ulceration, tenderness, tingling, and vomiting

Why should this drug not be prescribed?

If you have ever had an allergic reaction to or are sensitive to podofilox, you should not use this medication. Make sure your doctor is aware of any drug reactions you have experienced.

Special warnings about this medication

Remember that Condylox solution is for use only on the surface of your skin. If you should accidentally get the solution in your eye, flush it out immediately with plenty of water and call your doctor.

Do not use more than the recommended dosage. It is not known whether additonal medication will add to effectiveness, but additional applications of Condylox could be absorbed through the skin, causing an increase in side effects.

Possible food and drug interactions when taking this medication

No interactions with Condylox have been reported.

Special information
if you are pregnant or breastfeeding

The effects of Condylox during pregnancy have not been adequately studied. If you are pregnant or plan to become pregnant, tell your doctor immediately. Is is not known whether Condylox appears in breast milk. If you are nursing or plan to nurse, your doctor will decide whether you should stop nursing or discontinue the medication.

Recommended dosage

ADULTS

Apply Condylox twice daily, once in the morning and once in the evening (every 12 hours) for 3 consecutive days, then stop using the medication for 4 consecutive days. Repeat this cycle up to 4 times, until there is no visible art tissue.

CHILDREN

The safety and effectiveness of Condylox in children have not been determined.

Overdosage

Any medication taken in excess can have serious consequences. If too much Condylos is absorbed through the skin, it could cause the symptoms listed below. If you suspect an overdose, seek medical attention immediately.

■ *Symptoms of Condylox overdose may include:*
Abnormally fast breathing, blood in the urine, changes in mental attitude, coma, diarrhea, fever, kidney failure, lethargy (sluggishness), nausea, respiratory failure, seizures, vomiting

If you should accidentally apply too much Condylox solution, wash your skin thoroughly and call your doctor.

Generic name:

CONJUGATED ESTROGENS

See Premarin, page 722.

Brand name:

COTRIM

See Bactrim, page 523.

Brand name:

CO-TRIMOXAZOLE

See Bactrim, page 523.

Generic name:

CYCLOPHOSPHAMIDE

See Cytoxan, page 557.

Brand name:

CYCRIN

See Provera, page 727.

Brand name:

CYTOXAN

Pronounced: sigh-TOKS-an
Generic name: Cyclophosphamide

Why is this drug prescribed?

Cytoxan, an anticancer drug, works by interfering with the growth of malignant cells. It may be used alone but is often given with other anticancer medications.

Cytoxan is used in the treatment of the following types of cancer:

Breast cancer

Leukemias (cancers affecting the white blood cells)

Malignant lymphomas (Hodgkin's disease or cancer of the lymph nodes)

Multiple myeloma (a malignant condition or cancer of the plasma cells)

Advanced mycosis fungoides (cancer of the skin and lymph nodes)

Neuroblastoma (a malignant tumor of the adrenal gland or sympathetic nervous system)

Ovarian cancer (adenocarcinoma)

Retinoblastoma (a malignant tumor of the retina)

In addition, Cytoxan may sometimes be given to children who have "minimal change" nephrotic syndrome (kidney damage resulting in loss of protein in the urine) and who have not responded well to treatment with steroid medications.

Most important fact about this drug

Cytoxan may cause bladder damage, probably from toxic byproducts of the drug that are excreted in the urine. Potential problems include bladder infection with bleeding and fibrosis of the bladder.

While you are being treated with Cytoxan, drink 3 or 4 liters of fluid a day to help prevent bladder problems. The extra fluid will dilute your urine and make you urinate frequently, thus minimizing the Cytoxan byproducts' contact with your bladder.

How should you take this medication?

Take Cytoxan exactly as prescribed. You will undergo frequent blood tests, and the doctor will adjust your dosage depending on the evolution of your white blood cell count; a dosage reduction is necessary if the count drops below a certain level. You will also have frequent urine tests to check for

blood in the urine, a sign of bladder damage.

Take Cytoxan on an empty stomach. If you have severe stomach upset, then you may take it with food.

If you are unable to swallow the tablet form, you may be given an oral solution made from the injectable form of Cytoxan and Aromatic Elixir. This solution should be used within 14 days.

■ *If you miss a dose...*
Do not take the dose you missed. Go back to your regular schedule and contact your doctor. Do not take 2 doses at once.

■ *Storage instructions...*
Store tablets at room temperature. Store the oral solution in the refrigerator.

What side effects may occur?

Side effects cannot be anticipated. If any develop or change in intensity, inform your doctor immediately. Only your doctor can determine if it is safe for you to continue using Cytoxan.

One possible Cytoxan side effect is the development of a secondary cancer, typically of the bladder, lymph nodes, or bone marrow. A secondary cancer may occur up to several years after the drug is given.

Cytoxan can lower the activity of your immune system, making you more vulnerable to infection.

Noncancerous bladder problems may occur during Cytoxan therapy (see "Most important fact about this drug" section, above).

■ *More common side effects may include:*
Loss of appetite
Nausea and vomiting
Temporary hair loss

■ *Less common or rare side effects may include:*

Abdominal pain, anemia, bleeding, inflamed colon, darkening of skin and changes in fingernails, decreased sperm count, diarrhea, impaired wound healing, mouth sores, new tumor growth, prolonged impairment of fertility or temporary sterility in men, rash, severe allergic reaction, temporary failure to menstruate, yellowing of eyes and skin

Why should this drug not be prescribed?

Do not take this medication if you have ever had an allergic reaction to it.

Also, tell your doctor if you have ever had an allergic reaction to another alkylating anticancer drug such as Alkeran, CeeNU, Emcyt, Leukeran, Myleran, or Zanosar.

In adults, Cytoxan should not be given for "minimal change" nephrotic syndrome or any other kidney disease.

Also, Cytoxan should not be given to anyone who is unable to produce normal blood cells because the bone marrow— where blood cells are made—is not functioning well.

Special warnings about this medication

You are at increased risk for toxic side effects from Cytoxan if you have any of the following conditions:

Blood disorder (low white blood cell or platelet count)
Bone marrow tumors
Kidney disorder
Liver disorder
Past anticancer therapy
Past X-ray therapy

Possible food and drug interactions when taking this medication

If Cytoxan is taken with certain other drugs, the effects of either could be increased, decreased, or altered. It is especially important to check with your doctor before combining Cytoxan with the following:

Adriamycin (another anticancer drug)
Allopurinol (the gout medicine Zyloprim)
Anectine (used in anesthesia)
Digoxin (the heart medication Lanoxin)
Phenobarbital

If you take adrenal steroid hormones because you have had your adrenal glands removed, you are at increased risk for toxic effects from Cytoxan; your dosage of both steroids and Cytoxan may need to be modified.

Special information if you are pregnant or breastfeeding

If you are pregnant or plan to become pregnant, inform your doctor immediately. When taken during pregnancy, Cytoxan can cause defects in the unborn baby. Women taking Cytoxan should use effective contraception. Cytoxan does appear in breast milk. A new mother will need to choose between taking this drug and nursing her baby.

Recommended dosage

ADULTS AND CHILDREN

Malignant Diseases
Your doctor will tailor your dosage according to your condition and other drugs taken with Cytoxan.

The recommended oral dosage range is 1 to 5 milligrams per 2.2 pounds of body weight per day.

CHILDREN

"Minimal Change" Nephrotic Syndrome
The recommended oral dosage is 2.5 to 3
milligrams per 2.2 pounds of body weight
per day for a period of 60 to 90 days.

Overdosage

Although there is no specific information on
Cytoxan overdose, any medication taken in
excess can have serious consequences. If you
suspect an overdose of Cytoxan, seek
medical attention immediately.

Brand name:

DAYPRO

Pronounced: DAY-pro
Generic name: Oxaprozin

Why is this drug prescribed?

Daypro is a nonsteroidal anti-inflammatory
drug used to relieve the inflammation,
swelling, stiffness, and joint pain associated
with rheumatoid atrritis and osteoarthritis
(the most common kind of arthritis).

Most important fact about this drug

You should have frquent check-ups with
your doctor if you take Daypro regularly.
Ulcers and internal bleeding can occur
without warning.

How should you take this medication?

Take Daypro with a full glass of water. If
the drug upsets your stomach, your doctor
may recommend taking Daypro with food,
milk, or an antacid, even though food may
delay onset of relief.

It will also help to prevent irritation in your
upper digestive tract if you avoid lying down
for about 20 minutes after taking Daypro.

Take this medication exactly as prescribed.

■ *If you miss a dose...*
Try to take Daypro at the same time each
day, for example, after breakfast. If you
forget to take a dose and remember later
in the day, you can still take it. If you
completely forget to take your medication,
do *not* double the dose the next day to
make up for the missed dose. You should
get back on your normal schedule as soon
as possible.

■ *Storage instructions...*
Store at room temperature in a tightly
closed container, away from light.

What side effects may occur?

Side effects cannot be anticipated. If any
develop or change in intensity, tell your
doctor as soon as possible. Only your
doctor can decide if it is safe for you to
continue taking Daypro.

■ *More common side effects may include:*
Constipation
Diarrhea
Indigestion
Nausea
Rash

■ *Less common side effects may include:*
Abdominal pain, confusion, depression,
frequent or painful urination, gas, loss of
appetite, ringing in the ears, sleep
disturbances, sleepiness, vomiting

■ *Rare side effects may include:*
Anaphylaxis (a severe allergic reaction),
anemia, blood in the urine, blood pressure
changes, blurred vision, bruising, changes
in kidney and liver function, decreased
menstrual flow, fluid retention, general
feeling of illness, hemorrhoidal or rectal
bleeding, hepatitis, hives, inflammation of
the mouth, irritated eyes, itching, peptic
ulcerations, respiratory infection, sensitivity
to light, stomach and intestinal bleeding,
weight gain or loss, weakness

Why should this drug not be prescribed?

If you are sensitive to or have ever had an allergic reaction to Daypro, or if you have ever developed asthma, nasal tumors, or other allergic reactions due to aspirin or other nonsteroidal anti-inflammatory drugs, you should not take this medication. Make sure your doctor is aware of any drug reactions you have experienced.

Special warnings about this medication

Use Daypro with caution if you have kidney or liver disease.

Do not take aspirin or any other anti-inflammatory medications while taking Daypro, unless your doctor tells you to do so.

Daypro can increase water retention. Use with caution if you have heart disease or high blood pressure.

If you are taking Daypro for an extended period, your doctor should check your blood for anemia.

Daypro can prolong bleeding time. If you are taking a blood-thinning medication, use Daypro with caution.

Daypro may cause sensitivity to sunlight. Avoid prolonged exposure to the sun. Use sunscreens and wear protective clothing.

Do not use Daypro if you are planning to have surgery in the immediate future.

Possible food and drug interactions when taking this medication

If you take Daypro with certain other drugs, the effects of either medication could be increased, decreased, or altered. It is especially important to check with your doctor before combining Daypro with following medications:

Aspirin
Beta-blocking blood pressure medications
    such as Inderal and Tenormin
Blood thinners such as Coumadin
Diuretics such as Lasix and Midamor
Lithium (Lithonate)

Avoid alcoholic beverages while taking Daypro.

Special information if you are pregnant or breastfeeding

The effects of Daypro during pregnancy have not been adequately studied. If you are pregnant or plan to become pregnant, tell your doctor immediately. Since the effects of Daypro on nursing infants are not known, tell you doctor if you are nursing or plan to nurse. If Daypro treatment is necessary for your health, your doctor may tell you to discontinue nursing until your treatment is finished.

Recommended dosage

ADULTS

Your doctor will adjust the dose based on your needs.

Rheumatoid Arthritis
The usual daily dose is 1200 milligrams (two 600-milligram caplets) once a day.

Osteoarthritis
The usual starting dose for moderate to severe osteoarthritis is 1200 milligrams (two 600-milligram caplets) once a day.

The most you should take in a day is 1800 milligrams divided into smaller doses, or 26 milligrams per 2.2 pounds of body weight, whichever is lower.

CHILDREN

The safety and efficacy of Daypro in children have not been determined.

Overdosage

If you take too much of any medication, it can have serious consequences. If you suspect an overdose, seek medical attention immediately.

■ *Symptoms of Daypro overdose may include:*
Coma
Drowsiness
Fatigue
Nausea
Pain in the stomach
Stomach and intestinal bleeding
Vomiting

Acute kidney failure, high blood pressure, and a slow down in breathing have occurred rarely.

Brand name:

DEMULEN

See Oral Contraceptives, page 702.

Brand name:

DEPO-PROVERA

Pronounced: DE-po pro-VEH-ra
Generic name: Medroxyprogesterone acetate

Why is this drug prescribed?

Depo-Provera is an injection given in the buttock or upper arm to prevent pregnancy. It is more than 99 percent effective; your chances of becoming pregnant during the first year of use are less than 1 in 100. The injection is given every 3 months by your doctor. Depo-Provera works by preventing the release of hormones called gonadotropins from the pituitary gland in the brain. Without these hormones, the monthly release of an egg from the ovary cannot occur. If no egg is released, pregnancy is impossible. Depo-Provera also causes changes in the lining of the uterus that make pregnancy less likely even if an egg is released.

Depo-Provera is also used in the treatment of certain cancers including cancer of the endometrium (lining of the uterus) and kidney cancer.

Most important fact about this drug

Because Depo-Provera is a long-acting form of birth control, it will take a while for the effects of your last injection to wear off. In medical studies, only 68 percent of women became pregnant within 12 months after stopping Depo-Provera. However, within 18 months, 93 percent had become pregnant. If you think you will want to get pregnant right away when you stop using birth control, Depo-Provera may not be the ideal method for you. The amount of time you use Depo-Provera does not affect the delay in becoming pregnant when you stop.

How should you take this medication?

Depo-Provera is given by a doctor. To make sure you are not pregnant when you receive your first injection, it is given only during the first 5 days after your menstrual period, when it is very unlikely that you could be pregnant. If you are breastfeeding, Depo-Provera is given 6 weeks after childbirth to reduce the infant's exposure to the drug through breast milk. If you are not breastfeeding, it is given within 5 days of childbirth.

Depo-Provera must be taken every 3 months, on schedule. Although the birth-control effects of the drug generally take time to wear off, there is still a possibility of becoming pregnant right away if you miss your scheduled injection.

■ *If you miss a dose...*
After 3 months, if you allow more than 2 weeks to elapse before your next injection, your doctor will do a test to make sure you are not pregnant before giving you another injection.

■ *Storage instructions...*
Depo-Provera is always given at at doctor's office or clinic, never at home.

What side effects may occur?
Side effects cannot be anticipated. If any develop or change in intensity, inform your doctor as soon as possible. Only your doctor can determine if it is safe for you to continue taking Depo-Provera.

By far, the most common side effect of Depo-Provera is unpredictable menstrual bleeding. In fact, most women have some change in their menstrual pattern. For example, when first taking Depo-Provera, it is common to have spotting between menstrual periods, or an increase or decrease in the amount of bleeding when menstrual periods occur. With continued use, many women stop having their menstrual periods altogether. By 12 months (or four injections), 57 percent of women report not having periods, and by 24 months, 68 percent no longer have periods. Going without a menstrual period is not an indication that something is wrong, however.

■ *More common side effects may include:*
Abdominal pain or discomfort
Dizziness
Headaches
Nervousness
Unpredictable menstrual bleeding
Weakness or fatigue
Weight gain

■ *Less common side effects may include:*
Acne, backaches, bloating, breast pain, decreased sex drive, depression, fluid retention, hair loss, hot flashes, inability to have an orgasm, insomnia, leg cramps, nausea, pain in the pelvic area, rash, vaginal discharge, vaginal inflammation

■ *Rare side effects may include:*
Accidental pregnancy, allergic reactions, anemia, asthma, bleeding from the rectum or nipples, blood clots, blood clots in the lungs, breast cancer, breast lumps, cancer in the neck of the uterus, changes in appetite, change in breast size, chest pain, chills, convulsions, difficult or labored breathing, drowsiness, dry skin, excessive growth of hair, excessive or unusual flow of milk, excessive sweating and body odor, excessive thirst, fainting, feeling of being pregnant, fever, hoarseness, increased sex drive, infections of the reproductive and urinary tracts, lack of return to fertility, overgrowth of the uterus, pain at the injection site, pain during sexual intercourse, painful menstruation, paralysis, prevention of the flow of milk, rapid heartbeat, skin discoloration, stomach and intestinal problems, swelling in the armpit, thinning of bones, tingling or "pins and needles", toughening or hardening of the skin, vaginal cysts, varicose veins, yellowed eyes and skin

Why should this drug not be prescribed?
You should not use Depo-Provera if you know or suspect you are pregnant, or if you have vaginal bleeding that has not been diagnosed by a doctor.

Also avoid Depo-Provera if you know or suspect you have breast cancer, or if you have a disease of the liver.

Do not use this method of birth control if you have thrombophlebitis (inflammation of a vein with development of a blood clot), or have ever had any blood-clotting disorders or disease of the blood vessels in the brain.

You should not take Depo-Provera if you have ever had an allergic reaction to it or any of its ingredients.

Special warnings about this medication

Call your doctor immediately if any of these problems occur after an injection of Depo-Provera: sharp chest pain, coughing of blood, sudden shortness of breath, sudden severe headache or vomiting, dizziness or fainting, problems with your eyesight or speech, weakness in an arm or leg, severe pain or swelling in the calf, unusually heavy vaginal bleeding, severe pain or tenderness in the lower abdominal area, migraine headache, or persistent pain, pus, or bleeding at the injection site.

Studies indicate that using Depo-Provera may make you more prone to osteoporosis, or brittle bone disease. The rate at which bone loss occurs is greatest during the early years of Depo-Provera use, and the risk decreases to normal over time.

Studies of women who have used Depo-Provera for a long time have found no increased risk of cancers of the breast, ovaries, liver, or cervix (mouth of the uterus). Some studies do show a slight increased risk of breast cancer in women younger than 35 years old who have taken Depo-Provera for a short time, but the increase is about three additional cases of breast cancer per 10,000 women. At the same time, Depo-Provera helps *prevent* cancer of the endometrium, or lining of the uterus.

Depo-Provera may cause fluid retention, so if you have conditions that may be worsened by fluid retention, such as epilepsy, migraine headaches, asthma, heart disease, or kidney disease, make sure the doctor is aware of it.

Depo-Provera tends to alter levels of blood sugar, so diabetic women need to be carefully observed by their doctors when taking Depo-Provera.

If you develop jaundice (a yellowing of the skin and whites of the eyes caused by liver disease), you probably should not receive Depo-Provera again.

While it is an excellent birth control method, Depo-Provera does not protect you against AIDS or other sexually transmitted diseases. If you are concerned about AIDS or other STDs, be sure your partner uses a condom during intercourse (or, for absolute safety, abstain from sex).

Possible food and drug interactions when taking this medication

If Depo-Provera is taken with aminoglutethimide (Cytadren), a drug used to treat a disorder of the adrenal glands called Cushing's syndrome, it could make the Depo-Provera less potent, which could lead to accidental pregnancy. Check with your doctor before taking Cytadren if you are on Depo-Provera.

Special information if you are pregnant or breastfeeding

Depo-Provera is not given to pregnant women. If an accidental pregnancy occurs 1 to 2 months after a Depo-Provera injection, the baby is more likely to have low birth weight. Children born to women who were taking Depo-Provera show no signs of poor health or development. Because Depo-Provera does not prevent the breasts from producing milk, it can be used by women who are breastfeeding. However, to minimize the amount of Depo-Provera that is passed to the infant during the first weeks of life, the drug is not given until 6 weeks after childbirth. Studies show Depo-Provera is not harmful to the infant then or in later life.

Recommended dosage

Depo-Provera is given in 150-milligram doses every 3 months as a single injection.

Overdosage

An overdose of Depo-Provera is highly unlikely, since it is given as a single injection by your doctor. However, if you suspect you have received an overdose, seek medical attention immediately.

Generic name:

DESIPRAMINE

See Norpramin, page 694.

Brand name:

DESOGEN

See Oral Contraceptives, page 702.

Brand name:

DESQUAM-E

Pronounced: DES-kwam ee
Generic name: Benzoyl peroxide
Other brand names: Benzac W, Benzagel,
  BenzaShave, Theroxide

Why is this drug prescribed?

Desquam-E gel is used to treat various types of acne. It can be used alone or with other treatments, including antibiotics and products that contain retinoic acid, sulfur, or salicylic acid.

Most important fact about this drug

Significant clearing of the skin should occur after 2 to 3 weeks of treatment with Desquam-E. If used with sunscreens such as PreSun 15, which contain PABA (para-amino benzoic acid), it may cause temporary skin discoloration.

How should you use this medication?

Cleanse the affected area thoroughly before applying the medication. Desquam-E should then be gently rubbed in.

■ *If you miss a dose...*
  Apply it as soon as you remember. Then go back to your regular schedule.

■ *Storage instructions...*
  Store at room temperature.

What side effects may occur?

Side effects cannot be anticipated. If any develop or change in intensity, notify your doctor as soon as possible. Only your doctor can determine whether it is safe for you to continue using Desquam-E.

■ *Side effects may include:*
  Allergic reaction (itching, rash in area
    where the medication was applied)
  Excessive drying (red and peeling skin and
    possible swelling)

Why should this drug not be prescribed?

Do not use Desquam-E if you are sensitive to or allergic to benzoyl peroxide.

Special warnings about this medication

Desquam-E is for external use only. Avoid contact with your eyes, nose, or throat.

If you are sensitive to medications derived from benzoic acid (including certain topical anesthetics) or to cinnamon, you may also be sensitive to Desquam-E.

Desquam-E can bleach hair or colored fabric.

Possible food and drug interactions when taking this medication

When used with sunscreens containing PABA (para-amino benzoic acid), Desquam-E may cause temporary skin discoloration.

Special information if you are pregnant or breastfeeding

The effects of Desquam-E during pregnancy have not been adequately studied. It should be used only if clearly needed. If you are pregnant or plan to become pregnant, inform your doctor immediately. This medication may appear in breast milk and could affect a nursing infant. If this medication is essential to your health, your doctor may advise you to stop breastfeeding until your treatment with Desquam-E is finished.

Recommended dosage

ADULTS AND CHILDREN 12 YEARS AND OVER

Gently rub Desquam-E gel into all affected areas once or twice a day. If you are fair-skinned or live in an excessively dry climate, you should probably start with one application a day. You can continue to use Desquam-E for as long as your doctor thinks it is necessary.

Overdosage

Overdosage of Desquam-E can result in excessive scaling of the skin, reddening skin, or swelling due to fluid retention. Any medication taken in excess can have serious consequences. If you suspect an overdose, seek medical attention.

Brand name:

DESYREL

Pronounced: DES-ee-rel
Generic name: Trazodone hydrochloride

Why is this drug prescribed?

Desyrel is prescribed for the treatment of depression with or without anxiety.

Most important fact about this drug

Desyrel has been associated with priapism, a persistent, painful erection of the penis. Men who experience prolonged or inappropriate erections should stop taking this drug and consult their doctor.

How should you take this medication?

Take Desyrel shortly after a meal or light snack. You may be more apt to feel dizzy or light-headed if you take the drug before you have eaten.

Take Desyrel exactly as prescribed. It may take up to 4 weeks before you begin to feel better, although most patients notice improvement within 2 weeks.

Desyrel may cause dry mouth. Sucking on a hard candy, chewing gum, or melting bits of ice in your mouth can relieve the problem.

■ If you miss a dose...
Take it as soon as you remember. If it is within 4 hours of your next dose, skip the one you missed and go back to your regular schedule. Never take 2 doses at once.

■ Storage instructions...
Store at room temperature in a tightly closed container away from light and excessive heat.

What side effects may occur?

Side effects cannot be anticipated. If any develop or change in intensity, inform your doctor as soon as possible. Only your doctor can determine if it is safe for you to continue taking Desyrel.

■ *More common side effects may include:*
Abdominal or stomach disorder, aches or pains in muscles and bones, allergic skin reaction, anger or hostility, blurred vision, brief loss of consciousness, confusion, constipation, decreased appetite, diarrhea, dizziness or light-headedness, drowsiness, dry mouth, excitement, fast, fluttery heartbeat, fatigue, fluid retention and swelling, headache, impaired memory, inability to fall or stay asleep, low blood pressure, nasal or sinus congestion, nausea, nervousness, nightmares or vivid dreams, rapid heartbeat, sudden loss of strength or fainting, tremors, uncoordinated movements, vomiting, weight gain or loss

■ *Less common or rare side effects may include:*
Allergic reactions, anemia, bad taste in mouth, blood in the urine, chest pain, delayed urine flow, decreased concentration, decreased sex drive, disorientation, early menstruation, ejaculation problems, excess salivation, fullness or heaviness in the head, gas, general feeling of illness, hallucinations or delusions, high blood pressure, impaired memory, impaired speech, impotence, increased appetite, increased sex drive, missed menstrual periods, more frequent urination, muscle twitches, numbness, prolonged erections, red, tired, itchy eyes, restlessness, ringing in the ears, shortness of breath, sweating or clammy skin, tingling or pins and needles,

Why should this drug not be prescribed?
If you are sensitive to or have ever had an allergic reaction to Desyrel or similar drugs, you should not take this medication. Make sure your doctor is aware of any drug reactions you have experienced.

Special warnings about this medication
Desyrel may cause you to become drowsy or less alert and may affect your judgment. Therefore, you should not drive or operate dangerous machinery or participe in any hazardous activity that requires full mental alertness until you know how this drug affects you.

Notify your doctor or dentist that you are taking this drug if you have a medical emergency, and before you have surgery or dental treatment. Stop using the drug if you are going to have elective surgery.

Be careful taking this drug if you have heart disease. Disyrel can cause irregular heartbeats.

Possible food and drug interactions when taking this medication
Desyrel may intensify the effects of alcohol. Do not drink alcohol while taking this medication.

If Desyrel is taken with certain other drugs, the effects of either could be increased, decreased, or altered. It is especially important to check with your doctor before combining Desyrel with the following:

Antidepressant drugs known as MAO inhibitors, including Nardil and Parnate
Barbiturates such as Seconal
Central nervous system depressants such as Demerol and Halcion
Chlorpromazine (Thorazine)
Digoxin (Lanoxin)
Drugs for high blood pressure such as Catapres and Wytensin
Other antidepressants such as Prozac and Norpramim
Phenytoin (Dilantin)

Special information
if you are pregnant or breastfeeding

The effects of Desyrel during pregnancy have not been adequately studied. If you are pregnant or planning to become pregnant, inform your doctor immediately. This medication may appear in breast milk. If treatment with this drug is essential to your health, your doctor may advise you to discontinue breastfeeding your baby until your treatment is finished.

Recommended dosage

ADULTS

The usual starting dosage is a total of 150 milligrams per day, divided into 2 or more smaller doses. Your doctor may increase your dose by 50 milligrams per day every 3 or 4 days. Total dosage should not exceed 400 milligrams per day, divided into smaller doses. Once you have responded well to the drug, your doctor may gradually reduce your dose. Because this medication makes you drowsy, your doctor may tell you to take the largest dose at bedtime.

CHILDREN

The safety and effectiveness of Desyrel have not been established in children below 18 years of age.

Overdosage

Any medication taken in excess can have serious consequences. An overdose of Desyrel in combination with other drugs can be fatal.

- Symptoms of a Desyrel overdose may include:
  Breathing failure
  Drowsiness
  Irregular heartbeat
  Prolonged, painful erection
  Seizures
  Vomiting

If you suspect an overdose, seek medical attention immediately.

Generic name:

DIAZEPAM

See Valium, page 786.

Generic name:

DICLOFENAC

See Voltaren, page 790.

Generic name:

DIETHYLPROPION

See Tenuate, page 760.
Generic name:

DIETHYLSTILBESTROL (DES)

Pronounced: dye-ETH-il-stil-BESS-trole

Why is this drug prescribed?

Diethylstilbestrol (DES), a synthetic estrogen (female hormone), is often given to ease symptoms of some inoperable kinds of breast cancer and prostate cancer.

Most important fact about this drug

DES must not be taken during pregnancy. In the past it was sometimes given in early pregnancy to try to prevent miscarriage. Now we know that if the unborn child is female (a so-called DES daughter), she may grow up to develop cancer or other tissue abnormalities of the cervix or vagina. DES may also cause malformation of the fetal heart or limbs.

How should you take this medication?

Take DES exactly as prescribed. If you are being treated for inoperable prostate cancer, your initial dosage of DES may later be reduced.

- *If you miss a dose...*
  If you take DES once a day, take the dose you missed as soon as you remember. If you do not remember it until the next day, skip the dose you missed and go back to your regular schedule. If you take DES 2 or more times a day, take the dose you missed as soon as you remember. If it is almost time for your next dose, skip the one you missed and go back to your regular schedule. Never take 2 doses at once.

- *Storage instructions...*
  Store away from heat, light, and moisture.

What side effects may occur?

Side effects cannot be anticipated. If any develop or change in intensity, inform your doctor as soon as possible. Only your doctor can determine if it is safe for you to continue taking DES.

- *Serious potential side effects of DES include:*
  Blood clots, heart attack, stroke
  Blood sugar problems
  Endometrial cancer
  Gallbladder disease
  High blood pressure
  Liver tumor

- *Additional side effects you may experience include:*
  Abnormal uterine bleeding, fluid retention, jaundice

DES can produce many of the same side effects as oral contraceptives. Grouped by physical category, these include:

- Bladder irritation, breakthrough bleeding, cervical changes, menstrual changes, painful or missed periods, premenstrual syndrome, spotting, vaginal yeast infection;
- Breast enlargement, breast tenderness or pain, or secretion from the breasts;
- Abdominal cramps, bloating, jaundice, nausea, vomiting;
- Abnormal body hair growth, redness and skin eruptions, scalp hair loss, skin pigmentation;
- Intolerance to contact lenses;
- Depression, dizziness, headache, involuntary movements, migraine;
- Changed sex drive, swelling due to fluid retention, weight gain or loss.

Why should this drug not be prescribed?

Do not take this medication if you are sensitive to it or have ever had an allergic reaction to it.

You should have a complete physical before starting treatment with DES, and should not be given the drug if you are pregnant or have any of the following:

Abnormal, undiagnosed genital bleeding
Breast cancer (except in certain cases)
Estrogen-dependent tumor of any kind
History of a blood clot due to estrogen
Thrombophlebitis (blood clots and inflammation of part of a vein)

Special warnings about this medication

DES should never be used as a "morning-after pill" for birth control.

DES increases the risk of cancer of the endometrium (lining of the uterus).

If you are taking DES and you notice any unusual bleeding from the vagina, notify your doctor immediately.

There is some suspicion that DES may also be capable of triggering other kinds of cancer. If breast cancer runs in your family, or if you have ever had breast nodules, breast fibrocystic disease, or an abnormal mammogram, make sure you tell this to your doctor before you take DES.

If you are diabetic, you should monitor your blood or urine glucose level carefully, since DES decreases glucose tolerance.

DES causes fluid retention, and this may aggravate certain conditions, such as epilepsy, migraine, and heart or kidney disease.

Your doctor will be especially careful in prescribing DES for you if your liver is not functioning properly, if you have certain bone diseases, or if your kidney is not functioning adequately.

Estrogens can affect bone growth. Your doctor will be cautious in giving this drug to a child.

Possible food and drug interactions when taking this medication

If DES is taken with certain other drugs, the effects of either could be increased, decreased, or altered. It is especially important to check with your doctor before combining DES with the following:

Warfarin (Coumadin)
Vitamin C

Special information if you are pregnant or breastfeeding

As noted, DES must not be taken during pregnancy because of the high risk of harm to the unborn child. If you are pregnant and are taking DES, contact your doctor immediately to discuss your options. No specific information is available about DES and breastfeeding. In general, a nursing mother should not take drugs. It may be necessary to choose between taking DES and breastfeeding your baby.

Recommended dosage

ADULTS

Inoperable Progressing Prostate Cancer
The usual starting dose is 1 to 3 milligrams daily, more in advanced cases. The dosage may later be reduced to an average of 1 milligram daily.

Inoperable Progressing Breast Cancer
The usual dose is 15 milligrams daily.

Overdosage

An acute overdose of DES may cause abdominal cramps, loss of appetite, diarrhea, nausea, and vomiting. After a large dose, vaginal bleeding may occur.

Chronic overdosage with DES may cause facial skin darkening, fluid retention and swelling, headache, leg cramps, male breast development, and vertigo.

Any medication taken in excess can have serious consequences. If you suspect an overdose of DES, seek medical attention immediately.

Brand name:

DIFLUCAN

Pronounced: Dye-FLEW-can
Generic name: Fluconazole

Why is this drug prescribed?

Diflucan is used to treat fungal infections called candidiasis (also known as thrush or yeast infections). These include throat infections and fungal infections elsewhere in the body, such as infections of the urinary tract, peritonitis (inflammation of the lining of the abdomen), and pneumonia. This drug is also used to treat meningitis (brain or spinal cord inflammation) caused by another type of fungus.

In addition, Diflucan is now being prescribed for vaginal yeast infections, fungal infections in kidney and liver transplant patients, and fungal infections in patients with AIDS.

Most important fact about this drug

Strong allergic reactions to Diflucan, although rare, have been reported. Symptoms may include hives, itching, swelling, sudden drop in blood pressure, difficulty breathing or swallowing, diarrhea, or abdominal pain. If you experience any of these symptoms, notify your doctor immediately.

How should you take this medication?

You can take Diflucan with or without meals.

Take this medication exactly as prescribed, and continue taking it for as long as your doctor instructs. You may being to feel better after the first few days; but it takes weeks or even months of treatment to completely cure certain fungal infections.

- *If you miss a dose...*
  Take the forgotten dose as soon as you remeber. However, if it is almost time for your next dose, skip the one you missed and return to your regular schedule. Do not take double doses.

- *Storage instructions...*
  Diflucan tablets should be stored at normal room temperature. Avoid exposing them to temperatures above 86°F.

What side effects may occur?

Side effects cannot be anticipated. If any develop or change in intensity, inform your doctor as soon as possible. Only your doctor can determine if it is safe for you to continue taking Diflucan.

The most common side effect is nausea.

- *Less common side effects may include:*
  Abdominal pain, diarrhea, headache, skin rash, vomiting

Why should this drug not be prescribed?

Do not take Diflucan if you are sensitive to any of its ingredients or have ever had an allergic reaction to similar drugs, such as Nizoral. Make sure your doctor is aware of any drug reactions you have experienced.

Special warnings about this medication

Your doctor will watch your liver function carefully while you are taking Diflucan.

If your immunity is low and you develop a rash, your doctor should monitor your condition closely. You may have to stop taking Diflucan if the rash gets worse.

Possible food and drug interactions when taking this medication

If Diflucan is taken with certain other drugs, the effects of either could be increased, decreased, or altered. It is especially important to check with your doctor before combining Diflucan with the following:

Anticoagulants (Coumadin)
Antidiabetic drugs such as Orinase, DiaBeta and Glucotrol
Certain antihistamines, such as Hismanal
Cyclosporine (Sandimmune)
Hydrochlorothiazide (HydroDIURIL)
Phenytoin (Dilantin)
Rifampin (Rifadin)
Ulcer medications such as Tagamet

Special information if you are pregnant or breastfeeding

The effects of Diflucan during pregnancy have not been adequately studied. If you are pregnant or plan to become pregnant, inform your doctor immediately. Diflucan appears in breast milk and could affect a nursing infant. If this medication is essential to your health, your doctor may advise you to stop breastfeeding until your treatment with Diflucan is finished.

Recommended dosage

ADULTS

For throat infections
The usual dose for candidiasis of the mouth and throat is 200 milligrams on the first day, followed by 100 milligrams once a day. Treatment should continue for at least 2 weeks to avoid a relapse. For candidiasis of the esophagus (gullet) the usual dose is 200 milligrams on the first day, followed by 100 milligrams once a day. Treatment should continue for a minimum of 3 weeks and for at least 2 weeks after symptoms have stopped.

For systemic (bodywide) infections
The usual dose is 400 milligrams on the first day, followed by 200 milligrams once a day. Treatment should continue for a minimum of 4 weeks and for at least 2 weeks after symptoms have stopped.

For cryptococcal meningitis
The usual dose is 400 milligrams on the first day, followed by 200 milligrams once a day. Treatment should continue for 10 to 12 weeks once tests of spinal fluid come back negative. For AIDS patients, a 200-milligram dose taken once a day is recommended to prevent relapse.

If you have kidney disease, your doctor may have to reduce your dosage.

CHILDREN

Efficacy has not been established in children, although a small number of children have been treated safely with Diflucan.

Overdosage

Any medication taken in excess can have serious consequences. If you suspect an overdose, seek medical treatment immediately.

■ *Symptoms of Diflucan overdose may include:*
Hallucinations
Paranoia

Generic name:

DIFLUNISAL

See Dolobid, page 572.

Generic name:

DOCUSATE SODIUM

See Colace, page 554.

Brand name:

DOLOBID

Pronounced: DOLL-oh-bid
Generic name: Diflunisal

Why is this drug prescribed?

Dolobid, a nonsteroidal anti-inflammatory drug, is used to treat mild to moderate pain and relieve the inflammation, swelling, stiffness, and joint pain associated with rheumatoid arthritis and osteoarthritis (the most common form of arthritis).

Most important fact about this drug

You should have frequent check-ups with your doctor if you take Dolobid regularly. Ulcers or internal bleeding can occur without warning.

How should you take this medication?

Dolobid should be taken with food or food together with an antacid, and with a full glass of water or milk. Never take it on an empty stomach.

Tablets should be swallowed whole, not chewed or crushed.

Take this medication exactly as prescribed by your doctor. If you are using Dolobid for arthritis, it should be taken regularly.

■ *If you miss a dose...*
Take it as soon as you remember. If it is almost time for your next dose, skip the one you missed and go back to your regular schedule. Never take two doses at the same time.

■ *Storage instructions...*
Do not store in damp places, like the bathroom.

What side effects may occur?
Side effects cannot be anticipated. If any develop or change in intensity, inform your doctor as soon as possible. Only your doctor can determine if it is safe for you to continue taking Dolobid.

■ *More common side effects may include:*
Abdominal pain, constipation, diarrhea, dizziness, fatigue, gas, headache, inability to sleep, indigestion, nausea, rash, ringing in ears, sleepiness, vomiting

■ *Less common or rare side effects may include:*
Abdominal bleeding, anemia, blurred vision, confusion, depression, disorientation, dry mouth and nose, fluid retention, flushing, hepatitis, hives, inflammation of lips and tongue, itching, kidney failure, light-headedness, loss of appetite, nervousness, painful urination, peptic ulcer, pins and needles, protein or blood in urine, rash, sensitivity to light, skin eruptions, Stevens-Johnson syndrome, vertigo, weakness, yellow eyes and skin

Why should this drug not be prescribed?
If you are sensitive to or have had an allergic reaction to Dolobid, aspirin, or similar drugs, or if you have had asthma attacks caused by aspirin or other drugs of this type, you should not take this medication. Make sure that your doctor is aware of any drug reactions that you have experienced.

Special warnings about this medication
Peptic ulcers and bleeding can occur without warning.

This drug should be used with caution if you have kidney or liver disease; and it can cause liver inflammation in some people.

Do not take aspirin or any other anti-inflammatory medications while taking Dolobid, unless your doctor tells you to do so.

Nonsteroidal anti-inflammatory drugs such as Dolobid can hide the signs and symptoms of infection. Be sure your doctor knows about any infection you may have.

Dolobid can cause vision problems. If you experience any changes in your vision, inform your doctor.

Dolobid may prolong bleeding time. If you are taking blood-thinning medication, take Dolobid with caution.

If you have heart disease or high blood pressure, use Dolobid with caution. It can increase water retention.

Dolobid may cause you to become drowsy or less alert; therefore, driving or operating dangerous machinery or participating in any hazardous activity that requires full mental alertness is not recommended.

Possible food and drug interactions when taking this medication

If Dolobid is taken with certain other drugs, the effects of either could be increased, decreased, or altered. It is especially important to check with your doctor before combining Dolobid with the following:

Acetaminophen (Tylenol)
Antacids taken regularly
Aspirin
Cyclosporine (Sandimmune)
Methotrexate (Rheumatrex)
Naproxen (Naprosyn)
Oral anticoagulants (blood thinners)
The arthritis medication sulindac (Clinoril)
The diuretic hydrochlorothiazide

Special information if you are pregnant or breastfeeding

The effects of Dolobid during pregnancy have not been adequately studied. If you are pregnant or plan to become pregnant, inform your doctor immediately. Dolobid appears in breast milk and could affect a nursing infant. If this medication is essential to your health, your doctor may advise you to discontinue breastfeeding until your treatment with Dolobid is finished.

Recommended dosage

ADULTS

Mild to Moderate Pain
Starting dose is 1,000 milligrams, followed by 500 milligrams every 8 to 12 hours, depending on the individual. Your physician may adjust your dosage according to your age and weight, and the severity of your symptoms.

Osteoarthritis and Rheumatoid Arthritis
The usual dose is 500 to 1,000 milligrams per day in 2 doses of 250 milligrams or 500 milligrams.

The lowest dose that proves beneficial should be used.

The maximum recommended dosage is 1,500 milligrams per day.

CHILDREN

Safety and effectiveness of Dolobid have not been established in children under 12 years of age. However, your doctor may decide that the benefits of this medication may outweigh the potential risks.

Overdosage

Any medication taken in excess can cause symptoms of overdose. If you suspect an overdose, seek medical attention immediately.

■ *Symptoms of Dolobid overdose may include:*
Abnormally rapid heartbeat, coma, diarrhea, disorientation, drowsiness, hyperventilation, nausea, ringing in the ears, stupor, sweating, vomiting

Brand name:

DORYX

Pronounced: DORE-icks
Generic name: Doxycycline hyclate
Other brand names: Vibramycin, Vibra-Tabs

Why is this drug prescribed?

Doxycycline is a broad-spectrum tetracycline antibiotic used against a wide variety of bacterial infections, including Rocky Mountain spotted fever and other fevers caused by ticks, fleas, and lice; urinary tract infections; trachoma (chronic infections of the eye); and some gonococcal infections in adults. It is also used with other medications to treat severe acne and amoebic dysentery (diarrhea caused by severe parasitic infection of the intestines).

Doxycycline may also be taken for the prevention of malaria on foreign trips of less than 4 months duration.

Occasionally doctors prescribe doxycycline to treat early Lyme disease and to prevent "traveler's diarrhea". These are not yet officially approved uses for this drug.

Most important fact about this drug

Children under 8 years old and women in the last half of pregnancy should not take this medication. It may cause developing teeth to become permanently discolored (yellow-gray-brown).

How should you take this medication?

Take doxycycline with a full glass of water or other liquid to avoid irritating your throat or stomach. Doxycycline can be taken with or without food. However, if the medicine does upset your stomach, you may wish to take it with a glass of milk or after you have eaten. Doxycycline tablets should be swallowed whole.

Take this medication exactly as prescribed by your doctor, even if your symptoms have disappeared.

If you are taking an oral suspension form of doxycycline, shake the bottle well before using. Do not use outdated doxycycline.

■ *If you miss a dose...*
Take the forgotten dose as soon as you remember. If it is almost time for the next dose, put it off for several hours after taking the missed dose. Specifically, if you are taking one dose a day, take the next one 10 to 12 hours after the missed dose. If you are taking two doses a day, take the next one 5 to 6 hours after the missed dose. If you are taking three doses a day, take the next one 2 to 4 hours after the missed dose. Then return to your regular schedule.

■ *Storage instructions...*
Doxycycline can be stored at room temperature. Protect from light and excessive heat.

What side effects may occur?

Side effects cannot be anticipated. If any develop or change in intensity, inform your doctor as soon as possible. Only your doctor can determine if it is safe for you to continue taking doxycycline.

■ *More common side effects may include*:
Angioedema (chest pain; swelling of face, around lips, tongue and throat, arms and legs; difficulty swallowing), bulging foreheads in infants, diarrhea, difficulty swallowing, discolored teeth in infants and children (more common during long-term use of tetracycline), inflammation of the tongue, loss of appetite, nausea, rash, rectal or genital itching, severe allergic reaction (hives, itching, and swelling), skin sensitivity to light, vomiting

■ *Less common or rare side effects may include:*
Aggravation of lupus erythematosus (disease of the connective tissue), skin inflammation and peeling, throat inflammation and ulcerations

Why should this drug not be prescribed?

If you are sensitive to or have ever had an allergic reaction to doxycycline or drugs of this type, you should not take this medication. Make sure your doctor is aware of any drug reactions that you have experienced.

Special warnings about this medication

As with other antibiotics, treatment with doxycycline may result in a growth of bacteria that do not respond to this medication and can cause a secondary infection.

Bulging foreheads in infants and headaches in adults have occurred. These symptoms disappeared when doxycycline was discontinued.

You may become more sensitive to sunlight while taking doxycycline. Be careful if you are going out in the sun or using a sunlamp. If you develop a skin rash, notify your doctor immediately.

Birth control pills that contain estrogen may not be as effective while you are taking tetracycline drugs. Ask your doctor or pharmacist if you should use another form of birth control while taking doxycycline.

Doxycycline syrup (Vibramycin) contains a sulfite that may cause allergic reactions in certain people. This reaction happens more frequently to people with asthma.

Possible food and drug interactions when taking this medication

If doxycycline is taken with certain other drugs, the effects of either could be increased, decreased, or altered. It is especially important to check with your doctor before combining doxycycline with the following:

Antacids containing aluminum, calcium, or magnesium, and iron-containing preparations such as Maalox, Mylanta, and others
Barbiturates such a Phenobarbital
Bismuth subsalicylate (Pepto-Bismol)
Blood-thinning medications such as Coumadin and Panwarfin
Carbamazepine (Tegretol)
Oral Contraceptives
Penicillin (V-Cillin K, Pen VK, others)
Phenytoin (Dilantin)
Sodium bicarbonate

Special information
if you are pregnant or breastfeeding

Doxycycline should not be used during pregnancy. Tetracycline can damage developing teeth during the last half of pregnancy. If you are pregnant or plan to become pregnant, inform your doctor immediately. Tetracyclines such as doxycycline appear in breast milk and can affect a nursing infant. If this medication is essential to your health, your doctor may advise you to discontinue breastfeeding until your treatment is finished.

Recommended dosage

ADULTS

The usual dose of oral doxycycline is 200 milligrams on the first day of treatment (100 milligrams every 12 hours) followed by a maintenance dose of 100 milligrams per day. The maintenance dose may be taken as a single dose or as 50 milligrams every 12 hours.

Your doctor may prescribe 100 milligrams every 12 hours for severe infections such as chronic urinary tract infection.

For Uncomplicated Gonorrhea (Except Anorectal Infections in Men)
The usual dose is 100 milligrams by mouth, twice a day for 7 days. An alternate, single-day treatment is 300 milligrams, followed in 1 hour by a second 300-milligram dose.

For Primary and Secondary Syphilis
The usual dose is 200 milligrams a day, divided into smaller, equal doses for 14 days.

For Prevention of Malaria
The usual dose is 100 milligrams a day. Treatment should begin 1 to 2 days before travel to the area where malaria is found, then continued daily during travel in the area and 4 weeks after leaving.

CHILDREN

For children above 8 years of age, the recommended dosage schedule for those weighing 100 pounds or less is 2 milligrams per pound of body weight, divided into 2 doses, on the first day of treatment, followed by 1 milligram per pound of body weight given as a single daily dose or divided into 2 doses on subsequent days.

For more severe infections, up to 2 milligrams per pound of body weight may be used.

For prevention of malaria, the recommended dose is 2 milligrams per 2.2 pounds of body weight up to 100 milligrams.

For children over 100 pounds, the usual adult dose should be used.

Overdosage

Any medication taken in excess can have serious consequences. If you suspect an overdose, seek medical treatment immediately.

Generic name:

DOXEPIN

See *Sinequan, page 744.*

Generic name:

DOXYCYCLINE

See *Doryx, page 574.*

Brand name:

DUPHALAC

See *Chronulac Syrup, page 541.*

Brand name:

DYNACIN

See *Minocin, page 665.*

Brand name:

ECOTRIN

See *Aspirin, page 515.*

Brand name:

E.E.S.

See *Erythromycin, Oral, page 584.*

Brand name:

EFFER-SYLLIUM

See *Metamucil, page 653.*

Brand name:

EFFEXOR

Pronounced: *ef-ecks-OR*
Generic name: *Venlafaxine hydrochloride*

Why is this drug prescribed?

Effexor is prescribed for the treatment of major depression—that is, a continuing depression that interferes with daily functioning. The symptoms usually include changes in appetite, sleep habits, and mind/body coordination, decreased sex drive, increased fatigue, feelings of guilt or worthlessness, difficulty concentrating, slowed thinking, and suicidal thoughts.

Most important fact about this drug

Serious, sometimes fatal reactions have occurred when Effexor is used in combination with other antidepressant drugs known as MAO inhibitors, including Nardil, Parnate, and Marplan. Never take Effexor with one of these drugs; and do not begin therapy with Effexor within 14 days of discontinuing treatment with one of them. Also, allow at least 7 days between the last dose of Effexor and the first dose of an MAO inhibitor.

How should you take this medication?

Take Effexor with food, exactly as prescribed. It may take several weeks before you begin to feel better. Your doctor should check your progress periodically.

■ *If you miss a dose...*
It is not necessary to make it up. Skip the missed dose and continue with your next scheduled dose. Do not take 2 doses at once.

■ *Storage instructions...*
Store in a tightly closed container at room temperature. Protect from excessive heat and moisture.

What side effects may occur?

Side effects cannot be anticipated. If any develop or change in intensity, tell your doctor as soon as possible. Only your doctor can determine if it is safe for you to continue taking Effexor.

■ *More common side effects may include:*
Abnormal dreams, abnormal ejaculaton/orgasm, anxiety, blurred vision, chills, constipation, diarrhea, dizziness, dry mouth, extreme muscle tension, flushing, frequent urination, gas, headache, impotence, inability to sleep, indigestion, loss of appetite, nausea, nervousness, prickling or burning sensation, rash, sleepiness, sweating, tremor, vomiting, weakness, yawning

■ *Less common side effects may include:*
Abnormal thinking, abnormal vision, accidental injury, agitation, belching, blood in the urine, bronchitis, bruising, changeable emotions, chest pain, confusion, decreased sex drive, depression, difficult or painful urination, difficulty in breathing, difficulty swallowing, dilated pupils, ear pain, high or low blood pressure, inflammation of the vagina, injury, itching, lack of orgasm, light-headedness on standing up, lockjaw, loss of touch with reality, menstrual problems, migraine headache, neck pain, orgasm disturbance, rapid heartbeat, ringing in the ears, taste changes, twitching, uterine bleeding between menstrual periods, vague feeling of illness, vertigo, weight loss or gain

■ *Rare side effects may include:*
Abnormally slow movements, abnormal movements, abnormal sensitivity to sound, abnormal speech, abortion, abuse of alcohol, acne, alcohol intolerance, allergic reaction, anemia, angina pectoris (crushing chest pain), apathy, appendicitis, arthritis, asthma, bad breath, black stools, bleeding gums, blocked intestine, blood clots, blood clots in the lungs, blood disorders, bluish color to the skin, body odor, bone disease and/or pain, including osteoporosis, breast enlargement or swelling, breast pain, brittle nails, bulging eyes, cancerous growth, cataracts, changed sense of smell, chest congestion, cold hands and feet, colitis (inflamed bowel), confusion, conjunctivitis ("pinkeye"), coughing up blood, deafness, delusions, depression, diabetes, double vision, drug withdrawal symptoms, dry eyes, dry skin, ear infection, eczema, enlarged abdomen, enlarged thyroid gland, exaggerated feeling of well-being, excessive hair growth, excessive menstrual flow, eye disorders,

eye pain, fainting, fungus infection, gallstones, glaucoma, gout, hair discoloration, hair loss, hallucinations, hangover effect, heart disorders, hemorrhoids, hepatitis, herpes infections, high cholesterol, hives, hostility, hyperventilation (fast, deep breathing), inability to communicate, increased mucus, increased physical activity, increased salivation, increased sensitivity to touch, increased sex drive, inflammation of the stomach, intestines, anus and rectum, gums, tongue, eyelid, or inner ear, intolerance to light, involuntary eye movements, irregular or slow heartbeat, kidney disorders, lack of menstruation, large amounts of urine, laryngitis, loss of consciousness, loss of muscle movement, low or high blood sugar, menstrual problems, middle ear infection, mouth fungus, mouth sores, muscle spasms, muscle weakness, nosebleeds, over- and underactive thyroid gland, overdose, paranoia, pelvic pain, pinpoint pupils, "pins and needles" around the mouth, pneumonia, prolonged erection, psoriasis, rectal hemorrhage, reduced menstrual flow, restlessness, secretion of milk, sensitivity to light, skin disorders, skin eruptions or hemorrhage, skin inflammation, sleep disturbance, soft stools, stiff neck, stomach or peptic ulcer, stroke, stupor, sugar in the urine, swelling due to fluid retention, swollen or discolored tongue, taste loss, temporary failure to breathe, thirst, twisted neck, ulcer, unconsciousness, uncoordinated movements, urgent need to urinate, urination at night, uterine and vaginal hemorrhage, varicose veins, voice changes, vomiting blood, yellowed eyes and skin

Why should this drug not be prescribed?

There are no known conditions that preclude Effexor therapy.

Special warnings about this medication

Your doctor will prescribe Effexor with caution if you have high blood pressure, heart, liver, or kidney disease or a history of seizures or mania (extreme agitation or excitability). You should discuss all of your medical problems with your doctor before taking Effexor.

Effexor may cause you to feel drowsy or less alert and may affect your judgment. Therefore, avoid driving or operating dangerous machinery or participating in any hazardous activity that requires full mental alertness until you know how this drug affects you.

If you have every been addicted to drugs, tell your doctor before you start taking Effexor.

If you develop a skin rash or hives while taking Effexor, notify your doctor.

Do not stop taking the drug without consulting your doctor. If you stop suddenly, you may have withdrawal symptoms, even though this drug does not seem to be habit forming. Your doctor will have you taper off gradually.

Possible food and drug interactions when taking this medication

Combining Effexor with MAO inhibitors could cause a fatal reaction.

Although Effexor does not interact with alcohol, the manufacturer recommends avoiding alcohol while taking this medication.

If you have high blood pressure or liver disease, or are elderly, check with your doctor before combining Effexor with cimetidine (Tagamet).

Effexor does not interact with Lithium or Valium. However, you should consult your doctor before combing Effexor with other drugs that affect the central nervous system, including narcotic painkillers, sleep aids, tranquilizers, and other antidepressants.

Special information
if you are pregnant or breastfeeding

The effects of Effexor during pregnancy have not been adequately studied. If you are pregnant or are planning to become pregnant, tell your doctor immediately. Effexor should be used during pregnancy only if clearly needed. Effexor may appear in breast milk. If this medication is essential to your health, your doctor may tell your to discontinue breastfeeding your baby until your treatment with Effexor is finished.

Recommended dosage

ADULTS

The usual starting dose is 75 milligrams a day, divided into 2 or 3 smaller doses, and taken with food. If needed, your doctor may increase your dose to 150 to 225 milligrams a day. He or she will adjust the dose according to your response.

If you have kidney or liver disease or are taking other medications, your doctor will adjust your dosage accordingly.

CHILDREN

The safety and effectiveness of Effexor have not been established in children under 18 years of age.

Overdosage

Any medication taken in excess can have serious consequences. If you suspect an overdose, seek medical attention immediately.

■ *Symptoms of Effexor overdose include:*
Convulsions
Rapid heartbeat
Sleepiness

Brand name:

ELAVIL

Pronounced: ELL-uh-vil
Generic name: Amitriptyline hydrochloride
Other brand name: Endep

Why is this drug prescribed?

Elavil is prescribed for the relief of symptoms of mental depression. It is a member of the group of drugs called tricyclic antidepressants. Some doctors also prescribe Elavil to treat bulimia (an eating disorder), to control chronic pain, to prevent migraine headaches, and to treat a pathological weeping and laughing syndrome associated with multiple sclerosis.

Most important fact about this drug

You may need to take Elavil regularly for several weeks before it becomes fully effective. Do not skip doses, even if they seem to make no difference or you feel you don't need them.

How should you take this medication?

Take Elavil exactly as prescribed. You may experience side effects, such as mild drowsiness, early in therapy. However, they usually disappear after a few days.

Elavil may cause dry mouth. Sucking a hard candy, chewing gum or melting bits of ice in your mouth can provide relief.

■ *If you miss a dose...*
Take it as soon as you remember. If it is almost time for your next dose, skip the one you missed and go back to your

regular schedule. Never take 2 doses at the same time.

If you take a single daily dose at bedtime, do not make up for it in the morning. It may cause side effects during the day.

■ *Storage instructions...*
Keep Elavil in a tightly closed container. Store at room temperature. Protect from light and excessive heat.

What side effects may occur?
Side effects cannot be anticipated. If any develop or change in intensity, inform your doctor as soon as possible. Only your doctor can determine if it is safe for you to continue taking Elavil.

■ *Side effects may include:*
Abnormal movements, anxiety, black tongue, blurred vision, breast development in males, breast enlargement, coma, confusion, constipation, delusions, diarrhea, difficult or frequent urination, difficulty in speech, dilation of pupils, disorientation, disturbed concentration, dizziness on getting up, dizziness or light-headedness, drowsiness, dry mouth, excessive or spontaneous flow of milk, excitement, fatigue, fluid retention, hair loss, hallucinations, headache, heart attack, hepatitis, high blood pressure, high fever, high or low blood sugar, hives, impotence, inability to sleep, increased or decreased sex drive, increased perspiration, increased pressure within the eye, inflammation of the mouth, intestinal obstruction, irregular heartbeat, lack or loss of coordination, loss of appetite, low blood pressure, nausea, nightmares, numbness, rapid and/or fast, fluttery heartbeat, rash, red or purple spots on skin, restlessness, ringing in the ears, seizures, sensitivity to light, stomach upset, strange taste, stroke, swelling due to fluid retention in the face

and tongue, swelling of testicles, swollen glands, tingling and pins and needles in the arms and legs, tremors, vomiting, weakness, weight gain or loss, yellowed eyes and skin

■ *Side effects due to rapid decrease or abrupt withdrawal from Elavil include:*
Headache
Nausea
Vague feeling of bodily discomfort

■ *Side effects due to gradual dosage reduction may include:*
Dream and sleep disturbances
Irritability
Restlessness

These side effects do not signify an addiction to the drug.

Why should this drug not be prescribed?
If you are sensitive to or have ever had an allergic reaction to Elavil or similar drugs such as Norpramin and Tofranil, you should not take this medication. Make sure your doctor is aware of any drug reactions you have experienced.

Do not take Elavil while taking other antidepressants known as MAO inhibitors. Drugs in this category include Nardil, Parnate, and Marplan.

Unless you are directed to do so by your doctor, do not take this medication if you are recovering from a heart attack.

Special warnings about this medication
Do not stop taking Elavil abruptly, especially if you have been taking large doses for a long time. Your doctor probably will want to decrease your dosage gradually. This will help prevent a possible relapse and will reduce the possibility of withdrawl symptoms.

Elavil may make your skin more sensitive to sunlight. Try to stay out of the sun, wear protective clothing, and apply a sun block.

Elavil may cause you to become drowsy or less alert; therefore, you should not drive or operate dangerous machinery or participate in any hazardous activity that requires full mental alertness until you know how this drug affects you.

While taking this medication, you may feel dizzy or light-headed or actually faint when getting up from a lying or sitting position. If getting up slowly doesn't help or if this problem continues, notify your doctor.

Use Elavil with caution if you have ever had seizures, urinary retention, glaucoma or other chronic eye conditions, a heart or circulatory system disorder, or liver problems. Be cautious, too, if you are receiving thyroid medication. You should discuss all of your medical problems with your doctor before starting Elavil therapy.

Before having surgery, dental treatment or any diagnostic procedure, tell the doctor that you are taking Elavil. Certain drugs used during surgery, such as anesthetics and muscle relaxants, and drugs used in certain diagnostic procedures may react badly with Elavil.

Possible food and drug interactions when taking this medication

Elavil may intensify the effects of alcohol. Do not drink alcohol while taking this medication.

If Elavil is taken with certain other drugs, the effects of either could be increased, decreased, or altered. It is especially important that you consult with your doctor before taking Elavil in combination with the following:

Acetazolamide (Diamox)
Airway-opening drugs such as Proventil and Ventolin
Allergy and cold medicines such as Comtrex and Dristan
Antispasmodic drugs such as Bentyl
Antihistamines such as Benadryl and Tavist
Barbiturates such as phenobarbital
Certain blood pressure medicines such as Catapres
Cimetidine (Tagamet)
Disulfiram (Antabuse)
Estrogen drugs such as Premarin
Ethchlorvynol (Placidyl)
Fluoxetine (Prozac)
Guanethidine (Ismelin)
Levodopa (Larodopa)
Major tranquilizers such as Mellaril and Thorazine
Muscle relaxants such as Lioresal
Oral Contraceptives
Painkillers such as Demerol and Percocet
Parkinsonism drugs such as Cogentin
Quinidine (Quinidex)
Seizure medications such as Tegretol and Dilantin
Sleep medicines such as Halcion and Dalmane
Thyroid hormones (Synthroid)
Tranquilizers such as Librium and Xanax
Vitamin C in large doses
Warfarin (Coumadin)

Special information if you are pregnant or breastfeeding

The effects of Elavil during pregnancy have not been adequately studied. If you are pregnant or planning to become pregnant, inform your doctor immediately. This medication appears in breast milk. If Elavil is essential to your health, your doctor may advise you to discontinue breastfeeding until your treatment is finished.

Recommended dosage

ADULTS

The usual starting dosage is 75 milligrams per day divided into 2 or more smaller doses. Your doctor may gradually increase this dose to 150 milligrams per day. The total daily dose is generally never higher than 200 milligrams.

Alternatively, your doctor may want you to start with 50 milligrams to 100 milligrams at bedtime. He or she may increase this bedtime dose by 25 or 50 milligrams up to a total of 150 milligrams a day.

For long-term use, the usual dose ranges from 40 to 100 milligrams taken once daily, usually at bedtime.

CHILDREN

Use of Elavil is not recommended for children under 12 years of age.

The usual dose for adolescents 12 years of age and over is 10 milligrams, 3 times a day, with 20 milligrams taken at bedtime.

ELDERLY

The usual dose is 10 milligrams taken 3 times a day, with 20 milligrams taken at bedtime.

Overdosage

An overdose of Elavil can prove fatal.

■ *Symptoms of Elavil overdose may include:*
Abnormally low blood pressure
Congestive heart failure
Convulsions
Dilated pupils
Drowsiness
Rapid or irregular heartbeat
Reduced body temperature
Stupor
Unresponsiveness or coma

■ *Symptoms contrary to the effect of this medication, are:*
Agitation
Extremely high body temperature
Rigid muscles
Vomiting

If you suspect an overdose, seek medical attention immediately.

Brand name:

EMPIRIN

See Aspirin, page 515.

Brand name:

E-MYCIN

See Erythromycin, Oral, page 584.

Brand name:

ENDEP

See Elavil, page 580.

Generic name:

ERGOLOID MESYLATES

See Hydergine, page 616.

Generic name:

ERGOTAMINE WITH CAFFEINE

See Cafergot, page 529.

Brand name:

ERYC

See Erythromycin, Oral, page 584.

Brand name:

ERYCETTE

See Erythromycin, Topical, page 587.

Brand name:

ERY-TAB

See Erythromycin, Oral, page 584.

Brand name:

ERYTHROCIN

See Erythromycin, Oral, page 584.

Generic name:

ERYTHROMYCIN, ORAL

Pronounced: er-ITH-row MY-sin
Brand names: E.E.S., E-Mycin, ERYC, Ery-
    Tab, Erythrocin, Ilosone, PCE

Why is this drug prescribed?
Erythromycin is an antibiotic used to treat many kinds of infections, including:

Chlamydia
Diphtheria
Ear infections (along with sulfa drugs)
Gonorrhea
Intestinal infections
Legionnaires' disease
Rheumatic fever
Skin infections
Syphilis
Upper and lower respiratory tract infections
Urinary tract infections

Whooping cough
Prevention of infections of the heart (rheumatic fever and bacterial endocarditis) in people who are allergic to penicillin or who have congenital or rheumatic heart disease

Most important fact about this drug
Erythromycin, like any other antibiotic, works best when there is a constant amount of drug in the blood. To help keep the drug amount constant, it is important not to miss any doses. Also, it is advisable to take the doses at evenly spaced times around the clock.

How should you take this medication?
Most people can take erythromycin with or without meals. However, food may decrease the effectiveness of erythromycin in some people.

Your doctor may advise you to take erythromycin 30 minutes to 2 hours before or after meals. Take erythromycin exactly as prescribed.

Chewable forms of erythromycin should be crushed or chewed before being swallowed.

Delayed-release brands and tablets and capsules that are coated to slow their breakdown should be swallowed whole. Do not crush or break. If you are not sure about the form of erythromycin you are taking, ask your pharmacist.

The liquid should be shaken well before each use.

■ If you miss a dose...
    Take it as soon as you remember. If it is almost time for your next dose, skip the one you missed and go back to your regular schedule. Never take 2 doses at the same time.

■ *Storage instructions...*
The liquid form of erythromycin should be kept in the refrigerator. Do not freeze. Store tablets and capsules at room temperature.

What side effects may occur?

Side effects cannot be anticipated. If any develop or change in intensity, inform your doctor as soon as possible. Only your doctor can determine whether it is safe to continue taking this medication.

■ *More common side effects may include:*
Abdominal pain
Diarrhea
Loss of appetite
Nausea
Vomiting

■ *Less common side effects may include:*
Hives, rash, skin eruptions, yellow eyes and skin

■ *Rare side effects may include:*
Chest pain, confusion, dizziness, hallucinations, hearing loss (temporary), inflammation of the large intestine, palpitations, rapid heartbeat, seizures, severe allergic reaction, vertigo

Why should this drug not be prescribed?

You should not use erythromycin if you have ever had an allergic reaction or are sensitive to it. Erythromycin should not be used with Seldane or Hismanal.

Special warnings about this medication

If you have ever had liver disease, consult with your doctor before taking erythromycin.

If new infections (called superinfections) occur, talk to your doctor. You may need to be treated with a different antibiotic.

Possible food and drug interactions when taking this medication

If erythromycin is taken with certain other drugs, the effects of either could be increased, decreased, or altered. It is especially important to check with your doctor before combining erythromycin with the following:

Alfentanil (Alfenta)
Astemizole (Hisminal)
Blood-thinning drugs such as Coumadin
Bromocriptime (Parlodel)
Carbamazepine (Tegretol)
Cyclosporine (Sandimmune)
Digoxin (Lanoxin)
Disopyramide (Norpace)
Ergotamine (Cafergot)
Felodipine (Plendil)
Hexobarbital
Lovastatin (Mevacor)
Midazolam (Versed)
Other antibiotics
Penicillin (Amoxil, Omnipcn)
Phenytoin (Dilantin)
Terfenadine (Seldane)
Theophylline (Theo-Dur)
Triazolam (Halcion)

Special information if you are pregnant or breastfeeding

If you are pregnant or plan to become pregnant, inform your doctor immediately. Erythromycin appears in breast milk and could affect a nursing infant. If this medication is essential to your health, your doctor may advise you to discontinue breastfeeding until your treatment is finished.

Recommended dosage

Dosage instructions are determined by the type (and severity) of infection being treated and may vary slightly for different brands of erythromycin. The following are recommended dosages for PCE, one of the most commonly prescribed brands.

ADULTS

Streptococcal Infections

The usual dose is 250 milligrams every 6 hours, 333 milligrams every 8 hours, or 500 milligrams every 12 hours. Depending on the severity of the infection, the dose may be increased to a total of 4 grams a day. However, when the daily dosage is larger than 1 gram, twice-a-day doses are not recommended, and the drug should be taken more often in smaller doses.

To treat streptococcal infections of the upper respiratory tract (tonsillitis or strep throat), erythromycin should be taken for 10 days. The usual dosage in long-term prevention to prevent recurring attacks of rheumatic fever is 250 milligrams twice daily.

Gonorrhea

The usual dosage is 3 grams in a single oral dose.

To Prevent Bacterial Endocarditis (Inflammation and Infection of the Heart Lining and Valves) in Patients Who Are Allergic to Penicillin

The oral regimen is 1 gram of erythromycin taken one-half to 2 hours before dental surgery or surgical procedures of the upper respiratory tract, followed by 500 milligrams every 6 hours for 8 doses.

Urinary Tract Infections Due to Chlamydia Trachomatis During Pregnancy

Although the optimal dose and duration of therapy have not been established, the suggested treatment is 500 milligrams of erythromycin by mouth 4 times a day or 666 milligrams every 8 hours on an empty stomach for at least 7 days. For women who cannot tolerate this regimen, a decreased dose of 500 milligrams by mouth every 12 hours, 333 milligrams orally every 8 hours, or 250 milligrams by mouth 4 times a day should be used for at least 14 days.

For Patients with Uncomplicated Urinary, Reproductive Tract, or Rectal Infections Caused by Chlamydia Trachomatis When Tetracycline Cannot Be Taken

The usual dosage is 500 milligrams of erythromycin by mouth 4 times a day or 333 milligrams every 8 hours for at least 7 days.

For Patients with Nongonococcal Urethral Infections When Tetracycline Cannot Be Taken

The usual dosage is 500 milligrams of erythromycin by mouth 4 times a day or 666 milligrams orally every 8 hours for at least 7 days.

Syphilis

The usual dosage is 30 to 40 grams divided into smaller doses over a period of 10 to 15 days.

Intestinal Infections

The usual dosage is 500 milligrams every 12 hours, 333 milligrams every 8 hours, or 250 milligrams every 6 hours for 10 to 14 days.

Legionnaires' Disease

Although the optimal dosage has not been established, doses utilized in reported clinical data were 1 to 4 grams daily, divided into smaller doses.

CHILDREN

Age, weight, and severity of the infection determine the correct dosage.

The usual dosage is from 30 to 50 milligrams daily for each 2.2 pounds of body weight, divided into equal doses.

For more severe infections, this dosage may be doubled, but it should not exceed 4 grams per day.

Children weighing over 44 pounds should follow the recommended adult dose schedule.

The dosage for children weighing under 44 pounds is determined by their weight.

Conjunctivitis (Pinkeye) in the Newborn Caused by Chlamydia Trachomatis (a Sexually Transmitted Infection Passed on by the Mother)
The usual dosage of oral erythromycin suspension is 50 milligrams for each 2.2 pounds of body weight daily, divided into 4 doses, for at least 2 weeks.

Pneumonia in Infants Caused by Chlamydia Trachomatis
Although the most effective length of treatment has not been established, the recommended therapy is oral erythromycin suspension, 50 milligrams for each 2.2 pounds of body weight daily, divided into 4 doses, for at least 3 weeks.

Whooping Cough
Although the optimal dosage and duration have not been established, clinical studies utilized 40 to 50 milligrams for each 2.2 pounds of body weight daily, divided into smaller doses for 5 to 14 days.

ELDERLY

Erythromycin should be used with caution in elderly patients.

Overdosage

Any medication taken in excess can have serious consequences. If you suspect an overdose, seek medical help immediately.

■ *Symptoms of erythromycin overdose may include:*
Diarrhea
Nausea
Stomach cramps
Vomiting
Generic name:

ERYTHROMYCIN, TOPICAL

Pronounced: err-rith-ro-MY-sin
Brand names: A/T/S, Erycette, T-Stat

Why is this drug prescribed?
Erythromycin topical (applied directly to the skin) is used for the treatment of acne.

Most important fact about this drug
For best results, you should continue the treatment for as long as prescribed, even if your acne begins to clear up. This medicine is not an instant cure.

How should you use this medication?
Use exactly as prescribed by your doctor.

Thoroughly wash the affected area with soap and water and pat dry before applying medication.

Moisten the applicator or pad with the medication and lightly spread it over the affected area. A/T/S Topical Gel should not be rubbed in.

■ *If you miss a dose...*
Apply the forgotten dose as soon as you remember. If it is almost time for the next application, skip the one you missed and go back to your regular schedule.

■ *Storage instructions...*
This medicine can be stored at room temperature.

What side effects may occur?
Side effects cannot be anticipated. If any develop or change in intensity, inform your

doctor as soon as possible. Only your doctor can determine if it is safe for you to continue using erythromycin topical.

■ *Side effects may include:*
Burning sensation
Dryness
Hives
Irritation of the eyes
Itching
Oiliness
Peeling
Scaling
Tenderness
Unusual redness of the skin

Why should this drug not be prescribed?

Erythromycin topical should not be used if you are sensitive to or have ever had an allergic reaction to any of the ingredients.

Special warnings about this medication

This type of erythromycin is for external use only. Do not use is in or around the eyes, nose, or mouth.

The use of antibiotics can stimulate the growth of other bacteria that are resistant to the antibiotic you are taking. If new infections (called superinfections) occur, talk to your doctor. You may need to be treated with a different antibiotic drug.

The use of other topical acne medications in combination with erythromycin topical may cause irritation, especially with the use of peeling, scaling, or abrasive medications.

The safety and effectiveness of A/T/S has not been established in children.

Possible food and drug interactions when using this medication

If erythromycin topical is used with certain other drugs, the effects of either could be increased, decreased, or altered. It is especially important to check with your doctor before combining erythromycin topical with other topical acne medications.

Special information if you are pregnant or breastfeeding

The effects of erythromycin topical during pregnancy have not been adequately studied. If you are pregnant or plan to become pregnant, inform your doctor immediately. Erythromycin topical may appear in breast milk and could affect a nursing infant. If this medication is essential to your health, your doctor may advise you to stop breastfeeding until your treatment with erythromycin topical is finished.

Recommended dosage

A/T/S TOPICAL SOLUTION

Apply the solution to the affected area(s) 2 times a day, in the morning and at night. Moisten the applicator or a pad with A/T/S, then rub over the affected area(s). Make sure the area(s) is (are) thoroughly washed with soap and water and patted dry before applying medication.

A/T/S TOPICAL GEL

Apply a thin film of gel to the affected area(s). Spread the medication lightly. Do not rub it in. Make sure the area(s) is (are) thoroughly washed with soap and water and patted dry before applying medication. Thoroughly wash your hands after application of the medication.

ERYCETTE TOPICAL SOLUTION

Rub the pledget (pad) over the affected area(s) 2 times a day. Make sure the area(s) is (are) thoroughly washed with soap and water and patted dry before applying medication. Additional pledgets can be used, if needed. Each pledget should be used just once and then thrown away.

T-STAT TOPICAL SOLUTION

The solution or pads should be applied over the affected area(s) 2 times a day. Make sure the area(s) is (are) thoroughly washed with soap and water and patted dry before applying medication. Additional pads can be used, if needed. T-Stat should be applied with the applicator top or disposable pads. If you use the pads or your fingertips, wash your hands after application.

Reducing the frequency of applications may reduce peeling and drying.

Overdosage

Although overdosage is unlikely, any medication used in excess can have serious consequences. If you suspect an overdose, seek medical treatment immediately.

Generic name:

ERYTHROMYCIN WITH BENZOYL PEROXIDE

See Benzamycin, page 526.

Brand name:

ESGIC

See Fioricet, page 598.

Brand name:

ESGIC PLUS

See Fioricet, page 598.

Brand name:

ESIDRIX

See HydroDIURIL, page 617.

Brand name:

ESTRACE

See Estraderm, page 589.

Brand name:

ESTRADERM

Pronounced: ESS-tra-derm
Generic name: Estradiol
Other brand name: Estrace

Why is this drug prescribed?

Estraderm is an estrogen replacement drug. It is used to reduce symptoms of menopause, including feelings of warmth in face, neck, and chest, and the sudden intense episodes of heat and sweating known as "hot flashes." It is also used for other conditions caused by lack of estrogen, such as dry, itchy external genitals and vaginal irritation, and may be prescribed for teenagers who fail to mature at the usual rate.

Along with diet, calcium supplements, and exercise, Estraderm is also prescribed to prevent osteoporosis, a condition in which the bones become brittle and easily broken.

Estrace is also used to treat low levels of estrogen in certain people and to provide relief in breast or prostate cancer.

Most important fact about this drug

Because estrogens have been linked with increased risk of endometrial cancer (cancer in the lining of the uterus), it is essential to have regular checkups and to report any unusual vaginal bleeding to your doctor immediately.

How should you take this medication?

Each Estraderm patch is individually sealed in a protective pouch and is applied directly to the skin.

A stiff protective liner covers the adhesive side of the patch. Remove the liner by sliding it sideways between your thumb and index finger. Holding the patch at one edge, remove the protective liner and discard it. Try to avoid touching the adhesive. Use immediately after removing the liner.

Apply the adhesive side to a clean, dry area of your skin on the trunk of your body (including the buttocks and abdomen). Do not apply to your breasts or waist. Firmly press the patch in place with the palm of your hand for about 10 seconds, to make sure the edges are flat against your skin.

Contact with water during bathing, swimming, or showering will not affect the patch.

The application site must be rotated. Allow an interval of at least 1 week between apppications to a particular site.

Estrace Tablets are taken orally.

If you are using Estrace vaginal cream, follow these steps to apply:

1. Load the supplied applicator to the fill line.
2. Lie on your back with your knees drawn up.
3. Gently insert the applicator high into the vagina. Release the medicine by pushing the plunger.
4. Withdraw the applicator.
5. Wash the applicator with soap and water.

■ *If you miss a dose...*
 If you forget to apply a new patch when you are supposed to, do it as soon as you remember. If it is almost time to change patches anyway, skip the one you missed and go back to your regular schedule. Do not use more than one patch at a time.

 If you miss a dose of the tablets, take it as soon as you remember. If it is almost time for your next dose, skip the one you missed and go back to your regular schedule. Do not take 2 doses at once.

■ *Storage instructions...*
 Store Estraderm at room temperature, in its sealed pouch.

 Store Estrace at room temperature.

What side effects may occur?

Side effects cannot be anticipated. If any develop or change in intensity, notify your doctor as soon as possible. Only your doctor can determine if it is safe for you to continue taking Estraderm.

■ *The most common side effect is:*
 skin redness and irritation at the site of the patch.

■ *Less common or rare side effects may include:*
 Abdominal cramps, bloating, breakthrough bleeding, breast enlargement, breast tenderness, change in cervical secretions, change in menstrual flow, change in sex drive, change in weight, darkening of skin, dizziness, fluid retention, growth of benign fibroid tumors in the uterus, headache, intolerance to contact lenses, migraine, nausea, rash, severe allergic reaction, spotting, vomiting, yellowing of eyes and skin

■ *Other side effects reported with estradiol include:*
 Abnormal withdrawal bleeding
 Certain cancers
 Cardiovascular disease

Depression
Excessive growth of hair
Gallbladder disease
Hair loss
High blood pressure
Reddened skin
Skin discoloration
Skin eruptions
Twitching
Vaginal yeast infection

Why should this drug not be prescribed?

Estraderm should not be used if you are sensitive to or have ever had an allergic reaction to any of its components.

Estrogens should not be used if you know or suspect you have breast cancer or a tumor promoted by estrogen. Also avoid estrogens if you are pregnant or think you are pregnant, if you have abnormal, undiagnosed genital bleeding, if you have blood clots or a blood clotting disorder, or if you have a history of blood clotting disorders associated with previous estrogen use.

Special warnings about this medication

The risk of cancer of the uterus increases when estrogen is used for a long time or taken in large doses. There also may be increased risk of breast cancer in women who take estrogen for an extended period of time.

Women who take estrogen after menopause are more likely to develop gall bladder disease.

Estraderm also increases the risk of blood clots. These blood clots can cause stroke, heart attack, or other serious disorders.

While taking Estraderm, get in touch with your doctor right away if you notice any of the following:

Abdominal pain, tenderness, or swelling
Abnormal bleeding of the vagina
Breast lumps
Coughing up blood
Pain in your chest or calves
Severe headache, dizziness, or faintness
Sudden shortness of breath
Vision changes
Yellowing of the skin

A complete medical and family history should be taken by your doctor before starting any estrogen therapy.

In general, you should not take estrogen for more than 1 year without another physical examination by your doctor.

Estraderm may cause fluid retention in some people. If you have asthma, epilepsy, migraine, or heart or kidney disease, use this medication cautiously.

Estogen therapy may cause uterine bleeding or breast pain.

Possible food and drug interactions when taking this medication

If you take certain other drugs while using Estraderm, the effects of either could be increased, decreased, or altered. It is especially important to check with your doctor before taking the following:

Barbiturates such as phenobarbitol
Blood thinners such as Coumadin
Epilepsy drugs (Tegretol, Dilantin, others)
Rifampin (Rifadin)
Tricyclic antidepressants (Elavil, Tofranil, others)

Special information if you are pregnant or breastfeeding

Estrogens should not be used during pregnancy. If you are pregnant or plan to become pregnant, notify your doctor immediately. Estraderm may appear in breast milk and could affect a nursing infant. If this medication is essential to your health, your doctor may advise you to discontinue breastfeeding until your treatment is finished.

Recommended dosage

SYMPTOMS OF MENOPAUSE

Estraderm
The usual starting dose is 0.05 milligram applied to the skin 2 times a week. Dosage should be decreased at 3- to 6-month intervals.

Estrace
The usual starting dose is 1 or 2 milligrams a day; you will take the tablets for 3 weeks and then have 1 week off for each cycle.

PREVENTION OF OSTEOPOROSIS

Estraderm
The usual starting dose is 0.05 milligram per day.

Estrace
The usual dose is 0.5 milligram taken every day for 3 weeks, followed by 1 week off.

LOW ESTROGEN LEVELS

Estrace
The usual starting dose is 1 or 2 milligrams a day.

RELIEF IN BREAST CANCER

Estrace
The usual dose is 10 milligrams 3 times a day for at least 3 months.

RELIEF IN PROSTATE CANCER

Estrace
The usual dose is 1 to 2 milligrams 3 times a day.

VAGINAL ITCHING AND DRYNESS

Estrace Vaginal Cream
The usual dosage is 2 to 4 grams (marked on the applicator) inserted into the vagina once a day, for 1 to 2 weeks. The dosage and frequency may be reduced after your condition improves.

Overdosage

Any medication taken in excess can have serious consequences. If you suspect an overdose, seek medical attention immediately.

■ *Symptoms of Estraderm overdose may include:*
Nausea
Vomiting
Withdrawal bleeding

Generic name:

ESTRADIOL

See Estraderm, page 589.

Generic name:

ESTROPIPATE

See Ogen, page 697.

Generic name:

ETODOLAC

See Lodine, page 638.

Brand name:

FASTIN

Pronounced: FAS-tin
Generic name: Phentermine hydrochloride
Other brand name: Ionamin

Why is this drug prescribed?

Fastin, an appetite suppressant, is prescribed for short-term use (a few weeks) as part of an overall diet plan for weight reduction. Fastin should be used along with a behavior modification program.

Most important fact about this drug

Always remember that Fastin is an aid to, not a substitute for, good diet and exercise. Take Fastin only as directed by your doctor. Do not take it more often or for a longer time than your doctor has ordered. Fastin can lose its effectiveness after a few weeks.

How should you take this medication?

Take Fastin about 2 hours after breakfast. Do not take it late in the evening because it may keep you from sleeping.

Take Ionamin before breakfast or 10 to 14 hours before you go to bed. Ionamin capsules should be swallowed whole.

■ *If you miss a dose...*
Skip the missed dose completely; then take the next dose at the regularly scheduled time.

■ *Storage instructions...*
Store away from heat, light, and moisture.

What side effects may occur?

Side effects cannot be anticipated. If any develop or change in intensity, inform your doctor as soon as possible. Only your doctor can determine if it is safe for you to continue taking this medication.

■ *Side effects may include:*
Changes in sex drive, constipation, diarrhea, dizziness, dry mouth, exaggerated feelings of depression or elation, headache, high blood pressure, hives, impotence, inability to fall or stay asleep, increased heart rate, overstimulation, restlessness, stomach or intestinal problems, throbbing heartbeat, tremors, unpleasant taste

Why should this drug not be prescribed?

If you are sensitive to or have ever had an allergic reaction to phentermine hydrochloride or other drugs that stimulate the nervous system, you should not take this medication. Make sure your doctor is aware of any drug reactions you have experienced.

Do not take this drug if you have hardening of the arteries, symptoms of heart or blood vessel disease, an overactive thyroid gland, the eye condition known as glaucoma, or moderate to severe high blood pressure. Also avoid this drug if you are agitated, have ever abused drugs, or have taken an MAO inhibitor, including antidepressant drugs such as Nardil and Parnate, within the last 14 days.

Special warnings about this medication

Fastin may affect your ability to perform potentially hazardous activities. Therefore, you should be extremely careful if you have to drive a car or operate machinery.

You can become psychologically dependent on this drug. Consult your doctor if you rely on this drug to maintain a state of well-being.

If you stop taking Fastin suddenly after you have taken high doses for a long time, you may find you are extremely fatigued or depressed, or that you have trouble sleeping.

If you continually take too much of any appetite suppressant it can cause severe skin disorders, a pronounced inability to fall or stay asleep, irritability, hyperactivity, and personality changes.

Even if your blood pressure is only mildly high, be careful taking this drug.

Possible food and drug interactions when taking this medication

This drug may intensify the effects of alcohol. Avoid alcoholic beverages while you are taking it.

If Fastin is taken with certain other drugs, the effects of either can be increased, decreased, or altered. It is especially important that you check with your doctor before combining Fastin with the following:

Antidepressants classified as MAO inhibitors, including Nardil and Parnate
Diabetes medications such as insulin and Micronase
High blood pressure medications such as guanethidine (Ismelin)

Special information if you are pregnant or breastfeeding

The effects of Fastin during pregnancy have not been adequately studied. If you are pregnant, plan to become pregnant, or are breastfeeding, notify your doctor immediately.

Recommended dosage

ADULTS

Fastin
The usual dosage is 1 capsule approximately 2 hours after breakfast. One capsule should suppress your appetite for 12 to 14 hours.

Ionamin
The usual dose is 1 capsule a day, taken before breakfast or 10 to 14 hours before bedtime.

CHILDREN

This drug is not recommended for use in children under 12 years of age.

Overdosage

Any medication taken in excess can have serious consequences. An overdose of Fastin can be fatal. If you suspect an overdose, seek emergency medical treatment immediately.

■ *Symptoms of Fastin overdose may include:* Abdominal cramps, aggressiveness, confusion, diarrhea, exaggerated reflexes, hallucinations, high or low blood pressure, irregular heartbeat, nausea, panic states, rapid breathing, restlessness, tremors, vomiting

Fatigue and depression may follow the stimulant effects of Fastin.

In cases of fatal poisoning, convulsions and coma usually precede death.

Brand name:

FELDENE

Pronounced: FELL-deen
Generic name: Piroxicam

Why is this drug prescribed?

Feldene, a nonsteroidal anti-inflammatory drug, is used to relieve the inflammation, swelling, stiffness, and joint pain associated with rheumatoid arthritis and osteoarthritis (the most common form of arthritis). It is prescribed both for sudden flare-ups and for long term treatment.

Most important fact about this drug

In a few patients on long-term therapy, Feldene can cause stomach ulcers and bleeding. Warning signs include severe abdominal or stomach cramps, pain or burning in the stomach, and black, tarry stools. Inform your doctor immediately if you develop any of these symptoms.

How should you take this medication?

To avoid digestive side effects, take Feldene with food or an antacid, and with a full glass of water. Never take it on an empty stomach.

Take this medication exactly as prescribed by your doctor. Avoid alcohol and aspirin while taking this drug.

■ *If you miss a dose...*
If you forget to take a dose, take it as soon as you remember. If it is almost time for your next dose, skip the one you missed and go back to your regular schedule. Never take two doses at the same time.

■ *Storage instructions...*
Store at room temperature. Protect from light and heat.

What side effects may occur?

Side effects cannot be anticipated. If any develop or change in intensity, inform your doctor as soon as possible. Only your doctor can determine if it is safe for you to continue taking Feldene.

■ *More common side effects may include:*
Abdominal pain or discomfort, anemia, constipation, diarrhea, dizziness, fluid retention, gas, general feeling of ill health, headache, heartburn, indigestion, inflammation inside the mouth, itching, loss of appetite, nausea, rash, ringing in ears, sleepiness, stomach upset, vertigo

■ *Less common or rare side effects may include:*
Abdominal bleeding, severe allergic reactions, angioedema (swelling of lips, face, tongue and throat), black stools, blood in the urine, blurred vision, bruising, colicky pain, congestive heart failure (worsening of), depression, dry mouth, eye irritations, fatigue, fever, flu-like symptoms, hepatitis, high blood pressure, hives, inability to sleep, joint pain, labored breathing, low or high blood sugar, nervousness, nosebleed, serum sickness (fever, painful joints, enlarged lymph nodes, skin rash), skin allergy to sunlight, skin eruptions, Stevens-Johnson syndrome (blisters in the mouth and eyes), sweating, swollen eyes, vomiting, vomiting blood, weight loss or gain, wheezing, worsening of angina, yellow eyes and skin

Why should this drug not be prescribed?

If you are sensitive to or have ever had an allergic reaction to Feldene, aspirin, or similar drugs, or if you have had asthma attacks caused by aspirin or other drugs of this type, you should not take this medication. Make sure that your doctor is aware of any drug reactions that you have experienced.

Special warnings about this medication

If you have heart disease, or high blood pressure, or other conditions that cause fluid retention, use this drug with caution. Feldene can increase water retention.

This drug should be used with caution if you have kidney or liver disease; it can cause liver inflammation in some people.

Drugs such as Feldene may cause eye disturbances in some people. If you develop visual problems, notify your eye doctor.

Possible food and drug interactions when taking this medication

If Feldene is taken with certain other drugs, the effects of either could be increased, decreased, or altered. It is especially important to check with your doctor before combining Feldene with the following:

Anticoagulants (blood thinners such as
    Coumadin)
Aspirin
Lithium

Special information if you are pregnant or breastfeeding

Feldene is not recommended for use in nursing mothers or pregnant women. If you are pregnant or plan to become pregnant, inform your doctor immediately.

Recommended dosage

ADULTS

Rheumatoid Arthritis and Osteoarthritis:
The usual dose is 20 milligrams a day in one dose. Your doctor may want you to divide this dose into smaller ones. You will not feel Feldene's full effects for 7 to 12 days, although some relief of symptoms will start to occur soon after you take the medication.

CHILDREN

The safety and effectiveness of Feldene have not been established in children.

ELDERLY

Your doctor will determine your dosage according to your particular needs.

Overdosage

Although there are no specific symptoms of a Feldene overdose, any medication taken in excess can have serious consequences. If you suspect an overdose, seek medical attention immediately.

Brand name:

FEMSTAT

Pronounced: FEM-stat
Generic name: Butoconazole nitrate

Why is this drug prescribed?

Femstat Vaginal Cream is prescribed for the treatment of yeast-like fungal infections of the vulva and vagina.

Most important fact about this drug

To obtain maximum benefit, it is important that you continue to use Femstat Vaginal Cream during menstruation and that you finish using all of the medication, even if your symptoms have disappeared.

How should you use this medication?

Use this medication exactly as prescribed. To keep it from getting on your clothing, wear a sanitary napkin. Do not use a tampon; it will absorb the drug. Do not douche unless your doctor tells you to do so.

While using Femstat, wear cotton underwear or pantyhose with a cotton crotch. Avoid synthetic fabrics such as rayon and nylon.

To apply Femstat:
1. Fill the applicator that comes with the vaginal cream to the level indicated.
2. Lie on your back with your knees drawn up.
3. Gently insert the applicator high into vagina and push the plunger.
4. Withdraw the applicator and discard if disposable or wash with soap and water.

To avoid reinfection, refrain from intercourse during treatment or ask your partner to use a condom.

■ *If you miss a dose...*
Insert it as soon as you remember. If it is almost time for your next dose, skip the one you missed and go back to your regular schedule.

■ *Storage instructions...*
Store at room temperature, away from heat. Do not freeze.

What side effects may occur?
Side effects cannot be anticipated. If any develop or change in intensity, inform your doctor as soon as possible. Only your doctor can determine if it is safe for you to continue using Femstat.

■ *Side effects may include:*
Itching of the fingers
Soreness
Swelling
Vaginal discharge
Vulvar itching
Vulvar or vaginal burning

Why should this drug not be prescribed?
If you are sensitive to or have ever had an allergic reaction to butoconazole nitrate or any other ingredients in Femstat Cream, you should not use this medication. Make sure your doctor is aware of any drug reactions you have experienced.

Special warnings about this medication
If your symptoms persist, or if you become irritated or have an allergic reaction while using this medication, notify your doctor.

Possible food and drug interactions when taking this medication
No interactions with other drugs have been reported.

Special information if you are pregnant or breastfeeding
The effects of Femstat Cream during the first trimester (first 3 months) of pregnancy have not been adequately studied. However, women using this cream for 3 to 6 days during the second or third trimester of pregnancy have experienced no adverse effects or complications, nor have their infants. It is not known whether this drug appears in breast milk. If Femstat is essential to your health, your doctor may advise you to discontinue breastfeeding until your treatment is finished.

Recommended dosage

ADULTS

Non-pregnant Women
The recommended dose is 1 applicatorful of cream inserted in the vagina at bedtime for 3 days. Your doctor may extend your treatment for an additional 3 days if necessary.

Pregnant Women (Second and Third Trimesters Only)
The recommended dose is 1 applicatorful of cream inserted in the vagina at bedtime for 6 days.

CHILDREN

Safety and effectiveness have not been established in children.

Overdosage
No overdosage has been reported.

Generic name:

FENOPROFEN

See Nalfon, page 672.

Brand name:

FIBERALL

See Metamucil, page 653.

Brand name:

FIORICET

Pronounced: fee-OAR-i-set
Generic ingredients: Butalbital,
   Acetaminophen, Caffeine
Other brand names: Esgic, Esgic Plus

Why is this drug prescribed?

Fioricet, a strong, non-narcotic pain reliever and muscle relaxant, is prescribed for the relief of tension headache symptoms caused by muscle contractions in the head, neck, and shoulder area. It combines a non-narcotic, sedative barbiturate (butalbital), a non-aspirin pain reliever (acetaminophen), and caffeine.

Most important fact about this drug

Mental and physical dependence can occur with the use of barbiturates such as butalbital when these drugs are taken in higher than recommended doses over long periods of time.

How should you take this medication?

Take Fioricet exactly as prescribed. Do not increase the amount you take without your doctor's approval.

■ *If you miss a dose...*
Take it as soon as you remember. If it is almost time for your next dose, skip the one you missed and go back to your regular schedule. Never take 2 doses at the same time.

■ *Storage instructions...*
Store at room temperature in a tight, light-resistant container.

What side effects may occur?

Side effects cannot be anticipated. If any develop or change in intensity, inform your doctor as soon as possible. Only your doctor can determine if it is safe for you to continue taking Fioricet.

■ *More common side effects may include:*
Dizziness
Drowsiness

If these side effects occur, it may help if you lie down after taking the medication.

■ *Less common or rare side effects may include:*
Depression, gas, light-headedness, mental confusion, nausea, rash, skin peeling, vomiting

Why should this drug not be prescribed?

If you are sensitive to or have ever had an allergic reaction to barbiturates, acetaminophen, caffeine, or other drugs of this type, you should not take this medication. Make sure that your doctor is aware of any drug reactions that you have experienced.

Unless you are directed to do so by your doctor, do not take this medication if you have porphyria (an inherited metabolic disorder affecting the liver or bone marrow).

Special warnings about this medication

Fioricet may cause you to become drowsy or less alert; therefore, driving or operating dangerous machinery or participating in any hazardous activity that requires full mental alertness is not recommended until you know your response to this drug.

If you are being treated for severe depression or have a history of severe depression or drug abuse, consult with your doctor before taking Fioricet.

Possible food and drug interactions when taking this medication

Butalbital is a central nervous system (brain and spinal cord) depressant and intensifies the effects of alcohol. Use of alcohol with this drug may also cause overdose symptoms. Therefore, use of alcohol should be avoided.

If Fioricet is taken with certain other drugs, the effects of either could be increased, decreased, or altered. It is especially important to check with your doctor before combining Fioricet with the following:

Antihistamines such as Benadryl
Antipsychotics such as Haldol, Thorazine
Drugs to treat depression such as Elavil
Muscle relaxants such as Flexeril
Narcotic pain relievers such as Darvon
Sleep aids such as Halcion
Tranquilizers such as Xanax, Valium

Fioricet may decrease the effect of anticoagulants (blood thinners). If you are taking an anticoagulant, consult with your doctor before taking this drug.

Special information
if you are pregnant or breastfeeding

The effects of Fioricet during pregnancy have not been adequately studied. If you are pregnant or plan to become pregnant, inform your doctor immediately. Butalbital does appear in breast milk. If this medication is essential to your health, your doctor may advise you to discontinue breastfeeding your baby until your treatment is finished.

Recommended dosage

ADULTS

The usual dose of Fioricet is 1 or 2 tablets taken every 4 hours as needed. Do not exceed a total dose of 6 tablets per day.

The usual dose of Esgic-Plus is 1 tablet every 4 hours as needed. Do not take more than 6 tablets a day.

CHILDREN

The safety and effectiveness of Fioricet have not been established in children under 12 years of age.

ELDERLY

Fioricet may cause excitement, depression, and confusion in the elderly. Therefore, your doctor will prescribe a dose individualized to suit your needs.

Overdosage

Symptoms of Fioricet overdose are mainly due to its barbiturate component. These symptoms may include:

Coma
Confusion
Drowsiness
Low blood pressure
Shock
Slow or troubled breathing

Overdose due to the acctaminophen component of Fioricet may cause kidney and liver damage or coma due to low blood sugar. Massive doses may cause liver failure.

Symptoms of liver damage include:
　Excess perspiration
　Feeling of bodily discomfort
　Nausea
　Vomiting

If you suspect an overdose, seek emergency medical treatment immediately.

Brand name:

FIORINAL

Pronounced: *fee-OR-i-nahl*
Generic ingredients: *Butalbital, Aspirin,*
   Caffeine
Other brand name: *Isollyl Improved*

Why is this drug prescribed?

Fiorinal, a strong, non-narcotic pain reliever
and muscle relaxant, is prescribed for the
relief of tension headache symptoms caused
by stress or muscle contraction in the head,
neck, and shoulder area. It combines a non-
narcotic, sedative barbiturate (butalbital)
with a pain reliever (aspirin) and a stimulant
(caffeine).

Most important fact about this drug

Barbiturates such as butalbital can be habit-
forming if you take them over long periods
of time.

How should you take this medication?

For best relief, take Fiorinal as soon as a
headache begins.

Take the medication with a full glass of
water or food to reduce stomach irritation.
Do not take this medication if it has a
strong odor of vinegar.

Take Fiorinal exactly as prescribed. Do not
increase the amount you take without your
doctor's approval.

■ *If you miss a dose...*
   If you take Fiorinal on a regular schedule,
   take the forgotten dose as soon as you
   remember. If it is almost time for your
   next dose, skip the one you missed and
   go back to your regular schedule. Do not
   take 2 doses at once.

■ *Storage instructions...*
   Store at room temperature. Keep the
   container tightly closed.

What side effects may occur?

Side effects cannot be anticipated. If any
develop or change in intensity, inform your
doctor as soon as possible. Only your
doctor can determine if it is safe for you to
continue taking Fiorinal.

■ *More common side effects may include:*
   Dizziness
   Drowsiness

■ *Less common or rare side effects may*
   include:
   Gas, light-headedness, nausea, skin
   problems, vomiting

Why should this drug not be prescribed?

If you are sensitive to or have ever had an
allergic reaction to barbiturates, aspirin,
caffeine, or other sedatives and pain
relievers, you should not take this
medication. Make sure your doctor is aware
of any drug reactions you have experienced.

Unless you are directed to do so by your
doctor, do not take this medication if you
have porphyria (an inherited metabolic
disorder affecting the liver or bone marrow).

Because aspirin, when given to children and
teenagers suffering from flu or chickenpox,
can cause a dangerous neurological disease
called Reye's syndrome, do not use Fiorinal
under these circumstances.

Special warnings about this medication

Fiorinal may make you drowsy or less alert;
therefore, you should not drive or operate
dangerous machinery or participate in any
hazardous activity that requires full mental
alertness until you know your response to
this drug.

Fiorinal contains aspirin. If you have a
stomach (peptic) ulcer or a disorder affecting
the blood clotting process, consult your
doctor before taking Fiorinal. Aspirin may

irritate the stomach lining and may cause bleeding.

If you have chronic (long-lasting or frequently recurring) tension headaches and your prescribed dose of Fiorinal does not relieve the pain, consult with your doctor. Taking more of this drug than your doctor has prescribed may cause dependence and symptoms of overdose.

Possible food and drug interactions when taking this medication

Butalbital decreases the activity of the central nervous system and intensifies the effects of alcohol. Avoid drinking alcohol while you are taking Fiorinal.

If Fiorinal is taken with certain other drugs, the effects of either could be increased, decreased, or altered. It is especially important to check with your doctor before combining Fiorinal with the following:

Acetazolamide (Diamox)
Antidepressant drugs such as Elavil, Norpramin, Nardil, and Parnate
Beta-blocking blood pressure drugs such as Inderal and Tenormin
Blood-thinning drugs such as Coumadin
Insulin
Narcotic pain relievers such as Darvon and Percocet
Oral contraceptives
Oral diabetes drugs such as Micronase
Sleep aids such as Halcion, Nembutal, and phenobarbital
Steroid medications such as prednisone
Theophylline (Theo-Dur, others)
Tranquilizers such as Librium, Valium, and Xanax
Valproic acid (Depakene, Depakote)

Special information if you are pregnant or breastfeeding

The effects of Fiorinal during pregnancy have not been adequately studied. If you are pregnant or plan to become pregnant, inform your doctor immediately. Butalbital and aspirin appear in breast milk. If this medication is essential to your health, your doctor may advise you to discontinue breastfeeding until your treatment with this medication is finished.

Recommended dosage

ADULTS

The usual dose of Fiorinal is 1 or 2 tablets or capsules taken every 4 hours. You should not take more than 6 tablets or capsules in a day.

CHILDREN

The safety and effectiveness of Fiorinal have not been established in children under 12 years of age.

Overdosage

Any medication taken in excess can have serious consequences. If you suspect an overdose, seek medical attention immediately.

■ *Symptoms of an overdose of Fiorinal are mainly attributed to its barbiturate component. These symptoms may include:*
Coma
Confusion
Drowsiness
Low blood pressure
Shock
Slow or troubled breathing

■ *Symptoms attributed to the aspirin and caffeine components of Fiorinal may include:*
Abdominal pain
Deep, rapid breathing
Delirium
High fever
Inability to fall or stay asleep
Rapid or irregular heartbeat
Restlessness

Ringing in the ears
Seizures
Tremor
Vomiting

Brand name:

FIORINAL WITH CODEINE

Pronounced: fee-OR-i-nahl with KO-deen
Generic ingredients: Butalbital, Codeine
   phosphate, Aspirin, Caffeine

Why is this drug prescribed?

Fiorinal with Codeine, a strong narcotic pain
reliever and muscle relaxant, is prescribed
for the relief of tension headache caused by
stress and muscle contraction in the head,
neck, and shoulder area. It combines a
sedative-barbiturate (butalbital), a narcotic
pain reliever and cough suppressant
(codeine), a non-narcotic pain and fever
reliever (aspirin), and a stimulant (caffeine).

Most important fact about this drug

Barbiturates such as butalbital and narcotics
such as codeine can be habit-forming when
taken in higher than recommended doses
over long periods of time.

How should you take this medication?

Take Fiornal with Codeine with a full glass
of water or food to reduce stomach
irritation. Do not take this medication if it
has a strong odor of vinegar.

Take Fiorinal with Codeine exactly as
prescribed. Do not increase the amount you
take without your doctor's approval.

Do not take it more frequently than your
doctor has prescribed.

■ *If you miss a dose...*
If you take the drug on a regular
schedule, take the forgotten dose as soon
as you remember. If it is almost time for
your next dose, skip the one you missed
and go back to your regular schedule. Do
not take 2 doses at once.

■ *Storage instructions...*
Store at room temperature. Keep the
container tightly closed.

What side effects may occur?

Side effects cannot be anticipated. If any
develop or change in intensity, inform your
doctor as soon as possible. Only your
doctor can determine if it is safe for you to
continue taking Fiorinal with Codeine.

■ *More common side effects may include:*
Abdominal pain
Dizziness
Drowsiness
Nausea

■ *Additional side effects, which can be
caused by this drug's components, may
include:*
Anemia, blocked air passages, hepatitis,
high blood sugar, internal bleeding,
intoxicated feeling, irritability, kidney
damage, lack of clotting, light-headedness,
peptic ulcer, stomach upset, tremors

Why should this drug not be prescribed?

If you are sensitive to or have ever had an
allergic reaction to butalbital, codeine,
aspirin, caffeine, or other pain relievers, you
should not take this medication. Make sure
your doctor is aware of any drug reactions
you have experienced.

Unless you are directed to do so by your
doctor, do not take this medication if you
have: a tendency to bleed too much, severe
vitamin K deficiency, severe liver damage,
nasal polyps (growths or nodules), asthma
due to aspirin or other nonsteroidal anti-
inflammatory drugs such as Motrin, swelling
due to fluid retention, peptic ulcer, or

porphyria (an inherited metabolic disorder affecting the liver and bone marrow).

Because aspirin, when given to children and teenagers with chickenpox or flu, can cause a dangerous neurological disease called Reye's syndrome, do not use Fiorinal with Codeine under these circumstances.

Special warnings about this medication

Fiorinal with Codeine may make you drowsy or less alert; therefore, you should not drive or operate dangerous machinery or participate in any hazardous activity that requires full mental alertness until you know how this drug affects you.

Codeine may cause unusually slow or troubled breathing and may increase the pressure caused by fluid surrounding the brain and spinal cord in people with head injury. Codeine also affects brain and spinal cord function and makes it hard for the doctor to see how people with head injuries are doing.

If you have chronic (long-lasting or frequently recurring) tension headaches and your prescribed dose of Fiorinal with Codeine does not relieve the pain, consult with your doctor. Taking more of this drug than your doctor has prescribed may cause dependence and symptoms of overdose.

Aspirin can cause internal bleeding in people with ulcers or bleeding disorders.

Codeine can hide signs of severe abdominal problems.

If you have ever developed dependence on a drug, consult with your doctor before taking Fiorinal with Codeine.

If you are being treated for a kidney, liver, or blood clotting disorder, consult with your doctor before taking Fiorinal with Codeine.

If you are older or in a weakened condition, be very careful taking Fiornal with Codeine.

Possible food and drug interactions when taking this medication

Fiorinal with Codeine reduces the activity of the central nervous system and intensifies the effects of alcohol. Use of alcohol with this drug may also cause overdose symptoms. Therefore, use of alcohol should be avoided.

If Fiorinal with Codeine is taken with certain other drugs, the effects of either could be increased, decreased, or altered. It is especially important to check with your doctor before combining Fiorinal with Codeine with the following:

Acetazolamide (Diamox)
Antidepressant drugs such as Elavil, Sinequan, Nardil, and Parnate
Antigout medications such as Zyloprim
Antihistamines such as Benadryl
Beta-blocking blood pressure drugs such as Inderal and Tenormin
Blood-thinning drugs such as Coumadin
Insulin
6-Mercaptopurine
Methotrexate (Rheumatrex)
Narcotic pain relievers such as Darvon and Vicodin
Nonsteroidal anti-inflammatory drugs such as Motrin and Indocin
Oral contraceptives
Oral diabetes drugs such as Micronase
Sleep aids such as Nembutal and phenobarbital
Steroid drugs such as prednisone
Theophylline (Theo-Dur, others)
Tranquilizers such as Librium, Xanax, and Valium
Valproic acid (Depakone, Depakote)

Special information
if you are pregnant or breastfeeding

The effects of Fiorinal with Codeine during pregnancy have not been adequately studied. If you are pregnant or plan to become pregnant, inform your doctor immediately. Butalbital, aspirin, caffeine, and codeine appear in breast milk. If this medication is essential to your health, your doctor may advise you to discontinue breastfeeding until your treatment with this medication is finished.

Recommended dosage

ADULTS

The usual dose of Fiorinal with Codeine is 1 or 2 capsules taken every 4 hours. Do not take more than 6 capsules per day.

CHILDREN

The safety and effectiveness of butalbital have not been established in children under 12 years of age.

Overdosage

Symptoms of an overdose of Fiorinal with Codeine are mainly attributed to its barbiturate and codeine ingredients.

■ *Symptoms attributed to the barbiturate ingredient of Fiorinal with Codeine may include:*
Coma
Confusion
Dizziness
Drowsiness
Low blood pressure
Shock
Slow or troubled breathing

■ *Symptoms attributed to the codeine ingredient of Fiorinal with Codeine may include:*
Convulsions
Loss of consciousness

Pinpoint pupils
Troubled and slowed breathing

■ *Symptoms attributed to the aspirin ingredient of Fiorinal with Codeine may include:*
Abdominal pain
Deep, rapid breathing
Delirium
High fever
Restlessness
Ringing in the ears
Seizures
Vomiting

Though caffeine poisoning occurs only at very high doses, it can cause delirium, insomnia, irregular heartbeat, rapid heartbeat, restlessness, and tremor.

If you suspect an overdose of Fiorinal with Codeine, seek emergency medical treatment immediately.

Brand name:

FLAGYL

Pronounced: FLAJ-ill
Generic name: Metronidazole
Other brand name: Protostat

Why is this drug prescribed?

Flagyl is an antibacterial drug prescribed for certain vaginal and urinary tract infections in men and women; amebic dysentery and liver abscess; and infections of the abdomen, skin, bones and joints, brain, lungs, and heart caused by certain bacteria.

Most important fact about this drug

Do not drink alcoholic beverages while taking Flagyl. The combination can cause abdominal cramps, nausea, vomiting, headaches, and flushing. It can also change the taste of the alcoholic beverage. When you have stopped taking Flagyl, wait another 24 hours (one day) before consuming any alcohol. Also avoid over-the-counter medications containing alcohol, such as certain cough and cold products.

How should you take this medication?

Flagyl works best when there is a constant amount in the blood. Take your doses at evenly spaced intervals, day and night, and try to avoid missing any.

If you are being treated for the sexually transmitted genital infection called trichomoniasis, your doctor may want to treat your partner at the same time, even if there are no symptoms. Try to avoid sexual intercourse until infection is cured. If you do have sex, use a condom.

Flagyl can be taken with or without food. It may cause dry mouth. Hard candy, chewing gum, or bits of ice can help to relieve the problem.

- *If you miss a dose...*
  Take it as soon as you remember. If it is almost time for your next dose skip the one you missed and go back to your regular schedule. Do not take 2 doses at once.

- *Storage Instructions...*
  Store at room temperature. Protect from light.

What side effects may occur?

Side effects cannot be anticipated. If any develop or change in intensity, tell your doctor immediately. Only your doctor can determine whether it is safe for you to continue taking Flagyl.

Two serious side effects that have occurred with Flagyl are seizures and numbness or tingling in the arms, legs, hands, and feet. If you experience either of these symptoms,

stop taking the medication and call your doctor immediately.

- *More common side effects may include:*
  Abdominal cramps
  Constipation
  Diarrhea
  Headache
  Loss of appetite
  Nausea
  Upset stomach
  Vomiting

- *Less common side effects may include:*
  Blood disorders, confusion, dark urine, decreased sex drive, depression, difficulty sleeping, dizziness, dry mouth (or vagina or vulva), fever, flushing, furry tongue, hives, inability to hold urine, increased production of pale urine, inflamed mouth or tongue, inflammation of the rectum, irritability, lack of muscle coordination, metallic taste, occasional joint pain, pain during sexual intercourse, painful or difficult urination, pelvic pressure, rash, stuffy nose, vertigo, weakness, yeast infection (candida) in vagina

Why should this drug not be prescribed?

Flagyl should not be used during the first 3 months of pregnancy to treat vaginal infections. Do not take Flagyl if you have ever had an allergic reaction to or are sensitive to metronidazole or similar drugs. Tell your doctor about any drug reactions you have experienced.

Special warnings about this medication

If you experience seizures or numbness or tingling in your arms, legs, hands, or feet, remember that you should stop taking Flagyl and call your doctor immediately.

If you have liver disease, make sure the doctor is aware of it. Flagyl should be used with caution.

Active or undiagnosed yeast infections may appear or worsen when you take Flagyl.

Possible food and drug interactions when taking this medication

Do not drink alcohol while taking Flagyl and for another 24 hours after your last dose.

If Flagyl is taken with certain other drugs, the effects of either could be increased, decreased, or altered. It is especially important to check with your doctor before combining Flagyl with any of the following:

Blood thinners such as Coumadin
Cholestyramine (Questran)
Cimetidine (Tagamet)
Disulfiram (Antabuse)
Lithium (Lithonate)
Phenobarbital
Phenytoin (Dilantin)

Special information if you are pregnant or breastfeeding

The effects of Flagyl in pregnancy have not been adequately studied. If you are pregnant or plan to become pregnant, notify your doctor. This medication should be used during pregnancy only if it is clearly needed. Flagyl appears in breast milk and could affect a nursing infant. If Flagyl is essential to your health, your doctor may advise you to stop breastfeeding until your treatment is finished.

Recommended dosage

ADULT

Trichomoniasis
One-day treatment: 2 grams of Flagyl, taken as a single dose or divided into 2 doses (1 gram each) taken in the same day.

Seven-day course of treatment: 250 milligrams 3 times daily for 7 consecutive days.

Acute Intestinal Amebiasis (Acute Amebic Dysentery)
The usual dose is 750 milligrams taken by mouth 3 times daily for 5 to 10 days.

Amebic Liver Abscess
The usual dose is 500 milligrams or 750 milligrams taken by mouth 3 times daily for 5 to 10 days.

Anaerobic Bacterial Infections
The usual adult oral dosage is 7.5 milligrams per 2.2 pounds of body weight every 6 hours.

CHILDREN

Amebiasis
The usual dose is 35 to 50 milligrams for each 2.2 pounds of body weight per day, divided into 3 doses taken for 10 days.

The safety and efficacy of Flagyl for any other condition in children have not been established.

ELDERLY

Your doctor will test to see how much medication is in your blood and will adjust your dosage if necessary.

Overdosage

Any medication taken in excess can have serious consequences. If you suspect an overdose, seek medical treatment immediately.

■ *Symptoms of Flagyl overdose may include:*
Lack of muscle coordination
Nausea
Vomiting

Generic name:

FLAVOXATE

See Urispas, page 783.

Brand name:

FLOXIN

Pronounced: FLOCKS-in
Generic name: Ofloxacin

Why is this drug prescribed?

Floxin is an antibiotic. It has been used effectively to treat lower respiratory tract infections, including chronic bronchitis and pneumonia, sexually transmitted diseases (except syphilis), and infections of the urinary tract, prostate gland, and skin.

Most important fact about this drug

Floxin kills a variety of bacteria, and is frequently used to treat infections in many parts of the body. However, you should stop taking the drug and notify your doctor immediately at the first sign of a skin rash or any other allergic reaction. Although quite rare, serious and occasionally fatal allergic reactions have been reported, some after only one dose. Signs of an impending reaction include swelling of the face and throat, shortness of breath, difficulty swallowing, rapid heartbeat, tingling, itching, and hives.

How should you take this medication?

Do not take Floxin with food. Be sure to drink plenty of fluids while taking this medication.

Do not take mineral supplements, vitamins with iron or minerals, or antacids containing calcium, aluminum, or magnesium within 2 hours of taking Floxin.

Take Floxin exactly as prescribed. You need to complete the full course of therapy to obtain best results and decrease the risk of a recurrence of the infection.

■ *If you miss a dose...*
Take it as soon as you remember. If it is almost time for your next dose, skip the one you missed and go back to your regular schedule. Never take 2 doses at the same time.

■ *Storage instructions...*
Store at room temperature in a tightly closed container.

What side effects may occur?

Side effects cannot be anticipated. If any develop or change in intensity, inform your doctor as soon as possible. Only your doctor can determine if it is safe for you to continue taking Floxin.

■ *More common side effects may include:*
Diarrhea
Difficulty sleeping
Dizziness
Headache
Itching of genital area in women
Nausea
Vaginal inflammation
Vomiting

■ *Less common or rare side effects may include:*
Abdominal pain and cramps, aggressiveness or hostility, agitation, anemia, anxiety, asthma, blood in the urine, blurred vision, body pain, bruising, burning or rash of the female genitals, burning sensation in the upper chest, changeable emotions, changes in thinking and perception, chest pain, confusion, conjunctivitis (pinkeye), continual runny nose, constipation, cough, decreased appetite, depression, difficult or labored breathing, disorientation, disturbed dreams, disturbed sense of smell, double vision, dry mouth, exaggerated sense of well-being, excessive perspiration, fainting, fatigue, fear, fever, fluid retention, frequent urination, gas, hallucinations,

hearing disturbance or loss, hepatitis, hiccups, high or low blood pressure, high or low blood sugar, hives, inability to urinate, increased urination, indigestion, inflammation of the colon, inflammation or rupture of tendons, intolerance to light, involuntary eye movement, itching, joint pain, kidney problems, lack of coordination, light-headedness, liver problems, menstrual changes, muscle pain, nervousness, nightmares, nosebleed, pain, pain in arms and legs, painful or difficult urination, purple or red areas/spots on the skin, rapid heartbeat, rash, reddened skin, restlessness, ringing in the ears, seizures, sensitivity to light, severe allergic reaction, skin inflammation and flaking or eruptions, sleepiness, sleep problems, sore mouth or throat, speech difficulty, Stevens-Johnson syndrome (severe skin eruptions), stomach and intestinal upset or bleeding, taste distortion, thirst, throbbing or fluttering heartbeat, tingling or pins and needles, tremor, unexplained bleeding from the uterus, vaginal discharge, vaginal yeast infection, vague feeling of illness, vertigo, visual disturbances, weakness, weight loss, yellowing of eyes and skin

Why should this drug not be prescribed?

Do not take Floxin if you are sensitive to or have ever had an allergic reaction to it or other quinolone antibiotics such as Cipro and Noroxin.

Special warnings about this medication

Floxin, used in high doses for short periods of time, may hide or delay the symptoms of syphilis, but is not effective in treating syphilis. If you are taking Floxin for gonorrhea, your doctor will test you for syphilis and then perform a follow-up test after 3 months of treatment.

Convulsions, increased pressure in the head, psychosis, tremors, restlessness, light-headedness, nervousness, confusion, depression, nightmares, insomnia, and hallucinations have occasionally been reported with this type of antibiotic. If you experience any of these symptoms, stop taking the drug and contact your doctor immediately.

If you are prone to seizures due to kidney disease, a brain disorder, or epilepsy, make sure your doctor knows about it. Floxin should be used with caution under these conditions.

If you have liver or kidney disease, your doctor will watch you closely while you are taking Floxin.

Avoid being in the sun too much; you can develop sun poisoning while you are taking Floxin.

Floxin may make you feel dizzy or light-headed. Be careful driving, operating machinery, or doing any activity that requires full mental alertness until you know how you react to this medication.

Safety has not been established for children under 18 years of age.

Possible food and drug interactions when taking this medication

If Floxin is taken with certain other drugs, the effects of either could be increased, decreased, or altered. It is especially important to check with your doctor before combining Floxin with the following:

Antacids containing calcium, magnesium, or aluminum
Blood thinners such as Coumadin
Calcium supplements such as Caltrate
Cyclosporine (Sandimmune)
Insulin
Iron supplements such as Feosol
Multivitamins containing zinc

Nonsteroidal anti-inflammatory drugs such as Motrin and Naprosyn
Oral diabetes drugs such as Diabinese and Micronase
Sucralfate (Carafate)
Theophylline-containing drugs, such as Theo-Dur

Special information
if you are pregnant or breastfeeding

The effects of Floxin during pregnancy have not been adequately studied. If you are pregnant or plan to become pregnant, inform your doctor immediately. This medication should not be used during pregnancy unless your doctor has determined that the benefit to you outweighs the risk to the unborn baby. Floxin appears in breast milk and could affect a nursing infant. If this medication is essential to your health, your doctor may advise you to stop breastfeeding until your treatment with Floxin is finished.

Recommended dosage

LOWER RESPIRATORY TRACT INFECTIONS

Worsening of Chronic Bronchitis
The usual dose is 400 milligrams every 12 hours for 10 days, for a total daily dose of 800 milligrams.

Pneumonia
The usual dose is 400 milligrams every 12 hours for 10 days, for a total daily dose of 800 milligrams.

SEXUALLY TRANSMITTED DISEASES

Gonorrhea
The usual dose is 400 milligrams taken once.

Infections of the Cervix or Urethra
The usual dose is 300 milligrams every 12 hours for 7 days, for a total daily dose of 600 milligrams.

MILD TO MODERATE SKIN INFECTIONS

The usual dose is 400 milligrams every 12 hours for 10 days, for a total daily dose of 800 milligrams.

URINARY TRACT INFECTIONS

Bladder Infections
The usual dose is 200 milligrams every 12 hours for a total daily dose of 400 milligrams. This dose is taken for 3 days for infections due to *E. Coli* or *K. Pneumoniae.* For infections due to other microbes, it is taken for 7 days.

Complicated Urinary Tract Infections
The usual dose is 200 milligrams every 12 hours for 10 days, for a total daily dose of 400 milligrams.

Prostatitis
The usual dose is 300 milligrams every 12 hours for 6 weeks, for a total daily dose of 600 milligrams.

Overdosage

Although no specific information is available, any medication taken in excess can have serious consequences. If you suspect an overdose, seek medical treatment immediately.

Generic name:

FLUCONAZOLE

See Diflucan, page 570.

Generic name:

FLUOXETINE

See Prozac, page 729.

Generic name:

FLUOXYMESTERONE

See Halotestin, page 615.

Generic name:

FLURBIPROFEN

See Ansaid, page 510.

Generic name:

FUROSEMIDE

See Lasix, page 631.

Brand name:

GANTRISIN

Pronounced: GAN-tris-in
Generic name: Sulfisoxazole

Why is this drug prescribed?

Gantrisin is prescribed for the treatment of severe, repeated, or long-lasting urinary tract infections. These include pyelonephritis (bacterial kidney inflammation), pyelitis (inflammation of the part of the kidney that drains urine into the ureter), and cystitis (inflammation of the bladder).

This drug is also used to treat bacterial meningitis, and is prescribed as a preventive measure for people who have been exposed to meningitis.

Some middle ear infections are treated with Gantrisin in combination with penicillin or erythromycin.

Toxoplasmosis (parasitic disease transmitted by infected cats, their feces or litter boxes, and by undercooked meat) can be treated

with Gantrisin in combination with pyrimethamine (Daraprim).

Malaria that does not respond to the drug chloroquine (Aralen) can be treated with Gantrisin in combination with other drug treatment.

Gantrisin is also used in the treatment of bacterial infections such as trachoma and inclusion inflammation conjunctivitis (eye infections), nocardiosis (bacterial disease affecting the lungs, skin, and brain), and chancroid (venereal disease causing enlargement and ulceration of lymph nodes in the groin).

Most important fact about this drug

Notify your doctor at the first sign of a reaction such as skin rash, sore throat, fever, joint pain, cough, shortness of breath, or other breathing difficulties, abnormal skin paleness, reddish or purplish skin spots or yellowing of the skin or whites of the eyes.

Rare but severe reactions, sometimes fatal, have occurred with the use of sulfa drugs such as Gantrisin. These reactions include sudden and severe liver damage, agranulocytosis (a severe blood disorder), aplastic anemia (a lack of red and white blood cells because of a bone marrow disorder), and Stevens-Johnson syndrome (severe blistering).

Patients taking sulfa drugs such as Gantrisin should have frequent blood counts.

How should you take this medication?

Take Gantrisin exactly as prescribed. It is important that you drink plenty of fluids while taking this medication in order to prevent crystals in the urine and the formation of stones.

Gantrisin Pediatric Suspension should be shaken well before each dose. To assure an accurate dose, ask you pharmacist for a specially marked measuring spoon.

Gantrisin, like other antibacterials, works best when there is a constant amount in the blood and urine. To help keep a constant level, try not to miss any doses and take them at evenly spaced intervals, around the clock.

■ *If you miss a dose...*
Take it as soon as you remember. If it is almost time for your next dose, skip the one you missed and go back to your regular schedule. Never take 2 doses at the same time.

■ *Storage instructions...*
Keep this medication in the container it came in, tightly closed. Store it at room temperature, away from moist places and direct light.

What side effects may occur?
Side effects cannot be anticipated. If any develop or change in intensity, inform your doctor as soon as possible. Only your doctor can determine if it is safe for you to continue taking Gantrisin.

■ *Side effects may include:*
Abdominal bleeding, abdominal pain, allergic reactions, anemia and other blood disorders, angioedema (swelling of face, lips, tongue and throat), anxiety, bluish discoloration of the skin, chills, colitis, convulsions, cough, dark, tarry stools, depression, diarrhea, disorientation, dizziness, drowsiness, enlarged salivary glands, enlarged thyroid, exhaustion, fainting, fatigue, fever, flushing, gas, hallucinations, headache, hearing loss, hepatitis, hives, inability to fall or stay asleep, inability to urinate, increased urination, inflammation of the mouth or tongue, itching, joint pain, kidney failure, lack of feeling or concern, lack of muscle

coordination, lack or loss of appetite, low blood sugar, muscle pain, nausea, palpitations, presence of blood or crystals in urine, rapid heartbeat, reddish or purplish skin spots, retention of urine, ringing in the ears, sensitivity to light, serum sickness (fever, painful joints, enlarged lymph nodes, skin rash), severe skin welts or swelling, shortness of breath, skin eruptions, skin rash, swelling due to fluid retention, tingling or pins and needles, vertigo, vomiting, weakness, yellow eyes and skin

Why should this drug not be prescribed?
If you are sensitive to or have ever had an allergic reaction to Gantrisin or other sulfa drugs, you should not take this medication. Make sure that your doctor is aware of any drug reactions that you have experienced.

Except in rare cases, doctors do not prescribe Gantrisin for infants less than 2 months of age. Also, you should not take Gantrisin if you are at the end of your pregnancy or if you are nursing a baby under 2 months.

Special warnings about this medication
If you have impaired kidney or liver function, or if you have severe allergies or bronchial asthma make sure your doctor knows about it. Caution should be exercised when taking Gantrisin.

An analysis of your urine and kidney function should be performed by your doctor during treatment with Gantrisin, especially if you have a kidney problem.

If you develop diarrhea while taking Gantrisin notify your doctor.

Possible food and drug interactions when taking this medication
If Gantrisin is taken with certain other drugs, the effects of either could be

increased, decreased, or altered. It is especially important to check with your doctor before combining this drug with the following:

Blood-thinning drugs such as Coumadin
Methotrexate, an anticancer drug
Oral contraceptives
Oral diabetes drugs such as Micronase

Special information
if you are pregnant or breastfeeding
There are no adequate and well controlled studies in pregnant women. This medication should not be used during pregnancy unless your doctor has determined that the benefits outweigh the potential risks. Gantrisin appears in breast milk. If this medication is essential to your health, your doctor may advise you to discontinue breastfeeding until your treatment with this drug is finished.

Recommended dosage

ADULTS

The recommended starting dose is 2 to 4 grams. Later, regular dose of 4 to 8 grams per day, divided into 4 to 6 doses, is recommended.

CHILDREN

This medication should not be prescribed for infants under 2 months of age except in the treatment of congenital toxoplasmosis (a parasitic infection contracted by pregnant women and passed along to the fetus).

The usual dose for children 2 months of age or older is 150 milligrams per 2.2 pounds of body weight divided into 4 to 6 doses taken over 24 hours.

The usual starting dose is one-half of the regular dose, or 75 milligrams per 2.2 pounds of body weight divided into 4 to 6 doses taken over 24 hours. Doses should not exceed 6 grams over 24 hours.

Gantrisin tablets come in a half-gram (500 milligram) strength. Gantrisin pediatric suspension and syrup supply a half-gram (500 milligram) in each teaspoonful.

Overdosage
Any medication taken in excess can have serious consequences. If you suspect an overdose, seek emergency medical treatment immediately.

■ *Symptoms of an overdose of Gantrisin include:*
Blood or sediment in the urine, blue tinge to the skin, colic, dizziness, drowsiness, fever, headache, lack or loss of appetite, nausea, unconsciousness, vomiting, yellowing of skin and whites of eyes

Brand name:

GENORA 1/35-28
See Oral Contraceptives, page 702.

Brand name:

GENUINE BAYER
See Aspirin, page 515.

Brand name:

GYNE-LOTRIMIN
Pronounced: GUY-nuh-LOW-trim-in
Generic name: Clotrimazole
Other brand names: Lotrimin, Mycelex, Mycelex-7

Why is this drug prescribed?
Clotrimazole, the active ingredient in these medications, is used to treat fungal infections. In preparations for the skin, it is effective against ringworm, athlete's foot,

and jock itch. In vaginal creams and tablets, it is used against vaginal yeast infections. In lozenge form, it is taken for oral yeast infections (thrush).

Most important fact about this drug

Keep using this medicine for the full time of treatment, even if the infection seems to have disappeared. If you stop too soon, the infection could return. You should continue using the vaginal forms of this medicine even during your menstrual period.

How should you take this medication?

Keep all forms of this medicine away from your eyes.

Before applying the skin preparations, be sure to wash your hands. Massage the medication gently into the affected area and the surrounding skin.

If you are taking Mycelex troches, place the lozenge in your mouth and let it dissolve slowly for 15 to 30 minutes. Do not chew the lozenge or swallow it whole.

If you are using a vaginal cream or tablet, use the following administration technique:

1. Load the applicator to the fill line with cream, or unwrap a tablet, wet it with warm water, and place it in the applicator as shown in the instructions you receive with the product.
2. Lie on your back with your knees drawn up.
3. Gently insert the applicator high into the vagina and push the plunger.
4. Withdraw the applicator and discard it if disposable, or wash with soap and water.

To keep the vaginal medication from getting on your clothing, wear a sanitary napkin. Do not use a tampon because it will absorb the medicine. Wear underwear or pantyhose with a cotton crotch—avoid synthetic

fabrics such as nylon or rayon. Do not douche unless your doctor tells you to do so.

■ *If you miss a dose...*
Make up for it as soon as you remember. If it is almost time for the next dose, skip the one you missed and go back to your regular schedule.

■ *Storage instructions...*
Store at room temperature, away from heat, light, and moisture.

What side effects may occur?

Side effects cannot be anticipated. If any develop or change in intensity, inform your doctor as soon as possible. Only your doctor can determine if it is safe for you to continue using this medication.

■ *Side effects may include:*
Blistering
Burning
Hives
Irritated skin
Itching
Peeling
Reddened skin
Stinging
Swelling due to fluid retention

■ *Side effects of clotrimazole vaginal preparations may include:*
Abdominal/stomach cramps/pain
Burning/irritation of penis of sexual partner
Headache
Pain during sexual intercourse
Skin rash, hives
Vaginal burning
Vaginal irritation
Vaginal itching
Vaginal soreness during sexual intercourse

An unpleasant mouth sensation has been reported by some people taking Mycelex.

Why should this drug not be prescribed?

You should not be using this medication if you have had an allergic reaction to any of its ingredients.

Special warnings about this medication

Contact your doctor if you experience increased skin irritations (such as redness, itching, burning, blistering, swelling, or oozing).

Check with your doctor before using this medication on a child.

In general, if your symptoms have not improved within 2 to 4 weeks of treatment, notify your doctor.

Clotrimazole vaginal preparations should not be used if you have abdominal pain, fever, or a foul-smelling vaginal discharge. Contact your doctor immediately.

While using the vaginal preparations, either avoid sexual intercourse or make sure your partner uses a condom. This will prevent reinfection. Oils used in some vaginal preparations can weaken latex condoms or diaphragms. To find out whether you can use your medication with latex products, check with your pharmacist.

Possible food and drug interactions when taking this medication

None have been reported.

Special information if you are pregnant or breastfeeding

The use of clotrimazole during the first trimester of pregnancy has not been adequately studied. It should be used during the first trimester only if clearly needed. Do not use clotrimazole at any time during pregnancy without the advice and supervision of your doctor.

It is not known whether clotrimazole appears in breast milk. Nursing mothers should use this medication cautiously and only when clearly needed.

Recommended dosage

LOTRIMIN

Adults and Children
Wash your hands before and after you use Lotrimin. Apply in the morning and evening. Use enough Lotrimin to massage into the affected area.

Symptoms usually improve during the first week of treatment with Lotrimin.

GYNE-LOTRIMIN CREAM

Adults
Fill the applicator with the cream and insert 1 applicatorful into the vagina everyday, preferably at bedtime. Repeat this procedure for 7 consecutive days.

MYCELEX TROCHE

Adults
The recommended dosage is 1 troche slowly dissolved in the mouth 5 times daily for 14 consective days. To prevent recurrence, the recommended dose is 1 troche 3 times daily.

Overdosage

Although any medication used in excess can have serious consequences, an overdose of clotrimazole is unlikely. If you suspect an overdose, however, seek medical help immediately.

Brand name:

HABITROL

See Nicotine Patches, page 682.

Brand name:

HALOTESTIN

Pronounced: HA-lo-TES-tin
Generic name: Fluoxymesterone

Why is this drug prescribed?

Halotestin is a male hormone used to ease the symptoms of advanced, recurrent breast cancer in women who are between 1 and 5 years past menopause or who have a type of breast tumor that is promoted by female hormones. Halotestin is also proscribed for men who have too little of the male hormone testosterone.

Most important fact about this drug

Because it is a male hormone, Halotestin may cause women to develop male secondary sex characteristics, such as deepening of the voice, increased facial hair, and an enlarged clitoris. Unless the drug is stopped when symptoms are first noticed, the male sex characteristics will be permanent.

How should you take this medication?

Take this medication exactly as prescribed. Your doctor will divide your total daily dose into 3 or 4 smaller ones.

■ If you miss a dose...
   Take it as soon as you remember. If it is almost time for your next dose, skip the one you missed and go back to your regular schedule. Do not take 2 doses at once.

■ Storage instructions...
   Store away from heat, light, and moisture.

What side effects may occur?

Side effects cannot be anticipated. If any develop or change in intensity, inform your doctor as soon as possible. Only your doctor can determine if it is safe for you to continue taking Halotestin.

■ More common side effects may include:
   Development of male sex characteristics such as deepening of the voice and an enlarged clitoris
   Irregular menstrual periods
   Lack of menstrual periods

■ Less common side effects may include:
   Abnormal burning or prickling sensation of the skin, abnormal hairiness, acne, anxiety, bleeding when on blood-thinning medications, depression, fluid retention, headache, hair loss in men, increase in red blood cells (polycythemia), increased or decreased sex drive, inflammation of the liver, nausea, oily skin secretions, rash, yellowing of the skin and eyes

Why should this drug not be prescribed?

Do not take Halotestin if you are sensitive or allergic to it, if you know or suspect you are pregnant, or if you have serious heart, liver, or kidney disease.

Special warnings about this medication

You may develop an excess of calcium in the blood while taking Halotestin. If this happens, your doctor will discontinue the drug.

Tell your doctor at once if you have any nausea, vomiting, changes in skin color, or swelling of the ankles.

Long-term use of Halotestin can cause liver cancer.

Halotestin contains the coloring additive tartrazine, which may cause an allergic reaction in those sensitive to it.

You could develop liver problems such as hepatitis or jaundice while taking Halotestin. If you do, your doctor will discontinue the drug.

Fluid retention and swelling, possibly with congestive heart failure, can be a serious complication in people who already have heart, liver, or kidney disease.

Possible food and drug interactions when taking this medication

If Halotestin is taken with certain other drugs, the effects of either could be increased, decreased, or altered. It is especially important to check with your doctor before combining Halotestin with the following:

Blood thinners such as Coumadin
Cyclosporine (Sandimmune)
Insulin
Oxyphenbutazone, a nonsteroidal anti-inflammatory drug

Special information if you are pregnant or breastfeeding

Halotestin should not be taken during pregnancy because it may affect a female baby.

The drug is not recommended for use in women who are breastfeeding.

Recommended dosage

The usual dosage for women with breast cancer is 10 to 40 milligrams per day taken in 3 or 4 smaller doses. You will take the drug for at least 1 month.

Overdosage

There have been no reports of overdose with Halotestin. However, any medication taken in excess can have serious consequences. If you suspect an overdose, seek medical treatment immediately.

Generic name:

HUMAN CHORIONIC GONADOTROPIN

See Profasi, page 725.

Brand name:

HYDERGINE

Pronounced: HY-der-jeen
Generic name: Ergoloid mesylates

Why is this drug prescribed?

Hydergine helps relieve symptoms of declining mental capacity, thought to be related to aging or dementia, seen in some people over age 60. The symptoms include reduced understanding and motivation, and a decline in self-care and interpersonal skills.

Most important fact about this drug

It may take several weeks or more for Hydergine to produce noticeable results. In fact, your doctor may need up to 6 months to determine whether the drug is right for you. Keep taking your regular doses even if you feel no effect.

How should you take this medication?

Take Hydergine exactly as prescribed.

If you are taking sublingual tablets, allow them to dissolve completely under the tongue. Do not crush or chew them.

■ *If you miss a dose...*
Skip the dose you missed and go back to your regular schedule. Do not take 2 doses at once. If you miss 2 or more doses in a row, consult your doctor.

■ *Storage instructions...*
Store away from heat, light, and moisture. Do not freeze the oral solution.

What side effects may occur?

Side effects cannot be anticipated. If any develop or change in intensity, notify your doctor as soon as possible. Only your doctor can determine whether it is safe to continue taking Hydergine.

■ *Side effects may include:*
Irritation below the tongue (with
    sublingual tablets)
Stomach upset
Temporary nausea

Why should this drug not be prescribed?
Do not use Hydergine if you have ever had
an allergic reaction to or are sensitive to the
drug, or if you have a mental disorder.

Special warnings about this medication
Since the symptoms treated with Hydergine
are of unknown origin and may change or
evolve into a specific disease, your doctor
will make a careful diagnosis before
prescribing Hydergine and then watch
closely for any changes in your condition.

Possible food and drug interactions
when taking this medication
No interactions have been reported.

Special information
if you are pregnant or breastfeeding
Hydergine is not intended for use by
women of childbearing age.

Recommended dosage

ADULTS

The usual dose of Hydergine is 1 milligram,
3 times a day.

Overdosage
Any medication taken in excess can have
serious consequences. If you suspect an
overdose of Hydergine, seek medical
attention immediately.

Generic name:

HYDROCHLOROTHIAZIDE

See HydroDIURIL, page 617.

Brand name:

HYDROCIL INSTANT

See Metamucil, page 653.

Generic name:

HYDROCORTISONE

See Anusol-HC, page 512.

Brand name:

HYDRODIURIL

Pronounced: High-dro-DYE-your-il
Generic name: Hydrochlorothiazide
Other brand name: Esidrix

Why is this drug prescribed?
HydroDIURIL is used in the treatment of
high blood pressure and other conditions
that require the elimination of excess fluid
(water) from the body. These conditions
include congestive heart failure, cirrhosis of
the liver, corticosteroid and estrogen
therapy, and kidney disorders. When used
for high blood pressure, HydroDIURIL can
be used alone or with other high blood
pressure medications. HydroDIURIL contains
a form of thiazide, a diuretic that prompts
your body to produce and eliminate more
urine, which helps lower blood pressure.

Most important fact about this drug:
If you have high blood pressure, you must
take HydroDIURIL regularly for it to be
effective. Since blood pressure declines
gradually, it may be several weeks before
you get the full benefit of HydroDIURIL;
and you must continue taking it even if you
are feeling well. HydroDIURIL does not
cure high blood pressure; it merely keeps it
under control.

How should you take this medication?

Take HydroDIURIL exactly as prescribed by your doctor.

■ *If you miss a dose...*
 If you forget a dose, take it as soon as you remember. If it is almost time for your next dose, skip the one you missed and go back to your regular schedule. Never take two doses at the same time.

■ *Storage instructions...*
 Keep container tightly closed. Protect from light, moisture, and freezing cold. Store at room temperature.

What side effects may occur?

Side effects cannot be anticipated. If any develop or change in intensity, inform your doctor as soon as possible. Only your doctor can determine if it is safe for you to continue taking HydroDIURIL.

■ *Side effects may include:*
 Abdominal cramping
 Diarrhea
 Dizziness upon standing up
 Headache
 Loss of appetite
 Low blood pressure
 Low potassium leading to symptoms such as dry mouth, excessive thirst, weak or irregular heartbeat, muscle pain or cramps
 Stomach irritation
 Stomach upset
 Weakness

■ *Less common or rare side effects may include:*
 Anemia, blood disorders, changes in blood sugar, constipation, difficulty breathing, dizziness, fever, fluid in the lung, hair loss, high levels of sugar in the urine, hives, hypersensitivity reactions, impotence, inflammation of the lung, inflammation of the pancreas, inflammation of the salivary glands, kidney failure, muscle spasms, nausea, rash, reddish or purplish spots on the skin, restlessness, sensitivity to light, skin disorders including Stevens-Johnson syndrome (blisters in the mouthand eyes), skin peeling, tingling or pins and needles, vertigo, vision changes, vomiting, yellow eyes and skin

Why should this drug not be prescribed?

If you are unable to urinate, you should not take this medication.

If you are sensitive to or have ever had an allergic reaction to HydroDIURIL or similar drugs, or if you are sensitive to sulfa or other sulfonamide-derived drugs, you should not take this medication.

Special warnings about this medication

Diuretics can cause your body to lose too much potassium. Signs of an excessively low potassium level include muscle weakness and rapid or irregular heartbeat. To boost your potassium level, your doctor may recommend eating potassium-rich foods or taking a potassium supplement.

If you are taking HydroDIURIL, your kidney function should be given a complete assessment, and should continue to be monitored.

If you have liver disease, diabetes, gout, or lupus erythematosus (a form of rheumatism), HydroDIURIL should be used with caution.

If you have bronchial asthma or a history of allergies, you may be at greater risk for an allergic reaction to this medication.

Dehydration, excessive sweating, severe diarrhea or vomiting could deplete your body's fluids and cause your blood pressure to become too low. Be careful when exercising and in hot weather.

Possible food and drug interactions when taking this medication

HydroDIURIL may increase the effects of alcohol. Do not drink alcohol while taking this medication.

If HydroDIURIL is taken with certain other drugs, the effects of either could be increased, decreased, or altered. It is especially important to check with your doctor before combining HydroDIURIL with the following:

Barbiturates such as phenobarbital
Cholestyramine (Questran)
Colestipol (Colestid)
Corticosteroids such as prednisone and ACTH
Drugs to treat diabetes such as insulin or
    Micronase
Lithium
Narcotics such as Percocet
Nonsteroidal anti-inflammatory drugs such
    as Naprosyn
Norepinephrine (Levophed)
Other high blood pressure medications
Skeletal muscle relaxants, such as
    tubocurarine

Special information if you are pregnant or breastfeeding

The effects of HydroDIURIL during pregnancy have not been adequately studied. If you are pregnant or plan to become pregnant, inform your doctor immediately. HydroDIURIL appears in breast milk and could affect a nursing infant. If this medication is essential to your health, your doctor may advise you to discontinue breastfeeding until your treatment is finished.

Recommended dosage

Dosage should be adjusted to each individual's needs. The smallest dose that is effective should be used.

ADULTS

Water Retention

The usual dose is 25 milligrams to 100 milligrams per day. Your doctor may tell you to take the drug in a single dose or to divide the total amount into more than one dose. Your doctor may put you on a day on, day off schedule or some other alternate day schedule to suit your needs.

High Blood Pressure

The usual dose is 25 milligrams as a single dose. Your doctor may increase the dose to 50 milligrams, as a single dose or divided into 2 doses. Dosages should be adjusted when used with other high blood pressure medications.

CHILDREN

Dosages for children should be adjusted according to weight, generally 1 milligram per pound of body weight in 2 doses per day. Children with high blood pressure only rarely will benefit from doses larger than 50 milligrams per day. Infants under 6 months may need 1.5 milligrams per pound per day in 2 doses.

Under 2 years

Based on age and body weight, the dosage is 12.5 milligrams to 37.5 milligrams per day in 2 doses.

2 to 12 years

The dosage, based on body weight, is 37.5 milligrams to 100 milligrams in 2 doses.

HydroDIURIL tablets come in strengths of 25, 50 and 100 milligrams.

Overdosage

Any medication taken in excess can cause symptoms of overdose. If you suspect an overdose, seek medical attention immediately.

■ *The Symptoms of HydroDIURIL overdose may include:*
Dry mouth
Electrolyte imbalance
Excessive thirst
Muscle pain or cramps
Symptoms of low potassium such as dehydration
Weak or irregular heartbeat

Brand name:

HYTONE

See Anusol-HC, page 512.

Brand name:

ILOSONE

See Erythromycin, Oral, page 584.

Generic name:

IMIPRAMINE

See Tofranil, page 764.

Brand name:

IMITREX INJECTION

Pronounced: IM-i-trex
Generic name: Sumatriptan succinate

Why is this drug prescribed?

Imitrex Injection is prescribed for the treatment of a severe migraine attack with or without the presence of an aura (visual disturbances, usually sensations of halos or flickering lights, which precede an attack). This medication will not prevent or reduce the number of attacks you may experience.

Most important fact about this drug

Imitrex Injection should be used only to treat an acute, classic migraine attack. It should not be used for headaches or certain unusual types of migraine.

How should you take this medication?

Imitrex is injected just below the skin with an autoinjector (self-injection device). Your doctor should carefully instruct you on how to use the autoinjector and how to dispose of the empty syringes. You should carefully read the instruction pamphlet that comes with the medication.

Imitrex should be injected as soon as your migraine symptoms appear, but may be used at any time during an attack.

A second injection may be given if your migraine symptoms return; however, never take more than 2 injections within 24 hours, and be sure to wait 1 hour between doses.

■ *If you miss a dose...*
Imitrex is *not* for regular use. Take it only during an attack.

■ *Storage instructions...*
Store Imitrex Injection away from heat and light, at room temperature, in the case provided. If your medication has expired (the expiration date is printed on the treatment pack), throw it away as instructed, but keep the autoinjector. If your doctor decides to stop your treatment, do not keep any leftover medicine unless your doctor tells you to. Throw away your medicine as instructed.

What side effects may occur?

Side effects cannot be anticipated. If any develop or change in intensity, inform your doctor as soon as possible. Only your doctor can determine if it is safe for you to continue taking Imitrex Injection.

- *More common side effects may include:*
Burning sensation, dizziness or vertigo, feeling of heaviness, feeling of tightness, flushing, mouth and tongue discomfort, muscle weakness, neck pain and stiffness, numbness, pressure sensation, redness at the site of injection, sore throat, tingling, warm/hot sensation

- *Less common or rare side effects may include:*
Abdominal discomfort, anxiety, changes in heart rhythm, cold sensation, difficulty swallowing, drowsiness/calmness, fatigue, feeling strange, general feeling of illness, headache, jaw discomfort, muscle cramps, muscle pain or tenderness, pressure in chest, rise in blood pressure (temporary), sinus or nasal discomfort, sweating, tight feeling in head, tightness in chest, vision changes

Why should this drug not be prescribed?
If you are sensitive to or have an allergic reaction to sumatriptan or similar drugs, you should not use Imitrex Injection. Make sure your doctor is aware of any drug reactions you have experienced.

Imitrex Injection should not be used if you have certain types of heart disease, including angina (crushing chest pain) or a history of heart attack, if you suffer from irregular heartbeat, shortness of breath, or uncontrolled blood pressure, or if you are taking a medication containing ergotamine (often used in other migraine medications).

Special warnings about this medication
Your doctor may administer the first dose of Imitrex Injection in his office. Although extremely rare, serious heart problems have occurred in people with heart disease when receiving an injection of this medication, and you should be carefully observed after

the initial dose to make sure this medication is safe for you to use.

Do not use Imitrex Injection intravenously. This can cause a serious heart irregularity.

This medication should not be used for other types of migraine headache.

Use Imitrex Injection cautiously if you have liver or kidney disease.

Possible food and drug interactions while taking this medication
If Imitrex Injection is taken with certain other drugs, the effects of either may be increased, decreased, or altered. It is especially important to check with your doctor before combining Imitrex Injection with the following:

Ergotamine (Cafergot)
Other ergot containing drugs (Ergostat)

Special information if you are pregnant or breastfeeding
The effects of Imitrex Injection during pregnancy have not been adequately studied. If you are pregnant or plan to become pregnant, inform your doctor immediately. Imitrex Injection may appear in breast milk and could affect a nursing infant. If this medication is essential to your health, your doctor may advise you to discontinue breastfeeding until your treatment with Imitrex Injection is finished.

Recommended dosage

ADULTS

The maximum single recommended dose of Imitrex Injection is 6 milligrams injected under the skin.

The maximum recommended dose that may be given within 24 hours is two 6 milligram injections taken at least 1 hour apart.

CHILDREN

The safety and effectiveness of Imitrex Injection in children have not been established.

ELDERLY

The safety and effectiveness of Imitrex Injection in people 65 and older have not been established.

Overdosage

Any medication taken in excess can have serious consequences. If you suspect an overdose of Imitrex, seek medical attention immediately.

■ *Symptoms of Imitrex overdose may include:*
Bluish tinge to the skin
Convulsions
Dilated pupils
Inactivity
Lack of coordination
Paralysis
Redness in the arms and legs
Skin changes at the site of injection
Slow breathing
Tremor

Brand name:

INDERAL

Pronounced: IN-der-al
Generic name: Propranolol hydrochloride

Why is this drug prescribed?

Inderal, a type of medication known as a beta blocker, is used in the treatment of high blood pressure, angina pectoris (chest pain, usually caused by lack of oxygen to the heart due to clogged arteries), changes in heart rhythm, prevention of migraine headache, hereditary tremors, hypertrophic subaortic stenosis (a condition related to

exertional angina), and tumors of the adrenal gland. It is also used to reduce the risk of death from recurring heart attack. When used for the treatment of high blood pressure, it is effective alone or combined with other high blood pressure medications, particularly thiazide-type diuretics. Beta blockers decrease the force and rate of heart contractions, reducing the heart's demand for oxygen and lowering blood pressure.

Most important fact about this drug

If you have high blood pressure, you must take Inderal regularly for it to be effective. Since blood pressure declines gradually, it may be several weeks before you get the full benefit of Inderal; and you must continue taking it even it you are feeling well. Inderal does not cure high blood pressure; it merely keeps it under control.

How should you take this medication?

Inderal works best when taken before meals. Take it exactly as prescribed, even if your symptoms have disappeared.

Try not to miss any doses. If this medication is not taken regularly, your condition may worsen.

■ *If you miss a dose...*
Take it as soon as you remember. If it is within 8 hours of your next scheduled dose, skip the one you missed and go back to your regular schedule. Never take 2 doses at the same time.

■ *Storage instructions...*
Store at room temperature in a tightly closed, light-resistant container.

What side effects may occur?

Side effects cannot be anticipated. If any develop or change in intensity, inform your doctor as soon as possible. Only your doctor can determine if it is safe for you to continue taking Inderal.

■ *Side effects may include:*
Abdominal cramps, colitis, congestive heart failure, constipation, decreased sexual ability, depression, diarrhea, difficulty breathing, disorientation, dry eyes, fever with sore throat, hair loss, hallucinations, headache, light-headedness, low blood pressure, lupus erythematosus (a disease of the connective tissue), nausea, rash, reddish or purplish spots on the skin, short-term memory loss, slow heartbeat, tingling, prickling in hands, tiredness, trouble sleeping, upset stomach, visual changes, vivid dreams, vomiting, weakness, worsening of certain heartbeat irregularities

Why should this drug not be prescribed?

If you have inadequate blood supply to the circulatory system (cardiogenic shock), certain types of irregular heartbeat, a slow heartbeat, bronchial asthma, or severe congestive heart failure, you should not take this medication.

Special warnings about this medication

If you have a history of congestive heart failure, your doctor will prescribe Inderal cautiously.

Inderal should not be stopped suddenly. This can cause increased chest pain and heart attack. Dosage should be gradually reduced.

If you suffer from asthma or other bronchial conditions, coronary artery disease, or kidney or liver disease, this medication should be used with caution.

Ask your doctor if you should check your pulse while taking Inderal. This medication can cause your heartbeat to become too slow.

This medication may mask the symptoms of low blood sugar or alter blood sugar levels.

If you are diabetic, discuss this with your doctor.

Notify your doctor or dentist that you are taking Inderal if you have a medical emergency, and before you have surgery or dental treatment.

Possible food and drug interactions when taking this medication

If Inderal is taken with certain other drugs, the effects of either could be increased, decreased, or altered. It is especially important to check with your doctor before combining Inderal with the following:

Aluminum hydroxide gel (Amphojel)
Calcium-blocking blood pressure drugs such as Cardizem, Procardia, and Calan
Certain high blood pressure medications such as Diupres and Ser-Ap-Es
Chlorpromazine (Thorazine)
Cimetidine (Tagamet)
Epinephrine (Epipen)
Haloperidol (Haldol)
Insulin
Lidocaine (Xylocaine)
Nonsteroidal anti-inflammatory drugs such as Motrin and Naprosyn
Oral diabetes drugs such as Micronase
Phenobarbitone
Phenytoin (Dilantin)
Rifampin (Rifadin)
Theophylline (Theo-Dur, others)
Thyroid medications such as Synthroid

Special information
if you are pregnant or breastfeeding

The effects of Inderal during pregnancy have not been adequately studied. If you are pregnant or plan to become pregnant, inform your doctor immediately. Inderal appears in breast milk and could affect a nursing infant. If this medication is essential to your health, your doctor may advise you to discontinue breastfeeding until your treatment with this medication is finished.

Recommended dosage

ADULTS

All dosages of Inderal, for any problem, must be tailored to the individual. Your doctor will determine when and how often you should take this drug. Remember to take it exactly as directed.

Hypertension
The usual starting dose is 40 milligrams 2 times a day. This dose may be in combination with a diuretic. Dosages are gradually increased to between 120 milligrams and 240 milligrams per day for maintenance. In some cases, a dose of 640 milligrams per day may be needed. Depending on the individual, maximum effect of this drug may not be reached for a few days or even several weeks. Some people may do better taking this medication 3 times a day.

Angina Pectoris
The usual daily dosage is 80 milligrams to 320 milligrams, divided into 2, 3 or 4 smaller doses. When your treatment is being discontinued, your doctor will reduce the dosage gradually over a period of several weeks.

Irregular Heartbeat
The usual dose is 10 milligrams to 30 milligrams 3 or 4 times a day, before meals and at bedtime.

Heart Attack
The usual daily dosage is 180 milligrams to 240 milligrams divided into smaller doses. The usual maximum dose is 240 milligrams, although your doctor may increase the dose when treating heart attack with angina or high blood pressure.

Migraine
The usual starting dosage is 80 milligrams per day divided into smaller doses. Dosages can be increased gradually to between 160 milligrams and 240 milligrams per day. If this dose does not relieve your symptoms in 4 to 6 weeks, your doctor will slowly take you off the drug.

Tremors
The usual starting dose is 40 milligrams, 2 times per day. Symptoms will usually be relieved with a dose of 120 milligrams per day; however, on occasion, dosages of 240 milligrams to 320 milligrams per day may be necessary.

Hypertrophic Subaortic Stenosis
The usual dose is 20 milligrams to 40 milligrams, 3 to 4 times a day, before meals and at bedtime.

Before Adrenal Gland Surgery
The usual dose is 60 milligrams a day divided into smaller doses for 3 days before surgery in combination with an alpha-blocker drug.

Inderal may also be taken by people with inoperable tumors in doses of 30 milligrams a day, divided into smaller doses.

CHILDREN

Inderal will be carefully individualized for use in children and is used only for high blood pressure. Doses in children are calculated by body weight, and range from 2 milligrams to 4 milligrams per 2.2 pounds daily, divided into 2 equal doses. The maximum dose is 16 milligrams per 2.2 pounds per day.

If treatment is stopped, this drug must be gradually reduced over a 7- to 14-day period.

ELDERLY

Your doctor will determine the dosage according to your needs.

Inderal is also available in a sustained-release formulation, called Inderal LA, for once-a-day dosing.

Overdosage

No specific information on Inderal overdosage is available; however, overdose symptoms with other beta blockers include:

Extremely slow heartbeat
Irregular heartbeat
Low blood pressure
Severe congestive heart failure
Seizures
Wheezing

Any medication taken in excess can have serious consequences. If you suspect an overdose, seek medical attention immediately.

Brand name:

INDOCIN

Pronounced: IN-doh-sin
Generic name: Indomethacin

Why is this drug prescribed?

Indocin, a nonsteroidal anti-inflammatory drug, is used to relieve the inflammation, swelling, stiffness and joint pain associated with moderate or severe rheumatoid arthritis and osteoarthritis (the most common form of arthritis), and ankylosing spondylitis (arthritis of the spine). It is also used to treat bursitis, tendinitis (acute painful shoulder), acute gouty arthritis, and other kinds of pain.

Most important fact about this drug

You should have frequent checkups with your doctor if you take Indocin regularly. Ulcers or internal bleeding can occur without warning.

How should you take this medication?

Indocin should be taken with food or an antacid, and with a full glass of water. Never take on an empty stomach.

Take this medication exactly as prescribed by your doctor.

If you are using Indocin for arthritis, it should be taken regularly.

If you are taking the liquid form of this medicine, shake the bottle well before each use.

Indocin SR capsules should be swallowed whole, not crushed or broken.

Do not lie down for about 20 to 30 minutes after taking Indocin. This helps prevent irritation that could lead to trouble in swallowing.

If you are using suppository form of this medicine:

1. If the suppository is too soft to insert, hold it under cool water or chill it before removing the wrapper
2. Remove the foil wrapper and moisten your rectal area with cool tap water.
3. Lie down your side and use your finger to push the suppository well up into the rectum. Hold your buttocks together for a few seconds.
4. Indocin suppositories should be kept inside the rectum for at least one hour so that all of the medicine can be absorbed by your body.

■ *If you miss a dose...*
Take the forgotten dose as soon as you
remember. If it is time for your next dose,
skip the one you missed and return to
your regular schedule. Never take a
double dose.

■ *Storage instructions...*
The liquid and suppository forms of
Indocin may be stored at room
temperature. Keep both forms from
extreme heat, and protect the liquid from
freezing.

What side effects may occur?

Side effects cannot be anticipated. If any
develop or change in intensity inform your
doctor as soon as possible. Only your
doctor can determine if it is safe for you to
continue taking Indocin.

■ *More common side effects may include:*
Abdominal pain, constipation, depression,
diarrhea, dizziness, fatigue, headache,
heartburn, indigestion, nausea, ringing in
the ears, sleepiness or excessive
drowsiness, stomach pain, stomach upset,
vertigo, vomiting

■ *Less common or rare side effects may
include:*
Anemia, anxiety, asthma, behavior
disturbances, bloating, blurred vision,
breast changes, changes in heartrate, chest
pain, coma, congestive heart failure,
convulsions, decrease in white blood cells,
fever, fluid in lungs, fluid retention,
flushing, gas, hair loss, hepatitis, high or
low blood pressure, hives, itching, increase
in blood sugar, insomnia, kidney failure,
labored breathing, light-headedness, loss of
appetite, mental confusion, muscle
weakness, nosebleed, peptic ulcer,
problems in hearing, rash, rectal bleeding,
Stevens-Johnson syndrome (skin peeling),
stomach or intestinal bleeding, sweating,
twitching, unusual redness of skin, vaginal
bleeding, weight gain, worsening of
epilepsy, yellow eyes and skin

Why should this drug not be prescribed?

If you are sensitive to or have ever had an
allergic reaction to Indocin, aspirin, or
similar drugs, or if you have had asthma
attacks caused by aspirin or other drugs of
this type, you should not take this
medication. Make sure that your doctor is
aware of any drug reactions that you have
experienced.

Do not use Indocin suppositories if you
have a history of rectal inflammation or
recent rectal bleeding.

Special warnings about this medication

Indocin prolongs bleeding time. If you are
taking blood-thinning medication, this drug
should be taken with caution.

Your doctor should prescribe the lowest
possible effective dose. The incidence of
side effects increases as dosage increases.

Peptic ulcers and bleeding can occur
without warning.

This drug should be used with caution if
you have kidney or liver disease, and it can
cause liver inflammation in some people.

Do not take aspirin or any other anti-
inflammatory medications while taking
Indocin, unless your doctor tells you to do
so.

If you have heart disease or high blood
pressure, this drug can increase water
retention.

This drug can mask the symptoms of an
existing infection.

Indocin may cause you to become drowsy
or less alert; therefore, driving or operating

dangerous machinery or participating in any hazardous activity that requires full mental alertness is not recommended.

Possible food and drug interactions when taking this medication

If Indocin is taken with certain other drugs, the effects of either could be increased, decreased or altered. It is especially important to check with your doctor before combining Indocin with the following:

Aspirin
Beta-adrenergic blockers such as Tenormin, Inderal
Blood-thinning medicines such as Coumadin
Captopril (Capoten)
Cyclosporine (Sandimmune)
Diflunisal (Dolobid)
Digoxin (Lanoxin)
Lithium (Eskalith)
Loop diuretics (Lasix)
Potassium-sparing diuretics such as Aldactone
Probenecid (Benemid, ColBENEMID)
The anticancer drug methotrexate
Thiazide-type diuretics such as Diuril
Triamterene (Dyazide)

Special information if you are pregnant or breastfeeding

The effects of Indocin during pregnancy have not been adequately studied. If you are pregnant or plan to become pregnant inform your doctor immediately. Indocin appears in breast milk and could affect a nursing infant. If this medication is essential to your health, your doctor may advise you to discontinue breastfeeding until your treatment with this medication is finished.

Recommended dosage

ADULTS

This medication is available in liquid, capsule, and suppository form. The following dosages are for the capsule form.

If you prefer the liquid form ask your doctor to make the proper substitution. Do not try to convert the medication or dosage yourself.

Moderate to Severe Rheumatoid Arthritis, Osteoarthritis, Ankylosing Spondylitis
The usual dose is 25 milligrams 2 or 3 times a day, increasing to a total daily dose of 150 to 200 milligrams. Your doctor should monitor you carefully for side effects when you are taking this drug.

Your doctor may prescribe a single daily 75-milligram capsule of Indocin SR in place of regular Indocin.

Bursitis or Tendinitis
The usual dose is 75 to 150 milligrams daily divided into 3 to 4 small doses for 1 to 2 weeks, until symptoms disappear.

Acute Gouty Arthritis
The usual dose is 50 milligrams 3 times a day until pain is reduced to a tolerable level (usually 3 to 5 days). Your doctor will advise you when to stop taking this drug for this condition. Keep him informed of its effects on your symptoms.

CHILDREN

The safety and effectiveness of Indocin have not been established in children under 14 years of age. However, your doctor may decide that the benefits of this medication may outweigh the potential risks.

ELDERLY

Your doctor will adjust the dosage as needed.

Overdosage

Any medication taken in excess can cause symptoms of overdose. If you suspect an overdose seek medical attention immediately.

■ *The symptoms of Indocin overdose may include:*
Convulsions
Disorientation
Dizziness
Intense headache
Lethargy
Mental confusion
Nausea, vomiting
Numbness
Tingling or pins and needles

Generic name:

INDOMETHACIN

See Indocin, page 625.

Brand name:

IONAMIN

See Fastin, page 593.

Brand name:

ISOLLYL IMPROVED

See Fiorinal, page 600.

Generic name:

ISOMETHEPTENE MUCATE, DICHLORALPHENAZONE, AND ACETAMINOPHEN

See Midrin, page 664.

Generic name:

ISOTRETINOIN

See Accutane, page 497.

Brand name:

KEFLEX

Pronounced: KEF-lecks
Generic name: Cephalexin hydrochloride
Other brand name: Keftab

Why is this drug prescribed?
Keflex and Keftab are cephalosporin antibiotics. They are prescribed for bacterial infections of the respiratory tract including middle ear infection, bone, skin, and the reproductive and urinary systems. Because they are effective for only certain types of bacterial infections, before beginning treatment your doctor may perform tests to identify the organisms causing the infection.

Keflex is available in capsules and an oral suspension form for use in children. Keftab, available only in tablet form, is prescribed exclusively for adults.

Most important fact about this drug
If you are allergic to either penicillin or cephalosporin antibiotics in any form, consult your doctor *before taking Keflex.* There is a possibility that you are allergic to both types of medication and if a reaction occurs, it could be extremely severe. If you take the drug and feel signs of a reaction, seek medical attention immediately.

How should you take this medication?
Keflex may be taken with or without meals. However, if the drug upsets your stomach, you may want to take it after you have eaten.

Take Keflex at even intervals around the clock as prescribed by your doctor.

If you are taking the liquid form of Keflex, use the specially marked spoon to measure each dose accurately.

To obtain maximum benefit, it is important that you finish taking all of this medication, even if you are feeling better.

- *If you miss a dose...*
  Take it as soon as you remember. If it is almost time for the next dose, and you take 2 doses a day, take the one you missed and the next dose 5 to 6 hours later. If you take 3 or more doses a day, take the one you missed and the next dose 2 to 4 hours later, or double the next dose. Then go back to your regular schedule.

- *Storage instructions...*
  Store capsules and tablets at room temperature. Store the liquid suspension in a refrigerator; discard any unused medication after 14 days.

What side effects may occur?

Side effects cannot be anticipated. If any develop or change in intensity, inform your doctor as soon as possible. Only your doctor can determine if it is safe for you to continue taking Keflex.

- *More common side effects may include:*
  Diarrhea

- *Less common or rare side effects may include:*
  Abdominal pain, agitation, colitis (inflammation of the large intestine), confusion, dizziness, fatigue, fever, genital and rectal itching, hallucinations, headache, hepatitis, hives, indigestion, inflammation of joints, inflammation of the stomach, joint pain, nausea, rash, seizures, severe allergic reaction, skin peeling, skin redness, swelling due to fluid retention, vaginal discharge, vaginal inflammation, vomiting, yellowing of skin and whites of eyes

Why should this drug not be prescribed?

If you are sensitive to or have ever had an allergic reaction to the cephalosporin group of antibiotics, you should not use this medication. Make sure your doctor is aware of any drug reactions you have experienced.

Special warnings about this medication

If you have a history of stomach or intestinal disease, especially colitis, check with your doctor before taking Keflex.

If you have ever had an allergic reaction, particularly to drugs, be sure to tell your doctor.

If diarrhea occurs while taking cephalexin, check with your doctor before taking a remedy. Certain diarrhea medications (for instance, Lomotil) may increase your diarrhea or make it last longer.

Prolonged use of Keflex may result in an overgrowth of bacteria that do not respond to the medication, causing a secondary infection. Your doctor will monitor your use of this drug on a regular basis.

If you have a kidney disorder, check with your doctor before taking Keflex. You may need a reduced dose.

If you are diabetic, it is important to note that Keflex may cause false results in tests for urine sugar. Notify your doctor that you are taking this medication before being tested. Do not change your diet or dosage of diabetes medication without first consulting with your doctor.

If your symptoms do not improve within a few days, or if they get worse, notify your doctor immediately.

Do not give this medication to other people or use it for other infections before checking with your doctor.

Possible food and drug interactions when taking this medication

If Keflex is taken with certain other drugs, the effects of either could be increased, decreased, or altered. It is especially important to check with your doctor before combining Keflex with the following:

Certain diarrhea medications such as Lomotil
Oral contraceptives

Special information if you are pregnant or breastfeeding

The effects of Keflex during pregnancy have not been adequately studied. If you are pregnant or plan to become pregnant, notify your doctor immediately. Keflex appears in breast milk and could affect a nursing infant. If this medication is essential to your health, your doctor may advise you to discontinue breastfeeding until your treatment is finished.

Recommended dosage

ADULTS

Throat, Skin, and Urinary Tract Infections
The usual adult dosage is 500 milligrams taken every 12 hours. Cystitis (bladder infection) therapy should be continued for 7 to 14 days.

Other Infections
The usual recommended dosage is 250 milligrams taken every 6 hours. For more severe infections, larger doses may be needed, as determined by your doctor.

CHILDREN

Keflex
The usual dose is 25 to 50 milligrams for each 2.2 pounds of body weight per day, divided into smaller doses.

For strep throat in children over 1 year of age and for skin infections, the dose may be divided into 2 doses taken every 12 hours.

For strep infections, the medication should be taken for at least 10 days. Your doctor may double the dose if your child has a severe infection.

For middle ear infection, the dose is 75 to 100 milligrams per 2.2 pounds per day, divided into 4 doses.

Keftab
Safety and effectiveness have not been established in children.

Overdosage

Any medication taken in excess can have serious consequences.

If you suspect an overdose, seek emergency medical treatment immediately.

■ *Symptoms of Keflex overdose may include:*
Blood in the urine
Diarrhea
Nausea
Upper abdominal pain
Vomiting

Brand name:

KEFTAB

See Keflex, page 628.

Generic name:

KETOCONAZOLE

See Nizoral, page 685.

Generic name:

KETOPROFEN

See Orudis, page 705.

Brand name:

KONSYL

See Metamucil, page 653.

Generic name:

LACTULOSE

See Chronulac Syrup, page 541.

Brand name:

LASIX

Pronounced: LAY-six
Generic name: Furosemide

Why is this drug prescribed?

Lasix is used in the treatment of high blood pressure and other conditions that require the elimination of excess fluid (water) from the body. These conditions include congestive heart failure, cirrhosis of the liver, and kidney disease. When used to treat high blood pressure, Lasix is effective alone or in combination with other high blood pressure medications. Diuretics help your body produce and eliminate more urine, which helps lower blood pressure. Lasix is classified as a "loop diuretic" because of its point of action in the kidneys.

Most important fact about this drug

If you have high blood pressure, you must take Lasix regularly for it to be effective. Since blood pressure declines gradually, it may be several weeks before you get the full benefit of Lasix; and you must continue taking it even if you are feeling well. Lasix does not cure high blood pressure; it merely keeps it under control.

How should you take this medication?

Take this medication exactly as prescribed by your doctor.

■ *If you miss a dose...*
Take the forgotten dose as soon as you remember. If it is almost time for your next dose, skip the one you missed and go back to your regular schedule. Never take two doses at the same time.

■ *Storage instructions...*
Keep this medication in the container it came in, tightly closed, and away from moist places and direct light. Store Lasix tablets at room temperature. Store the oral solution in the refrigerator; discard an open bottle after 60 days.

What side effects may occur?

Side effects cannot be anticipated. If any develop or change in intensity, inform your doctor as soon as possible. Only your doctor can determine if it is safe for you to continue taking Lasix.

■ *Side effects may include:*
Anemia, blood disorders, blurred vision, constipation, cramping, diarrhea, dizziness, dizziness upon standing, fever, headache, hearing loss, high blood sugar, hives, itching, loss of appetite, low potassium (leading to symptoms like dry mouth, excessive thirst, weak or irregular heartbeat, muscle pain or cramps), muscle spasms, nausea, rash, reddish or purplish spots on the skin, restlessness, ringing in the ears, sensitivity to light, skin eruptions, skin inflammation and flaking, stomach or mouth irritation, tingling or pins and needles, vertigo, vision changes, vomiting, weakness, yellow eyes and skin

Why should this drug not be prescribed?

If you are sensitive to or have ever had an allergic reaction to Lasix or diuretics, or if you are unable to urinate, you should not take this medication.

Special warnings about this medication

Lasix can cause your body to lose too much potassium. Signs of an excessively low potassium level include muscle weakness and rapid or irregular heartbeat. To improve your potassium level, your doctor may prescribe a potassium supplement or recommend potassium-rich foods, such as bananas, prunes, raisins, orange juice and whole and skim milk.

Make sure the doctor knows if you have kidney disease, liver disease, diabetes, gout, or the connective tissue disease, lupus erythematosus. Lasix should be used with caution.

If you are allergic to sulfa drugs, you may also be allergic to Lasix.

If you have high blood pressure, avoid over-the-counter medications that may increase blood pressure, including cold remedies and appetite suppressants.

Your skin may be more sensitive to the effects of sunlight.

Possible food and drug interactions when taking this medication

If Lasix is taken with certain other drugs, the effects of either could be increased, decreased, or altered. It is especially important to consult with your doctor before taking Lasix with any of the following:

Aminoglycoside antibiotics such as
   Garamycin
Aspirin
Barbiturates such as phenobarbital
Ethacrynic acid (Edecrin)
Indomethacin (Indocin)
Lithium (Lithonate)

The muscle-relaxing drug Tubocurarine
Narcotics such as Darvon and Percocet
Nonsteroidal anti-inflammatory drugs such
   as Advil and Naprosyn
Norepinephrine (Levophed)
Other high blood pressure medications such
   as Vasotec and Aldomet
Succinylcholine (Anectine)
Sucralfate (Carafate)

Special information if you are pregnant or breastfeeding

The effects of Lasix during pregnancy have not been adequately studied. If you are pregnant or plan to become pregnant, inform your doctor immediately. Lasix appears in breast milk and could affect a nursing infant. If this medication is essential to your health, your doctor may advise you to discontinue breastfeeding until your treatment is finished.

Recommended dosage

Your doctor will adjust the dosages of this medication, which is a strong diuretic, to meet your specific needs. It is available in both oral and injectable form. The injectable form is used only in emergency situations or in cases where patients cannot take oral medication. Dosages shown here are for the oral form only.

ADULTS

Edema Fluid Retention

You will be started at a single dose of 20 to 80 milligrams. If needed, the same dose can be repeated 6 to 8 hours later. Your doctor may raise the dosage by 20 milligrams or 40 milligrams with each successive administration— each 6 to 8 hours after the previous dose—until the desired effect is achieved. This dosage is then taken once or twice daily thereafter. Your doctor will monitor you carefully using laboratory tests. The maximum daily dose is 600 milligrams.

High Blood Pressure

The usual starting dose is 80 milligrams per day divided into 2 doses. Your doctor will adjust the dosages and may add other high blood pressure medications if Lasix is not enough.

CHILDREN

The usual initial dose is 2 milligrams per 2.2 pounds of body weight. The doctor may increase subsequent doses by 1 to 2 milligrams per 2.2 pounds. Doses are spaced 6 to 8 hours apart. A child's dosage will be adjusted to the lowest needed to achieve maximum effect, and should not exceed 6 milligrams pcr 2.2 pounds.

ELDERLY

The doctor will determine thc dosage based on the particular needs of the individual.

Overdosage

Any medication taken in excess can cause symptoms of overdose. If you suspect an overdose, seek medical attention immediately.

■ *The symptoms of Lasix overdose may include:*
Dehydration
Dry mouth
Excessive thirst
Low blood pressure
Muscle pain or cramps
Weak or irregular heartbeat

Generic name:

LEUPROLIDE

See Lupron Depot (3.75 mg), page 642.

Brand name:

LEVLEN

See Oral Contraceptives, page 702.

Generic name:

LEVONORGESTREL IMPLANTS

See Norplant, page 691.

Brand name:

LEVOTHROID

See Synthroid, page 756.

Generic name:

LEVOTHYROXINE

See Synthroid, page 756.

Brand name:

LEVOXINE

See Synthroid, page 756.

Brand name:

LIBRITABS

See Librium, page 634.

Brand name:

LIBRIUM

Pronounced: LIB-ree-um
Generic name: Chlordiazepoxide
Other brand name: Libritabs

Why is this drug prescribed?

Librium is used in the treatment of anxiety disorders. It is also prescribed for short-term relief of the symptoms of anxiety, symptoms of withdrawl in acute alcoholism, and anxiety and apprehension before surgery. It belongs to a class of drugs known as benzodiazepines.

Most important fact about this drug

Librium is habit-forming and you can become dependent on it. You could experience withdrawal symptoms if you stopped taking it abruptly (See "What side effects may occur?"). Discontinue or change your dose only on advice of your doctor.

How should you take this medication?

Take this medication exactly as prescribed.

■ *If you miss a dose...*
Take it as soon as you remember if it is within an hour or so of your scheduled time. If you do not remember until later, skip the dose you missed and go back to your regular schedule. Do not take 2 doses at once.

■ *Storage instructions...*
Store away from heat, light, and moisture.

What side effects may occur?

Side effects cannot be anticipated. If any develop or change in intensity, inform your doctor as soon as possible. Only your doctor can determine if it is safe for you to continue taking Librium.

■ *Side effects may include:*
Confusion, constipation, drowsiness, fainting, increased or decreased sex drive, liver problems, lack of muscle coordination, minor menstrual irregularities, nausea, skin rash or eruptions, swelling due to fluid retention, yellow eyes and skin

■ *Side effects due to rapid decrease or abrupt withdrawal from Librium include:*
Abdominal and muscle cramps
Convulsions
Exaggerated feeling of depression
Sleeplessness
Sweating
Tremors
Vomiting

Why should this drug not be prescribed?

If you are sensitive to or have ever had an allergic reaction to Librium or similar tranquilizers, you should not take this medication.

Anxiety or tension related to everyday stress usually does not require treatment with Librium. Discuss your symptoms thoroughly with your doctor.

Special warnings about this medication

Librium may cause you to become drowsy or less alert; therefore, you should not drive or operate dangerous machinery or participate in any hazardous activity that requires full mental alertness until you know how you react to this drug.

If you are severely depressed or have suffered from severe depression, consult with your doctor before taking this medication.

This drug may cause children to become less alert.

If you have a hyperactive, aggressive child taking Librium, inform your doctor if you notice contrary reactions such as excitement, stimulation, or acute rage.

Consult with your doctor before taking Librium if you are being treated for porphyria (a rare metabolic disorder) or kidney or liver disease.

Possible food and drug interactions when taking this medication

Librium is a central nervous system depressant and may intensify the effects of alcohol or have an additive effect. Do not drink alcohol while taking this medication.

If Librium is taken with certain other drugs, the effects of either can be increased, decreased, or altered. It is especially important to check with your doctor before combining Librium with the following:

Antacids such as Maalox and Mylanta
Antidepressant drugs known as MAO
   inhibitors, including Nardil and Parnate
Barbiturates such as phenobarbital
Blood-thinning drugs such as Coumadin
Cimetidine (Tagamet)
Disulfiram (Antabuse)
Levodopa (Laradopa)
Major tranquilizers such as Stelazine and
   Thorazine
Narcotic pain relievers such as Demerol and
   Percocet
Oral contraceptives

Special information if you are pregnant or breastfeeding

Do not take Librium if you are pregnant or planning to become pregnant. There may be an increased risk of birth defects. This drug may appear in breast milk and could affect a nursing infant. If the medication is essential to your health, your doctor may advise you to discontinue breastfeeding until your treatment with the drug is finished.

Recommended dosage

ADULTS

Mild or Moderate Anxiety
The usual dose is 5 or 10 milligrams, 3 or 4 times a day.

Severe Anxiety
The usual dose is 20 to 25 milligrams, 3 or 4 times a day.

Apprehension and Anxiety before Surgery
On days preceding surgery, the usual dose is 5 to 10 milligrams, 3 or 4 times a day.

Withdrawal Symptoms of Acute Alcoholism
The usual starting oral dose is 50 to 100 milligrams; the doctor will repeat this dose, up to a maximum of 300 milligrams per day, until agitation is controlled. The dose will then be reduced as much as possible.

CHILDREN

The usual dose for children 6 years of age and older is 5 milligrams, 2 to 4 times per day. Some children may need to take 10 milligrams, 2 or 3 times per day. The drug is not recommended for children under 6.

ELDERLY

Your doctor will limit the dose to the smallest effective amount in order to avoid oversedation or lack of coordination. The usual dose is 5 milligrams, 2 to 4 times per day.

Overdosage

Any medication taken in excess can cause symptoms of overdose. If you suspect an overdose, seek medical attention immediately.

■ *The symptoms of Librium overdose may include:*
Coma
Confusion

Slow reflexes
Sleepiness

Brand name:

LIMBITROL

Pronounced: LIM-bit-roll
Generic ingredients: Chlordiazepoxide,
    Amitriptyline hydrochloride

Why is this drug prescribed?

Limbitrol is a combination of an
antidepressant and an antianxiety drug. It is
used in the treatment of moderate to severe
depression associated with moderate to
severe anxiety.

Most important fact about this drug

Limbitrol is habit-forming and you can
become dependent on it. You could
experience withdrawal symptoms if you
stopped taking it abruptly (see "What side
affects may occur?"). Discontinue or change
your dose only on advice of your doctor.

How should you take this medication?

Take this medication exactly as prescribed.

- *If you miss a dose...*
  Skip the dose you missed and go back to
  your regular schedule. Do not take 2
  doses at once.

- *Storage instructions...*
  Store away from heat, light, and moisture.

What side effects may occur?

Side effects cannot be anticipated. If any
develop or change in intensity, inform your
doctor as soon as possible. Only your
doctor can determine if it is safe for you to
continue taking Limbitrol.

- *More common side effects may include:*
  Bloating
  Blurred vision

Constipation
Dizziness
Drowsiness
Dry mouth

- *Less common or rare side effects may
  include:*
  Confusion, fatigue, impotence, lack or loss
  of appetite, liver problems, nasal
  congestion, restlessness, sluggishness,
  unresponsiveness, tremors, vivid dreams,
  weakness, yellow eyes and skin

- *Side effects from rapid decrease or abrupt
  withdrawal from Limbitrol include:*
  Abdominal and muscle cramps,
  convulsions, exaggerated feeling of
  depression, headache, inability to fall
  asleep or stay asleep, nausea, restlessness,
  sweating, tremors, vague bodily
  discomfort, vomiting

Why should this drug not be prescribed?

If you are sensitive to or have ever had an
allergic reaction to related drugs—
benzodiazepine tranquilizers and tricyclic
antidepressants—you should not take
Limbitrol.

Do not take this medication if you have just
had a heart attack.

If you are taking an antidepressant drug
known as an MAO inhibitor (Nardil, Parnate,
others), consult with your doctor before
taking Limbitrol. Convulsions and death
have occurred when the drugs were
combined.

Special warnings about this medication

Limbitrol may cause you to become drowsy
or less alert; therefore, you should not drive
or operate dangerous machinery or
participate in any hazardous activity that
requires full mental alertness until you know
how this drug affects you.

This drug, especially when given in high doses, can cause irregular heartbeat, an increase in heart rate, heart attack, or stroke. If you are being treated for a heart or circulatory disorder, consult with your doctor before taking Limbitrol.

Also consult with your doctor before taking this medication if you are severely depressed or have been treated for severe depression.

Double check with your doctor before taking this medication if you are being treated for the eye condition known as angle-closure glaucoma or for inability to pass urine.

If you are planning elective surgery, your doctor will take you off Limbitrol several days prior to the operation. Limbitrol should be used with caution if you are getting electroconvulsive therapy.

Possible food and drug interactions when taking this medication
Limbitrol is a central nervous system depressant and may intensify the effects of alcohol. Do not drink alcohol while taking this medication.

If Limbitrol is taken with certain other drugs, the effects of either could be increased, decreased, or altered. It is especially important to check with your doctor before combining Limbitrol with the following:

Antidepressant drugs known as MAO
    inhibitors, including Nardil and Parnate
Barbiturates such as phenobarbital
Cimetidine (Tagamet)
Disulfiram (Antabuse)
Levodopa (Larodopa)
Oral contraceptives
Other mood-altering drugs
The blood-pressure medication guanethidine
    (Ismelin)

Severe constipation may occur if you take Limbitrol in combination with antispasmodic drugs such as Donnatal or Bentyl.

**Special information
if you are pregnant or breastfeeding**
Do not take Limbitrol if you are pregnant or planning to become pregnant. There is an increased risk of birth defects. This drug may appear in breast milk and could affect a nursing infant. If this medication is essential to your health, your doctor may advise you to discontinue breastfeeding until your treatment is finished.

Recommended dosage

ADULTS

Limbitrol Tablets
The usual starting dosage is a total of 3 or 4 tablets per day divided into smaller individual doses. The larger portion of the daily dose may be taken at bedtime. A single bedtime dose may be sufficient.

Limbitrol DS (double-strength)
The usual starting dosage is a total of 3 or 4 tablets per day divided into smaller individual doses. Your doctor may increase the dose to 6 tablets per day or decrease it to 2 tablets per day, depending on your response.

CHILDREN

Safety and effectiveness have not been established in children under 12 years old.

ELDERLY

Your doctor will have you take the smallest amount possible in order to avoid side effects such as oversedation, confusion, and loss of muscle control.

Overdosage
Any medication taken in excess can cause symptoms of overdose. If you suspect an

overdose, seek medical attention immediately.

■ *The symptoms of Limbitrol overdose may include*:
Abnormally fast heart rate, agitation, coma, confusion, congestive heart failure, convulsions, dilated pupils, disturbed concentration, drowsiness, exaggerated reflexes, hallucinations, high fever, irregular heartbeat, muscle rigidity, reduction of body temperature, severe low blood pressure, stupor, vomiting

Brand name:

LODINE

Pronounced: LOW-deen
Generic name: Etodolac

Why is this drug prescribed?
Lodine, a nonsteroidal anti-inflammatory drug, is used to relieve the inflammation, swelling, stiffness, and joint pain associated with acute and long-term treatment of osteoarthritis (the most common form of arthritis).

Most important fact about this drug
You should have frequent checkups with your doctor if you take Lodine regularly. Ulcers or internal bleeding can occur without warning.

How should you take this medication?
Your doctor may ask you to take Lodine with food or an antacid, and with a full glass of water. Never take it on an empty stomach.

Take this medication exactly as prescribed by your doctor.

If you are using Lodine for arthritis, it should be taken regularly.

■ *If you miss a dose...*
Take the forgotten dose as soon as you remember. If it is almost time for the next dose, skip the one you missed and go back to your regular schedule. Never try to "catch up" by doubling the dose.

■ *Storage instructions...*
Store at room temperature. Protect from moisture.

What side effects may occur?
Side effects cannot be anticipated. If any develop or change in intensity, inform your doctor as soon as possible. Only your doctor can determine if it is safe for you to continue taking Lodine.

■ *More common side effects may include:*
Abdominal pain, black stools, blurred vision, chills, constipation, depression, diarrhea, dizziness, fever, gas, increased frequency of urination, indigestion, itching, nausea, nervousness, rash, ringing in ears, painful or difficult urination, vomiting, weakness

■ *Less common or rare side effects may include:*
Abdominal bleeding, abnormal intolerance of light, anemia, asthma, blood disorders, congestive heart failure, dry mouth, fainting, flushing, hepatitis, high blood pressure, high blood sugar in some diabetics, hives, inability to sleep, inflammation of mouth, kidney problems, including kidney failure, loss of appetite, peptic ulcer, rapid heartbeat, rash, skin disorders, including increased pigmentation, sleepiness, Stevens-Johnson syndrome (peeling skin), sweating, swelling (fluid retention), thirst, visual disturbances, yellowed skin and eyes

Why should this drug not be prescribed?
If you are sensitive to or have ever had an allergic reaction to Lodine, aspirin, or similar

drugs, or if you have had asthma attacks caused by aspirin or other drugs of this type, you should not take this medication. Make sure that your doctor is aware of any drug reactions that you have experienced.

Special warnings about this medication

Peptic ulcers and bleeding can occur without warning.

This drug should be used with caution if you have kidney or liver disease; and it can cause liver inflammation in some people.

Do not take aspirin or any other anti-inflammatory medications while taking Lodine, unless your doctor tells you to do so.

If you are taking Lodine over an extended period of time, your doctor should check your blood for anemia.

This drug can increase water retention. Use with caution if you have heart disease or high blood pressure.

Possible food and drug interactions when taking this medication

If Lodine is taken with certain other drugs, the effects of either could be increased, decreased, or altered. It is especially important to check with your doctor before combining Lodine with the following:

Aspirin
Cyclosporine (Sandimmune)
Diuretics such as HydroDIURIL
Digoxin (Lanoxin)
Lithium (Lithobid, others)
Methotrexate
Phenylbutazone (Butazolidin)
The blood-thinning drug warfarin
   (Coumadin)

Special information if you are pregnant or breastfeeding

The effects of Lodine during pregnancy have not been adequately studied. If you are pregnant or plan to become pregnant, inform your doctor immediately. Lodine may appear in breast milk and could affect a nursing infant. If this medication is essential to your health, your doctor may advise you to discontinue breastfeeding until your treatment with this medication is finished.

Recommended dosage

ADULTS

General Pain Relief
Take 200 to 400 milligrams every 6 to 8 hours as needed. Do not take more than 1,200 milligrams a day. For individuals weighing less than 132 pounds, the maximum dose is 20 milligrams per 2.2 pounds.

Osteoarthritis
Starting dose is a total of 800 to 1,200 milligrams per day divided into smaller doses, followed by 600 to 1,200 milligrams per day in divided doses (i.e., 400 milligrams 2 or 3 times a day; 300 milligrams 2, 3 or 4 times a day). For those weighing less than 132 pounds the maximum dose is 20 milligrams per 2.2 pounds.

The lowest dose that proves beneficial should be used.

CHILDREN

The safety and effectiveness of Lodine have not been established in children.

Overdosage

Any medication taken in excess can cause symptoms of overdose. If you suspect an overdose, seek medical attention immediately.

■ *The symptoms of Lodine overdose may include:*
Drowsiness
Lethargy
Nausea
Stomach pain
Vomiting

Brand name:

LOESTRIN

See Oral Contraceptives, page 702.

Brand name:

LO/OVRAL

See Oral Contraceptives, page 702.

Generic name:

LORAZEPAM

See Ativan, page 517.

Brand name:

LOTRIMIN

See Gyne-Lotrimin, page 612.

Brand name:

LUDIOMIL

Pronounced: LOO-dee-oh-mill
Generic name: Maprotiline hydrochloride

Why is this drug prescribed?
Ludiomil is used to treat depression and anxiety associated with depression. It is also used for depression in people with manic-depressive illness.

Ludiomil is classified as a tetracyclic antidepressant. It is thought to work by boosting sensitivity at nerve junctions in the brain.

Most important fact about this drug
Seizures have been associated with Ludiomil, particularly when the drug was taken in amounts larger than prescribed, the dosage was increased too fast, or it was taken with certain other drugs such as Stelazine and Thorazine. To reduce the risk of seizures, be sure to follow your doctor's instructions for taking this medication.

How should you take this medication?
Your doctor may prescribe a single daily dose or several smaller doses.

You may not feel any improvement for 2 to 3 weeks. Do not become discouraged and discontinue Ludiomil therapy unless instructed by your doctor.

■ *If you miss a dose...*
If you take 1 dose at bedtime, check with your doctor. Taking it in the morning may cause side effects during the day.

If you take more than 1 dose a day, take the forgotten dose as soon as you remember. If it is almost time for the next dose, skip the one you missed and go back to your regular schedule. Never try to "catch up" by doubling the dose.

■ *Storage instructions...*
Store at room temperature in a tightly closed container.

What side effects may occur?
Side effects cannot be anticipated. If any develop or change in intensity, inform your doctor as soon as possible. Only your doctor can determine if it is safe for you to continue taking Ludiomil.

■ *More common side effects may include:*
Anxiety, blurred vision, constipation, dizziness, drowsiness, dry mouth, fatigue, headache, nervousness, tremors, weakness

■ *Less common or rare side effects may include:*
Abdominal cramps, agitation, allergies, bitter taste in the mouth, black tongue, bleeding sores, blocked intestine, breast development in the male, breast enlargement in the female, confusion (especially in elderly people), decreased memory, delusions, diarrhea, difficulty swallowing, difficulty urinating, dilated pupils, disorientation, excessive or spontaneous milk excretion, excessive sweating, fainting, feeling of unreality, fever, flushing, frequent urination, hair loss, hallucinations, heart attack, high blood pressure, impotence, inability to fall or stay asleep, increased or decreased sex drive, increased psychotic symptoms, increased salivation, inflammation of the mouth, involuntary movement, irregular heart rate, itching, low blood pressure, low or high blood sugar, mania, nasal congestion, nausea, nightmares, numbness, overactivity, palpitations, rapid heartbeat, red, black and blue, or purple spots on skin, restlessness, ringing in the ears, seizures, sensitivity to light, skin itching, skin rash, speech disorder, stomach pain, stroke, swelling due to fluid retention, swelling of testicles, tingling, twitches, unstable movements and gait, visual problems, vomiting, weight loss or gain, yellowish skin tone

Why should this drug not be prescribed?
Ludiomil should not be used if you have had a recent heart attack.

Do not take Ludiomil if you have taken one of the antidepressant drugs known as MAO inhibitors, including Parnate, Nardil, and Marplan, within the preceding 14 days.

Ludiomil should not be used by people who have had seizures.

Do not take Ludiomil if you are known to be hypersensitive to it.

Special warnings about this medication
Use Ludiomil cautiously if you have ever had glaucoma (excessive pressure in the eyes), heart disease, heart attacks, irregular heartbeats, strokes, thyroid disease or difficulty urinating.

This drug may impair your ability to drive a car or operate potentially dangerous machinery. Do not participate in any activities that require full alertness if you are unsure of your response to the drug.

Ludiomil may cause sensitivity to light. Avoid prolonged exposure to the sun. Use sunscreens and wear protective clothing until you learn your tolerance.

Possible food and drug interactions when taking this medication
If you take antidepressants such as Nardil, do not take Ludiomil.

If Ludiomil is taken with certain other drugs, the effects of either could be increased, decreased, or altered. It is especially important to check with your doctor before combining Ludiomil with the following:

Antispasmodic drugs such as Bentyl
Choline
Cimetidine (Tagamet)
Fluoxetine (Prozac)
Guanethidine (Ismelin)
Major tranquilizers such as Stelazine and
    Thorazine
Phenytoin (Dilantin)

Sympathomimetics such as Ventolin
Thyroid medications such as Synthroid
Tranquilizers such as Valium and Xanax

Extreme drowsiness and other potentially
serious effects can result if Ludiomil is
combined with alcohol, sleeping medications
such as Seconal, and other central nervous
system depressants.

Special information
if you are pregnant or breastfeeding
The effects of Ludiomil during pregnancy
have not been adequately studied. If you are
pregnant or plan to become pregnant,
inform your doctor immediately. Pregnant
women should use Ludiomil only if clearly
needed. Ludiomil appears in breast milk and
could affect a nursing infant. Women who
nurse infants should use the drug cautiously
and only when the potential benefits clearly
outweigh the potential risks.

Recommended dosage

ADULTS

For Mild to Moderate Depression
Dosages usually start at 75 milligrams a day,
taken as a single daily dose or divided into
smaller doses. Your doctor may increase the
dose gradually to a maximum of 150
milligrams daily.

For Moderate to Severe Depression
For those who are hospitalized, dosages as
high as 225 milligrams daily may be
prescribed.

CHILDREN

Safety and effectiveness for children under
18 years old has not been established.

ELDERLY

For Mild to Moderate Depression
Dosages usually start at 25 milligrams a day
and may range up to 50 to 75 milligrams
daily.

Overdosage
Any medication taken in excess can have
serious consequences. An overdose of
Ludiomil can be fatal. If you suspect an
overdose, seek medical help immediately.

■ *Symptoms of Ludiomil overdose may
include:*
Agitation, bluish skin, convulsions, dilated
pupils, drowsiness, heart failure, high
fever, irregular heart rate, lack of
coordination, loss of consciousness, low
blood pressure, muscle rigidity, rapid
heartbeat, restlessness, shock, vomiting,
writhing movement of the hands

Brand name:

LUPRON DEPOT (3.75 MG)

Pronounced: LU-pron DEE-poe
Generic name: Leuprolide acetate

Why is this drug prescribed?
Lupron is a synthetic version of the
naturally occurring gonadotropin releasing
hormone (GnRH). Lupron suppresses
shedding of the endometrium (lining of the
uterus) during menstruation and is used to
treat endometriosis, a condition in which
cells from the endometrium grow outside of
the uterus. Endometriosis causes painful
growths to form around the outside of the
uterus, fallopian tubes, and ovaries. Lupron
Depot 3.75 relieves the pain and reduces the
growths. In other forms and strengths,
Lupron is also used to treat prostate cancer
and early puberty. Some doctors also use
Lupron as a treatment for infertility.

Most important fact about this drug

Lupron lowers estrogen levels, which can lead to a decrease in bone density. Decreased bone density could increase your risk of osteoporosis, or brittle bone disease, later in life. Consequently, the drug is not usually given for longer than 6 months at at time.

How should you take this medication?

Lupron must be given under the supervision of a physician. It is given by injection once a month. Lupron comes in powder form and must be mixed with a special vial of sterile water before it is injected.

■ *If you miss a dose...*
Missing your monthly injections can lead to a resumption of menstrual bleeding.

■ *Storage instructions...*
Lupron does not need to be refrigerated. Protect from freezing.

What side effects may occur?

Side effects cannot be anticipated. If any develop or change in intensity, inform your doctor as soon as possible. Only your doctor can determine if it is safe for you to continue taking Lupron.

Lupron stops menstruation and reduces estrogen levels in your body. Reduced estrogen may cause side effects such as acne, decreased sex drive, headaches, hot flashes, mood swings, muscle pain, a reduction in breast size, and vaginal dryness. Your menstrual periods and estrogen levels will return to normal when you stop taking Lupron.

■ *Other more common side effects may include:*
Breast tenderness or pain, depression, fluid retension, development of male characteristics, dizziness, inflammation of the vagina (vaginitis), insomnia or other

sleep disorders, joint pain, muscle pain, nausea and vomiting, nervousness, skin reactions, stomach or intestinal disorders, unusual burning or prickling sensation of the skin, weakness, weight gain or loss

■ *Less common side effects may include:*
Anxiety, appetite changes, bruising, delusions, difficult or painful urination, dry mouth, eye problems, fainting, hair loss, hair problems, memory problems, palpitations (throbbing heartbeat), rapid heartbeat, secretion of milk, thirst

Why should this drug not be prescribed?

Lupron should not be used if you are known to be hypersensitive to it, or to any drug containing a form of GnRH.

If you have undiagnosed abnormal vaginal bleeding, you should not take Lupron.

If you are pregnant or might become pregnant, you should not take Lupron. The drug could harm a developing baby. Also avoid Lupron if you are breastfeeding.

Special warnings about this medication

Your doctor will want to make sure you are not pregnant before giving you Lupron. If you become pregnant while taking the drug, stop taking it and notify your doctor immediately.

Even though your menstrual periods stop while you are taking Lupron for endometriosis, there is still a chance you could become pregnant and you should take birth control measures. Use condoms or diaphragms rather than hormonal methods such a birth control pills or Norplant, because hormones will interfere with Lupron treatment.

Notify your doctor if you continue to have a menstrual period. If you miss succesive doses of Lupron you may have some bleeding.

Possible food and drug interactions when taking this medication

If Lupron is taken with certain other drugs, the effects of either could be increased, decreased, or altered. It is especially important to check with your doctor before combining Lupron with any type of hormones, such as birth control pills.

Special information if you are pregnant or breastfeeding

Do not take Lupron if you are pregnant or breastfeeding.

Recommended dosage

For endometriosis, Lupron is given as a single intramuscular injection once a month in a dose of 3.75 mg.

Overdosage

It is not known if an overdose of Lupron will cause harmful side effects, and an overdose is extremely unlikely. However, if you suspect overdosage, call your doctor immediately.

Brand name:

MAALOX DAILY FIBER THERAPY

See Metamucil, page 653.

Brand name:

MACROBID

See Macrodantin, page 644.

Brand name:

MACRODANTIN

Pronounced: *Mack-row-DAN-tin*
Generic name: *Nitrofurantoin*
Other brand name: *Macrobid*

Why is this drug prescribed?

Nitrofurantoin, an antibacterial drug, is prescribed for the treatment of urinary tract infections caused by certain strains of bacteria.

Most important fact about this drug

Breathing disorders have occurred in patients taking nitrofurantoin. The drug can cause inflammation of the lungs characterized by coughing, difficulty breathing, and wheezing. Pulmonary fibrosis (an abnormal increase in fibrous tissue of the lungs) can develop gradually without symptoms and can cause death. An allergic reaction to this drug is also possible and may occur without warning. Symptoms include a feeling of ill health and a persistent cough. However, these reactions occur rarely and generally in those receiving nitrofurantoin therapy for 6 months or longer.

Sudden and severe lung reactions are characterized by fever, chills, cough, chest pain, and difficulty breathing. These acute reactions usually occur within the first week of treatment and subside when therapy with nitrofurantoin is stopped.

Your doctor should monitor your condition closely, especially if you are receiving long-term treatment with this medication.

How should you take this medication?

To improve absorption of the drug, nitrofurantoin should be taken with food.

Follow your doctor's instructions carefully. Take the full amount prescribed, even if you are feeling better.

This medication works better if your urine is acidic. Ask your doctor whether you should be taking special measures to assure its acidity.

Nitrofurantoin may turn the urine brown.

■ *If you miss a dose...*
Take the forgotten dose as soon as you remember, then space out the rest of the day's doses at equal intervals.

■ *Storage instructions...*
Store at room temperature. Protect from light and keep the container tightly closed.

What side effects may occur?
Side effects cannot be anticipated. If any develop or change in intensity, inform your doctor as soon as possible. Only your doctor can determine if it is safe for you to continue taking nitrofurantoin.

■ *More common side effects may include:*
Lack or loss of appetite
Nausea
Vomiting

■ *Less common or rare side effects may include:*
Abdominal pain/discomfort, chills, confusion, cough, chest pain, depression, diarrhea, difficulty breathing, dizziness, drowsiness, exaggerated sense of well being, fever, hair loss, headache, hepatitis, hives, inflammation of the nerves causing symptoms of numbness, tingling, pain, or muscle weakness, involuntary eye movement, itching, itchy, red skin patches, joint pain, muscle pain, peeling skin, psychotic reactions, rash, severe allergic reactions, skin inflammation with flaking, skin swelling or welts, vertigo, yellowing of the skin and whites of the eyes, weakness

Why should this drug not be prescribed?
If you are sensitive to or have ever had an allergic reaction to nitrofurantoin or other drugs of this type, you should not take this medication. Make sure that your doctor is aware of any drug reactions that you have experienced.

Unless you are directed to do so by your doctor, do not take this medication if your kidneys are not functioning properly, if they are unable to produce urine or produce only a small amount.

Nitrofurantoin should not be taken at term of pregnancy or during labor and delivery; it should not be given to infants under 1 month of age.

Special warnings about this medication
Tell your doctor if you have any unusual symptoms while you are taking this drug.

Fatalities have been reported from hepatitis (liver disease) during treatment with nitrofurantoin. Long-lasting, active hepatitis can occur without symptoms; therefore, if you are receiving long-term treatment with this drug, your doctor should check you periodically for changes in liver function.

Fatalities from peripheral neuropathy— disease of the nerves—have been reported in people taking nitrofurantoin.

If you have a kidney disorder, anemia, diabetes mellitus, a debilitating disease, or a vitamin B deficiency, caution should be exercised when taking this medication. These conditions make peripheral neuropathy more likely. Consult with your doctor.

Hemolytic anemia (below-normal hemoglobin content in the blood caused by the destruction of red blood cells) has occurred in people taking nitrofurantoin.

Continued or prolonged use of this drug may result in growth of bacteria that do not respond to it. This can cause a secondary infection, so it is important that your doctor monitor your condition on a regular basis.

Possible food and drug interactions when taking this medication
If nitrofurantoin is taken with certain other drugs, the effects of either could be increased, decreased, or altered. It is especially important to check with your doctor before combining nitrofurantoin with the following:

Drugs for spasms of the digestive tract, such as Bentyl and Donnatal
Magnesium trisilicate (Gaviscon), an antacid
Uricosuric drugs (medications that increase the amount of the uric acid eliminated in the urine, such as the antigout drug, Benemid)

Special information if you are pregnant or breastfeeding
The safety of nitrofurantoin during pregnancy and breastfeeding has not been established. If you are pregnant or breastfeeding or you plan to become pregnant or breastfeed, inform your doctor immediately.

Recommended dosage
Treatment with nitrofurantoin should be continued for 1 week or for at least 3 days after obtaining a urine specimen free of infection. If your infection has not cleared up, your doctor should re-evaluate your case.

ADULTS

The recommended dosage of Macrodantin is 50 to 100 milligrams taken 4 times a day. For long-term treatment, your doctor may reduce your dosage to 50 to 100 milligrams taken at bedtime.

The recommended dosage of Macrobid is one 100-milligram capsule every 12 hours for 7 days.

CHILDREN

This medication should not be prescribed for children under 1 month of age.

The recommended dosage of Macrodantin for infants and children over 1 month of age is 5 to 7 milligrams per 2.2 pounds of body weight, divided into 4 doses in 24 hours.

For the long-term treatment of children, the doctor may prescribe daily doses as low as 1 milligram per 2.2 pounds of body weight taken in 1 or 2 doses per day.

The dosage of Macrobid for children over 12 years of age is one 100-milligram capsule every 12 hours for 7 days. Safety and effectiveness have not been established for children under 12.

Overdosage
An overdose of nitrofurantoin has not resulted in any specific symptoms other than vomiting. If vomiting does not occur soon after an excessive dose, it should be induced.

If you suspect an overdose, seek emergency medical treatment immediately.

Generic name:

MAPROTILINE

See Ludiomil, page 640.

Brand name:

MATERNA

See Stuartnatal Plus, page 746.

Generic name:

MECLOFENAMATE

See Meclomen, page 647.

Brand name:

MECLOMEN

Pronounced: MEH-cloh-men
Generic name: Meclofenamate sodium

Why is this drug prescribed?

Meclomen, a nonsteroidal anti-inflammatory drug, is used for the relief of mild to moderate pain. It is also used in the treatment of menstrual pain and heavy menstrual blood loss (when the cause is unknown) and to relieve the inflammation, swelling, stiffness, and joint pain associated with rheumatoid arthritis and osteoarthritis (the most common form of arthritis).

Most important fact about this drug

You should have frequent checkups with your doctor if you use Meclomen regularly. Ulcers or internal bleeding can occur without warning.

How should you take this medication?

Your doctor may ask you to take Meclomen with food or milk to avoid stomach upset. Try to avoid taking it on an empty stomach.

Take this medication exactly as prescribed. If you are using Meclomen for arthritis, it should be taken regularly.

■ *If you miss a dose...*
Take it as soon as you remember. If it is almost time for your next dose, skip the one you missed and go back to your regular schedule. Never take 2 doses at the same time.

■ *Storage instructions...*
Store at room temperature, away from moisture and light.

What side effects may occur?

Side effects cannot be anticipated. If any develop or change in intensity, inform your doctor as soon as possible. Only your doctor can determine if it is safe for you to continue taking Meclomen.

■ *More common side effects may include:*
Abdominal pain, diarrhea, dizziness, gas, headache, heartburn, nausea, rash, stomach and intestinal problems, vomiting

■ *Less common or rare side effects may include:*
Abdominal bleeding, anemia, colitis (inflammation of the bowel), constipation, hives, inflammation of the mouth, itching, kidney failure, loss of appetite, lupus (a disease of the immune system), peptic ulcer, red or purple areas on the skin, ringing in the ears, scaling of skin, skin inflammation and flaking, skin peeling, swelling due to fluid retention, yellow eyes and skin

Why should this drug not be prescribed?

If you are sensitive to or have ever had an allergic reaction to Meclomen, aspirin, or other nonsteroidal anti-inflammatory drugs, or if you have had asthma attacks, hay fever, or hives caused by aspirin or other drugs of this type, you should not take this medication. Make sure your doctor is aware of any drug reactions you have experienced.

Special warnings about this medication

Remember, if you must use Meclomen regularly, there is a possibility of peptic ulcers and bleeding occuring without warning.

This drug should be used with caution if you have kidney or liver disease.

If you develop severe nausea, vomiting, diarrhea, or abdominal pain, stop taking the drug and contact your doctor.

If you are taking this medication for an extended period of time, your doctor will probably check your blood for anemia.

If you are taking Meclomen for heavy menstrual blood loss and the bleeding gets worse, stop taking the drug and contact your doctor.

This medication should not be used for spotting or bleeding between menstrual cycles. If these occur while you are taking Meclomen, stop taking the drug and contact your doctor.

This medication may cause vision problems. If you experience any changes in your vision, inform your doctor.

Meclomen may mask the usual signs of infection. Your doctor will prescribe it cautiously if you have an existing infection.

This drug can cause water retention. It should be used with caution if you have high blood pressure or poor heart function.

Possible food and drug interactions when taking this medication

Meclomen may prolong bleeding. If you are taking blood-thinning medication, use this drug with caution.

If Meclomen is taken with certain other drugs, the effects of either could be increased, decreased, or altered. It is especially important to check with your doctor before taking Meclomen with the following:

Aspirin
Methotrexate
Probenecid (The gout medication Benemid)

Special information
if you are pregnant or breastfeeding

The effects of Meclomen during pregnancy have not been adequately studied. If you are pregnant or plan to become pregnant, inform your doctor immediately. Meclomen appears in breast milk and could affect a nursing infant. If this medication is essential to your health, your doctor may advise you to discontinue breastfeeding until your treatment with this medication is finished.

Recommended dosage

ADULTS

Mild to Moderate Pain
The usual dose is 50 milligrams every 4 to 6 hours. Some people will need doses of 100 milligrams, but you should not take more than 400 milligrams per day.

Excessive Menstrual Blood Loss and Pain
The usual dose is 100 milligrams 3 times a day for up to 6 days, starting at the onset of your period.

Rheumatoid Arthritis and Osteoarthritis
The usual dose is a total of 200 to 400 milligrams a day divided into 3 or 4 equal

doses. The maximum daily dose is 400 milligrams.

CHILDREN

The safety and effectiveness of Meclomen have not been established in children under 14 years of age.

ELDERLY

Side effects are seen more commonly in the elderly, so an older person will probably be prescribed a lower dose.

Overdosage

Any medication taken in excess can cause symptoms of overdose. If you suspect an overdose, seek medical attention immediately.

■ *The most common symptoms of Meclomen overdose are:*
Agitation
Irrational behavior
Little or no urine
Seizures

Generic name:

MEDROXYPROGESTERONE

See Depo-Provera, page 562, and Provera, page 727.

Generic name:

MEFENAMIC ACID

See Ponstel, page 720.

Brand name:

MEGACE

Pronounced: MEG-ace
Generic name: Megestrol acetate

Why is this drug prescribed?

Megace is a synthetic progestational drug (a drug that has the same effect as the female hormone progesterone). In tablet form it is used to treat cancer of the breast and uterus. Megace is usually prescribed when a tumor cannot be removed by surgery or has recurred after surgery, or when other drugs or radiation therapy are ineffective. Megace Oral Suspension is used to treat lack or loss of appetite, malnutrition and wasting away, and unexplained, significant weight loss in AIDS patients.

Most important fact about this drug

Drugs in the same category as Megace have sometimes been used to prevent miscarriage. However, Megace is not effective for this purpose. In the vast majority of women, the cause of miscarriage is a defective egg, which cannot be corrected with medication. Furthermore, several reports suggest that the use of progestational drugs such as Megace in the early months of pregnancy can cause birth defects.

How should you take this medication?

Take this medication exactly as prescribed by your doctor.

Megace Oral Suspension comes with a plastic dosage cup marked at 10 milliliters and 20 milliliters.

Shake Megace Oral Suspension well before you use it.

Megace works best when taken on an empty stomach, but it can be taken with food if it upsets your stomach.

■ *If you miss a dose...*
Take it as soon as you remember. If it is almost time for your next dose, skip the one you missed and go back to your regular schedule. Do not take 2 doses at once.

■ *Storage instructions...*
Store at room temperature; protect from extreme heat. Keep the suspension bottle tightly closed.

What side effects may occur?
Side effects cannot be anticipated. If any develop or change in intensity, inform your doctor as soon as possible. Only your doctor can determine if it is safe for you to continue taking Megace.

■ *A frequent side effect of Megace tablets is:*
Weight gain

■ *Less common side effects of Megace tablets may include:*
Breakthrough bleeding, carpal tunnel syndrome, fluid retention, hair loss, high blood pressure, increase in blood sugar, labored breathing, nausea, rash, vomiting

■ *Rare side effects of Megace tablets may include:*
Blood clots in lungs or veins

■ *Side effects of Megace oral suspension may include:*
Abdominal pain, abnormal sensitivity to touch, abnormal thinking, anemia, breast development in males, chest pain, confusion, constipation, convulsions, cough, decreased sex drive, depression, diarrhea, dimmed vision, dry mouth, fever, fluid retention, fluttery or throbbing heartbeat, frequent urination, gas, hair loss, headache, herpes infection, high blood pressure, impotence, inability to hold urine, inability to sleep, increase in blood sugar, increased salivation,

indigestion, infection, itching, labored breathing, lung problems, nausea, pain, pneumonia, rash, sarcoma (cancerous tumor), skin problems, sore throat, sweating, tingling or pins and needles, urinary tract infection, vomiting, weakness, yeast infection of the skin and membranes or the mouth

Why should this drug not be prescribed?
Neither Megace Tablets nor Megace Oral Suspension should be used as a diagnostic test for pregnancy. Do not use Megace Oral Suspension if you are pregnant.

Special warnings about this medication
Avoid becoming pregnant while taking this medication. Megace can cause damage to a developing baby. Megace Tablets should not be used during the first 4 months of pregnancy; Megace Oral Suspension should not be used at all during pregnancy. Use a contraceptive while you are taking this medication. If you do become pregnant, notify your doctor immediately.

If you have ever had a problem with blood clots, take Megace Oral Suspension cautiously.

This drug is not for use in children.

Possible food and drug interactions when taking this medication
No interactions have been reported.

Special information if you are pregnant or breastfeeding
The use of Megace Tablets during the first 4 months of pregnancy is not recommended. Megace Oral Suspension is not to be used during pregnancy. If you are pregnant or plan to become pregnant, notify your doctor immediately. Because there is the possibility of harmful effects on the newborn, your doctor will have you stop nursing if you need to take Megace.

Recommended dosage

MEGACE TABLETS

Breast Cancer
The usual dose is 160 milligrams per day (a dose of 40 milligrams taken 4 times a day).

Uterine Cancer
The usual dose is 40 to 320 milligrams per day, divided into smaller doses.

It takes at least 2 months of continuous treatment with Megace Tablets before your doctor can determine whether or not it is effective.

MEGACE ORAL SUSPENSION

The usual starting dose is 800 miligrams (20 milliliters) a day. Your doctor may have you take 400 or 800 milligrams for the rest of your treatment.

Overdosage

Although no specific information about Megace is available, any medication taken in excess can have serious consequences. If you suspect an overdose, seek medical treatment immediately.

Generic name:

MEGESTROL

See Megace, page 649.

Brand name:

MELLARIL

Pronounced: MEL-ah-rill
Generic name: Thioridazine hydrocholoride

Why is this drug prescribed?

Mellaril is used to reduce the symptoms of psychotic disorders such as schizophrenia, and to treat depression and anxiety in adults. Mellaril is also used in the treatment of agitation, fears, sleep disturbances, tension, depression, and anxiety in elderly people, and for certain behavior problems in children.

Most important fact about this drug

Mellaril may cause tardive dyskinesia—a condition marked by involuntary muscle spasms and twitches in the face and body. This condition may be permanent, and appears to be most common among the elderly, especially women. Ask your doctor for information about this possible risk.

How should you take this medication?

If you are taking Mellaril in a liquid concentrate form, you can dilute it with a liquid such as distilled water, soft tap water, or juice just before taking it.

Do not change from one brand to another without consulting your doctor.

■ *If you miss a dose...*
If you take 1 dose a day and remember later in the day, take the dose immediately. If you don't remember until the next day, skip the dose and go back to your regular schedule.

If you take more than 1 dose a day and remember the forgotten dose within an hour or so after its scheduled time, take it immediately. If you don't remember until later, skip the dose and go back to your regular schedule.

Never try to "catch up" by doubling a dose.

■ *Storage instructions...*
Store at room temperature, tightly closed, in the container the medication came in.

What side effects may occur?
Side effects cannot be anticipated. If any develop or change in intensity, inform your doctor as soon as possible. Only your doctor can determine if it is safe for you to continue taking Mellaril.

■ *Side effects may include:*
Abnormal and excessive secretion of milk, agitation, anemia, asthma, blurred vision, body spasm, breast development in males, changed mental state, changes in sex drive, chewing movements, confusion (especially at night), constipation, diarrhea, discolored eyes, drowsiness, dry mouth, excitement, eyeball rotation, fever, fluid accumulation and swelling, headache, inability to hold urine, inability to urinate, inhibition of ejaculation, intestinal blockage, involuntary movements, irregular blood pressure, pulse, and heartbeat, irregular or missed menstrual periods, jaw spasm, loss of appetite, loss of muscle movement, mouth puckering, muscle rigidity, nasal congestion, nausea, overactivity, painful muscle spasm, paleness, pinpoint pupils, protruding tongue, psychotic reactions, puffing of cheeks, rapid heartbeat, redness of the skin, restlessness, rigid and masklike face, sensitivity to light, skin pigmentation and rash, sluggishness, stiff, twisted neck, strange dreams, sweating, swelling in the throat, swelling or filling of breasts, swollen glands, tremors, vomiting, weight gain, yellowing of the skin and whites of eyes

Why should this drug not be prescribed?
Never combine this drug with excessive amounts of central nervous system depressants such as alcohol, barbiturates, or narcotics. Do not take Mellaril if you have heart disease accompanied by severe high or low blood pressure.

Special warnings about this medication
This drug may impair your ability to drive a car or operate potentially dangerous machinery. Do not participate in any activities that require full alertness until you are certain the drug will not interfere.

If you have ever had breast cancer, make sure your doctor is aware of it.

Mellaril may cause false positive results in tests for pregnancy.

Possible food and drug interactions when taking this medication
If Mellaril is taken with certain other drugs, the effects of either could be increased, decreased, or altered. It is especially important to check with your doctor before combining Mellaril with the following:

Epinephrine (EpiPen)
Phosphorus insecticides
Pindolol (Visken)
Propranolol (Inderal)

Extreme drowsiness and other potentially serious effects can result if Mellaril is combined with alcohol or other central nervous system depressants such as narcotics, painkillers, and sleeping medications.

Special information if you are pregnant or breastfeeding
Pregnant women should use Mellaril only if clearly needed. If you are pregnant or plan to become pregnant, inform your doctor immediately.

Recommended dosage
Your doctor will tailor your dose to your needs, using the smallest effective amount.

ADULTS

Psychotic Disorders
The starting dose ranges from 150 to 300 milligrams a day, divided into 3 equal doses.

Your doctor may increase your dosage to as much as 800 milligrams a day, taken in 2 to 4 small doses. Once your symptoms improve, your doctor will decrease the dosage to the lowest effective amount.

Depression and Anxiety
The initial dose is 75 milligrams a day, divided into 3 doses per day. Dosage may range from 20 to 200 milligrams a day, divided into 2 to 4 doses.

CHILDREN

Behavior Problems
Mellaril should not be given to children younger than 2 years old. For children 2 to 12 years old, doses are determined by body weight. Total daily doses range from 0.5 milligram to 3 milligrams for every 2.2 pounds of body weight.

The usual beginning dose for children with moderate disorders is from 20 to 30 milligrams a day, divided into 2 or 3 doses.

ELDERLY

In general, elderly people take dosages of Mellaril in the lower range. Elderly people (especially elderly women) may be more susceptible to tardive dyskinesia—a possibly irreversible condition marked by involuntary muscle spasms and twitches in the face and body. Elderly people should consult their doctor for information about these potential risks.

Depression, Anxiety and Sleep Disturbances
The starting dose is 75 milligrams a day, divided into 3 doses per day. The dosage may range from 20 to 200 milligrams a day, divided into 2 to 4 doses.

Overdosage
Any medication taken in excess can have serious consequences. An overdose of

Mellaril can be fatal. If you suspect an overdose, seek medical help immediately.

- *Symptoms of Mellaril overdose may include:*
  Agitation
  Coma
  Convulsions
  Dry mouth
  Extreme drowsiness
  Extreme low blood pressure
  Fever
  Intestinal blockage
  Irregular heart rate
  Restlessness

Generic name:

MENOTROPINS

See Pergonal, page 717.

Brand name:

METAMUCIL

Pronounced: MET-uh-MEW-sil
Generic name: Psyllium
Other brand names: Effer-Syllium, Fiberall, Hydrocil Instant, Konsyl, Maalox Daily Fiber Therapy, Perdiem Fiber, Reguloid, Syllact, Serutan

Why is this drug prescribed?
Metamucil is used to treat constipation and irritable bowel syndrome (pain the the lower abdomen accompanied by diarrhea, usually stress-related). Metamucil is also prescribed to help treat the constipation of diverticular disease (development of pouches in the wall of the lower bowel). It is also used to clean the bowel in people with hemorrhoids and to treat the constipation that often accompanies convalescence, old age, and pregnancy.

Some doctors also prescribe Metamucil to aid in reducing high cholesterol levels.

Most important fact about this drug

Contact your doctor before using Metamucil if you have any of the following conditions:

Abdominal pain
Difficulty in swallowing
Nausea
Sudden change in bowel habits that has lasted at least 2 weeks
Rectal bleeding
Vomiting

How should you take this medication?

If you are just starting on Metamucil, take 1 dose per day, gradually increasing to 3 times a day if needed, or recommended by your doctor. If you experience any gas or bloating, slightly reduce the amount of Metamucil until your system adjusts to the additional fiber in your diet. Never attempt to swallow dry powder or wafers, mix Metamucil with an 8-ounce glass of water, fruit juice, or milk. Drink an additional glass of liquid if you can, and try to drink at least 6 to 8 full glasses of liquid daily to aid in stool softening. You may have to take Metamucil for 2 to 3 days to get the most benefit from it.

■ *If you miss a dose...*
Resume your regular schedule with the next dose.

■ *Storage instructions...*
Store at room temperature. Protect from heat, light, and moisture.

What side effects may occur?

Side effects are unlikely.

Why should this drug not be prescribed?

If you are sensitive to or have ever had an allergic reaction to psyllium, you should not take this medication. Also avoid Metamucil if you have either of the following conditions:

Intestinal obstruction
Fecal impaction (an accumulation of hardened stool in the rectum or colon that cannot be passed)

Special warnings about this medication

If your constipation lasts longer than 1 week, call your doctor. This could be a sign of a more serious condition.

If you suffer from phenylketonuria (an enzyme-deficit disorder preventing the body's use of phenylalanine and resulting in harmful levels of this amino acid), avoid taking Sugar-Free Metamucil because it contains phenylalanine.

Possible food and drug interactions when taking this medication

None have been reported.

Special information if you are pregnant or breastfeeding

If you are pregnant or plan to become pregnant, or if you are breastfeeding, consult your doctor before starting on Metamucil.

Recommended dosage

ADULTS

Metamucil is generally taken 1 to 3 times daily, mixed with an 8-ounce glass of liquid. The amount per dose depends on the flavor type, and form of Metamucil you are using. Follow the package directions.

CHILDREN (6 to 12 YEARS OLD)

Use one-half the adult dose.

Overdosage

An overdose of Metamucil is unlikely. However, any medication taken in excess can have serious consequences.

If you suspect an overdose, seek medical attention immediately.

Generic name:

METHENAMINE

See Urised, page 782.

Brand name:

METHERGINE

Pronounced: METH-er-jin
Generic name: Methylergonovine maleate

Why is this drug prescribed?
Methergine, a blood-vessel constrictor, is given to prevent or control excessive bleeding following childbirth. It works by causing the uterine muscles to contract, therefore reducing the mother's blood loss.

Methergine comes in tablet and injectable forms.

Most important fact about this drug
Some blood-vessel disorders and certain infections make the use of Methergine dangerous. Make sure your doctor is aware of any medical conditions you may have.

How should you take this medication?
Take Methergine tablets exactly as prescribed.

- If you miss a dose...
  Do not take the missed dose at all and do not double the next one. Instead, go back to your regular schedule.

- Storage instructions...
  Store at room temperature in a tightly closed container, away from light.

What side effects may occur?
Side effects cannot be anticipated. If any develop or change in intensity, inform your doctor as soon as possible. Only your doctor can determine if it is safe for you to continue taking Methergine.

The most common side effect is high blood pressure, which may cause a headache or even a seizure. In some people, however, Methergine may cause low blood pressure.

- Less common or rare side effects may include:
  Bad taste, blood clots, blood in urine, chest pains (temporary), diarrhea, difficult or labored breathing, dizziness, edema, hallucinations, leg cramps, nasal congestion, nausea, palpitations (throbbing heartbeat), ringing in the ears, sweating, vomiting

Why should this drug not be prescribed?
You should not take Methergine if you are allergic to it, if you are pregnant, or if you have high blood pressure or toxemia (poisons circulating in the blood).

Special warnings about this medication
It may be dangerous to take Methergine if you have an infection, certain blood vessel disorders, or a liver or kidney problem. Inform your doctor if you think you have any such condition.

Possible food and drug interactions when taking this medication
If Methergine is taken with certain other drugs, the effects of either may be increased, decreased, or altered. It is especially important to check with your doctor before combining Methergine with the following:

Other blood-vessel constrictors such as EpiPen
Other ergot-derived medications such as Ergotrate

Special information
if you are pregnant or breastfeeding

Methergine should not be taken during pregnancy. Methergine appears in breast milk. Although no specific information is available about possible effects of Methergine on a nursing baby, the general rule is that a mother who is breastfeeding should not take any drug unless it is clearly needed.

Recommended dosage

The usual dose is 1 tablet, 0.2 milligram, 3 or 4 times daily after childbirth for a maximum of 1 week.

Overdosage

Any medication taken in excess can have serious consequences. If you suspect symptoms of a Methergine overdose, seek medical attention immediately.

■ *Symptoms of Methergine overdose may include:*
Abdominal pain, coma, convulsions, elevated blood pressure, hypothermia (drop in body temperature), lowered blood pressure, nausea, numbness, slowed breathing, tingling of the arms and legs, vomiting

Generic name:

METHOTREXATE

Pronounced: meth-oh-TREX-ate
Brand name: Rheumatrex

Why is this drug prescribed?

Methotrexate is an anticancer drug used in the treatment of lymphoma (cancer of the lymph nodes) and certain forms of leukemia. It is also given to treat some forms of cancers of the uterus, breast, lung, head, neck, and ovary. Methotrexate is also given to treat rheumatoid arthritis when other treatments have proved ineffective, and is sometimes used to treat very severe and disabling psoriasis (a skin disease characterized by thickened patches of red, inflamed skin often covered by silver scales).

Most important fact about this drug

Be certain to remember that in the treatment of psoriasis and rheumatoid arthritis, methotrexate is taken once a *week*, not once a day. Accidentally taking the recommended weekly dosage on a daily basis can lead to fatal overdosage. Be sure to read the patient instructions that come with the package.

How should you take this medication?

Take methotrexate exactly as prescribed, and promptly report to your doctor any new symptoms that may develop.

Methotrexate is given at a higher dosage for cancer than for psoriasis or rheumatoid arthritis. After high-dose methotrexate treatment, a drug called leucovorin may be given to limit the toxic effects.

■ *If you miss a dose...*
Skip it and go back to your regular schedule. Do not take 2 doses at once.

■ *Storage instructions...*
Store at room temperature, away from light.

What side effects may occur?

Side effects cannot be anticipated. If any develop or change in intensity, inform your doctor as soon as possible. Only your doctor can determine whether it is safe for you to continue taking methotrexate.

■ *More common side effects may include:*
Abdominal pain and upset
Chills and fever
Decreased resistance to infection
Dizziness
Fatigue
General feeling of illness

Mouth ulcers
Nausea

■ *Less common side effects may include:*
Abortion, acne, anemia, birth defects, black or tarry stool, blurred vision, boils, bruises, changes in skin coloration, convulsions, diarrhea, drowsiness, fatigue, hair loss, headaches, hives, inability to speak, infection of hair follicles, infertility, inflammation of the gums or mouth, intestinal inflammation, kidney failure, loss of appetite, lung disease, menstrual problems, partial or complete paralysis, rash or itching, red patches on skin, sensitivity to light, sore throat, stomach and intestinal ulcers and bleeding, stomach pain, vaginal discharge, vomiting, vomiting blood

■ *Rare side effects may include:*
Diabetes, impotence, infection, joint pain, loss of sexual desire, muscular pain, osteoporosis, ringing in the ears, severe allergic reaction, shortness of breath, sleepiness, sudden death, sweating

If you are taking methotrexate for psoriasis, you may also experience hair loss and/or sun sensitivity, and your patches of psoriasis may give a burning sensation.

Methotrexate can sometimes cause serious lung damage that makes it necessary to limit the treatment. If you experience a dry cough, fever, or breathing difficulties while taking methotrexate, be sure to tell your doctor right away.

During and immediately after treatment with methotrexate, fertility may be impaired. Men may have an abnormally low sperm count; women may have menstrual irregularities.

Why should this drug not be prescribed?

Do not take this medication if you are sensitive to it or it has given you an allergic reaction.

Do not take this medication if you are pregnant.

Methotrexate treatment is not suitable for you if you suffer from psoriasis or rheumatoid arthritis and also have one of the following conditions:

Abnormal blood cell count
Alcoholic liver disease or other chronic liver
    disease
Alcoholism
Anemia
Immune-system deficiency

Special warnings about this medication

Before you start taking methotrexate, your doctor will do a chest X-ray plus blood tests to determine your blood cell counts, liver enzyme levels, and the efficiency of your kidney function. While you are taking methotrexate, the blood tests will be repeated at regular intervals; if you develop a cough or chest pain, the chest X-ray will be repeated.

Older or physically debilitated people are particularly vulnerable to toxic effects from methotrexate.

Your doctor will prescribe methotrexate with great caution if you have any of the following:

Active infection
Liver disease
Peptic ulcer
Ulcerative colitis

Possible food and drug interactions when taking this medication

If you are being given methotrexate for the treatment of cancer or psoriasis, you should not take aspirin or other nonsteroidal painkillers such as Advil or Naprosyn; this combination could increase the toxic effects of methotrexate. If you are taking methotrexate for rheumatoid arthritis, you may be able to continue taking aspirin or a nonsteroidal painkiller, but your doctor should monitor you carefully.

Other drugs that may increase the toxic effects of methotrexate include:

Cisplatin (Platinol)
Phenylbutazone (Butazolidin)
Phenytoin (Dilantin)
Probenecid (Benemid)
Sulfa drugs such as Bactrim and Gantrisin

Sulfa drugs may increase methotrexate's toxic effect on the bone marrow, where new blood cells are made.

Certain antibiotics, including tetracycline (Achromycin) and chloramphenicol (Chloromycetin) may reduce the effectiveness of methotrexate. This is also true of vitamin preparations that contain folic acid.

Special information if you are pregnant or breastfeeding

A woman should not start methotrexate therapy until the doctor is sure she is not pregnant. Because methotrexate causes birth defects and miscarriages, it must not be taken during pregnancy by women with psoriasis or rheumatoid arthritis. It should be taken by women being treated for cancer only if the potential benefit outweighs the risk to the developing baby. In fact, a couple should avoid pregnancy if either the man or the woman is taking methotrexate. After the end of methotrexate treatment, a man should wait at least 3 months, and a woman should wait for the completion of at least one menstrual cycle, before attempting to conceive a child.

Methotrexate should not be taken by a woman who is breastfeeding; it does pass into breast milk and may harm a nursing baby.

Recommended dosage

Treatment with methotrexate is highly individualized. Your doctor will carefully tailor your dosage of methotrexate in order to avoid serious side effects and possible under- or overdosing.

Overdosage

Taken in excess, methotrexate can cause serious and even fatal damage to the liver, kidneys, bone marrow, lungs, or other parts of the body. Symptoms of overdosage may include lung or breathing problems, mouth ulcers, or diarrhea. Initially, however, serious damage caused by methotrexate may be apparent only in the results of blood tests. For this reason, careful, regular monitoring by your doctor is necessary. If for any reason you suspect symptoms of an overdose of methotrexate, seek medical attention immediately.

Generic name:

METHYLERGONOVINE

See Methergine, page 655.

Generic name:

METHYLTESTOSTERONE

See Android, page 508.

Generic name:

METHYSERGIDE

See Sansert, page 739.

Brand name:

METRODIN

Pronounced: MEH-troh-deen
Generic name: Urofollitropin

Why is this drug prescribed?

Metrodin is a synthetic version of the female hormone called follicle-stimulating hormone (FSH). It is used to trigger ovulation, or release of an egg by the ovary, in women who have difficulty ovulating on their own. Metrodin therapy is followed by 1 injection of another drug, human chorionic gonadotropin (Profasi). Metrodin is also given to produce many eggs in women going through in vetro fertilization.

Most important fact about this drug

While you are undergoing Metrodin therapy, you'll be asked to record your basal body temperature daily. You should do this at approximately the same time each morning before getting out of bed. Beginning on the last day you receive Metrodin, you should have intercourse daily until ovulation occurs, so that sperm will be present when the egg is released.

How should you take this medication?

Metrodin comes as a powder and must be mixed with the sterile salt solution that comes with it. The drug is given as an injection into the buttock for 7 to 12 days per month, followed by a single injection of Profasi one day after the last dose of Metrodin. Some women must take Metrodin longer than 12 days if their ovaries do not respond enough to the drug.

The injection can be given by your partner or another reliable person. Your doctor should show you and your partner how to give Metrodin at home.

■ *If you miss a dose...*
Be sure to take an injection every day for the exact number of days your doctor prescribes.

■ *Storage instructions...*
Store the powder at room temperature. Protect from light. After you mix the powder and saline solution, use it immediately. Discard any that is left over.

What side effects may occur?

Side effects cannot be anticipated. If any develop or change in intensity, inform your doctor as soon as possible. Only your doctor can determine if it is safe for you to continue taking Metrodin.

■ *Side effects may include:*
Abdominal cramps or bloating, abdominal pain, birth defects in infants, blood clotting, bone aches, breast tenderness, chills, collapsed lung or other problems with your respiratory system, diarrhea, dizziness, dry skin, fatigue, fever, general feeling of illness, hair loss, headache, hives, muscle aches, joint pain, nausea, ovarian cysts, pain or irritation at the place of injection, rash, stroke, vomiting

Why should this drug not be prescribed?

Do not take Metrodin if you:

■ Are sensitive to or have had an allergic reaction to it
■ Have high levels of FSH in your blood
■ Have untreated problems with your thyroid or adrenal glands
■ Have a tumor in your pituitary gland, or any other type of brain tumor
■ Have unusual vaginal bleeding of unknown cause

■ Have ovarian cysts or ovarian enlargement not caused by polycystic ovarian syndrome
■ Are pregnant

Special warnings about this medication

There have been reports of multiple births occurring after Metrodin therapy, including triplets and quintuplets. Studies show that 17 percent of births among women taking Metrodin were multiple.

In about 6 percent of women taking Metrodin, a serious condition called "ovarian hyperstimulation syndrome" occurs, in which the ovaries become enlarged and fluid gathers in the chest, abdomen, and around the heart. You will need to be hospitalized if this happens. Early warning signs of the syndrome are severe pelvic pain, nausea, vomiting, and weight gain. Other symptoms are: abdominal pain and swelling, diarrhea, weight gain, labored breathing, and decreased amount of urine. Breathing may be very difficult and you may have blood clotting problems. If you experience any of these symptoms while on Metrodin, seek medical attention immediately. Your doctor will give you frequent ultrasound tests while you are taking Metrodin to check for this syndrome.

Possible food and drug interactions when taking this medication

There have been no drug or food interactions reported during studies of Metrodin.

Special information if you are pregnant or breastfeeding

Metrodin should not be used during pregnancy because it may harm the developing baby.

It is not known whether Metrodin appears in breast milk. Because many drugs do appear in breast milk, your doctor may have you stop breastfeeding while you are taking Metrodin.

Recommended dosage

For women who have difficulty ovulating, the ususal dose is 75 international units of Metrodin per day for 7 ot 12 days, followed by 5,000 to 10,000 international units of Profasi the day after the last dose of Metrodin. Metrodin may be used for longer than 12 days if complete ovulation does not occur (as determined by ultrasound examination of the ovaries or a blood test for estrogen). To prevent ovarian hyperstimulation syndrome, Profasi should not be taken if the ovaries appear abnormally enlarged on the last day of Metrodin therapy. If you do not become pregnant after 3 cycles, the dose of Metrodin may be increased to 150 international units per day for 7 to 12 days.

For women undergoing in vitro fertilization, the usual dosage is 150 international units per day beginning on the second or third day of their cycle until the follicles of the ovaries develop, indicating that ovulation is going to occur. Women undergoing in vitro fertilization should not take Metrodin for more than 10 days.

Overdosage

The most likely result of a Metrodin overdose is ovarian hyperstimulation syndrome. If you suspect this is happening, contact your doctor immediately.

Brand name:

METROGEL-VAGINAL

Pronounced: MET-roh-jell VA-jin-al
Generic name: Metronidazole

Why is this drug prescribed?

Metrogel-Vaginal is used to treat bacterial vaginosis, a bacteria-caused inflammation of the vagina accompanied by pain and a vaginal discharge.

Most important fact about this drug

Keep using Metrogel for the full time of treatment even if your symptoms begin to clear up after a few days. You could have a relapse if you stop using the medication too soon. Continue using Metrogel during your menstrual period if necessary.

How should you take this medication?

To apply Metrogel-Vaginal, follow these steps:

1. Load the applicator to the fill line with gel as shown in the instructions you receive with the product.
2. Lie on your back with knees drawn up.
3. Gently insert the applicator high in the vagina and push the plunger.
4. Withdraw the applicator and wash it with soap and water.

To keep the medication from getting on your clothing, wear a sanitary napkin. Do not use a tampon because it will absorb the medicine. Wear cotton underwear; avoid synthetic fabrics such as rayon or nylon.

Do not scratch if you can help it. Scratching can cause more irritation and can spread the infection.

■ *If you miss a dose...*
Apply it as soon as you remember. If it is almost time for your next dose, skip the one you missed and go back to your regular schedule.

■ *Storage instructions...*
Store at room temperature; protect from freezing.

What side effects may occur?

Side effects cannot by anticipated. If any do develop or change in intensity, be sure to call your doctor as soon as possible. Only your doctor can determine if it is safe for you to continue taking Metrogel-Vaginal.

■ *More common side effects may include:*
Cramps/pain in the abdomen or uterus
Inflammation of the cervix (the neck of the uterus) or vagina

■ *Less common side effects may include:*
Itching of the vagina and surrounding areas
Metallic or bad taste
Nausea

■ *Rare side effects may include:*
Burning or irritation of the vagina and external genitals, constipation, decreased appetite, diarrhea, dizziness, frequent urination, headache, light-headedness, rash, swelling of the external genitals, vaginal discharge

Why should this drug not be prescribed?

If you have ever had an allergic reaction to or are sensitive to metronidazole, you should not use this medication.

You should not begin using this medication if you have taken Antabuse (a medication used to help alcohol withdrawal) within the previous 2 weeks.

Be sure to tell your doctor about any drug reactions you have experienced.

Special warnings about this medication

Metrogel-Vaginal contains ingredients that may cause burning and irritation in the eye. If you accidentally get Metrogel-Vaginal in your eye, rinse it with plenty of cool tap water.

You should avoid having intercourse while using Metrogel-Vaginal.

If you have severe liver disease or have a seizure disorder, use Metrogel-Vaginal with caution. Metrogel-Vaginal can cause seizures.

You should discontinue using Metrogel-Vaginal if you begin to feel any numbness, tingling, or burning in your arms or legs. Tell your doctor if you notice any of these symptoms.

Possible food and drug interactions when taking this medication

Do not use Metrogel-Vaginal if you are taking blood thinners such as Coumadin.

If you are taking Antabuse, do not begin treatment with Metrogel-Vaginal.

Do not drink alcohol while using Metrogel-Vaginal.

Special information if you are pregnant or breastfeeding

No information is available about the safety of Metrogen-Vaginal during pregnancy. If you are pregnant or plan to become pregnant, tell your doctor immediately.

It is not known whether Metrogel-Vaginal is absorbed through the skin in sufficient amounts to appear in breast milk. If your doctor thinks Metrogel-Vaginal is essential to your health, he or she may tell you to stop breastfeeding until your treatment is completed.

Recommended dosage

The recommended dose for Metrogel-Vaginal is 1 applicatorful (5 grams) inserted into the vagina twice daily, morning and evening, for 5 consecutive days.

Overdosage

There are no reported overdoses with this medication. However, if you use too much of any medication, you may experience serious problems. If you suspect an overdose of Metrogel-Vaginal, seek medical attention immediately.

Generic name:

METRONIDAZOLE

See Flagyl, page 604, and Metrogel-Vaginal, page 661.

Generic name:

MICONAZOLE

See Monistat, page 667.

Brand name:

MIDOL

Pronounced: MY-dol
Generic ingredients: Acetaminophen, Caffeine, Pamabrom, Pyrilamine maleate

Why is this drug used?

Midol is available in a variety of formulations. Regular Strength Midol is used for the temporary relief of cramps, headaches, backaches, and muscular aches. Maximum Strength and PMS Midol relieve these symptoms plus bloating and water-weight gain. In addition to relieving menstrual symptoms, Midol PM helps ease the sleeplessness that often accompanies the menstrual cycle. Teen Midol is a specially designed milder formula to help relieve teenage menstrual symptoms.

Most important fact about this drug
Do not take Midol for pain for more than 10 days unless you check with your doctor. If your pain persists or gets worse, or new symptoms develop, call your doctor.

How should you take this medication?
Follow the dosing instructions on the outside of the box. Do not take more medication than recommended. Take Midol with water.

■ *If you miss a dose...*
If you take this medicine on a regular schedule, take the dose you missed as soon as you remember. If it is almost time for your next dose, skip the one you missed and go back to your regular schedule. Do not take 2 doses at once.

■ *Storage instructions...*
Store at room temperature. Protect from excessive heat, direct light, and moisture.

What side effects may occur?
Side effects for Midol cannot be anticipated. If any become troublesome, call your doctor.

Regular Strength, Maximum Strength and PMS Midol may cause drowsiness.

Why should this drug not be prescribed?
Do not take Midol PM if you are taking sedatives or tranquilizers without discussing it with your doctor. Do not take Regular Strength Midol, PMS Midol, or Midol PM if you have asthma, glaucoma (abnormal pressure within the eye), emphysema (a lung condition marked by labored breathing), other chronic lung disease, shortness of breath, or difficulty in breathing.

Do not give Midol to children under 12 years of age unless directed by your doctor.

Special warnings about this medication
Regular Strength, Maximum Strength and PMS Midol may cause drowsiness. Be careful when driving or operating machinery. Alcohol, sedatives, or tranquilizers may increase this drowsiness.

If you are taking Midol PM and your symptoms persist or get worse, new symptoms appear, or you have not been able to sleep for more than 2 weeks, consult your doctor.

Possible food and drug interactions when taking this medication
Do not drink alcohol when taking Midol PM. If you are taking Regular Strength, Maximum Strength, or PMS Midol, alcohol, sedatives, or tranquilizers may increase the drug's drowsiness effect.

Maximum Strength Midol contains as much caffeine as a cup of coffee. Limit your intake of caffeine-containing medications, foods, or beverages while taking Maximum Strength Midol, as too much caffeine can make you nervous and irritable, cause rapid heart beat, and give you trouble sleeping.

Special information if you are pregnant or breastfeeding
As with all medications, ask your doctor or pharmacist whether it is safe for you to use Midol while you are pregnant or breastfeeding.

Recommended dosage
REGULAR STRENGTH MIDOL

Adults and Children 12 Years and Older
Take 2 caplets every 4 hours up to a maximum of 12 caplets per day.

MAXIMUM STRENGTH, PMS, AND TEEN
MIDOL

Adults and Children 12 Years and Older
Take 2 caplets every 4 hours up to a
maximum of 8 caplets per day.

MIDOL PM

Adults and Children 12 Years and Older
Take 2 caplets at bedtime as needed. Do
not take more than the recommended
dosage.

Children under 12 Years Old
Consult your physician or pharmacist.

Overdosage

In case of accidental overdose, seek
professional assistance or contact a poison
control center immediately, even if you do
not notice any signs or symptoms.

Brand name:

MIDRIN

Pronounced: MID-rin
Generic ingredients: Isometheptene mucate,
   Dichloralphenazone, Acetaminophen

Why is this drug prescribed?

Midrin is prescribed for the treatment of
tension headaches. It is also used to treat
vascular headaches such as migraine.

Most important fact about this drug

Midrin can be used only after the headache
starts. It does not prevent headaches.

How should you take this medication?

You should start taking Midrin at the first
sign of a migraine attack.

Do not take more than the maximum dose
of Midrin.

Take this medication exactly as prescribed
by your doctor.

■ *If you miss a dose...*
   Take this medication only as needed.

■ *Storage instructions...*
   Store at room temperature in a dry place.

What side effects may occur?

Side effects cannot be anticipated. If any
develop or change in intensity, tell your
doctor immediately. Only your doctor can
determine whether it is safe for you to
continue taking Midrin.

■ *Side effects may include:*
   Short periods of dizziness
   Skin rash

Why should this drug not be prescribed?

Unless directed to do so by your doctor, do
not take Midrin if you have the eye
condition called glaucoma or severe kidney
disease, high blood pressure, a physical
defect of the heart, or liver disease, or if
you are currently taking antidepressant drugs
known as MAO inhibitors, including Nardil
and Parnate.

Special warnings about this medication

Take Midrin cautiously if you have high
blood pressure or any abnormal condition
of the blood vessels outside of the heart, or
have recently had a cardiovascular attack
such as a heart attack or stroke.

Possible food and drug interactions
when taking this medication

Avoid alcoholic beverages.

If Midrin is taken with certain other drugs,
the effects of either drug could be
increased, decreased, or altered. It is
especially important to check with your
doctor before combining Midrin with the
following:

Acetaminophen-containing pain relievers such as Tylenol
Antidepressants classified as MAO inhibitors, including Nardil and Parnate
Antihistamines such as Benadryl
Central nervous system depressants such as Halcion, Valium and Xanax

Special information if you are pregnant or breastfeeding

If you are pregnant, plan to become pregnant, or are breastfeeding your baby, check with your doctor before taking Midrin.

Recommended dosage

ADULTS

Relief of Migraine Headache
The usual dosage is 2 capsules at once, followed by 1 capsule every hour until the headache is relieved; do not take more than 5 capsules within a 12-hour period.

Relief of Tension Headache
The usual dosage is 1 or 2 capsules every 4 hours up to a maximum of 8 capsules a day.

Overdosage

Any medication taken in excess can have serious consequences. If you suspect a Midrin overdose, seek emergency medical treatment immediately.

Brand name:

MINOCIN

Pronounced: MIN-o-sin
Generic name: Minocycline hydrochloride
Other brand name: Dynacin

Why is this drug prescribed?

Minocin is a form of the antibiotic tetracycline.

It is given to help treat many different kinds of infection, including:

Acne
Amebic dysentery
Anthrax (a rare skin infection)
Cholera
Gonorrhea (when penicillin cannot be given)
Plague
Respiratory infections such as pnuemonia
Rocky Mountain spotted fever
Syphilis (when penicillin cannot be given)
Urinary tract infections caused by certain microbes

Most important fact about this drug

To help clear up your infection completely, keep taking minocin for the full time of treatment, even if you begin to feel better after a few days. Minocin, like other antibiotics, works best when there is a constant amount in the body. To help keep the level constant, take the doses at evenly spaced times around the clock.

How should you take this medication?

You may take the capsules with or without food. Take Minocin exactly as directed. Your doctor will prescribe it for a specific number of days according to the condition you are being treated for; keep taking the medication until you have used it all up.

To reduce the risk of throat irritation, take the capsule form of Minocin with plenty of fluids.

You should avoid use of antacids that contain aluminum, calcium, or magnesium, such as Maalox and Mylanta, and iron preparations such as Feosol. If you must take these medicines, take them 2 to 3 hours before or after taking Minocin.

■ *If you miss a dose...*
    Take it as soon as you remember, then space out evenly any remaining doses for

that day. Never take 2 doses at the same time.

■ *Storage instructions...*
Store capsules at room temperature, away from moist places and direct light. The liquid form of Minocin may be kept in the refrigerator. Do not freeze. Shake well before using.

What side effects may occur?
Side effects cannot be anticipated. If any develop or change in intensity, inform your doctor as soon as possible. Only your doctor can determine if it is safe for you to continue taking Minocin.

■ *Side effects may include:*
Aching, inflamed joints, anal or genital sores with fungus infection, anaphylaxis (life-threatening allergic reaction), anemia, appetite loss, blurry vision, bulging of soft spots in infants' heads, decreased hearing, diarrhea, difficulty swallowing, discoloration of children's teeth, fluid retention, headache, hepatitis, hives, inflammation of the head of the penis, inflammation of the intestines, inflammation of the tongue, nausea, rash, sensitivity to light, skin coloration, skin inflammation and peeling, throat irritation, vomiting

Why should this drug not be prescribed?
Do not take Minocin if you have ever had an allergic reaction to it or to any other tetracycline antibiotic.

Although Minocin may be given to kill meningococcal (spinal) bacteria in people who are carriers, it should not be given to treat actual meningococcal meningitis (inflammation in the spinal canal).

Minocin is not a first-choice drug for treating any staphylococcal ("staph") infection.

Special warnings about this medication
If you have a kidney problem, a normal dose of Minocin may amount to an overdose for you. It is likely that you will need a lower-than-average dosage; if you need to take Minocin for an extended period of time, your doctor may order frequent blood tests to make sure you are not getting too much of the drug.

Because Minocin may make you dizzy or light-headed or cause a whirling feeling, do not drive, climb, or perform hazardous tasks until you know how the medication affects you.

Minocin should not be given to children 8 years old or younger, since it may cause discoloration of the teeth. Occasionally, Minocin has also caused tooth discoloration in adults.

Like other tetracycline antibiotics, Minocin may cause a sensitivity to light, and you may sunburn very easily. Be careful in sun and under sunlamps. If your skin turns red and hot, stop taking Minocin immediately.

While taking Minocin you may be especially susceptible to fungus infections such as vaginal yeast infection. If you do get a fungus infection, check with your doctor immediately.

If you get a headache and blurry vision while taking Minocin, or if an infant receiving Minocin develops bulging of the "soft spots" (fontanels) on the head, this could mean that the drug is causing a buildup of fluid within the skull. It is important to stop taking Minocin and see a doctor immediately.

Possible food and drug interactions when taking this medication
If Minocin is taken with certain other drugs, the effects of either could be increased,

decreased, or altered. It is especially important to check with your doctor before combining Minocin with the following:

Antacids containing aluminum, calcium, or
    magnesium, such as Mylanta
Blood thinners such as Coumadin
Iron-containing preparations such as Feosol
Oral contraceptives
Penicillin (Pen-Veek)

Special information
if you are pregnant or breastfeeding

If you are pregnant or plan to become pregnant, inform your doctor immediately. If you take Minocin during the second half of pregnancy, it may cause permanent yellow, gray, or brown discoloration of your baby's teeth.

There is reason to believe that taking Minocin during pregnancy could also harm the baby in other ways. Therefore, Minocin should be taken during pregnancy only if an antibiotic is clearly needed and only if a non-tetracycline antibiotic cannot be used instead. Because Minocin appears in breast milk and could harm the baby, it should not be taken by a woman who is breastfeeding. If this drug is essential to your health, your doctor may advise you to discontinue breastfeeding until treatment is finished.

Recommended dosage

Minocin differs from the other tetracyclines in the usual dosage and number of times it is taken per day.

You may experience more side effects if you take more than the recommended dosage.

ADULTS

The usual dosage of Minocin is 200 milligrams to start with, followed by 100 milligrams every 12 hours. If your doctor wants you to take more frequent doses, he or she may prescribe two or four 50-milligram capsules initially, and then one 50-milligram capsule 4 times daily.

CHILDREN ABOVE 8 YEARS OF AGE

The usual dosage of Minocin is 4 milligrams per 2.2 pounds of body weight to start, followed by 2 milligrams per 2.2 pounds every 12 hours.

Overdosage

Although no specific information is available, any medication taken in excess can have serious consequences. If you suspect symptoms of an overdose of Minocin, seek medical attention immediately.

Generic name:

MINOCYCLINE

See Minocin, page 665.

Brand name:

MODICON

See Oral Contraceptives, page 702.

Brand name:

MONISTAT

Pronounced: MON-ih-stat
Generic name: Miconazole nitrate

Why is this drug prescribed?

Monistat is available in several formulations, including Monistat 3 vaginal suppositories, Monistat 7 vaginal cream and suppositories, and Monistat-Derm skin cream. Monistat's active ingredient, Miconazole, fights fungal infections.

Monistat 3 and Monistat 7 are used for vaginal yeast infections. Monistat-Derm is used for skin infections such as athlete's foot, ringworm, jock itch, yeast infection on the skin (cutaneous candidiasis), and tinea versicolor (a common skin condition that produces patches of white, tan, or brown finely flaking skin over the neck and trunk).

Most important fact about this drug

Keep using this medicine regularly for the full time of the treatment, even if the infection seems to have disappeared. If you stop too soon, the infections could return. You should continue using the vaginal forms of the medicine even during your menstrual period.

How should you use this medication?

Use this medication exactly as prescribed.

Keep all forms of this medicine away from your eyes.

Before applying Monistat-Derm to your skin, be sure to wash your hands. Massage the medication gently into the affected area and the surrounding skin.

If you are using the vaginal cream or suppository, follow these steps:

1. Load the applicator to the fill line with cream, or unwrap a tablet, wet it with warm water, and place it in the applicator as shown in the instructions you received with the product.
2. Lie on your back with your knees drawn up.
3. Gently insert the application high into the vagina and push the plunger.
4. Withdraw the applicator and discard it if disposable, or wash with soap and water.

To keep the vaginal medication from getting on your clothing, wear a sanitary napkin. Do not use tampons because they will absorb the medicine. Wear cotton underwear—avoid synthetic fabrics such as rayon or nylon. Do not douche unless your doctor tells you to do so.

Dry the genital area thoroughly after a shower, bath, or swim. Change out of a wet bathing suit or damp workout clothes as soon as possible. Yeast is less likely to flourish in a dry environment.

Do not scratch if you can help it. Scratching can cause more irritation and can spread the infection.

■ *If you miss a dose...*
 Make up for it as soon as you remember. However, if it is almost time for your next dose, skip the one you missed and go back to your regular schedule.

■ *Storage instructions...*
 Store at room temperature.

What side effects may occur?

Side effects cannot be anticipated. If any develop or change in intensity, inform your doctor. Only your doctor can determine whether it is safe for you to continue taking Monistat.

■ *Side effects may include:*
 Burning sensation
 Cramping
 Headaches
 Hives
 Irritation
 Rash
 Vulval or vaginal itching

Why should this drug not be prescribed?

If you have ever had an allergic reaction to or are sensitive to miconazole nitrate, you should not use this medication. Make sure your doctor is aware of any drug reactions you have experienced.

Special warnings about this medication

If symptoms persist, or if an irritation or allergic reaction develops while you are using Monistat, notify your doctor.

The hydrogenated vegetable oil base of Monistat 3 may interact with the latex in vaginal diaphragms, so concurrent use of these two products is not recommended.

Your doctor may recommend Monistat 7 Vaginal Cream if you are using a diaphragm. However, you should be aware that the mineral oil in the vaginal cream can weaken the latex in condoms and diaphragms, making them less reliable for prevention of pregnancy or sexually transmitted disease.

If you are using Monistat 3 or Monistat 7 suppositories, you should either avoid sexual intercourse or make sure your partner uses a condom.

Do not give Monistat 7 to girls less than 12 years of age. Also avoid using Monistat 7 if you have any of the following symptoms:

Fever above 100°F orally
Foul-smelling vaginal discharge
Pain in the lower abdomen, back, or either
   shoulder

If these symptoms develop while you are using Monistat 7, stop treatment and contact your doctor right away. You may have a more serious infection.

If the infection fails to improve or worsens within 3 days, or you do not obtain complete relief within 7 days, or symptoms return within two months, you may have something other than a yeast infection.

Possible food and drug interactions when taking this medication

No interactions have been reported.

Special information if you are pregnant or breastfeeding

Unless you are directed to do so by your doctor, do not use Monistat during the first trimester (three months) of pregnancy because it is absorbed in small amounts from the vagina. It is not known whether miconazole appears in breast milk. If Monistat is essential to your health, your doctor may advise you to discontinue breastfeeding until your treatment with this medication is finished.

Recommended dosage

MONISTAT-7 VAGINAL CREAM

The usual daily dose is 1 applicatorful inserted into the vagina at bedtime for 7 consecutive days.

MONISTAT-7 VAGINAL SUPPOSITORIES

The usual daily dose is 1 suppository inserted into the vagina at bedtime for 7 consecutive days.

MONISTAT-DERM

For jock itch, ringworm, athlete's foot, or yeast infection of the skin, apply a thin layer of Monistat-Derm over the affected area morning and night. For tinea versicolor, apply a thing layer over the affected area once daily.

Overdosage

Overdose of Monistat has not been reported. However any medication used in excess can have serious consequences. If you suspect an overdose, seek medical attention immediately.

Brand name:

MYCELEX

See Gyne-Lotrimin, page 612.

Brand name:

MYCELEX-7

See Gyne-Lotrimin, page 612.

Brand name:

MYCOLOG-II

Pronounced: MY-koe-log too
Generic ingredients: Nystatin, Triamcinolone
*   acetonide*
Other brand names: Myco-Triacet II, Mytrex

Why is this drug prescribed?

Mycolog-II Cream and Ointment are prescribed for the treatment of candidiasis (a yeast-like fungal infection) of the skin. The combination of an antifungal (nystatin) and a steroid (triamcinolone acetonide) provides greater benefit than nystatin alone during the first few days of treatment. Nystatin kills the fungus or prevents its growth; triamcinolone helps relieve the redness, swelling, itching, and other discomfort that can accompany a skin infection.

Most important fact about this drug

Absorption of this drug through the skin can affect the whole body instead of just the surface of the skin being treated. Although unusual, it is possible that you could experience symptoms of steroid excess such as weight gain, reddening and rounding of the face and neck, growth of excess body and facial hair, high blood pressure, emotional disturbances, increased blood sugar, and urinary excretion of glucose (marked by an increase in frequency of urination).

Use of this medication over large surface areas, for prolonged periods, or with airtight dressings or bandages, could cause these problems. Your doctor will watch your condition and periodically check for symptoms.

How should you use this medication?

Use this medicine for the full course of treatment, even if your symptoms are gone. Apply a thin layer to the affected area and gently rub it in. Do not bandage or wrap the area being treated, unless your doctor tells you to. Keep the area cool and dry.

Use this medication exactly as prescribed by your doctor. Do not use it more often or for a longer time. It is for external use only. Avoid contact with the eyes.

■ *If you miss a dose...*
Apply it as soon as you remember. If it is almost time for your next dose, skip the one you missed and go back to your regular schedule.

■ *Storage instructions...*
Store away from heat and light. Do not freeze.

What side effects may occur?

Side effects cannot be anticipated. If any develop or change in intensity, inform your doctor as soon as possible. Only your doctor can determine if it is safe for you to continue taking Mycolog-II.

■ *Side effects may include:*
Blistering, burning, dryness, eruptions resembling acne, excessive discoloring of the skin, excessive growth of hair (especially on the face), hair loss (especially on the scalp), inflammation around the mouth, inflammation of hair follicles, irritation, itching, peeling, prickly heat, reddish purple lines on skin, secondary infection, severe inflammation of the skin, softening of the skin, stretch marks, stretching or thinning of the skin

Why should this drug not be prescribed?

If you are sensitive to or have ever had an allergic reaction to nystatin, triamcinolone acetonide, or other antifungals or steroids, you should not take this medication. Make sure your doctor is aware of any drug reactions you have experienced.

Special warnings about this medication

Do not use this drug for any disorder other than the one for which it was prescribed.

Remember to avoid wrapping or bandaging the affected area. The use of tight-fitting diapers or plastic pants is not recommended for a child being treated in the diaper area with Mycolog-II. These garments may act in the same way as airtight dressings or bandages.

If an irritation or allergic reaction develops while using Mycolog-II, notify your doctor.

If used in the groin area, apply Mycolog-II sparingly and wear loose-fitting clothing.

If your condition does not show improvement after 2 to 3 weeks, or if it gets worse, consult your doctor.

Possible food and drug interactions when taking this medication

No interactions have been reported.

Special information if you are pregnant or breastfeeding

The effects of Mycolog-II in pregnancy have not been adequately studied. If you are pregnant or plan to become pregnant, inform your doctor before using Mycolog-II.

It is not known whether this medication appears in breast milk. If this drug is essential to your health, your doctor may advise you to discontinue breastfeeding until your treatment with this medication is finished.

Recommended dosage

ADULTS

Mycolog-II Cream

Mycolog-II Cream is usually applied to the affected areas 2 times a day, in the morning and evening, by gently and thoroughly massaging the preparation into the skin. Your doctor will have you stop using the cream if your symptoms persist after 25 days of treatment.

Mycolog-II Ointment

A thin film of Mycolog-II Ointment is usually applied to the affected areas 2 times a day, in the morning and the evening. Your doctor will have you stop using the ointment if your symptoms persist after 25 days of treatment.

CHILDREN

Your doctor will limit use of Mycolog-II for children to the least amount that is effective. Long-term treatment may interfere with the growth and development of children.

Overdosage

An acute overdosage is unlikely with the use of Mycolog-II; however, long-term or prolonged use can produce reactions throughout the body. See "Most important fact about this drug."

Brand name:

MYCO-TRIACET II

See Mycolog-II, page 670.

Brand name:

MYTREX

See Mycolog-II, page 670.

Generic name:

NABUMETONE

See Relafen, page 733.

Generic name:

NAFARELIN

See Synarel, page 753.

Brand name:

NALFON

Pronounced: NAL-fahn
Generic name: Fenoprofen calcium

Why is this drug prescribed?

Nalfon, a nonsteroidal anti-inflammatory drug, is used to relieve the inflammation, swelling, stiffness, and joint pain associated with rheumatoid arthritis and osteoarthritis (the most common form of arthritis). It is also used to relieve mild to moderate pain.

Most important fact about this drug

You should have frequent checkups with your doctor if you take Nalfon regularly. Ulcers or internal bleeding can occur without warning.

How should you take this medication?

Your doctor will ask you to take Nalfon with food, an antacid, or a full glass of milk.

If you are using Nalfon for arthritis, it should be taken regularly. Take it exactly as prescribed.

■ *If you miss a dose...*
If you take Nalfon on a regular schedule, take it as soon as you remember. If it is almost time for your next dose, skip the one you missed and go back to your regular schedule. Never take 2 doses at the same time.

■ *Storage instructions...*
Store at room temperature.

What side effects may occur?

Side effects cannot be anticipated. If any develop or change in intensity, inform your doctor as soon as possible. Only your doctor can determine if it is safe for you to continue taking Nalfon.

■ *More common side effects may include:*
Constipation, dizziness, fluid retention, headache, indigestion, itching, nausea, nervousness, rapid heartbeat, rash, ringing in ears, sleepiness, sweating, weakness

■ *Less common or rare side effects may include:*
Abdominal bleeding, abdominal pain, anemia, blood in urine, bloody stools, blurred vision, bruising, confusion, diarrhea, difficult or labored breathing, dry mouth, fatigue, gas, general feeling of illness, hearing loss, hemorrhage, hepatitis, hives, inability to sleep, inflammation of the nose and throat, little or no urine, loss of appetite, painful or difficult urination, peptic ulcer, rapid heartbeat, red or purple spots on the skin, severe allergic reaction, stomach inflammation, throbbing heartbeat, tremor, upper respiratory infection, vomiting, yellow eyes and skin

Why should this drug not be prescribed?

If you are sensitive to or have ever had an allergic reaction to Nalfon, aspirin, or other anti-inflammatories, or if you have had asthma, nasal inflammation, or hives caused by aspirin or other nonsteroidal anti-inflammatory drugs, you should not take this medication. If you have ever had kidney problems, you should not take this medication. Make sure your doctor is aware of any drug reactions you have experienced.

Special warnings about this medication

Remember that peptic ulcers and bleeding can occur without warning. Call your doctor if you suspect a problem.

This drug should be prescribed with caution if you have kidney or liver disease. It can cause liver inflammation in some people.

Nalfon may cause vision problems. If you experience any changes in your vision, inform your doctor.

Nalfon may prolong bleeding time. If you are taking blood-thinning medication, your doctor will prescribe Nalfon with caution.

This drug can increase water retention. Your doctor will be cautious if you have heart disease or high blood pressure.

Nalfon may cause you to become drowsy or less alert; therefore, you should not drive, operate dangerous machinery, or participate in any hazardous activity that requires full mental alertness until you know how this drug affects you.

Possible food and drug interactions when taking this medication

If Nalfon is taken with certain other drugs, the effects of either could be increased, decreased, or altered. It is especially important to check with your doctor before combining Nalfon with the following:

Aspirin
Blood-thinning drugs such as Coumadin
Certain diuretics such as Lasix
Oral diabetes drugs such as Diabinese and
    Micronase
Phenobarbital
Phenytoin (Dilantin)
Steroids such as Decadron and Deltasone
Sulfa drugs such as Gantrisin and Azulfidine

Special information if you are pregnant or breastfeeding

The effects of Nalfon during pregnancy have not been adequately studied. If you are pregnant or plan to become pregnant, inform your doctor immediately. Nalfon appears in breast milk and could affect a nursing infant. If this medication is essential to your health, your doctor may advise you to discontinue breastfeeding until your treatment with this medication is finished.

Recommended dosage

ADULTS

Mild to Moderate Pain
The usual dose is 200 milligrams every 4 to 6 hours.

Rheumatoid Arthritis and Osteoarthritis
Your dosage will be tailored to your needs; however, people with rheumatoid arthritis generally seem to need larger doses than do those with osteoarthritis. Your doctor will prescribe the smallest dosage that provides control of pain. The usual dosage is 300 to 600 milligrams, 3 to 4 times per day. You should not take more than 3,200 milligrams in a day.

CHILDREN

The safety and effectiveness of Nalfon have not been established in children.

Overdosage

Any medication taken in excess can cause symptoms of overdose. If you suspect an overdose, seek medical attention immediately.

■ *The most common symptoms of Nalfon overdose may include:*
Abdominal pain, acute kidney failure, confusion, difficulty breathing, dizziness, drowsiness, extremely high temperature, headache, indigestion, lack of coordination, low blood pressure, nausea,

rapid heartbeat, ringing in ears, tremors, vomiting

The symptoms can appear within several hours of taking the drug.

Brand name:

NAPROSYN

Pronounced: NA-proh-sinn
Generic name: Naproxen

Why is this drug prescribed?
Naprosyn, a nonsteroidal anti-inflammatory drug, is used to relieve the inflammation, swelling, stiffness, and joint pain associated with rheumatoid arthritis, osteoarthritis (the most common form of arthritis), juvenile arthritis, ankylosing spondylitis (spinal arthritis), tendinitis, bursitis, and acute gout; it is also used to relieve menstrual cramps and other types of mild to moderate pain.

Most important fact about this drug
You should have frequent checkups with your doctor if you take Naprosyn regularly. Ulcers or internal bleeding can occur without warning.

How should you take this medication?
Naprosyn may be taken with food or an antacid, and with a full glass of water to avoid stomach upset. Avoid taking it on an empty stomach.

If you are using Naprosyn for arthritis, it should be taken regularly; take it exactly as prescribed.

■ If you miss a dose...
And you take the drug on a regular schedule, take the dose as soon as you remember. If it is almost time for your next dose, skip the one you missed and go back to your regular schedule. Do not take 2 doses at once.

■ Storage instructions...
Store Naprosyn tablets at room temperature in a well-closed container, away from light. Store Naprosyn suspension at room temperature; Protect from light and extreme heat.

What side effects may occur?
Side effects cannot be anticipated. If any develop or change in intensity, inform your doctor as soon as possible. Only your doctor can determine if it is safe for you to continue taking Naprosyn.

■ More common side effects may include:
Abdominal pain, bruising, constipation, difficult or labored breathing, dizziness, drowsiness, headache, heartburn, itching, nausea, ringing in ears, skin eruptions, swelling due to fluid retention

■ Less common or rare side effects may include:
Abdominal bleeding, black stools, blood in the urine, changes in liver function, chills and fever, colitis, congestive heart failure, depression, diarrhea, dream abnormalities, general feeling of illness, hair loss, hearing disturbances or loss, inability to concentrate, inability to sleep, indigestion, inflammation of the lungs, inflammation of the mouth, kidney disease or failure, light-headedness, menstrual disorders, muscle pain and weakness, peptic ulcer, red or purple spots on the skin, severe allergic reaction, skin inflammation due to sensitivity to light, skin rashes, sweating, thirst, throbbing heartbeat, vertigo, visual disturbances, vomiting, vomiting of blood, yellow skin and eyes

Why should this drug not be prescribed?
If you are sensitive to or have ever had an allergic reaction to Naprosyn, Anaprox or

Anaprox DS, you should not take this drug. Also, if aspirin, or other nonsteroidal anti-inflammatory drugs have ever given you asthma or nasal inflammation or tumors, you should not take this medication. Make sure your doctor is aware of any drug reactions you have experienced.

Special warnings about this medication
Remember that peptic ulcers and bleeding can occur without warning. Call your doctor immediately if you suspect a problem.

Use this drug with caution if you have kidney or liver disease; it can cause liver inflammation in some people.

Naprosyn may prolong bleeding time. If you are taking blood-thinning medication, your doctor will prescribe Naprosyn with caution.

This medication may cause vision problems. If you experience any changes in your vision, inform your doctor.

This drug can increase water retention. It will be prescribed with caution if you have heart disease or high blood pressure. Naprosyn suspension contains a significant amount of sodium. If you are on a low-sodium diet, discuss this with your doctor.

Naprosyn may cause you to become drowsy or less alert; therefore, avoid driving, operating dangerous machinery, or participating in any hazardous activity that requires full mental alertness until you are sure of the drug's effect on you.

Possible food and drug interactions when taking this medication
If Naprosyn is taken with certain other drugs, the effects of either could be increased, decreased, or altered. It is especially important to check with your doctor before combining Naprosyn with the following:

Aspirin
Beta blockers such as Tenormin
Blood-thinning drugs such as Coumadin
Furosemide (Lasix)
Lithium (Lithonate)
Methotrexate
Naproxen sodium (Anaprox)
Phenytoin (Dilantin)
Probenecid (Benemid)
Sulfa drugs such as Bactrim and Septra
Oral diabetes drugs such as Diabinese and
    Micronase

**Special information
if you are pregnant or breastfeeding**
The effects of Naprosyn during pregnancy have not been adequately studied. If you are pregnant or plan to become pregnant, inform your doctor immediately. Naprosyn appears in breast milk and could affect a nursing infant. If this medication is essential to your health, your doctor may advise you to discontinue breastfeeding until your treatment with this medication is finished.

Recommended dosage
Naprosyn is available in tablet and liquid form. When taking the liquid, use a teaspoon or the measuring cup, marked in one-half teaspoon and 2.5 milliliter increments, that comes with Naprosyn.

ADULTS

Rheumatoid Arthritis, Osteoarthritis, and Ankylosing Spondylitis
The usual dose is 250 milligrams (10 milliliters or 2 teaspoons of suspension), 375 milligrams (15 milliliters or 3 teaspoons), or 500 milligrams (20 milliliters or 4 teaspoons) 2 times a day (morning and evening). Your dose may be adjusted by your doctor over your period of treatment. Improvement of symptoms should be seen in 2 to 4 weeks.

Acute Gout
Starting dose is 750 milligrams (30 milliliters or 6 teaspoons), followed by 250 milligrams (10 milliliters or 2 teaspoons) every 8 hours until the symptoms are relieved.

Mild to Moderate Pain, Menstrual Cramps, Acute Tendinitis and Bursitis
Starting dose is 500 milligrams (20 milliliters or 4 teaspoons of suspension), followed by 250 milligrams (10 milliliters or 2 teaspoons) every 6 to 8 hours as needed. The most you should take in a day is 1,250 milligrams (50 milliliters or 10 teaspoons).

CHILDREN

Juvenile Arthritis
The usual dose is 10 milligrams per 2.2 pounds of body weight, 2 times a day. Follow your doctor's directions carefully when giving a child this medicine.

The safety and effectiveness of Naprosyn have not been established in children under 2 years of age.

Overdosage

Any medication taken in excess can have serious consequences. If you suspect an overdose seek medical attention immediately.

■ *The Symptoms of Naprosyn overdose may include:*
　Drowsiness
　Heartburn
　Indigestion
　Nausea
　Vomiting

Generic name:

NAPROXEN

See Naprosyn, page 674.

Generic name:

NAPROXEN SODIUM

See Anaprox, page 505.

Brand name:

NARDIL

Pronounced: NAHR-dill
Generic name: Phenelzine sulfate

Why is this drug prescribed?

Nardil is a monoamine oxidase (MAO) inhibitor used to treat depression as well as anxiety or phobias mixed with depression. MAO is an enzyme responsible for breaking down certain neurotransmitters (chemical messengers) in the brain. By inhibiting MAO, Nardil helps restore more normal mood states. Unfortunately, MAO inhibitors such as Nardil also block MAO activity throughout the body, an action that can have serious, even fatal, side effects—especially if MAO inhibitors are combined with other foods or drugs containing a substance called tyramine.

Most important fact about this drug

Avoid the following foods, beverages, and medications while taking Nardil and for 2 weeks thereafter:

Beer (including alcohol-free or reduced-alcohol beer)
Caffeine (in excessive amounts)
Cheese (except for cottage cheese and cream cheese)
Chocolate (in excessive amounts)
Dry sausage (including Genoa salami, hard salami, pepperoni, and Lebanon bologna)
Fava bean pods
Liver
Meat extract
Pickled herring
Pickled, fermented, aged, or smoked meat,

fish, or dairy products
Sauerkraut
Spoiled or improperly stored meat, fish, or
    dairy products
Wine (including alcohol-free or reduced-
    alcohol wine)
Yeast extract (including large amounts of
    brewer's yeast)
Yogurt

Medications to avoid:
    Amphetamines
    Appetite suppressants such as Tenuate
    Antidepressants and related medications
        such as Prozac, Elavil, Triavil, Tegretol,
        and Flexeril
    Asthma inhalants such as Proventil and
        Ventolin
    Cold and cough preparations including
        those with dextromethorphan, such as
        Robitussin DM
    Hay fever medications such as Contac,
        Dristan, and Sudafed
    L-tryptophan-containing products
    Nasal decongestants in tablet, drop, or
        spray form
    Sinus medications
    Weight-loss medications

Taking Nardil with any of the above foods,
beverages, or medications can cause serious,
potentially fatal, high blood pressure.
Therefore, when taking Nardil you should
immediately report the occurrence of a
headache, heart palpitations, or any other
unusual symptom. In addition, make certain
that you inform any other physician or
dentist you see that you are currently taking
Nardil or have taken Nardil within the last
2 weeks.

How should you take this medication?
Nardil may be taken with or without food.
Take it exactly as prescribed. It can take up
to 4 weeks for the drug to begin working.

Use of Nardil may complicate other medical
treatment. Always carry a card that says you
take Nardil, or wear a Medic Alert bracelet.

■ *If you miss a dose...*
Take it as soon as you remember. If it is
within 2 hours of your next dose, skip
the one you missed and go back to your
regular schedule. Do not take 2 doses at
once.

■ *Storage instructions...*
Store at room temperature.

What side effects may occur?
Side effects cannot be anticipated. If any
develop or change in intensity, inform your
doctor as soon as possible. Only your
doctor can determine if it is safe for you to
continue taking Nardil.

■ *More common side effects may include:*
Constipation, disorders of the stomach
and intestines, dizziness, drowsiness, dry
mouth, excessive sleeping, fatigue,
headache, insomnia, low blood pressure
(especially when rising quickly from lying
down or sitting up), muscle spasms, sexual
difficulties, strong reflexes, swelling due to
fluid retention, tremors, twitching,
weakness, weight gain

■ *Less common or rare side effects may
include:*
Anxiety, blurred vision, coma, convulsions,
delirium, exaggerated feeling of well-being,
fever, glaucoma, inability to urinate,
involuntary eyeball movements, jitteriness,
lack of coordination, liver damage, mania,
muscular rigidity, onset of the mental
disorder schizophrenia, rapid breathing,
rapid heart rate, repetitious use of words
and phrases, skin rash, sweating, swelling
in the throat, tingling sensation, yellowed
skin and whites of eyes

Why should this drug not be prescribed?

You should not take this drug if you have pheochromocytoma (a tumor of the adrenal gland), congestive heart failure, or a history of liver disease, or if you have had an allergic reaction to it.

You should not take Nardil if you are taking medications that may increase blood pressure (such as amphetamines, cocaine, allergy and cold medications, or Ritalin), other MAO inhibitors, L-dopa, methyldopa (Aldomet), phenylalanine, L-tryptophan, L-tyrosine, fluoxetine (Prozac), buspirone (BuSpar), bupropion (Wellbutrin), guanethidine (Ismelin), meperidine (Demerol), dextromethorphan, or central nervous system depressants such as alcohol and narcotics; or if you must consume the foods, beverages, or medications listed above in the "Most important fact about this drug" section.

Special warnings about this medication

You must follow the food and drug limitations established by your physician; failure to do so may lead to potentially fatal side effects. While taking Nardil, you should promptly report the occurrence of a headache or any other unusual symptoms.

If you are diabetic, your doctor will prescribe Nardil with caution, since it is not clear how MAO inhibitors affect blood sugar levels.

If you are taking Nardil, talk to your doctor before you decide to have elective surgery.

If you stop taking Nardil abruptly, you may have withdrawl symptoms. They may include nightmares, agitation, strange behavior, and convulsions.

Possible food and drug interactions when taking this medication

If Nardil is taken with certain other drugs, the effects of either could be increased, decreased, or altered. It is important that you closely follow your doctor's dietary and medication limitations when taking Nardil. Consult the "Most important fact about this drug" and "Why should this drug not be prescribed?" sections for lists of the foods, beverages, and medications that should be avoided while taking Nardil.

In addition, you should use blood pressure medications (including diuretics and beta blockers) with caution when taking Nardil, since excessively low blood pressure may result. Symptoms of low blood pressure include dizziness when rising from a lying or sitting position, fainting, and tingling in the hands or feet.

Special information if you are pregnant or breastfeeding

The effects of Nardil during pregnancy have not been adequately studied. Nardil should be used during pregnancy only if the benefits of therapy clearly outweigh the potential risks to the fetus. If you are pregnant or plan to become pregnant, inform your doctor immediately. Nursing mothers should use Nardil only after consulting their physician, since it is not known whether Nardil appears in human milk.

Recommended dosage

ADULTS

The usual starting dose is 15 milligrams (1 tablet) 3 times a day. Your doctor may increase the dosage to 90 milligrams per day.

It may be 4 weeks before the drug starts to work.

Once you have had good results, your doctor may gradually reduce the dose, possibly to as low as 15 milligrams daily or every 2 days.

CHILDREN

Nardil is not recommended, since safety and efficacy for children under the age of 16 have not been determined.

Overdosage

Any medication taken in excess can have serious consequences. An overdose of Nardil can be fatal. If you suspect an overdose, seek medical help immediately.

■ *Symptoms of overdose may include:*
Agitation, backward arching of the head, neck, and back, cool, clammy skin, coma, convulsions, difficult breathing, dizziness, drowsiness, faintness, hallucinations, high blood pressure, high fever, hyperactivity, irritability, jaw muscle spasms, low blood pressure, pain in the heart area, rapid and irregular pulse, severe headache, sweating

Brand name:

NATALINS

See Stuartnatal Plus, page 746.

Brand name:

NICODERM

See Nicotine Patches, page 682.

Brand name:

NICORETTE

Pronounced: Nik-ho-RET
Generic name: Nicotine polacrilex

Why is this drug prescribed?

Nicorette and Nicorette DS (double strength) are used as a temporary aid by cigarette smokers who want to stop.

Nicorette is most effective when used in a medically supervised behavior modification program offering education, counseling, and psychological support.

Most important fact about this drug

Nicorette contains nicotine—an addicting and toxic substance. Nicorette is a powerful, potentially addicting medication that must be used according to your doctor's instructions.

How should you take this medication?

The following are general, medically approved guidelines for taking Nicorette, but you should carefully follow your doctor's instructions to avoid side effects and addiction to Nicorette.

1) You must give up smoking completely and immediately when you start using Nicorette.

2) When you want to smoke, put 1 piece of Nicorette in your mouth.

3) Chew Nicorette very slowly; chewing Nicorette too fast may release the nicotine in the product too quickly, causing the same effects as inhaling for the first time or smoking too fast (e.g., light-headedness, nausea, vomiting, throat and mouth soreness, hiccups, and upset stomach).

4) Stop chewing when you get a peppery taste or feel a slight tingling in your mouth. This usually happens after about 15 chews.

5) "Park" the gum by placing it between your cheek and gums.

6) Start slowly chewing again when the peppery taste or tingling feeling is almost gone (about 1 minute). Stop chewing when the peppery taste or tingling returns.

7) "Park" the gum again in a different part of the mouth.

8) Repeat this procedure until most of the nicotine is gone from the gum (about 30 minutes).

9) Do not use more than 30 pieces of Nicorette or 20 pieces of Nicorette DS a day.

10) As your urge to smoke fades, gradually use fewer pieces of Nicorette. This may be possible in 2 to 3 months.

11) Stop using Nicorette when you are satisfied with 1 or 2 pieces a day, unless your doctor tells you otherwise. If you have trouble reducing your use of Nicorette, contact your doctor. Do not use Nicorette for more than 6 months.

12) Carry Nicorette with you at all times in case you feel the urge to smoke again.

The effects of Nicorette may be reduced by many foods or drinks such as coffee, juices, wine or soft drinks. Do not eat or drink 15 minutes before or while chewing Nicorette.

■ *If you miss a dose...*
 With Nicorette, the goal is to take as few doses as possible. Don't make up a missed dose, and never double the dose.

■ *Storage instructions...*
 Keep Nicorette below 86 degrees. (Remember, the inside of a parked car can get much hotter than this.) Protect the chewing pieces from light.

What side effects may occur?
Side effects cannot be anticipated. If any develop or change in intensity, inform your doctor as soon as possible. Only your doctor can determine if it is safe for you to continue taking this medication.

■ *More common side effects may include:*
 Bleeding gums, excessive saliva in mouth, hiccups, indigestion, inflammation of the mouth, injury to teeth or cheeks, nausea, stomach and intestinal discomfort, throat soreness, tingling or pins and needles

■ *Less common or rare side effects may include:*
 Diarrhea, dry mouth, inflammation of the gums, tongue, throat, mouth sores, muscle pain, rash, sweating, tongue sores,

Why should this drug not be prescribed?
Do not use Nicorette if you are sensitive to or have ever had an allergic reaction to nicotine or any of the other ingredients of Nicorette.

Special warnings about this medication
Using Nicorette on a long-term basis is not recommended because nicotine, if consumed for a long enough time, can be harmful and addicting.

You must chew Nicorette slowly and follow your doctor's instructions carefully to avoid side effects and addiction.

If you develop an allergic reaction such as hives or rash, stop using Nicorette and contact your doctor.

Before using Nicorette, tell your doctor if you have ever had angina (severe chest pain), Buerger's disease (disease of the arteries), diabetes or other endocrine (hormone) diseases, dental problems, difficulty swallowing, drug allergies, heartburn, heart disease, high blood pressure, kidney or liver disease, peptic ulcer, throat or mouth inflammation, or overactive thyroid or TMJ (disease at the joint of the jaw).

Nicorette should be used with caution if you have recently had a heart attack or have a seriously irregular heart beat.

Nicorette may stick to dentures; if this becomes a problem, stop chewing Nicorette and tell your doctor.

Possible food and drug interactions when taking this medication

If Nicorette is taken with certain other drugs, the effects of either could be increased, decreased, or altered. It is especially important to check with your doctor before combining Nicorette with the following:

Acetaminophen (Tylenol)
Caffeine
Furosemide (Lasix)
Glutethimide (the sedative drug Doriden)
Imipramine (Tofranil)
Insulin
Isoproterenol (Isuprel)
Labetalol (Normodyne)
Oxazepam (Serax)
Pentazocine (Talwin)
Phenacetin, the pain and fever reducer
Phenylephrine (Entex)
Prazosin (Minipress)
Propoxyphene (Darvon)
Propranolol (Inderal)
Theophylline (Theo-Dur)

Special information
if you are pregnant or breastfeeding

If you are pregnant or nursing your baby, you should not use Nicorette. If you become pregnant while using Nicorette, contact your doctor immediately.

Nicotine, either from smoking or from chewing Nicorette, does appear in breast milk and can affect the baby.

Recommended dosage

ADULTS

Nicorette-2 milligram
Chew 1 piece of Nicorette every 1 to 2 hours. Most adults require 9 to 12 pieces of Nicorette a day during the first month of treatment. Follow your doctor's advice to be sure you are using Nicorette correctly. Do not use more than 30 pieces a day. After 2 to 3 months, follow your doctor's plan for gradual withdrawal of Nicorette.

Nicorette DS-4 milligram
Chew 1 piece of Nicorette every 1 to 2 hours. Most adults require 9 to 12 pieces of Nicorette a day during the first months of treatment. Follow your doctor's advice to be sure you are using Nicorette correctly. Do not use more than 20 pieces a day. After 2 to 3 months, follow your doctor's plan for gradual withdrawal of Nicorette.

Gradual withdrawal of Nicorette is recommended to avoid the return of symptoms that may lead you to start smoking again. Suggested procedures are as follows:

1. Decrease the total number of pieces of Nicorette used per day by 1 or more pieces every 4 7 days.
2. Decrease the chewing time with each piece of Nicorette from the normal 30 minutes to 10 to 15 minutes. Then gradually decrease the total number of pieces used per day. You can also chew each piece longer than 30 minutes and cut down the number of pieces you chew a day.
3. Substitute 1 or more pieces of sugarless gum for an equal number of pieces of Nicorette. Increase the number of pieces of sugarless gum substituted for Nicorette every 4 to 7 days.

CHILDREN

Safety and effectiveness for children and adolescents who smoke have not been established. If a child swallows a piece of Nicorette accidentally, contact your doctor or local poison control center immediately.

ELDERLY

Elderly individuals should use Nicorette cautiously.

Overdosage

Any medication taken in excess can have serious consequences. Overdose may occur if you chew many pieces of Nicorette at one time or in rapid succession, or if you smoke while you are using Nicorette. Accidentally swallowing a piece of Nicorette will probably not cause side effects, but if you have any reason to suspect an overdose, seek medical help immediately.

Symptoms of Nicorette overdose are similar to symptoms of acute nicotine poisoning and may include:

Abdominal pain, blurred vision, cold sweat, diarrhea, difficulty breathing, disturbed hearing, dizziness, exhaustion, fainting, headache, low blood pressure, mental confusion, nausea, paleness, rapid and irregular pulse, salivation, tremor, upset stomach, vomiting, weakness

A large overdose can result in prostration and respiratory failure.

Category:

NICOTINE PATCHES

Brand names: Habitrol, Nicoderm, Nicotrol, Prostep

Why is this drug prescribed?

Nicotine patches, which are available under several brand names, are designed to help you quit smoking by reducing your craving for tobacco. Each adhesive patch contains a specific amount of nicotine embedded in a pad or gel.

Nicotine, the habit-forming ingredient in tobacco, is a stimulant and a mood lifter.

When you give up smoking, lack of nicotine makes you crave cigarettes and may also cause anger, anxiety, concentration problems, irritability, frustration, or restlessness.

When you wear a nicotine patch, a specific amount of nicotine steadily travels out of the patch, through your skin, and into your bloodstream, keeping a constant low level of nicotine in your body. Although the resulting level of nicotine is less than you would get from smoking, it may be enough to keep you from craving cigarettes or experiencing other withdrawal symptoms.

Habitrol patches are round and come in three strengths: 21, 14, or 7 milligrams of nicotine per patch. You wear a Habitrol patch 24 hours a day.

Nicoderm patches are rectangular and come in three strengths: 21, 14, or 7 milligrams of nicotine per patch. You wear a Nicoderm patch 24 hours a day.

Nicotrol patches are rectangular and come in three strengths: 15, 10, or 5 milligrams of nicotine per patch. You put on a Nicotrol patch in the morning, wear it all day, and remove it at bedtime. You do not use it when you sleep.

ProStep patches are round and come in two strengths: 22 or 11 milligrams of nicotine per patch. You wear a Prostep patch 24 hours a day.

Most important fact about this drug

Nicotine patch therapy should be part of an overall stop-smoking program that also includes behavior modification, counseling, and support. The goal of the therapy should be complete cessation of smoking, not just "cutting down."

How should you use this medication?

Use nicotine patches exactly as prescribed. The general procedure is as follows:

- Take a fresh patch out of its packaging and remove the protective liner from the adhesive. Save the wrapper for later disposal of the used patch.
- Stick the patch onto your outer upper arm or any clean, non-hairy part of your trunk.
- Press the patch firmly onto your skin for about 10 seconds, making sure that the edges are sticking well.
- Wash your hands. Any nicotine sticking to your hands could get into your eyes or nose, causing irritation.
- After 16 or 24 hours (depending on the brand), remove that patch and apply a fresh patch to a different spot on your body. To reduce the chances of irritation, do not return to a previously used spot for at least a week.
- Fold the used patch in half, place it back in its own wrapper, and throw it in a trash container that cannot be reached by children or pets.

Water will not harm the nicotine patch. You may keep wearing your patch while bathing, showering, swimming, or using a hot tub.

If your patch does fall off, dispose of it carefully and apply a new patch.

As a memory aid, pick a specific time of day and always apply a fresh patch at that time. You may change the schedule if you need to. Just remember not to wear any single patch for more than the recommended time (16 or 24 hours), since after that time the patch will begin to lose strength and may begin to irritate your skin.

Do not change brands without consulting your doctor.

If you are unable to stop smoking by your fourth week of wearing nicotine patches, it is likely that patch treatment will not work for you. At this point, your doctor may stop prescribing the patches for you.

- *If you miss a dose...*
  Apply the patch as soon as you remember. Never use 2 patches at once.

- *Storage instructions.*
  Do not remove a patch from its wrapping until you are ready to use it. Store your supply of patches at temperatures no higher than 86 degrees Fahrenheit; remember that in warm weather the inside of a car can get much hotter than this.

What side effects may occur?

Side effects cannot be anticipated. If any develop or change in intensity, inform your doctor as soon as possible. Only your doctor can determine if it is safe for you to continue using nicotine patches.

- *Most common side effects may include:*
  Itching and burning at the application site
  Rash
  Redness of the skin

- *Less common side effects may include:*
  Abnormal dreaming, allergic reactions, back pain, chest pain, constipation, cough, diarrhea, dizziness, drowsiness, dry mouth, headache, high blood pressure, impaired concentration, indigestion, inflammation of sinuses, menstrual irregularities, nausea, nervousness, numbness, pain, pins and needles sensation, sleeplessness, sore throat, stomach pain, sweating, taste changes, tingling, vomiting, weakness

Why should this drug not be prescribed?

Do not take this medication if you are sensitive to or have ever had an allergic reaction to nicotine. Be cautious if you have ever had a bad reaction to a different brand of nicotine patch or to adhesive tape or other adhesive material.

Special warnings about this medication

Do not smoke any form of tobacco while wearing a patch; doing so could give you an overdose of nicotine. Be aware that for several hours after you remove a patch, nicotine from the patch is still in your skin and passing into your bloodstream.

The use of nicotine patches may aggravate certain medical conditions. Before you use any brand of nicotine patch, make sure your doctor knows if you have, or have ever had, any of the following conditions:

Allergies to drugs, adhesive tape, or
    bandages
Chest pain from a heart condition (angina)
Diabetes requiring insulin injections
Heart attack
High blood pressure (severe)
Irregular heartbeat (heart arrhythmia)
Kidney disease
Liver disease
Overactive thyroid
Skin disease
Stomach ulcer

Nicotine, from any source, can be toxic and addictive. Thoroughly discuss with your doctor the benefits and risks of nicotine replacement therapy.

Because a used nicotine patch still contains enough nicotine to poison a child or a pet, you must dispose of used patches with special care. Wrap each patch in the opened pouch or aluminum foil in which it came and throw it in a trash receptacle that is out of the reach of youngsters and animals.

Possible food and drug interactions when taking this medication

If nicotine patches are used with certain other drugs, the effects of either could be increased, decreased, or altered. It is especially important to check with your doctor before combining nicotine patches with the following:

Acetaminophen-containing drugs such as
    Tylenol
Caffeine-containing drugs such as No Doz
Certain airway-opening drugs such as Isuprel,
    Dristan, and Neo-Synephrine
Certain blood pressure medicines such as
    Minipress, Trandate, and Normodyne
Cimetidine (Tagamet)
Haloperidol (Haldol)
Imipramine (Tofranil)
Insulin
Lithium (Lithonate)
Oxazepam (Serax)
Pentazocine (Talwin)
Propranolol (Inderal)
Theophylline (Theo-Dur)

Special information if you are pregnant or breastfeeding

If you are pregnant or plan to become pregnant, inform your doctor immediately. Ideally, a pregnant woman should not take nicotine in any form. Do your best to quit smoking with the aid of counseling and support and without drug therapy. If you are unable to quit, you and your doctor should discuss which is more likely to harm your unborn baby: continued smoking or use of nicotine patches to help you quit smoking. Because nicotine passes very readily into breast milk, ideally it should not be taken in any form during breastfeeding. If you are breastfeeding and are unable to quit smoking, discuss with your doctor the pros and cons of using nicotine patches.

Remember that if you smoke while wearing a patch, you are giving your body a "double dose" of nicotine; if you are pregnant or breastfeeding, your baby will get the "double dose", too.

Recommended dosage
Nicotine patches come in two or three strengths, depending on the brand; larger patches contain higher doses of nicotine. The usual starting dose is 1 high-strength patch per day. If you weigh less than 100 pounds, however, or if you smoke less than half a pack of cigarettes a day or have heart disease, your doctor may start you on a lower-dose patch.

Your doctor will work closely with you to determine the best product and the most effective cessation program.

Overdosage
Any medication used in excess, including nicotine patches, can have serious consequences. If you suspect symptoms of an overdose of nicotine, either from a patch or from smoking while wearing a patch, seek medical attention immediately.

■ *Symptoms of nicotine overdose may include:*
Abdominal pain, blurred vision, breathing abnormalities, cold sweat, confusion, diarrhea, dizziness, drooling, fainting, hearing difficulties, heart palpitations, low blood pressure, nausea, pallor, salivation, severe headaches, sweating, tremor, upset stomach, vision problems, vomiting, weakness

Generic name:

NICOTINE POLACRILEX

See Nicorette, page 679.

Brand name:

NICOTROL

See Nicotine Patches, page 682.

Generic name:

NITROFURANTOIN

See Macrodantin, page 644.

Brand name:

NIZORAL

Pronounced: NYE-zore-al
Generic name: Ketoconazole

Why is this drug prescribed?
Nizoral, a broad-spectrum antifungal drug available in tablet form, may be given to treat several fungal infections within the body, including oral thrush and candidiasis.

It may also be given to treat severe, hard-to-treat fungal skin infections that have not cleared up after treatment with the drug griseofulvin, including Fulvicin, Grisactin, and others.

Most important fact about this drug
In some people, Nizoral may cause serious or even fatal damage to the liver. Before starting to take Nizoral, and at frequent intervals while you are taking it, you should have blood tests to evaluate your liver function. Tell your doctor immediately if you experience any signs or symptoms that could mean liver damage: these include

unusual fatigue, loss of appetite, nausea or vomiting, jaundice, dark urine, or pale stools.

Rare, but sometimes fatal reactions involving the heart have been reported in people taking Nizoral and Seldane. You must not take these two drugs together.

How should you take this medication?
Take Nizoral exactly as prescribed.

You should keep taking the drug until tests show that your fungal infection has subsided. If you stop too soon, the infection might return.

You may want to take Nizoral Tablets with meals to avoid stomach upset.

Avoid alcohol and do not take with antacids. If necessary, you should wait 2 to 3 hours before taking antacids.

■ *If you miss a dose...*
  Take the forgotten dose as soon as you remember. This will help to keep the proper amount of medicine in the body. However, if it is almost time for your next dose, skip the one you missed and go back to your regular schedule. Do not take double doses.

■ *Storage instructions...*
  Nizoral should be stored at room temperature.

What side effects may occur?
Side effects from Nizoral cannot be anticipated. If any develop or change in intensity, inform your doctor as soon as possible. Only your doctor can determine if it is safe for you to continue taking Nizoral.

■ *More common side effects may include:*
  Nausea
  Vomiting

■ *Less common side effects may include:*
  Abdominal pain
  itching

■ *Rare side effects may include:*
  Breast swelling (in men), bulging fontanel (soft areas on a baby's scalp), depression, diarrhea, dizziness, drowsiness, fever and chills, headache, hives, impotence, light-sensitivity, rash

Why should this drug not be prescribed?
Do not take Nizoral if you are sensitive to it or have ever had an allergic reaction to it. Never take Nizoral together with Seldane or Hismanal.

Special warnings about this medication
A few people have had anaphylaxis (a life-threatening allergic reaction) after taking their first dose of Nizoral.

Observe caution when driving or performing other tasks requiring alertness, due to potential side effects of headache, dizziness, and drowsiness.

Possible food and drug interactions when taking this medication
If Nizoral is taken with certain other drugs, the effects of either could be increased, decreased, or altered. It is especially important to check with your doctor before combining Nizoral with the following:

Alcoholic beverages
Antacids such as Di-Gel, Maalox, Mylanta, and others
Anticoagulants such as Coumadin, Dicumarol, and others
Anti-ulcer medications such as Axid, Pepcid, Tagamet, and Zantac
Astemizole (Hismanal)
Corticosteroids such as Prednisone and Medrol
Cyclosporine (Sandimmune)
Isoniazid (Nydrazid)

Phenytoin (Dilantin)
Rifampin (Rifadin, Rifamate, and Rimactane)
Terfenadine (Seldane)
Theophyllines such as Theo 24, Slo-Phyllin, Theo-Dur, and others

Special information if you are pregnant or breastfeeding

If you are pregnant or plan to become pregnant, inform your doctor immediately. Nizoral should be taken during pregnancy only if the benefit outweighs the possible harm to your unborn child.

Since Nizoral can probably make its way into breast milk, it should not be taken during breastfeeding. If you are a new mother, check with your doctor. You may need to stop breastfeeding while you are taking Nizoral.

Recommended dosage

ADULTS

The recommended starting dose of Nizoral is a single daily dose of 200 milligrams (1 tablet).

In very serious infections, or if the problem does not clear up within the expected time, the dose of Nizoral may be increased to 400 milligrams (2 tablets) once daily. Treatment lasts at least 1 to 2 weeks, and for some infections much longer.

CHILDREN

In small numbers of children over 2 years of age, a single daily dose of 3.3 to 6.6 milligrams per 2.2 pounds of body weight has been used.

Nizoral has not been studied in children under 2 years of age.

Overdosage

Although no specific information is available, any medication taken in excess can have serious consequences. If you suspect an overdose of Nizoral, seek medical attention immediately.

Brand name:

NOLVADEX

Pronounced: NOLL-vah-decks
Generic name: Tamoxifen citrate

Why is this drug prescribed?

Nolvadex, an anticancer drug, may be given after mastectomy to help delay a recurrence of breast cancer. It also has proved effective when cancer has spread to other parts of the body. Nolvadex is most effective in stopping the kind of breast cancer that thrives on estrogen.

Most important fact about this drug

If you are taking Nolvadex, you should have routine gynecological examinations and report any abnormal vaginal bleeding to your doctor immediately.

How should you take this medication?

Take Nolvadex exactly as prescribed. Do not stop taking this medication without first consulting your doctor. It may be necessary to continue taking the drug for several years.

Birth control measures are recommended during treatment with Nolvadex. However, methods other than "the Pill" must be employed.

■ *If you miss a dose...*
Do not try to make it up. Go back to your regular schedule with the next dose.

■ *Storage instructions...*
Nolvadex should be stored away from heat and light.

What side effects may occur?

Side effects from Nolvadex are usually mild and rarely require the drug to be stopped. If any develop or change in intensity, inform your doctor as soon as possible. Only your doctor can determine if it is safe for you to continue taking Nolvadex.

- *More common side effects may include:*
  Hot flashes
  Nausea
  Vomiting

- *Less common side effects may include:*
  Bone pain, diarrhea, menstrual irregularities, skin rash, tumor pain, vaginal bleeding, vaginal discharge

- *Rare side effects may include:*
  Depression, distaste for food, dizziness, hair thinning or partial loss, headache, light-headedness, liver disorders, swelling of arms or legs, vaginal itching, visual problems

Why should this drug not be prescribed?

Do not take Nolvadex if you are sensitive to it or have ever had an allergic reaction to it.

Special warnings about this medication

If you experience visual problems while taking Nolvadex, notify your doctor immediately.

In a few women Nolvadex may raise the level of cholesterol and other fats in the blood. Your doctor may periodically do blood tests to check your cholesterol and triglyceride levels.

Nolvadex may produce an abnormally high level of calcium in the blood. Symptoms include muscle pain and weakness, loss of appetite, and, if severe, kidney failure. If you experience any of these symptoms, notify your doctor as soon as possible.

If tests show that your blood contains too few white blood cells or platelets while you are taking Nolvadex, your doctor should monitor you with special care. These problems have sometimes been found in women taking Nolvadex; whether the drug caused the blood-cell abnormalities is uncertain.

Possible food and drug interactions when taking this medication

If Nolvadex is taken with certain other drugs, the effects of either could be increased, decreased, or altered. It is especially important to check with your doctor before combining Nolvadex with the following:

Blood-thinning drugs such as Coumadin
Bromocriptin (Parlodel)
Phenobarbital

Special information if you are pregnant or breastfeeding

It is important to avoid pregnancy while taking Nolvadex, because the drug could harm the unborn child. Since Nolvadex is an anti-estrogen drug, you will need to use a non-hormonal form of contraception, such as a condom and/or diaphragm, and not birth control pills. If you accidentally become pregnant while taking Nolvadex, discuss this with your doctor immediately.

Because Nolvadex might cause serious harm to a nursing infant, you should not breastfeed your baby while taking this drug. If this medication is essential to your health, your doctor may advise you to discontinue breastfeeding until your treatment is finished.

Recommended dosage

ADULTS

The recommended dosage is one or two 10-milligram tablets in the morning and evening.

Overdosage

Any medication taken in excess can have serious consequences. If you suspect an overdose of Nolvadex, seek medical attention immediately.

- *Symptoms of Nolvadex overdose may include:*
  Dizziness
  Overactive reflexes
  Tremor
  Unsteady gait

Brand name:

NORDETTE

See Oral Contraceptives, page 702.

Brand name:

NORETHIN

See Oral Contraceptives, page 702.

Generic name:

NORFLOXACIN

See Noroxin, page 689.

Brand name:

NORINYL

See Oral Contraceptives, page 702.

Brand name:

NOROXIN

Pronounced: Nor-OX-in
Generic name: Norfloxacin

Why is this drug prescribed?

Noroxin is an antibacterial used to treat infections of the urinary tract, including cystitis (inflammation of the inner lining of the bladder caused by a bacterial infection), and certain sexually transmitted diseases, such as gonorrhea.

Most important fact about this drug

Noroxin is not given for the treatment of syphilis. When used in high doses for a short period of time to treat gonorrhea, it may actually mask or delay the symptoms of syphilis. Your doctor may perform certain tests for syphilis at the time of diagnosing gonorrhea, and after treatment with Noroxin.

How should you take this medication?

Noroxin should be taken, with a glass of water, either 1 hour *before* or 2 hours *after* eating a meal. Do not take more than the dosage prescribed by your doctor.

It is important to drink plenty of fluids while taking Noroxin.

Take all the Noroxin your doctor prescribes. If you stop taking the medicine too soon, you may have a relapse.

- *If you miss a dose...*
  Be sure to take it as soon as possible. This will help to keep a constant amount of Noroxin in your body. However, if it is almost time for your next dose, skip the one you missed and go back to your regular schedule. Do not take two doses at the same time.

■ *Storage instructions...*
Store at room temperature. Keep container tightly closed. Store out of reach of children.

What side effects may occur?

Side effects cannot be anticipated. If any develop or change in intensity, inform your doctor as soon as possible. Only your doctor can determine whether it is safe for you to continue taking Noroxin.

■ *More common side effects may include:*
Dizziness
Fatigue
Headache
Nausea

■ *Other side effects may include:*
Abdominal cramping, arthritis, back pain, bitter taste, blood abnormalities, confusion, constipation, convulsions, dead skin, depression, diarrhea, dizziness, dry mouth, double vision, extreme sleepiness, fever, flushing, reddish skin, gas, hallucinations, headache, heartburn, hives, indigestion, insomnia, itching, joint pain, kidney failure (symptoms may include reduced amount of urine, drowsiness, nausea, vomiting and coma), lack of coordination, light-headedness, loss of appetite, low blood sugar, muscle pain, nausea, peeling skin, psychotic reactions, rash (such as pimples, blisters, and nodules) on skin and mucous membranes, reduced blood platelets causing bleeding disorders (such as bleeding into the skin), restlessness, severe blisters and bleeding in genitals and in mucous membranes of eyes, lips, mouth, and nasal passages, severe skin reaction to sun, shock, shortness of breath, stomach pain, sweating, temporary hearing loss, tingling (pins and needles sensation), vomiting, weakness, yellow eyes and skin

Why should this drug not be prescribed?

You should not be using Noroxin if you are sensitive to it or to other drugs of the same type, such as Cipro.

Special warnings about this medication

Noroxin is not recommended for:

Children (under the age of 18)
Nursing mothers
Pregnant women

People with disorders such as epilepsy, severe cerebral arteriosclerosis, and other conditions that might lead to seizures should use Noroxin cautiously. There have been reports of convulsions in some people taking Noroxin.

Some people taking drugs chemically similar to Noroxin have experienced severe, sometimes fatal reactions, occasionally after only one dose.

These reactions may include:
Confusion, convulsions, difficulty breathing, hallucinations, heart collapse, hives, increased pressure in the head, itching, light-headedness, loss of consciousness, psychosis, rash, restlessness, shock, swelling in the face or throat, tingling, tremors.

If you experience any of these reactions you should immediately stop taking Noroxin and seek medical help.

Some people find needle-shaped crystals in their urine after taking Noroxin. Drink plenty of fluids while taking Noroxin. This will increase urine output and reduce crystalization.

Noroxin may cause dizziness or light-headedness and might impair your ability to drive a car or operate potentially dangerous machinery. Use caution when undertaking any activities that require full alertness if you are unsure of your ability.

You should avoid excessive exposure to direct sunlight while taking Noroxin. Stop taking Noroxin immediately if you have a severe reaction to sunlight, such as a skin rash.

Possible food and drug interactions when taking this medication

If Noroxin is taken with certain other drugs, the effects of either could be increased, decreased, or altered. It is especially important to check with your doctor before combining Noroxin with the following:

Antacids such as Maalox and Tums
Caffeine (including coffee, tea, and some soft drinks)
Calcium supplements
Cyclosporine (Sandimmune)
Multivitamins and other products containing iron or zinc
Nitrofurantoin (Macrodantin, Macrobid)
Oral anticoagulants, such as warfarin (Coumadin)
Probenecid (Benemid)
Sucralfate (Carafate)
Theophylline (Theo-Dur)

Special information if you are pregnant or breastfeeding

The effects of Noroxin during pregnancy have not been adequately studied. Inform your doctor if you are pregnant or planning a pregnancy.

Do not take Noroxin while breastfeeding. There is a possibility of harm to the infant.

Recommended dosage

Take Noroxin with a full glass of water 1 hour before, or 2 hours after, eating a meal. Drink plenty of liquids while taking Noroxin.

Uncomplicated Urinary Tract Infections
The suggested dose is 800 milligrams per day. 400 milligrams should be taken twice a day for 3 to 10 days, depending upon the kind of bacteria causing the infection. People with impaired kidney function may take 400 milligrams once a day for 3 to 10 days.

Complicated Urinary Tract Infections
The suggested dose is 800 milligrams per day. 400 milligrams should be taken twice a day for 10 to 21 days.

Sexually Transmitted Diseases (Gonorrhea)
The usual recommended dose is one single dose of 800 milligrams for 1 day.

The maximum total daily dosage of Noroxin should not be more than 800 milligrams.

Overdosage

The symptoms of overdose with Noroxin are not known. However, any medication taken in excess can have serious consequences. If you suspect a Noroxin overdose, seek medical help immediately.

Brand name:

NORPLANT

Pronounced: NOR-plant
Generic name: Levonorgestrel implants

Why is this drug prescribed?

Norplant is a birth control method consisting of 6 thin, flexible plastic capsules implanted just beneath the skin in a woman's upper, inner arm. The implants are inserted by your doctor. Each set prevents pregnancy for 5 years, but can be removed by your doctor at any time. The Norplant capsules contain progestin, a synthetic version of a naturally occurring female hormone progesterone, which they release slowly and continuously into the bloodstream. This constant release of progestin prevents the ovaries from releasing eggs for fertilization. Norplant also works by thickening the mucus in the vagina near the opening of the uterus. The thick mucus makes it difficult for sperm to enter the uterus during sexual intercourse.

Norplant is more than 99 percent effective in preventing pregnancy. Overall, fewer than one woman per 100 women become pregnant during the first year of Norplant use.

Most important fact about this drug

Norplant contains the same type of hormone, progestin, found in many birth control pills. Women taking birth control pills, which also contain the hormone estrogen, are at slightly increased risk of serious heart-related problems such as stroke, heart attack, and blood clots. The risk of heart problems is greater among women who smoke more than 15 cigarettes per day, especially those older than age 35. Although the heart problems associated with birth control pills are thought to be related to the estrogen in the pills, rather than the progestin, the possibility of a similar risk with progestin-only birth control methods such as Norplant has not been ruled out. To be on the safe side, women who use Norplant are advised not to smoke, particularly if they are over 35 years of age.

How should you take this medication?

Your doctor inserts the Norplant capsules directly under the skin of the upper, inner arm, just above the elbow crease. The procedure takes about 15 minutes. Because a local anesthetic is injected into the area beforehand, there is very little discomfort; and since only one small, shallow incision is made in the arm, very little bleeding occurs. Each of the six Norplant capsules is about

the size of a thin matchstick, and they are inserted in a fan-shaped configuration. After 5 years, you will need to get a new set of Norplant implants or choose another method of birth control.

To make certain you are not pregnant when receiving Norplant, the capsules are usually inserted during the first 7 days after the beginning of menstruation or immediatly following an abortion. If you have the insertion performed at any other time during the menstrual cycle, you should use a nonhormonal contraceptive, such as diaphragm or condom, for the remainder of that cycle.

What side effects may occur?

Side effects cannot be anticipated. If any develop or change in intensity, inform your doctor as soon as possible. Only your doctor can determine if it is safe for you to continue using Norplant.

■ *More common side effects may include:*
Abdominal discomfort
Breast discharge
Infection at the implant site
Inflammation of the opening of the uterus
Irregular periods
Missed or light menstrual periods
Pain in the muscles or bones
Pain or itching near the implant site
(usually temporary)
Prolonged menstrual bleeding
Spotting (bleeding between periods)
Vaginal discharge
Vaginal inflammation

■ *Less common side effects may include:*
Abnormal hair growth, acne, anxiety, breast pain, change in appetite, dizziness, headache, inflammation of the skin, nervousness, rash, scalp-hair loss, weight gain

Why should this drug not be prescribed?
While the Norplant System can be used by the majority of women, there are some who should not use it for medical reasons. These include pregnancy, acute liver disease, unexplained vaginal bleeding, breast cancer, and blood clots in the lungs, eyes, or legs.

Special warnings about this medication
In rare instances, one of the Norplant capsules may be expelled due to improper insertion or infection. If you notice any of the capsules comming out, or if you have an infection with redness, swelling, or pus at the insertion site, contact your doctor immediately. Loss of a capsule makes Norplant less potent, and increases the risk of pregnancy.

Since some Norplant users stop having menstrual periods, it is impossible to tell whether a missed period is due to the drug or pregnancy. Your doctor will give you a pregnancy test if you go for 6 weeks or more without any menstrual bleeding after a pattern of regular bleeding. However, if menstrual bleeding starts tapering off and stops over time, chances are that it is an effect of Norplant rather thatn an indication of prenancy. If pregnancy occurs, Norplant must be removed by your doctor. However, when left in accidentally during pregnancy, Norplant does not increase the risk of birth defects.

The heavier you are, the greater your chances of becoming pregnant while on Norplant. For instance, among women weighing less than 110 pounds, only 2 in 1,000 become pregnant over 5 years, while among women weighing more than 154 pounds, the pregnancy rate rises to 8.5 out of 100.

Occasionally, a follicle, or egg sac, in an ovary may grow beyond its normal size while a women is using Norplant. These enlarged follicles are usually harmless, and generally disappear on their own. Rarely, an enlarged follicle may twist or burst, causing abdominal pain. In that case, surgery will be done to remove it.

The risk of ectopic (outside of the uterus) pregnancy increases with the length of time a woman is using Norplant, and among women who are overweight. If you have unexplained pain in your lower abdomen, your doctor will want to check you for ectopic pregnancy.

If you develop any blood-clotting disorders while on Norplant, the capsules should be removed.

Also, because Norplant could affect your blood-clotting ability, your doctor may want to remove the capsules if you are going to be confined in bed for any length of time due to surgery or other illnesses.

Norplant may increase your blood pressure. If you have high blood pressure, make sure the doctor is aware of it. If you have high blood pressure and you smoke, you should not use Norplant, because it could increase your risk of stroke.

Norplant may alter your blood sugar levels; if you are diabetic, your doctor will want to watch you closely.

Norplant may cause fluid retention, so it may not be recommended if you have a problem that could be aggravated by fluid retention, such as migraine headaches, heart or kidney disease, or epilepsy.

If you notice a yellow tint to your skin or the whites of your eyes, tell your doctor immediately.

If you develop any problems with your vision, notify your doctor at once.

Although Norplant is a very effective method of birth control, it does not protect you against AIDS or other sexually transmitted diseases. If you are concerned about AIDS or other STDs, make sure your partner uses a latex condom during sexual intercourse. (For total safety, refrain from sex.)

Possible food and drug interactions when taking this medication

If other medications are taken with Norplant, the effects of either could be increased, decreased, or altered. It is especially important to check with your doctor if you use Norplant and take any of the following:

Carbamazepine (Tegretrol, Atretol)
Phenytoin (Dilantin)

Special information if you are pregnant or breastfeeding

If you are pregnant, you should not use Norplant. If you are breastfeeding, Norplant is not considered the best birth control method, because it does appear in breast milk. However, in studies on women who breastfed their babies and received Norplant 6 weeks after childbirth, there were no problems found with the growth or health of their infants. There are no studies on the safety of Norplant in women who breastfed their infants during the 6 weeks immediately following childbirth.

Recommended dosage

The 6 Norplant capsules are implanted by your doctor once every 5 years.

Overdosage

When implanting a new set of Norplant capsules, your doctor should make sure that all 6 of the previous capsules are removed

first. This is the only way an overdose could occur.

■ *Symptoms of Norplant overdose may include:*
Fluid retention
Uterine bleeding irregularities

Brand name:

NORPRAMIN

Pronounced: NOR-pram-in
Generic name: Desipramine hydrochloride

Why is this drug prescribed?

Norpramin is used in the treatment of depression. It is one of a family of drugs called tricyclic antidepressants. Drugs in this class are thought to work by affecting the levels of the brain's natural chemical messengers (called neurotransmitters), and adjusting the brain's response to them.

Norpramin has also been used to treat bulimia and attention deflicit disorders, and to help with cocaine withdrawal.

Most important fact about this drug

Serious, sometimes fatal, reactions have been known to occur when drugs such as Norpramin are taken with another type of antidepressant called and MAO inhibitor. Drugs in this category include Nardil, Marplan, and Parnate. Do not take Norpramin within two weeks of taking one of these drugs. Make sure your doctor and pharmacist know of all the medications you are taking.

How should you take this medication?

Norpramin should be taken exactly as prescribed.

Do not stop taking Norpramin if you feel no immediate effect. It can take up to 2 or 3 weeks for improvement to begin.

Norpramin can cause dry mouth. Sucking hard candy or chewing gum can help this problem.

■ *If you miss a dose...*
If you take several doses per day, take the forgotten dose as soon as you remember, then take any remaining doses for the day at evenly spaced intervals. If you take Norpramin once a day at bedtime and don't remember until morning, skip the missed dose. Never try to "catch up" by doubling the dose.

■ *Storage instructions...*
Norpramin can be stored at room temperature. Protect it from excessive heat.

What side effects may occur?
Side effects cannot be anticipated. If any develop or change in intensity, inform your doctor as soon as possible. Only your doctor can determine if it is safe for you to continue taking Norpramin.

■ *Side effects may include:*
Abdominal cramps, agitation, anxiety, black tongue, black, red, or blue spots on skin, blurred vision, breast development in males, breast enlargement in females, confusion, constipation, delusions, diarrhea, dilated pupils, disorientation, dizziness, drowsiness, dry mouth, excessive or spontaneous flow of milk, fatigue, fever, flushing, frequent urination or difficulty or delay in urinating, hallucinations, headache, heart attack, heartbeat irregularities, hepatitis, high or low blood pressure, high or low blood sugar, hives, impotence, increased or decreased sex drive, inflammation of the mouth, insomnia, intestinal blockage, lack of coordination, light-headedness (especially when rising from lying down), loss of appetite, loss of hair, mild elation, nausea, nightmares, odd taste in mouth, painful ejaculation, palpitations, purplish spots on the skin, rapid heartbeat, restlessness, ringing in the ears, seizures, sensitivity to light, skin itching and rash, sore throat, stomach pain, stroke, sweating, swelling due to fluid retention (especially in face or tongue), swelling of testicles, swollen glands, tingling, numbness and pins and needles in hands and feet, tremors, urinating at night, visual problems, vomiting, weakness, weight gain or loss, worsening of psychosis, yellowed skin and whites of eyes

Why should this drug not be prescribed?
Norpramin should not be used if you are known to be hypersensitive to it, or if you have had a recent heart attack.

People who take antidepressant drugs known as MAO inhibitors (including Nardil, Parnate, and Marplan) should not take Norpramin.

Special warnings about this medication
Before using Norpramin, tell your doctor if you have heart or thyroid disease, a seizure disorder, a history of being unable to urinate, or glaucoma.

Nausea, headache, and uneasiness can result if you suddenly stop taking Norpramin. Consult your doctor and follow instructions closely when discontinuing Norpramin.

This drug may impair your ability to drive a car or operate potentially dangerous machinery. Do not participate in any activities that require full alertness if you are unsure about your ability.

Norpramin may increase your skin's sensitivity to sunlight. Overexposure could cause rash, itching, redness, or sunburn. Avoid direct sunlight or wear protective clothing.

If you are planning to have elective surgery, make sure that your doctor is aware that you are taking Norpramin. It should be discontinued as soon as possible prior to surgery.

Tell your doctor if you develop a fever and sore throat while you are taking Norpramin. He may want to do some blood tests.

Possible food and drug interactions when taking this medication

People who take antidepressant drugs known as MAO inhibitors (including Nardil, Parnate, and Marplan) should not take Norpramin.

If Norpramin is taken with certain other drugs, the effects of either could be increased, decreased, or altered. It is especially important to check with your doctor before combining Norpramin with the following:

Cimetidine (Tagamet)
Drugs that improve breathing, such as
    Proventil
Drugs that relax certain muscles, such as
    Bentyl
Fluoxetine (Prozac)
Guanethidine (Ismelin)
Sedatives/hypnotics (Halcion, Valium)
Thyroid medications (Synthroid)

Extreme drowsiness and other potentially serious effects can result if Norpramin is combined with alcohol or other depressants, including narcotic painkillers such as Percocet and Demerol, sleeping medications such as Halcion and Nembutal, and tranquilizers such as Valium and Xanax.

Special information if you are pregnant or breastfeeding

Pregnant women or mothers who are nursing an infant should use Norpramin only when the potential benefits clearly outweigh the potential risks. If you are pregnant or planning to become pregnant, inform your doctor immediately.

Recommended dosage

Your doctor will tailor the dose to your individual needs.

ADULTS

The usual dose ranges from 100 to 200 milligrams per day, taken in 1 dose or divided into smaller doses. If needed, dosages may gradually be increased to 300 milligrams a day. Dosages above 300 milligrams per day are not recommended.

CHILDREN

Norpramin is not recommended for children.

ELDERLY AND ADOLESCENTS

The usual dose ranges from 25 to 100 milligrams per day. If needed, dosages may gradually be increased to 150 milligrams a day. Doses above 150 milligrams per day are not recommended.

Overdosage

Any medication taken in excess can have serious consequences. An overdosage of Norpramin can be fatal. If you suspect an overdose, seek medical help immediately.

■ *Symptoms of overdose may include:* Agitation, coma, confusion, delirium, difficult breathing, dilated pupils, extremely low blood pressure, fever, inability to urinate, irregular heart rate, kidney failure, restlessness, rigid muscles, seizures, shock, stupor, vomiting

Generic name:

NORTRIPTYLINE

See Pamelor, page 708.

Generic name:

NYSTATIN WITH TRIAMCINOLONE

See Mycolog-II, page 670.

Generic name:

OFLOXACIN

See Floxin, page 607.

Brand name:

OGEN

Pronounced: OH-jen
Generic name: Estropipate
Other brand name: Ortho-Est 1.25

Why is this drug prescribed?

Ogen and Ortho-Est are estrogen replacement drugs. The tablets are used to reduce symptoms of menopause, including feelings of warmth in face, neck, and chest, and the sudden intense episodes of heat and sweating known as "hot flashes." They also may be prescribed for teenagers who fail to mature at the usual rate.

In addition, either the tablets or Ogen vaginal cream can be used for other conditions caused by lack of estrogen, such as dry, itchy external genitals and vaginal irritation.

Along with diet, calcium supplements, and exercise, Ogen tablets are also prescribed to prevent osteoporosis, a condition in which the bones become brittle and easily broken.

Most important fact about this drug

Because estrogens have been linked with increased risk of endometrial cancer (cancer in the lining of the uterus) in women who have had their menopause, it is essential to have regular check-ups and to report any unusual vaginal bleeding to your doctor immediately.

How should you take this medication?

Be careful to follow the cycle of administration your doctor establishes for you. Take the medication exactly as prescribed.

When using Ogen Vaginal Cream, follow the instructions printed on the carton. It is for short-term use only. Remove the cap from the tube and make sure the plunger of the applicator is all the way into the barrel. Screw the nozzle of the applicator onto the tube and squeeze the cream into the applicator. The number on the plunger, which indicates the dose you should take, should be level with the top of the barrel. Unscrew the applicator and replace the cap on the tube. Insert the applicator into the vagina and push the plunger all the way down. Between uses, take the plunger out of the barrel and wash the applicator with warm, soapy water. Never use hot or boiling water.

■ If you miss a dose...
  Take the forgotten dose as soon as you remember. If it is almost time for the next dose, skip the one you missed and go back to your regular schedule. Never try to "catch up" by doubling the dose.

■ Storage instructions...
  Store at room temperature.

What side effects may occur?

Side effects cannot be anticipated. If any develop or change in intensity, notify your doctor as soon as possible. Only your doctor can determine if it is safe for you to continue taking estrogen.

■ *Side effects may include:*
Abdominal cramps, bloating, breakthrough bleeding, breast enlargement, breast tenderness, change in amount of cervical secretion, change in menstrual flow, changes in sex drive, changes in vaginal bleeding patterns, chorea (irregular, rapid, jerky movements, usually affecting the face and limbs), depression, dizziness, enlargement of benign tumors (fibroids), excessive hairiness, fluid retention, hair loss, headache, inability to use contact lenses, lack of menstruation, migraine, nausea, painful menstruation, secretion from the breasts, spotting, spotty darkening of the skin, especially around the face, skin eruptions (especially on the legs and arms), skin irritation, vaginal yeast infection, vision problems, vomiting, weight gain or loss, yellow eyes and skin

Why should this drug not be prescribed?
Estrogens should not be used if you know or suspect you have breast cancer or other cancers promoted by estrogen. Also, do not use estrogen if you are pregnant or think you may be pregnant, if you have abnormal, undiagnosed genital bleeding, or if you have blood clots or a blood clotting disorder or a history of blood clotting disorders associated with previous estrogen use.

Ogen Vaginal Cream should not be used if you are sensitive to or have ever had an allergic reaction to any of its components.

Special warnings about this medication
The risk of cancer of the uterus increases when estrogen is used for a long time or taken in large doses. There also may be increased risk of breast cancer in women who take estrogen for an extended period of time.

Women who take estrogen after menopause are more likely to develop gallbladder disease.

Ogen also increases the risk of blood clots. These blood clots can cause stroke, heart attack, or other serious disorders.

While taking estrogen, get in touch with your doctor right away if you notice any of the following:

Abdominal pain, tenderness, or swelling
Abnormal bleeding from the vagina
Breast lumps
Coughing up blood
Pain in your chest or calves
Severe headache, dizziness, or faintness
Sudden shortness of breath
Vision changes
Yellowing of the skin

Ogen may cause fluid retention in some people. If you have asthma, epilepsy, migraine or heart or kidney disease, use this medication with care.

Estrogen therapy may cause uterine bleeding or breast pain.

Possible food and drug interactions when taking this medication
If Ogen is taken with certain other drugs, the effects of either could be increased, decreased, or altered. It is especially important to check with your doctor before combining Ogen with the following:

Barbiturates such as pheobarbital
Blood thinners such as Coumadin
Epilepsy drugs (Tegretol, Dilantin, others)
Insulin
Tricyclic antidepressants (Elavil, Tofranil, others)
Rifampin (Rifadin)

Special information
if you are pregnant or breastfeeding

Estrogens should not be used during pregnancy. If you are pregnant or plan to become pregnant, notify your doctor immediately. These drugs may appear in breast milk and could affect a nursing infant. If this medication is essential to your health, your doctor may advise you to discontinue breastfeeding until your treatment is finished.

Recommended dosage

ADULTS

Hot flashes and night sweats
Ogen Tablets: The usual dose ranges from one 0.625 tablet to two 2.5 tablets per day. Tablets should be taken in cycles, according to your doctor's instructions.

Ortho-Est 1.25 Tablets: The usual dose ranges from ½ tablet to 4 tablets per day. Tablets should be taken in cycles, according to your doctor's instructions.

Vaginal inflammation and dryness
Ogen Tablets: The usual dose ranges from one 0.625 tablet to two 2.5 tablets per day. Tablets should be taken in cycles, according to your doctor's instructions.

Ortho-Est 1.25 Tablets: The usual dose ranges from ½ tablet to 4 tablets per day. Tablets should be taken in cycles, according to your doctor's instructions.

Ogen Vaginal Cream: The usual dose is 2 to 4 grams daily. Cream should be used in cycles, and only for limited periods of time.

Estrogen hormone deficiency
Ogen Tablets: The usual dose ranges from one 1.25 tablet to three 2.5 tablets per day, taken for 3 weeks, followed by a rest period of 8 to 10 days.

Ortho-Est 1.25 Tablets: The usual dose ranges from 1 to 6 tablets per day, given for 3 weeks, followed by a rest period of 8 to 10 days.

Hysterectomy or ovarian failure
Ogen Tablets: The usual dose ranges from one 1.25 tablet to three 2.5 tablets per day for 3 weeks, followed by a rest period of 8 to 10 days. Your doctor may increase or decrease your dosage according to your response.

Ortho-Est 1.25 Tablets: The usual dose ranges from 1 to 6 tablets per day for 3 weeks, followed by a rest period of 8 to 10 days. Your doctor may increase or decrease your dosage according to your response.

Prevention of osteoporosis
Ogen Tablets: The usual dose is one 0.625 tablet per day for 25 days of a 31-day cycle.

Overdosage

Any medication taken in excess can have serious consequences. If you suspect an overdose, seek emergency medical treatment immediately.

■ *Symptoms of Ogen overdose may include:*
   Nausea
   Vomiting
   Withdrawal bleeding

Brand name:

OMNIPEN

Pronounced:AHM-nee-pen
Generic name: Ampicillin
Other Brands: Polycillin, Principen, Totacillin

Why is this drug prescribed?

Omnipen is a penicillin-like antibiotic that treats a wide variety of infections, including gonorrhea and other genital and urinary infections, and gastrointestinal infections.

Most important fact about this drug

If you are allergic to either penicillin or cephalosporin antibiotics in any form, consult your doctor *before taking Omnipen*. There is a possibility that you are allergic to both types of medication; and if a reaction occurs, it could be extremely severe. If you take the drug and feel signs of a reaction, seek medical attention immediately.

How should you use this medication?

Take Omnipen capsules with a full glass of water, a half hour before or 2 hours after a meal.

Omnipen Oral Suspension should be shaken well before using.

Take Omnipen exactly as prescribed. It works best when there is a constant amount in the body. Take your doses at evenly spaced times around the clock, and try not to miss a dose.

■ *If you miss a dose...*
Take it as soon as you remember. If it is almost time for the next dose, and you take 2 doses a day, take the one you missed and the next dose 5 to 6 hours later. If you take 3 or more doses a day, take the one you missed and the next dose 2 to 4 hours later. Then go back to your regular schedule. Do not take 2 doses at once.

■ *Storage information...*
Store Omnipen Capsules at room temperature in a tightly closed container.

Keep Omnipen Oral Suspension in the refrigerator, in a tightly closed container. Discard the unused portion after 14 days.

What side effects may occur?

Side effects cannot be anticipated. If any develop or change in intensity, inform your doctor as soon as possible. Only your

doctor can determine whether it is safe for you to continue taking Omnipen.

■ *Side effects may include:*
Anemia, colitis (inflammation of the bowel), diarrhea, fever, hives, itching, nausea, hives, rash, skin redness, peeling, or flaking, sore or inflamed tongue or mouth, vomiting

Why should this drug not be prescribed?

You should not take Omnipen if you are allergic to penicillin or cephalosporin antibiotics.

Special warnings about this medication

If you have an allergic reaction, stop taking Omnipen and contact your doctor immediately.

After you have taken Omnipen for a long time, you may get a new infection (called a superinfection) due to an organism this medication cannot treat. Consult your doctor if you develop any symptoms of infection.

Omnipen sometimes causes diarrhea. Some diarrhea medications can make the diarrhea worse. Check with your doctor before taking any diarrhea remedy.

Oral contraceptives may not work properly while you are taking Omnipen. For greater certainty, use other measures while taking Omnipen.

If you are diabetic, be aware that Omnipen may cause a *false positive* urine glucose test. You should talk to your doctor about using different tests while you are taking Omnipen.

For infections such as strep throat, it is important to take Omnipen for the entire amount of time your doctor has prescribed. Even if you feel better, you need to continue taking the medication. If you stop taking Omnipen before your treatment time is complete, you may get other infections, such as glomerulonephritis (a kidney infection) or rheumatic fever.

Possible food and drug interactions when taking this medication

If Omnipen is taken with certain other drugs the effects of either could be increased, decreased, or altered. It is especially important to check with your doctor before combining Omnipen with any oth the following:

Allopurinol (Zyloprim)
Atenolol (Tenormin)
Chloroquine (Aralen)
Mefloquine (Lariam)
Other antibiotics such as chloramphenicol, tetracycline, erythromycin, and sulfonamides
Oral contraceptives
Probenecid (Benemid)

Special information if you are pregnant or breastfeeding

The effects of Omnipen during pregnancy have not been adequately studied. If you are pregnant or plan to become pregnant, inform your doctor immediately. Omnipen should be used during pregnancy only if the potential benefit justifies the potential risk to the developing baby.

Omnipen appears in breast milk and could affect a nursing infant. If this medication is essential to your health, your doctor may advise you to stop breastfeeding until your treatment with Omnipen is finished.

Recommended dosage

Unless you are being treated for gonnorhea, your doctor will have you continue taking Omnipen for 2 to 3 days after your symptoms have disappeared. Dosages are for capsules and oral suspension.

ADULTS

Infections of the Genital, Urinary or Gastrointestinal Tracts
The usual dose is 500 milligrams, taken 4 times a day.

Gonorrhea
The usual dose is 3.5 grams in a single oral dose along with 1 gram of probenecid

Respiratory Tract Infections
The usual dose is 250 milligrams, taken 4 times a day.

CHILDREN

Children weighing over 44 pounds should follow the adult dose schedule.

Children weighing 44 pounds or less should have their dosage determined by their weight.

Infections of the Genital, Urinary or Gastrointestinal Tracts
The usual dose is 100 milligrams for each 2.2 pounds of body weight daily, divided into 4 doses for the capsules, and 3 to 4 doses for the suspension.

Respiratory Tract Infections
The usual dose is 50 milligrams for each 2.2 pounds of body weight daily, divided into 3 to 4 doses.

Overdosage

Although no specific symptoms have been reported, any medication taken in excess can have serious consequences. If you suspect an overdose of Omnipen, seek medical attention immediately.

Category:

ORAL CONTRACEPTIVES

Brand names: Demulen, Desogen, Genora 1/35-28, Levlen, Loestrin, Lo/Ovral, Modicon, Nordette, Norethin, Norinyl, Ortho-Cept, Ortho-Cyclen, Ortho-Novum, Ortho Tri-Cyclen, Ovcon, Ovral, Triphasil

Why is this drug prescribed?

Oral contraceptives (also known as "The Pill") are highly effective means of preventing pregnancy. Oral contraceptives consist of synthetic forms of two hormones produced naturally in the body: either progestin alone or estrogen and progestin. Estrogen and progestin regulate a woman's menstrual cycle, and the fluctuating levels of these hormones play an essential role in pregnancy.

To reduce side effects, oral contraceptives are available in a wide range of estrogen and progestin concentrations. Progestin-only products (such as Micronor) are usually prescribed for women who should avoid estrogens; however, they may not be as effective as estrogen/progestin contraceptives.

Most important fact about this drug

Cigarette smoking increases the risk of serious heart-related side effects (stroke, heart attack, blood clots, etc.) in women who use oral contraceptives. This risk increases with heavy smoking (15 or more cigarettes per day) and with age. There is an especially significant increase in heart disease risk in women over 35 years old who smoke and use oral contraceptives.

How should you take this medication?

Oral contraceptives should be taken every day, no more than 24 hours apart, and according to your physician's instructions. Ideally, you should take your pill at the same time every day to reduce the chance of forgetting a dose.

■ *If you miss a dose...*
If you neglect to take only one estrogen/progestin pill, take it as soon as you remember and continue taking the rest of the medication cycle. The risk of pregnancy is small if you miss only one combination pill per cycle. If you miss more than one tablet, do not take the missed tablets; instead resume the normal medication cycle while *employing another form of contraceptive for the duration of that medication cycle.*

Missing a single progestin-only tablet increases the chance of pregnancy. Therefore, you should consult with your doctor immediately if you miss a single dose.

■ *Storage instructions...*
To help keep track of your doses, use the original container. Store at room temperature.

What side effects may occur?

Side effects cannot be anticipated. If any develop or change in intensity, inform your doctor as soon as possible. Only your doctor can determine if it is safe for you to continue taking an oral contraceptive.

■ *Side effects may include:*
Abdominal cramps, acne, appetite changes, bladder infection, bleeding in spots during a menstrual period, bloating, blood clots, breast tenderness or enlargement, cataracts, chest pain, contact lens discomfort, decreased flow of milk when given immediately after birth, depression, difficulty breathing, dizziness, fluid retention, gallbladder disease, growth of face, back, chest, or stomach hair, hair loss, headache, heart attack, high blood pressure, inflammation of the large

intestine, kidney trouble, lack of menstrual periods, liver tumors, lumps in the breast, menstrual pattern changes, migraine, muscle, joint, or leg pain, nausea, nervousness, premenstrual syndrome (PMS), secretion of milk, sex drive changes, skin infection, skin rash or discoloration, stomach cramps, stroke, swelling, temporary infertility, unexplained bleeding in the vagina, vaginal discharge, vaginal infections (and/or burning and itching), visual disturbances, vomiting, weight gain or loss, yellow skin or whites of eyes

Why should this drug not be prescribed?

You should not take oral contraceptives if you have had an allergic reaction to them or if you are pregnant (or think you might be).

If you have ever had breast cancer or cancer in the reproductive organs or liver tumors, you should not take oral contraceptives.

If you have or have ever had a stroke, heart disease, angina (severe chest pain), or blood clots, you should not take oral contraceptives. Women who have had pregnancy-related jaundice or jaundice stemming from previous use of oral contraceptives should not take them.

If you have undiagnosed and/or unexplained abnormal genital bleeding, do not take oral contraceptives.

Special warnings about this medication

Oral contraceptives should be used with caution if you are over 40 years old; smoke tobacco; have liver, heart, gallbladder, kidney, or thyroid disease; have high blood pressure, high cholesterol, diabetes, epilepsy, asthma, or porphyria (a blood disorder); or are obese.

In addition, you should use oral contraceptives with caution if you have a family history of breast cancer or other cancers, or you have a personal history of depression, migraine or other headaches, irregular menstrual periods, or visual disturbances.

Since the blood's clotting ability may be affected by oral contraceptives, your doctor may take you off them prior to surgery. If bleeding lasts more than 8 days while you are on a progestin-only oral contraceptive, be sure to let your doctor know.

Oral contraceptives do not protect against HIV infection (AIDS) or any other sexually transmitted disease.

If you miss a menstrual period but have taken your pills regularly, contact your doctor but do not stop taking your pills. If you miss a period and have not taken your pills regularly, or if you miss two consecutive periods, you may be pregnant; stop taking your pills and check with your doctor immediately to see if you are pregnant. Use another form of birth control while you are not taking your pills.

Possible food and drug interactions when taking this medication

If oral contraceptives are taken with certain other drugs, the effects of either could be increased, decreased, or altered. It is especially important to check with your doctor before combining oral contraceptives with the following:

Amitriptyline (Elavil, Endep)
Ampicillin (Polycillin, Principen)
Barbiturates (phenobarbital)
Carbamazepine (Tegretol)
Chloramphenicol (Chloromycetin)
Clomipramine (Anafranil)
Diazepam (Valium)
Doxepin (Sinequan)
Glipizide (Glucotrol)

Griseofulvin (Fulvicin, Grisactin)
Imipramine (Tofranil, Janimine)
Lorazepam (Ativan)
Metoprolol (Lopressor)
Oxazepam (Serax)
Penicillin (Veetids, Pen-Vee K)
Phenylbutazone (Butazolidin)
Phenytoin (Dilantin)
Prednisolone (Delta-Cortef, Prelone)
Prednisone (Deltasone)
Primidone (Mysoline)
Propranolol (Inderal)
Rifampin (Rifadin, Rimactane)
Sulfonamides (Bactrim, Septra)
Tetracycline (Achromycin V)
Theophylline (Theo-Dur)
Warfarin (Coumadin, Panwarfin)

In addition, oral contraceptives may affect tests for blood sugar levels and thyroid function and may cause an increase in blood cholesterol levels.

Special information if you are pregnant or breastfeeding

If you are pregnant (or think you might be), you should not use oral contraceptives, since they are not safe during pregnancy.

In general, nursing mothers should not use oral contraceptives, since these drugs can appear in breast milk and may cause jaundice and enlarged breasts in nursing infants. Your doctor may advise you to use a different form of contraception while you are nursing your baby.

Recommended dosage

If you have any questions about how you should take oral contraceptives, consult your doctor or the patient instructions that come in the drug package. The following is a partial list of instructions for taking oral contraceptives; it should not be used as a substitute for consultation with your doctor.

Some brands can be started on the first day of your menstrual cycle or on the first Sunday afterwards. Others must be started on the fifth day of the cycle or the first Sunday afterwards. The instructions below are for the first-Sunday schedule.

Oral contraceptives are supplied in 21-day and 28-day packages.

For a 21-day schedule
Oral contraceptives are taken for a 3-week period, followed by 1 week of no oral contraceptives.

1) Starting on the first Sunday after the beginning of your menstrual period, take one tablet daily (at the same time each day) for the next 20 or 21 days (depending upon the brand of oral contraceptive used). Note: If your period begins on Sunday, take the first tablet that day.

2) Wait 1 week before taking any tablets. Your menstrual period should occur during this time.

3) Following this 1-week waiting time, begin taking tablets again for the next 20 or 21 days.

For a 28-day schedule
Starting on the first Sunday after the beginning of your menstrual period, take one tablet daily (at the same time each day) for the next 28 days. Continue taking the oral contraceptives according to your physician's instructions. Note: If your period begins on Sunday, take the first tablet that day.

For both 21- and 28-day regimens
If the first Sunday falls more than 5 days after the beginning of your period, it is important to use an alternate means of contraception while taking oral

contraceptives until your physician indicates it is no longer necessary.

Progestin-only tablets should be taken every day of the year.

Overdosage

While any medication taken in excess can cause overdose, the risk associated with oral contraceptives is minimal. Even young children who have taken large amounts of oral contraceptives have not experienced serious adverse effects. However, if you suspect an overdose, seek medical help immediately.

■ *Symptoms of overdose may include:*
  Nausea
  Withdrawal bleeding in females

Brand name:

ORETON METHYL

See Android, page 508.

Brand name:

ORTHO-CEPT

See Oral Contraceptives, page 702.

Brand name:

ORTHO-CYCLEN

See Oral Contraceptives, page 702.

Brand name:

ORTHO-EST 1.25

See Ogen, page 697.

Brand name:

ORTHO-NOVUM

See Oral Contraceptives, page 702.

Brand name:

ORTHO TRI-CYCLEN

See Oral Contraceptives, page 702.

Brand name:

ORUDIS

Pronounced: Oh-ROO-dis
Generic name: Ketoprofen
Other brand name: Oruvail

Why is this drug prescribed?

Orudis, a nonsteroidal anti-inflammatory drug, is used to relieve the inflammation, swelling, stiffness, and joint pain associated with rheumatoid arthritis and osteoarthritis (the most common form of arthritis). It is also used to relieve mild to moderate pain, as well as menstrual pain. Oruvail, an extended-release form of the drug, is used to treat the signs and symptoms of rheumatoid arthritis and osteoarthritis over the long term, not severe attacks that come on suddenly.

Most important fact about this drug

You should have frequent check-ups with your doctor if you take Orudis regularly Ulcers or internal bleeding can occur without warning.

How should you take this medication?

To minimize side effects, your doctor may recommend that you take Orudis with food, an antacid, or milk.

Take this medication exactly as prescribed by your doctor.

If you are using Orudis for arthritis, it should be taken regularly.

■ *If you miss a dose...*
If you take Orudis on a regular schedule, take the forgotten dose as soon as you remember. If it is almost time for your next dose, skip the one you missed and go back to your regular schedule. Do not take 2 doses at once.

■ *Storage instructions...*
Store at room temperature in a tightly closed container.

What side effects may occur?
Side effects cannot be anticipated. If any develop or change in intensity, inform your doctor as soon as possible. Only your doctor can determine if it is safe for you to continue taking Orudis.

■ *More common side effects may include:*
Abdominal pain, changes in kidney function, constipation, diarrhea, dreams, fluid retention, gas, headache, inability to sleep, indigestion, nausea

■ *Less common or rare side effects may include:*
Allergic reaction, amnesia, anemia, asthma, belching, blood in the urine, bloody or black stools, change in taste, chills, confusion, congestive heart failure, coughing up blood, conjunctivitis (pinkeye), depression, difficult or labored breathing, dizziness, dry mouth, eye pain, facial swelling due to fluid retention, general feeling of illness, hair loss, high blood pressure, hives, impaired hearing, impotence, increase in appetite, increased salivation, infection, inflammation of the mouth, irregular or excessive menstrual bleeding, itching, kidney failure, loosening of fingernails, loss of appetite, migraine, muscle pain, nasal inflammation, nosebleed, pain, peptic or intestinal ulcer, rapid heartbeat, rash, rectal bleeding, red or purple spots on the skin, ringing in the ears, sensitivity to light, skin discoloration, skin eruptions, skin inflammation and flaking, sleepiness, sore throat, stomach inflammation, sweating, swelling of the throat, thirst, throbbing heartbeat, tingling or pins and needles, vertigo, visual disturbances, vomiting, vomiting blood, weight gain or loss

Why should this drug not be prescribed?
If you are sensitive to or have ever had an allergic reaction to Orudis, or if you have had asthma attacks, hives, or other allergic reactions caused by aspirin or other nonsteroidal anti-inflammatory drugs, you should not take this medication. Make sure your doctor is aware of any drug reactions you have experienced.

Special warnings about this medication
Remember that stomach ulcers and bleeding can occur without warning.

This drug should be used with caution if you have kidney or liver disease.

If you are taking Orudis for an extended period of time, your doctor will check your blood for anemia.

This drug can increase water retention. Use with caution if you have heart disease or high blood pressure.

Possible food and drug interactions when taking this medication
If Orudis is taken with certain other drugs, the effects of either could be increased, decreased, or altered. It is especially important to check with your doctor before combining Orudis with the following:

Aspirin
Blood thinners such as Coumadin
Diuretics such as hydrochlorothiazide
  (HydroDIURIL)
Lithium (Lithonate)
Methotrexate
Probenecid (the gout medication Benemid)

Orudis can prolong bleeding time. If you are taking blood-thinning medication, use this drug cautiously.

Special information if you are pregnant or breastfeeding

The effects of Orudis during pregnancy have not been adequately studied. If you are pregnant or plan to become pregnant, inform your doctor immediately. Orudis may appear in breast milk and could affect a nursing infant. If this medication is essential to your health, your doctor may advise you to discontinue breastfeeding until your treatment with this medication is finished.

Recommended dosage

ADULTS

Rheumatoid Arthritis and Osteoarthritis
The starting dose of Orudis is 75 milligrams 3 times a day or 50 milligrams 4 times a day; for Oruvail, 200 milligrams taken once a day. The most you should take in a day is 300 milligrams. Some side effects, such as headache or upset stomach, increase in severity as the dose gets higher. Smaller people may need smaller doses.

Mild to Moderate Pain and Menstrual Pain
The usual dose of Orudis is 25 to 50 milligrams every 6 to 8 hours as needed. Your doctor may adjust the dosage if you are small or if you have kidney or liver disease.

CHILDREN

The safety and effectiveness of Orudis have not been established in children.

ELDERLY

You may need a lower dosage.

Overdosage

Any medication taken in excess can have serious consequences. If you suspect an overdose of Orudis, seek medical attention immediately.

- *Signs and symptoms of Orudis overdose may include:*
  Breathing difficulty
  Coma
  Convulsions
  Drowsiness
  High blood pressure
  Kidney failure
  Low blood pressure
  Nausea
  Sluggishness
  Stomach and intestinal bleeding
  Stomach pain
  Vomiting

Brand name:

ORUVAIL

See Orudis, page 705.

Brand name:

OS-CAL 500

See Caltrate 600, page 533.

Brand name:

OVCON

See Oral Contraceptives, page 702.

Brand name:

OVRAL

See Oral Contraceptives, page 702.

Generic name:

OXAPROZIN

See Daypro, page 560.

Generic name:

OXAZEPAM

See Serax, page 742.

Brand name:

OYSTERCAL 500

See Caltrate 600, page 533.

Generic name:

PACLITAXEL

See Taxol, page 758.

Brand name:

PAMELOR

Pronounced: PAM-eh-lore
Generic name: Nortriptyline hydrochloride
Other brand name: Aventyl

Why is this drug prescribed?

Pamelor is prescribed for the relief of symptoms of depression. Pamelor is in the class of drugs known as tricyclic antidepressants.

Some doctors also prescribe Pamelor to treat chronic hives, premenstrual depression, attention deficit hyperactivity disorder in children, and bedwetting.

Most important fact about this drug

Pamelor must be taken regularly to be effective and it may be several weeks before you begin to feel better. Do not skip doses, even if they seem to make no difference.

How should you take this medication?

Take Pamelor exactly as prescribed. Pamelor may make your mouth dry. Sucking on hard candy, chewing gum, or melting ice chips in your mouth can provide relief.

■ *If you miss a dose...*
Take it as soon as you remember. If it is almost time for the next dose, skip the one you missed and go back to your regular schedule. If you take Pamelor once a day at bedtime and you miss a dose, do not take it in the morning, since disturbing side effects could occur. Never take 2 doses at once.

■ *Storage instructions...*
Keep Pamelor in the container it came in, tightly closed and away from light. Be sure to keep this drug out of reach of children; an overdose is particularly dangerous in the young. Store at room temperature.

What side effects may occur?

Side effects cannot be anticipated. If any develop or change in intensity, inform your doctor as soon as possible. Only your doctor can determine if it is safe for you to continue taking Pamelor.

- *Side effects may include:*
  Abdominal cramps, agitation, anxiety, black tongue, blurred vision, breast development in males, breast enlargement, confusion, constipation, delusions, diarrhea, dilation of pupils, disorientation, dizziness, drowsiness, dry mouth, excessive or spontaneous flow of milk, excessive urination at night, fatigue, fever, fluid retention, flushing, frequent urination, hair loss, hallucinations, headache, heart attack, high or low blood pressure, high or low blood sugar, hives, impotence, inability to sleep, inability to urinate, increased or decreased sex drive, inflammation of the mouth, intestinal blockage, itching, loss of appetite, loss of coordination, nausea, nightmares, numbness, panic, perspiration, pins and needles in the arms and legs, rapid, fluttery, or irregular heartbeat, rash, reddish or purplish spots on skin, restlessness, ringing in the ears, seizures, sensitivity to light, stomach upset, strange taste, stroke, swelling of the testicles, swollen glands, tingling, tremors, vision problems, vomiting, weakness, weight gain or loss, yellow eyes and skin

- *Side effects due to rapid decrease or abrupt withdrawal from Pamelor after a long term of treatment include:*
  Headache
  Nausea
  Vague feeling of bodily discomfort

These side effects do not indicate addiction to this drug.

Why should this drug not be prescribed?

If you are sensitive to or have ever had an allergic reaction to Pamelor or similar drugs, you should not take this medication. Make sure your doctor is aware of any drug reactions you have experienced.

Do not take Pamelor if you are taking—or have taken one within the past 14 days—an antidepressant drug classified as an MAO inhibitor. Drugs in this category include Nardil, Parnate, and Marplan. Combining these drugs with Pamelor can cause fever and convulsions, and could even be fatal.

Unless you are directed to do so by your doctor, do not take this medication if you are recovering from a heart attack or are taking any other antidepressant drugs.

Special warnings about this medication

Pamelor may cause you to become drowsy or less alert; therefore, you should not drive or operate dangerous machinery or participate in any hazardous activity that requires full mental alertness until you know how this drug affects you.

Use Pamelor with caution if you have a history of seizures, difficulty urinating, diabetes, or chronic eye conditions such as glaucoma. Be careful, also, if you have heart disease, high blood pressure, an overactive thyroid, or are receiving thyroid medication. You should discuss all of your medical problems with your doctor before taking this medication.

If you are being treated for a severe mental disorder (schizophrenia or manic depression), tell your doctor before taking Pamelor.

Pamelor may make your skin more sensitive to sunlight. Try to stay out of the sun, wear protective clothing, and apply a sun block.

Before having surgery, dental treatment or any diagnostic procedure, tell your doctor that you are taking Pamelor. Certain drugs used during these procedures, such as anesthetics and muscle relaxants, may interact with Pamelor.

Possible food and drug interactions when taking this medication

Combining Pamelor and MAO inhibitors can be fatal.

Pamelor may intensify the effects of alcohol. Do not drink alcohol while taking this medication.

If Pamelor is taken with certain other drugs, the effects of either can be increased, decreased, or altered. It is especially important to check with your doctor before combining Pamelor with the following:

Acetazalomide (Diamox)
Airway-opening drugs such as Ventolin and
    Proventil
Amphetamines such as Dexedrine
Antispasmodic drugs such as Donnatal and
    Bentyl
Blood pressure medications such Catapres
    and Esmulin
Cimetidine (Tagamet)
Levodopa (Laradopa)
Other antidepressants such as Prozac
Quinidine (Quinaglute)
Reserpine (Diupres)
Thyroid medication such as Synthroid
Vitamin C (in large doses)
Warfarin (Coumadin)

Special information
if you are pregnant or breastfeeding

The effects of Pamelor during pregnancy have not been adequately studied. If you are pregnant or planning to become pregnant, inform your doctor immediately. Also consult your doctor before breastfeeding.

Recommended dosage

This medication is available in tablet and liquid form. Only tablet dosages are listed. Consult your doctor if you cannot take the tablet form of this medication.

ADULTS

Your doctor will monitor your response to this medication carefully and will gradually increase or decrease the dose to suit your needs.

The usual starting dosage is 25 milligrams, 3 or 4 times per day.

Alternatively, your doctor may prescribe that the total daily dose be taken once a day.

Doses above 150 milligrams per day are not recommended.

Your doctor may want to perform a blood test to help in deciding the best dose you should receive.

CHILDREN

The safety and effectiveness of Pamelor have not been established for children and its use is not recommended. However, adolescents may be given 30 to 50 milligrams per day, either in a single dose or divided into smaller doses, as determined by your doctor.

ELDERLY

The usual dose is 30 to 50 milligrams taken in a single dose or divided into smaller doses, as determined by your doctor.

Overdosage

An overdose of this type of antidepressant can be fatal. If you suspect an overdose, seek medical help immediately.

■ *Symptoms of Pamelor overdose may include:*
Agitation, coma, confusion, congestive heart failure, convulsions, decreased breathing, excessive reflexes, extremely high fever, rapid heartbeat, restlessness, rigid muscles, shock, stupor, vomiting

If you suspect a Pamelor overdose, seek medical attention immediately.

Brand name:

PANADOL

See Tylenol, page 777.

Brand name:

PARLODEL

Pronounced: PAR-luh-del
Generic name: Bromocriptine mesylate

Why is this drug prescribed?
Parlodel inhibits the secretion of the hormone prolactin from the pituitary gland, thereby preventing production of breast milk. It also mimics the action of dopamine, a chemical lacking in the brain of someone with Parkinson's disease. It is used to treat a variety of medical conditions, including:

■ Infertility in some women
■ Menstrual problems such as the abnormal stoppage or absence of flow
■ Excessive or spontaneous flow of milk
■ Growth hormone overproduction leading to acromegaly, a condition characterized by an abnormally large skull, jaw, hands, and feet
■ Parkinson's disease
■ Pituitary gland tumors

Parlodel is also used to interrupt milk production in women who do not want to breastfeed or should not breastfeed for medical reasons.

Some doctors also prescribe Parlodel to treat cocaine addiction, the eye condition known as glaucoma, erection problems in certain men, restless leg syndrome, and a dangerous reaction to major tranquilizers called neuroleptic malignant syndrome.

Most important fact about this drug
Since Parlodel can restore fertility and pregnancy can result, women who do not want to become pregnant should use a "barrier" method of contraception during treatment with this medication. Do not use the "Pill" or oral contraceptives, as they may prevent Parlodel from working properly.

If you become pregnant while taking Parlodel, notify your doctor immediately.

How should you take this medication?
Parlodel should be taken with food in your stomach. Take the first dose while lying down. You may faint or become dizzy due to a lower blood pressure, especially following the first dose.

You may not feel the full effect of this medication for a few weeks. Do not stop taking Parlodel without first checking with your doctor.

■ *If you miss a dose...*
Take it as soon as you remember if it is within 4 hours of the scheduled time. Otherwise, skip the dose you missed and go back to your regular schedule. Do not take 2 doses at once.

■ *Storage information...*
Store at room temperature in a tightly closed, light-resistant container. Protect from excessive heat.

What side effects may occur?

The number and severity of side effects depend on many factors, including the condition being treated, dosage, and duration of treatment. Side effects cannot be anticipated. If any develop or change in intensity, inform your doctor as soon as possible. Only your doctor can determine if it is safe for you to continue taking Parlodel.

■ *More common side effects may include:*
Abdominal cramps or discomfort, confusion, constipation, depression, diarrhea, dizziness, drop in blood pressure, drowsiness, dry mouth, fainting, fatigue, hallucinations (particularly in Parkinson's patients), headache, inability to sleep, indigestion, light-headedness, loss of appetite, loss of coordination, nasal congestion, nausea, shortness of breath, uncontrolled body movement, vertigo, visual disturbance, vomiting, weakness

■ *Less common side effects may include:*
Abdominal bleeding, anxiety, difficulty swallowing, frequent urination, heart attack, inability to hold urine, inability to urinate, nightmares, nervousness, rash, seizures, splotchy skin, stroke, swelling/fluid retention in feet and ankles, twitching of eyelids

Some of the above side effects are also symptoms of Parkinson's disease.

■ *Rare side effects may include:*
Abnormal heart rhythm, blurred vision or temporary blindness, cold feet, fast or slow heartbeat, hair loss, heavy headedness, increase in blood pressure, lower back pain, muscle cramps, muscle cramps in feet and legs, numbness, pale face, paranoia, prickling or tingling, reduced tolerance to cold, severe or continuous headache, shortness of breath, sluggishness, tingling of ears or fingers

Why should this drug not be prescribed?

You should not be using Parlodel if you have high blood pressure that is not being treated or or blood poisoning called toxemia of pregnancy. You should also not take Parlodel if you are allergic to it or to any other drugs considered to be ergot alkaloids, such as Bellergal-S or Cafergot.

Special warnings about this medication

Your doctor will check your pituitary gland thoroughly before you are treated with Parlodel.

Notify your doctor immediately if you become pregnant while you are being treated with Parlodel.

If you have kidney or liver disease, consult your doctor before taking Parlodel.

If you are being treated with Parlodel for endocrine problems related to a tumor and stop taking this medication, the tumor may grow back rapidly.

If you are being treated for Parkinson's disease, the use of Parlodel alone or Parlodel with levodopa may cause hallucinations, confusion, and low blood pressure. If this happens, notify your doctor immediately.

If you have an abnormal heartbeat rhythm caused by a previous heart attack, consult your doctor before taking Parlodel.

If you experience a persistent watery nasal discharge while taking Parlodel, notify your doctor.

This drug may impair your ability to drive a car or operate potentially dangerous machinery. Do not participate in any activities that require full alertness if you are unsure about your ability to do so.

Your first dose of Parlodel may cause dizziness. If so, check with your doctor.

If you are taking Parlodel to stop your milk production, notify your doctor immediately if you develop a severe headache that does not let up or continues to get worse. It could be a warning of the possibility of other dangerous reactions, including seizure, stroke, or heart attack.

Possible food and drug interactions when taking this medication

Combining alcohol with Parlodel can cause blurred vision, chest pain, pounding heartbeat, throbbing headache, confusion, and other problems. Do not drink alcoholic beverages while taking this medication.

Certain drugs used for psychotic conditions, including Thorazine or other phenothiazines and Haldol, inhibit the action of Parlodel. It is important that you consult your doctor before taking these drugs while on Parlodel therapy.

Other drugs that may interact with Parlodel include:

Blood pressure lowering drugs such as Aldomet and Catapres
Erythromycin (E.E.S., ERYC, PCE, others)
Metoclopramide (Reglan)
Oral contraceptives
Other ergot derivatives such as Hydergine
Progesterone (Provera)

Special information if you are pregnant or breastfeeding

The use of Parlodel during pregnancy should be discussed thoroughly with your doctor. If Parlodel is essential to your treatment, your doctor will carefully monitor you throughout your pregnancy.

Because Parlodel can be used to prevent milk flow, it should not be used by mothers who wish to breastfeed their infants.

Recommended dosage

ADULTS

Parlodel is available as 2.5-milligram tablets and 5-milligram capsules. Dosage information given is for 2.5-milligram tablets.

Prevention of Milk Production after Delivery
The usual dose is 1 tablet twice daily for 14 days. If necessary your doctor may continue therapy for up to 21 days.

Excess Prolactin Hormone
If you are being treated for conditions associated with excess prolactin, such as excessive milk production, menstrual problems, infertility, or pituitary gland tumors, the usual starting dose is one-half to 1 tablet daily. Your doctor may add a tablet every 3 to 7 days, until the treatment works. The usual longer term dose is 5 to 7.5 milligrams per day and ranges from 2.5 to 15 milligrams per day.

Growth Hormone Overproduction
Treatment for the over-production of growth hormones is usually one-half to 1 tablet with food at bedtime for 3 days. Your doctor may add one-half to 1 tablet every 3 to 7 days. The usual treatment dose varies from 20 to 30 milligrams per day. The dose should not exceed 100 milligrams per day. Your doctor will do a monthly re-evaluation.

Parkinson's Disease
Parlodel taken in combination with levodopa may provide additional treatment benefits if you are currently taking high doses of levodopa, are beginning to develop a tolerance to levodopa, or are experiencing "end of dose failure" on levodopa therapy.

The usual starting dose of Parlodel is one-half tablet twice a day with meals. Your dose will be monitored by your doctor at 2-week intervals. If necessary, your doctor may increase the dose every 14 to 28 days by 1 tablet per day.

CHILDREN

The safety and effectiveness of Parlodel have not been established in children under 15 years of age.

Overdosage

Any medication taken in excess can have serious consequences. If you suspect an overdose of Parlodel, contact your doctor immediately or seek other medical attention.

Generic name:

PAROXETINE

See Paxil, page 714.

Brand name:

PAXIL

Pronounced: PACKS-ill
Generic name: Paroxetine hydrochloride

Why is this drug prescribed?

Paxil is prescribed for a serious, continuing depression that interferes with your abilty to function. Symptoms of this type of depression often include changes in appetite and sleep patterns, a persistent low mood, loss of interest in people and activities, decreased sex drive, feelings of guilt or worthlessness, suicidal thoughts, difficulty concentrating, and slowed thinking.

Most important fact about this drug

Do not take Paxil if, within the past two weeks, you have taken another type of antidepressant medication known as an MAO inhibitor. Drugs in this category include Nardil, Parnate, and Marplan. When medications like Paxil are combined with MAO inhibitors, serious and sometimes fatal reactions can occur.

How should you take this medication?

Take this medication exactly as prescribed by your doctor. Inform your doctor if you are taking or plan to take any prescription or over-the-counter drugs, since they may interact unfavorably with Paxil.

Your depression may seem to lessen within 1 to 4 weeks after beginning treatment with Paxil. Even if you feel better, continue to take the medication as long as your doctor tells you to do so.

- *If you miss a dose...*
  Skip the forgotten dose and go back to your regular schedule with the next dose. Do not take a double dose to make up for the one you missed.

- *Storage instructions...*
  Paxil can be stored at room temperature.

What side effects may occur?

Side effects cannot be anticipated. If any develop or change in intensity, inform your doctor as soon as possible. Only your doctor can determine whether it is safe for you to continue taking this medication.

Over a 4 to 6 week period, you may find some side effects less troublesome (nausea and dizziness, for example) than others (dry mouth, drowsiness, and weakness).

- *More common side effects may include:*
  Abdominal pain, amnesia, anxiety, blurred vision, breathing disorders, burning sensation, chills, cold symptoms, constipation, decreased appetite, decreased sex drive, depression, diarrhea, difficulty

concentrating, dizziness, drowsiness, dry mouth, emotional instability, fainting, feeling of general discomfort, fluid retention, frequent urination, headache, high blood pressure, increased coughing, inflammation of the nose, intestinal gas, itching, male genital disorders, nausea, nervousness, prickling and tingling, rapid heartbeat, sleepiness, sleeplessness, stomach pain, stuffy nose, sweating, tremor, trouble ejaculating, vertigo, weight gain, weight loss, yawning

■ *Less common side effects may include:*
Abnormal thinking, abortion, acne, agitation, alcohol abuse, allergic reactions, altered sense of taste, anemia, arthritis, asthma, back pain, belching, blood disorders, boils, breast pain, bronchitis, bruises, cessation of menstruation, chest pain, confusion, convulsions, difficulty swallowing, dilation of the pupils, dizziness on standing up, drugged feeling, dry skin, ear pain, eczema, excessive menstrual bleeding, excessive muscular activity, excessive urination, eye pain, feeling of persecution, feeling of unreality, female genital disorders, fevers, grinding of teeth, hair loss, hallucinations, high blood sugar, hives, hyperventilation, incoordination, increased appetite, increased salivation, indigestion, infection of hair follicles, infection of the middle ear, infection of skin and mucous membranes, inflammation of the bladder, stomach, throat, tongue, urethra, or vagina, joint pain, lack of coordination, lack of emotion, loss of muscle movement, loss of taste, low blood pressure, lump in throat, manic reaction, menstrual difficulties, migraine headache, mouth ulcers, mouth ulcers, muscle disease, muscle pain, muscle rigidity, muscle twitching, muscle weakness, neck pain, nosebleeds, overactivity, painful or

difficult urination, pneumonia, pounding heartbeat, rash, rectal bleeding, red or purple spots on the skin, respiratory flu, ringing in the ears, shortness of breath, sinusitis, slow heartbeat, swelling of the arms and legs, swelling of the face, thirst, tightness in throat, tumor, urinary incontinence, urinary retention, urinary urgency, urinating at night, vision problems, vomiting

■ *Rare side effects may include:*
Abnormal gait, abnormal kidney function, abscesses, antisocial reaction, blood in the urine, bloody diarrhea, breast cancer, bulimia, bursitis, cataract, chest pain, congestive heart failure, dark, tarry, bloody stools, decreased reflexes, decreased urination, dehydration, delirium, delusions, diabetes, difficulty performing voluntary movements, difficulty speaking, dimmed vision, double vision, drug dependence, elevated cholesterol, exaggerated feeling of well-being, extreme sensitivity to painful stimuli, eye hemorrhage, gout, grand mal epileptic convulsions, heart attack, hepatitis, hiccups, hostility, hysteria, impacted stool, inability to control bowel movements, increased eye pressure (glaucoma), increased reflexes, increased sexual appetite, increased sputum, inflammation of the breast, gums, lining of the eyelid, lining of the stomach and intestine, outer ear, skin, or esophagus, intestinal blockage, intolerance of light, irregular heartbeat, jerky movement, kidney pain, kidney stone, low blood sugar, lung cancer, neck rigidity, osteoporosis, paralysis, pelvic pain, peptic or stomach ulcer, protruding eyeballs, rapid movement of the eyeballs, red and painful spots on the legs, salivary gland enlargement, sensitivity to light, sensitivity to sound, skin discoloration, skin tumor, spasms in

the arms and legs, stomach ulcer, stomach pain, stroke, stupor, swelling of the thyroid, swelling of the tongue, tooth cavities, ulcer on the cornea, ulcers, vaginal yeast infection, varicose veins, vomiting blood, yellowed eyes and skin

Why should this drug not be prescribed?

Do not take Paxil if you are also taking an MAO inhibitor antidepressant or within 14 days after you discontinue treatment with this type of medication.

Special warnings about this medication

Paxil should be used cautiously by people with a history of manic disorders.

If you have a history of seizures, make sure your doctor knows about it. Paxil should be used with caution in this situation. If you develop seizures once therapy has begun, the drug should be discontinued.

If you have a disease or condition that affects your metabolism or blood circulation, make sure your doctor is aware of it. Paxil should be used cautiously in this situation.

Paxil may impair your judgment, thinking, or motor skills. Do not drive, operate dangerous machinery, or participate in any hazardous activity that requires full mental alertness until you are sure the medication is not affecting you in this way.

Possible food and drug interactions when taking this medication

Do not drink alcohol during your treatment with Paxil.

If Paxil is taken with certain other drugs, the effects of either could be increased, decreased, or altered. It is especially important to check with your doctor before combining Paxil with any of the following:

Amitriptyline (Elavil)
Cimetidine (Tagamet)
Desipramine (Norpramin)
Diazepam (Valium)
Digoxin (Lanoxin)
Flecainide (Tambocor)
Fluoxetine (Prozac)
Imipramine (Tofranil)
Lithium (Lithonate)
MAO inhibitors (antidepressant drugs such as Nardil, Marplan, and Parnate)
Nortriptyline (Pamelor)
Phenobarbital
Phenytoin (Dilantin)
Procyclidine (Kemadrin)
Propafenone (Rythmol)
Propranolol (Inderal, Inderide)
Quinidine (Quinaglute)
Thioridazine (Mellaril)
Tryptophan
Warfarin (Coumadin)

Special information if you are pregnant or breastfeeding

The effects of Paxil during pregnancy have not been adequately studied. If you are pregnant or plan to become pregnant, inform your doctor immediately. Paxil appears in breast milk and could affect a nursing infant. If this medication is essential to your health, your doctor may advise you to discontinue breastfeeding until your treatment with Paxil is finished.

Recommended dosage

ADULTS

The usual starting dose is 20 milligrams a day, taken as a single dose, usually in the morning. Your physician may increase your dosage by 10 milligrams a day, up to a maximum of 50 milligrams a day.

CHILDREN

The safety and effectiveness of this drug in children have not been established.

ELDERLY

The recommended initial dose for elderly or weak individuals or those with severe kidney or liver disease is 10 milligrams a day. Your doctor may increase the dosage if needed, but it should not exceed 40 milligrams a day.

Overdosage

Any medication taken in excess can have serious consequences. If you suspect an overdose, seek medical attention immediately.

■ *The symptoms of Paxil overdose may include:*
Drowsiness
Enlarged pupils
Nausea
Rapid heartbeat
Vomiting

Brand name:

PCE

See Erythromycin, Oral, page 584.

Brand name:

PERDIEM FIBER

See Metamucil, page 653.

Brand name:

PERGONAL

Pronounced: PER-go-nal
Generic name: Menotropins

Why is this drug prescribed?

Pergonal is a synthetic version of two female hormones, luteinizing hormone (LH) and follicle-stimulating hormone (FSH). It is used to stimulate the follicles in the ovaries to cause ovulation, or release of an egg, in women who are having difficulty getting pregnant. It is usually followed by 1 injection of human chorionic gonadotropin (Profasi). In addition, Pergonal is given to produce many eggs in women undergoing in vitro fertilization.

Pergonal is also used to stimulate the production of sperm in men with some forms of male infertility.

Most important fact about this drug

While undergoing Pergonal therapy, you'll be asked to record your basal body temperatures daily. You should do this at approximately the same time each morning before getting out of bed. Beginning on the last day of receiving Pergonal, you should have intercourse daily until ovulation occurs, so that sperm will be present when the egg is released.

How should you take this medication?

Pergonal comes in powder form in a glass vial. It must be mixed with a special vial of sterile salt water that comes with it. The drug is given by injection in the buttock. Your partner or another reliable person can give you the injection. Your doctor should show you and your partner on how to give the injection at home.

■ *If you miss a dose...*
Be certain to take this drug every day for the exact number of days prescribed.

■ *Storage instructions...*
Store the powder in the refrigerator or at room temperature. Protect from light. Use it immediately after it has been mixed with the saline solution. Discard any that has not been used.

What side effects may occur?

Side effects cannot be anticipated. If any appear or change in intensity, inform your doctor as soon as possible. Only your doctor can determine if it is safe for you to continue taking Pergonal.

■ *Side effects may include:*
Abdominal pain, abdominal bloating or cramps, aching muscles and bones, birth defects in infants, blood clots, chills, collapsed lung or other breathing problems, diarrhea, difficult or labored breathing, dizziness, ectopic (tubal) pregnancy, fast heartbeat or breathing, fever, general feeling of illness, headaches, joint pain, multiple births, nausea, pain or irritation at the place where the injection was given, rash, stroke, vomiting

Why should this drug not be prescribed?

Do not take Pergonal if you:

■ Are sensitive to or have had an allergic reaction to it
■ Are told you have a high FSH level
■ Have an uncontrolled thyroid or adrenal gland problem
■ Have a tumor in your pituitary gland, or any other type of brain tumor
■ Have irregular vaginal bleeding of unknown cause
■ Have ovarian cysts or enlarged ovaries not due to polycystic ovarian syndrome (a condition characterized by hormonal imbalance)
■ Are pregnant

Special warnings about this medication

A number of women who take Pergonal have mild to moderate enlargement of the ovaries that causes abdominal swelling and pain, but is not otherwise serious. It will generally disappear without treatment in 2 to 3 weeks.

In a few women taking Pergonal, a condition called "ovarian hyperstimulation syndrome" occurs. Throughout Pergonal treatment, your doctor will perform ultrasound examinatins of your ovaries to see if ovulation is occurring. These exams will also tell if your ovaries are becoming abnormally large.

If ovarian hyperstimulation syndrome occurs, you can have serious problems with fluid gathering in your chest, abdomen, and around your heart, and you will need to be hospitalized. Early warning signs of the syndrome are severe pelvic pain, nausea, vomiting, and weight gain. Other symptoms are: swelling of the abdomen, abdominal pain, nausea, vomiting, diarrhea, weight gain, difficulty breathing, and decreased amount of urine. You may have serious breathing problems and blood clot formations.

If your doctor finds that your ovaries are abnormally enlarged on the last day of your Pergonal therapy, you may be developing ovarian hyperstimulation syndrome, and you will not receive Profasi to complete your treatment.

About 20 percent of women who take Pergonal who get pregnant have multiple births: about 15 percent resulting in twins, and 5 percent resulting in 3 or more babies.

Possible food and drug interactions when taking this medication

There have been no drug or food interactions reported during Pergonal therapy.

Special information if you are pregnant or breastfeeding

Pergonal should not be taken during pregnancy because it is suspected of increasing the risk of birth defects.

It is not known whether Pergonal appears in breast milk. Therefore, it is not certain if the drug is safe to use by women who are breastfeeding.

Recommended dosage

For women who have difficulty ovulating, the first dose of Pergonal should be 75 international units per day. It is given as an injection in the buttock for 7 to 12 days and is followed by Profasi, 5,000 units to 10,000 international units 1 day after the last dose of Pergonal. Pergonal should not be taken for more than 12 days at a time. However, if after 3 cycles pregnancy does not occur, your doctor may want to increase the dose of Pergonal to 150 international units per day for 7 to 12 days. If you are undergoing in vitro fertilization, you will receive the higher dose of Pergonal as well.

Overdosage

Ovarian hyperstimulation syndrome is the most likely result of a Pergonal overdose. If you suspect an overdose, seek medical attention immediately.

Brand name:

PHENAPHEN WITH CODEINE

See Tylenol with Codeine, page 779.

Generic name:

PHENAZOPYRIDINE

See Pyridium, page 732.

Generic name:

PHENELZINE

See Nardil, page 676.

Generic name:

PHENTERMINE

See Fastin, page 593.

Generic name:

PIROXICAM

See Feldene, page 594.

Generic name:

PODOFILOX

See Condylox, page 555.

Brand name:

POLYCILLIN

See Omnipen, page 699.

Brand name:

POLY-VI-FLOR

Pronounced: pol-ee-VIE-floor
Generic ingredients: Vitamins, Fluoride

Why is this drug prescribed?

Poly-Vi-Flor is a multivitamin and fluoride supplement with 10 essential vitamins plus the mineral fluoride. It is prescribed for children aged 2 and older to provide fluoride where the drinking water contains less than the amount recommended by the American Dental Association to build strong teeth and prevent cavities. Poly-Vi-Flor supplies significant amounts of other vitamins to avoid deficiencies. The American Academy of Pediatrics recommends that children up to age 16 take a fluoride supplement if they live in areas where the drinking water contains less than the recommended amount of fluoride.

Most important fact about this drug

Do not give your child more than the recommended dose. Too much fluoride can cause discoloration and pitting of teeth.

How should you take this medication?

Do not give your child more than your doctor prescribes.

Poly-Vi-Flor should be chewed or crushed before swallowing.

■ *If you miss a dose...*
Take it as soon as you remember. If it is almost time for the next dose, skip the one you missed and go back to your regular schedule. Do not take 2 doses at once.

■ *Storage instructions...*
Store away from heat, light, and moisture.

What side effects may occur?

Rarely, an allergic rash has occurred.

Why should this drug not be prescribed?

Children should not take Poly-Vi-Flor if they are getting significant amounts of fluoride from other medications or sources.

Special warnings about this medication

Do not give your child more than the recommended dosage. Your child's teeth should be checked periodically for discoloration or pitting. Notify your doctor if white, brown, or black spots appear on your child's teeth.

The fluoride level of your drinking water should be determined before Poly-Vi-Flor is prescribed.

Let your doctor know if you change drinking water or filtering systems.

Fluoride does not replace proper dental habits, such as brushing, flossing, and having dental checkups.

Recommended dosage

The usual dose is 1 tablet every day as prescribed by the doctor.

Overdosage

Although overdose is unlikely, any medication taken in excess can have serious consequences. If you suspect an overdose, seek medical treatment immediately.

Brand name:

PONSTEL

Pronounced: PON-stel
Generic name: Mefenamic acid

Why is this drug prescribed?

Ponstel, a nonsteroidal anti-inflammatory drug, is used for the relief of moderate pain (when treatment will not last for more than 7 days) and for the treatment of menstrual pain.

Most important fact about this drug

You should have frequent checkups with your doctor if you take Ponstel regularly. Ulcers or internal bleeding can occur without warning.

How should you take this medication?

Take Ponstel with food if possible. If it upsets your stomach, be sure to take it with food or an antacid or with a full glass of milk.

Take Ponstel exactly as prescribed by your doctor.

■ *If you miss a dose...*
If you take Ponstel on a regular schedule, take the forgotten dose as soon as you remember. If it is almost time for your

next dose, skip the one you missed and go back to your regular schedule. Do not take 2 doses at once.

■ *Storage instructions...*
Store away from heat, light, and moisture.

What side effects may occur?

Side effects cannot be anticipated. If any develop or change in intensity, inform your doctor as soon as possible. Only your doctor can determine if it is safe for you to continue taking Ponstel.

■ *More common side effects may include:*
Abdominal pain
Diarrhea
Nausea
Stomach and intestinal upset
Vomiting

■ *Less common or rare side effects may include:*
Anemia, blurred vision, blood in the urine, changes in liver function, constipation, difficult or painful urination, dizziness, drowsiness, ear pain, eye irritation, facial swelling due to fluid retention, fluttery or throbbing heartbeat, gas, headache, heartburn, hives, inability to sleep, increased need for insulin in a diabetic, kidney failure, labored breathing, loss of appetite, loss of color vision, nervousness, rash, red or purple spots on the skin, sweating, ulcers and internal bleeding

Why should this drug not be prescribed?

Do not take Ponstel if you are sensitive to or have ever had an allergic reaction to it. You should not take it, either, if you have had asthma attacks, hay fever, or hives caused by aspirin or other nonsteroidal anti-inflammatory drugs, such as Motrin and Nuprin. Make sure your doctor is aware of any drug reactions you have experienced.

Do not take Ponstel if you have ulcerations or frequently recurring inflammation of your stomach or intestines.

Avoid this drug if you have serious kidney disease.

Special warnings about this medication

If you develop a rash, diarrhea, or other stomach problems, stop taking this medication and contact your doctor.

Ponstel should be used with caution if you have kidney disease, heart failure, or liver disease; it can cause liver inflammation in some people.

This drug may prolong bleeding time. If you are taking blood-thinning medication, take Ponstel with caution.

Possible food and drug interactions when taking this medication

If Ponstel is taken with certain other drugs, the effects of either can be increased, decreased, or altered. It is especially important to check with your doctor before combining Ponstel with the following:

Aspirin
Blood-thinning medications such as
    Coumadin
Diuretics such as Lasix and HydroDIURIL
Lithium (Lithonate)
Methotrexate

Special information if you are pregnant or breastfeeding

The effects of Ponstel during pregnancy have not been adequately studied. If you are pregnant or plan to become pregnant, inform your doctor immediately. You should not use Ponstel in late pregnancy because nonsteroidal anti-inflammatory drugs affect the heart and blood vessels of the developing baby. Ponstel may appear in breast milk and could affect a nursing infant. If this medication is essential to your health, your doctor may advise you to discontinue breastfeeding until your treatment is finished.

Recommended dosage

ADULTS AND CHILDREN OVER 14

Moderate Pain
The usual starting dose is 500 milligrams, followed by 250 milligrams every 6 hours, if needed, for 1 week.

Menstrual Pain
The usual starting dose, once symptoms appear, is 500 milligrams, followed by 250 milligrams every 6 hours for 2 to 3 days.

CHILDREN

The safety and effectiveness of Ponstel have not been established in children under 14.

Overdosage
Although there is no information available on overdosage with Ponstel, any medication taken in excess can have serious consequences. If you suspect an overdose of Ponstel, seek medical attention immediately.

Generic name:

PRAZEPAM

See Centrax, page 538.

Brand name:

PREMARIN

Pronounced: PREM-uh-rin
Generic name: Conjugated estrogens

Why is this drug prescribed?
Premarin is an estrogen replacement drug. The tablets are used to reduce symptoms of menopause, including feelings of warmth in face, neck, and chest, and the sudden intense episodes of heat and sweating known as "hot flashes." They also may be prescribed for teenagers who fail to mature at the usual rate, and to relieve the symptoms of certain types of cancer, including some forms of breast and prostate cancer.

In addition, either the tablets or Premarin vaginal cream can be used for other conditions caused by lack of estrogen, such as dry, itchy external genitals and vaginal irritation.

Along with diet, calcium supplements, and exercise, Premarin tablets are also prescribed to prevent osteoporosis, a condition in which the bones become brittle and easily broken.

Most important fact about this drug
Because estrogens have been linked with increased risk of endometrial cancer (cancer in lining of the uterus), it is essential to have regular checkups and to report any unusual vaginal bleeding to your doctor immediately.

How should you take this medication?
Take Premarin exactly as prescribed. Do not share it with anyone else.

If you are taking calcium supplements as a part of the treatment to help prevent brittle bones, check with your doctor about how much to take.

You should take a few moments to read the patient package insert provided with your prescription.

If you are using Premarin vaginal cream, apply it as follows:

1. Remove cap from tube.

2. Screw nozzle end of applicator onto tube.
3. Gently squeeze tube from the bottom to force sufficient cream into the barrel to provide the prescribed dose.
4. Unscrew applicator from tube.
5. Lie on back with knees drawn up. Gently insert applicator deeply into the vagina and press plunger downward to its original position.

To cleanse the applicator, pull the plunger out of the barrel, then wash with mild soap and warm water. Do not boil or use hot water.

■ *If you miss a dose...*
Take the forgotten dose as soon as you remember. If it is almost time for the next dose, skip the one you missed and go back to your regular schedule. Never try to "catch up" by doubling the dose.

■ *Storage instructions...*
Store at room temperature.

What side effects may occur?
Side effects cannot be anticipated. If any develop or change in intensity, inform your doctor immediately. Only your doctor can determine whether it is safe to continue taking Premarin.

■ *Side effects may include:*
Abdominal cramps, abnormal vaginal bleeding, bloating, breast swelling and tenderness, depression, dizziness, enlargement of benign tumors in the uterus, fluid retention, gallbladder disease, hair loss from the scalp, increased body hair, intolerance to contact lenses, migraine headache, nausea, vomiting, sex-drive changes, skin darkening, especially on the face, skin rash or redness, swelling of wrists and ankles, vaginal yeast infection, weight gain or loss, yellow eyes and skin

Why should this drug not be prescribed?
Do not take Premarin if you have ever had a bad reaction to it, or have undiagnosed abnormal vaginal bleeding.

Except in certain special circumstances, you should not be given Premarin if you have breast cancer or any other "estrogen-dependent" cancer.

Do not take Premarin if you have had any heart or circulation problem including a tendency for abnormal blood clotting.

Special warnings about this medication
The risk of cancer of the uterus increases when estrogen is used for a long time or taken in large doses.

There may be an increased risk of breast cancer in women who take estrogen for a long time. If you have a family history of breast cancer or have ever had an abnormal mammogram, you need to have more frequent breast examinations.

Women who take Premarin after menopause are more likely to develop gallbladder disease.

Premarin also increases the risk of blood clots. These blood clots can cause stroke, heart attack, or other serious disorders.

While taking Premarin, get in touch with your doctor right away if you notice any of the following:

Abdominal pain, tenderness, or swelling
Abnormal bleeding from the vagina
Breast lumps
Coughing up blood
Pain in your chest or calves
Severe headache, dizziness, or faintness
Sudden shortness of breath
Vision changes
Yellowing of the skin

Possible food and drug interactions when taking this medication

If Premarin is taken with certain other drugs, the effects of either could be increased, decreased, or altered. It is especially important to check with your doctor before combining Premarin with the following:

Barbiturates such as phenobarbital
Blood thinners such as Coumadin
Drugs used for epilepsy, such as Dilantin
Major tranquilizers such as Thorazine
Oral diabetics such as Micronase
Rifampin (Rifadin)
Thyroid preparations such as Synthroid
Tricyclic antidepressants such as Elavil and
  Tofranil
Vitamin C

Special information if you are pregnant or breastfeeding

If you are pregnant or plan to become pregnant, notify your doctor immediately. Premarin should not be taken during pregnancy because of the possibility of harm to the unborn child. Premarin cannot prevent a miscarriage.

Recommended dosage

Your doctor will start therapy with Premarin at a low dose. He or she will want to check you periodically at 3- to 6-month intervals to determine the need for continued therapy.

PREMARIN TABLETS

Vasomotor Symptoms (Hot Flashes Associated with Menopause)
The usual recommended dosage is 0.3 to 1.25 milligrams daily. If the woman has not menstruated within the last two months or more, therapy is started arbitrarily. If the woman is menstruating, cyclic (3 weeks on and 1 week off) therapy is started on day 5 of bleeding.

Atrophic Vaginitis (Tissue Degeneration in the Vagina)
The usual recommended dosage is 0.3 to 1.25 milligrams or more daily, depending upon the response of the individual. The drug is taken cyclically (3 weeks on and 1 week off).

Hypoestrogenism (Low Estrogen Levels) Due to Reduced Ovary Function
The usual dosage is 2.5 to 7.5 milligrams daily, in divided doses for 20 days, followed by a 10-day rest period. If bleeding does not occur by the end of this period, the same dosage schedule is repeated. The number of courses of estrogen therapy necessary to produce bleeding may vary depending on the responsiveness of the endometrium (lining of the uterus).

If bleeding occurs before the end of the 10-day period, a 20-day estrogen-progestin cyclic regimen should be begun with Premarin: 2.5 to 7.5 milligrams daily in divided doses for 20 days. During the last 5 days of estrogen therapy, an oral progestin should be given.

If bleeding occurs before this course is concluded, therapy is discontinued and may be resumed on the 5th day of bleeding.

Ovary Removal or Ovarian Failure
The usual dosage is 1.25 milligrams daily, cyclically (3 weeks on and 1 week off). Dosage is adjusted upward or downward, according to severity of symptoms and your response to treatment. For maintenance, the dosage should be adjusted to the lowest level that will provide effective control.

Osteoporosis (Loss of Bone Mass)
The usual dosage is 0.625 milligram daily. Administration should be cyclic (3 weeks on and 1 week off).

Advanced Androgen-Dependent Cancer of the Prostate, for Relief of Symptoms Only
The usual dosage is 1.25 to 2.5 milligrams 3 times daily. The effectiveness of therapy can be judged by laboratory tests as well as by improvement of symptoms.

Breast Cancer (for Relief of Symptoms Only) in Appropriately Selected Women and Men with Metastatic Disease
The suggested dosage is 10 milligrams 3 times daily for a period of at least 3 months. Women with an intact uterus are monitored closely for signs of endometrial cancer, and appropriate diagnostic tests are run to rule out malignancy in the event of persistent or recurring abnormal vaginal bleeding.

PREMARIN VAGINAL CREAM
Given cyclically for short-term use only.

Atrophic Vaginitis or Kraurosis Vulva (Degeneration of Genital Tissue or Severe Itching in the genital area)
The lowest dose that will control symptoms should be used, with treatment discontinued as soon as possible. Administration should be cyclic (3 weeks on and 1 week off). Attempts to discontinue or taper medication should be made at 3- to 6-month intervals.

The recommended dosage is 2 to 4 grams (one-half to 1 applicator of cream) daily, inserted into the vagina, depending on the severity of the condition. Women with an intact uterus should be monitored closely for signs of endometrial cancer, with appropriate diagnostic measures taken to rule out malignancy in the event of persistent or recurring abnormal vaginal bleeding.

Overdosage
Any medication taken in excess can have serious consequences. If you suspect an overdose of Premarin, seek medical attention immediately.

Brand name:

PRINCIPEN

See Omnipen, page 699.

Brand name:

PROFASI

Pronounced: PRO-fah-see
Generic name: Human chorionic gonadotropin

Why is this drug prescribed?
Profasi is an infertility treatment that brings an ovulation, or release of an egg from the ovary, in women who do not ovulate on their own. It is used after therapy with another drug, Pergonal (menotropins).

Profasi is also given to boys to treat undescended or underdeveloped testicles. It is also used in men to stimulate the production of testosterone.

Some doctors also use chorionic gonadotropin in men with erection problems or lack of sexual desire, and in the therapy of male "menopause".

Most important fact about this drug
Your doctor will ask you to record your basal body temperatures daily during your treatment. This should be done at approximately the same time each morning before getting out of bed. Beginning on the day prior to taking Profasi you should start having intercourse daily to ensure the presence of sperm when ovulation takes place.

How should you take this medication?

Profasi is available as a powder in a glass vial. It must be mixed with a special vial of water that comes with it. Profasi is given by injection in the buttock after you receive your last dose of Pergonal. The injection can be given by your partner or another reliable person. Your doctor should show you and your partner how to give the injection at home.

■ *If you miss a dose...*
Profasi is taken only once at the end of each treatment cycle.

■ *Storage instructions...*
Store the dry powder at room temperature. After it has been mixed with water, refrigerate and use within 30 days.

What side effects may occur?

Side effects cannot be anticipated. If any develop or change in intensity, inform your doctor as soon as possible. Only your doctor can determine if it is safe for you to continue taking Profasi.

■ *Side effects may include:*
Breast development in males, depression, difficult or labored breathing, early puberty (if given to adolescent boys or girls), fatigue, fluid retention, headache, hives, irritability, pain at the injection site, rash, redness, restlessness, shortness of breath, swelling

Why should this drug not be prescribed?

During the 1960s and 1970s, some doctors gave human chorionic gonadotropin (HCG) injections to overweight women. The theory behind the injections was that HCG decreased the appetite and led to more even fat distribution throughout the body. However, there is not proof that HCG helps women lose weight faster or more easily. Profasi is not intended to treatment of obesity.

Profasi should not be taken by girls going through puberty at an unusually early age. Also avoid Profasi if you have had an allergic reaction to it in the past.

Special warnings about this medication

Because Profasi may cause fluid retention, it should be used with caution in women with heart or kidney disease, epilepsy, migraine headache, or asthma. Women taking this drug risk developing blood clots. After taking this drug, you may have a multiple birth.

Possible food and drug interactions when taking this medication

No interactions have been reported.

Special information if you are pregnant or breastfeeding

The effects of Profasi during pregnancy have not been adequately studied; and is not known whether Profasi could harm a developing baby. In any event, the drug is not needed if you are already pregnant. There is not information available on the effect of Profasi during breastfeeding.

Recommended dosage

Profasi is given in a dose of 5,000 to 10,000 international units on the day after the last dose of Pergonal.

Overdosage

While an onverdose of Profasi is highly unlikely, any medication taken in excess can have serious consequences. If you suspect an overdose, seek medical attention immediately.

Generic name:

PROPRANOLOL

See Inderal, page 622.

Brand name:

PROSTEP

See Nicotine Patches, page 682.

Brand name:

PROTOSTAT

See Flagyl, page 604.

Brand name:

PROVERA

Pronounced: pro-VAIR-uh
Generic name: Medroxyprogesterone acetate
Other brand name: Cycrin

Why is this drug prescribed?

Provera is derived from the female hormone progesterone. You may be given Provera if your menstrual periods have stopped or a female hormone imbalance is causing your uterus to bleed abnormally.

Other forms of medroxyprogesterone, such as Depo-Provera, are used as a contraceptive injection and prescribed in the treatment of endometrial cancer.

Some doctors prescribe Provera to treat endometriosis, menopausal symptoms, premenstrual tension, sexual aggressive behavior in men, and sleep apnea (temporary failure to breath while sleeping).

Most important fact about this drug

You should never take Provera during the first 4 months of pregnancy. During this formative period, even a few days of treatment with Provera might put your unborn baby at increased risk for birth defects. If you take Provera and later discover that you were pregnant when you took it, discuss this with your doctor right away.

How should you take this medication?

Provera may be taken with or between meals.

Do not change from one brand to another without consulting your doctor or pharmacist.

Your doctor will probably have you take Provera for 5 to 10 days and then stop; you should have your period within 3 to 7 days after the last dose.

If you are being treated for lack of regular menstrual periods, your doctor may have you start taking Provera at any time. If you are being treated for abnormal uterine bleeding due to a female-hormone imbalance, your doctor will probably have you start taking Provera on day 16 or 21 of your menstrual cycle (i.e., 16 or 21 days after the start of your last period). You should have your period within 3 to 7 days after the last dose.

■ *If you miss a dose...*
  Take it as soon as you remember. If it is almost time for your next dose, skip the one you missed and go back to your regular schedule. Never take 2 doses at the same time.

■ *Storage instructions...*
  Store at room temperature.

What side effects may occur?

Side effects cannot be anticipated. If any develop or change in intensity, inform your doctor as soon as possible. Only your doctor can determine if it is safe for you to continue taking Provera.

■ *Side effects may include:*

Acne, anaphylaxis (life-threatening allergic reaction), blood clot in a vein, lungs, or brain, breakthrough bleeding (between menstrual periods), breast tenderness or sudden or excessive flow of milk, cervical erosion or changes in secretions, depression, excessive growth of hair, fever, fluid retention, hair loss, headache, hives, insomnia, itching, lack of menstruation, menstrual flow changes, spotting, nausea, rash, skin discoloration, sleepiness, weight gain or loss, yellowed eyes and skin

Why should this drug not be prescribed?

Do not take Provera if you are sensitive to it or have ever had an allergic reaction to it.

If you suspect you may have become pregnant, do not take Provera as a test for pregnancy. Doctors once prescribed Provera for this purpose, but no longer do so for 2 reasons:

■ Quicker, safer pregnancy tests are now available.
■ If you are in fact pregnant, Provera might injure the baby.

Do not take Provera during your first 4 months of pregnancy. In the past, Provera was sometimes given to try to prevent miscarriage. However, doctors now believe that this treatment is not only ineffective but also potentially harmful to the baby.

Do not take Provera if you have:

■ Cancer of the breast or genital organs
■ Liver disease or a liver condition
■ A dead fetus still in the uterus
■ Undiagnosed bleeding from the vagina

Do not take Provera if you have, or have ever developed, blood clots.

Special warnings about this medication

Before you start to take Provera, your doctor will give you a complete physical exam, including examination of your breasts and pelvic organs. You should also have a cervical smear (Pap test).

Provera may cause some degree of fluid retention. If you have a medical condition that could be made worse by fluid retention—such as epilepsy, migraine, asthma, or a heart or kidney problem—make sure your doctor knows about it.

Provera may mask the onset of menopause. In other words, while taking Provera you may continue to experience regular menstrual bleeding even if your menopause has started.

Provera may make you depressed, especially if you have suffered from depression in the past. If you become seriously depressed, tell your doctor; you should probably stop taking Provera.

If you are diabetic, Provera could make your diabetes worse; your doctor will want to watch you closely while you are taking this drug.

There is some concern that Provera, like birth control pills, may increasen your risk for a blood clot in a vein. If you experience any symptoms that might suggest the onset of such a condition—pain with swelling, warmth, and redness in a leg vein, coughing or shortness of breath, vision problems, migraine, or weakness or numbness in an arm or leg—see your doctor immediately.

Tell your doctor right away if you lose some or all of your vision or you start seeing double. You may have to stop taking the medication.

Possible food and drug interactions when taking this medication

If Provera is taken with certain other drugs, the effects of either may be increased, decreased, or altered. It is especially important to check with your doctor before combining Provera with aminoglutethimide (Cytadren).

Special information if you are pregnant or breastfeeding

You should not take Provera during pregnancy. If you are pregnant or plan to become pregnant, inform your doctor immediately.

Provera appears in breast milk. If you are a new mother, you may need to choose between taking Provera and breastfeeding your baby.

Recommended dosage

ADULTS

To Restore Menstrual Periods
Provera Tablets are taken in dosages of 5 to 10 milligrams daily for 5 to 10 days. Make sure you discuss what effect this will have on your menstrual cycle with your doctor. You should have bleeding 3 to 7 days after you stop taking Provera.

Abnormal Uterine Bleeding Due to Hormonal Imbalance
Beginning on the 16th or 21st day of your menstrual cycle, you will take 5 to 10 milligrams daily for 5 to 10 days. Make sure you discuss what effect this will have on your menstrual cycle with your doctor. You should have bleeding 3 to 7 days after you stop taking Provera.

Overdosage

Although no specific information is available, any medication taken in excess can have serious consequences. If you suspect an overdose of Provera, seek medical attention immediately.

Brand name:

PROZAC

Pronounced: PRO-zak
Generic name: Fluoxetine hydrochloride

Why is this drug prescribed?

Prozac is prescribed for the treatment of major depression, that is, a continuing depression that interferes with daily functioning. The symptoms of major depression often include changes in appetite, sleep habits and mind/body coordination; decreased sex drive; increased fatigue; feelings of guilt or worthlessness; difficulty concentrating; slowed thinking; and suicidal thoughts.

Prozac is thought to work by adjusting the balance of the brain's natural chemical messengers. It also has been used to treat obesity, eating disorders, and obsessive-compulsive disorders.

Most important fact about this drug

Serious, sometimes fatal reactions have been known to occur when Prozac is used in combination with other antidepressant drugs known as MAO inhibitors, including Nardil, Parnate, and Marplan; and when Prozac is discontinued and a MAO inhibitor is started. Never take Prozac with one of these drugs or within 14 days of discontinuing therapy with one of them; and allow 5 weeks or more between stopping Prozac and starting a MAO inhibitor. Be especially cautious if you have been taking Prozac in high doses or for a long time.

If you are taking any prescription or nonprescription drugs, notify your doctor before taking Prozac.

How should you take this medication?

Prozac should be taken exactly as prescribed by your doctor.

Prozac usually is taken once a day, in the morning. It should be taken regularly to be effective. Make a habit of taking it at the same time you do some other daily activity.

■ *If you miss a dose...*
Take the forgotten dose as soon as you remember. If several hours have passed, skip the dose. Never try to "catch up" by doubling the dose.

■ *Storage instructions...*
Store at room temperature.

What side effects may occur?

Side effects cannot be anticipated. If any develop or change in intensity, inform your doctor as soon as possible. Only your doctor can determine if it is safe for you to continue taking Prozac.

■ *More common side effects may include:*
Abnormal dreams, agitation, anxiety, bronchitis, chills, diarrhea, dizziness, drowsiness and fatigue, hay fever, inability to fall or stay asleep, increased appetite, lack or loss of appetite, light-headedness, nausea, nervousness, sweating, tremors, weakness, weight loss, yawning

■ *Less common side effects may include:*
Abnormal ejaculation, abnormal gait, abnormal stoppage of menstrual flow, acne, amnesia, apathy, arthritis, asthma, belching, bone pain, breast cysts, breast pain, brief loss of consciousness, bursitis, chills and fever, conjunctivitis, convulsions, dark, tarry stool, difficulty in swallowing, dilation of pupils, dimness of vision, dry skin, ear pain, eye pain, exaggerated feeling of well-being, excessive bleeding, facial swelling due to fluid retention, fluid retention, hair loss, hallucinations,

hangover effect, hiccups, high or low blood pressure, hives, hostility, impotence, increased sex drive, inflammation of the esophagus, inflammation of the gums, inflammation of the stomach lining, inflammation of the tongue, inflammation of the vagina, intolerance of light, involuntary movement, irrational ideas, irregular heartbeat, jaw or neck pain, lack of muscle coordination, low blood pressure upon standing, low blood sugar, migraine headache, mouth inflammation, neck pain and rigidity, nosebleed, ovarian disorders, paranoid reaction, pelvic pain, pneumonia, rapid breathing, rapid heartbeat, ringing in the ears, severe chest pain, skin inflammation, skin rash, thirst, twitching, uncoordinated movements, urinary disorders, vague feeling of bodily discomfort, vertigo, weight gain

■ *Rare side effects may include:*
Antisocial behavior, blood in urine, bloody diarrhea, bone disease, breast enlargement, cataracts, colitis, coma, deafness, decreased reflexes, dehydration, double vision, drooping of eyelids, duodenal ulcer, enlarged abdomen, enlargement of liver, enlargement or increased activity of thyroid gland, excess growth of coarse hair on face, chest etc., excess uterine or vaginal bleeding, extreme muscle tension, eye bleeding, female milk production, fluid accumulation and swelling in the head, fluid buildup in larynx and lungs, gallstones, glaucoma, gout, heart attack, hepatitis, high blood sugar, hysteria, inability to control bowel movements, increased salivation, inflammation of eyes and eyelids, inflammation of fallopian tubes, inflammation of testes, inflammation of the gallbladder, inflammation of the small intestine, inflammation of tissue below skin, kidney disorders, lung inflammation, menstrual

disorders, miscarriage, mouth sores, muscle inflammation or bleeding, muscle spasms, painful sexual intercourse for women, psoriasis, rashes, reddish or purplish spots on the skin, reduction of body temperature, rheumatoid arthritis, seborrhea, shingles, skin discoloration, skin inflammation and disorders, slowing of heart rate, slurred speech, spitting blood, stomach ulcer, stupor, suicidal thoughts, taste loss, temporary cessation of breathing, tingling sensation around the mouth, tongue discoloration and swelling, urinary tract disorders, vomiting blood, yellow eyes and skin

Why should this drug not be prescribed?

If you are sensitive to or have ever had an allergic reaction to Prozac or similar drugs, you should not take this medication. Make sure that your doctor is aware of any drug reactions that you have experienced.

Do not take this drug while using a MAO inhibitor. (See "Most important fact about this drug.")

Special warnings about this medication

Unless you are directed to do so by your doctor, do not take this medication if you are recovering from a heart attack or if you have kidney or liver disease or diabetes.

Prozac may cause you to become drowsy or less alert and may affect your judgment. Therefore, driving or operating dangerous machinery or participating in any hazardous activity that requires full mental alertness is not recommended.

While taking this medication, you may feel dizzy or light-headed or actually faint when getting up from a lying or sitting position. If getting up slowly doesn't help or if this problem continues, notify your doctor.

If you develop a skin rash or hives while taking Prozac, discontinue use of the medication and notify your doctor immediately.

Prozac should be used with caution if you have a history of seizures. You should discuss all of your medical problems with your doctor before taking this medication.

Possible food and drug interactions when taking this medication

Combining Prozac with MAO inhibitors is dangerous.

Do not drink alcohol while taking this medication.

If Prozac is taken with certain other drugs, the effects of either could be increased, decreased, or altered. It is especially important to check with your doctor before combining Prozac with the following:

Carbamazepine (Tegretol)
Diazepam (Valium)
Digitalis (Lanoxin)
Drugs that act on the central nervous system (brain and spinal cord) such as Xanax and Valium
Flecainide (Tambocor)
Lithium (Eskalith)
Other antidepressants (Elavil)
Tryptophan
Vinblastine (Velban)
Warfarin (Coumadin)

Special information if you are pregnant or breastfeeding

The effects of Prozac during pregnancy have not been adequately studied. If you are pregnant or plan to become pregnant, inform your doctor immediately. This medication may appear in breast milk. If this medication is essential to your health, your doctor may advise you to discontinue breastfeeding your baby until your treatment with Prozac is finished.

Recommended dosage

ADULTS

The usual starting dose is 20 milligrams per day, taken in the morning. Your doctor may increase your dose after several weeks if no improvement is observed. Patients with kidney or liver disease and those taking other drugs may have their dosages adjusted by their doctor.

Dosages above 20 milligrams daily should be divided into 2 doses per day. Dosage should not exceed 80 milligrams per day.

CHILDREN

The safety and effectiveness of Prozac have not been established in children.

ELDERLY

Your dose should be determined by your doctor.

Overdosage

Any medication taken in excess or in combination with other drugs can cause symptoms of overdose. If you suspect an overdose, seek medical attention immediately.

- *Symptoms of Prozac overdose include:*
  Agitation
  Nausea
  Restlessness
  Vomiting

Generic name:

PSYLLIUM

See Metamucil, page 653.

Brand name:

PYRIDIUM

Pronounced: pie-RI-di-um
Generic name: Phenazopyridine hydrochloride

Why is this drug prescribed?

Pyridium is a urinary tract analgesic that helps relieve the pain, burning, urgency, frequency, and irritation caused by infection, trauma, catheters, or various surgical procedures in the lower urinary tract. Pyridium is indicated for short-term use and can only relieve symptoms; it is not a treatment for the underlying cause of the symptoms.

Most important fact about this drug

Pyridium produces an orange to red color in urine, and may stain fabric. Staining of contact lenses has also been reported.

How should you take this medication?

Take Pyridium after meals, exactly as prescribed.

- *If you miss a dose...*
  Take it as soon as you remember. If it is almost time for your next dose, skip the one you missed and go back to your regular schedule. Never take 2 doses at the same time.

- *Storage instructions...*
  Store at room temperature.

What side effects may occur?

Side effects cannot be anticipated. If any occur or change in intensity, inform your doctor as soon as possible. Only your doctor can determine if it is safe for you to continue taking Pyridium.

- *Side effects may include:*
  Abdominal upset
  Headache
  Itching

Rash
Severe allergic reaction (rash, difficulty
breathing, fever, rapid heartbeat,
convulsions)

Why should this drug not be prescribed?
Pyridium should be avoided if you have
kidney disease, or if you are sensitive to or
have ever had an allergic reaction to it.

Special warnings about this medication
If your skin or the whites of your eyes
develop a yellowish tone, it may indicate
that your kidneys are not eliminating the
medication as they should. Notify your
doctor immediately.

Possible food and drug interactions
when taking this medication
No interactions have been reported.

Special information
if you are pregnant or breastfeeding
The effects of Pyridium during pregnancy
have not been adequately studied. If you are
pregnant or plan to become pregnant,
inform your doctor immediately. To date,
there is no information on whether Pyridium
appears in breast milk. If this medication is
essential to your health, your doctor may
advise you to stop breastfeeding until your
treatment with Pyridium is finished.

Recommended dosage

ADULTS

The usual dose is two 100-milligram tablets
or one 200-milligram tablet 3 times a day
after meals.

You should not take Pyridium for more
than 2 days if you are also taking an
antibiotic for the treatment of a urinary
tract infection.

Overdosage
Any medication taken in excess can have
serious consequences. If you suspect an
overdose, seek medical treatment
immediately.

■ *Symptoms of Pyridium overdose may
include:*
Changes in kidney, liver, and blood
functioning

Brand name:

REGULOID

See Metamucil, page 653.

Brand name:

RELAFEN

Pronounced: REL-ah-fen
Generic name: Nabumetone

Why is this drug prescribed?
Relafen, a nonsteroidal anti-inflammatory
drug, is used to relieve the inflammation,
swelling, stiffness, and joint pain associated
with rheumatoid arthritis and osteoarthritis
(the most common form of arthritis).

Most important fact about this drug
You should have frequent checkups with
your doctor if you take Relafen regularly.
Ulcers or internal bleeding can occur with
or without warning.

How should you take this medication?
Relafen can be taken with or without food.
Take it exactly as prescribed.

■ *If you miss a dose...*
Take the forgotten dose as soon as you
remember. If it is almost time for your
next dose, skip the one you mised and go

back to your regular schedule. Never take a double dose.

■ *Storage instructions...*
Keep this medication in the container it came in, tightly closed, and away from moist places and direct light. It can be stored at room temperature.

What side effects may occur?
Side effects cannot be anticipated. If any develop or change in intensity, inform your doctor as soon as possible. Only your doctor can determine whether it is safe for you to continue taking Relafen.

■ *More common side effects may include:*
Abdominal pain, constipation, diarrhea, dizziness, fluid retention, gas, headache, indigestion, itching, nausea, rash, ringing in ears

■ *Less common side effects may include:*
Dry mouth, fatigue, inability to fall or stay asleep, increased sweating, inflammation of the mouth, inflammation of the stomach, nervousness, sleepiness, vomiting

■ *Rare side effects may include:*
Agitation, anxiety, confusion, dark, tarry, bloody stools, depression, difficult or labored breathing, difficulty swallowing, fluid retention, general feeling of illness, hives, increase or loss of appetite, large blisters, pins and needles, pneumonia or lung inflammation, sensitivity to light, severe allergic reactions, skin peeling, stomach and intestinal inflammation and/or bleeding, tremor, ulcers, vaginal bleeding, vertigo, vision changes, weakness, weight gain, yellow eyes and skin

Why should this drug not be prescribed?
Do not take this medication if you are sensitive to or have ever had an allergic reaction to Relafen, or if you have had asthma attacks, hives or other allergic reactions caused by Relafen, aspirin, or other nonsteroidal anti-inflammatory drugs.

Special warnings about this medication
Stomach and intestinal ulcers can occur without warning. Remember to get regular check-ups.

Make sure the doctor knows if you have kidney or liver disease. Relafen should be used with caution.

This drug can cause fluid retention and swelling. It should be used with caution if you have congestive heart failure or high blood pressure.

Relafen can cause increased sensitivity to sunlight.

Possible food and drug interactions when taking this medication
If Relafen is taken with certain other drugs, the effects of either could be increased, decreased, or altered. It is especially important to check with your doctor before combining Relafen with blood-thinning drugs such as Coumadin and aspirin.

Other drugs with which Relafen could possibly interact include:

Diuretics (HydroDiuril, Lasix)
Lithium (Lithonate)
Methotrexate

Special information if you are pregnant or breastfeeding
The effects of Relafen during pregnancy have not been adequately studied. If you are pregnant or plan to become pregnant, inform your doctor immediately. Relafen may appear in breast milk and could affect a nursing infant. If this medication is essential to your health, your doctor may advise you to discontinue breastfeeding until your treatment with Paxil is finished.

Recommended dosage

ADULTS

The usual starting dose is 1000 milligrams taken as a single dose. Dosage may be increased up to 2000 milligrams per day, taken once or twice a day.

CHILDREN

The safety and effectiveness of this drug in children have not been established.

Overdosage

Any medication taken in excess can have serious consequences. If you suspect an overdose, seek medical attention immediately.

Brand name:

RETIN-A

Pronounced: Ret-in-A
Generic name: Tretinoin

Why is this drug prescribed?

Retin-A is prescribed for the treatment of acne vulgaris (an inflammatory disease of the skin, usually affecting persons in puberty or early adult years).

Most important fact about this drug

While using Retin-A, exposure to sunlight, including sunlamps, should be kept to a minimum. If you have a sunburn, do not use this medication until you have fully recovered. Use of sunscreen products and protective clothing over treated areas is recommended when exposure to the sun cannot be avoided. Weather extremes, such as wind and cold, should also be avoided while using Retin-A.

How should you use this medication?

Retin-A gel, cream, or liquid should be applied once a day, at bedtime, to the skin where acne appears, using enough to cover lightly the affected area. The liquid may be applied using a fingertip, gauze pad, or cotton swab. If you use gauze or cotton, avoid oversaturation, which might cause the liquid to run into areas where treatment is not intended.

You may use cosmetics while being treated with Retin-A; however, you should thoroughly cleanse the areas to be treated before applying the medication.

■ *If you miss a dose...*
Resume your regular schedule the next day.

■ *Storage instructions...*
Store at ordinary room temperature. Protect from extreme heat. Keep the cream or gel tube tightly capped.

What side effects may occur?

If you have sensitive skin, the use of this medication may cause your skin to become excessively red, puffy, blistered, or crusted. If this happens, notify your doctor, who may recommend that you discontinue Retin-A until your skin returns to normal, or adjust the medication to a level that you can tolerate.

An unusual darkening of the skin or lack of color of the skin may occur temporarily with repeated application of Retin-A.

Why should this drug not be prescribed?

If you are sensitive to or have ever had an allergic reaction to any of the ingredients in Retin-A, you should not use this medication. Make sure that your doctor is aware of any drug reactions that you have experienced.

The safety and effectiveness of long-term use of this product in the treatment of disorders other than acne have not been established.

Special warnings about this medication

Retin-A should be kept away from the eyes, mouth, angles of the nose, and mucous membranes.

If use of this medication causes an abnormal redness or peeling of the skin where it has been applied, notify your doctor. He may suggest that you use Retin-A less frequently, discontinue use temporarily, or discontinue use altogether.

If you have eczema (skin inflammation consisting of itching and small blisters that ooze and crust over), use this medication with extreme caution, as it may cause severe irritation.

If a sensitivity reaction or chemical irritation occurs, notify your doctor. He may suggest that you discontinue using this medication.

Retin-A may cause a brief feeling of warmth or slight stinging when applied.

During the early weeks of therapy, a worsening of acne may occur due to the action of the medication on deep, previously unseen areas of inflammation. This is not a reason to discontinue therapy, but do notify your doctor if it occurs.

Retin-A gel is flammable and should be kept away from heat and flame.

Possible food and drug interactions when taking this medication

If Retin-A is taken with certain other drugs, the effects of either could be increased, decreased, or altered. It is especially important to check with your doctor before combining Retin-A with the following:

Preparations containing sulfur (ointments and other preparations used to treat skin disorders and infections)
Resorcinol (a drug, used in ointments to treat acne, that causes skin to peel)
Salicylic acid (a drug that kills bacteria and fungi and causes skin to peel)

"Resting" your skin is recommended between use of the above preparations and treatment with Retin-A.

Caution should be exercised when using Retin-A in combination with other topical medications, medicated or abrasive soaps and cleansers, soaps and cosmetics that have a strong drying effect, and products with high concentrations of alcohol, astringents, spices, or lime.

Special information if you are pregnant or breastfeeding

There are no adequate and well-controlled studies in pregnant women. If you are pregnant or plan to become pregnant, inform your doctor immediately. It is not known if this drug appears in breast milk. If Retin-A is essential to your treatment, your doctor may advise you to discontinue breastfeeding until your treatment is finished.

Recommended dosage

ADULTS

Apply once a day at bedtime.

Results should be noticed after 2 to 3 weeks of treatment. More than 6 weeks of treatment may be needed before definite beneficial effects are seen.

Once acne has responded satisfactorily, it may be possible to maintain the improvement with less frequent applications or other dosage forms. However, any change in formulation, drug concentration, or dose frequency should be closely monitored by your doctor to determine your tolerance and response.

Overdosage

Applying this medication excessively will not produce faster or better results, and marked redness, peeling, or discomfort could occur.

Brand name:

RETROVIR

Pronounced: reh-troh-VEER
Generic name: Zidovudine

Why is this drug prescribed?

Retrovir is prescribed for adults infected with human immunodeficiency virus (HIV). HIV causes the immune system to break down so that it can no longer respond effectively to infection. This virus leads to the fatal disease known as acquired immune deficiency syndrome (AIDS). Retrovir slows down the progress of HIV.

This drug is also prescribed for HIV-infected children over 3 months of age who have symptoms of HIV or who have no symptoms but, through testing, have shown evidence of impaired immunity.

Signs and symptoms consistent with HIV disease are significant weight loss, fever, diarrhea, infections, and problems with the nervous system.

Most important fact about this drug

The long-term effects of treatment with zidovudine are unknown. However, treatment with this drug may lead to blood diseases, including granulocytopenia (a severe blood disorder characterized by a sharp decrease of certain types of white blood cells called granulocytes) and severe anemia requiring blood transfusions. This is especially true in people with more advanced HIV and those who start treatment later in the course of their infection.

Also, because Retrovir is not a cure for HIV infections or AIDS, those who are infected may continue to develop complications, including opportunistic infections (infections not usually seen in humans that develop when the immune system falters). Therefore, frequent blood counts by your doctor are strongly advised. Notify your doctor immediately of any changes in your general health.

How should you take this medication?

Take this medication exactly as prescribed by your doctor. Do not share this medication with anyone and do not exceed your recommended dosage. Take it at even intervals every 4 hours around the clock (children every 6 hours).

■ *If you miss a dose...*
Take it as soon as you remember. If it is almost time for your next dose, skip the one you missed and go back to your regular schedule. Do not take 2 doses at once.

■ *Storage instructions...*
Capsules should be stored at room temperature, away from light and moisture. Syrup should be stored at room temperature, away from light.

What side effects may occur?

Side effects cannot be anticipated. If any develop or change in intensity, inform your doctor as soon as possible. Only your doctor can determine if it is safe for you to continue taking Retrovir.

The frequency and severity of side effects associated with the use of Retrovir are greater in people whose infection is more advanced when treatment is started. Sometimes it is difficult to distinguish side effects from the underlying signs of HIV disease or the infections caused by HIV.

■ *More common side effects may include:*
Change in sense of taste, constipation, diarrhea, difficult or labored breathing, dizziness, fever, general feeling of illness, inability to fall or stay asleep, indigestion, loss of appetite, muscle pain, nausea, rash, severe headache, sleepiness, stomach and intestinal pain, sweating, tingling or pins and needles, vomiting, weakness

■ *Less common side effects may include:*
Acne, anxiety, back pain, belching, bleeding from the rectum, bleeding gums, body odor, changeable emotions, chest pain, chills, confusion, cough, decreased mental sharpness, depression, difficulty swallowing, dimness of vision, excess sensitivity to pain, fainting, fatigue, flu-like symptoms, frequent urination, gas, hearing loss, hives, hoarseness, increase in urine volume, inflammation of the sinuses or nose, itching, joint pain, light intolerance, mouth sores, muscle spasm, nervousness, nosebleed, painful or difficult urination, sore throat, swelling of the lip, swelling of the tongue, tremor, twitching, vertigo

Why should this drug not be prescribed?

If you have ever had a life-threatening allergic reaction to Retrovir or any of its ingredients, you should not take this drug.

Special warnings about this medication

This drug has been studied for only a limited period of time. Long-term safety and effectiveness are not known, especially for people who are in a less advanced stage of AIDS or AIDS-related complex (the condition that precedes AIDS), and for those using the drug over a prolonged period of time.

If you develop a blood disease, you may require a blood transfusion, and your doctor may reduce your dose or take you off the drug altogether. Make sure your doctor monitors your blood count on a regular basis.

The use of Retrovir has *not* been shown to reduce the risk of transmission of HIV to others through sexual contact or blood contamination.

Retrovir should be used with extreme caution by people who have a bone marrow disease.

Some people taking Retrovir develop a sensitization reaction, often signaled by a rash. If you notice a rash developing, notify your doctor.

Because little data are available concerning the use of this drug in people with impaired kidney or liver function, check with your doctor before using Retrovir if you have either problem.

Possible food and drug interactions when taking this medication

If Retrovir is taken with certain other drugs, the effects of either could be increased, decreased, or altered. It is especially important to check with your doctor before combining Retrovir with the following:

Acetaminophen (Tylenol)
Amphotericin B (Fungizone, a drug used to treat fungal infections)
Doxorubicin (Adriamycin, a cancer drug)
Aspirin
Dapsone (a drug used to treat leprosy)
Flucytosine (Ancobon)
Indomethacin (Indocin)
Interferon (Intron A, Roferon)
Pentamidine (NebuPent, Pentam)
Phenytoin (Dilantin, an anticonvulsant)
Probenecid (Benemid, an antigout drug)
Vinblastine (Velban, a cancer drug)
Vincristine (Oncovin, a cancer drug)

The combined use of phenytoin and Retrovir will be monitored by your doctor because of the possibility of seizures.

Special information if you are pregnant or breastfeeding

The effects of Retrovir during pregnancy are under study. Use during pregnancy has been shown to protect the developing baby from contracting HIV. If you are pregnant or plan to become pregnant, inform your doctor immediately. This drug may appear in breast milk and could affect a nursing infant. If this medication is essential to your health, your doctor may advise you to discontinue breastfeeding until your treatment is finished.

Recommended dosage

ADULTS

All dosages of Retrovir must be very closely monitored by your physician. The following dosages are general; your physician will tailor the dose to your specific condition.

Capsules and Syrup
For adults who have symptoms of HIV infection, including AIDS, the usual starting dose is 200 milligrams (two 100-milligram capsules or 4 teaspoonfuls of syrup) taken every 4 hours. After 1 month, your doctor may reduce your dose to 100 milligrams taken every 4 hours.

For adults who have HIV infection but no symptoms, the usual dose is 100 milligrams taken every 4 hours while awake.

CHILDREN

The usual starting dose for children 3 months to 12 years of age is determined by body size. While the dose should not exceed 200 milligrams every 6 hours, it must still be individually determined. Safety and efficacy have not been determined for infants under 3 months of age.

Overdosage

Any medication taken in excess can have serious consequences. If you suspect an overdose, seek emergency medical treatment immediately.

■ *Symptoms of Retrovir overdose may include:*
Nausea
Vomiting

Brand name:

RHEUMATREX

See Methotrexate, page 656.

Generic name:

RITRODRINE

See Yutopar, page 798.

Brand name:

SANSERT

Pronounced: SAN-surt
Generic name: Methysergide maleate

Why is this drug prescribed?

Sansert tablets are prescribed to prevent or reduce the intensity and frequency of severe "vascular" headaches (the kind caused by constriction and dilation of arteries within the head). Your doctor may consider treating you with Sansert if you have one or more severe headaches per week, or if your headaches are extremely severe and uncontrollable.

Sansert is preventive medication. Sansert is not a painkiller and cannot diminish a headache that has already developed.

Most important fact about this drug

Long-term treatment with Sansert may cause abnormal tissue growth in the lungs, or around the blood vessels. This may result in cold, numb, painful hands and feet, chest or hip pain, or leg cramps. Therefore, Sansert is used as a preventive measure in people whose headaches are frequent or severe and uncontrollable, and who are under close medical supervision. Report any symptoms you develop to your doctor.

How should you take this medication?

To avoid stomach upset, take Sansert with meals.

Sansert may cause weight gain. You should watch your caloric intake.

Take Sansert exactly as prescribed. To reduce the risk of serious side effects, your doctor will tell you to take Sansert no longer than 6 consecutive months, gradually reducing the dosage during the last 2 or 3 weeks to prevent "rebound" headaches. After completing the 6-month course of treatment, you should take a 3- or 4-week break and then begin taking Sansert for another 6-month stretch, if your doctor advises.

■ *If you miss a dose...*
 Skip the one you missed and go back to your regular schedule. Do not take 2 doses at once.

■ *Storage instructions...*
 Store away from heat, light, and moisture.

What side effects may occur?

Side effects cannot be anticipated. If any develop or change in intensity, inform your doctor as soon as possible. Only your

doctor can determine if it is safe for you to continue taking Sansert.

Diarrhea, nausea, vomiting, abdominal pain, and heartburn are typical early reactions to Sansert; you can avoid these symptoms if you start with a lower dosage of Sansert and increase the amount gradually, and if you always take the medication with meals.

■ *Other potential side effects include:*
 Aching joints or muscles, blood cell abnormalities, constipation, dizziness, drowsiness, exaggerated feeling of well-being, fluid retention, flushing, hair loss (may be temporary), hallucinations or "disconnected" feelings, increased sensitivity to touch, lack of muscular coordination, light-headedness, rapid heartbeat, rash, sleeplessness, weakness, weight gain

If you retain fluid, it may help to lower your dosage, follow a low-salt diet, or take diuretics (water pills).

If you use Sansert for a long time, there is a risk that fibrotic tissue will develop within the abdomen, lungs, heart valves, or other parts of the body. Because of this danger, you should immediately contact your doctor if you experience any of the following:

Abdominal pain
Backache
Breathing difficulty
Chest pain or tightness
Cold, numb, painful hands or feet
Fatigue
General feeling of illness
Intermittent limping because of pain in the
   thigh or buttocks
Leg swelling or pain
Low-grade fever
Painful or difficult urination
Weight loss

Why should this drug not be prescribed?

Do not take Sansert if you have any of the following conditions:

Connective tissue disease
Coronary artery disease
Debilitation from chronic illness
Fibrotic conditions
Hardening of the arteries
Heart valve disease
High blood pressure (severe)
Infection (serious)
Kidney problems
Liver problems
Lung disease
Phlebitis or cellulitis in the legs
Pregnancy

Special warnings about this medication

Remember that long-term use of Sansert may cause unwanted fibrotic changes in various body tissues. Be especially alert for the following symptoms:

Cold, numb, painful hands and feet
Cramps in the legs while walking
Pain in the chest, side, or groin

If you develop any of these symptoms, stop taking Sansert and see your doctor right away.

If fibrotic changes do occur, there is a good chance the condition will disappear when you stop taking Sansert. Thus, corrective surgery may not be necessary.

Sansert tablets contain a food coloring agent called FD&C Yellow No. 5. In some people, it may cause an allergic reaction that includes bronchial asthma. You are at increased risk for this reaction if you are allergic to aspirin.

Possible food and drug interactions when taking this medication

No information is available regarding interactions with Sansert.

Special information if you are pregnant or breastfeeding

Sansert should not be used during pregnancy. If you are pregnant or plan to become pregnant, inform your doctor immediately. It is not known whether Sansert appears in breast milk. If this drug is essential to your health, your doctor may advise you to stop breastfeeding until your treatment is finished.

Recommended dosage

ADULTS

The usual dose is 4 to 8 milligrams daily, taken with meals.

CHILDREN

Sansert is not recommended for use in children.

Overdosage

Although no specific information is available, any medication taken in excess can have serious consequences. If you suspect an overdose of Sansert, seek medical attention immediately.

Brand name:

SEPTRA

See Bactrim, page 523.

Brand name:

SERAX

Pronounced: SER-aks
Generic name: Oxazepam

Why is this drug prescribed?

Serax is used in the treatment of anxiety disorders, including anxiety associated with depression.

This drug seems to be particularly effective for anxiety, tension, agitation, and irritability in older people. It is also prescribed to relieve symptoms of acute alcohol withdrawal.

Serax belongs to a class of drugs known as benzodiazepines.

Most important fact about this drug

Serax can be habit-forming or addicting and can lose its effectiveness over time, as you develop a tolerance for it. You may experience withdrawal symptoms if you stop using the drug abruptly. When discontinuing the drug, your doctor will reduce the dose gradually.

How should you take this medication?

Take Serax exactly as prescribed.

■ *If you miss a dose...*
If you remember within an hour or so, take the dose immediately. If you do not remember until later, skip the dose you missed and go back to your regular schedule. Do not take 2 doses at once.

■ *Storage instructions...*
Store at room temperature in a tightly closed container.

What side effects may occur?

Side effects cannot be anticipated. If any develop or change in intensity, inform your doctor as soon as possible. Only your

doctor can determine if it is safe for you to continue taking Serax. Your doctor should periodically reassess the need for this drug.

■ *More common side effects may include:*
Drowsiness

■ *Less common or rare side effects may include:*
Blood disorders, change in sex drive, dizziness, excitement, fainting, headache, hives, liver problems, loss or lack of muscle control, nausea, skin rashes, sluggishness or unresponsiveness, slurred speech, swelling due to fluid retention, tremors, vertigo, yellowed eyes and skin

■ *Side effects due to rapid decrease or abrupt withdrawal from Serax:*
Abdominal and muscle cramps, convulsions, depressed mood, inability to fall or stay asleep, sweating, tremors, vomiting

Why should this drug not be prescribed?

If you are sensitive to or have ever had an allergic reaction to Serax or other tranquilizers such as Valium, you should not take this medication. Make sure your doctor is aware of any drug reactions you have experienced.

Anxiety or tension related to everyday stress usually does not require treatment with Serax. Discuss your symptoms thoroughly with your doctor.

Serax should not be prescribed if you are being treated for mental disorders more serious than anxiety.

Special warnings about this medication

Serax may cause you to become drowsy or less alert; therefore, you should not drive or operate dangerous machinery or participate in any hazardous activity that requires full mental alertness until you know how this drug affects you.

This medication may cause your blood pressure to drop. If you have any heart problems, consult your doctor before taking this medication.

The 15-milligram tablet of this drug contains the coloring agent FD&C Yellow No. 5, which may cause an allergic reaction. If you are sensitive to aspirin or susceptible to allergies, consult your doctor before taking the tablet.

Possible food and drug interactions when taking this medication

Serax may intensify the effects of alcohol. It may be better not to drink alcohol while taking this medication.

If Serax is taken with certain other drugs, the effects of either could be increased, decreased, or altered. It is especially important to check with your doctor before combining Serax with the following:

Antihistamines such as Benadryl
Narcotic painkillers such as Percocet and
    Demerol
Sedatives such as Seconal and Halcion
Tranquilizers such as Valium and Xanax

Special information
if you are pregnant or breastfeeding

Do not take Serax if you are pregnant or planning to become pregnant. There is an increased risk of birth defects. Serax may appear in breast milk and could affect a nursing infant. If this drug is essential to your health, your doctor may advise you to stop breastfeeding until your treatment with this medication is finished.

Recommended dosage

ADULTS

Mild to Moderate Anxiety with Tension, Irritability, Agitation
The usual dose is 10 to 15 milligrams 3 or 4 times per day.

Severe Anxiety, Depression with Anxiety, or Alcohol Withdrawl
The usual dose is 15 to 30 milligrams, 3 or 4 times per day.

CHILDREN

This medication is not intended for use in children under 6 years of age. Dosage guidelines for children 6 to 12 years of age have not been established. Your doctor will adjust the dosage to fit the child's needs.

ELDERLY

The usual starting dose is 10 milligrams, 3 times a day. Your doctor may increase the dose to 15 milligrams 3 or 4 times a day, if needed.

Overdosage

Although no specific information is available, any medication taken in excess can have serious consequences. If you suspect an overdose of Serax, seek medical attention immediately.

Brand name:

SEROPHENE

See Clomiphene Citrate, page 550.

Generic name:

SERTRALINE

See Zoloft, page 801.

Brand name:

SERUTAN

See Metamucil, page 653.

Brand name:

SINEQUAN

Pronounced: SIN-uh-kwan
Generic name: Doxepin hydrochloride
Other brand name: Adapin

Why is this drug prescribed?

Sinequan is used in the treatment of depression and anxiety. It helps relieve tension, improve sleep, elevate mood, increase energy, and generally ease the feelings of fear, guilt, apprehension, and worry most people experience. It is effective in treating people whose depression and/or anxiety is psychological, associated with alcoholism, or a result of another disease (cancer, for example) or psychotic depressive disorders (severe mental illness). It is in the family of drugs called tricyclic antidepressants.

Most important fact about this drug

Serious, sometimes fatal, reactions have occurred when Sinequan is used in combination with another type of antidepressant called MAO inhibitors. Any drug of this type should be discontinued at least 2 weeks prior to starting treatment with Sinequan, and you should be carefully monitored by your doctor.

If you are taking any prescription or nonprescription drugs, consult with your doctor before taking Sinequan.

How should you take this medication?

Take this medication exactly as prescribed. It may take several weeks for you to feel better.

■ *If you miss a dose...*
If you are taking several doses a day, take the missed dose as soon as you remember, then take any remaining doses for that day at evenly spaced intervals. If it is almost time for your next dose, skip the one you missed and go back to your regular schedule. Never take 2 doses at the same time.

If you are taking a single dose at bedtime and do not remember until the next morning, skip the dose. Do not take a double dose to make up for a missed one.

■ *Storage instructions...*
Store at room temperature.

What side effects may occur?

Side effects cannot be anticipated. If any develop or change in intensity, inform your doctor as soon as possible. Only your doctor can determine if it is safe for you to continue taking Sinequan.

The most common side effect is drowsiness

■ *Less common or rare side effects may include:*
Blurred vision, breast development in males, bruises, buzzing or ringing in the ears, changes in sex drive, chills, confusion, constipation, diarrhea, difficulty urinating, disorientation, dizziness, dry mouth, enlarged breasts, fatigue, fluid retention, flushing, fragmented or incomplete movements, hair loss, hallucinations, headache, high fever, high or low blood sugar, inappropriate breast milk secretion, indigestion, inflammation of the mouth, itching and skin rash, lack of muscle control, loss of appetite, loss of coordination, low blood pressure, nausea, nervousness, numbness, poor bladder control, rapid heartbeat, red or brownish spots on the skin, seizures, sensitivity to

light, severe muscle stiffness, sore throat, sweating, swelling of the testicles, taste disturbances, tingling sensation, tremors, vomiting, weakness, weight gain, yellow eyes and skin

Why should this drug not be prescribed?

If you are sensitive to or have ever had an allergic reaction to Sinequan or similar antidepressants, you should not take this medication. Make sure that your doctor is aware of any drug reactions that you have experienced.

Unless you are directed to do so by your doctor, do not take this medication if you have the eye condition known as glaucoma or difficulty urinating.

Special warnings about this medication

Sinequan may cause you to become drowsy or less alert; driving or operating dangerous machinery or participating in any hazardous activity that requires full mental alertness is not recommended.

Notify your doctor or dentist that you are taking Sinequan if you have a medical emergency, and before you have surgery or dental treatment.

Possible food and drug interactions when taking this medication

Alcohol increases the danger in a Sinequan overdose. Do not drink alcohol while taking this medication.

Never combine Sinequan with the other antidepressants known as MAO inhibitors. Drugs in this category include Navdil, Parnate, and Marplan.

If Sinequan is taken with certain other drugs, the effects of either could be increased, decreased, or altered. It is especially important to check with your doctor before combining Sinequan with the following:

Amphetamines such as Dexedrine
Antihistamines such as Benadryl and Tavist
Baclofen (Lioresal)
Benztropine (Cogentin)
Carbamazepine (Tegretol)
Central nervous system depressants such as
    Darvon, Valium, and Xanax
Cimetidine (Tagamet)
Clonidine (Catapres)
Epinephrine (Epipen)
Fluoxetine (Prozac)
Guanethidine (Ismelin)
Quinidine (Quinidex)
Tolazamide (Tolinase)

Special information if you are pregnant or breastfeeding

The effects of Sinequan during pregnancy have not been adequately studied. If you are pregnant or planning to become pregnant, inform your doctor immediately. Sinequan may appear in breast milk and could affect a nursing infant. If this medication is essential to your health, your doctor may advise you to discontinue breastfeeding your baby until your treatment is finished.

Recommended dosage

ADULTS

The starting dose for mild to moderate illness is usually 75 milligrams per day. This dose can be increased or decreased by your doctor according to individual need. The usual ideal dose ranges from 75 milligrams per day to 150 milligrams per day, although it can be as low as 25 to 50 milligrams per day. The total daily dose can be given once a day or divided into smaller doses. If you are taking this drug once a day, the recommended dose is 150 milligrams at bedtime.

The 150-milligram capsule strength is intended for long-term therapy only and is not recommended as a starting dose.

For more severe illness, gradually increased doses of up to 300 milligrams may be required as determined by your doctor.

CHILDREN

Safety and effectiveness have not been established for use in children under 12 years of age.

ELDERLY

A once-a-day dosage should be carefully adjusted by your doctor, depending upon the severity of your illness.

Overdosage

■ *Symptoms of Sinequan overdose may include:*
Blurred vision, coma, convulsions, decreased intestinal movement, dilated pupils, drowsiness, excessive dryness of mouth, high or low body temperature, irregular or rapid heartbeat, low or high blood pressure, overactive reflexes, severe breathing problems, stupor, urinary problems

If you experience any of these symptoms, seek medical attention immediately.

Brand name:

STUARTNATAL PLUS

Pronounced: STU-art NAY-tal plus
Generic ingredients: Supplemental vitamins and minerals
Other brand name: Materna, Natalins

Why is this drug prescribed?

Stuartnatal Plus contains vitamins and minerals including iron, calcium, zinc, and folic acid. The tablets are given during pregnancy and after childbirth to ensure an adequate supply of these critical nutrients. They may also be prescribed to improve a woman's nutritional status before she becomes pregnant.

Most important fact about this drug

Nutritional supplementation is especially important during pregnancy. Be sure to take Stuartnatal Plus regularly as prescribed.

How should you take this medication?

Take Stuartnatal Plus exactly as prescribed. The usual dosage is 1 tablet per day with or without food.

■ *If you miss a dose...*
Take it as soon as you remember, then return to your regular schedule.

■ *Storage instructions...*
Store at room temperature, away from light or excessive heat, in a tightly closed container.

Why should this drug not be prescribed?

There are no known reasons to avoid this preparation.

Special information
if you are pregnant or breastfeeding

Pregnancy and breastfeeding impose special nutritional demands on the mother. A vitamin and mineral supplement can help ensure that there are enough nutrients for both you and your baby.

Recommended dosage

ADULTS

Before, during, and after pregnancy, take 1 tablet daily, or as directed by your doctor.

Overdosage

Although no specific overdose information is available, even a nutritional supplement in extremely large amounts can have serious consequences. If you suspect an overdose of

Stuartnatal Plus, seek medical attention immediately.

Generic name:

SULFANILAMIDE

See AVC, page 521.

Generic name:

SULFISOXAZOLE

See Gantrisin, page 610.

Generic name:

SULINDAC

See Clinoril, page 548.

Brand name:

SULTRIN

Pronounced: *SUL-trin*
Generic ingredients: *Sulfathiazone,*
  Sulfacetamide, Sulfabenzamide
Other brand name: *Triple Sulfa*

Why is this drug prescribed?

Sultrin vaginal cream and vaginal tablets are used to treat bacterial vaginitis (bacteria-caused inflammation of the vagina with a gray or yellow discharge like a thin flour paste and a fishy odor).

Because Sultrin is effective only against one type of bacteria, your doctor may run tests before prescribing this medication.

Most important fact about this drug

Keep using Sultrin for the full time of treatment, even if the infection seems to have disappeared. If you stop too soon, the infection could return. Keep using Sultrin even if you have a period.

How should you take this medication?

Use this medication exactly as prescribed.

To administer, follow these steps:

1. Load the applicator to the fill line with cream, or unwrap a tablet, wet it with warm water, and place it in the applicator as shown in the instructions you received with the product.
2. Lie on your back with knees drawn up.
3. Gently insert the applicator high into the vagina and push the plunger.
4. Withdraw the applicator and discard it if disposable, or wash with soap and water.

To keep the medication from getting on your clothing, wear a sanitary napkin. Do not use a tampon because it will absorb the medicine. Wear cotton underwear; avoid synthetic fabrics such as rayon or nylon.

Do not scratch if you can help it. Scratching can cause more irritation and can spread the infection.

■ *If you miss a dose...*
Apply it as soon as you remember. If it is almost time for your next dose, skip the one you missed and go back to your regular schedule.

■ *Storage instructions...*
Store away from heat and light. Do not store the tablets near moisture; protect the cream from freezing.

What side effects may occur?

Side effects cannot always be predicted. If any do develop, be sure to tell your doctor as soon as possible. Only your doctor can determine if it is safe for you to continue taking Sultrin.

■ *Side effects may include:*
Irritation in the vagina or external genitals
In rare cases, severe blistering in the
mouth, throat, nose, and the area
between the vagina and the rectum

Why should this drug not be prescribed?

Do not use Sultrin vaginal cream or vaginal
tablets if you have kidney disease or have
ever had an allergic reaction to sulfa drugs
of any kind.

You should not start using Sultrin if you are
in the final weeks of pregnancy or are
nursing.

Be sure to tell your doctor about any drug
reactions you have experienced.

Special warnings about this medication

While using Sultrin, avoid vaginal
intercourse.

Sultrin vaginal cream and vaginal tablets are
for use only within the vagina. You should
not take the vaginal tablets or the vaginal
cream by mouth.

Sultrin may be absorbed through the lining
of the vagina and can affect your whole
body instead of just the area being treated.
If you begin to feel any reactions or develop
a rash, stop using the medication at once
and call your doctor.

If you experience a sore throat, fever,
paleness, red or purple areas on the skin, or
yellowing of the skin or eyes, call your
doctor immediately; these symptoms may
indicate a serious blood disorder.

Possible food and drug interactions when taking this medication

No interactions have been reported.

Special information if you are pregnant or breastfeeding

The safety of Sultrin during pregnancy has
not been confirmed, and its use is generally
avoided, especially at the end of pregnancy.

If you are nursing, do not begin treatment
with Sultrin since its effects may be harmful
to your baby. If your doctor considers this
medication essential to your health, he or
she may have you stop breastfeeding until
your treatment is finished.

Recommended dosage

ADULTS

Sultrin Vaginal Cream
The usual dose is 1 applicatorful twice a
day for 4 to 6 days.

If your discharge does not clear up, your
doctor may have you repeat the treatment,
using one-half to one-quarter the original
dose.

Sultrin Vaginal Tablets
Insert 1 tablet into the vagina morning and
evening for 10 days, using the applicator
that comes in the package. Your doctor may
have you repeat the treatment if necessary.

Overdosage

There are no reports of overdosage with this
medication. If you use too much of any
medidation, however, you may develop
serious problems. If you suspect an overdose
of Sultrin, seek medical attention
immediately.

Generic name:

SUMATRIPTAN

See Imitrex Injection, page 620.

Brand name:

SUMYCIN

See Achromycin V Capsules, page 499.

Generic name:

SUPPLEMENTAL VITAMINS AND MINERALS

See Stuartnatal Plus, page 746.

Brand name:

SUPRAX

Pronounced: SUE-praks
Generic name: Cefixime

Why is this drug prescribed?

Suprax, a cephalosporin antibiotic, is prescribed for bacterial infections of the chest, ears, urinary tract, and throat and for uncomplicated gonorrhea.

Most important fact about this drug

If you are allergic to either penicillin or cephalosporin antibiotics in any form, consult your doctor *before taking* Suprax. There is a possibility that you are allergic to both types of medication; and if a reaction occurs, it could be extremely severe. If you take the drug and feel signs of a reaction, seek medical attention immediately.

How should you take this medication?

Suprax can be taken with or without food. If the medication causes stomach upset, take it with meals. Food, however, will slow down the rate at which medication is absorbed into your bloodstream.

If you are taking a liquid form of Suprax, use the specially marked measuring spoon to measure each dose accurately. Shake well before using.

It is important that you finish taking all of this medication even if you are feeling better, in order to obtain the medicine's maximum benefit.

■ *If you miss a dose...*
If you are taking this medication once a day and you forget to take a dose, take it as soon as you remember. Wait at least 10 to 12 hours before taking your next dose. Then return to your regular schedule.

If you are taking this medication 2 times a day and you forget to take a dose, take it as soon as you remember and take your next dose 5 to 6 hours later. Then go back to your regular schedule.

If you are taking this medication 3 times a day and you forget to take a dose, take it as soon as you remember and take your next dose 2 to 4 hours later. Then return to your regular schedule.

■ *Storage instructions...*
Suprax liquid may be kept for 14 days, either at room temperature or in the refrigerator. Keep the bottle tightly closed. Do not store in damp places. Keep out of reach of children and away from direct light and heat. Discard any unused portion after 14 days.

What side effects may occur?

Side effects cannot be anticipated. If any develop or change in intensity, inform your doctor as soon as possible. Only your doctor can determine if it is safe for you to continue taking Suprax.

■ *More common side effects may include:*
Abdominal pain
Gas

Indigestion
Loose stools
Mild diarrhea
Nausea
Vomiting

- *Less common side effects may include:*
Colitis, dizziness, fever, headaches, hives, itching, skin rashes, vaginitis

- *Rare side effects may include:*
Bleeding, decrease in urine output, seizures, severe abdominal or stomach cramps, severe diarrhea (sometimes accompanied by blood), shock, skin redness

Why should this drug not be prescribed?

If you are sensitive to or have ever had an allergic reaction to Suprax, other cephalosporin antibiotics, or any form of penicillin, you should not take this medication. Make sure that your doctor is aware of any drug reactions that you have experienced.

Special warnings about this medication

Notify your doctor if you have had allergic reactions to penicillins or other cephalosporin antibiotics.

If you have a history of stomach or intestinal disease such as colitis, check with your doctor before taking Suprax.

If your symptoms of infection do not improve within a few days, or if they get worse, notify your doctor immediately.

If you suffer nausea, vomiting, or severe diarrhea while taking Suprax, check with your doctor before taking a diarrhea medication. Some of these medications, such as Lomotil and Paregoric, may make your diarrhea worse or cause it to last longer.

If you are a diabetic, it is important to note that Suprax may cause false urine-sugar test results. Notify your doctor that you are taking this medication before being tested for sugar in the urine. Do not change diet or dosage of diabetes medication without first consulting with your doctor.

When prescribing Suprax, your doctor may perform laboratory tests to make certain it is effective against the bacteria causing the infection. Some bacteria do not respond to Suprax, so do not give it to other people or use it for other infections.

If you have a kidney disorder, check with your doctor before taking Suprax. You may need a reduced dose of this medication because of your medical condition.

Repeated use of Suprax may result in an overgrowth of bacteria that do not respond to the medication and can cause a secondary infection. Therefore, do not save this medication for use at another time. Take this medication only when directed to do so by your doctor.

Possible food and drug interactions when taking this medication

No interactions with food or other drugs have been reported.

Special information if you are pregnant or breastfeeding

The effects of Suprax during pregnancy have not been adequately studied. If you are pregnant or plan to become pregnant, inform your doctor immediately. Suprax may appear in breast milk and could affect a nursing infant. If this medication is essential to your health, your doctor may advise you to discontinue breastfeeding your baby until your treatment with this medication is finished.

Recommended dosage

ADULTS

Infections Other Than Gonorrhea
The usual adult dose is 400 milligrams daily. This may be taken as a single 400 milligram tablet once a day or as a 200-milligram tablet every 12 hours. If you have kidney disease, the dose may be lower.

Uncomplicated Gonorrhea
A single 400-milligram oral dose is usually prescribed.

CHILDREN

The safety and effectiveness of Suprax in children less than 6 months old have not been established. The usual child's dose is 8 milligrams of liquid per 2.2 pounds of body weight per day. This may be given as a single dose or in 2 half doses every 12 hours. Children weighing more than 110 pounds or older than 12 years of age should be treated with an adult dose.

If your child has a middle ear infection (otitis media), your doctor will probably prescribe Suprax suspension. The tablet form is less effective against this type of infection.

ELDERLY

Your doctor may start you on a low dosage because this drug is eliminated from your body by the kidneys and kidney function tends to decrease with age.

Overdosage

Any medication taken in excess can cause symptoms of overdose. If you suspect an overdose, seek medical attention immediately.

■ *Symptoms of Suprax overdose may include:*
Blood in the urine
Diarrhea

Nausea
Upper abdominal pain
Vomiting

Brand name:

SURMONTIL

Pronounced: SIR-mon-til
Generic name: Trimipramine maleate

Why is this drug prescribed?
Surmontil is used to treat depression. It is a member of the family of drugs known as tricyclic antidepressants.

Most important fact about this drug
Serious, sometimes fatal, reactions ahve been known to occur when drugs such as Surmontil are taken with another type of antidepressant called an MAO inhibitor. Drugs in this category include Nardil, Marplan, and Parnate. Do not take Surmontil within 2 weeks of taking one of these drugs. Make sure your doctor and pharmacist know of all the medications you are taking.

How should you take this medication?
Surmontil may be taken in 1 dose at bedtime. Alternatively, the total daily dosage may be divided into smaller amounts taken during the day. If you are on long-term therapy with Surmontil, the single bedtime dose is preferred.

It is important to take Surmontil exactly as prescribed, even if the drug seems to have no effect. It may take up to 4 weeks for its benefits to appear.

Surmontil can make your mouth dry. Sucking hard candy or chewing gum can help this problem.

■ *If you miss a dose...*
Take it as soon as you remember. If it is almost time for the next dose, skip the one you missed and go back to your regular schedule. Do not take 2 doses at once. If you take Surmontil once a day at bedtime and you miss a dose, do not take it in the morning. It could cause disturbing side effects during the day.

■ *Storage instructions...*
Store at room temperature in a tightly closed container. Capsules in blister strips should be protected from moisture.

What side effects may occur?
Side effects cannot be anticipated. If any develop or change in intensity, inform your doctor as soon as possible. Only your doctor can determine if it is safe for you to continue taking Surmontil.

■ *Side effects may include:*
Abdominal cramps, agitation, anxiety, black tongue, blocked intestine, blood disorders, blurred vision, breast development in the male, confusion (especially in elderly people), constipation, delusions, diarrhea, difficulty urinating, dilated pupils, disorientation, dizziness, drowsiness, dry mouth, excessive or spontaneous milk excretion, fatigue, fever, flushing, fluttery or throbbing heartbeat, frequent urination, hair loss, hallucinations, headache, heart attack, high blood pressure, high blood sugar, hives, impotence, increased or decreased sex drive, inflammation of the mouth, insomnia, irregular heart rate, lack of coordination, loss of appetite, low blood pressure, low blood sugar, nausea, nightmares, numbness, peculiar taste in mouth, purple or reddish-brown spots on skin, rapid heartbeat, restlessness, ringing in the ears, seizures, sensitivity to light, skin itching, skin rash, sore throat, stomach upset, stroke, sweating, swelling of breasts, swelling of face and tongue, swelling of testicles, swollen glands, tingling, pins and needles, tremors, visual problems, vomiting, weakness, weight gain or loss, yellowing of the skin and whites of the eyes

Why should this drug not be prescribed?
Surmontil should not be used if you are recovering from a recent heart attack.

You should not take Surmontil if you are sensitive to it or have ever had an allergic reaction to it or to other similar drugs such as Tofranil.

Special warnings about this medication
Use Surmontil cautiously if you have a seizure disorder, the eye condition known as glaucoma, heart disease, or a liver disorder. Also use caution if you have thyroid disease or are taking thyroid medication. People who have had problems urinating should also be careful about taking Surmontil.

Nausea, headache, and a general feeling of illness may result if you suddenly stop taking Surmontil. This does not mean you are addicted, but you should follow your doctor's instructions closely when discontinuing the drug.

This drug may impair your ability to drive a car or operate potentially dangerous machinery. Do not participate in any activities that require full alertness if you are unsure of the drug's effect on you.

Possible food and drug interactions when taking this medication
People who are taking antidepressants known as MAO inhibitors (Parnate, Nardil, or Marplan) should not take Surmontil. Wait 2 weeks after stopping an MAO inhibitor before you begin taking Surmontil.

If Surmontil is taken with certain other drugs, the effects of either could be increased, decreased, or altered. It is especially important to check with your doctor before combining Surmontil with the following:

Antispasmodic drugs such as Cogentin
Cimetidine (Tagamet)
Guanethidine (Ismelin)
Local anesthetics
Local decongestants such as Dristan Nasal
   Spray
Oral nasal decongestants such as Sudafed
Stimulants such as EpiPen
Thyroid medications such as Synthroid

Extreme drowsiness and other potentially serious effects may result if you drink alcoholic beverages while you are taking Surmontil.

Special information
if you are pregnant or breastfeeding
The effects of Surmontil in pregnancy have not been adequately studied. Pregnant women should use Surmontil only when the potential benefits clearly outweigh the potential risks.

Recommended dosage

ADULTS

The usual starting dose is 75 milligrams per day, divided into equal smaller doses. Your doctor may gradually increase your dose to 150 milligrams per day, divided into smaller doses. Doses over 200 milligrams a day are not recommended. Doses in long-term therapy may range from 50 to 150 milligrams daily. You can take this total daily dosage at bedtime or spread it throughout the day.

CHILDREN

Safety and effectiveness of Surmontil in children have not been established.

ELDERLY AND ADOLESCENTS

Dosages usually start at 50 milligrams per day. Your doctor may increase the dose to 100 milligrams a day, if needed.

Overdosage
Any medication taken in excess can have serious consequences. An overdose of Surmontil can be fatal. If you suspect an overdose, seek medical help immediately.

■ *Symptoms of Surmontil overdose may include:*
Agitation, coma, convulsions, difficulty breathing, dilated pupils, discolored bluish skin, drowsiness, heart failure, high fever, involuntary movement, irregular heart rate, lack of coordination, low blood pressure, muscle rigidity, rapid heartbeat, restlessness, shock, stupor, sweating, vomiting

Brand name:

SYLLACT
See Metamucil, page 653.

Brand name:

SYNAREL
Pronounced: SIN-er-el
Generic name: Nafarelin acetate

Why is this drug prescribed?
Synarel is used to relieve the symptoms of endometriosis, including menstrual cramps or low back pain during menstruation, painful intercourse, painful bowel movements, and abnormal and heavy menstrual bleeding.

Endometriosis is a condition in which fragments of the tissue that lines the uterus are found in the other parts of the pelvic cavity. Synarel is also used to treat unusually early puberty in children of both sexes.

Some doctors prescribe Synarel as a contraceptive for both men and women.

Most important fact about this drug

Although Synarel usually stops ovulation and menstruation, there is still a possibility of becoming pregnant while taking the medication. Since Synarel could harm a fetus, be sure to use a nonhormonal, barrier form of birth control such as condoms and diaphragms. If you should become pregnant, stop the drug and tell your doctor immediately.

How should you take this medication?

Take this medication exactly as prescribed.

Synarel is sprayed into one nostril in the morning and the other nostril in the evening. If your doctor increases the dose, you will spray Synarel into both nostrils morning and evening.

Try not to sneeze during or immediately after spraying Synarel into your nostrils.

Wait 2 hours after taking Synarel before using a decongestant spray or drops.

You should not use Synarel for more than 6 months. If your symptoms recur after you have finished taking the medication, your doctor will usually not prescribe it again.

Before you use each new bottle of Snyarel for the first time, you have to prime the spray pump. Remove the plastic wrap from the spray bottle and hold it in an upright position pointed away from you. Applying pressure evenly to the "shoulders," push down quickly and firmly 7 to 10 times.

Usually the spray will appear after about 7 pumps. Priming need only be done once.

To use the Synarel Nasal Spray Unit, follow these steps:

1. Gently blow your nose to clear both nostrils.
2. Remove the safety clip and clear plastic dust cover from the spray bottle.
3. Bend your head forward a little and put the spray tip into one nostril. Close the other nostril with your finger.
4. Applying pressure evenly to the "shoulders," quickly and firmly pump the sprayer one time while gently sniffing in.
5. Remove the sprayer from your nose and tilt your head backwards for a few seconds. Do not take additional sprays unless your doctor has specifically instructed you to do so.
6. Wipe tip of the pump with a soft cloth or tissue after each use.

■ *If you miss a dose...*
Take it as soon as you remember. If it is almost time for your next dose, skip the one you missed and go back to your regular schedule. Never try to "catch up" by doubling the dose.

Try not to miss any doses. If you miss successive doses, bleeding and ovulation can start again, and you could become pregnant.

■ *Storage instructions...*
Store the Synarel bottle upright at room temperature. Protect from excessive heat and freezing. Keep away from light.

What side effects may occur?

Side effects cannot be anticipated. If any develop or change in intensity, inform your doctor as soon as possible. Only your doctor can determine whether it is safe for you to continue taking Synarel.

■ *More common side effects may include:*
Acne, decreased in breast size, decreased sex drive, depression, dry skin, hair growth, headaches, hot flashes, insomnia, muscle pain, nasal inflammation, nasal irritation, oily skin, rapidly shifting or changing emotions, swelling due to fluid retention, vaginal dryness, weight gain

■ *Less common or rare side effects may include:*
Burning or prickling sensation, discharge of milk from the breast, distension of breast milk, eye pain, flat or bumpy skin rash, fluttery or throbbing heartbeat, hives, increased sex drive, severe joint pain, yellowish-brown spots on the skin, weakness, weight loss

When Synarel is used in the treatment of early puberty, it causes body odor and a transient increase in the amount of pubic hair.

Why should this drug not be prescribed?
Do not take Synarel is you are sensitive to it or have ever had an allergic reaction to it or to any of its ingredients.

Your doctor should not prescribe Synarel if you have undiagnosed vaginal bleeding between menstrual periods.

You should not take Synarel if you are pregnant or breastfeeding.

Special warnings about this medication
Because Synarel works by temporarily reducing the body's production of estrogen, you may experience some of the same changes that normally occur at the time of menopause when the body's production of estrogen decreases naturally. For the first 2 months after you start using Synarel, you may have some irregular vaginal bleeding. This will stop by itself.

Your menstrual periods should stop completely during Synarel therapy. If you continue to bleed regularly, or if you spot or bleed between periods, inform your physician immediately. Vaginal bleeding can occur if you are not following your doctor's instructions carefully or if you need a higher dosage of the medication.

Synarel can cause vaginal dryness. If this is a problem, especially during sexual intercourse, you may want to use vaginal lubricant. Ask your doctor or pharmacist for a recommendation.

Synarel may cause a small amount of bone loss over the course of your treatment. If you consume large amounts of alcohol, smoke, have a strong family history of osteoporosis, or use drugs that can reduce bone mass such as anticonvulsants or steroids, discuss your condition with your doctor before using Synarel. It may be wiser for you to take another medication.

If your nasal passages become inflamed, your doctor may prescribe a medication to relieve your congestion while you are taking Synarel.

Possible food and drug interactions when taking this medication
No interactions have been reported.

Special information if you are pregnant or breastfeeding
Although the effects of Synarel during pregnancy have not been adequately studied, it is known that the medication could cause harm to a developing baby. If you are pregnant, inform your doctor immediately. Use a barrier method of birth control to prevent pregnancy while you are taking this medication.

It is not known whether Synarel appears in breast milk. If this drug is essential to your health, your doctor will advise you to discontinue breastfeeding until your treatment with the medication if finished.

Recommended dosage

The recommended dosage of Synarel is 400 micrograms daily, divided into 2 doses—one spray (200 micrograms) into one nostril in the morning and one spray into the other nostril in the evening. Start your treatment between days 2 and 4 of your menstrual cycle.

If the above dosage does not stop your menstrual period after 2 months of treatment, your doctor may increase your dosage to 800 micrograms daily—one spray into each nostril in the morning and one spray into each nostril in the evening.

Treatment should last no more than 6 months.

Overdosage

Although there is no information on Synarel overdose, any medication taken in excess can have serious consequences. If you suspect an overdose, seek medical attention immediately.

Brand name:

SYNTHROID

Pronounced: SINTH-roid
Generic name: Levothyroxine
Other brand names: Levothroid, Levoxine

Why is this drug prescribed?

Synthroid, a synthetic thyroid hormone available in tablet or injectable form, may be given in any of the following cases:

If your own thyroid gland is not making enough hormone;

If you have a goiter or are at risk for developing goiter;

If you need a "suppression test" to determine whether your thyroid gland is making too much hormone;

If you have received neck irradiation for cancer, to prevent development of thyroid gland cancer.

Most important fact about this drug

Although Synthroid will speed up your metabolism, it is not effective as a weight-loss drug and should not be used as such. An overdose may cause life-threatening side effects, especially if you take Synthroid with an appetite-suppressant medication.

How should you take this medication?

Take Synthroid exactly as directed. Take no more or less than the prescribed amount. Take your dose at the same time every day for consistent effect.

If a child cannot swallow whole tablets, you may crush a Synthroid tablet and mix it into a spoonful of liquid or sprinkle it over a small amount of food such as cooked cereal or applesauce. Give this mixture while it is very fresh; never store it for future use.

If you are taking Synthroid because your thyroid gland does not make enough hormone, you may need the medication indefinitely.

While taking Synthroid, your doctor will perform periodic blood tests to determine whether you are getting the right amount.

■ *If you miss a dose...*
  Take it as soon as you remember. If it is almost ime for your next dose, skip the one you missed and go back to your regular schedule. Never take 2 doses at the same time.

■ *Storage instructions...*
Keep this medication in a tightly closed container. Store it at room temperature.

What side effects may occur?
Side effects from Synthroid, other than overdose symptoms, are rare. Children who are treated with Synthroid may initially lose some hair, but this effect is temporary. However, excessive dosage or a too rapid increase in dosage may lead to over stimulation of the thyroid gland.

■ *Symptoms of overstimulation may include:*
Abdominal cramps, changes in appetite, chest pain, diarrhea, fever, headache, heat intolerance, increased heart rate, irregular heartbeat, irritability, nausea, nervousness, palpitations, sleeplessness, sweating, tremors, weight loss

Why should this drug not be prescribed?
You should not be treated with Synthroid if you have ever had an allergic reaction to it; your thyroid gland is making too much thyroid hormone; or your adrenal glands are not making enough corticosteroid hormone.

Special warnings about this medication
You should receive low doses of Synthroid, under very close supervision, if you are an older person, or if you suffer from angina (chest pain caused by a heart condition).

If you have diabetes mellitus or diabetes insipidus, or if your body makes insufficient adrenal corticosteroid hormone, Synthroid will tend to make your symptoms worse. If you take medication for any of these disorders, the dosage will probably have to be adjusted once you begin taking Synthroid.

Possible food and drug interactions when taking this medication
If Synthroid is taken with certain other drugs, the effects of either could be increased, decreased, or altered. It is especially important to check with your doctor before combining Synthroid with the following:

Antacids such as Mylanta
Antidiabetic drugs such as Diabinese and Glucotrol
Blood thinners such as Coumadin
Cholestyramine drugs such as Questran
Colestipol (Colestid)
Epinephrine (Epipen)
Estrogen or contraceptive pills with estrogen such as Ortho-Novum, Ovral, and Premarin
Insulin
Lovastatin (Mevacor)
Phenytoin (Dilantin)
Tricyclic antidepressants such as Elavil and Tofranil

If you are having a blood test to determine whether your dosage of Synthroid is correct, make sure your doctor knows about other medications you may be taking. Any of the following drugs may interfere with the results of the thyroid-level test:

Androgens
Corticosteroids such as Decadron and prednisone
Estrogens such as Premarin
Iodine-containing drugs
Oral contraceptive pills containing estrogen
Salicylate-containing drugs such as aspirin

Special Information
if you are pregnant or breastfeeding
If you need to take synthroid because of a thyroid hormone deficiency, you can continue to take the medication during pregnancy. Once your baby is born, you may breastfeed while continuing to take Synthroid.

Recommended dosage

Your doctor will tailor the dosage to meet your individual requirements, taking into consideration the status of your thyroid gland and other medical conditions you may have.

Overdosage

If you suspect a Synthroid overdose, seek medical attention immediately. Taken in excess, the drug may have serious consequences.

■ *Symptoms of Synthroid overdose may include:*
Abdominal cramps, chest pain, diarrhea, excessive sweating, fever, headaches, heat intolerance, irregular heartbeat, nervousness, palpitations, rapid heartbeat, tremors, trouble sleeping, weight loss

Generic name:

TACRINE

See Cognex, page 552.

Generic name:

TAMOXIFEN

See Nolvadex, page 687.

Brand name:

TAXOL

Pronounced: TACKS-all
Generic name: Paclitaxel

Why is this drug prescribed?

Taxol is used to treat cancer of the ovary. An extract of the bark of the Pacific yew tree, it works by interfering with the growth of cancer cells.

Some doctors also prescribe Taxol to treat breast cancer and certain kinds of lung cancer.

Most important fact about this drug

Taxol interferes with the growth of normal body cells as well as cancer cells. This can cause serious side effects. Be sure to keep your regular appointments with the doctor, so that any dangerous conditions that may be developing can be corrected before they become severe.

How should you take this medication?

To prevent allergic reactions, your doctor will treat you with steroids (Deltasone, Medrol, Decadron), diphenhydramine (Benadryl), and H2 antagonists (Tagamet, Zantac) before giving you Taxol.

Taxol must be given intravenously by a doctor, medical technician, or nurse, usually in a hospital or clinic. It is a powerful drug and must be handled carefully.

■ *If you miss a dose...*
Call your doctor for instructions as soon as you remember.

■ *Storage instructions...*
Taxol is not for use at home.

What side effects may occur?

Side effects cannot be anticipated. If any develop or change in intensity, inform your doctor immediately. Only your doctor can determine if it is safe for you to continue using Taxol.

■ *More common side effects may include:*
Allergic reactions, anemia, bleeding, blood infections, burning or tingling sensations, chest pains, diarrhea, difficult or labored breathing, fever, flushing, hair loss, imflammation of internal membranes, joint pain, low blood pressure, muscular pain, nausea, rash, slow heartbeat, upper

respiratory tract infections, urinary tract infections, vomiting

■ *Less common or rare side effects may include:*
Fainting, grand mal epileptic seizures, heart attack, irregular or rapid heartbeat

Why should this drug not be prescribed?
Your doctor will not give you Taxol if you are sensitive to it or have ever had an allergic reaction to it or to other medications that contain Cremophor EL, a type of castor oil.

Taxol can destroy white blood cells necessary to fight infection. If you have too few white blood cells, you may develop severe infections or diseases such as acute leukemia, and rheumatoid arthritis. Before prescribing Taxol, your doctor will test your blood. If your white cell count is abnormally low, the doctor will not use Taxol.

Special warnings about this medication
A few women have had severe reactions such as shortness of breath, low blood pressure, swelling, and widespread hives while taking Taxol. To prevent these symptoms from occurring, your doctor should start you on medicine for them *before* giving you Taxol. If you have a severe reaction to this drug, you should stop taking it immediately and get prompt medical treatment.

Taxol temporarily impairs the body's ability to produce infection-fighting white blood cells. Avoid people with infections and check with your doctor immediately if you think you have caught something or if you have fever, chills, muscle aches, lower back pain and pain when urinating.

Taxol can lower the number of platelets in your blood, interfering with normal blood clotting. Avoid contact sports or other situations where injury could occur. Report unusal bleeding or bruising, bloody stools, or blood in the urine. Be careful with sharp objects and even items such as your toothbrush, toothpicks or dental floss.

Possible food and drug interactions when taking this medication
If Taxol is used with certain other drugs, the effect of either medication could be increased, decreased, or altered.

If you take Taxol *after* taking cisplatin (Platinol, another anticancer drug), your blood may not be able to produce enough disease-fighting white blood cells. If both these drugs are necessary for your treatment, your doctor may prescribe Taxol *before* cisplatin.

Ketoconazole (Nizoral) may prevent Taxol from working as effectively as it should. If you are taking both these medications, your physician will monitor your condition carefully.

Because of the danger of severe reactions, your doctor will avoid giving you medications—such as cyclosporine (Sandimmune) given by injection—that contain Cremophor EL, a type of castor oil.

Special information if you are pregnant or breastfeeding
The effects of Taxol during pregnancy have not been adequately studied, but it is thought that the medication could harm a developing baby. If you are pregnant or plan to become pregnant, inform your doctor immediately. Your physician will probably suggest that you use some form of contraception to prevent pregnancy while you are taking Taxol.

It is not known whether Taxol appears in breast milk. Your doctor may advise you to discontinue breastfeeding until your treatment with Taxol is finished.

Recommended dosage

At approximately 6 and 12 hours before taking Taxol, you will be given a 20-milligram oral dose of dexamethasone (Decadron). Then, 30 to 60 minutes before Taxol, you will get 50 milligrams of diphenhydramine (Benadryl) and either 300 milligrams of cimetidine (Tagamet) or 50 milligrams of ranitidine (Zantac) by intravenous injection.

The usual dosage of Taxol is 135 milligrams per square meter of body surface given intravenously over a 24-hour period every 3 weeks. Larger doses have not proved more effective. Your doctor will carefully monitor your blood counts while you are taking the medication to make sure that you have enough white blood cells to fight a possible infection. If your white blood cell count is low, your dosage may be decreased, or your treatment may be temporarily stopped.

Overdosage

If you suspect an overdose, call your doctor immediately.

■ *Symptoms of Taxol overdose may include:*
   Burning, prickling, or tingling in the hands or feet
   Inflammation of internal membranes such as those in the mouth and throat

Brand name:

TENUATE

Pronounced: TEN-you-ate
Generic name: Diethylpropion hydrochloride

Why is this drug prescribed?

Tenuate, an appetite suppressant, is prescribed for short-term use (a few weeks)

as part of an overall diet plan for weight reduction. It is available in two forms: immediate-release tablets (Tenuate) and controlled-release tablets (Tenuate Dospan). Tenuate should be used with a behavior modification program.

Most important fact about this drug

Tenuate will lose its effectiveness within a few weeks. When this begins to happen, you should discontinue the medicine rather than increase the dosage.

How should you take this medication?

Take this medication exactly as prescribed. Tenuate may be habit-forming and can be addicting.

If you are taking Tenuate Dospan (the controlled release formulation), do not crush or chew the tablets. Swallow the medication whole.

■ *If you miss a dose...*
   If you are taking the immediate-release form of Tenuate, go back to your regular schedule at the next meal.

   If you are taking Tenuate Dospan, take the missed dose as soon as you remember. If you do not remember until the next day, skip the dose. Never take 2 doses at once.

■ *Storage instructions...*
   Store at room temperature in a tightly closed container. Protect from excessive heat.

What side effects may occur?

Side effects cannot be anticipated. If any develop or change in intensity, inform your doctor as soon as possible. Only your doctor can determine if it is safe for you to continue using Tenuate.

■ *Side effects may include:*
Abdominal discomfort, abnormal redness of the skin, anxiety, blood pressure elevation, blurred vision, breast development in males, bruising, changes in sex drive, chest pain, constipation, depression, diarrhea, difficulty with voluntary movements, dizziness, drowsiness, dryness of the mouth, feelings of discomfort, feelings of elation, feeling of illness, hair loss, headache, hives, impotence, inability to fall or stay asleep, increased heart rate, increased seizures in epileptics, increased sweating, increased volume of diluted urine, irregular heartbeat, jitteriness, menstrual upset, muscle pain, nausea, nervousness, overstimulation, painful urination, palpitations, pupil dilation, rash, restlessness, shortness of breath or labored breathing, stomach and intestinal disturbances, tremors, unpleasant taste, vomiting

Why should this drug not be prescribed?

If you are sensitive to or have ever had an allergic reaction to Tenuate or other appetite suppressants, you should not take this medication. Make sure your doctor is aware of any drug reactions you have experienced.

Do not take this drug if you have severe hardening of the arteries, an overactive thyroid, glaucoma, or severe high blood pressure, or if you are agitated, have a history of drug abuse or are taking an MAO inhibitor (antidepressant drug such as Nardil) or have taken one within the last 14 days.

Special warnings about this medication

Tenuate or Tenuate Dospan may impair your ability to engage in potentially hazardous activities. Therefore, make sure you know how you react to this medication before you drive, operate dangerous

machinery, or do anything else that requires alertness or concentration.

If you have heart disease or high blood pressure, use caution when taking this medication.

This drug may increase convulsions in some epileptics. Your doctor should monitor you carefully if you have epilepsy.

Psychological dependence has occurred while taking this drug. Talk with your doctor if you find you are relying on this drug to maintain a state of well-being.

The abrupt withdrawal of this medication following prolonged use at high doses may result in extreme fatigue, mental depression, and sleep disturbances.

Possible food and drug interactions when taking this medication

Tenuate or Tenuate Dospan may interact with alcohol unfavorably. Do not drink alcohol while taking this medication.

If Tenuate or Tenuate Dospan is taken with certain other drugs, the effects of either could be increased, decreased, or altered. It is especially important that you consult your doctor before combining Tenuate with the following:

Blood pressure medications such as Ismelin
Insulin
Phenothiazine drugs such as the major
  tranquilizer Thorazine

**Special information
if you are pregnant or breastfeeding**

The effects of Tenuate or Tenuate Dospan during pregnancy have not been adequately studied. If you are pregnant or plan to become pregnant, inform your doctor immediately. This drug appears in breast milk. If the medication is essential to your health, your doctor may advise you to discontinue breastfeeding until your treatment is finished.

Recommended dosage

ADULTS

Tenuate Immediate-Release

The usual dosage is one 25-milligram tablet taken 3 times a day, 1 hour before meals; you may take 1 tablet in the middle of the evening, if you want, to overcome night hunger.

Tenuate Dospan Controlled-Release

The usual dosage is one 75-milligram tablet taken once daily, swallowed whole, in midmorning.

CHILDREN

Safety and effectiveness have not been established in children below 12 years of age.

Overdosage

Any medication taken in excess can have serious consequences. If you suspect an overdose, seek emergency medical treatment immediately.

■ *Symptoms of Tenuate overdose may include:*
Abdominal cramps, assaultiveness, confusion, depression, diarrhea, elevated blood pressure, fatigue, hallucinations, irregular heartbeat, lowered blood pressure, nausea, overreactive reflexes, panic state, rapid breathing, restlessness, tremors, vomiting

Brand name:

TERAZOL 3

Pronounced: TER-uh-zawl
Generic name: Terconazole

Why is this drug prescribed?
Terazol 3 Vaginal Cream and Suppositories are prescribed to treat candidiasis (a yeast-like fungal infection) of the vulva and vagina.

Most important fact about this drug
Keep using Terazol 3 for the full time of treatment, even if the infection seems to have disappeared. If you stop too soon, the infection could return. You should continue using this medicine during your menstrual period.

How should you use this medication?
Follow these steps to apply Terazol 3:

1. Load the applicator to the fill line with cream, or unwrap a suppository, wet it with warm water, and place it in the applicator as shown in the instructions you received with the product.
2. Lie on your back with knees drawn up.
3. Gently insert the applicator high into the vagina and push the plunger.
4. Withdraw the applicator and wash with soap and water.

To protect your clothing, wear a sanitary napkin. Do not use tampons because they will absorb the medicine. Wear cotton underwear—avoid synthetic fabrics such as rayon or nylon. Do not douche unless your doctor tells you to do so.

Dry the genital area thoroughly after a shower, bath, or swim. Change out of a wet bathing suit or damp workout clothes as soon as possible. Moisture encourages the growth of yeast.

Try not to scratch. It can cause more irritation and can spread the infection.

- *If you miss a dose...*
Apply it as soon as you remember. If it is almost time for your next dose, skip the one you missed and go back to your regular schedule.

- *Storage instructions...*
Store at room temperature.

What side effects may occur?

Side effects cannot be anticipated. If any develop or change in intensity, inform your doctor as soon as possible. Only your doctor can determine if it is safe for you to continue using Terazol 3.

- *More common side effects may include:*
Body pain
Burning
Genital pain
Headache
Menstrual pain

- *Less common side effects may include:*
Abdominal pain, chills, fever, itching

Why should this drug not be prescribed?

If you have ever had an allergic reaction to or are sensitive to terconazole or any other ingredients of Terazol 3, you should not use this medication. Make sure your doctor is aware of any drug reactions you have experienced.

Special warnings about this medication

If irritation, an allergic reaction, fever, chills, or flu-like symptoms develop while using this medication, notify your doctor.

To avoid re-infection while using Terazol 3, either avoid sexual intercourse or make sure your partner uses a non-latex condom.

Terazol 3 suppositories can interact with latex products such as diaphragms and

certain type of condoms. Use some other method of birth control while you are taking Terazol 3.

Possible food and drug interactions when taking this medication

No interactions have been reported.

Special information if you are pregnant or breastfeeding

Since Terazol 3 is absorbed from the vagina, it should not be used during the first trimester (first 3 months) of pregnancy unless your doctor considers it essential to your health. It is not known whether this drug appears in breast milk. Your doctor may advise you to discontinue breastfeeding your baby while using this medication.

Recommended dosage

ADULTS

Terazol 3 Vaginal Cream
The recommended dose is 1 full applicator (5 grams) of cream inserted into the vagina once daily at bedtime for 3 consecutive days.

Terazol 3 Vaginal Suppositories
The recommended dose is 1 suppository inserted into the vagina once daily at bedtime for 3 consecutive days.

CHILDREN

Safety and effectiveness have not been established in children.

Overdosage

There has been no reported overdose of this medication. Any medication used in excess, however, can have serious consequences. If you suspect an overdose of Terazol 3, seek medical attention immediately.

Generic name:

TERCONAZOLE

See Terazol 3, page 762.

Brand name:

TESTRED

See Android, page 508.

Generic name:

TETRACYCLINE

See Achromycin V Capsules, page 499.

Brand name:

THEROXIDE

See Desquam-E, page 565.

Generic name:

THIORIDAZINE

See Mellaril, page 651.

Generic name:

TIOCONAZOLE

See Vagistat-1, page 785.

Brand name:

TOFRANIL

Pronounced: toe-FRAY-nil
Generic name: Imipramine hydrochloride

Why is this drug prescribed?

Tofranil is used to treat depression. It is a member of the family of drugs called tricyclic antidepressants.

Tofranil is also used on a short term basis, along with behavioral therapies, to treat bedwetting in children aged 6 and older. Its effectiveness may decrease with longer use.

Some doctors also prescribe Tofranil to treat bulimia, attention deficit disorder in children, obsessive-compulsive disorder, and panic disorder.

Most important fact about this drug

Serious, sometimes fatal, reactions have been known to occur when drugs such as Tofranil are taken with another type of antidepressant called an MAO inhibitor. Drugs in this category include Nardil, Marplan, and Parnate. Do not take Tofranil within 2 weeks of taking one of these drugs. Make sure your doctor and pharmacist know of all the medications you are taking.

How should you take this medication?

Tofranil may be taken with or without food.

You should not take Tofranil with alcohol.

Do not stop taking Tofranil if you feel no immediate effect. It can take from 4 to 6 weeks for improvement to begin.

Tofranil can cause dry mouth. Sucking hard candy or chewing gum can help this problem.

■ *If you miss a dose...*
If you take 1 dose a day at bedtime, contact your doctor. Do not take the dose in the morning because of possible side effects.

If you take 2 or more doses a day, take the forgotten dose as soon as you remember. If it is almost time for your next dose, skip the one you missed and go back to your regular schedule. Do not take 2 doses a once.

■ *Storage instructions...*
Store at room temperature in a tightly closed container.

What side effects may occur?
Side effects cannot be anticipated. If any develop or change in intensity, inform your doctor as soon as possible. Only your doctor can determine if it is safe for you to continue taking Tofranil.

■ *Side effects may include:*
Abdominal cramps, agitation, anxiety, black tongue, bleeding sores, blood disorders, blurred vision, breast development in males, confusion, congestive heart failure, constipation or diarrhea, cough, fever, sore throat, delusions, dilated pupils, disorientation, dizziness, drowsiness, dry mouth, episodes of elation or irritability, excessive or spontaneous flow of milk, fatigue, fever, flushing, frequent urination or difficulty or delay in urinating, hair loss, hallucinations, headache, heart attack, heart failure, high blood pressure, high or low blood sugar, high pressure of fluid in the eyes, hives, impotence, increased or decreased sex drive, inflammation of the mouth, insomnia, intestinal blockage, irregular heartbeat, lack of coordination, light-headedness (especially when rising from lying down), loss of appetite, nausea,

nightmares, odd taste in mouth, palpitations, purple or reddish-brown spots on skin, rapid heartbeat, restlessness, ringing in the ears, seizures, sensitivity to light, skin itching and rash, stomach upset, stroke, sweating, swelling due to fluid retention (especially in face or tongue), swelling of breasts, swelling of testicles, swollen glands, tendency to fall, tingling, pins and needles, and numbness in hands and feet, tremors, visual problems, vomiting, weakness, weight gain or loss, yellowed skin and whites of eyes

■ *The most common side effects in children being treated for bed wetting are:*
Nervousness, sleep disorders, stomach and intestinal problems, tiredness

■ *Other side effects in children are:*
Anxiety, collapse, constipation, convulsions, emotional instability, fainting

Why should this drug not be prescribed?
Tofranil should not be used if you are recovering from a recent heart attack

People who take antidepressant drugs known as MAO inhibitors, such as Nardil and Parnate, should not take Tofranil. You should not take Tofranil if you are sensitive or allergic to it.

Special warnings about this medication
You should use Tofranil cautiously if you have or have ever had: narrow-angle glaucoma (increased pressure in the eye); difficulty in urinating; heart, liver, kidney, or thyroid disease; or seizures. Also be cautious if you are taking thyroid medication.

General feelings of illness, headache, and nausea can result if you suddenly stop taking Tofranil. Follow your doctor's instructions closely when discontinuing Tofranil.

Tell your doctor if you develop a sore throat or fever while taking Tofranil.

This drug may impair your ability to drive a car or operate potentially dangerous machinery. Do not participate in any activities that require full alertness if you are unsure about your ability.

This drug can make you sensitive to light. Try to stay out of the sun as much as possible while you are taking it.

If you are going to have elective surgery, your doctor will take you off Tofranil.

Possible food and drug interactions when taking this medication

If Tofranil is taken with certain other drugs, the effects of either could be increased, decreased, or altered. It is especially important to check with your doctor before combining Tofranil with the following:

Albuterol (Proventil, Ventolin)
Anticholinergics such as Cogentin
Antihypertensives such as Wytensin
Barbiturates such as Nembutal and Seconal
Carbamazepine (Tegretol)
Central nervous system depressants such as
    Xanax and Valium
Cimetidine (Tagamet)
Clonidine (Catapres)
Decongestants such as Sudafed
Epinephrine (Epipen)
Fluoxetine (Prozac)
Guanethidine (Ismelin)
Methylphenidate (Ritalin)
Norepinephrine
Phenytoin (Dilantin)
Thyroid medications

Extreme drowsiness and other potentially serious effects can result if Tofranil is combined with alcohol or other mental depressants, such as narcotic painkillers (Percocet), sleeping medications (Halcion), or tranquilizers (Valium).

Special information if you are pregnant or breastfeeding

The effects of Tofranil during pregnancy have not been adequately studied. Pregnant women should use Tofranil only when the potential benefits clearly outweigh the potential risks. If you are pregnant or plan to become pregnant, inform your doctor immediately. Tofranil may appear in breast milk and could affect a nursing infant. If this medication is essential to your health, your doctor may advise you to stop breastfeeding until your treatment is finished.

Recommended dosage

ADULTS

The usual starting dose in 75 milligrams a day. The doctor may increase this to 150 milligrams a day. The maximum daily dose is 200 milligrams.

Tofranil is not to be used in children to treat any condition but bedwetting, and its use will be limited to short-term therapy. Safety and effectiveness in children under the age of 6 have not been established.

Total daily dosages for children should not exceed 2.5 milligrams for each 2.2 pounds of the child's weight.

Doses usually begin at 25 milligrams per day. This amount should be taken an hour before bedtime. If needed, this dose may be increased after 1 week to 50 milligrams (ages 6 through 11) or 75 milligrams (ages 12 and up), taken in one dose at bedtime or divided into 2 doses, 1 taken at mid-afternoon and 1 at bedtime.

ELDERLY AND ADOLESCENTS

People in these two age groups should take lower doses. Dosage starts out at 30 to 40 milligrams per day and can go up to no more than 100 milligrams a day.

Overdosage

Any medication taken in excess can have serious consequences. An overdose of Tofranil can cause death. It has been reported that children are more sensitive than adults to overdoses of Tofranil. If you suspect an overdose, seek medical help immediately.

■ *Symptoms of Tofranil overdose may include:*
Agitation, bluish skin, coma, convulsions, difficulty breathing, dilated pupils, drowsiness, heart failure, high fever, involuntary writhing or jerky movements, irregular or rapid heartbeat, lack of coordination, low blood pressure, overactive reflexes, restlessness, rigid muscles, shock, stupor, sweating, vomiting

Brand name:

TOLECTIN

Pronounced: *toe-LEK-tin*
Generic name: *Tolmetin sodium*

Why is this drug prescribed?

Tolectin is a nonsteroidal anti-inflammatory drug used to relieve the inflammation, swelling, stiffness, and joint pain associated with rheumatoid arthritis and osteoarthritis (the most common form of arthritis). It is used for both acute episodes and long-term treatment. It is also used to treat juvenile rheumatoid arthritis.

Most important fact about this drug

You should have frequent checkups with your doctor if you take Tolectin regularly.

Ulcers or internal bleeding can occur without warning.

How should you take this medication?

If Tolectin upsets your stomach, it may be taken with food or an antacid, and with a full glass of water. It may also help to prevent upset if you avoid lying down for 20 to 30 minutes after taking the drug.

Take this medication exactly as prescribed by your doctor.

■ *If you miss a dose...*
Take it as soon as you remember. If it is almost time for your next dose, skip the one you missed and go back to your regular schedule. Never take 2 doses at the same time.

■ *Storage instructions...*
Store at room temperature in a tightly closed container, away from light.

What side effects may occur?

Side effects cannot be anticipated. If any develop or change in intensity, inform your doctor as soon as possible. Only your doctor can determine if it is safe for you to continue taking Tolectin.

■ *More common side effects may include:*
Abdominal pain, change in weight, diarrhea, dizziness, gas, headache, heartburn, high blood pressure, indigestion, nausea, stomach and intestinal upset, swelling due to fluid retention, vomiting, weakness

■ *Less common or rare side effects may include:*
Anemia, blood in urine, chest pain, congestive heart failure, constipation, depression, drowsiness, fever, hepatitis, hives, inflammation of the mouth or tongue, kidney failure, painful urination, peptic ulcer, purple or reddish spots on

skin, ringing in the ears, severe allergic reactions, skin irritation, stomach inflammation, stomach or intestinal bleeding, urinary tract infection, visual disturbances, yellow eyes or skin

Why should this drug not be prescribed?

If you are sensitive to or have ever had an allergic reaction to Tolectin, aspirin, or other nonsteroidal anti-inflammatory drugs, or if you have had asthma, hives, or nasal inflammation caused by aspirin or other nonsteroidal anti-inflammatory drugs, you should not take this medication. Make sure your doctor is aware of any drug reactions you have experienced.

Special warnings about this medication

Tolectin can cause kidney problems, especially if you are elderly, suffer from heart failure or liver disease, or take diuretics.

This drug can also affect the liver. If you develop symptoms such as yellow skin and eyes, notify your doctor. You should be taken off Tolectin.

Do not take aspirin or any other anti-inflammatory medications while taking Tolectin unless your doctor tells you to do so.

Tolectin can cause visual disturbances. If you experience a change in your vision, inform your doctor.

Tolectin prolongs bleeding time. If you are taking blood-thinning medication, this drug should be taken with caution.

This drug can increase water retention. Use with caution if you have heart disease or high blood pressure.

Tolectin causes some people to become drowsy or less alert. If it has this effect on you, driving or operating dangerous machinery or participating in any hazardous activity that requires full mental alertness is not recommended.

Possible food and drug interactions when taking this medication

If Tolectin is taken with certain other drugs, the effects of either could be increased, decreased, or altered. It is especially important to check with your doctor before combining Tolectin with the following:

Aspirin
Blood thinners such as Coumadin
Carteolol (Cartrol)
Diuretics such as Lasix
Glyburide (Micronase)
Lithium (Lithonate)
Methotrexate

Special information if you are pregnant or breastfeeding

The effects of Tolectin during pregnancy have not been adequately studied. If you are pregnant or plan to become pregnant, inform your doctor immediately. Tolectin appears in breast milk and could affect a nursing infant. If this medication is essential to your health, your doctor may advise you to discontinue breastfeeding until your treatment is finished.

Recommended dosage

ADULTS

Rheumatoid Arthritis or Osteoarthritis
The starting dosage is usually 1,200 milligrams a day divided into 3 doses of 400 milligrams each. Take 1 dose when you wake up and 1 at bedtime, and 1 sometime in between. Your doctor may adjust the dosage after 1 to 2 weeks. Most people will take a total daily dosage of 600 to 1,800 milligrams usually divided into 3 doses.

You should see the benefits of Tolectin in a few days to a week.

CHILDREN

The starting dose for children 2 years and older is usually a total of 20 milligrams per 2.2 pounds of body weight per day, divided into 3 or 4 smaller doses. Your doctor will advise you on use in children. The usual dose ranges from 15 to 30 milligrams per 2.2 pounds per day.

The safety and effectiveness of Tolectin have not been established in children under 2 years of age.

Overdosage

Although no specific information is available, any medication taken in excess can have serious consequences. If you suspect an overdose of Tolectin, seek medical attention immediately.

Generic name:

TOLMETIN

See Tolectin, page 767.

Brand name:

TOTACILLIN

See Omnipen, page 699.

Brand name:

TRANXENE

Pronounced: TRAN-zeen
Generic name: Clorazepate dipotassium
Other brand names: Tranxene-SD, Tranxene-SD Half Strength

Why is this drug prescribed?

Tranxene belongs to a class of drugs known as benzodiazepines. It is used in the treatment of anxiety disorders and for short-term relief of the symptoms of anxiety.

It is also used to relieve the symptoms of acute alcohol withdrawal and to help in treating certain convulsive disorders such as epilepsy.

Most important fact about this drug

Tranxene can be habit-forming if taken regularly over a long period. You may experience withdrawal symptoms if you stop using this drug abruptly. Consult your doctor before discontinuing Tranxene or making any change in your dose.

How should you take this medication?

Tranxene should be taken exactly as prescribed by your doctor.

■ *If you miss a dose...*
   Take it as soon as you remember if it is within an hour or so of your scheduled time. If you do not remember until later, skip the dose you missed and go back to your regular schedule. Do not take 2 doses at once.

■ *Storage instructions...*
   Store at room temperature. Protect from excessive heat.

What side effects may occur?

Side effects cannot be anticipated. If any develop or change in intensity, inform your doctor as soon as possible. Only your doctor can determine if it is safe for you to continue taking Tranxene.

■ *More common side effects may include:*
Drowsiness

■ *Less common or rare side effects may include:*
Blurred vision, depression, difficulty in sleeping or falling asleep, dizziness, dry mouth, double vision, fatigue, genital and urinary tract disorders, headache, irritability, lack of muscle coordination, mental confusion, nervousness, tremors, skin rashes, slurred speech, stomach and intestinal disorders, tremor

■ *Side effects due to rapid decrease or abrupt withdrawal from Tranxene include:*
Diarrhea, difficulty in sleeping or falling asleep, hallucinations, impaired memory, irritability, muscle aches, nervousness, tremors

Why should this drug not be prescribed?
If you are sensitive to or have ever had an allergic reaction to Tranxene, you should not take this medication. Make sure your doctor is aware of any drug reactions you have experienced.

Do not take this medication if you have the eye condition known as acute narrow-angle glaucoma.

Anxiety or tension related to everyday stress usually does not require treatment with such a strong drug. Discuss your symptoms thoroughly with your doctor.

Tranxene is not recommended for use in more serious conditions such as depression or severe psychological disorders.

Special warnings about this medication
Tranxene may cause you to become drowsy or less alert; therefore, you should not drive or operate dangerous machinery or participate in any hazardous activity that requires full mental alertness until you know how this drug affects you.

If you are being treated for anxiety associated with depression, your doctor will have you take a low dose of this medication. Do not increase your dose without consulting your doctor.

The elderly and people in a weakened condition are more apt to become unsteady or oversedated when taking Tranxene.

Possible food and drug interactions when taking this medication
Tranxene slows down the central nervous system and may intensify the effects of alcohol. Do not drink alcohol while taking this medication.

If Tranxene is taken with certain other drugs, the effects of either could be increased, decreased, or altered. It is especially important to check with your doctor before combining Tranxene with the following:

Antidepressant drugs known as MAO inhibitors (Nardil, Parnate) and other antidepressants such as Elavil and Prozac
Barbiturates such as Nembutal and Seconal
Narcotic pain relievers such as Demerol and Percodan
Major tranquilizers such as Mellaril and Thorazine

Special information if you are pregnant or breastfeeding
The effects of Tranxene during pregnancy have not been adequately studied. However, because there is an increased risk of birth defects associated with this class of drug, its use during pregnancy should be avoided. Tranxene may appear in breast milk and could affect a nursing infant. If this

medication is essential to your health, your doctor may advise you to discontinue breastfeeding until your treatment with this medication is finished.

Recommended dosage

ADULTS

Anxiety
The usual daily dosage is 30 milligrams divided into several smaller doses. A normal daily dose can be as little as 15 milligrams. Your doctor may increase the dosage gradually to as much as 60 milligrams, according to your individual needs.

Tranxene can also be taken in a single bedtime dose. The initial dose is 15 milligrams, but your doctor will adjust the dosage to suit your individual needs.

Tranxene-SD, a 22.5-milligram tablet, can be taken once every 24 hours. This form of the drug should not be used when starting treatment.

Tranxene-SD Half Strength, an 11.25-milligram tablet, can be taken once every 24 hours. This form of the drug should not be used when starting treatment.

Acute Alcohol Withdrawal:
Tranxene can be used in a multi-day program for relief of the symptoms of acute alcohol withdrawal.

Dosages are usually increased in the first 2 days from 30 to 90 milligrams and then reduced over the next 2 days to lower levels. After that, your doctor will gradually lower the dose still further, and will take you off the drug when you are ready. This medication should be used for this purpose only under strict medical supervision.

When Used With Antiepileptic Drugs
Tranxene can be used in conjunction with antiepileptic drugs. Follow the recommended dosages carefully to avoid drowsiness.

ADULTS AND CHILDREN OVER 12 YEARS OLD

The starting dose is 7.5 milligrams 3 times a day. Your doctor may increase the dosage by 7.5 milligrams per week to a maximum of 90 milligrams a day.

CHILDREN 9 TO 12 YEARS OLD

The starting dose is 7.5 milligrams twice a day. Your doctor may increase the dosage by 7.5 milligrams a week to a maximum of 60 milligrams a day.

Safety and effectiveness in children under 9 years of age have not been established.

ELDERLY

The usual starting dose for elderly people with anxiety is 7.5 to 15 milligrams per day.

Overdosage

Any medication taken in excess can have serious consequences. If you suspect an overdose, seek medical treatment immediately.

■ *Symptoms of Tranxene overdose may include:*
   Coma
   Low blood pressure
   Sedation

Brand name:

TRANXENE-SD

See Tranxene, page 769.

Brand name:

TRANXENE-SD Half Strength

See Tranxene, page 769.

Generic name:

TRAZODONE

See Desyrel, page 566.

Generic name:

TRETINOIN

See Retin-A, page 735.

Brand name:

TRIAVIL

Pronounced: TRY-uh-vill
Generic ingredients: Amitriptyline
  hydrochloride, Perphenazine

Why is this drug prescribed?

Triavil is used to treat anxiety, agitation,
and depression. Triavil is a combination of a
tricyclic antidepressant (amitriptyline) and a
tranquilizer (perphenazine).

Triavil can also help people with
schizoprenia (distorted sense of reality) who
are depressed and people with insomnia,
fatigue, loss of interest, loss of appetite, or
a slowing of physical and mental reactions.

Most important fact about this drug

Triavil may cause tardive dyskinesia—a
condition marked by involuntary muscle
spasms and twitches in the face and body.
This condition may be permanent and
appears to be most common among the
elderly, especially women. Ask your doctor
for information about this possible risk.

How should you take this medication?

Triavil may be taken with or without food.
You should not take it with alcohol.

■ *If you miss a dose...*
Take it as soon as you remember. If it is
within 2 hours of your next dose, skip
the one you missed and go back to your
regular schedule. Do not take 2 doses at
once.

■ *Storage instructions...*
Store at room temperature in a tightly
closed container. Protect Triavil 2-10
tablets from light.

What side effects may occur?

Side effects cannot be anticipated. If any
develop or change in intensity, inform your
doctor as soon as possible. Only your
doctor can determine if it is safe for you to
continue taking Triavil.

■ *Side effects may include:*
Abnormal secretion of milk, abnormalities
of movements and posture, anxiety,
asthma, black tongue, blood disorders,
blurred vision, body rigidly arched
backward, breast development in males,
change in pulse rate, chewing movements,
coma, confusion, constipation, convulsions,
delusions, diarrhea, difficulty breathing,
difficulty concentrating, difficulty
swallowing, dilated pupils, disorientation,
dizziness, drowsiness, dry mouth, eating
abnormal amounts of food, ejaculation
failure, episodes of elation or irritability,
excessive or spontaneous flow of milk,
excitement, exhaustion, eye problems, eye
spasms, eyes in a fixed position, fatigue,
fever, fluid accumulation and swelling
(including throat and brain, face and
tongue, arms and legs), frequent urination,
hair loss, hallucinations, headache, heart
attacks, hepatitis, high blood pressure,
high fever, high or low blood sugar, hives,

impotence, inability to stop moving, inability to urinate, increased or decreased sex drive, inflammation of the mouth, insomnia, intestinal blockage, intolerance to light, involuntary jerky movements of tongue, face, mouth, lips, jaw, body, or arms and legs, irregular blood pressure, pulse, and heartbeat, irregular menstrual periods, lack of coordination, light-headedness upon standing up, liver problems, lockjaw, loss or increase of appetite, low blood pressure, muscle stiffness, nasal congestion, nausea, nightmares, odd taste in the mouth, overactive reflexes, pain and stiffness around neck, palpitations, protruding tongue, puckering of the mouth, puffing of the cheeks, purple-reddish-brown spots on skin, rapid heartbeat, restlessness, rigid arms, feet, head, and muscles, ringing in the ears, salivation, sedation, seizures, sensitivity to light, severe allergic reactions, skin rash or inflammation, scaling, spasms in the hands and feet, speech problems, stomach upset, stroke, sweating, swelling of breasts, swelling of testicles, swollen glands, tingling, pins and needles, and numbness in hands and feet, tremors, twisted neck, twitching in the body, neck, shoulders, and face, uncontrollable and involuntary urination, urinary problems, visual problems, vomiting, weakness, weight gain or loss, writhing motions, yellowed skin and whites of eyes

Why should this drug not be prescribed?

You should not be using Triavil if you are taking drugs that slow down the central nervous system, including alcohol, barbiturates, analgesics, antihistamines, or narcotics.

Triavil should not be used if you are recovering from a recent heart attack, or if you have an abnormal bone marrow condition. Avoid Triavil if you have ever had an allergic reaction to phenothiazines or amitriptyline.

People who are taking antidepressant drugs known as MAO inhibitors (including Nardil and Parnate) should not take Triavil.

Special warnings about this medication

Before using Triavil, tell your doctor if you have ever had: the eye condition known as glaucoma; difficulty urinating; breast cancer; seizures; heart, liver, or thyroid disease; or if you are exposed to extreme heat or pesticides. Be aware that Triavil may mask signs of brain tumor, intestinal blockage, and overdose of other drugs.

Nausea, headache, and a general ill feeling can result if you suddenly stop taking Triavil. Follow your doctor's instructions closely when discontinuing Triavil. If your dose is gradually reduced, you may experience irritability, restlessness, and dream and sleep disturbances, but these effects will not last.

This drug may impair your ability to drive a car or operate potentially dangerous machinery. Do not participate in any activities that require full alertness if you are unsure about your ability.

If you develop a fever that has no other cause, stop taking Triavil and call your doctor.

Possible food and drug interactions when taking this medication

If Triavil is taken with certain other drugs, the effects of either could be increased, decreased, or altered. It is especially important to check with your doctor before combining Triavil with the following:

Airway-opening drugs such as Proventil
Anticonvulsants such as Dilantin
Antidepressant drugs classified as MAO

inhibitors, including Nardil and Parnate
Antihistamines such as Benadryl
Antispasmodic drugs such as Bentyl
Atropine (Donnatal)
Barbiturates such as phenobarbital
Blood-thinning drugs such as Coumadin
Cimetidine (Tagamet)
Disulfiram (Antabuse)
Epinephrine (Epifen)
Ethchlorvynol (Placidyl)
Fluoxetine (Prozac)
Furazolidone (Furoxone)
Guanethidine (Ismelin)
Major tranquilizers such as Haldol
Narcotic analgesics such as Percocet
Thyroid medications such as Synthroid

Extreme drowsiness and other potentially serious effects can result if Triavil is combined with alcohol or other central nervous system depressants such as narcotics, painkillers, and sleep medications.

Special Information
if you are pregnant or breastfeeding
Triavil may cause false-positive results on pregnancy tests. Triavil should not be used by pregnant women or mothers who are breastfeeding.

Recommended dosage
Your doctor will individualize your dose.

You should not take more than 4 tablets of Triavil 4-50 or 8 tablets of any other strength in one day. It may be a few days to a few weeks before you notice any improvement.

ADULTS

For Non-Psychotic Anxiety and Depression
The usual dose is 1 tablet of Triavil 2-25 or 4-25 taken 3 or 4 times a day, or 1 tablet of Triavil 4-50 taken twice a day.

For Anxiety in People with Schizophrenia
The usual dose is 2 tablets of Triavil 4-25 taken 3 times a day. Your doctor may tell you to take another tablet of Triavil 4-25 at bedtime, if needed.

If you need to keep taking Triavil, your doctor will probably have you take 1 tablet of Triavil 2-25 or 4-25 from 2 to 4 times a day or 1 tablet of Triavil 4-50 twice a day.

CHILDREN

Children should not use Triavil.

ELDERLY AND ADOLESCENTS

For Anxiety
The usual dose is 1 tablet of Triavil 4-10, taken 3 or 4 times a day. People in these age groups usually take Triavil at lower doses.

Overdosage
Any medication taken in excess can have serious consequences. An overdose of Triavil can be fatal. If you suspect an overdose, seek medical help immediately.

■ *Symptoms of Triavil overdose may include:* Abnormalities of posture and movements, agitation, coma, convulsions, dilated pupils, drowsiness, extreme low body temperature, eye movement problems, high fever, heart failure, overactive reflexes, rapid or irregular heartbeat, rigid muscles, stupor, very low blood pressure, vomiting

Brand name:

TRILISATE

Pronounced: TRILL-ih-sate
Generic name: Choline magnesium
  trisalicylate

Why is this drug prescribed?

Trilisate, a nonsteroidal, anti-inflammatory medication, is prescribed for the relief of the signs and symptoms of rheumatoid arthritis (chronic joint inflammation disease), osteoarthritis (degenerative joint disease), and other forms of arthritis. This drug is used in the long-term management of these diseases and especially for flare-ups of severe rheumatoid arthritis.

Trilisate may also be prescribed for the treatment of acute painful shoulder, for mild to moderate pain in general, and for fever.

In children, this medication is prescribed for severe conditions—such as juvenile rheumatoid arthritis—that require relief of pain and inflammation.

Most important fact about this drug

Because there is a possible association between the development of the rare but serious neurological disorder known as Reye's syndrome and the use of medicines containing salicylates or aspirin, Trilisate should not be used by children or teenagers who have chickenpox or flu symptoms unless otherwise advised by their doctor.

How should you take this medication?

Trilisate is available in tablet or liquid form. Take Trilisate exactly as prescribed by your doctor.

■ *If you miss a dose...*
  If you take Trilisate on a regular schedule, take the forgotten dose as soon as you remember. If it is almost time for your next dose, skip the one you missed and go back to your regular schedule. Do not take 2 doses at once.

■ *Storage instructions...*
  Store at room temperature.

What side effects may occur?

Side effects cannot be anticipated. If any develop or change in intensity, inform your doctor as soon as possible. Only your doctor can determine if it is safe for you to continue taking Trilisate.

■ *More common side effects may include:*
  Constipation
  Diarrhea
  Heartburn
  Indigestion
  Nausea
  Ringing in the ears
  Stomach pain and upset
  Vomiting

■ *Less common side effects may include:*
  Dizziness, drowsiness, headache, hearing impairment, light-headedness, sluggishness

■ *Rare side effects may include:*
  Asthma, blood in the stool, bruising, confusion, distorted sense of taste, hallucinations, hearing loss, hepatitis, hives, inflammation of the upper gastric tract, itching, loss of appetite, nosebleed, rash, skin eruptions or discoloration, stomach or intestinal ulcers, swelling due to fluid accumulation, weight gain

Why should this drug not be prescribed?

If you are sensitive to or have ever had an allergic reaction to Trilisate or drugs of this type, such as aspirin, you should not take this medication. Make sure your doctor is aware of any drug reactions you have experienced.

Special warnings about this medication

Use Trilisate with caution if you have severe or recurring kidney or liver disorder, gastritis (inflammation of the stomach lining), or a stomach or intestinal ulcer. Consult your doctor regarding any medical problems you may have.

If you are an asthmatic allergic to aspirin, tell your doctor before taking Trilisate.

It may be 2 to 3 weeks before you feel the effect of this medication.

Possible food and drug interactions when taking this medication

If Trilisate is taken with certain other drugs, the effects of either could be increased, decreased, or altered. It is especially important to check with your doctor before combining Trilisate with the following:

Antacids such as Gaviscon and Maalox
Antigout medications
Blood-thinners such as Coumadin
Carbonic anhydrase inhibitors such as
    acetazolamide (Diamox) used to treat
    heart failure, the eye condition called
    glaucoma, and certain convulsive disorders
Diabetes medications such as insulin,
    Micronase, and Tolinase
Methotrexate, an anticancer drug
Other salicylates used to reduce fever,
    inflammation, and pain such as aspirin
Phenytoin (the anticonvulsant Dilantin)
Steroids such as prednisone
Valproic acid (the anticonvulsant Depakene)

Special information if you are pregnant or breastfeeding

The effects of Trilisate during pregnancy have not been adequately studied. If you are pregnant or plan to become pregnant, inform your doctor immediately. This drug does appear in breast milk and could affect a nursing infant. If this medication is essential to your health, your doctor may advise you not to breastfeed until your treatment is finished.

Recommended dosage

ADULTS

In rheumatoid arthritis, osteoarthritis, more severe arthritis, and acute painful shoulder, the recommended starting dose is 1,500 milligrams taken 2 times a day or 3,000 milligrams taken once a day. Your doctor will adjust the dosage based on your response to this medication.

If you have a kidney disorder, your doctor will monitor you and adjust your dose accordingly.

For mild to moderate pain or to reduce a high fever, the usual dosage is 2,000 to 3,000 milligrams per day divided into 2 equal doses as recommended by your doctor.

CHILDREN

For reduction of inflammation or pain, the recommended dose for children is determined by weight. The usual dose for children who weigh 81 pounds or less is 50 milligrams per 2.2 pounds of body weight, taken twice a day. For heavier children, the usual dose is 2,250 milligrams per day, divided into 2 doses.

Trilisate liquid can be taken by younger children and by adults who are unable to swallow a tablet.

ELDERLY

The usual dosage is 2,250 milligrams divided into 3 doses of 750 milligrams each.

Overdosage

Any medication taken in excess can have serious consequences. If you suspect an overdose, seek medical treatment immediately. An overdose of Trilisate can be fatal.

■ *Symptoms of Trilisate overdose may include:*
Confusion, diarrhea, dizziness, drowsiness, headache, hearing impairment, rapid breathing, ringing in the ears, sweating, vomiting

Generic name:

TRIMETHOPRIM WITH SULFAMETHOXAZOLE

See Bactrim, page 523.

Generic name:

TRIMIPRAMINE

See Surmontil, page 751.

Brand name:

TRIMOX

See Amoxil, page 503.

Brand name:

TRIPHASIL

See Oral Contraceptives, page 702.

Brand name:

TRIPLE SULFA

See Sultrin, page 747.

Brand name:

T-STAT

See Erythromycin, Topical, page 587.

Brand name:

TYLENOL

TIE-len-all
Generic name: *Acetaminophen*
Other brand names: *Panadol, Aspirin Free Anacin*

Why is this drug prescribed?

Tylenol is a fever- and pain-reducing medication that is widely used to relieve simple headaches and muscle aches; the minor aches and pains of bursitis, arthritis, rheumatism, neuralgia (nerve inflammation), sprains, overexertion, and menstrual cramps; and the discomfort of fever due to colds and the flu.

Tylenol Headache Plus contains an antacid to treat heartburn, indigestion or upset stomach that may accompany minor aches and pains.

Children's Tylenol is used to relieve fever, pain and discomfort due to colds, flu, teething, immunizations and tonsillectomy.

Most important fact about this drug

Do not use Tylenol to relieve pain for more than 10 days, or to reduce fever for more than 3 days unless your doctor has specifically told you to do so.

How should you take this medication?

Follow the dosing instructions on the label. Do not take more Tylenol than is recommended.

■ *If you miss a dose...*
Take this medication only as needed.

■ *Storage instructions...*
Store at room temperature. Keep the liquid form from freezing.

What side effects may occur?
Tylenol is relatively free of side effects. Rarely, an allergic reaction may occur. If you develop any allergic symptoms such as rash, hives, swelling, or difficulty breathing, stop taking Tylenol immediately.

Special warnings about this medication
Tylenol should not be used for more than 10 days for pain, or 3 days for fever. Children's Tylenol should not be used for more than 5 days for pain, or 3 days for fever. If fever remains, or pain persists, contact your doctor. These symptoms could indicate a more serious illness.

If a rare sensitivity reaction (allergic reaction) occurs, stop using Tylenol and notify your doctor.

Do not give Tylenol Headache Plus to children under 12 years of age.

Possible food and drug interactions when taking this medication
If Tylenol is taken with certain other drugs the effects of either could be increased, decreased, or altered. It is especially important to check with your doctor before combining Tylenol with the following:

Alcohol
Cholestyramine (Questran)
Isoniazid (Nydrazid)
Nonsteroidal anti-inflammatory drugs such as Dolobid and Motrin
Oral Contraceptives
Phenytoin (Dilantin)
Warfarin (Coumadin)
Zidovudine (Retrovir)

Special information if you are pregnant or breastfeeding
As with all medications, ask your doctor or health care professional whether it is safe for you to use Tylenol while you are pregnant or breastfeeding.

Recommended dosage
ADULTS AND CHILDREN 12 YEARS AND OLDER

Tylenol Regular Strength
The usual dose is 1 to 2 tablets, 3 or 4 times daily.

Extra Strength Tylenol Headache Plus
The usual dose is 2 caplets every 6 hours, not to exceed 8 caplets in any 24 hour period.

CHILDREN 6 TO 12 YEARS OLD

Tylenol Regular Strength
One-half to 1 tablet 3 or 4 times a day.

Children's Tylenol
All doses of Children's Tylenol may be repeated every 4 hours, but not more than 5 times daily.

Chewable Tablets
The usual dose for children 6 to 8 years of age is 4 tablets; 9 to 10 years, 5 tablets; 11 to 12 years, 6 tablets·

Elixir and Suspension Liquid
(A special cup for measuring dosage is provided.) The usual dose for children 6 to 8 years of age is 2 teaspoons; 9 to 10 years, 2½ teaspoons; 11 to 12 years, 3 teaspoons.

CHILDREN UNDER 6 YEARS OLD

Children under 2 years old should be given Children's Tylenol only on the advice of a physician.

Regular Strength Tylenol
Consult your physician or health care professional

Children's Tylenol
All doses of Children's Tylenol may be repeated every 4 hours, but not more than 5 times daily.

Chewable Tablets
The usual dose for children 2 to 3 years of age is 2 tablets; 4 to 5 years, 3 tablets.

Elixir and Suspension Liquid
(A special cup for measuring dosage is provided.) The usual dose for children 4 to 11 months of age is ½ teaspoon; 12 to 23 months, ¾ teaspoon; 2 to 3 years, 1 teaspoon; 4 to 5 years 1½ teaspoons.

Infants' Tylenol Drops and Suspension Drops
The usual dose for children 0 to 3 months of age is 0.4 milliliter; 4 to 11 months, 0.8 milliliter; 12 to 23 months, 1.2 milliliters; 2 to 3 years, 1.6 milliliters; 4 to 5 years, 2.4 milliliters.

Overdosage

Any medication taken in excess can have serious consequences. If you suspect an overdose, seek medical attention immediately. Massive doses of Tylenol may cause liver poisoning.

■ *Symptoms of Tylenol overdose may include:*
Excessive perspiration
Exhaustion
Nausea
Vomiting

Brand name:

TYLENOL WITH CODEINE

Pronounced: TIE-len-awl with CO-deen
Generic ingredients: Acetaminophen, Codeine phosphate
Other brand name: Phenaphen with Codeine

Why is this drug prescribed?

Tylenol with Codeine, a narcotic analgesic, is used to treat mild to moderately severe pain. It contains two drugs—acetaminophen and codeine. Acetaminophen, an antipyretic (fever-reducing) analgesic, is used to reduce pain and fever. Codeine, a narcotic analgesic, is used to treat pain that is moderate to severe.

People who are allergic to aspirin can take Tylenol with Codeine.

Most important fact about this drug

Tylenol with Codeine contains a narcotic (codeine) and, even if taken in prescribed amounts, can cause physical and psychological addiction if taken for a long enough time.

Addiction may be more of a risk for a person who has been addicted to alcohol or drugs. Be sure to follow your doctor's instructions carefully when taking Tylenol with Codeine (or any other drugs that contain a narcotic).

How should you take this medication?

Tylenol with Codeine may be taken with meals or with milk (but not with alcohol).

■ *If you miss a dose...*
If you take this medication on a regular schedule, take the forgotten dose as soon as you remember. If it is almost time for your next dose, skip the one you missed and go back to your regular schedule. Do not take 2 doses at once.

■ *Storage instructions...*
Store away from heat, light, and moisture. Keep the liquid from freezing.

What side effects may occur?
Side effects cannot be anticipated. If any develop or change in intensity, inform your doctor as soon as possible. Only your doctor can determine if it is safe for you to continue taking Tylenol with Codeine.

■ *More common side effects may include:*
Dizziness
Light-headedness
Nausea
Sedation
Shortness of breath
Vomiting

■ *Less common side effects may include:*
Abdominal pain, allergic reactions, constipation, depressed feeling, exaggerated feeling of well-being, itchy skin

■ *Rare side effects may include:*
Decreased breathing (when Tylenol with Codeine is taken at higher doses)

Why should this drug not be prescribed?
You should not use Tylenol with Codeine if you are sensitive to either acetaminophen (Tylenol) or codeine.

Special warnings about this medication
You should take Tylenol with Codeine cautiously and only according to your doctor's instructions, as you would take any medication containing a narcotic. Make sure your doctor is aware of any problems you have had with drug or alcohol addiction.

Tylenol with Codeine tablets contain a sulfite that may cause allergic reactions in some people. These reactions may include shock and severe, possibly life-threatening, asthma attacks. People with asthma are more likely to be sensitive to sulfites.

If you have experienced a head injury, consult your doctor before taking Tylenol with Codeine.

If you have stomach problems, such as an ulcer, check with your doctor before taking Tylenol with Codeine. Tylenol with Codeine may obscure the symptoms of stomach problems, making them difficult to diagnose and treat.

If you have ever had liver, kidney, thyroid, or adrenal disease, difficulty urinating, or an enlarged prostate, consult your doctor before taking Tylenol with Codeine.

This drug may cause drowsiness and impair your ability to drive a car or operate potentially dangerous machinery. Do not participate in any activities that require full attention when using this drug until you are sure of its effect on you.

Possible food and drug interactions when taking this medication
Alcohol may increase the sedative effects of Tylenol with Codeine. Therefore, do not drink alcohol while you are taking this medication.

If Tylenol with Codeine is taken with certain other drugs, the effects of either could be increased, decreased, or altered. It is especially important to check with your doctor before combining Tylenol with Codeine with the following:

Antipsychotic drugs such as Clozaril and
    Thorazine
Anticholinergic drugs such as Cogentin
General anesthetics
MAO inhibitors such as Nardil and Eldepryl
Other narcotic painkillers such as Darvon
Tranquilizers such as Xanax and Valium
Tricyclic antidepressants such as Elavil and
    Tofranil

Special information
if you are pregnant or breastfeeding

It is not known if Tylenol with Codeine could injure a fetus, or if it could affect a woman's reproductive capacity. Using any medication that contains a narcotic during pregnancy may cause babies to be born with a physical addiction to the narcotic. If you are pregnant or plan to become pregnant, you should not take Tylenol with Codeine unless the potential benefits clearly outweigh the possible dangers. As with other narcotic painkillers, taking Tylenol with Codeine shortly before delivery (especially at higher dosages) may cause some degree of breathing difficulty in the mother and newborn.

Some studies (but not all) have reported that codeine appears in breast milk and may affect a nursing infant. Therefore, nursing mothers should use Tylenol with Codeine only if the potential gains are greater than the potential hazards.

Recommended dosage

ADULTS

Dosage will depend on how severe your pain is and how you respond to the drug.

To Relieve Pain
A single dose may contain from 15 milligrams to 60 milligrams of codeine phosphate and from 300 to 1,000 milligrams of acetaminophen. The maximum dose in a 24-hour period should be 360 milligrams of codeine phosphate and 4,000 milligrams of acetaminophen. Your doctor will determine the amounts of codeine phosphate and acetaminophen taken in each dose. Doses may be repeated up to every 4 hours.

Single doses above 60 milligrams of codeine do not give enough pain relief to balance the increased number of side effects.

Adults may also take Tylenol with Codeine elixir (liquid). Tylenol with Codeine elixir contains 120 milligrams of acetaminophen and 12 milligrams of codeine phosphate per teaspoonful.

The usual adult dose is 1 tablespoonful every 4 hours as needed.

CHILDREN

The safety of Tylenol with Codeine elixir has not been established in children under 3 years old.

Children 3 to 6 years old may take 1 teaspoonful 3 or 4 times daily.

Children 7 to 12 years old may take 2 teaspoonsful 3 or 4 times daily.

ELDERLY

The elderly and anyone in a weakened or rundown condition should use Tylenol with Codeine cautiously.

Overdosage

Any medication taken in excess can cause symptoms of overdose. Severe overdosage of Tylenol with Codeine can cause death. If you suspect an overdose, seek medical attention immediately.

■ *Symptoms of Tylenol with Codeine overdose may include:*
Bluish skin, cold and clammy skin, coma due to low blood sugar, decreased, irregular, or stopped breathing, extreme sleepiness progressing to stupor or coma, general bodily discomfort, heart attack, kidney failure, liver failure, low blood pressure, muscle weakness, nausea, slow heartbeat, sweating, vomiting

Brand name:

URISED

Pronounced: YOUR-i-said
Generic ingredients: Methenamine, Methylene
  blue, Phenyl salicylate, Benzoic acid,
  Atropine sulfate, Hyoscyamine

Why is this drug prescribed?

Urised relieves lower urinary tract discomfort
caused by inflammation or diagnostic
procedures. It is used to treat urinary tract
infections including cystitis (inflammation of
the bladder and ureters), urethritis
(inflammation of the urethra), and trigonitis
(inflammation of the mucous membrane of
the bladder). Methenamine, the major
component of this drug, acts as a mild
antiseptic by changing into formaldehyde in
the urinary tract when it comes in contact
with acidic urine.

Most important fact about this drug

Urised may give a blue to blue-green color
to urine and discolor stools as well.

How should you take this medication?

If dry mouth occurs, hard candy or gum,
saliva substitute, or crushed ice may provide
temporary relief.

Take this medication exactly as prescribed;
do not take more than the recommended
dose.

Drinking plenty of fluids will help the
medication work better and relieve
discomfort.

■ If you miss a dose...
  Take it as soon as you remember. If it is
  almost time for your next dose, skip the
  one you missed and go back to your
  regular schedule. Never take 2 doses at
  the same time.

■ Storage instructions...
  Store Urised at room temperature, in a
  dry place.

What side effects may occur?

Side effects cannot be anticipated. If any
develop or change in intensity, inform your
doctor as soon as possible. Only your
doctor can determine if it is safe for you to
continue taking Urised.

■ Side effects with long-term use may
  include:
  Acute urinary retention (in men with an
    enlarged prostate)
  Blurry vision
  Difficulty urinating
  Dizziness
  Dry mouth
  Flushing
  Rapid pulse
  Skin rash

Why should this drug not be prescribed?

Urised should be avoided if you have
glaucoma, a bladder blockage, cardiospasm,
or a disorder that obstructs the passage of
food through the stomach. Also avoid
Urised if you are sensitive to or have ever
had an allergic reaction to any of its
ingredients.

Special warnings about this medication

Urised should be used cautiously if you have
heart disease or have ever had a reaction to
medications that are chemically similar to
atropine.

Your doctor may ask you to check your
urine with phenaphthazine paper to see if it
is acidic. Urine acidifiers, such as vitamin C,
may be recommended if the urine is not
acidic enough.

Possible food and drug interactions when taking this medication

If Urised is taken with certain other drugs, the effects of either could be increased, decreased, or altered. It is especially important to check with your doctor before combining Urised with the following:

Acetazolamide (Diamox)
Potassium supplements such as Slow-K
Sodium bicarbonate antacids such as Alka-Seltzer
Sulfa drugs such as Gantrisin, Gantanol, Bactrim, and Septra

Drugs and foods that produce alkaline urine (such as sodium bicarbonate, antacids, and orange juice) should be limited.

Special Information if you are pregnant or breastfeeding

The effects of Urised during pregnancy have not been adequately studied. If you are pregnant or plan to become pregnant, inform your doctor immediately. Urised may appear in breast milk and could affect a nursing infant. If this medication is essential to your health, your doctor may advise you to stop breastfeeding until your treatment with Urised ends.

Recommended dosage

ADULTS

The usual dose is 2 tablets, 4 times a day.

CHILDREN 6 YEARS AND OLDER

The dosage must be determined by your doctor.

CHILDREN UNDER 6 YEARS

Use is not recommended in children under 6 years old.

Overdosage

Any medication taken in excess can have serious consequences. If you suspect an overdose, seek medical treatment immediately.

■ *Symptoms of Urised overdose may include*: Abdominal pain, bladder and abdominal irritation, bloody diarrhea, bloody urine, burning pain in throat and mouth, circulatory collapse, coma, dilated pupils (large pupils), dizziness, dry nose, mouth, and throat, elevated blood pressure, extremely high body temperature, headache, hot, dry, flushed skin, painful and frequent urination, pallor (paleness), pounding heartbeat (pounding sensation against the chest), rapid heartbeat (increased pulse rate), respiratory failure, ringing in ears, sweating, vomiting, weakness, white sores in mouth

Brand name:

URISPAS

Pronounced: YOUR-eh-spaz
Generic name: Flavoxate hydrochloride

Why is this drug prescribed?

Urispas prevents spasms in the urinary tract and relieves the painful or difficult urination, urinary urgency, excessive nighttime urination, pubic area pain, frequency of urination, and inability to hold urine caused by urinary tract infections. Urispas is taken in combination with antibiotics to treat the infection.

Most important fact about this drug

Urispas can cause blurred vision and drowsiness. Be careful driving, operating machinery, or performing any activity that requires complete mental alertness until you know how you will react to this medication.

How should you take this medication?

Take this medication exactly as prescribed. Urispas may make your mouth dry. Sucking on a hard candy, chewing gum, or melting bits of ice in your mouth can provide relief.

■ *If you miss a dose...*
Take it as soon as you remember. If it is almost time for your next dose, skip the one you missed and go back to your regular schedule. Do not take 2 doses at once.

■ *Storage instructions...*
Store away from heat, light, and moisture.

What side effects may occur?
Side effects cannot be anticipated. If any develop or change in intensity, notify your doctor as soon as possible. Only your doctor can determine whether it is safe for you to continue taking Urispas.

■ *Side effects may include:*
Allergic skin reactions, including hives, blurred vision and vision changes, drowsiness, dry mouth, fluttery heartbeat, headache, high body temperature, mental confusion (especially in the elderly), nausea, nervousness, painful or difficult urination, rapid heartbeat, vertigo, vomiting

Why should this drug not be prescribed?
You should not take Urispas if you have stomach or intestinal blockage, muscle relaxation problems (especially the sphincter muscle), abdominal bleeding, or urinary tract blockage.

Special warnings about this medication
Use Urispas cautiously if you have the eye condition known as glaucoma.

Possible food and drug interactions when taking this medication
No interactions involving Urispas have been noted.

Special information if you are pregnant or breastfeeding
The effects of Urispas during pregnancy have not been adequately studied. If you are pregnant or plan to become pregnant, inform your doctor immediately. Urispas may appear in breast milk and could affect a nursing infant. If this medication is essential to your health, your doctor may advise you to stop breastfeeding until your treatment is finished.

Recommended dosage

ADULTS AND CHILDREN OVER AGE 12

The usual dose of Urispas is one or two 100-milligram tablets 3 or 4 times a day.

When your symptoms have improved, your doctor may reduce the dosage.

CHILDREN

Safety and effectiveness of Urispas in children under 12 years of age have not been established.

Overdosage
Any medication taken in excess can have serious consequences. If you suspect an overdose of Urispas, seek medical attention immediately.

■ *Symptoms of Urispas overdose may include:*
Convulsions
Decreased ability to sweat
(warm, red skin, dry mouth, and increased body temperature)
Hallucinations
Increased heart rate and blood pressure
Mental confusion

Generic name:

UROFOLLITROPIN

See Metrodin, page 659.

Brand name:

VAGISTAT-1

Pronounced: VAG-i-stat
Generic name: Tioconazole

Why is this drug prescribed?

Vagistat-1 vaginal ointment is used to treat candidiasis, a yeast-like fungal infection, of the vulva (external genitals) and vagina.

Before starting you on Vagistat-1 therapy, your doctor should do a culture or smear to confirm the diagnosis.

Most important fact about this drug

If your infection does not clear up, notify your doctor. Further tests will be needed to confirm the diagnosis.

How should you take this medication?

Vagistat-1 vaginal ointment is to use only within the vagina.

Insert the ready-to-use, prefilled applicator preferably just before going to bed. To avoid possible contamination, do not open the applicator package until you are ready to use it.

Instructions on how to insert the applicator are on the back of the foil envelope in the Vagistat-1 box. If you have any questions or do not understand the directions, check with your doctor.

■ *If you miss a dose...*
   Vagistat-1 is a single-dose treatment. Do not apply more than once.

■ *Storage instructions...*
   Store at room temperature. Protect from freezing.

What side effects may occur?

Side effects cannot be anticiapted. If any develop or change in intensity, notify your doctor as soon as possible.

■ *More common side effects may include:*
   Burning
   Itching

■ *Rare side effects may include:*
   Burning sensation, discharge, dryness of the vagina, frequent urination during the night, irritation, pain with sexual intercourse, painful urination, swelling of the vulva, vaginal pain

Why should this drug not be prescribed?

Do not use Vagistat-1 if you have ever had an allergic reaction to or are sensitive to tioconazole. Be sure to tell your doctor about any drug reactions you have experienced.

Special warnings about this medication

If you are diabetic, tell your doctor before using Vagistat-1. He or she will decide whether it is safe for you.

Do not use condoms or vaginal contraceptive diaphragms for 72 hours after treatment with Vagistat-1. The Vagistat-1 ointment base may interact with rubber or latex products and cause them to weaken or break.

To avoid future episodes of fungal infection, choose cotton underwear or pantyhose with a cotton crotch instead of nylon or rayon.

The safety and effectiveness of the product have not been established in children.

Possible food and drug interactions when taking this medication

No interactions have been reported.

Special information if you are pregnant or breastfeeding

If you are pregnant or plan to become pregnant, tell your doctor before using Vagistat-1. The effects of this drug in pregnant women have not been adequately studied. It is not known whether Vagistat-1 appears in breast milk. If you are breastfeeding or plan to breastfeed, you may need to stop nursing or forego the medication.

Recommended dosage

ADULTS

Using the prefilled applicator, insert one applicator-full into the vagina, preferably just before going to bed. Only 1 dose is needed.

Overdosage

Although an overdose of Vagistat-1 is extremely unlikely, any medication taken in excess can have serious consequences. If you suspect an overdose, seek medical attention immediately.

Brand name:

VALIUM

Pronounced: VAL-ee-um
Generic name: Diazepam

Why is this drug prescribed?

Valium is used in the treatment of anxiety disorders and for short-term relief of the symptoms of anxiety. It belongs to a class of drugs known as benzodiazepines.

It is also used to relieve the symptoms of acute alcohol withdrawal, to relax muscles, to relieve the uncontrolled muscle movements caused by cerebral palsy and

paralysis of the lower body and limbs, to control involuntary movement of the hands (athetosis), to relax tight, aching muscles, and, along with other medications, to treat convulsive disorders such as epilepsy.

Most important fact about this drug

Valium can be habit-forming or addictive. You may experience withdrawal symptoms if you stop using this drug abruptly. Discontinue or change your dose only on your doctor's advice.

How should you take this medication?

Take this medication exactly as prescribed. If you are taking Valium for epilepsy, make sure you take it every day at the same time.

■ *If you miss a dose...*
Take it as soon as you remember if it is within an hour or so of the scheduled time. If you do not remember until later, skip the dose you missed and go back to your regular schedule. Never take 2 doses at the same time.

■ *Storage instructions...*
Store away from heat, light, and moisture.

What side effects may occur?

Side effects cannot be anticipated. If any develop or change in intensity, inform your doctor as soon as possible. Only your doctor can determine if it is safe for you to continue taking Valium.

■ *More common side effects may include:*
Drowsiness
Fatigue
Light-headedness
Loss of muscle coordination

■ *Less common or rare side effects may include:*
Anxiety, blurred vision, changes in salivation, changes in sex drive, confusion, constipation, depression, difficulty

urinating, dizziness, double vision, hallucinations, headache, inability to hold urine, low blood pressure, nausea, overstimulation, rage, seizures (mild changes in brain wave patterns), skin rash, sleep disturbances, slow heartbeat, slurred speech and other speech problems, stimulation, tremors, vertigo, yellowing of eyes and skin

■ *Side effects due to rapid decrease in dose or abrupt withdrawal from Valium:* Abdominal and muscle cramps, convulsions, sweating, tremors, vomiting

Why should this drug not be prescribed?

If you are sensitive to or have ever had an allergic reaction to Valium, you should not take this medication.

Do not take this medication if you have the eye condition known as acute narrow-angle glaucoma.

Anxiety or tension related to everyday stress usually does not require treatment with such a powerful drug as Valium. Discuss your symptoms thoroughly with your doctor.

Valium should not be prescribed if you are being treated for mental disorders more serious than anxiety.

Special warnings about this medication

Valium may cause you to become drowsy or less alert; therefore, you should not drive or operate dangerous machinery or participate in any hazardous activity that requires full mental alertness until you know how this drug affects you.

If you have liver or kidney problems, use this medication cautiously.

Possible food and drug interactions when taking this medication

Valium slows down the central nervous system and may intensify the effects of alcohol. Do not drink alcohol while taking this medication.

If Valium is taken with certain other drugs, the effects of either could be increased, decreased, or altered. It is especially important to check with your doctor before combining Valium with any of the following:

Anticonvulsants such as Dilantin
Antidepressant drugs such as Elavil and Prozac
Barbiturates such as phenobarbital
Cimetidine (Tagamet)
Digoxin (Lanoxin)
Disulfiram (Antabuse)
Fluoxetine (Prozac)
Isoniazid (Rifamate)
Levodopa (Larodopa, Sinemet)
Major tranquilizers such as Mellaril and Thorazine
MAO inhibitors (antidepressant drugs such as Nardil)
Narcotics such as Percocet
Omeprazole (Prilosec)
Oral contraceptives
Propoxyphene (Darvon)
Ranitidine (Zantac)
Rifampin (Rifadin)

Special information if you are pregnant or breastfeeding

Do not take Valium if you are pregnant or planning to become pregnant. There is an increased risk of birth defects.

If this medication is essential to your health, your doctor may advise you to discontinue breastfeeding until your treatment is finished.

Recommended dosage

ADULTS

Treatment of Anxiety Disorders and Short-Term Relief of the Symptoms of Anxiety
The usual dose, depending upon severity of symptoms, is 2 milligrams to 10 milligrams 2 to 4 times daily.

Acute Alcohol Withdrawal
The usual dose is 10 milligrams 3 or 4 times during the first 24 hours, then 5 milligrams 3 or 4 times daily as needed.

Relief of Muscle Spasm
The usual dose is 2 milligrams to 10 milligrams 3 or 4 times daily.

Convulsive Disorders
The usual dose is 2 milligrams to 10 milligrams 2 to 4 times daily.

CHILDREN

Valium should not be given to children under 6 months of age.

The usual starting dose for children over 6 months is 1 to 2.5 milligrams 3 or 4 times a day. Your doctor may increase the dosage gradually if needed.

ELDERLY

The usual dosage is 2 milligrams to 2.5 milligrams once or twice a day, which your doctor will increase as needed. Your doctor will limit the dosage to the smallest effective amount because older people are more apt to become oversedated or uncoordinated.

Overdosage

Any medication taken in excess can have serious consequences. If you suspect an overdose, seek medical attention immediately.

■ *Symptoms of Valium overdose may include:*
Coma
Confusion
Diminished reflexes
Sleepiness

Brand name:

VELOSEF

Pronounced: VELL-oh-seff
Generic name: Cephradine

Why is this drug prescribed?

Velosef, a broad-spectrum cephalosporin antibiotic available in capsule or liquid form, is similar to oral penicillin. Velosef is given to treat certain infections of the upper or lower respiratory tract, including pharyngitis (strep throat) and pneumonia, as well as middle ear, skin, or urinary tract infections.

Most important fact about this drug

If you are allergic to either penicillin or cephalosporin antibiotics in any form, consult your doctor *before taking Velosef.* There is a possibility that you are allergic to both types of medicines; and if a reaction occurs, it could be extremely severe. If you take the drug and feel signs of a reaction, seek medical attention immediately.

How should you take this medication?

Take Velosef exactly as prescribed. You will usually be instructed to take a dose every 6 hours or every 12 hours. You may take the medication with meals or between meals.

Do not stop taking Velosef when you start feeling better; it is important to keep taking it on your usual schedule until you have finished all of the medicine.

■ *If you miss a dose...*
If you take 1 dose a day, take the missed dose as soon as you remember and the next dose 10 to 12 hours later.

If you take 2 doses a day, take the missed dose immediately and the next dose 5 to 6 hours later.

If you take 3 or more doses a day, take the missed dose immediately and the next dose 2 to 4 hours later.

Go back to your regular schedule after the second dose.

■ *Storage instructions...*
Store away from heat, light, and moisture. Store the liquid in the refrigerator, but do not allow to freeze.

What side effects may occur?
Side effects cannot be anticipated. If any develop or change in intensity, inform your doctor immediately. Only your doctor can determine if it is safe you to continue taking Velosef.

Velosef may cause diarrhea, which has the potential to become serious.

■ *Other potential side effects include:*
Abdominal pain, blistering or peeling of skin, confusion, convulsions, decreased urine output, difficulty breathing, dizziness, fever, headache, hives, itching, joint pain, loss of appetite, muscle aches, nausea, rash, redness, swelling, tightness in the chest, vaginal yeast infection, vomiting

Why should this drug not be prescribed?
You may be at increased risk of an allergic reaction to Velosef if you have a history of allergies, asthma, hay fever, or hives.

If you have impaired kidney function or gastrointestinal disease, your doctor will evaluate your condition before prescribing Velosef.

Special warnings about this medication
You should be aware that Velosef may produce false positive results in tests for sugar in the urine. If you are diabetic, you should use TesTape or Clinistix rather than Clinitest tablets while taking Velosef.

Possible food and drug interactions when taking this medication
If Velosef is taken with certain other drugs, the effects of either could be increased, decreased, or altered. It is especially important to check with your doctor before combining Velosef with the following:

Diuretics such as Lasix and Bumex
Other antibiotics such as Garamycin
Probenecid (Benemid)

Special information if you are pregnant or breastfeeding
The effects of Velosef in pregnancy have not been adequately studied.

If you are pregnant or plan to become pregnant, inform your doctor immediately. Velosef should be taken in pregnancy only if clearly needed. Caution is also advised for nursing mothers, since Velosef does appear in breast milk.

Recommended dosage

ADULTS

Respiratory Tract Infections (Other than Lobar Pneumonia) and Skin and Skin Structure Infections
The usual dose is 250 milligrams every 6 hours or 500 milligrams every 12 hours.

Lobar Pneumonia
The usual dose is 500 milligrams every 6 hours or 1 gram every 12 hours.

Urinary Tract Infections
The usual dose is 500 milligrams every 12 hours for uncomplicated urinary tract infections. In more serious urinary tract infections, including prostatitis, your doctor may prescribe 500 milligrams every 6 hours or 1 gram every 12 hours.

Severe or Chronic Infections
You may take larger doses (up to 1 gram four times a day) for severe or chronic infections. As with antibiotic therapy in general, you should continue treatment for a minimum of 48 to 72 hours after you feel better.

CHILDREN

The usual dose in children over 9 months of age is 25 to 50 milligrams for each 2.2 pounds of body weight per day, divided into equal doses and taken every 6 or 12 hours.

Otitis Media Due to H. influenzae
The recommended dose ranges from 75 to 100 milligrams for each 2.2 pounds of body weight per day, divided into equal doses and taken every 6 or 12 hours; the daily total should not exceed 4 grams.

Overdosage
Although no specific information is available regarding overdose, any medication taken in excess can have serious consequences. If you suspect a Velosef overdose, seek medical attention immediately.

Generic name:

VENLAFAXINE

See *Effexor*, page 577.

Brand name:

VIBRAMYCIN

See *Doryx*, page 574.

Brand name:

VIBRA-TABS

See *Doryx*, page 574.

Generic name:

VITAMINS WITH FLUORIDE

See *Poly-Vi-Flor*, page 719.

Brand name:

VOLTAREN

Pronounced: *vol-TAR-en*
Generic name: *Diclofenac sodium*
Other brand name: *Cataflam (Diclofenac Potassium)*

Why is this drug prescribed?
Voltaren and Cataflam, nonsteroidal anti-inflammatory drugs, are used to relieve the inflammation, swelling, stiffness, and joint pain associated with rheumatoid arthritis, osteoarthritis (the most common form of arthritis), and ankylosing spondylitis (arthritis and stiffness of the spine). Cataflam is also used in the treatment of menstral pain.

Most important fact about this drug
You should have frequent checkups with your doctor if you take Voltaren regularly. Ulcers or internal bleeding can occur without warning.

How should you take this medication?
To minimize stomach upset and related side effects, your doctor may recommend taking

this medicine with food, milk, or an antacid. However, this may delay onset of relief.

Take this drug with a full glass of water. Also, do not lie down for about 20 minutes after taking it. This will help to prevent irritation in your upper digestive tract.

Take this medication exactly as prescribed.

■ *If you miss a dose...*
If you take this medicine on a regular schedule, take it as soon as you remember. If it is almost time for your next dose, skip the one you missed and go back to your regular schedule. Do not take 2 doses at once.

■ *Storage instructions...*
Store at room temperature. Keep the container tightly closed and protect from moisture.

What side effects may occur?
Side effects cannot be anticipated. If any develop or change in intensity, inform your doctor as soon as possible. Only your doctor can determine if it is safe for you to continue taking Voltaren.

■ *More common side effects may include:*
Abdominal pain or cramps
Constipation
Diarrhea
Dizziness
Headache
Indigestion
Nausea

■ *Less common side effects may include:*
Abdominal bleeding, abdominal swelling, fluid retension, gas, itching, peptic ulcers, rash, ringing in the ears

■ *Rare side effects may include:*
Anaphylaxis (severe allergic reaction), anemia, anxiety, appetite change, asthma, black stools, blood disorders, bloody diarrhea, blurred vision, changes in taste, colitis, congestive heart failure, decrease in white blood cells, decreased urine production, depression, double vision, drowsiness, dry mouth, hair loss, hearing loss (temporary), hepatitis, high blood pressure, hives, inability to sleep, inflammation of mouth, irritability, kidney failure, low blood pressure, nosebleed, red or purple skin discoloration, rash, itching, sensitivity to light, skin eruptions, inflammation, scaling, or peeling, Stevens-Johnson syndrome (a severe form of skin eruption), swelling of eyelids, lips, and tongue, swelling of the throat due to fluid retention, vague feeling of illness, vision changes, vomiting, yellow eyes and skin

Why should this drug not be prescribed?
If you are sensitive to or have ever had an allergic reaction to Voltaren or Cataflam, or if you have had asthma attacks, hives, or other allergic reactions caused by aspirin or other nonsteroidal anti-inflammatory drugs, you should not take this medication. Make sure your doctor is aware of any drug reactions you have experienced.

Special warnings about this medication
Remember this medication has been known to cause peptic ulcers and bleeding. Contact your doctor immediately if you suspect a problem.

This drug should be used with caution if you have heart failure, kidney problems, or liver disease, and it can cause liver inflammation in some people.

If you are taking blood-thinning medication or diuretics, use this drug with caution.

Use with caution if you have heart disease or high blood pressure. This drug can increase water retention.

If you experience nausea, fatigue, lethargy, itching, yellowed eyes and skin, tenderness in the upper right area of your abdomen, or flu-like symptoms, notify your doctor at once.

Possible food and drug interactions when taking this medication

If Voltaren or Cataflam are taken with certain other drugs, the effects of either could be increased, decreased, or altered. It is especially important to check with your doctor before combining Voltaren with the following:

Aspirin
Blood thinners such as Coumadin
Carteolol (Cartrol)
Cyclosporine (Sandimmune)
Digitalis drugs such as Lanoxin
Diuretics such as Dyazide, Midamur, and Lasix
Insulin or oral antidiabetes medications such as Micronase
Lithium (Lithonate)
Methotrexate

Special information if you are pregnant or breastfeeding

The effects of Voltaren during pregnancy have not been adequately studied. If you are pregnant or plan to become pregnant, inform your doctor immediately. Voltaren appears in breast milk and could affect a nursing infant. If this medication is essential to your health, your doctor may advise you to discontinue breastfeeding until your treatment with Voltaren is finished.

Recommended dosage

ADULTS

Osteoarthritis
The usual dose is 100 to 150 milligrams a day, divided into smaller doses of 50 milligrams 2 or 3 times a day (for Voltaren or Cataflam) or 75 milligrams twice a day (for Voltaren).

Rheumatoid Arthritis
The usual dose is 150 to 200 milligrams a day, divided into smaller doses of 50 milligrams 3 or 4 times a day (for Voltaren or Cataflam) or 75 milligrams twice a day (for Voltaren).

People with rheumatoid arthritis should not take more than 225 milligrams a day.

Ankylosing Spondylitis
The usual dose is 100 to 125 milligrams a day, divided into smaller doses of 25 milligrams 4 times a day, with another 25 milligrams at bedtime if necessary.

Menstral pain and discomfort
The usual starting dose of Cataflam is 50 milligrams 3 times a day, although some women will take 100 milligrams for the first dose, followed by 50-milligram doses. After the first day, you should not take more than 150 milligrams in a day.

CHILDREN

The safety and effectiveness of Voltaren have not been established in children.

Overdosage

Any medication taken in excess can have serious consequences. If you suspect an overdose, seek medical attention immediately.

■ *The symptoms of Voltaren overdose may include:*
   Acute kidney failure
   Drowsiness
   Loss of consciousness
   Lung inflammation
   Vomiting

Brand name:

WELLBUTRIN

Pronounced: Well-BEW-trin
Generic name: Bupropion hydrochloride

Why is this drug prescribed?

Wellbutrin, a relatively new antidepressant medication, is given to help relieve certain kinds of major depression.

Major depression involves a severely depressed mood (for 2 weeks or more) accompanied by sleep and appetite disturbances, agitation or lack of energy, feelings of guilt or worthlessness, decreased sex drive, inability to concentrate, and perhaps thoughts of suicide.

Unlike the more familiar tricyclic antidepressants, such as Elavil, Tofranil, and others, Wellbutrin tends to have a somewhat stimulating effect.

Most important fact about this drug

Although Wellbutrin occasionally causes weight gain, a more common effect is weight loss. Some 28 percent of people who take this medication lose 5 pounds or more. If depression has already caused you to lose weight, and if further weight loss would be detrimental to your health, Wellbutrin may not be the best antidepressant for you.

How should you take this medication?

Take Wellbutrin exactly as prescribed by your doctor. The usual dosing regimen is 3 equal doses spaced evenly throughout the day. Allow at least 6 hours between doses. Your doctor will probably start you at a low dosage and gradually increase it; this helps minimize side effects.

Since Wellbutrin may impair your coordination or judgment, do not drive or operate dangerous machinery until you find out how the medication affects you.

If Wellbutrin does work for you, your doctor will probably have you continue taking it for at least several months.

Avoid alcoholic beverages.

■ If you miss a dose...
Take it as soon as you remember. If it is within 4 hours of your next dose, skip the one you missed and go back to your regular schedule. Never take two doses at the same time.

■ Storage instructions...
Store at room temperature.

What side effects may occur?

Side effects cannot be anticipated. If any develop or change in intensity, inform your doctor as soon as possible. Only your doctor can determine if it is safe for you to continue taking Wellbutrin.

Seizures are perhaps the most worrisome side effect.

■ More common side effects may include:
Agitation
Constipation
Dizziness
Dry mouth
Excessive sweating
Headache
Nausea, vomiting
Skin rash
Sleep disturbances
Tremor

■ Other side effects may include:
Acne, bed-wetting, blisters in the mouth and eyes (Stevens-Johnson syndrome), blurred vision, breathing difficulty, chest pain, chills, complete or almost complete loss of movement, confusion, dry skin,

episodes of over-activity, elation, or irritability, extreme calmness, fatigue, fever, fluid retention, flu-like symptoms, gum irritation and inflammation, hair color changes, hair loss, hives, impotence, incoordination and clumsiness, indigestion, itching, increased libido, menstrual complaints, mood instability, muscle rigidity, painful ejaculation, painful erection, retarded ejaculation, ringing in the ears, sexual dysfunction, suicidal ideation, thirst disturbances, toothache, urinary disturbances, weight gain or loss

Why should this drug not be prescribed?

Do not take Wellbutrin if you are sensitive to or have ever had an allergic reaction to it.

Since Wellbutrin causes seizures in some people, do not take it if you have any type of seizure disorder.

You should not take Wellbutrin if you currently have, or formerly had, an eating disorder. For some reason, people with a history of anorexia nervosa or bulimia seem to be more likely to experience Wellbutrin-related seizures.

Do not take Wellbutrin if, within the past 14 days, you have taken a monoamine oxidase inhibitor (MAO inhibitor) type of antidepressant, such as Nardil, Marplan, or Parnate. This particular drug combination could cause you to experience a sudden, dangerous rise in blood pressure.

Special warnings about this medication

If you take Wellbutrin, you may be vulnerable to seizures if your dosage is too high or if you ever suffered brain damage or experienced seizures in the past.

Do not take other medications that might help trigger seizures (e.g., antipsychotics, other antidepressants).

If you have been taking Valium or a similar tranquilizer but are ready to stop, taper off gradually rather than quitting abruptly.

Possible food and drug interactions when taking this medication

Do not drink alcohol while you are taking Wellbutrin; an interaction between alcohol and Wellbutrin could increase the possibility of a seizure.

If Wellbutrin is taken with certain other drugs, the effects of either could be increased, decreased, or altered. It is especially important to check with your doctor before combining Wellbutrin with the following:

Antipsychotics such as Thorazine
Dilantin
Levodopa (Larodopa and others)
MAO inhibitors (antidepressants such as Parnate and Nardil)
Phenobarbital (Luminal and others)
Tagamet
Tegretol
Tricyclic antidepressants such as Elavil and Tofranil

Special information if you are pregnant or breastfeeding

If you are pregnant or plan to become pregnant, notify your doctor immediately. Wellbutrin should be taken during pregnancy only if clearly needed.

Wellbutrin may pass into breast milk and cause serious reactions in a nursing baby; therefore, if you are a new mother, you may need to discontinue breastfeeding while you are taking this medication.

Recommended dosage

No single dose of Wellbutrin should exceed 150 milligrams.

ADULTS

At the beginning, your dose will probably be 200 miligrams per day, taken as 100 milligrams 2 times a day. After at least 3 days at this dose, your doctor may increase the dosage to 300 milligrams per day, taken as 100 milligrams 3 times a day, with at least 6 hours between doses. This is the usual adult dose. The maximum recommended dose is 150 milligrams taken 3 times a day.

CHILDREN

The safety and effectiveness in children under 18 years old have not been established.

ELDERLY

Because they are more sensitive to antidepressant drugs, older people may find smaller doses satisfactory.

Overdosage

Any medication taken in excess can have serious consequences. If you suspect an overdose of Wellbutrin, seek medical attention immediately.

- *Symptoms of Wellbutrin overdose may include:*
  Hallucinations
  Heart failure
  Loss of consciousness
  Rapid heartbeat
  Seizures

- *An overdose that involves other drugs in combination with Wellbutrin may also cause these symptoms:*
  Breathing difficulties
  Coma
  Fever
  Rigid muscles
  Stupor

Brand name:

WYMOX

See Amoxil, page 503.

Brand name:

XANAX

Pronounced: ZAN-ax
Generic name: Alprazolam

Why is this drug prescribed?

Xanax is a tranquilizer used in the short-term relief of symptoms of anxiety or the treatment of anxiety disorders. Anxiety disorder is marked by unrealistic worry or excessive fears and concerns.

Xanax is also used in the treatment of panic disorder, which appears as unexpected panic attacks and may be accompanied by a fear of open spaces called agoraphobia. Only your doctor can diagnose panic disorder and best advise you about treatment. Anxiety associated with depression is also responsive to Xanax.

Some doctors prescribe Xanax to treat alcohol withdrawal, fear of open spaces and strangers, depression, irritable bowel syndrome, and premenstrual syndrome.

Most important fact about this drug

Tolerance and dependence can occur with the use of Xanax. You may experience withdrawal symptoms if you stop using the drug abruptly. Only your doctor should advise you to discontinue or change your dose.

How should you take this medication?

Xanax may be taken with or without food. Take it exactly as prescribed.

■ *If you miss a dose...*
If you are less than 1 hour late, take it as soon as you remember. Otherwise skip the dose and go back to your regular schedule. Never take 2 doses at the same time.

■ *Storage instructions...*
Store Xanax at room temperature.

What side effects may occur?

Side effects cannot be anticipated. If any develop or change in intensity, inform your doctor as soon as possible. Only your doctor can determine if it is safe for you to continue taking Xanax. Your doctor should periodically reassess the need for this drug.

Side effects to Xanax are usually seen at the beginning of treatment and disappear with continued medication. However, if dosage is increased, side effects will be more likely.

■ *More common side effects may include:*
Abdominal discomfort, abnormal involuntary movement, agitation, allergies, anxiety, blurred vision, chest pain, confusion, constipation, decreased or increased sex drive, depression, diarrhea, difficult urination, dream abnormalities, drowsiness, dry mouth, fainting, fatigue, fluid retention, headache, hyperventilation (too frequent or too deep breathing), inability to fall asleep, increase or decrease in appetite, increased or decreased salivation, impaired memory, irritability, lack of coordination, light-headedness, low blood pressure, menstrual problems, muscular twitching, nausea and vomiting, nervousness, palpitations, rapid heartbeat, rash, restlessness, ringing in the ears, sexual dysfunction, skin inflammation, speech difficulties, stiffness, stuffy nose, sweating, tiredness/sleepiness, tremors, upper respiratory infections, weakness, weight gain or loss

■ *Less common or rare side effects may include:*
Abnormal muscle tone, concentration difficulties, decreased coordination, dizziness, double vision, fear, hallucinations, inability to control urination or bowel movements, infection, itching, loss of appetite, muscle cramps, muscle spasticity, rage, sedation, seizures, sleep disturbances, slurred speech, stimulation, talkativeness, taste alterations, temporary memory loss, tingling or pins and needles, uninhibited behavior, urine retention, warm feeling, weakness in muscle and bone, weight gain or loss, yellow eyes and skin

■ *Side effects due to decrease or withdrawal from Xanax:*
Blurred vision, decreased concentration, decreased mental clarity, diarrhea, heightened awareness of noise or bright lights, impaired sense of smell, loss of appetite, loss of weight, muscle cramps, seizures, tingling sensation, twitching

Why should this drug not be prescribed?

If you are sensitive to or have ever had an allergic reaction to Xanax or other tranquilizers, you should not take this medication. Make sure that your doctor is aware of any drug reactions that you have experienced.

Do not take this medication if you have been diagnosed with the eye condition called narrow-angle glaucoma.

Anxiety or tension related to everyday stress usually does not require treatment with Xanax. Discuss your symptoms thoroughly with your doctor.

Special warnings about this medication

Xanax may cause you to become drowsy or less alert; therefore, driving or operating dangerous machinery or participating in any hazardous activity that requires full mental alertness is not recommended.

If you are being treated for panic disorder, you may need to take a higher dose of Xanax than for anxiety alone. High doses of this medication taken for long intervals may cause emotional and physical dependence. It is important that your doctor supervise you carefully when you are using this medication.

Remember that withdrawal symptoms can occur when Xanax is stopped suddenly.

Possible food and drug interactions when taking this medication

Xanax may intensify the effect of alcohol. Do not drink alcohol while taking this medication.

If Xanax is taken with certain other drugs, the effects of either could be increased, decreased, or altered. It is important to check with your doctor before combining Xanax with the following:

Antihistamines such as Benadryl and Tavist
Carbamazepine (Tegretol)
Certain antidepressant drugs, includng
    Elavid, Norpramin, and Tofranil
Cimetidine (Tagamet)
Digoxin (Lanoxin)
Disulfiram (Antabuse)
Major tranquilizers such as Mellaril and
    Thorazine
Oral contraceptives
Other central nervous system depressants
    such as Valium and Demerol

Special information if you are pregnant or breastfeeding

Do not take this medication if you are pregnant or planning to become pregnant. There is an increased risk of respiratory problems and muscular weakness in your baby. Infants may also experience withdrawal symptoms. Xanax may appear in breast milk and could affect a nursing infant. If this medication is essential to your health, your doctor may advise you to stop breastfeeding until your treatment with this medication is finished.

Recommended dosage

ADULTS

Anxiety disorder
The usual starting dose of Xanax is 0.25 to 0.5 milligram taken 3 times a day. The dose may be increased every 3 to 4 days to a maximum daily dose of 4 milligrams, divided into smaller doses.

Panic disorder
You may be given a dose from 1 up to a total of 10 milligrams, according to your needs. The typical dose is 5 to 6 milligrams a day.

The usual starting dose is 0.5 milligram 3 times a day. This dose can be increased by 1 milligram a day every 3 or 4 days.

CHILDREN

Safety and effectiveness have not been established in children under 18 years of age.

ELDERLY

The usual starting dose for an anxiety disorder is 0.25 milligram, 2 or 3 times daily. This dose may be gradually increased if needed and tolerated.

Overdosage

Any medication taken in excess can have serious consequences. If you suspect an overdose, seek medical attention immediately.

■ *Symptoms of Xanax overdose may include:*
Confusion
Coma
Impaired coordination
Sleepiness
Slowed reaction time

An overdose of Xanax, alone or after combining it with alcohol, can be fatal.

Brand name:

YUTOPAR

Pronounced: YOU-tow-par
Generic name: Ritrodrine hydrochloride

Why is this drug prescribed?
Yutopar tablets are used as maintenance medication to prevent recurrence of premature labor after it has been stopped by Yutopar intravenous therapy, which is usually administered by your doctor in the hospital.

Most important fact about this drug
Before you start on Yutopar, your doctor needs to know all medications—both prescription or nonprescription—that you are taking. If you are taking steroids (cortisone-like medicines), there is an increased chance that too much fluid may accumulate in your lungs when you take Yutopar.

If you are taking beta-blocking blood pressure medicatons such as atenolol (Tenormin), propranolol (Inderal), or metroprolol (Lopressor), Yutopar may not be as effective.

How should you take this medication?
Take Yutopar tablets exactly as prescribed. You will receive your first dose of Yutopar tablets in the hospital, 30 minutes before you are taken off Yutopar intravenous

therapy. Before you leave the hospital, your doctor should tell you exactly how to take the medication at home. If you have any questions about your medication, be sure to ask your doctor.

■ *If you miss a dose...*
Take it as soon as you remember if it is within an hour or so of the scheduled time. If you do not remember until later, skip the dose and go back to your regular schedule. Do not take 2 doses at once.

■ *Storage instructions...*
Store at room temperature. Protect from excessive heat.

What side effects may occur?
Side effects cannot be anticipated. If any develop or change in intensity, tell your doctor as soon as possible. Only your doctor can determine if it is safe for you to continue using Yutopar.

■ *More common side effects may include:*
Faster heartbeat
Fluttery or throbbing heartbeat
Jitteriness
Nausea
Rash
Tremor

■ *Less common or rare side effects may include:*
Irregular heart beat, liver problems

Why should this drug not be prescribed?
Do not take Yutopar tablets if you have ever had an allergic reaction to or are sensitive to this medication. Tell your doctor if you have any medical problems. Your doctor will not prescribe Yutopar if you are suffering from any of the following conditions:

Asthma
Diabetes

Eclampsia (a rare condition of late
   pregnancy characterized by seizures)
Heart disease
Hemorrhaging
High blood pressure
Hypovolemia (abnormally low circulating
   blood volume)
Inflammation of the membranes surrounding
   the unborn baby caused by bacteria in
   the amniotic fluid
Migraine headaches
Overactive thyroid
Pulmonary hypertension (high blood pressure
   in the arteries supplying the lungs)
Tumor on the adrenal gland

Your doctor may suggest an
electrocardiogram (ECG), which will detect
any possible heart problems, before he or
she treats you with Yutopar.

Yutopar therapy is not given before the
20th week of pregnancy.

Special warnings about this medication

Pulmonary edema (the accumulation of fluid
in lung tissue and air sacs) may occur during
and after receiving Yutopar therapy. If you
experience any unusual symptoms such as
rapid breathing, nervousness, rapid heartbeat,
or any swelling in your arms or legs, call
your doctor immediately.

After you return from the hospital, should
your water break or contractions begin
again, call your doctor.

Possible food and drug interactions when taking this medication

If Yutopar is taken with certain other drugs,
the effects of either could be increased,
decreased, or altered. It is especially
important to check with your doctor before
combining Yutopar with the following:

Antidepressant drugs classified as MAO
   inhibitors, including Nardil, Parnate, and

Marplan
Beta-blocking blood pressure medicines, such
   as Inderal, Lopressor, and Tenormin
Cyclosporine (Sandimmune)
Steroids such as prednisone and Decadron

Special information about Yutopar and the baby

There are no studies of the effects of
Yutopar in pregnant women before the 20th
week of pregnancy. Studies of Yutopar given
to pregnant women after the 20th week of
pregnancy do not show an increased risk of
abnormalities in the unborn baby, but the
possibility cannot be totally ruled out. Your
doctor will decide whether the benefits of
taking Yutopar outweigh the risks to the
unborn child.

Recommended dosage

You will receive one 10-milligram tablet
approximately 30 minutes before the end of
your intravenous therapy. The usual dosage
schedule for the first 24 hours is one 10-
milligram tablet every 2 hours. After that
you will take 1 or 2 tablets (10 to 20
milligrams) every 4 to 6 hours. You should
not take more than 120 milligrams in a day.
Your doctor will decide how long you need
to stay on Yutopar.

Overdosage

If you suspect an overdose of Yutopar, call
your doctor immediately.

■ *Symptoms of Yutopar overdose may
   include:*
   Difficult or labored breathing
   Fluttery or throbbing heartbeat
   Irregular heartbeat
   Low blood pressure
   Nausea
   Nervousness
   Rapid heartbeat (in mother and baby)
   Tremors
   Vomiting

Generic name:

ZIDOVUDINE

See Retrovir, page 737.

Brand name:

ZITHROMAX

Pronounced: ZITH-roh-macks
Generic name: Azithromycin

Why is this drug prescribed?
Zithromax is an antibiotic related to erythromycin. It is prescribed to treat certain mild to moderate skin infections; upper and lower respiratory tract infections, including pharyngitis (strep throat), tonsillitis, and pneumonia; and sexually transmitted infections of the cervix or urinary tract.

Most important fact about this drug
There is a possibility of rare but very serious reactions to Zithromax, including angioedema (swelling of the face, lips, and neck that impedes speaking, swallowing, and breathing) and anaphylaxis (a violent, even fatal allergic reaction). If you develop these symptoms, stop taking Zithromax and call you doctor immediately.

How should you take this medication?
Take Zithromax at least 1 hour before or 2 hours after a meal. Do not take this medication with food, or with an antacid that contains aluminum or magnesium, such as Di-Gel, Gelusil, Maalox, and others.

Be sure to take all the Zithromax your doctor prescribes.

■ *If you miss a dose...*
Take the forgotten dose as soon as you remember. If you don't remember until the next day, skip the dose and go back to your regular schedule. Never try to "catch up" by doubling the dose.

■ *Storage instructions...*
Zithromax should be stored at room temperature.

What side effects may occur?
Side effects cannot be anticipated. If any develop or change in intensity, inform your doctor as soon as possible. Only your doctor can determine if it is safe for you to continue taking Zithromax.

■ *More common side effects may include:*
Abdominal pain
Diarrhea or loose stools
Nausea
Vomiting

■ *Less common side effects may include:*
Blood in the stools, chest pain, dizziness, drowsiness, fatigue, gas, headache, heart palpitations, indigestion, jaundice (yellowing of the skin and the whites of the eyes), kidney infection, light sensitivity, rash, severe allergic reaction including swelling (as in hives), sleepiness, vaginal inflammation, vertigo, yeast infection

The single large dose (4 capsules) of Zithromax that is prescribed to treat sexually transmitted infection of the cervix or urinary tract is more likely to cause stomach and bowel side effects than the smaller doses prescribed for a skin or respiratory tract infection.

Why should this drug not be prescribed?
Do not take Zithromax if you have ever had an allergic reaction to it or to similar antibiotics such as erythromycin (E.E.S., PCE, and others).

Special warnings about this medication
Like certain other antibiotics, Zithromax may cause a potentially life-threatening form

of diarrhea called pseudomembranous colitis. Pseudomembranous colitis may clear up spontaneously when the drug is stopped; if it does not, hospital treatment may be required. If you develop diarrhea, check with your doctor immediately.

If you have a liver problem, your doctor should monitor you very carefully while you are taking Zithromax.

Possible food and drug interactions when taking this medication

If Zithromax is taken with certain other drugs, the effects of either could be increased, decreased, or altered. It is especially important to check with your doctor before combining Zithromax with antacids containing aluminum or magnesium, such as Maalox and Mylanta.

The following interactions can occur with erythromycin, a similar drug.

Carbamazepine (Tegretol)
Certain antihistamines such as Hismanal and
   Seldane
Cyclosporine (Sandimmune)
Digoxin (Lanoxin, Lanoxicaps)
Ergot-containing drugs such as Cafergot and
   D.H.E.
Hexobarbital
Lovastatin (Mevacor)
Phenytoin (Dilantin)
Theophylline drugs such as Bronkodyl, Slo-
   Phyllin, Theo-Dur, and others
Triazolam (Halcion)
Warfarin (Coumadin)

Special information if you are pregnant or breastfeeding

If you are pregnant or plan to become pregnant, inform your doctor immediately. You should take Zithromax during pregnancy only if it is clearly needed. It is not known whether Zithromax can make its way into breast milk. If the drug is essential to your health, your doctor may advise you to stop breastfeeding until your treatment is finished.

Recommended dosage

ADULTS

The usual dose of Zithromax for patients age 16 years and older is 500 milligrams in a single dose the first day. This is followed by 250 milligrams one time each day for the next 4 days. The total amount taken should be 1.5 grams.

For treatment of non-gonococcal urethritis and cervitis (sexually transmitted disease) due to the organism *Chlamydia trachomatis*, the usual dose is a single gram (1,000 milligrams) one time only.

CHILDREN

This medication is not recommended for children under age 16.

Overdosage

Although no specific information on Zithromax overdose is available, any medication taken in excess can have serious consequences. If you suspect an overdose, seek medical attention immediately.

Brand name:

ZOLOFT

Pronounced: ZOE-loft
Generic name: Sertraline

Why is this drug prescribed?

Zoloft is prescribed for major depression—a persistently low mood that interferes with everyday living. Symptoms may include loss of interest in your usual activities, disturbed sleep, change in appetite, constant fidgeting or lethargic movement, fatigue, feelings of worthlessness or guilt, difficulty thinking or concentrating, and recurrent thoughts of suicide.

Some doctors also prescribe Zoloft for obsessive-compulsive disorders.

Zoloft is thought to work by adjusting the balance of the brain's natural chemical messengers.

Most important fact about this drug

Do not take Zoloft if, within the past two weeks, you have taken another type of antidepressant medication known as an MAO inhibitor. Drugs in this category include Nardil, Parnate, and Marplan. When medication like Zoloft are combined with MAO inhibitors, serious and sometimes fatal reactions can occur.

How should you take this medication?

Take Zoloft exactly as prescribed: once a day, in either the morning or the evening.

Improvement with Zoloft may not be seen for several days to a few weeks.

Zoloft may make your mouth dry. For temporary relief suck a hard candy, chew gum, or melt bits of ice in your mouth.

■ *If you miss a dose...*
Take the forgotten dose as soon as you remember. If several hours have passed, skip the dose. Never try to "catch up" by doubling the dose.

■ *Storage instructions...*
Store at room temperature.

What side effects may occur?

Side effects cannot be anticipated. If any develop or change in intensity, inform your doctor as soon as possible. Only your doctor can determine if it is safe for you to continue taking Zoloft.

■ *More common side effects may include:*
Agitation, confusion, constipation, diarrhea or loose stools, difficulty with ejaculation, dizziness, dry mouth, fatigue, fluttery or throbbing heartbeat, gas, headache, increased sweating, indigestion, insomnia, nausea, nervousness, sleepiness, tremor, vomiting,

■ *Less common or rare side effects may include:*
Abdominal pain, abnormal hair growth, abnormal skin odor, acne, altered taste, anxiety, back pain, bad breath, breast development in males, breast pain or enlargement, bruise-like marks on the skin, changeable emotions, chest pain, cold, clammy skin, conjunctivitis (pinkeye), coughing, difficulty breathing, difficulty concentrating, difficulty swallowing, double vision, dry eyes, enlarged abdomen, excessive menstrual bleeding, eye pain, fainting, feeling faint upon arising from a sitting or lying position, female sexual problems, fever, fluid retention, flushing, frequent urination, hair loss, heart attack, hemorrhoids, hiccups, high blood pressure, hot flushes, increased appetite, increased salivation, inflammation of nose or throat, inflammation of the penis, intolerance to light, itching, joint pains, lack of coordination, lack of menstruation, lack of sensation, loss of appetite, low blood pressure, menstrual problems, middle ear infection, migraine, movement problems, muscle cramps or weakness, muscle pain, need to urinate during the night, nosebleed, pain upon urination, painful menstruation, purple or red spots on the skin, racing heartbeat, rash, ringing in the ears, sensitivity to light, sinus inflammation, skin eruptions or inflammation, sleepwalking, sores on tongue, speech problems, stomach and intestinal inflammation, swelling of the

face, swollen wrists and ankles, thirst, tingling or pins and needles, twitching, urinary trouble, vaginal inflammation or discharge, varicose veins, vision problems, weight loss or gain, yawning

■ *Zoloft may also cause mental or emotional symptoms such as:*
Abnormal dreams or thoughts, aggressiveness, exaggerated feeling of well-being, depersonalization ("unreal" feeling), hallucinations, memory loss, paranoia, rapid mood shifts, suicidal thoughts, tooth-grinding, worsened depression

Many people lose a pound or two of body weight while taking Zoloft. This usually poses no problem but may be a concern if your depression has already caused you to lose a great deal of weight.

In a few people, Zoloft may trigger the grandiose, inappropriate, out-of-control behavior called mania or the similar, but less dramatic, "hyper" state called hypomania.

Why should this drug not be prescribed?
There are no known reasons to limit the use of this medication.

Special warnings about this medication
If you have a kidney or liver disorder, take Zoloft cautiously and under close medical supervision.

Possible food and drug interactions when taking this medication
You should not drink alcoholic beverages while taking Zoloft.

If Zoloft is taken with certain other drugs, the effects of either could be increased, decreased, or altered. It is especially important to check with your doctor before combining Zoloft with the following:

Cimetidine (Tagamet)
Diazepam (Valium, Valrelease)
Digitoxin (Crystodigin)
Lithium (Lithonate)
MAO inhibitors (antidepressant drugs such as Nardil, Parnate, and Marplan)
Other psychiatric drugs such as Elavil and Mellaril
Over-the-counter drugs such as cold remedies
Tolbutamide (Orinase)
Warfarin (Coumadin)

Special information if you are pregnant or breastfeeding
The effects of Zoloft during pregnancy have not been adequately studied. If you are pregnant or plan to become pregnant, inform your doctor immediately. Zoloft should be taken during pregnancy only if it is clearly needed. It is not known whether Zoloft appears in breast milk. Caution is advised when using Zoloft during breastfeeding.

Recommended dosage

ADULTS

The usual starting dose is 50 milligrams once a day, taken either in the morning or in the evening.

Your doctor may increase your dose depending upon your response. You should not take more than 200 milligrams in a day.

Overdosage
Any medication taken in excess can have serious consequences. If you suspect an overdose, seek medical attention immediately.

■ *Symptoms of Zoloft overdose may include:*
Anxiety
Dilated pupils
Nausea
Rapid heartbeat

Sleepiness
Vomiting

Brand name:

ZOVIRAX

Pronounced: zoh-VIGH-racks
Generic name: Acyclovir

Why is this drug prescribed?
Zovirax liquid, capsules, and tablets, are
used in the treatment of certain infections
with herpes viruses. These include genital
herpes, shingles, and chickenpox. This drug
may not be appropriate for everyone, and its
use should be thoroughly discussed with
your doctor. Zovirax ointment is used to
treat initial episodes of genital herpes and
certain herpes simplex infections of the skin
and mucous membranes.

Some doctors use Zovirax, along with other
drugs, in the treatment of AIDS, and for
unusual herpes infections such as those
following kidney and bone marrow
transplants.

Most important fact about this drug
Zovirax does not cure herpes. However, it
does reduce pain and may help the sores
caused by herpes to heal faster. Genital
herpes is a sexually transmitted disease. To
avoid infecting your partner, forego
intercourse and other sexual contact when
visible lesions are present.

How should you take this medication?
Your medication should not be shared with
others, and the prescribed dose should not
be exceeded. Zovirax ointment should not
be used in or near the eyes.

To reduce the risk of spreading the
infection, use a rubber glove to apply the
ointment.

■ If you miss a dose...
Take it as soon as you remember. If it is
almost time for your next dose, skip the
one you missed and go back to your
regular schedule. Never take 2 doses at
the same time.

If you are using the ointment, apply it as
soon as you remember and continue your
regular schedule.

■ Storage instructions...
Store Zovirax at room temperature in a
dry place.

What side effects may occur?
Side effects cannot be anticipated. If any
develop or change in intensity, inform your
doctor as soon as possible. Only your
doctor can determine if it is safe for you to
continue taking Zovirax.

■ More common side effects may include:
Confusion, constipation, diarrhea,
dizziness, fever, fluid retention, general
feeling of bodily discomfort, gland
enlargement in the groin, hair loss,
hallucinations, headache, hives, itching,
muscle pain, nausea, pain, skin rash,
sleepiness, stomach and intestinal
problems, visual abnormalities, vomiting

■ Less common or rare side effects may
include:
Abdominal pain, anaphylasix (severe
allergic reaction), diarrhea, dizziness,
fatigue, gas, headache, inability to sleep,
leg pain, loss of appetite, medicinal taste,
rash, retention of fluid, sore throat,
tingling or pins and needles, vomiting,
weakness

■ Common side effects of Zovirax ointment
may include:
Burning
Itching
Mild pain

Skin rash
Stinging
Vaginal inflammation

Why should this drug not be prescribed?

If you are sensitive to or have ever had an allergic reaction to Zovirax or similar drugs, you should not take this medication. Make sure that your doctor is aware of any drug reactions that you have experienced.

Special warnings about this medication

If you are being treated for a kidney disorder, consult with your doctor before taking Zovirax.

Although decreased sperm count has been reported in animals given high doses of Zovirax, this effect has not been documented to occur in humans.

Possible food and drug interactions when taking this medication

If Zovirax is taken with certain other drugs, the effects of either could be increased, decreased, or altered. It is especially important to check with your doctor before combining Zovirax with the following:

Cyclosporine (Sandimmune)
Interferon (Roferon)
Probenecid (Benemid)
Zidovudine (Retrovir)

Special information if you are pregnant or breastfeeding

The effects of Zovirax during pregnancy have not been adequately studied. If you are pregnant or plan to become pregnant, inform your doctor immediately. Zovirax appears in breast milk and could affect a nursing infant. If this medication is essential to your health, your doctor may advise you to discontinue breastfeeding your baby until your treatment with Zovirax is finished.

Recommended dosage

ADULTS

For Genital Herpes

The usual dose is one 200-milligram capsule or 1 teaspoonful of liquid every 4 hours, 5 times daily for 10 days. If the herpes is recurrent, the usual adult dose is 400 milligrams (two 200-milligram capsules, one 400-milligram tablet or 2 teaspoonfuls) 2 times daily for up to 12 months.

If genital herpes is intermittent, the usual adult dose is one 200-milligram capsule or 1 teaspoon of liquid every 4 hours, 5 times a day for 5 days. Therapy should be started at the earliest sign or symptom.

Ointment

Apply ointment to affected area every 3 hours, 6 times per day, for 7 days. Use enough ointment (approximately one-half inch ribbon of ointment per 4 square inches of surface area) to cover the affected area.

For Herpes Zoster (Shingles)

The usual adult dose is 800 milligrams (four 200-milligram capsules, two 400-milligram tablets, or 4 teaspoonfuls of liquid) every 4 hours, 5 times daily for 7 to 10 days.

If you have a kidney disorder, the dose will need to be adjusted by your doctor.

CHILDREN

The usual dose for chickenpox is 20 milligrams per 2.2 pounds of body weight, not to exceed 800 milligrams, taken orally 4 times daily for 5 days. Therapy should be initiated at the earliest sign or symptom.

The safety and effectiveness of Zovirax have not been established in children under 2 years of age. However, your doctor may decide that the benefits of this medication outweigh the potential risks.

ELDERLY

No special considerations apply.

Overdosage

Zovirax is generally safe; however, there have been cases of kidney disorder in patients taking Zovirax orally.

Any medication taken in excess can have serious consequences.

If you suspect an overdose, seek medical attention immediately.

Drug Risks in Pregnancy

Virtually no medications are certified completely safe in pregnancy. On the other hand, very few drugs are sure to do the baby harm. Most fall into a gray area where the threat of damage varies, but can never be entirely ruled out. Risks range from minimal to severe. And to make the situation even more confusing, there's no predictable pattern to the degree of danger.

To make sense of the situation, the U.S. Food and Drug Administration has established a rating system designed to show exactly what is known about each drug's potential for harm. Doctors use the system as a guide when prescribing. The table on the following pages gives these same ratings for all the most frequently prescribed drugs in the United States.

The FDA's system divides drugs into five categories, ranging from completely safe to absolutely forbidden in pregnancy. To qualify for a particular category, a drug must pass (or fail) certain scientific tests in animals, humans, or both. Here are the exact standards for each category.

A: Proved Safe

A drug in this category has been carefully tested in pregnant women and has done no harm. Almost no drugs meet this requirement because, if scientists think that there is even a remote chance that a drug will hurt a developing baby, they will not give it to the mother. The drug could, in fact, be perfectly safe; but without test results to *prove* its harmlessness, this rating doesn't apply.

B: No Proven Risk

A drug can achieve this rating without human tests. It simply needs to pass all animal tests without causing damage. If animal tests do sound an alarm, a drug can still qualify for this rating if studies in humans fail to uncover any risk. Although reassuring, this rating does not provide you with *absolute* certainty of safety. The effects of a drug sometimes differ between animals and humans; and even if the drug has never done harm in humans, animal tests can still leave some lingering doubt.

C: Possible Risk

Drugs in this category have not been tested in pregnant women, and may not have been tested in animals either. Whatever testing has been done in animals *has* uncovered a chance of harm. However, the likelihood is considered small enough to justify taking the drug if it's essential to your health.

D: Proven Risk

Drugs with this rating are known to have caused babies harm, but still may be needed in certain cases. Not every child whose mother takes the drug will suffer damage; and drugs in this category have no safer alternative. Despite the possible threat to the baby, the drug may be so important to the mother's health that not taking it is even more dangerous.

X: Do Not Use

This rating means that there is absolutely no reason to risk using the drug while pregnant. There is clear evidence that the drug can do harm, and it is either not essential to your health or can be replaced with a safer alternative.

Except for "A" and "X", you can see that these ratings do require a judgment call. Harm to the baby is never a certainty, and some drugs, such as epilepsy medications, may be so crucial to the *mother's* safety as to make taking them the least risky choice.

If a drug is rated "X" there's no question: Avoid it at all costs if you even *think* you're pregnant. But if it falls into the "B", "C", or "D" categories, check with your doctor before discontinuing it. Its risks may be low enough, and its benefits sufficiently high, to make its continued use the wisest course.

In any event, don't hesitate to voice your concern. In many cases, another drug–or no drug–may be a reasonable, medically sound alternative.

Profile Name	A Proved Safe	B No Proven Risk	C Possible Risk	D Proven Risk	X Do Not Use	Comments
Accupril			■	■		Not recommended in 1st trimester; do not use in 2nd & 3rd trimesters
Accutane					■	High risk of birth defects
Achromycin V						Unrated; a possible risk
Aci-Jel			■			
Aclovate			■			Do not use in large amounts or for prolonged periods
Actigall		■				Not recommended in pregnancy
AeroBid			■			
Aldactazide						Unrated; use only if necessary
Aldactone						Unrated; use only if necessary
Aldomet		■				Use only if clearly needed
Altace			■	■		2nd trimester—can be injurious; 3rd trimester—is injurious
Alupent			■			
Ambien		■				Use only if clearly needed
Amoxil						Unrated; safety not established
Anafranil			■			Withdrawal side effects; use only if necessary
Anaprox		■				Avoid in late pregnancy
Android					■	Causes masculinization of female fetus
Ansaid		■				Not recommended in pregnancy
Antivert		■				Use only if clearly needed
Anusol HC			■			Do not use in large amounts or for prolonged periods
Artane						Unrated
Asendin			■			
Aspirin						Avoid in 3rd trimester
Atarax						Unrated; avoid in early pregnancy
Ativan						Unrated; avoid in early pregnancy
Atrovent		■				Use only if clearly needed
Augmentin		■				Use only if clearly needed
Auralgan			■			
AVC			■			
Axid			■			

Profile Name	A Proved Safe	B No Proven Risk	C Possible Risk	D Proven Risk	X Do Not Use	Comments
Azmacort			■			Treatment may not be needed during pregnancy
Azulfidine		■				Use only if clearly needed
Bactrim			■			
Bactroban		■				Use only if clearly needed
Beconase			■			
Benadryl		■				Use only if clearly needed
Bentyl		■				Use only if clearly needed
Benzamycin Gel			■			
Betagan			■			
Betoptic			■			
Biaxin			■			
Brethine		■				For injections; tablets unrated; use only if clearly needed
Bronkometer						Unrated; use only if necessary
Bumex			■			
BuSpar		■				Use only if clearly needed
Cafergot					■	
Calan			■			
Calcimar Injection			■			
Caltrate 600						Unrated; no warning
Capoten			■	■		1st trimester—possible risk; 2nd & 3rd trimester—definite risk
Capozide			■	■		1st trimester—possible risk; 2nd & 3rd trimester—definite risk
Carafate		■				Use only if clearly needed
Cardene			■			
Cardizem			■			
Cardura			■			
Cartrol			■			
Catapres			■			
Ceclor		■				Use only if clearly needed
Ceftin		■				Use only if clearly needed
Cefzil		■				Use only if clearly needed

Profile Name	A Proved Safe	B No Proven Risk	C Possible Risk	D Proven Risk	X Do Not Use	Comments
Centrax						Unrated; not recommended in pregnancy
Choledyl			■			
Chronulac		■				Use only if necessary
Cipro			■			Use only if necessary
Claritin		■				Use only if clearly needed
Cleocin T		■				Use only if clearly needed
Cleocin Vaginal Cream		■				Use only if clearly needed
Clinoril						Unrated; not recommended in pregnancy, avoid in 3rd trimester
Clomid						Unrated; not recommended in pregnancy
Clozaril		■				Use only if clearly needed
Cogentin						Unrated; safety not established
Cognex			■			
Colace						Unrated
ColBenemid						Unrated; do not use in pregnancy
Colestid						Unrated; safety not established
Coly-Mycin S Otic						Unrated
Colyte			■			
Compazine						Unrated; use only if necessary
Condylox			■			
Corgard			■			
Cortisporin Ophthalmic			■			
Corzide			■			
Coumadin					■	Possible hemorrhaging and malformations or fetal death
Cutivate			■			
Cyclocort			■			
Cylert		■				Use only if necessary
Cytotec					■	
Cytoxan				■		May cause sterility in both genders
Dalmane						Unrated; do not use in pregnancy

Profile Name	A Proved Safe	B No Proven Risk	C Possible Risk	D Proven Risk	X Do Not Use	Comments
Dantrium						Unrated; safety not established
Darvocet-N						Unrated; withdrawal symptoms in newborns
Darvon						Unrated; withdrawal symptoms in newborns
Daypro			■			
DDAVP		■				
Decadron in Tubinaire						Unrated; may affect adrenal function of newborns
Decadron Tablets						Unrated; may affect adrenal function of newborns
Deltasone						Unrated; may affect adrenal function of newborns
Demerol						Unrated; not recommended in pregnancy
Depakene				■		Not recommended in pregnancy
Depakote				■		Not recommended in pregnancy
Depo-Provera						Unrated; avoid in 1st 4 months
Desquam-E			■			
Desyrel			■			
Dexedrine			■			
Diabinese			■			Can cause low blood sugar in newborns
Diamox			■			
Diethylstilbestrol					■	Can cause cancer in reproductive organs of offspring
Diflucan			■			
Dilantin						Unrated; not recommended in pregnancy
Dilaudid			■			Can cause dependency in newborns
Dimetane-DC			■			
Dipentum			■			
Diprolene			■			Do not use in large amounts or for prolonged periods
Disalcid			■			
Ditropan		■				

Profile Name	A Proved Safe	B NoProven Risk	C Possible Risk	D Proven Risk	X Do Not Use	Comments
Diuril			■			
Dolobid			■			Not recommended in 3rd trimester
Donnatal			■			
Doral					■	
Doryx				■		Can cause discoloration of baby's teeth
Duricef		■				Use only if necessary
Dyazide			■			
DynaCirc			■			
Effexor			■			
Efudex						Unrated; safety not established
Elavil						Unrated; use only if necessary
Eldepryl			■			
Elocon			■			Do not use in large amounts or for prolonged periods
Empirin with Codeine			■			Can cause complications in 3rd trimester
Enduron		■				Use only if necessary
Entex LA			■			
Erythromycin, Oral		■				Use only if necessary
Erythromycin Topicals						Unrated; safety not established
Estraderm					■	
Ethmozine		■				Use only if necessary
Eulexin				■		
Fastin						Unrated; use only if necessary
Felbatol			■			
Feldene						Unrated; not recommended in pregnancy
Femstat			■			
Fioricet						Unrated; use only if necessary
Fiorinal						Unrated; use only if necessary
Fiornal with Codeine			■			

Profile Name	A Proved Safe	B No Proven Risk	C Possible Risk	D Proven Risk	X Do Not Use	Comments
Flagyl		■				Do not use in 1st trimester; use in 2nd & 3rd trimester only if necessary
Flexeril		■				Use only if clearly needed
Floxin			■			
FML			■			
Gantrisin			■			Higher risk at term
Garamycin Ophthalmic						Unrated; safety not established
Glucotrol			■			Discontinue 1 month before term, can cause low blood sugar in newborns
Gris-PEG						Unrated; may cause birth defects
Halcion					■	
Haldol			■			
Halotestin					■	
Hismanal			■			
Humulin N						Unrated; important for healthy pregnancy
Hydergine						Unrated
HydroDIURIL		■				May cause jaundice in newborns
Hytrin			■			
Imdur		■				Use only if clearly needed
Imitrex			■			
Imodium		■				Use only if clearly needed
Inderal			■			
Inderide			■			
Indocin						Unrated; not recommended in pregnancy
Intal		■				Use only if necessary
Ionamin						Unrated; use only if necessary
Isordil			■			
Keflex		■				Use only if clearly needed
Keftab		■				Use only if clearly needed
Klonopin						Unrated; not recommended in pregnancy
Lanoxin			■			

Profile Name	A Proved Safe	B NoProven Risk	C Possible Risk	D Proven Risk	X Do Not Use	Comments
Larodopa						Unrated; safety not established
Lasix			■			
Lescol					■	
Levsin			■			
Librax						Unrated; not recommended in pregnancy
Librium						Unrated; not recommended in pregnancy
Lidex			■			Do not use in large amounts or for prolonged periods
Limbitrol						Unrated; not recommended in pregnancy
Lioresal						Unrated; use only if necessary
Lithonate						Unrated; avoid use, especially in 1st trimester
Lodine			■			Avoid in late pregnancy
Lomotil			■			
Lopid			■			
Lopressor			■			
Loprox		■				Use only if clearly needed
Lorabid		■				Use only if clearly needed
Lorelco		■				Use only if clearly needed
Lotensin			■	■		Risk possible in 1st trimester, definite in 2nd and 3rd trimesters
Lotrimin		■				Use only if necessary in 1st trimester; avoid in 2nd and 3rd trimesters
Lotrisone			■			Do not use in large amounts or for prolonged periods
Lozol		■				May cause jaundice in newborns
Ludiomil		■				Use only if clearly needed
Lupron Depot 3.75					■	
Luride Lozi-Tabs						Unrated
Macrodantin		■				Use only if necessary
Maxaquin			■			
Maxzide			■			Can cause jaundice in newborns

Profile Name	A Proved Safe	B No Proven Risk	C Possible Risk	D Proven Risk	X Do Not Use	Comments
Meclomen						Unrated; not recommended in pregnancy
Medrol						Unrated, may affect adrenal function in newborns
Megace				■		
Mellaril						Unrated; use only if necessary
Metamucil		■				
Methergine			■			Do not use in pregnancy
Methotrexate					■	
Metrodin					■	May cause multiple births
Metrogel-Vaginal		■				Use only if clearly needed
Mevacor					■	
Mexitil			■			
Micro-K			■			
Micronase		■				Use only if clearly needed
Midol						Unrated; check with your doctor
Midrin						Unrated
Miltown						Unrated, not recommended in pregnancy
Minipress			■			
Minocin				■		Can cause discoloration of baby's teeth
Moduretic		■				Use only if clearly needed
Monistat						Unrated; do not use in 1st trimester unless necessary
Monopril			■	■		Possible risk in 1st trimester, definite risk in 2nd & 3rd trimester
Motrin						Unrated; not recommended in pregnancy
MS Contin			■			Use only if necessary; can cause withdrawal symptoms in newborns
Mycolog II			■			Do not use in large amounts or for prolonged periods
Mysoline						Unrated; may cause birth defects
Nalfon						Unrated, not recommended in pregnancy
Naphcon A			■			

Profile Name	A Proved Safe	B NoProven Risk	C Possible Risk	D Proven Risk	X Do Not Use	Comments
Naprosyn		■				Not recommended in late pregnancy
Nardil			■			
Navane						Unrated; use only if necessary
Nembutal				■		Can cause withdrawal symptoms in newborns
Neodecadron Topical Cream			■			Do not use in large amounts or for prolonged periods
Neptazane			■			
Nicorette			■			
Nicotine Patches				■		
Nimotop			■			
Nitroglycerin			■			
Nizoral			■			
Nolamine						Unrated
Nolvadex				■		Not recommended in pregnancy
Norgesic Forte						Unrated; safety not established
Normodyne			■			
Noroxin			■			
Norpace			■			
Norplant					■	Risk of tubal pregnancy
Norpramin						Unrated; safety not established
Norvasc			■			
Ogen					■	
Omnipen		■				Use only if clearly needed
Oral Contraceptives					■	
Orap			■			
Orinase			■			Not recommended in pregnancy
Orudis		■				Use only if necessary
Oxistat		■				Use only if clearly needed
Pamelor						Unrated; safety not established
Pancrease			■			
Parafon Forte DSC						Unrated; safety not established
Parlodel						Unrated
Pathocil						Unrated; safety not established

Profile Name	A Proved Safe	B No Proven Risk	C Possible Risk	D Proven Risk	X Do Not Use	Comments
Paxil		■				Use only if clearly needed
PBZ						Unrated; safety not established
Pediapred			■			
Pediazole			■			Do not use at term
Penetrex			■			
Penicillin V Potassium						Unrated
Pepcid		■				Use only if clearly needed
Percocet			■			Can cause dependence in newborns
Pergonal				■		Risk of fetal harm, multiple births
Periactin		■				Use only if clearly needed
Peridex		■				Use only if necessary
Permax		■				Use only if necessary
Persantine		■				Use only if clearly needed
Phenergan			■			
Phenergan with Codeine			■			Can cause dependence in newborns
Phenobarbital				■		Can cause withdrawal symptoms in newborns
Phospholine Iodide			■			
Pilocar			■			
Plaquenil						Unrated; use only if necessary to counter malaria
Plendil			■			Unrated
Ponstel			■			Not recommended in late pregnancy
Pravachol				■		
Pred Forte			■			
Premarin					■	
Prilosec			■			
Procan SR			■			
Procardia			■			
Profasi			■			May cause multiple births
Prolixin						Unrated; use only if necessary
Propine		■				Use only if clearly needed
Proscar					■	

Profile Name	A Proved Safe	B NoProven Risk	C Possible Risk	D Proven Risk	X Do Not Use	Comments
ProSom					■	
Proventil			■			
Provera						Unrated; not recommended in last 4 months of pregnancy
Prozac		■				Use only if clearly needed
Psorcon Ointment			■			
Pyridium		■				Use only if clearly needed
Questran Powder						Unrated; not considered harmful
Quinamm					■	
Quinidex			■			
Reglan		■				Use only if clearly needed
Relafen			■			Avoid in 3rd trimester
Restoril					■	
Retin-A			■			
Retrovir			■			
Ridaura			■			Not recommended in pregnancy
Rifadin			■			Can cause hemorrhaging if used in last few weeks of pregnancy
Risperal			■			
Ritalin						Unrated; use only if necessary
Robaxin						Unrated; use only if necessary
Rocaltrol			■			
Rogaine			■			Not recommended in pregnancy
Rondec			■			
Rowasa		■				Use only if clearly needed
Ru-Tuss						Unrated; not recommended in pregnancy
Rynatan			■			
Rythmol			■			
Sandimmune			■			
Sansert						Unrated; do not use in pregnancy
Seconal Sodium				■		Can cause withdrawal symptoms
Sectral		■				Can cause growth problems in newborns
Seldane			■			

Profile Name	A Proved Safe	B No Proven Risk	C Possible Risk	D Proven Risk	X Do Not Use	Comments
Ser-Ap-Es			■			
Serax						Unrated; not recommended in pregnancy
Silvadene Cream 1%		■				Use only if necessary
Sinemet CR			■			
Sinequan						Unrated; safety not established
Sodium Sulamyd						Unrated
Soma						Unrated; use only if necessary
Spectazole			■			
Sporanex			■			
Stelazine						Unrated; can cause jaundice in newborns
Stuartnatal Plus						Unrated; recommended for use in pregnancy
Sultrin			■			Do not use at term
Suprax		■				Use only if clearly needed
Surmontil			■			
Symmetrel			■			
Synalgos-DC						Unrated
Synarel				■		
Synthroid	■					
Tagamet		■				Use only if clearly needed
Talwin						Unrated; use only if necessary, especially in premature delivery
Tambocor			■			
Tavist		■				Syrup rated B; tablets unrated
Taxol				■		
Tegretol			■			
Temovate			■			Do not use in large amounts or for prolonged periods
Tenex		■				Use only if clearly needed
Tenoretic				■		
Tenormin				■		
Tenuate		■				Use only if clearly needed
Terazol 3 Cream			■			Use only if necessary, in 1st trimester

Profile Name	A Proved Safe	B NoProven Risk	C Possible Risk	D Proven Risk	X Do Not Use	Comments
Tessalon			■			
Theo-Dur			■			
Thorazine						Unrated; can cause jaundice in newborns
Tigan						Unrated; safety not established
Tilade		■				Use only if clearly needed
Timoptic			■			
Tobrex		■				Use only if clearly needed
Tofranil						Unrated; use only if necessary
Tolectin			■			Can cause lung problems in newborns
Tolinase			■			Not recommended in pregnancy
Tonocard			■			
Topicort			■			Do not use in large amounts or for prolonged periods
Toradol			■			Do not use during labor and delivery
Tranxene						Unrated; not recommended in pregnancy
Trental			■			
Triavil						Unrated; not recommended in pregnancy
Tridesilon			■			Do not use in large amounts or for prolonged periods
Tridione						Unrated; does cause birth defects
Trilisate			■			Avoid in late pregnancy
Trinalin			■			Not recommended in 3rd trimester
Tussi-Organidin				■		
Tussionex			■			
Tylenol						Unrated
Tylenol with Codeine			■			Can cause withdrawal symptoms in newborns
Urised			■			
Urispas		■				Use only if clearly needed
Vagistat			■			
Valium						Unrated; not recommended in pregnancy
Vascor			■			

Profile Name	A Proved Safe	B No Proven Risk	C Possible Risk	D Proven Risk	X Do Not Use	Comments
Vaseretic			■	■		Not recommended in 1st trimester; do not use in 2nd & 3rd trimesters
Vasotec			■	■		Not recommended in 1st trimester; do not use in 2nd & 3rd trimesters
Vicodin			■			Can cause dependency in newborns
Visken		■				Use only if necessary
Voltaren		■				Not recommended in 3rd trimester
VoSoL HC						Unrated
Wellbutrin		■				Use only if clearly needed
Wytensin			■			
Xanax				■		
Yocon						Unrated; not recommended for women
Yutopar		■				Do not use before 20th week
Zantac		■				
Zaroxolyn		■				
Zestoretic			■	■		Not recommended in 1st trimester; do not use in 2nd & 3rd trimesters
Zestril			■	■		Not recommended in 1st trimester, do not use in 2nd & 3rd trimesters
Zithromax		■				Use only if clearly needed
Zocor					■	
Zofran		■				Use only if clearly needed
Zoloft		■				Use only if clearly needed
Zovirax			■			
Zyloprim			■			

Appendix and Index Section

APPENDIX 1

Directory of Support Groups

Organizations in this directory are listed alphabetically by problem or concern. The subject headings are:

AIDS
Anxiety
Breastfeeding
Cancer
Chronic Fatigue Syndrome
Depression
Eating Disorders
Fertility and Family Planning
Headache
Heart Disease
Hysterectomy
Miscarriage and Stillbirth
Rape
Sexually Transmitted Disease
Women's Health

Only national headquarters are listed. Many can put you in contact with local chapters. All offer information on their area of concern.

AIDS

Agency for Health Care Policy and Research, U.S. Public Health Service
P.O. Box 8547
Silver Spring, MD 20907
Phone: 800-358-9295
Hours: Monday through Friday,
9 AM to 5 PM EST.

Description: AHCPR researches and publishes free booklets for consumers that explain the benefits and risks of tests and treatments available for specific health problems such as depression, HIV infection, and cancer pain.
Information: Free booklets are available by mail or by calling toll-free.

AIDS Clinical Trials Information Service.
P.O. Box 6421
Rockville, MD 20849-6421
Phone: 800-874-2572;
800-243 7012
Fax: 301-738-6616
Hours: Monday through Friday,
9 AM to 7 PM EST.
Description: Provides current information on federally and privately sponsored clinical trials evaluating experimental therapies for adults and children with HIV, AIDs, and related conditions.
Information: Free information is available by calling toll-free.

CDC National AIDS Hotline
P.O. Box 13827
Research Triangle Park, NC 27709
Phone: 800-342-AIDS (English line)
800-344-SIDA (Spanish line)
800-243-7889 (TTY)

Hours: English line: 7 days a week, 24 hours a day; Spanish line: 7 days a week, 8 AM to 2 AM EST; Toll-free line: Monday through Friday, 10 AM to 10 PM EST.
Description: Provides free information and referrals related to HIV/AIDS.

Center for Women Policy
2000 P St., NW
Washington, DC 20036
Phone: 202-872-1770
Fax: 202-296-8962
Description: The center sponsors 3 programs: The National Resource Center on Women and Aids; Women's Health Decision Making Project; and The Law and Pregnancy-Implementing Policies for Women's Reproductive Rights and Health.
Information: Associate Member annual fee of $50.00 includes complimentary copies of the center's newest fact sheets on *Violence Against Women* and *Girls & Violence*. Members also receive a copy of the CWPS report, a 30 percent discount on new publications, and a subscription to the quarterly newsletter.

Project Inform
1965 Market Street #220
San Francisco, CA 94103
Phone: 415-558-8669
        800-822-7422
Fax: 415-558-0684
Hours: Monday through Saturday, 10 AM to 4 PM EST.
Description: Provides HIV/AIDS treatment information via hotline or mail as well as treatment advocacy for AIDS funding and research improvement.
Information: Information is available by mail or by calling toll-free.

ANXIETY

The Anxiety Disorders Association of America
6000 Executive Boulevard, Suite 513
Rockville, MD 20852
Phone: 301-231-9350
Fax: 301-231-7392
Hours: Monday through Friday, 9 AM to 5 PM EST.
Description: The ADAA is an information clearing house for all kinds of anxiety disorders, offering local referrals and a general information packet. A caring staff will tailor information to specific needs or inquiries, such as panic disorders, phobias, or diet-related therapies.

BREASTFEEDING

La-Leche League International
1400 N. Meacham Road
Schaumburg, IL 60173
Phone: 708-519-7730
Fax: 708-455-0035
Hours: Monday through Friday, 8 AM to 5 PM CST.
Description: Provides information and support to breastfeeding women.
Information: Membership is $30.00 annually. Offers publications, meetings, telephone help, biannual catalogue, seminars, and conferences.

CANCER

Agency for Health Care Policy and Research, U.S. Public Health Service
P.O. Box 8547
Silver Spring, MD 20907
Phone: 800-358-9295

Hours: Monday through Friday,
9 AM to 5 PM EST.

Description: AHCPR researches and publishes free booklets for consumers that explain the benefits and risks of tests and treatments available for specific health problems such as depression, HIV infection, and cancer pain.

Information: Free booklets are available by mail or by calling toll-free.

The American Cancer Society

1599 Clifton Road NE
Atlanta, GA 30329
Phone: 404-320-3333
        800-ACS-2345
(routes calls to local societies)
Hours: 8:30 AM to 5 PM EST
(national office)

Description: ACS sends individuals free materials on the different kinds of cancer, their signs and symptoms, and diagnostic procedures; questions about financial resources, support groups, and patient services will be referred to local cancer societies.

National Cancer Institute

Cancer Information Services (CIS)
Building 31, Room 10A24
Bethesda, MD 20892
Phone: (CIS) 800-4-CANCER
Hours: Monday through Friday,
9 AM to 7 PM EST.

Description: Offers publications, including Cancer Facts, that keep one informed on the latest treatment options and the stages of the disease; information on smoking is also available.

CHRONIC FATIGUE SYNDROME

The CFIDS Association of America, Inc.

P.O. Box 220398
Charlotte, NC 28222
Phone: 800-442-3437
Fax: 704-365-9755
Hours: 7 days a week, 24 hours a day.

Description: A nonprofit organization which sponsors CFIDS (Chronic Fatigue and Immune Dysfunction Syndrome) research, education, and public policy programs.

Information: A free information packet may be obtained by calling toll-free. Annual membership fee of $30.00 is fully tax-deductible.

National Chronic Fatigue Syndrome and Fibromyalgia Association

3521 Broadway, Suite 222
Kansas City, MO 64111
Phone: (816) 931-4777
Hours: Monday through Friday,
8 AM to 5 PM CST.

Description: Nonprofit organization which educates and informs the public about the nature and impact of Chronic Fatigue Syndrome and related disorders.

Information: $15.00 annual membership dues include 24-hour information line and quarterly newsletter.

DEPRESSION

Agency for Health Care Policy and Research, U.S. Public Health Service

P.O. Box 8547
Silver Spring, MD 20907
Phone: 800-358-9295
Hours: Monday through Friday,
9 AM to 5 PM EST.

Description: AHCPR researches and publishes free booklets for consumers that explain the

benefits and risks of tests and treatments available for specific health problems such as depression, HIV infection, and cancer pain.
Information: Free booklets are available by mail or by calling toll-free.

National Depressive and Manic-Depressive Association

730 Franklin St., #501
Chicago, IL 60610
Phone: 800-826-3632;
312-642-0049
Fax: 312-642-7243
Description: Nonprofit organization advocates research and educates patients, families, professionals and the general public concerning the nature of depressive and manic-depressive illnesses.
Information: Free information packets and a list of chapters nationwide are available by calling toll-free.

The National Foundation for Depressive Illness, Inc.

P.O. Box 2257
New York, NY 10116
Phone: 212-268-4260
800-248-4344
Fax: 212-268-4434
Hours: 7 days a week, 24 hours a day.
Description: Provides a recorded announcement with information about the symptoms and treatment of depressive illness, instructions on how to send for an information packet and physician referral list, as well as a list of local support groups.
Information: Information can be obtained by calling toll-free. To defray the cost of the packet, a contribution of $5.00 or more is requested along with a business-sized, self-addressed envelope with $0.98 postage affixed.

EATING DISORDERS

Anorexia Nervosa & Related Eating Disorders, Inc.

P.O. Box 5102
Eugene, OR 97405
Phone: 503-344-1144
Hours: 7 days a week, 24 hours a day.
Description: Provides information and support to people who have eating disorders, as well as to their families and friends.
Information: Free packet of information available by calling. Monthly newsletter: $15.00 per year.

National Association of Anorexia and Associated Disorders

Box 7
Highland Park, IL 60035
Phone: 708-831-3438
Fax: 708-433-4632
Hours: Monday through Friday,
9 AM to 5 PM CST.
Description: A nonprofit organization which offers educational materials, free health-professional referral services, advocacy programs, self-help groups, and hotline services for those with eating disorders.
Information: ANAD services are free. There is a $25.00 annual membership fee, but free memberships are available to those who cannot afford it.

National Eating Disorders Organization

445 E. Granville Road
Worthington, OH 43085
Phone: 614-436-1112
Fax: 614-785-7471
Hours: Monday through Wednesday, and Friday: 8 AM to 5 PM EST; Thursday, 8 AM to 9 PM EST.

Description: Provides education, consultation, research, and treatment referral services, nationally and internationally, related to eating disorders.

Information: Sponsors a national conference on eating disorders; maintains a support group registry; publishes an international treatment directory, educational pamphlets, and newsletters.

Overeaters Anonymous

Check the telephone book for chapters in your area.

Description: This organization has thousands of local chapters. It is modeled on the 12-step program of Alcoholics Anonymous and seeks to help members overcome compulsive eating.

Information: Free newsletters, booklets, and pamphlets are available. No dues or membership fees.

Weight Watchers International

The Jericho Atrium
500 N. Broadway
Jericho, NY 11753-2196
Phone: 516-939-0400

Description: This is a commercial organization that holds weekly meetings to teach members how to modify their behavior and maintain weight loss. It has many local chapters; check the telephone book for local listings.

FERILITY AND FAMILY PLANNING

American College of Obstetricians and Gynecologists Resource Center

409 12th St., SW
Washington, DC 20024-2188
Phone: 202-638-5577
Hours: Monday through Friday,
    9 AM to 4: 30 PM EST.

Description: National professional organization for obstetrician-gynecologists.
Information: Offers a free physician referral service and consumer information materials.

The American Fertility Society

1209 Montgomery Highway
Birmingham, AL 35216-2809
Phone: 205-978-5000
Fax: 205-978-5005
Hours: Monday through Friday,
    8 AM to 5 PM CST.

Description: Private, nonprofit, professional medical organization devoted to advancing knowledge and expertise in reproductive medicine for both professionals and the public. Publishes patient education brochures, maintains a bibliography, and provides physician referrals.

Information: Nominal fee for publications; no fee for bibliography, resource lists, or referrals. Membership limited to professionals.

Center for Women Policy

2000 P St., NW
Washington, DC 20036
Phone: 202-872-1770
Fax: 202-296-8962

Description: The center sponsors 3 programs: The National Resource Center on Women and Aids; Women's Health Decision Making Project; and The Law and Pregnancy-Implementing Policies for Women's Reproductive Rights and Health.

Information: Associate Member annual fee of $50.00 includes complimentary copies of the center's newest fact sheets on *Violence Against Women* and *Girls & Violence*. Members also receive a copy of the CWPS report, a 30 percent discount on new publications, and a subscription to the quarterly newsletter.

March of Dimes Birth Defects Foundation

1275 Mamaroneck Avenue
White Plains, NY 10605
Phone: 914-428-7100
Fax: 914-428-8203
Hours: Monday through Friday,
   9 AM to 5 PM EST.
Description: Sponsors fundraising campaigns for research programs, community services, education, and advocacy related to birth defects.
Information: Information available by phone.

Planned Parenthood Federation of America, Inc.

810 Seventh Avenue
New York, NY 10019
Phone: 212-541-7800
         800-230-PLAN
Fax: 212-765-4711
Hours: Monday through Friday,
   9 AM to 5 PM EST.
Description: Nonprofit affiliates operate nearly 1,000 clinics, providing medical and educational services to 5 million Americans each year. Services include contraception, reproductive cancer screenings, abortion, sexuality education, and testing and treatment of sexually transmitted infections.
Information: Call toll-free to locate the nearest clinic.

RESOLVE, INC.

1310 Broadway
Somerville, MA 02144-1731
Phone: 617-623-1156 (business)
         617-623-0744 (helpline)
Fax: 617-623-0252

Hours: Monday through Friday,
   9:00 AM to 12:00 PM,
   1:00 PM to 4:00 PM EST.
Description: Provides support and information to people who are experiencing infertility.
Information: Information is available by phone.

Sidelines National Support Network

P.O. Box 1808
Laguna Beach, CA 92651
Phone: 714-497-2265
Description: National nonprofit support group for women experiencing a complicated pregnancy, and their families. Provides counseling by trained volunteers, publishes an annual magazine, and provides booklets and information packets.
Information: For patients no dues or fees, except for educational packet if requested. Physicians, hospitals, and healthcare companies pay for magazines.

HEADACHE

American Council for Headache Education

875 Kings Highway, Suite 200
Woodbury, NJ 08096
Phone: 609-845-0322
         800-255-ACHE
Hours: Monday through Friday,
   8:30 AM to 5 PM EST.
Description: A membership organization which provides support for headache sufferers, ACHE also works to increase public awareness of headache. The quarterly newsletter contains information on new developments in treatments, news of legislative efforts, and a question-and-answer column. ACHE also provides a list of headache specialists in local areas, as well as a list of nationally known treatment and research centers.

HEART DISEASE

American Heart Association
National Center
7272 Greenville Avenue
Dallas, TX 75231-4596
Phone: 800-634-1242
Hours: Monday through Friday,
9 AM to 5 PM CST.
Description: AHA answers basic questions on heart health, including diet and exercise. It makes no specific physician referrals, but has a referral service for those in need of funding. Educational materials are available, some at no cost; the AHA also certifies CPR training.

HYSTERECTOMY

Hysterectomy Educational Resources & Services Foundation
422 Bryn Mawr Avenue
Bala Cynwyd, PA 19004
Phone: 610 667 7757
Fax: 215-667-8096
Hours: Monday through Friday,
9 AM to 5 PM EST.
Description: HERS provides information about the alternatives to hysterectomy and coping with the consequences of the surgery.
Information: Offers a 24-hour hotline for emergencies and a free physician referral service. Free counseling by telephone appointment is available. Newsletter subscription is $20.00 annually.

MISCARRIAGE AND STILLBIRTH

RTS Bereavement Services
1910 Southern Avenue
LaCrosse, WI 54601
Phone: 608-791-4747
800-362-9567 x 4747

Hours: Monday through Friday,
8 AM to 4:30 PM CST.
Description: Provides referrals to local counselors and support groups trained by its own teaching team. Helps parents deal with miscarriage, ectopic pregnancies, stillbirths and newborn death.

SHARE–Pregnancy & Infant Loss Support, Inc.
National SHARE Office
St. Joseph Health Center
300 First Capitol Drive
St. Charles, MO 63301
Phone: 314-947-6164
Fax: 314-947-7486
Hours: Monday through Friday,
9 AM to 5 PM EST.
Description: Provides those who have lost a baby through miscarriage, stillbirth, or newborn death with a network of groups, resource materials, and bimonthly newsletters.
Information: No fees for bereaved parents/families; newsletter subscription, $12 a year; annual fee for groups.

RAPE

Center for Women Policy
2000 P St., NW
Washington, DC 20036
Phone: 202-872-1770
Fax: 202-296-8962
Description: The center sponsors 3 programs: The National Resource Center on Women and Aids; Women's Health Decision Making Project; and The Law and Pregnancy-Implementing Policies for Women's Reproductive Rights and Health.
Information: Associate Member annual fee of $50.00 includes complimentary copies of the center's newest fact sheets on *Violence*

Against Women and *Girls & Violence.* Members also receive a copy of the CWPS report, a 30 percent discount on new publications, and a subscription to the quarterly newsletter.

SEXUALLY TRANSMITTED DISEASE

The Herpes Resource Center

American Social Health Organization
P.O. Box 13827
Research Triangle Park, NC 27709
Phone: 919-361-8488;
  STD hotline: 800-227-8922
Hours: Monday through Friday,
  9 AM to 7 PM EST.
Description: ASHA provides referrals to public health clinics, other hotlines, and support groups for herpes and HPV. It also offers written information on sexually transmitted diseases.

Planned Parenthood Federation of America, Inc.

810 Seventh Avenue
New York, NY 10019
Phone: 212-541-7800
         800-230-PLAN
Fax: 212-765-4711
Hours: Monday through Friday,
  9 AM to 5 PM EST.
Description: Nonprofit affiliates operate nearly 1,000 clinics, providing medical and educational services to 5 million Americans each year. Services include contraception, reproductive cancer screenings, abortion, sexuality education, and testing and treatment of sexually transmitted infections.
Information: Call toll-free to locate the nearest clinic.

WOMEN'S HEALTH

Center for Women Policy

2000 P St., NW
Washington, DC 20036
Phone: 202-872-1770
Fax: 202-296-8962
Description: The center sponsors 3 programs: The National Resource Center on Women and Aids; Women's Health Decision Making Project; and The Law and Pregnancy-Implementing Policies for Women's Reproductive Rights and Health.
Information: Associate Member annual fee of $50.00 includes complimentary copies of the center's newest fact sheets on *Violence Against Women* and *Girls & Violence.* Members also receive a copy of the CWPS report, a 30 percent discount on new publications, and a subscription to the quarterly newsletter.

National Women's Health Resource Center

2440 M Street, NW, Suite 325
Washington, DC 20037
Phone: 202-293-6045
Fax: 202-293-7256
Hours: Monday through Friday,
  8 AM to 4 PM EST.
Description: Nonprofit education organization dedicated to helping women make informed decisions about their health.
Information: Individual membership of $25.00 annually includes subscription to bimonthly *National Women's Health Report,* discounts on publications, and access to women's health information.

APPENDIX 2

Common Words in Women's Health

ACE inhibitors (ayss in–HIB–it–ers): Type of drug that supresses the production of angiotensin, a chemical that the body produces to raise blood pressure.

Acupuncture (ak–yoo–PUNK–chur): Pain–relieving technique in which thin needles are inserted in the body at specific points.

AIDS (ades): Acquired immunodeficiency syndrome, a fatal disease characterized by an impaired immune system that allows a variety of infections to take hold.

Amenorrhea (a–men–o–REE–a): Absence of menstruation.

Amniotic fluid (am–nee–OT–ik FLU–id): Fluid in which the developing baby is suspended inside the uterus.

Angina pectoris (an–JI–na PEK–te–res): Chest pain that results when the heart does not receive an adequate supply of blood; usually occurring during activity requiring exertion or during emotional excitement.

Angiogram (AN–jee–o–gram): Diagnostic tool in which dye is injected into a tube that has been inserted into a large blood vessel and threaded up to the heart. Allows doctors to see the interior of the heart and blood vessels through x–rays.

Angioplasty (AN–jee–o–plas–tee): Procedure in which a tiny balloon, attached to a tube, is threaded into a partially blocked segment of an artery, then inflated to squeeze the obstruction aside.

Anovulatory cycle (an–OV–yoo–lo–tor–ee SI–kel): Menstrual cycle in which no egg is produced.

Antibiotic (AN–tee–bi–ot–ik): A drug used to fight bacterial infections. These drugs have no effect on infections with viruses.

Anxiety disorder (ang–ZI–e–tee dis–ORD–er): Psychiatric illness characterized by excessive concern or uneasiness that interferes with daily life or that causes incapacitating fear.

Arrhythmia (a–RITH–mee–a): Irregular heartbeat.

Artificial menopause (art–e–FISH–el MEN–e–poz): Brought on by surgical removal of the ovaries or radiation therapy that renders the ovaries nonfunctional; also known as induced menopause.

Asymptomatic (A–sim–to–mat–ik): Absence of symptoms in the presence of a disease.

Atherosclerosis (ath–er–o–skler–O–sis): Build–up of fatty plaque on the walls of an artery, stiffening the artery and reducing the flow of blood.

Atrial fibrillation (A–tree–al fib–re–LAY–shun): Rapid, uncoordinated twitching movements that replace the normally rhythmic contractions of the upper chambers of the heart.

Bacteria (bak–TEER–ee–a): Microscopic single–celled organisms that can infect any part of the body. Many harmelss types of bacteria inhabit the body routinely.

Bacterial endocarditits (bak–TEER–ee–al EN–doe–kar–DI–tis): Infection of the inside of the heart by bacteria.

Bacterial vaginosis (bak–TEER–ee–al vaj–e–NO–sis): Inflammation of the vagina caused by bacteria.

Basal thermometer BAY–sel ther–MOM–e–ter): Specially calibrated instrument to measure body temperature in relation to ovulation.

BBT (Basal Body Temperature) (Bee–Bee–Tee [BAY–sel BOD–ee TEM–per–chure]): The body's average temperature, charted over the long–term; a change may indicate ovulation.

Benign (bee–NINE): Noncancerous.

Benign cystic teratoma (bee–NINE sis–tik ter–ah–TOE–ma): Another name for a dermoid cyst.

Benign uterine fibroids (bee–NINE YOOT–e–reen FI–broyds): Noncancerous abnormal growth composed of fibrous tissue in the uterine wall.

Beta blockers (BAY–ta BLOK–ers): Type of drug that reduces the force and speed of the heart's pumping action and lowers blood pressure.

Biofeedback (BI–o–FEED–bak): Technique that uses equipment to monitor and provide information on ordinarily involuntary body functions such as heart rate or blood circulation, to help the patient gain control over those functions. Often used to help reduce stress or control pain.

Biopsy (BI–op–see): Removal of a small piece of tissue for microscopic examination by a specialist in diseased tissue.

Blood pressure (blud PRESH–er): Measure of the force of blood flow through the circulatory system.

Bone density (boen DEN–set–ee): Measurement of bone mass or how light or heavy one's bones are.

Bone density screening (boen DEN–set–ee SKREE–ning): Low dose x–ray procedures that allow a doctor to measure bone density throughout the body or at specific points in the body such as the arm or heel.

Bradycardia (brad–ee–KAR–dee–a): Slow heart rate (less than 60 beats per minute).

Breakthrough bleeding (BRAYK–throo BLEE–ding): Menstrual bleeding that occurs despite a medication to suppress menstruation.

Broad–spectrum antibiotic (BROD–spek–trum AN–tee–bi–ot–ik): A drug designed to work against many types of bacteria.

Bypass surgery (BI–pas SERJ–e–ree): Operation in which a clogged portion of an artery serving the heart is replaced.

Calcium (KAL–see–um): Mineral necessary for strong bones.

Calcium channel blockers (KAL–see–um CHAN–al BLOK–ers): Type of drug that slows rapid heartbeat and reduces blood pressure.

Cancer (KAN–ser): Uncontrolled growth of invasive malignant cells.

Candidiasis (kan–dee–DI–a–sis): Vaginal yeast infection caused by the *candida* organism.

Carcinoma (KARS–in–o–ma): Cancer of the tissue that covers body surfaces, both external and internal.

Carcinoma in situ (KARS–in–o–ma in SI–tyoo): A carcinoma that has not yet invaded surrounding tissue.

Cardiomyopathy (KAR–dee–o–mi–OP–a–thee): Any disease of the heart muscle.

Cardiovascular (KAR–dee–o–VAS–kyoo–lar): Referring to the heart and blood vessels.

Catheter (KATH–e–ter): A tube that transports fluids into or out of the body.

Cautery (KAW–ter–ee): The burning away of damaged cell tissue.

CD4 cells (CEE–DEE–four sells): Specific type of T–lymphocyte cells (a form of white blood cell); the measure of these cells is often indicative of the stage of HIV infection.

Cervical cap (SER–ve–kel cap): A small rubber dome designed to fit snugly over the cervix (passage to the uterus), holding spermicide in place.

Cervicitis (SER–vi–site–us): Inflammation of the cervix caused by infection, injury, or irritation.

Cerviography (SER–vee–OG–ra–fee): Diagnostic technique using photographs of the cervix.

Cervix (SER–viks): The lower, narrow end of the uterus opening into the vagina.

Chancroid (SHANG–kroyd): Infectious venereal sore or ulcer.

Chemotherapy (KEE–mo–THER–a–pee): Treatment of cancer with specific chemical agents or drugs that are destructive to malignant tissue and cells.

Chlamydia (kla–MID–ee–a): An organism causing a widespread gonorrhea-like veneral disease.

Cholesterol (ko–LES–ter–ol): A substance that is both manufactured in the liver and supplied by animal food items. Involved in a number of functions in the body including producing some hormones and building a protective cell membrane, it travels through the bloodstream attached to lipoproteins.

Chromosomes (KRO–mo–somes): Rod–shaped bodies carrying the genes that convey inherited characteristics.

Chronic Fatigue Syndrome (KRON–ik fa–TEEG SIN–drome): Physical illness characterized by debilitating tiredness and a combination of flu–like symptoms.

Clomiphene citrate (KLO–me–feen SIT–rayt): A drug used to induce release of an egg from the ovaries.

Colposcopy (kol–POS–ko–pee): Diagnostic technique allowing a doctor to look at a magnified view of the surface of the cervix through a binocular–like instrument called a colposcope.

Columnar tissue (ko–LUM–ner TISH–yoo): Lining composed of tall, narrow cells; another name for glandular tissue in the cervix.

Combination therapy (KOM–be–nay–shun THER–a–pee): Another name for hormone replacement therapy in which both estrogen and progestin are taken.

Condom (KON–dum): A sheath made of latex or animal membrane that is placed on the erect penis before intercourse; it is used to prevent both pregnancy and sexually transmitted diseases.

Congenital (kon–JEN–e–tel): Existing at or dating from birth but not due to heredity.

Congestive heart failure (kon–JES–tive HART FAYL–yer): Condition that occurs when the heart muscle is unable to maintain normal blood flow throughout the body.

Conization of the cervix (ko–ni–ZAY–shun of the SER–viks): A minor surgical procedure in which a part of the cervix surrounding the cervical canal is removed.

Coronary arteries (KOR–e–nayr–ee ART–uh–rees): The vessels that supply blood to the heart muscle tissue.

Coronary artery disease (KOR–e–nayr–ee ART–e–ree diz–EEZ): The build–up of plaque in the coronary arteries.

Corpus luteum (KOR–pus LOO–te–um): A yellow progesterone–secreting sac that forms from an ovarian follicle after the release of a mature egg; if the egg is fertilized, the corpus luteum helps support the developing embryo; if not, it disintegrates.

Corpus luteum cyst (KOR–pus LOO–te–um sist): An abnormal sac that develops on the corpus luteum.

Cryosurgery (KRY–o–serj–e–ree): Use of a cold source to freeze damaged cell tissue.

Cyst (sist): An abnormal sac containing gas, fluid, or semisolid material, with a membranous lining.

Cystadenoma (SIST–ad–e–NO–ma): Cyst that develops as new growth from ovarian tissue.

Cystitis (sis–TI–tis): Bladder infection; the term is sometimes used interchangeably with urinary tract infection.

Cystocele (sis–TOE–sel): Protrusion of the bladder into the vaginal wall.

Cystometry (sis–TOM–e–tree): Test to measure bladder function based on the bladder's ability to expand and contract.

Cystoscope (SIS–toe–skope): Instrument which allows a doctor to look at the inside of the bladder.

Cystourethrography (SIS–toe–YOOR–eeth–ROG–ra–fee): Test to determine if urine is backing up into the urethra.

Cytologist (si–TOL–o–jist): One who studies cell structure.

Cytology (si–TOL–o–jee): Study of the formation, structure, and function of cells.

Cytomegalovirus (CMV) (si–toe–MEG–a–lo–VI–rus): An infection which often causes blindness in AIDS patients.

Defibrillator (dee–FIB–rill–ayt–er): A device that provides an electrical shock to correct rapid, uncontrolled heartbeat.

Depression (dee–PRESH–en): Psychiatric illness with a set of specific symptoms, such as feelings of despondency or worthlessness, that affect one's body, behavior and emotions.

Dermoid cyst (DER–moyd sist): A cyst that develops as new growth from ovarian tissue; contains skin–related tissues such as teeth.

DES (Diethylstilbestrol) (di–ETH–il–stil–BES–trol): A synthetic estrogen that was once given in early pregnancy to prevent miscarriage; if the unborn child was female, it was later discovered, she had a higher risk of developing cervical or vaginal cancer as an adult; DES is no longer prescribed for pregnant women.

Diaphragm (DI–a–fram): A shallow rubber dome that is placed over the cervix, or entrance to the uterus, between the pubic bone and the rear wall of the vagina, to hold spermicide against the cervix; it offers a measure of protection against certain types of sexually transmittted disease.

Diastolic pressure (di–AS–stal–ik PRESH–er): Force of blood flow when heart is at rest.

Diurotic (di–yoo–RET–ik): Prescription medication that helps the body eliminate excess fluid through the kidneys; often prescribed to relieve PMS bloating and to lower high blood pressure.

Diverticula (di–ver–TIK–yoo–la): Pouches in the walls of organs such as the intestines or urethra.

DNA (Deoxyribonucleic acid) (de–OK–see–RI–bo–nyoo–KLEE–ik ASS–id): The substance in living cells that carries the genetic message.

Duct (dukt): A tube in the body for carrying natural fluid.

Dysmenorrhea (dis–men–o–REE–a): Painful menstrual cramps.

Dyspareunia (dis–par–ee–OO–nee–uh): Pain or bleeding during sexual intercourse.

Dysplasia (dis–PLAY–zee–a): Abnormal growth or development of cells, sometimes a precursor of cancer.

Dysuria (dis–YOOR–ee–a): Painful urination.

Echocardiogram (ek–o–KAR–dee–o–gram): Diagnostic tool that uses ultrasound waves to create echoes on the heart's surface showing the size, shape, and movement of the heart.

Eclampsia (ee–KLAMP–see–a): Convulsions during pregnancy or labor in someone prone to high blood pressure or swelling.

Ectopic pregnancy (ec–TOP–ik PREG–nan–see): Condition in which the fertilized egg implants itself outside the uterus, usually in the fallopian tube. Ectopic (or tubal) pregnancies are dangerous and require immediate medical attention.

Electrocardiogram (ee–lek–tro–KAR–dee–o–gram): Diagnostic tool that provides graphic representation of the heart's action by tracing variations in the electrical current that runs through the heart as it pumps (EKG or ECG).

Electroconvulsive therapy (ee–LEK–tro–con–VUL–siv THER–a–pee): Administration of electric currents to the brain used in the treatment of certain mental disorders.

ELISA (Enzyme–linked immunosorbent assay) (EN–zime linked IM–yoo–no–SOR–bent ass–ay): Test to detect the presence of HIV antibodies.

Endometrial biopsy (en–doe–MEE–tree–al BI–op–see): The extraction of a small piece of tissue from the lining of the uterus for microscopic examination.

Endometrial hyperplasia (en–doe–MEE–tree–al hi–per–PLAY–zee–a): Abnormally rapid growth of the lining of the uterus.

Endometrioma (EN–doe–mee–tree–O–ma): A cyst that forms as the result of endometriosis, the disease in which endometrial tissue (or tissue of the uterine lining) implants outside the uterus.

Endometriosis (EN–doe–mee–tree–O–sis): Condition in which uterine tissue is found outside the uterus; can cause pain in the lower abdomen and can lead to infertility.

Endometrium (EN–doe–mee–tree–um): The lining of the uterus, shed each month during menstruation; during pregnancy, the endometrium provides a site for the implantation of the fertilized egg.

Endorphins (EN–door–finz): Hormones found in the brain that affects emotions and sensations of pain.

Enzyme (EN–zime): A complex protein that causes chemical reactions in cells without being changed itself.

Epilepsy (EP–ill–ep–see): Neurological disorders characterized by sudden, recurring attacks of motor, sensory or mental malfunction, sometimes with loss of consciousness or with seizures.

Epithelial cells (ep–e–THEE–lee–al sells): Cells that make up the tissue covering most internal and external surfaces of the body and its organs.

Estrogen (ES–tro–jen): Hormone produced by the ovaries.

Estrogen replacement therapy (ES–tro–jen re–PLAY–sment THER–a–pee): Use of the female hormone estrogen alone to restore hormonal balance after menopause; typically not recommended for women who still have their uteruses because the therapy can increase the risk of uterine cancer.

Fallopian tubes (fa–LO–pee–an toobs): A pair of tubes, each leading from an ovary to one side of the uterus, down which the egg travels to meet the sperm in normal conception.

False negative (fawls NEG–a–tiv): In the case of a Pap test, when analysis of the test fails to detect an existing cell abnormality that is present; in general, an erroneous diagnostic test.

False positive (fawls POS–it–iv): In the case of a Pap test, when analysis of the test reports a cell abnormality that is not there; in general, an erroneous test result indicating a disease that isn't there.

Female condom (FEE–mayl KON–dum): A thin, flexible sheath that covers the cervix and vaginal walls. A newly introduced birth control method, it is also effective for the prevention of sexually transmitted disease and HIV. Also called vaginal pouch.

Fetal alcohol syndrome (FEE–tal AL–ko–hol SIN–drome): Birth defects including physical and mental growth retardation and abnormalities of the heart, head, face, and nerves that occur as a result of the mother consuming excess alcohol during pregnancy.

Fiboradenoma (FI–bro–ad–e–NO–ma): Noncancerous glandular tumor containing some fibroid material.

Fibrocystic breast disease (FI–bro–sis–tik brest diz–EEZ): Noncancerous lumps in the breast; usually occurs in tandem with the menstrual cycle.

Fibroid (FI–broyd): A lump or tumor make up of fiber–like (fibrous) tissue.

Folic acid (FOE–lik ASS–ud): One of the vitamin B complex group which is believed to help prevent neural tube defects in the newborn, especially in cases where a woman has previously given birth to a baby with this condition.

Follicle (FOL–ik–el): Ovarian sac containing immature eggs and fluids.

Follicle cyst (FOL–ik–el sist): A material–filled sac that develops in an ovarian follicle.

Follicle–stimulating hormone (FOL–ik–el STIM–yoo–layt–ing HOR–moan): Also known as FSH, this hormone from the pituitary gland triggers monthly growth of an egg in one of the ovaries' follicles.

Formication (for–mee–KA–shun): Prickling, itching sensation on the skin that occurs during menopause.

Functional cyst (FUNK–shun–al sist): A material–filled sac that develops as part of the ovary's natural cycle.

Galactorrhea (ga–lak–toe–REE–a): Condition in which hormones governing lactation (milk production) are out of balance, causing spontaneous milk flow not associated with childbirth or nursing.

Genetic (je–NET–ik): A quality or condition determined by the genes.

Genetic diseases (je–NET–ik diz–EEZES): Conditions caused by abnormalities in specific genes inherited from one or both parents; carrying a gene for a disease does not mean you or your baby will necessarily develop the disorder; there are tests for some genetic diseases which can tell you and your partner whether or not you are carriers, and the odds of your baby developing the disease.

Germ cells (jerm sells): Egg (or sperm) cells and their precursors.

Gland: An organized group of cells often secreting hormones.

Glandular tissue (GLAN–je–ler TISH–yoo): In the cervical canal, tissue filled with mucous–producing groups of cells.

Gonorrhea (gon–o–REE–a): A contagious inflammation of the genital membranes, transmitted by sexual contact.

HDL : High–density lipoproteins, known as the "good" cholesterol because it has a cleansing effect in the blood.

Hemorrhoids (HEM–o–royds): Dilated veins in swollen rectal tissue which cause pain and itching.

Herpes simplex virus (HSV) (HER–peez SIM–pleks VI–rus): Infection marked by watery blisters on the skin (especially by the lips) or on a mucous membranes (especially in the genital area).

Hirsutism (HER–se–tiz–em): Growth of excess coarse hair; sometimes seen as a result of hormonal changes during menopause.

HIV (Human immunodeficiency virus)
[HYOO–man IM–yoo–no–dee–FISH–en–see VI–rus]: The virus that causes AIDS (Acquired immunodeficiency syndrome), a disease that can be spread by sexual contact and eventually results in death.

HIV disease, HIV/AIDS, ARC (AIDS related complex): Terms used for the various progressive stages of HIV infection.

Hormone (HOR–moan): Glandular secretion that controls activity of an organ or tissue.

Hormone replacement therapy (HOR–moan ree–PLAY–sment THER–a–pee): Use of a combination of estrogen and progestin to replace hormones no longer produced after menopause; also known as HRT, it has shown beneficial results in preventing osteoporosis and heart disease, and in relieving menopausal symptoms.

Hot flashes (haht FLASH–ez): One of the most common symptoms of menopause characterized by a warming sensation throughout the body; hot flashes sometimes begin with pressure in the head and may be followed by profuse sweating.

Human papilloma virus (HPV) (HYOO–man pap–ill–OHM–uh VI–rus): The cause of infectious genital warts.

Hydatidiform mole (hi–da–TID–i–form moal): Results of a pregnancy in which developing fetal tissue degenerates into a disorganized mass.

Hypertension (HI–per–ten–shun): High blood pressure.

Hypothalamus (HI–po–THAL–e–mas): Part of the brain that regulates body temperature and certain metabolic functions.

Hysterectomy (HISS–te–rek–te–mee): Surgical removal of the uterus.

Hysterosalpingogram
(HISS–ter–o–sal–ping–O–gram): An x–ray procedure in which a special dye is inserted to delineate the inner shape of the uterus and the degree of openness of the fallopian tubes.

Hysteroscopy (hiss–ter–OS–ko–pee): A diganostic procedure in which a lighted scope (hysteroscope) is inserted through the cervix into the uterus to enable the doctor to view the inside of the uterus.

Idiopathic (ID–ee–o–PATH–ik): Term describing a disease of unknown origin or cause.

Immune (im–YOON): Resistant to infection.

Immune dysfunction (im–YOON dis–FUNK–shun): Term referring to an inability of the immune system to fight off certain infections.

Incompetent cervix (in–KOM–pet–ent SER–viks): A cervix (the passage to the uterus) that is incapable of holding a pregnancy without surgical correction.

Infarction (in–FARK–shun): The area of tissue that dies due to a lack of oxygenated blood.

Infection (in–FEK–shun): Multiplication of parasitic organisms within the body.

Inherent error (in–HARE–ent AYR–er): Unavoidable mistakes in interpreting diagnostic tests due to technical limitations.

Instillation (in–sti–LA–shun): To pour in medicine drop by drop.

Interstitial cystitis (int–er–STISH–al sis–TIE–tis): Scarred or ulcerated bladder lining.

Intraductal papilloma (IN–tra–DUK–tal pap–ill–OHM–uh): Lumps in the breast ducts.

Intravenous pyelogram (in–tra–VEE–nes PIE–el–o–gram): A test that traces through the veins to identify any blockage or anatomic variations in the urinary tract.

Invasive (in–VA–siv): Describing a test or procedure requiring an incision or skin puncture or insertion of an instrument.

In vitro fertilization (in VEE–tro fert–al–e–ZA–shun): A procedure in which a woman's egg is fertilized with her husband's sperm in the laboratory; the fertilized ovum is then placed directly into the woman's uterus.

Ionizing radiation (I–uh–nize–ing rade–ee–A–shun): The type of radiation found in x–rays; it can harm a developing baby.

Ischemic heart disease (is–KEE–mik hart diz–EEZ): A heart condition caused by obstructed blood flow.

Kegel exercises (KAY–gell EK–ser–size–ez): Exercises done to strengthen the pelvic muscles and control urination.

Lactose intolerance (LAK–toce in–TAL–e–rents): A deficiency of the enzyme lactase, which aids in the digestion of dairy products.

Laparoscopy (lap–a–ROS–ko–pee): Surgical procedure in which a fiberoptic scope and other instruments are inserted into the abdomen through a small incision; used for a variety of operations, including evaluation of the fallopian tubes and pelvic cavity endometriosis.

Laparotomy (LAP–a–ROT–o–mee): General term used to describe abdominal surgery.

Laser treatment (LAY–zer TREET–ment): Use of an intense, focused beam of light to evaporate damaged cell tissue.

LDL: Low–density lipoproteins, known as the "bad" cholesterol because it leaves deposits on the interior walls of the arteries as it travels through the blood stream.

Lipoproteins (lip–o–PRO–teenz): Compounds made of fats (lipids), proteins and triglycerides (another kind of fat) that are categorized according to their weight (very low density, VLDL; low density, LDL; high density, HDL; and very high density, VHDL); cholesterol travels through the bloodstream attached to lipoproteins.

Luteal phase (LYOO–tee–al fayz): The second half of the menstrual cycle after ovulation during which the corpus luteum secretes progesterone, the production of which is important to prepare the endometrium to receive an embryo.

Luteinizing hormone (LH) (LYOO–tee–en–ize–ing HOR–moan): Hormone secreted by the pituitary gland; it stimulates the ovaries in females and the testes in males.

Luteinizing hormone releasing factor (LH–RF) (LYOO–tee–en–ize–ing HOR–moan ree–LEES–ing FAK–ter): Hormone produced by the hypothalamus in females to control release of LH from the pituitary.

Lymph nodes (limf noedz): Also called lymph glands, these tissues supply lymphocytes (white blood cells that help in developing immunity) to the bloodstream and take bacteria and foreign particles out of the fluid (lymph) that contains the white blood cells.

Malignant (ma–LIG–nent): Cancerous.

Mammary duct ectasia (MAM–e–ree dukt ek–TAY–zee–a): Inflammation of tissue beneath the nipple caused by a rupture in dilated breast ducts.

Menopause (MEN–e–poz): Cessation of menstruation.

Menstruation (men–STRAY–shun): The shedding of the endometrium (uterine lining) if an egg has not been fertilzed during the cycle; days 1 to 4 of a "normal" cycle.

Metastasis (me–TAS–te–sis): Spread of cancer from one part of the body to another.

Miscarriage (mis–KARE–ij): Also called spontaneous abortion, premature expulsion of a nonviable fetus from the uterus; commonly used to describe any pregnancy that does not go to term.

Mitral valve prolapse (MI–tral valv pro–LAPS): Valvular disease in which the valve between the upper and lower chambers of the heart does not shut tightly, allowing a partial two–way flow called regurgitation.

Mitral valve stenosis (MI–tral valv ste–NO–sis): Narrowing of the opening of the valve between the upper and lower chambers of the heart.

Mittelschmerz (MITT–al–shmarts): A German word meaning "middle pain," referring to the pain some women experience when they ovulate.

Molluscum (mo–LUS–kum): A smooth, skin–colored bump, often contracted sexually.

Monoclonal antibodies (mon–o–KLOE–nal AN–tee–bod–ees): Chemicals that mark foreign invaders for attack by other elements of the body's immune system; monoclonal when artificaly produced by cultures derived from a single cell.

Monogamous (mah–NAHG–e–mus): Having sexual relations with only one person.

Mucinous cystadenoma (MYOO–si–nus SIST–ad–e–NO–ma): A cyst that develops as new growth from ovarian tisue, filled with a thick slicky gelatinous material.

Mycobaterium avium–intracellulare (MAI) (MI–ko–bak–TEER–ee–um A–vee–um in–tra–SEL–yoo–lar–eh): Tuberculosis–like organism that causes generalized infection.

Mycoplasma (mi–ko–PLAZ–ma): A class of bacteria that lacks cell walls and may cause diseases that effect reproduction.

Myocardial infarction (mi–o–KARD–ee–al in–FARK–shun): Heart attack, when the blood supply to part of the heart is severely reduced or stopped, resulting in the death of an area of heart muscle due to a lack of oxygenated blood.

Myocardium (mi–o–KARD–ee–um): Muscle tissue of the heart.

Myometrium (MI–o–mee–tree–um): The muscular wall of the uterus.

Neoplasm (NEE–o–plaz–em): New growth of tissue serving no physiological function.

Non–ionizing radiation (non–I–uh–nize–ing rade–ee–A–shun): The type of radiation emitted by video display terminals, color televisions and microwave ovens; it is not believed to cause harm to a developing baby.

Nonoxynol–9 (no–NOX–ee–nol–NINE): A spermicide.

Obsessive–Compulsive Disorder (ob–SES–iv kom–PUL–siv dis–ORD–er): A form of anxiety disorder characterized by uncontrollable intrusion of unwanted thoughts and repetitive actions to deal with the thoughts.

Oocyte (O–o–site): A developing ovum (egg).

Opportunistic infections (OP–or–too–NIS–tik in–FEK–shuns): Diseases, especially those not usually found in humans, that take advantage of a weakened immune system, as in AIDS.

Os (ahss): Opening of the cervical canal.

Osteoporosis (OS–tee–o–po–RO–sis): Condition causing severe loss of bone mass, making the bones brittle; typically strikes postmenopausal women.

OTC: Over–the–counter; abbreviation for medications sold without a prescription.

Ovarian cyst (o–VAR–ee–en sist): Sac or pouch containing liquid or solid material that develops on or in the ovary.

Ovarian cystectomy (o–VAR–ee–en sis–TEK–toe–mee): Surgical removal of an ovarian cyst.

Ovaries (O–va–reez): the two female reproductive organs that store and release eggs; the female hormones estrogen and progesterone are secreted here.

Ovulation (ov–yoo–LAY–shun): Release of a mature egg from a follicle in the ovary.

Ovum (O–vum): An egg released from the ovary; plural: ova.

Pacemaker (PAYSS–mayk–er): Surgically implanted device used to electrically regulate the contractions of the heart muscle.

Palpate (pal–PAYT): To examine an organ directly by feeling it.

Pap test (pap test): Also called Pap smear; screening method for cancer or precancer of the cervix by looking for abnormalities in the cervical cells.

Partial oophorectomy (PAR–sahl o–of–or–EK–toe–mee): Surgical removal of an ovarian cyst that includes removal of part of the ovary.

Pathologist (pa–THOL–o–jist): One who interprets and diagnoses the changes in diseased tissues.

Perimenopause (pehr–ee–MEN–e–poz): Period during which menstruation slowly tapers off (complete cessation of menstruation is called menopause).

Periodontal disease (per–ee–o–DANT–el diz–eez): Loss of tooth–holding bone and tissue.

pH paper (pee–aitch PAY–per): Strip of paper that is chemically treated to measure acidity or alkalinity.

Phobias (FO–bee–as): Fear reactions inappropriate to the situation causing them: for example, agoraphobia is a complex set of fears about being alone or being trapped in a public place.

Pituitary gland (pit–OO–it–ayr–ee gland): A cell structure at the base of the brain; secretes two hormones that govern release of an egg from the ovaries: LH and FSH

Placenta (pla–SENT–a): A disk–shaped organ attached to the wall of the uterus during pregnancy; supplies nourishment to the developing baby via the umbilical cord.

Plaque (plak): In heart disease, a build–up of fats and calcium on the interior walls of the coronary arteries.

Plasma (PLAZ–ma): The fluid portion of the blood.

Pneumocystis carinii pneumonia (PCP) (noo–mo–SIS–tis ka–REE–nee–eye noo–MO–nee–a): A type of pneumonia seen frequently in AIDS patients; it is caused by a common organism that immune systems of healthy people readily resist.

Polycystic ovaries (pol–ee–SIS–tik O–va–reez): Condition in which the ovaries produce many cysts due to a hormonal imbalance; also called Stein–Leventhal Syndrome and Sclerocystic Ovarian Disease.

Portio (POR–shee–o): Outside part of the cervix.

Precancer (pree–KANT–ser): Uncontrolled cell growth preceding development of cancer.

Prednisone (PRED–ni–zone): A steroid prescribed to bolster the immune system on a short term basis.

Preeclampsia (pree–ee–KLAMP–see–a): Condition of high blood pressure and swelling due to pregnancy, especially in first–time mothers; can lead to eclampsia, a dangerous condition characterized by convulsions.

Premature ovarian failure (PREE–ma–tyoor o–VAR–ee–en FAYL–yer): Cessation of ovulation and the menstrual cycle prior to age 40; also known as premature menopause.

Premenstrual dysphoric disorder (PMDD) (pree–MEN–stroo–al dis–FIR–ik dis–ORD–er): Depressive disorder characterized by severe recurrent symptoms of sadness that occur during the last week of the menstrual cycle and that interfere with daily living.

Premenstrual syndrome (pree–MEN–stroo–al SIN–drome): Physical or behavioral changes that occur before the onset of the menstrual period.

Prodromal symptoms (pro–DRO–mal SIMP–toms): Warnings of impending disease or disorder; for example, the itching or tingling sensation in the genital area that occurs prior to the outbreak of sores caused by herpes simplex virus.

Progesterone (pro–JES–ter–own): Hormone secreted by the corpus luteum that prepares the uterus for implantation of the fertilized egg; also secreted by the placenta to maintain the pregnancy.

Prolactin (pro–LAK–tin): A pituitary hormone that stimulates milk secretion.

Psychotherapy (SI–ko–THER–a–pee): Treatment of mental and emotional disorders using techniques designed to encourage communication of conflicts and insights into problems; the goals are personality growth and behavior modification.

Pubic lice (PYOO–bik LIESS): Parasitic infestation of the outer genital region.

Pyelonephritus (PI–eh–lo–neh–fry–tis): Kidney infection characterized by lower back pain, fever, chills, nausea, vomiting, and painful urination.

Rad (rahd): Measurement of exposure to radiation.

Radioimmunoassay (RADE–ee–o–im–myoo–no–AS–ay): A test used to measure small amounts of a substance, such as a hormone; antibodies and radioactive tracers are used to quantify the amount of substance.

Radionuclide studies
(rade–ee–o–NYOO–klyd STUD–eez):
Diagnostic tool that uses radioactive substances injected into the bloodstream to assess blood flow.

Radiotherapy (rade–ee–o THER–a–pee):
Treatment of cancer with radiation to kill malignant cells and tissues.

Recurrent miscarriage (re–KER–ent mis–KARE–ij): Three consecutive pregnancy losses before 20 weeks gestation with fetuses weighing less than one pound.

Rh factor (are–aitch FAK–ter): A type of blood protein that is inherited: if you have it your blood type is positive; if not, it is negative.

Salpingo–oophorectomy
(sal–PING–go–o–of–o–REK–toe–mee):
Surgical removal of the fallopian tube along with the ovary.

Sarcoma (sar–KO–ma): Cancer of the connective tissue.

Scabies (SKAY–heez): Itch or mange caused by parasitic mite infestation.

Sclerocystic ovarian disease
(SKLER–o–sist–ik o–VAR–ee–en diz–EEZ):
Another name for polycystic ovaries; it refers to enlarged, thickened ovaries.

Septate uterus (SEP–tayt YOOT–e–rus): A uterus with a dividing membrane protruding into the uterine cavity.

Septum (SEP–tum): Thin membrane that divides two cavities or soft masses of tissue.

Serotonin (seer–o–TOE–nin): A natural body chemical with a role in constricting blood vessels, stimulating smooth muscles and transmitting impulses between nerve cells; concentrated in the nervous system.

Serous cystadenoma (SEE–rus SIST–ad–e–NO–ma): A cyst that develops as new growth from ovarian tissue, filled with a thin watery fluid.

Sexually transmitted disease (STD)
(SEKSH–oo–a–lee trans–MIT–ed diz–EEZ):
Class of viral, bacterial, and skin infestation diseases transmitted from one person to another through sexual contact. Formerly called venereal disease.

Sonogram (SON–o–gram): Another name for an ultrasound test.

Speculum (SPEK–yoo–lum): Instrument inserted into the vagina to hold the vaginal walls apart; permits examination of the cervix and vaginal lining.

Spermicide (SPER–mi–side): A chemical that kills sperm; some also offer limited protection against certain types of sexually transmitted disease.

Sphygmomanometer
(sfig–mo–ma–NOM–e–ter): Blood pressure cuff.

Squamo–columnar junction (skwa-mo-KOL-um-nar JUNK-shun): Point at which the glandular tissue of the cervix and squamous tissue of the vagina meet; also point at which cancerous or precancerous cells are most likely to arise.

Squamous metaplasia (skwa–mus met–a–PLAY–zee–a): Process in which the squamous tissue of the vagina slowly replaces the glandular tissue that grows out of the cervical canal.

Squamous tissue (skwa–mus TISH–yoo): Flat, smooth tissue that covers many interior and exterior body surfaces.

Stein–Leventhal syndrome (stine–LEV–en–thol SIN–drome): Another name for polycystic ovaries.

Stress incontinence (stres in–KANT–en–ents): Inability to hold in urine during sudden pressure brought on by sneezing, laughing, jogging, etc.

Stroke (stroek): A condition that results when one of the arteries leading to the brain bursts or is clogged by a blood clot or particle, depriving a section of the brain of oxygen and killing nerve cells in the area.

Stromal cells (STRO–mal sells): Cells that make up the connective tissue framework of an organ.

Superinfection (SOO–pe–rin–FEK–shun): Infection that no longer responds to the antibiotics which were designed to treat it.

Syphilis (SIF–i–lis): Chronic, contagious sexually transmitted disease caused by a spirochete (a form of bacteria).

Systemic lupus erythematosis (SIS–tem–ik LOO–pus er– ith–EEM–ah–TOE–sis): A chronic disease of unknown origin that principally affects the skin and the joints causing arthritis–like symptoms and pimply rashes.

Systolic pressure (sis–TOL–ik PRESH–er): Force of blood flow when the heart contracts.

Tachycardia (tak–ee–KAR–dee–a): Fast heart rate (more than 100 beats per minute).

Teratoma (ter–a–TOE–ma): Tumor consisting of various tissues not found in the organ in which it appears, such as the tumors of skin and hair tissue found in the ovary.

Thrombolytic (throm–bo–LIT–ik): Type of drug injected into the bloodstream to dissolve blood clots.

Thrush (thruhsh): A fungus infection of the mouth or throat caused by the *candida* organism, which also causes yeast infections in the vagina. The disease is very common in HIV/AIDS patients.

Thyroid gland (THI–royd gland): A large gland that lies in front and on one side of the windpipe and secretes a hormone that regulates body growth and metabolism.

T–lymphocyte cells (tee–LIM–fo–site sells): A group of white blood cells that attack infections.

Torsion (TORE–shun): Process in which the stem of an ovarian cyst becomes twisted.

Total abdominal hysterectomy with bilateral salpingo–oophorectomy (TOTE–al ab–DOM–en–al HISS–te–rek–te–mee with by–LAT–e–ral sal–PING–go–o–of–o–REK–toe–mee): Surgical removal of the uterus, both fallopian tubes and both ovaries.

Transient ischemic attacks (TIAs) (TRANS–yent is–KEE–mik a–TAKS): Little strokes that occur when an artery leading to the brain is temporarily clogged.

Tubal infertility (TOO–bal in–fer–TILL–et–ee): Obstructions in or adhesions on the fallopian tubes which prevent an egg from reaching the uterus, thus preventing implantation and a viable pregnancy.

Tumor (TOO–mor): Abnormal mass of tissue arising without obvious cause and having no natural function.

Ultrasound (UL–tra–sownd): Diagnostic technique using echoes to provide a picture of tissue and organs inside the body.

"Unopposed" estrogen (UN–o–pozed ES–tro–jen): The hormone taken without the addition of progestin.

Urethra (yoo–REE–thra): Tube that carries urine (waste fluid and dissolved substances excreted by the kidney) out of the body.

Urethral stenosis (yoo–REE–thral ste–NO–sis): Narrowing of the urethra.

Urethritis (yoo–ree–THRI–tis): Inflammation of the urethra, usually due to infection.

Urge incontinence (erj in–KANT–en–ents): Sensation of needing to urinate even though the bladder may be empty.

Urinalysis (yoor–in–AL–iss–iss): Analysis of urine sample to determine presence of infection or other conditions.

Urinary stones (YOOR–in–ayr–ee stoenz): Made primarily of calcium, stones can be anywhere in the urinary system and the condition can require surgery if stones are not passed on their own; better known as kidney stones.

Urine culture (yoor–in KUL–cher): Analysis of urine to determine presence of specific bacteria.

Urologist (yoor–ROL–o–jist): Physician who specializes in the urinary system.

Uterine fibroids (YOO–ter–reen FI–broyds): Benign (noncancerous) tumors in the uterus (womb).

Uterus (YOO–ter–us): The hollow, muscular organ where the fetus develops during pregnancy; the monthly menstrual blood flow originates here when the lining of the uterus is shed in absence of a fertilized egg.

UTI: Urinary tract infection.

Vagina (ve–JI–na): The canal leading from the uterus to the external genital area.

Vaginal atrophy (VAJ–in–al AT–ro–fee): The vaginal walls lose elasticity and strength, and begin to shrink, becoming shorter and narrower at the opening.

Vaginal discharge (VAJ–in–al DISH–charj): Unusual mucous or other substance coming from the vagina; frequently accompanied by pain, burning, itching, and painful urination.

Vaginal sponge (VAJ–in–al spunj): A soft, absorbent plug that is saturated with spermicide and inserted into the vagina to cover the cervix.

Vaginal suppository (VAJ–in–al se–PAHZ–it–or–ee): A solid but meltable cone of medicated material inserted into the vagina.

Vaginismus (vaj–e–NIZZ–mus): Unintentional muscle spasms in the thighs, pelvis, and vagina.

Vaginitis (vaj–e–NI–tis): Inflammation of the vagina usually caused by infection; also atrophic vaginitis, where inflammation is caused by a lack of estrogen.

Valvuloplasty (VALV–yoo–lo–plas–tee): A procedure in which a tiny balloon attached to a tube is used to open an obstructed portion of a heart valve; similar to angioplasty.

Vascular (VAS–kyoo–ler): Relating to blood vessels.

Vasectomy (va–SEK–te–mee): Surgical removal of the duct (vas deferens) that carries semen, resulting in permanent male sterilization.

Vasodilators (VAY–so–die–LAY–torz): Type of drug that relaxes the arteries to ease blood flow.

Virus (VI–russ): A type of microorganism responsible for certain infectious diseases. Unlike bacteria, viruses are unaffected by antibiotics.

Western blot (WEST–urn blaht): Test for infection with the HIV virus that causes AIDS, used to confirm another test called ELISA; looks specifically for HIV proteins.

Wet smear (wet smeer): Small amount of tissue placed on a slide for microscopic examination.

Withdrawal bleeding (with–DRA–wel BLEED–ing): Menstrual–like discharge that occurs during the scheduled monthly withdrawal of progestin from a regimen of combined hormonal therapy.

X–ray (EKS–raye): Short wavelength radiation that can penetrate solid forms, leaving an image on photosensitive plates or film.

Yeast infection (yeest in–FEK–shun): Disease caused by fungus–like parasitic micoorganisms.

Zidovudine (AZT or Retrovir) (zie–DOE–voo–deen): The first drug found to slow the progress of AIDS. Other drugs in this category are didanosine (ddL or Videx) and zalcitabine (ddC or Hivid).

APPENDIX 3

Safe Medication Use

Using medications safely is largely a matter of common sense and caution. Remember that the effects of a drug can vary from one person to another, so don't rely on others for drug information. Seek the advice of trained professionals such as your doctor or pharmacist before making any changes in the way you take a medication. The following are general guidelines for most situations:

You and your doctor

■ Always tell your doctor everything about your medical history, including reactions to medications you've used in the past. In fact, it may be a good idea to keep a family medication log to help your doctor.

■ Tell the doctor about any medications you are using now, even if they are over-the-counter drugs like antacids or cold medications. They may contain ingredients that could cause a reaction with the drugs your doctor prescribes.

■ Keep track of your reactions to a medication—both positive and negative—and report them to your doctor at a follow-up visit.

■ Ask your doctor what you can or cannot do when given a new drug. For example, are there any foods to avoid when taking the drug? Should you avoid alcohol? Is it safe to drive a car? Is it alright to go out in bright sunlight?

■ Never change your dose schedule unless your doctor tells you to do so.

■ Ask about the addiction or dependence potential of any new drug.

■ Don't be shy—ask your doctor ANY question you may have in mind and report any side effect, even if it seems trivial or embarrassing.

You and your pharmacist

■ Your pharmacist is a medication specialist. Don't be afraid to ask questions you might have forgotten to ask your doctor. See if there are any written instructions that you can take with you.

■ Ask the pharmacist to explain clearly when and how to take the drug, or to translate into plain English any information you don't understand, such as "milliliters" or "kilograms."

■ Check the ingredients of over-the-counter drugs you may be taking to ensure that your prescription doesn't interact with them.

■ If you are starting a new medication, ask your pharmacist to fill only half the prescription in case you have an adverse reaction and the drug is stopped.

■ Ask how long the medication remains effective. Don't take it after its expiration date.

■ If you are going on a vacation, make sure your drug can be used in different climates.

You and your medications
■ Never take someone else's medication; and don't share your own medicines with anyone else.

■ Check the label each time you take a drug. Don't take a drug in the dark.

■ Keep your medications in a dry, safe spot.

■ Avoid confusion: If the label falls off, tape it back on or replace it. Keep each medicine in the bottle from the drug store. Don't mix medicines together in a single bottle.

■ If you think you are pregnant or plan to become pregnant, consult with your doctor before using any medication.

■ Destroy any unused portions of a drug and throw out the bottle.

■ If you need a certain medicine (for instance, insulin) in case of emergency, carry the information with you or obtain a special bracelet from an organization such as Medic Alert. This will help a paramedic or emergency room doctor treat you properly.

Your medicines and your children
■ Keep all medications in a locked cabinet or in a spot that is well out of the reach of children.

■ Ask the pharmacist to use child-proof safety bottles.

■ To ensure that you're giving the proper dose, be alert and awake when giving a child medication.

■ Make sure that children know medications are only to be taken when sick and can be dangerous if misused.

■ Keep antidotes such as Syrup of Ipecac on hand.

■ Keep the numbers of your EMS and poison control centers handy.

Your medicines and the elderly
■ The elderly are no different than anyone else when it comes to safe medication use. They are, however, more likely to suffer a side effect or adverse reaction if proper dosing is not followed. The elderly should always be aware of any potential side effects from a medication and should report them to a doctor or family member whenever they occur.

Sources

Section 1: Common Disorders of the Reproductive System

Guide to Typical Symptoms and Their Meaning

Danforth, David N; Scott, James R (eds.): *Obstetrics and Gynecology, ed 5*. Philadelphia, JB Lippincott Co, 1986.

Mead, PB; Hager, WD (eds.): *Infection Protocols for Obstetrics and Gynecology*. Montvale, NJ, Medical Economics Publishing, 1992.

Wilson, Jean D; Braunwald, Eugene; Isselbacher, Kurt H; et al (eds.): *Harrison's Principles of Internal Medicine, ed 12*. New York, McGraw–Hill Inc, Health Professions Division, 1991.

What a Menstrual Problem Could Mean

Ayvazian, Andrea: Women in sport: a changing sense of self, in: *1982 Medical and Health Annual*. Chicago, Encyclopaedia Brittanica Inc, 1982, 285–290.

Barber, Hugh RK; Fields, David H; Kaufman, Sherwin A: *Quick Reference to OB–GYN Procedures, ed 3*. Philadelphia, JB Lippincott Co, 1990.

Benassi, L, et al: Effectiveness of magnesium pidolate in the prophylactic treatment of primary dysmenorrhea. *Clinical & Experimental Obstetrics & Gynecology* 1992; 19(#3): 176–179.

Bergdoll, Merlin S: Infectious diseases, in: *1985 Medical and Health Annual*. Chicago, Encyclopaedia Brittanica Inc, 1985, 263–266.

Connell, Elizabeth B: Gynecology and obstetrics, in: *1982 Medical and Health Annual*. Chicago, Encyclopaedia Brittanica Inc, 1982, 230–234.

Connell, Elizabeth B: Contraception, in: *1985 Medical and Health Annual*. Chicago, Encyclopaedia Brittanica Inc, 1985, 208–213.

Coupey, SM; Ahlstrom, P: Common menstrual disorders. *Pediatric Clinics of North America* 1989; 36(#3): 551–571.

Dawood, M Yusoff; Ramos, Josefina: Transcutaneous electric nerve stimulation (TENS) for the treatment of primary dysmenorrhea: a randomized crossover comparison with placebo TENS and ibuprofren. *Obstetrics and Gynecology* 1990; 75(#4): 6546–6560.

Fontana–Klaiber, H; Hogg, B: Therapeutic effects of magnesium in dysmenorrhea. *Schweizerische Rundschau fur Medizen Praxis* 1980; 79(16): 491–494.

Galle, PC; McRae, MA: Amenorrhea and chronic anovulation. Finding and addressing the underlying cause. *Postgraduate Medicine* 1992; 92(#2): 255–260.

Mansfield, MJ; Evans, SJ: Anorexia nervosa, athletics, and amenorrhea. *Pediatric Clinics of North America* 1989; 36(#3): 533–549.

Mishell, Daniel R, Jr; Brenner, Paul R (eds.): *Management of Common Problems in Obstetrics and Gynecology, ed 2*. Oradell, NJ, Medical Economics Books, 1988.

The New Encyclopaedia Brittanica, ed 15. Chicago, Encyclopaedia Brittanica Inc, 1978.

Pryor, Jerilynn C; Vigna, Yvette M; Schecter, Martin T; et al: Spinal bone loss & ovulatory disturbances. *New England Journal of Medicine* 1990; 323(#18): 1221.

Rogers, Robert E: Gynecology, in: *1981 Medical and Health Annual*. Chicago, Encyclopaedia Brittanica Inc, 1981, 229–232.

Shangold, Mona: Exercise and female reproductive health, in: *1985 Medical and Health Annual*. Chicago, Encyclopaedia Brittanica Inc, 1985, 369–372.

Shangold, M; Rebar, RW; Wentz, AC; et al: Evaluation and management of menstrual dysfunction in athletes. *Journal of the American Medical Association* 1990; 263(#12): 1665–1669.

Sheinin, James C: Eating disorders, in: *1985 Medical and Health Annual*. Chicago, Encyclopaedia Brittanica Inc, 1985, 232–235.

Sifton, David W (ed.): *The PDR Family Guide to Prescription Drugs*. Montvale, NJ, Medical Economics Data, 1993.

PMS: Sorting Fact from Fiction

American College of Obstetricians and Gynecologists Committee Opinion: *Premenstrual Syndrome*, No. 66. Washington, DC, American College of Obstetricians and Gynecologists, January 1989.

Facts About Dysmenorrhea and Premenstrual Syndrome. Washington, DC, U.S. Department of Health and Human Services, 1983.

Freeman, Ellen; Rickels, Karl; Sondheimer, Steven J; et al: Ineffectiveness of progesterone suppository treatment for premenstrual syndrome. *Journal of the American Medical Association* 1990; 264: 349–353.

Friedrich, Jo Ann; Hubbard, Rex; Schuman, Edward C; et al: *Premenstrual Syndrome: Breaking Through the PMS Cloud.* San Bruno, Calif, Krames Communications, 1990.

Harrison, Michelle: *Self-Help for Premenstrual Syndrome.* New York, Random House, 1985. (Revised)

Lamb, Lawrence E: Update on premenstrual syndrome, in : *The Health Letter.* New York, North America Syndicate Inc, 1992.

MacMahon, Alice: *Women & Hormones.* Maitland, Fla, Family Publications, 1990.

Osofsky, Howard J: Efficacious treatments of PMS: a need for further research. *Journal of the American Medical Association* 1990; 264: 387.

Premenstrual Syndrome. Washington, DC, American College of Obstetricians and Gynecologists, January 1985.

Psychiatric Diagnosis and the Diagnostic and Statistical Manual of Mental Disorders (DSM-IV), ed 4. Washington, DC, American Psychiatric Association, August 1993.

Psychiatrists set to approve DSM-IV. *Journal of the American Medical Association* 1993; 270: 13–15.

Rubinow, David R: The premenstrual syndrome: new views. *Journal of the American Medical Association* 1992; 268: 1908–1912.

Curing Vaginal Infections

Clarke–Pearson, Daniel; Dawood, M Yusoff (eds.): *Green's Gynecology: Essentials of Clinical Practice,* ed 4. Boston, Little, Brown & Co, 1990, 269–273.

Herbst, AL, et al (eds.): *Comprehensive Gynecology,* ed 2. St. Louis, Mosby–Year Book Inc, 1992, 657–668.

Mead, Philip B (ed.): Advances in the management of vulvo-vaginal disease: a symposium. *The Journal of Reproductive Medicine* 1989; 34(#8): 553–604.

Reed, Barbara; Eyler, Ann: Vaginal infections: diagnosis and management. *American Family Physician* 1993; 47(#8): 1805–1817.

Cervicitis: Causes and Cures

Benson, Ralph C; Pernoll, Martin L: *Handbook of Obstetrics & Gynecology,* ed 9. New York, McGraw–Hill, 1994.

Chang, AR: "Erosion" of the uterine cervix: an anachronism. *Australia & New Zealand Journal of Obstetrics & Gynaecology* 1991; 31(#4): 358–362.

Corrado, Michael L: The clinical experience with ofloxacin in the treatment of sexually transmitted diseases. *American Journal of Obstetrics and Gynecology* 1991; 164(#5, Pt 2): 1396–1399.

Doherty, Mark G; Van Dinh, Tung; Payne, Deborah; et al: Chronic plasma cell cervicitis simulating a cervical malignancy: a case report. *Obstetrics & Gynecology* 1993; 82(#4, Pt 2 suppl): 646–650.

Faro, Sebastian; Martens, Mark G; Maccato, Maurizio; et al: Effectiveness of ofloxacin in the treatment of chlamydia. *American Journal of Obstetrics and Gynecology* 1991; 164(#5, Pt 2): 1380–1383.

Ferris, Daron G; Payne, Peter; Frisch, Lawrence E: Cervicography: an intermediate triage test for the evaluation of cervical atypia. *The Journal of Family Practice* 1993; 37(#5): 463–467.

Malotte, C Kevin; Wiesmeier, Edward; Gelineau, Kristin J: Screening for chlamydial cervicitis in a sexually active university population. *American Journal of Public Health* 1990; 80(#4): 469–471.

Martin, David H; Mroczkowski, Tomasz F; Dalu, ZA; et al: A controlled trial of a single dose of azithromycin for the treatment of chlamydial urethritis and cervicitis. *The New England Journal of Medicine* 1992; 327(#13): 921–925.

Mogabgab, William J: Single–dose oral temafloxacin versus parenteral ceftriaxone in the treatment of gonococcal urethritus/cervicitis. *The American Journal of Medicine* 1991; (#6A): 145S–149S.

Parsons, Wanda L; Godwin, Marshall; Robbins, Carl; et al: Prevalence of cervical pathogens in women with and without inflammatory changes on smear testing. *British Medical Journal* 1993; 306(#6886): 1173–1174.

Pernoll, Martin (ed.): *Current Obstetric & Gynecologic Diagnosis & Treatment,* ed 7. East Norwalk, Conn, Appleton & Lange, 1991.

Potts, Jerome F: Chlamydial infection: screening and management update, 1992. *Postgraduate Medicine* 1992; 91(#1): 120–126.

Rabel, Robert E: *Conn's Current Therapy.* Philadelphia, WB Saunders,1993.

Rosenfeld, Walter D; Clark, Jill: Vulvovaginitis and cervicitis. *Pediatric Clinics of North America* 1989; 36(#3): 489–511.

Scott, James R; DiSaia, Philip J; Hammond, Charles B; et al (eds.): *Danforth's Obstetrics and Gynecology,* ed 6. Philadelphia, JB Lippincott Co, 1990.

Segreti, K: Fluoroquinolones for the treatment of nongono-coccal urethritis/cervicitis. *The American Journal of Medicine* 1991; (#6A): 150S–152S.

Sellors, John W; Pickard, Laura; Gafni, Amira; et al: Effectiveness and efficiency of selective vs. universal screening for chlamydial infection in sexually active young women. *Archives of Internal Medicine* 1992; 152(#9): 1837–1844.

Southgate, Lesley: The diagnosis and management of chlamydial cervicitis: a test of cure. *The Journal of Family Practice* 1990; 31(#1): 33–35.

Stamm, Walter E: Azithromycin in the treatment of uncomplicated genital chlamydia; infections. *The American Journal of Medicine* 1991; (#3a): 19–22.

Tierney, Lawrence M; et al: *Current Medical Diagnosis and Treatment*. East Norwalk, Conn, Appleton & Lange, 1993.

Workowski, Kimberly A; Lampe, Mary F; Wong, Kim G; et al: Long–term eradication of chlamydia trachomatis genital infection after antimicrobial therapy. *Journal of the American Medical Association* 1993; 270(#17): 2071–2075.

The Dangers of Pelvic Inflammatory Disease

Buchan, H, et al: Morbidity following pelvic inflammatory disease. *British Journal of Obstetrics & Gynaecology* 1993; 100: 558–562.

Cates, W, et al: Atypical pelvic inflammatory disease: can we identify clinical predictors? *American Journal of Obstetrics and Gynecology* 1993; 169: 341–346.

Eschenbach, DA: Acute pelvic inflammatory disease (Vol I), in: *Gynecology and Obstetrics*. Philadelphia, Harper & Row, 1985.

Grimes, David A: The intrauterine device, pelvic inflammatory disease, and infertility: the confusion between hypothesis and knowledge. *Fertility and Sterility* 1992; 58(#4): 670–673.

Herbst, AL, et al (eds.): *Comprehensive Gynecology*, ed 2. St. Louis, Mosby–Year Book Inc, 1992.

Hillis, Susan D; Joesoef, Riduan; Marchbanks, Polly A; et al: *Delayed Care of Pelvic Inflammatory Disease as a Risk Factor for Impaired Fertility*. Atlanta, Ga, Centers for Disease Control and Prevention, 1992.

Hillis, SD, et al: Delayed care of pelvic inflammatory disease as a risk factor for impaired fertility. *American Journal of Obstetrics and Gynecology* 1993; 168: 1503–1509.

Jacobsen, LJ: (table). *American Journal of Obstetrics and Gynecology* 1980; 138: 1008.

Morbidity and Mortality Weekly Report. (Centers for Disease Control and Prevention) 1989; 38(#8S): 29.

Morbidity and Mortality Weekly Report. (Centers for Disease Control and Prevention) 1993; 42(#14): 78–80.

Washington, E; Katz, P: Cost of and payment source for pelvic inflammatory disease. *Journal of the American Medical Association* 1991; 266: 2565–2569.

Wilson, JD, et al: *Harrison's Principles of Internal Medicine*, ed 12. New York, McGraw–Hill Inc, Health Professions Division, 1991.

Witkin, SS; Ledger, WJ: New directions in the diagnosis and treatment of pelvic inflammatory disease. *Journal of Antimicrobial Chemotherapy* 1993; 31: 197–199.

Your Treatment Options for Fibroids

Adamson, GD: Treatment of uterine fibroids: current findings with gonadotropin–releasing hormone agonists. *American Journal of Obstetrics and Gynecology* 1992; 166(#2): 746–751.

Benagiano, G, et al: Fibroids: overview of current and future treatment options. *British Journal of Obstetrics & Gynaecology* 1992; 99(suppl 7): 18–22.

Burton, CA, et al: Surgical management of leiomyomata during pregnancy. *Obstetrics & Gynecology* 1989; 74(#5): 707–709.

Cheng, C, et al: Leiomyomata of the female urethra: a case report and review. *Journal of Urology* 1992; 148(#5): 1526–1527.

Coddington, CC, et al: Short term treatment with leuprolide acetate is a successful adjunct to surgical therapy of leiomyomas of the uterus. *Surgery, Gynecology & Obstetrics* 1992; 175(#1): 57–63.

Davis, JL, et al: Uterine leiomyomas in pregnancy: a prospective study. *Obstetrics & Gynecology* 1990; 75(#1): 41–44.

Donnez, J, et al: The place of GnRH agonists in the treatment of endometriosis and fibroids by advanced endoscopic techniques. *British Journal of Obstetrics & Gynaecology* 1992; 99(suppl 7): 31–33.

Exacoustòs, C, et al: Ultrasound diagnosis of uterine myomas and complications in pregnancy. *Obstetrics & Gynecology* 1993; 82(#1): 97–101.

Fayez, JA, et al: Short hospital stay for gynecological reconstructive surgery via laparotomy. *Obstetrics & Gynecology* 1993; 81(#4): 598–600.

Friedman, AJ, et al: Should uterine size be an indication for surgical intervention in women with myomas? *American Journal of Obstetrics and Gynecology* 1993; 168(#3, Pt 1): 751–755.

Hardiman, MK: Routine hysterectomy for large asymptomatic uterine leiomyomata: a reappraisal [letter]. *Obstetrics & Gynecology* 1992; 80(#3, Pt 1): 475;[discussion] 475–476.

Hasson, HM, et al: Laparoscopic myomectomy. *Obsterics & Gynecology* 1992; 80(#5): 884–888.

Healy, DL, et al: The role of GnRH agonists in the treatment of uterine fibroids. *British Journal of Obstetrics & Gynaecology* 1992; 99(suppl 7): 23–26.

Karasick, S, et al: Imaging of uterine leiomyomas. *American Journal of Roentgenology* 1992; 158(#4): 799–805.

Mayheux, R, et al: Treatment of peri–menopausal women: potential long–term therapy with a depot GnRH agonist combined with hormonal replacement therapy. *British Journal of Obstetrics & Gynaecology* 1992; 99(suppl 7): 13–17.

Miller, RM, et al: Zoladex (goserelin) in the treatment of benign gynaecological disorders: an overview of safety and efficacy. *British Journal of Obstetrics & Gynaecology* 1992; 99(suppl 7): 37–41.

Mroueh, J, et al: Tubal pregnancy associated with ampullary tubal leiomyoma. *Obstetrics & Gynecology* 1993; 81(#5, Pt 2): 880–882.

Murphy, AA, et al: Regression of uterine leiomyomata in response to the antiprogesterone RU 486. *Journal of Clinical Endocrinology & Metabolism* 1993; 76(#2): 513–517.

Parazzini, F, et al: Oral contraceptive use and risk of uterine fibroids. *Obstetrics & Gynecology* 1992; 79(#3): 430–433.

Reiter, RC, et al: Routine hysterectomy for large asymptomatic uterine leiomyomaya: a reappraisal. *Obstetrics & Gynecology* 1992; 79(#4): 481–484.

Smith, DC, et al: Mymectomy as a reproductive procedure. *American Journal of Obstetrics and Gynecology* 1990; 162(#6): 1476–1479.

Soderstrom, RM: Routine hysterectomy for large asymptomatic uterine leiomyomata: a reappraisal [letter]. *Obstetrics & Gynecology* 1992; 80(#3, Pt 1): 474–475.

Tulandi, T, et al: Adhesion formation and reproductive outcome after myomectomy and second–look laparoscopy. *Obstetrics & Gynecology* 1993; 82(#2): 213–215.

Vollenhaven, BJ, et al: Uterine fibroids: a clinical review. *British Journal of Obstetrics & Gynaecology* 1990; 97(#4): 285–298.

West, CP, et al: Goserelin (Zoladex) in the treatment of fibroids. *British Journal of Obstetrics & Gynaecology* 1992; 99(suppl 7): 27–30.

Keeping Endometriosis at Bay

Ballweg, ML: *Overcoming Endometriosis*. Chicago, Congdon & Weed Inc, 1987.

Ballweg, Mary Lou: Endometriosis and hysterectomy. *Newsletter of the Endometriosis Association* 1993; 14: 3.

Berger, Gary: Endometriosis: how many women are affected? *Newsletter of the Endometriosis Association* 1993; 14: 4.

Clarke–Pearson, Daniel; Dawood, M Yusoff (eds.): *Green's Gynecology: Essentials of Clinical Practice*, ed 4. Boston, Little, Brown & Co, 1990.

Endometriosis linked to environmental pollutants. *Newsletters of the Endometriosis Association* 1993; 13: 2.

Exciting findings in dioxin monkey colony. *Newsletters of the Endometriosis Association* 1993; 13: 3.

Olive, DL; and Schwartz, LB: Endometriosis. *New England Journal of Medicine* 1993; 328: 1759.

Rice, Sherry: Research findings: dioxins. *Newsletter of the Endometriosis Association* 1993; 13: 4.

Schusebach, Lynn S: Learning to cope with endometriosis. *Newsletter of the Endometriosis Association* 1993; 14: 2.

Thylan, Sharyon; Redoine, David: *Statistics on Endometriosis: What Do They Mean?* (Bulletin) New York, Endometriosis Alliance of Greater New York, 1992.

Yap, AL: Endometriosis and the urinary tract. *Newsletter of the Endometriosis Association* 1993; 13: 1.

What You Need to Know About Ovarian Cysts

Caillouette and Koehler: Phasic contraceptive pills and functional ovarian cysts. *American Journal of Obsterics and Gynecology* 1987; 156: 1538–1542.

Clarke–Pearson, Daniel; Dawood, M Yusoff (eds.): *Green's Gynecology: Essentials of Clinical Practice*, ed 4. Boston, Little, Brown & Co, 1990.

Danforth, David N; Scott, James R (eds.): *Obstetrics and Gynecology*, ed 5. Philadelphia, JB Lippincott Co, 1986.

Dunnihoo, Dale R: *Fundamentals of Gynecology and Obstetrics*. Philadelphia, JB Lippincott Co, 1990.

Griffith–Kenney, Janet: *Contemporary Women's Health*. Menlo Park, Calif, Addison–Wesley Publishing Co, 1986.

Holt, Victoria, et al: Functional ovarian cysts in relation to the use of monophasic and triphasic oral contraceptives. *Obstetrics & Gynecology* 1992; 79: 529–33.

Lichtman, Ronnie; Papera, Susan: *Gynecology: Well Woman Care*. East Norwalk, Conn, Appleton & Lange, 1990.

Speroff, L, et al: *Clinical Gynecologic Endocrinology and Infertility*, ed 4. Baltimore, Williams & Wilkins, 1989.

Putting an End to Urinary Tract Infections

Berries battle bladder bugs. *Science News* 1991; 139(#23): 365.

Foxman, B: Recurring urinary tract infection: incidence and risk factors. *American Journal of Public Health* 1990; 80: 331–333.

Gillespie, L: *You Don't Have to Live with Cystitis!* New York, Rawson, 1986.

Kilmartin, A: *Cystitis: The Complete Self–Help Guide*. New York, Warner, 1981.

Martens, MG: Cystitis, in: Mead, PB; Hager, WD (eds.): *Infection Protocols for Obstetrics and Gynecology*. Montvale, NJ, Medical Economics Publishing, 1992, chap 53.

McNeeley, S. Gene, Jr: Lower urinary tract infections in pregnancy, in: *Infection Protocols for Obstetrics and Gynecology*. Montvale, NJ, Medical Economics Publishing, 1992; chap 4.

Mead, P; Cox, S; Crombleholme, W; et al: Urinary tract infection: is it reinfection or recurrence? *Contemporary Ob/Gyn* 1993; 35: 84–108.

Ofek, I; Goldhar, J; Zafriri, D; et al: Anti–*escherichia coli* adhesion activity of cranberry and blueberry juices. *New England Journal of Medicine* 1991; 324(#22): 1599.

Rind, P: Use of barrier methods with spermicides may increase vaginal flora. *Family Planning Perspectives* 1991; 23(#3): 142–143.

Rosenfeld, I: *The Best Treatment*. New York, Simon & Schuster, 1991, 274–275.

Schrotenberg, K: *The Woman Doctor's Guide to Overcoming Cystitis*. New York, New American Library, 1987.

Shephard, BD; Shephard, CA: *The Complete Guide to Women's Health*. Tampa, Fla, Mariner, 1982, 367–373.

Shreeve, C: *Cystitis, the New Approach*. Rochester, Vt, Thorsons, 1986.

Smith, W: *Overcoming Cystitis*. Toronto, Bantam Books, 1987.

Sobel, DS; Ferguson, T: *The People's Book of Medical Tests*. New York, Summit, 1985, 323–325, 373–375, 428–431.

Solomon, HS: *Beat the Odds*. New York, Villard, 1986, 243–244.

Spodnik, JP; Cogan, DP: *The 35–plus Good Health Guide for Women*. New York, Harper & Row, 1989, 208–209.

Tucker, MS: Self–medication protocol for UTI patients. *Contemporary Ob/Gyn* 1993; 35: 75–78.

Urinary Tract Infections. Washington, DC, American College of Obstetricians and Gynecologists, 1984.

Urinary tract infections. Part 1: in women. *Mayo Clinic Health Letter* 1992; 10(#6): 1–3.

Coming to Terms with Sexually Transmitted Disease

Chang, YL; Lin, CY; Tseng, CJ; et al: Prevalence of genital human papillomavirus infections in patients at a sexually transmitted diseases clinic. *European Journal of Clinical Microbiology & Infectious Diseases* 1992; 11: 454–457.

Chase, A: *The Truth About STD*. New York, William Morrow Co Inc, 1983.

Gibbons, W: Clueing in on chlamydia. *Science News* 1991; 139: 250–252.

Grodstein, F; Goldman, MB; Cramer, DW: Relation of tubal infertility to history of sexually transmitted diseases. *American Journal of Epidemiology* 1993; 137: 577–584.

Han, Y; Morse, DL; Lawrence, CE; et al: Risk profile for chlamydia infection in women from public health clinics in New York State. *Journal of Community Health* 1993; 18: 1–9.

The Helper. Research Triangle Park, NC, American Social Health Association, 1993, 15(#3).

Herpes Questions and Answers. Research Triangle Park, NC, American Social Health Association, 1991.

Hook, EW; Marra, CM: Acquired syphilis in adults. *The New England Journal of Medicine* 1992; 326: 1060–1069.

HPV News. Research Triangle Park, NC, American Social Health Association, 1992; 3(#2).

Infectious diseases society for obstetrics and gynecology, in: Mead, PB; Hager, WD (eds.): *Infection Protocols for Obstetrics and Gynecology*. Medical Economics Publishing, Montvale, NJ, 1992.

Jha, PKS; Beral, V; Peto, J; et al: Antibodies to human papillomavirus and to other genital infectious agents and invasive cervical cancer risk. *The Lancet* 1993; 341: 1116–1118.

Kulhanjian, JA; Soroush, V; Au, DS; et al: Identification of women at unsuspected risk of primary infection with herpes simplex virus type 2 during pregnancy. *The New England Journal of Medicine* 1992; 326: 916–920.

Mason, V: Acyclovir: Changing the course of herpes infections. *Contraceptive Technology Update* 1993; 14: 43–44.

Mason, V: CDC says chancroid may be underreported. *Contraceptive Technology Update* 1993; 14: 90–92.

Mason, V: High cost of one–dose chlamydia treatment will limit use. *Contraceptive Technology Update* 1993; 14: 41–44.

Mason, V: HPV–related warts often disappear without treatment. *Contraceptive Technology Update* 1992; 13: 184–186.

Meltzer, AS: *The ABCs of STD: A Guide to Sexually Transmitted Diseases*. Montreal, Eden Press, 1983.

Morbidity and Mortality Weekly Report. (Centers for Disease Control and Prevention) 1993; 42(#6).

1993 Sexually Transmitted Diseases Treatment Guidelines. Atlanta, Ga, Centers for Disease Control and Prevention, 1993.

Opaneye, AA; Jayaweera, DT; Walzman, M; et al: Pediculosis pubis: a surrogate marker for sexually transmitted diseases. *Nursing Times* 1993; 89: 12.

Psychosocial and Medical Aspects of Genital HSV Infection: The Proceedings of a Conference. Research Triangle Park, NC, American Social Health Association, 1993.

Some Questions and Answers About HPV and Genital Warts. Research Triangle Park, NC, American Social Health Association, 1992.

STD Handbook: Sexually Transmitted Diseases. Montreal, Montreal Health Press, 1991.

Telling Your Partner About Herpes. Research Triangle Park, NC, American Social Health Association, 1990.

Touchstone, DM; Davis, DD: Consider chlamydia. *RN*, February 1992; 32–35.

Webster, LA; Berman, SM; Greenspan, JR: Surveillance for gonorrhea and primary syphilis among adolescents—1981–1991. *Morbidity and Mortality Weekly Report* (Centers for Disease Control and Prevention) 1993; 42: 1–11.

Webster LA; Greenspan, JR; Nakashima, AK; et al: An evaluation of surveillance for chlamydia trachomatis infections in the United States, 1987–1991. *Morbidity and Mortality Weekly Report* (Centers for Disease Control and Prevention) 1993; 42: 22–27.

Webster, LA; Rolfs, RT: Surveillance for primary syphilis—United States 1991. *Morbidity and Mortality Weekly Report* (Centers for Disease Control and Prevention) 1993; 42: 13–19.

Wimalawansa, SJ: Sexually transmitted diseases in the age of AIDS. *Ceylon Medical Journal* 1993; 38: 12–14.

Section 2:
General Health Concerns

Heart Disease:
The Greatest Threat of All

Amsterdam, E, et al: Women and heart disease. *Patient Care* 1993; 27: 71–74.

Amsterdam, E; Legato, M: What's unique about CHD in women? *Patient Care* 1993; 27: 21–35.

Appel, L; Bush, T: Preventing heart disease in women: another role for aspirin? *Journal of the American Medical Association* 1991; 266: 565–567.

Ayanian, J; Epstein, A: Differences in the use of procedures between women and men hospitalized for coronary heart disease. Abstracted. *New England Journal of Medicine* 1991; 325: 221–226.

Barrett–Connor, E; et al: Why is diabetes mellitus a stronger risk factor in women than in men? *Journal of the American Medical Association*, 1991; 265: 627–632.

Barrett–Connor, E; Bush, T: Estrogen and coronary heart disease in women. *Journal of the American Medical Association* 1991; 265: 1861–1868.

Baxi, L; Rho, R: Pregnancy after cardiac transplantation. Abstracted. *American Journal of Obstetrics and Gynecology* 1993; 169: 33–35.

Bower, B: Women take un–type A behavior to heart. *Science News* 1993; 144: 244.

Coronary artery disease and lipid levels in women. *American Family Physician* 1992; 45: 2364.

Coronary heart disease incidence, by sex. *Journal of the American Medical Association* 1992; 268: 964–967.

Coronary risk factors in women: two reports. *Nutrition Research Newsletter*, April 1992.

Douglas, PS (ed.): *Cardiovascular Health and Disease in Women.* Philadelphia, WB Saunders Co, 1993.

Eaker, E, et al: Cardiovascular disease in women. *American Heart Association Medical/Scientific Statement*, February 17, 1993.

Eaker, E, et al: Heart disease in women: how different? *Patient Care* 1992; 26: 191.

Eaker, E: Myocardial infarction and coronary death among women: psychosocial predictors from a 20–year follow–up of women in the Framingham Study. Abstracted. *Journal of the American Medical Association* 1992; 268: 1854.

Effects of monounsaturated fatty acids on plasma lipoproteins in women. *Nutrition Research Newsletter*, July–August 1992.

Eysmann, S; Douglas, P: Reperfusion and revascularization strategies for coronary artery disease in women. *Journal of the American Medical Association* 1992; 268: 1903.

Fats and cholesterol. *Johns Hopkins Women's Health* 1993; 1: 1.

Garg, D, et al: Alcohol consumption and risk of ischemic heart disease in women. Abstracted. *Archives of Internal Medicine* 1993; 153: 1211–1217.

Gazaway, P, et al: Cardiac and respiratory drugs in pregnancy. *Patient Care* 1993; 27: 1197.

Heart and Stroke Facts. Dallas, Tex, American Heart Association, 1992.

Heart disease in women. *Johns Hopkins Women's Health* 1993; 1: 1.

Hong, M, et al: Effects of estrogen replacement therapy on serum lipid values and angiographically defined coronary artery disease in women. Abstracted. *American Journal of Cardiology* 1991; 69: 176.

Isles, C, et al: Relation between coronary mortality in women of the Renfrew and Paisley survey: comparison with men. *The Lancet* 1992; 339: 702–707.

Keil, J, et al: Mortality rates and risk factors for coronary disease in black as compared with white men and women. Abstracted. *New England Journal of Medicine* 1993; 329: 73.

Kris–Etherton, P; Krummel, D: Role of nutrition in the prevention and treatment of coronary heart disease in women. *Journal of the American Dietetic Association* 1993; 93: 987–994.

Krummel, D, et al: Prediction of plasma lipids in a cross–sectional sample of young women. *Journal of the American Dietetic Association* 1992; 92: 942–949.

Kupari, M; Koskinen, P: Comparison of the cardiotoxicity of ethanol in women versus men. Abstracted. *American Journal of Cardiology* 1992; 70: 645–650.

Lao, T, et al: Congenital aortic stenosis and pregnancy—a reappraisal. Abstracted. *American Journal of Obstetrics and Gynecology* 1993; 169: 540–546.

Largest trial on women's health targets heart disease and cancer. *Health News & Review* 1993; 3: A1.

Liao, Y, et al: Survival rates with coronary artery disease for black women compared with black men. *Journal of the American Medical Association* 1992; 268: 1867–1872.

Management of coronary artery disease in women. *American Family Physician* 1991; 44: 1867–1869.

Manson, J, et al: A prospective study of aspirin use and primary prevention of cardiovascular disease in women. *Journal of the American Medical Association* 1991; 266: 521–528.

Manson, J, et al: A prospective study of maturity–onset diabetes mellitus and risk of coronary heart disease and stroke in women. Abstracted. *Archives of Internal Medicine* 1991; 151: 1141.

Menegakis, N; Amstey, M: Case report of myocardial infarction in labor. Abstracted. *American Journal of Obstetrics and Gynecology* 1991; 165: 1383.

Mishra, M, et al: Murmurs in pregnancy: an audit of echocardiography. *British Medical Journal* 1992; 304: 1413–1415.

No haven in housework. *East West Natural Health* 1992; 22: 15.

Noninvasive diagnosis of coronary artery disease in women: ST–segment analysis on 24–hour ECG monitoring or exercise ECG? Abstracted. *Journal of the American Medical Association* 1991; 266: 1197.

Petticrew, M, et al: Coronary artery surgery: are women discriminated against? *British Medical Journal* 1993; 306: 1164.

Risk factors for coronary mortality in women. *American Family Physician* 1992; 46: 921.

Rosemond, R; Peterson, A: Cardioversion during pregnancy. *Journal of the American Medical Association* 1993; 269: 3167.

Sifton, David (ed.): *The PDR Family Guide to Prescription Drugs.* Medical Economics Data, 1993.

Silent Epidemic: The Truth About Women and Heart Disease. Dallas, Tex, American Heart Association, 1992.

Stampfer, M, et al: Postmenopausal estrogen therapy and cardiovascular disease: ten–year follow–up from the Nurse's Health Study. Abstracted. *New England Journal of Medicine* 1991; 325: 756.

Stampfer, M, et al: Vitamin E consumption and the risk of coronary artery disease in women. Abstracted. *New England Journal of Medicine* 1993; 328: 1444.

Steingart, R, et al: Sex differences in the management of coronary artery disease. Abstracted. *New England Journal of Medicine* 1991; 325: 226.

Sullivan, JL, et al: Estrogen and coronary heart disease in women. *Journal of the American Medical Association* 1991; 266: 1358.

Sullivan JM, et al: Estrogen replacement and coronary artery disease: effect on survival in postmenopausal women. Abstracted. *Archives of Internal Medicine* 1990: 265: 2244.

Wender, N, et al: Cardiovascular Health and Disease in Women. *New England Journal of Medicine* 1993; 329: 247–256.

Willett, W, et al: Intake of trans fatty acids and the risk of coronary heart disease among women. *The Lancet* 1993; 341: 581–587.

Wing, R, et al: Weight gain at the time of menopause. Abstracted. *Archives of Internal Medicine* 1991; 151: 97.

Women and heart disease. *Berkeley Wellness Letter* 1992; 8: 4–6.

Women and heart disease: another gender gap. *Patient Care* 1991; 25: 18–20.

The Growing Danger of AIDS

AIDS affects men, women differently. *AIDS Alert* 1991; 6: 111.

AIDS in women—United States. *Morbidity and Mortality Weekly Report* (Centers for Disease Control and Prevention) 1990; 39: 845–847.

AIDS increasing four times faster among women than among men. *AIDS Weekly*, August 9, 1993, 9.

AIDS on rise in women. *FDA Consumer* 1991; 25: 6.

Bastian, Lori, et al: Differences between men and women with HIV–related Pneumocystic carinii pneumonia. *Journal of Acquired Immune Deficiency Syndromes* 1993; 6: 617–624.

Berkelman, Ruth, L, et al: Clarification of AIDS mortality in women. *Journal of the American Medical Association* 1991; 265: 1952.

Biannual Pap smears urged for HIV–infected women. *AIDS Alert* 1991; 6: 13–16.

Carpenter, Charles CJ, et al: Human immunodeficiency virus infection on North American women: experience with 200 cases and a review of the literature. *Medicine* 1991; 70: 307–325.

Characteristics of, and HIV infection among, women served by publicly funded HIV counseling and testing services. *Morbidity and Mortality Weekly Report* (Centers for Disease Control and Prevention) 1991; 40; 195–200.

Clark, Rebecca, et al: HIV: What's different for women? *Patient Care* 1993; 27: 119–138.

Corea, Gena: *The Invisible Epidemic: The Story of Women and AIDS.* New York, HarperCollins, 1992.

Current trends: AIDS in women. *CDC AIDS Weekly*, December 10, 1990, 23.

Ellerbrock, Timothy, et al: Epidemiology of women with AIDS in the United States, 1981 through 1990. *Journal of the American Medical Association* 1991; 265: 2971–2977.

Erben, Rosemarie: The special threat to women. *World Health*, November–December 1990, 7–10.

Goldsmith, Marsha F: Specific HIV–related problems of women gain more attention at a price—affecting more women. *Journal of the American Medical Association* 1992; 268: 1814–1817.

Guinan, Mary E: HIV, heterosexual transmission, and women. *Journal of the American Medical Association* 1992; 268: 520–521.

Gwinn, Marta, et al: Prevalence of HIV infection in child-bearing women in the United States. *Journal of the American Medical Association* 1991; 265: 1704–1709.

Hankins, Catherine A: A research agenda for the 1990s. *World Health*, November–December 1990, 24–27.

HIV/AIDS pandemic in women and children. *American Family Physician* 1991; 43: 299–301.

HIV disease and AIDS in women: current knowledge and a research agenda. *AIDS Weekly* October 19, 1992, 20–23.

HIV–infected women threatened by cervical cancer. *AIDS Alert* 1992; 7: 17–22.

HIV infection, pregnant women, and newborns: a policy proposal for information and testing. *Journal of the American Medical Association* 1990; 264: 2416–2421.

Holmberg, Scott D, et al: AIDS Commentary: Biologic Factors in the Sexual Transmission of Human Immunodeficiency Virus. *The Journal of Infectious Diseases* 1989; 160: 1.

Jones, Laurie: AIDS definition needs broadening, congressional panel told. American Medical News 1991; 34: 3–5.

Kerr, Dianne L: Women with AIDS and HIV infection. *Journal of School Health* 1991; 61: 139–141.

Lifson, Alan R: Sentinel surveillance and prevention of HIV in women. *The Western Journal of Medicine* 1993; 158: 77–79.

Liskin, Laurie; Sakondhavat, C: The female condom: a new option for women, in: *Aids in the World*. Cambridge, Mass, Harvard University Press, 1992.

Many providers ignoring HIV risk in women. *AIDS Alert* 1991; 6: 26–31.

Mayes, Susan Dickerson, et al: Sexual practices and AIDS knowledge among women partners of HIV–infected hemophiliacs. *Public Health Reports* 1992; 107: 504–515.

Men much more likely to pass AIDS to women than women are to men. *AIDS Weekly*, April 6, 1992, 4.

Merson speaks about AIDS and women. *CDC AIDS Weekly*, December 10, 1990, 5.

Minkoff, Howard L; and DeHovitz, Jack A: Care of women infected with the human immunodeficiency virus. *Journal of the American Medical Association* 1991; 266: 2253–2259.

Minorities, women are fastest growing AIDS population. *AIDS Alert* 1993; 8: A1–A4.

Miranda–Maniquis, Estrella: The silence about women. *World Press Review* 1993; 40: 26.

Modeling the impact of breast feeding by HIV–infected women on child survival. *CDC AIDS Weekly*, December 17, 1990, 25–27.

More women diagnosed with AIDS, different symptoms emerging. *AIDS Alert* 1992; 7: S2.

1993 Revised Classification System for HIV Infection and Expanded Surveillance Case Definition for AIDS Among Adolescents and Adults. *Morbidity and Mortality Weekly Report* (Centers for Disease Control and Prevention) 1992; 41(#RR–17).

Novello warns physicians of hidden epidemics among women. *AIDS Weekly*, January 20, 1992, 7–9.

Padian, Nancy S, et al: Female–to–male transmission of human immunodeficiency virus. *Journal of the American Medical Association* 1991; 266: 1664–1668.

Peterman, Thomas A, et al: Prevention of the transmission of HIV, in: *AIDS—Etiology, Diagnosis, Treatment and Prevention*. Philadelphia, JB Lippincott Co, 1992.

Research on women and HIV featured at conference. *AIDS Weekly*, June 28, 1993, 13–16.

Research slow to meet needs of HIV infected women. *AIDS Alert* 1991; 6: 34–36.

Risk for cervical disease in HIV infected women—New York City. *CDC AIDS Weekly*, December 10, 1990, 23–26.

Schilling, Robert F, et al: Building skills of recovering women drug users to reduce heterosexual AIDS transmission. *Public Health Reports* 1991; 106: 297–305.

Scientists show changing face of AIDS in first comprehensive review of research on infected women. *AIDS Weekly*, January 27, 1992, 6–9.

Screening for HIV infection—benefits and costs. *New England Journal of Medicine* 1992; 327: 7.

Sifton, David (ed.): *The PDR Family Guide to Prescription Drugs*. Montvale, NJ, Medical Economics Data, 1993.

Sperling, Rhoda S: A survey of zidovudine use in pregnant women with human immunodeficiency virus infection. *New England Journal of Medicine* 1992; 268: 463.

Staver, Sari: Take AIDS message to white women, researcher urges. *American Medical News* 1991; 34: 5.

Stricof, Rachel L, et al: HIV seroprevalence in clients of sentinel family planning clinics. *The American Journal of Public Health* 1991; 81: 41–46.

Study reveals gender differences in AIDS treatment. *AIDS Weekly* June 29, 1992, 11–13.

Tannenbaum, Ilene: Women and HIV. *RN* 1993; 56: 34–41.

Update: Mortality attributable to HIV infection. *Morbidity and Mortality Weekly Report*. (Centers for Disease Control and Prevention) 1993; 42: 45.

Williams, Ann B: The epidemiology, clinical manifestations and health–maintenance needs of women infected with HIV. *Nurse Practitioner* 1992; 17: 27–42.

Women claim discrimination in AIDS matters, *AIDS Weekly*, August 10, 1992, 9–11.

Women with AIDS: what is cause of lower survival? *AIDS Alert* 1992; 7: 142–145.

Women's interagency HIV study begins. *AIDS Weekly*, July 12, 1993, 3–5.

Taking Control of Headache

A Clinical Demonstration of Migraine Relief You Can See in Minutes. Research Triangle Park, NC, Glaxo Pharmaceuticals, 1993.

Abraham, GE; Lubran, MM: Serum and red cell magnesium levels in patients with premenstrual tension. *American Journal of Clinical Nutrition* 1981; 34: 2364–2366.

Benedittis, G; Lorenzetti, A: Minor stressful life events (daily hassles) in chronic primary headache: relationship with MMPR personality patterns. *Headache* 1992; 32: 330–332.

Current Trends: Prevalence of chronic migraine headaches— United States, 1980–1989. *Morbidity and Mortality Weekly Report* (Centers for Disease Control and Prevention) 1991; 40: 331, 337–338.

Do You Suffer From Migraine? Research Triangle Park, NC, Glaxo Pharmaceuticals, 1992.

Glueck, CJ, et al: Amelioration of severe migraine with omega–3 fatty acids: A double–blind, placebo–controlled clinical trial. *American Journal of Clinical Nutrition* 1986; 43: 710.

Headache Q & A. West Deptford, NJ, The American Council for Headache Education.

Johnson, ES, et al: Efficacy of feverfew as prophylactic treatment of migraine. *British Medical Journal* 1982; 291: 653–660.

Kidd, RF; Nelson, R: Musculoskeletal dysfunction of the neck in migraine and tension headache. *Headache* 1993; 33: 566–569.

Lockett, DMC, Campbell, JF: The effects of aerobic exercise on migraine. *Headache* 1992; 32: 50–54.

Martin, PR; Milech, D; Nathan, PR: Towards a functional model of chronic headaches: investigation of antecedents and consequences. *Headache* 1993; 33: 461–470.

Mason, V: Headaches: OCS are "guilty by association." *Contraceptive Technology Update* 1993; 14: 109–112.

Mathew, NT: Cluster headache. *Neurology* 1992; 42(suppl 2): 22–31.

Murphy, JJ, et al: Randomized double–blinded placebo– controlled trial of feverfew in migraine prevention. *The Lancet* 1988; 2: 188–192.

Physician's Desk Reference. Montvale, NJ, Medical Economics Data, 1994.

Rapoport, AM: The diagnosis of migraine and tension–type headache, then and now. *Neurology* 1992; (suppl 2): 11–15.

Saper, JR: *Help for Headaches*. New York, Warner Books Inc, 1987.

Schulman, EA; Silberstein, SD: Symptomatic and prophylactic treatment of migraine and tension–type headache. *Neurology* 1992; 42(suppl 2): 16–21.

Sheftell, FD: Chronic daily headache. *Neurology* 1992; 42(suppl 2): 32–36.

Silberstein, SD: Advances in understanding the pathophysiology of headache. *Neurology* 1992; 42(suppl 2): 6–10.

Silberstein, SD: Headaches and women: Treatment of the pregnant and lactating migraineur. *Headache* 1993; 33: 533–540.

Silberstein, SD: The role of sex hormones in headache. *Neurology* 1992; 42(suppl 2): 37–42.

Stewart, WF; Lipton, RB; Celentano, DD; et al: Prevalence of migraine headache in the United States: Relation to age, income, race and other sociodemographic factors. *Journal of the American Medical Association* 1992; 267: 64–69.

Tschannen, TA; Duckro, PN; Margolis, RB; et al: The relationship of anger, depression, and perceived disability among headache patients. *Headache* 1992; 32: 501–503.

Weaver, K: Magnesium and its role in vascular reactivity and coagulation. *Contemporary Nutrition* 1987; 12(#3).

Werbach, M: *Healing Through Nutrition*. New York, HarperCollins Publishers Inc, 1993.

What Every Headache Patient Should Know About Migraine Headaches. West Deptford, NJ, The American Council for Headache Education.

You are not alone. West Deptford, NJ, The American Council for Headache Education.

A Common Sense Look at Diet and Health

Achieving and Maintaining Physical Fitness. Indianapolis, American College of Sports Medicine, 1990.

An introduction to free radicals. *Vitamin Nutrition Information Service* 1993; 1: 1–4.

Beal, Virginia: *Nutrition in The Lifespan*. New York, John Wiley and Sons Inc, 1980.

Bender, Mary M: Trends in prevalence and magnitude of vitamin and mineral supplement usage and correlation with health status. *American Dietetic Association* 1992; 92: 1096–1101.

Berning, Jacqueline R: *Sports Nutrition for the 90's*. Gaithersburg, Md, Aspen Publishers, 1991.

Bittman, M; Willoughby, J: Nature's food by design. *Eating Well*, March/April 1992; 37–43.

Blumberg, J: Recent Advances on Vitamins and Aging. *Vitamin Nutrition Information Service* 1993; 1–7.

Calcium: A Summary of Current Research for the Health Professional, ed 2. Rosemont, Ill, National Dairy Council, 1989.

Calvert–Finn, S: ADA's nutrition and health campaign for women. *American Dietetic Association* 1993; 93: 986.

Coleman, E: *Eating for Endurance*. Palo Alto, Calif, Bull Publishing Co, 1992.

Diplock, A: The protective role of antioxidant nutrients in disease prevention. *Vitamin Nutrition Information Service* 1993; 3: 1–9.

Grundy, S: Summary of the second report of the National Cholesterol Education Program Expert Panel on detection, evaluation, and treatment of high blood cholesterol in adults. *Journal of the American Medical Association* 1993; 269: 3015–3023.

Gurr, Michael: Dietary lipids and coronary heart disease: old evidence, new perspective. *Progressive Lipid Research* 1992; 31: 195–243.

Hankin, J: Role of nutrition in women's health: diet and breast cancer. *American Dietetic Association* 1993; 93: 994–999.

Havel, JH: *Recommended Dietary Allowances*, ed 10. Washington, DC, National Academy Press, 1989.

Hennekens, C: The role of antioxidant vitamins in the prevention of cardiovascular disease. *Vitamin Nutrition Information Service*. 1993; 4: 1–6.

Jaret, P: Bet on broccoli. *Health*, September/October, 1991; 59–62.

Kris–Etherton, PM: Role of nutrition in the prevention and treatment of cardiovascular disease in women. *American Dietetic Association* 1993; 93: 987–993.

Manson, GE: A prospective study of antioxidant vitamins and the incidence of coronary heart disease. *Circulation* 1991; 84(suppl 2): 546.

Margen, S: *The Wellness Encyclopedia of Food and Nutrition*. New York, Random House, 1992.

National Research Council: *Diet and Health*. Washington, DC, National Academy Press, 1989.

Osteen, R: *Cancer Manual*, ed 8. Boston, Mass, American Cancer Society, 1990.

Pennington, JA: *Food Values of Portions Commonly Consumed*. Philadelphia, JB Lippincott Co, 1994.

Position of the ADA: vegetarian diets. *American Dietetic Association* 1993; 93: 1317–1319.

Public Health Service: *Eat More Fruits and Vegetables: Five a Day for Better Health*. Rockville, Md, US Department of Health and Human Services, 1991.

Ross, AC: Vitamin A as a hormone: recent advances in understanding the actions of retinol, retinoic acid, and beta carotene. *American Dietetic Association* 1993; 93: 1285–1290.

Roufs, JB: Review of L–tryptophan and eosinophilia–mylagia syndrome. *American Dietetic Association* 1992; 92: 844–849.

Shils, M; Olson, J; Shike, M: *Modern Nutrition in Health and Disease*. Philadelphia, Lea and Febiger, 1994.

Tolstoi, L; Levin, R; Osteoporosis—the treatment controversy. *Nutrition Today*, July/August 1992; 6–12.

Plastic Surgery: What To Expect

Aston, Sherell J; Thorne, Charles HM: Aesthetic surgery of the aging face, in: Smith, James W; Aston Sherill G (eds.): *Grabb and Smith's Plastic Surgery*, ed 4. Boston, Little, Brown & Co, 1991, 609–631.

Baroudi, Ricardo: Body contour surgery, in: Smith, James W; Aston Sherill G (eds.): *Grabb and Smith's Plastic Surgery*, ed 4. Boston, Little, Brown & Co, 1991, 1319–1333.

Biggs, Thomas M; Humphreys, David H: Augmentation mammoplasty, in: Smith, James W; Aston Sherill G (eds.): *Grabb and Smith's Plastic Surgery*, ed 4. Boston, Little, Brown & Co, 1991, 1145–1156.

Georgiade, Nicholas G: Reconstructive and aesthetic breast surgery, in: Sabiston, David C Jr (ed.): *Textbook of Surgery: The Biological Basis of Modern Practice*, ed 13. Philadelphia, WB Saunders Co, 1986, 573–577.

Hinderer, Urich T: Aesthetic surgery of the eyelids and periocular region, in: Smith, James W; Aston Sherill G (eds.): *Grabb and Smith's Plastic Surgery*, ed 4. Boston, Little, Brown & Co, 1991, 565–608.

Sheen, Jack H; Constantian, Mark B: Primary and secondary aesthetic rhinoplasty, in: Smith, James W; Aston Sherill G (eds.): *Grabb and Smith's Plastic Surgery*, ed 4. Boston, Little, Brown & Co, 1991, 649–672.

Section 3:
Fertility and Family Planning

How the Reproductive System Works

Herbst, AL, et al (eds.): *Comprehensive Gynecology*, ed 2. St. Louis, Mosby–Year Book, 1992.

Speroff, L, et al: *Clinical Gynecologic Endocrinology and Infertility*, ed 4. Baltimore, Williams & Wilkins, 1989.

Wilson, JD, et al: *Harrison's Principles of Internal Medicine*, ed 12. New York, McGraw–Hill Inc, Health Professions Division, 1991.

Overcoming Infertility:
Tactics and Techniques

Herbst, AL, et al (eds.): *Comprehensive Gynecology*, ed 2. St. Louis, Mosby–Year Book, 1992.

Mishell, DR, et al: *Infertility, Contraception & Reproductive Endocrinology*, ed 3. Cambridge, Mass, Blackwell Scientific Publications, 1991.

Speroff, L, et al: *Clinical Gynecologic Endocrinology and Infertility*. Baltimore, Williams & Wilkins, 1989.

Barrier Contraceptives:
A Growing Array of Options

Allen, DC: Latex allergies and condom use [letter]. *Nursing* 1993; 23(#10): 4.

Campbell, P: Efficacy of female condom [letter]. *The Lancet* 1993; 341: 1155.

Heath, CB: Helping patients choose appropriate contraception. *American Family Physician* 1993; 48(#6): 1115–1124.

Henderson, R: Female condoms. *Johns Hopkins Women's Health Newsletter*, January 1994.

Johnson, MA: The cervical cap as a contraceptive alternative. *Nurse Practitioner* 1985; 10(#1): 37, 41–42, 45.

Liskin, LS; Sakondhavat, C: The female condom: a new option for women, in: Mann, JM; Tarantola, DJM; Netter, TW (eds.): *AIDS in the World: The Global AIDS Policy Coalition*. Cambridge, Mass, Harvard University Press, 1992, 700–707.

Physicians' Desk Reference. Montvale, NJ, Medical Economics Data, 1993, 1719–1720.

Prentif Cavity–Rim Cervical Cap. (Package insert) Luton, England, Lamberts (Dalston) Ltd, 1988.

Reality, the female condom: Questions and answers. (Information sheet) Jackson, Wis, Wisconsin Pharmacal Company, 1993.

Robertson, WH: *An Illustrated History of Contraception: A Concise Account of the Quest for Fertility Control*. Park Ridge, NJ, Parthenon Publishing Group, 1990, 23–35, 112–116.

Wisconsin Pharmacal: *Reality, the Female Condom: Questions and Answers*. (Information sheet) Jackson, Wis, Wisconsin Pharmacal Co, 1993.

IUDs: Still Worth Considering

Boschert, S: Bad reputation aside, IUDs "deserve another look." *OB GYN News* 1993; 28(#14): 2, 38.

Farley, TMM; Rowe, PJ; Rosenberg, MJ; et al: Intrauterine devices and pelvic inflammatory disease: an international perspective. *The Lancet* 1992; 339: 785–788.

Hatcher, RA; Trussell, J; Stewart, F; et al: *Contraceptive Technology*. New York, Irvington Publishers, 1994.

Kronmal, RA; Whitney, CW; Mumford, SD: The intrauterine device and pelvic inflammatory disease: the women's health study reanalyzed. *Journal of Clinical Epidemiology* 1991; 44: 109–122.

Mason, V: Changing attitudes may mean good news for IUD users. *Contraceptive Technology Update* 1992; 12: 93–96.

McIntosh, N; Kinzie, B; Blouse, A: *IUD Guidelines for Family Planning Service Programs: A Problem–Solving Reference Manual*. Baltimore, JHPIEGP Corp, 1992.

Mumford, SD; Kessel, E: Was the Dalkon Shield a safe and effective intrauterine device? *Fertility & Sterility* 1992; 57: 1151–1176.

Painter, K: IUDs have improved, but their image hasn't. *USA Today*, April 1, 1992.

Petitti, DB: Reconsidering the IUD. *Family Planning Perspective* 1992; 24: 33–35.

Rivera, R; Farr, G; Chi, I: *The copper IUD: Safe and effective*. Research Triangle Park, NC, Family Health International, 1992.

Roan, S: The quiet rebirth of the IUD. *Los Angeles Times*, July 22, 1993.

Sivin, I; Greenslade, F; Schmidt, F; et al: *The copper T 380 intrauterine device: a summary of scientific data*. New York, The Population Council, 1992.

Speroff, L; Darney, P: *Clinical Guide for Contraception*. Baltimore, Williams & Wilkins, 1992.

Zhang, J; Chi, I; Feldblum, PJ; et al: Risk factors for copper T IUD expulsion: an epidemiologic analysis. *Contraception* 1992; 46: 427–433.

Hormonal Options:
Pills, Shots, and Implants

Cancer and DMPA injectable contraceptive: latest evidence reassuring, says WHO. (Press release) Geneva, World Health Organization, June 1993.

Cachrimanidou, A–C; Hellberg, D; Nilsson, S; et al: Long–interval treatment regimen with a desogestrel–containing oral contraceptive. *Contraception* 1993; 48: 205–15.

Creinin, MD: Norplant can be given immediately postpartum. *Contraceptive Technology Update* 1993; 14: 114–115.

Depo–Provera Contraceptive Injection. (Package insert) Kalamazoo, Mich, The Upjohn Company, October 1992.

Goldzieher, JW: *Hormonal Contraception: Pills, Injections and Implants*. Dallas, Tex, Essential Medical Information Systems Inc, 1989.

Hatcher, RA; Schnare, S: Ask the experts: progestin–only contraceptives. *Contraceptive Technology Update* 1993; 14:114–115.

Hatcher, RA; Trussell, J Stewart, F; et al: *Contraceptive Technology*. New York, Irvington Publishers, 1994.

Injectable contraceptives: safe, effective but neglected. (Population policy information kit) Washington, DC, Population Crisis Committee, October 1992.

Irwin, KL; Rosero–Bixby, L; Oberle, MW; et al: Oral contraceptive use and risk of invasive cervical cancer in Costa Rica: Detection bias or causal association? *Journal of the American Medical Association* 1988; 259: 59.

Karlsson, R; Linden, A; von Shoultz, B: Suppression of 24–hour cholecystokinin secretion by oral contraceptives. *American Journal of Obstetrics and Gynecology* 1992; 167: 58–59.

Mason, V: Depo–Provera: A new contraceptive option for family planners. Special report. *Contraceptive Technology Update* 1993; 14: 1–11.

Mason, V: OCs are implicated in increased HIV transmission risk. *Contraceptive Technology Update* 1993; 14: 117–119.

Mason, V: Postcoital pills could cut unplanned pregnancies by half. *Contraceptive Technology Update* 1993; 14: 33–39.

Mason, V: Switch pills for headaches and mood swing, but not weight gain, say readers. *Contraceptive Technology Update* 1993; 14: 173–178.

Mason, V: Too much or too little—access to Norplant implants fuels ethics debate. *Contraceptive Technology Update* 1993; 14: 133–136.

Mason V: Two experts say no weight limit for Norplant implants. *Contraceptive Technology Update* 1993; 14: 138.

The most recent innovation in birth control. (Booklet) Philadelphia, Wyeth–Ayerst Laboratories, August 1991.

New—Depo–Provera Contraception. (Brochure) Kalamazoo, Mich, The Upjohn Company, October 1992.

Norplant System. (Package insert) Philadelphia, Wyeth–Ayerst Laboratories, December 1990.

The Ortho annual birth control study, 25th anniversary. Raritan, NJ, Ortho Pharmaceutical Corporation, 1994.

Population Council: *First year comparison of IUD and implant condition rates: Conditions for which percentages with condition were significantly higher for implant subjects. Table 21.* Presented at public hearings on Norplant subdermal implants before the Fertility and Maternal Health Drugs Advisory Committee of the US Food and Drug Administration, Rockville, Md, April 1989.

Population Information Program: Decisions for Norplant programs. *Population Reports* 1992; 20(#3).

Speroff, L; Darney, P: *Clinical Guide for Contraception.* Baltimore, Williams & Wiklins, 1992.

Trussell, J; Stewart, F: The effectiveness of postcoital hormonal contraception. *Family Planning Perspectives* 1992; 24: 262–264.

Waldron, T: Not FDA–approved, but experts recommend Depo–Provera. *Contraceptive Technology Update* 1992; 13: 1–7.

Waldron, T: Study links Depo–Provera to LBW, higher infant mortality. *Contraceptive Technology Update* 1992; 13: 52–54.

Those Other Approaches to Family Planning

DaVanzo, Julie; Parnell, Allan M; Foege, William H: Health consequences of contraceptive use and reproductive patterns: summary of a report from the US National Research Council. *Journal of the American Medical Association* 1991; 265: 2692–2696.

Female sterilization: answers to your questions about permanent birth control. New York, Association for Voluntary Surgical Contraception, 1986.

Guay, Terrie: *The Personal Fertility Guide: How to Avoid or Achieve Pregnancy Naturally.* San Francisco, Harbor Publishing Inc, 1980.

Hankinson, Susan E; Hunter, David J; Colditz, Graham A; et al: Tubal ligation, hysterectomy, and risk of ovarian cancer: a prospective study. *Journal of the American Medical Association.* 1993; 270: 2813–2818.

Hatcher, Robert A; Josephs, Nancy; Stewart, Felicia H; et al: *It's Your Choice: A Personal Guide to Birth Control Methods for Women...and Men Too!* New York, Irvington Publishers Inc, 1982.

Hatcher, Robert A; Stewart, Felicia; Trussel, James; et al: *Contraceptive Technology 1990–92,* ed 15. New York, Irvington Publishers, 1990.

Hatcher, Robert A; Trussell, James; Stewart, Felicia; et al: *Contraceptive Technology,* ed 16. Decatur, Ga, Bridging the Gap Communications, 1993.

Shulman, Lee P; Elias, Sherman: Second–trimester pregnancy termination by dilation and evacuation after detection of fetal abnormalities. *Journal of Women's Health* 1992; 1(#4): 255–258.

Speroff, Leon, et al. *Clinical Gynecologic Endocrinology and Infertility,* ed 3. Baltimore, Williams & Wilkins, 1983.

Spitz, Irving M; Bardin, CW: Mifepristone (RU 486)—a modulator of progestin and glucocorticoid action. *The New England Journal of Medicine* 1993; 329: 404–411.

Stergachis, Andy; Shy, Kirkwood K; Grothaus, Louis C; et al: Tubal sterilization and the long-term risk of hysterectomy. *Journal of the American Medical Association.* 1990; 264: 2893–2898.

Stevenson, R; King, Carole; Haynes, Twilla Locklear: Common problems of the female reproductive system, in: *Adult Nursing in Hospital and Community Settings.* East Norwalk, Conn, Appleton & Lange, 1992.

Winstein, Merryl: *Your Fertility Signals: Using Them to Achieve or Avoid Pregnancy Naturally.* St. Louis, Mo, Smooth Stone Press, 1990.

Section 4:
Toward Successful Pregnancies

Strategies for a Healthy Pregnancy

Brody, JE: Fitness and the Fetus: A turnabout in advice. *The New York Times*, February 2, 1994, C13.

Brody, JE: Personal health: exercising during pregnancy. *The New York Times*, February 2, 1994, C13.

Cunningham, FG; MacDonald, PC; Gant, NF; et al (eds.): *Williams Obstetrics*, ed 19. East Norwalk, Conn, Appleton & Lange, 1993.

*Nutrition During Pregnancy.*Washington, DC, American College of Obstetricians and Gynecologists Technical Bulletin, April 1993.

Pernoll, ML (ed.):*Current Diagnosis and Treatment, Obstetrics and Gynecology,* ed 7. East Norwalk, Conn, Appleton & Lange, 1991.

Queenan, JT; Leslie, KK (eds.): *Preconceptions: Preparation for Pregnancy.* Boston, Little, Brown & Co, 1989.

Smoking and Reproductive Health. Washington, DC, American College of Obstetricians and Gynecologists Technical Bulletin, May 1993.

Todd, DW; Tapley DF (eds.): *The Columbia University College of Physicians and Surgeons Complete Guide to Pregnancy.* New York, Crown Publishers Inc, 1988.

Travel During Pregnancy. Washington, DC, American College of Obstetricians and Gynecologists, June 1993.

Working During Your Pregnancy. Washington, DC, American College of Obstetricians and Gynecologists, September 1992.

Prenatal Tests to Consider

Danforth, David N; Scott, James R (eds.): *Obstetrics and Gynecology,* ed 5. Philadelphia, JB Lippincott Co, 1986.

Eisenberg, Arlene: *What to Expect When You're Expecting.* New York, Workman Publishing Co, 1991.

Pernoll, Martin (ed.): *Current Obstetric & Gynecologic Diagnosis & Treatment,* ed 7. East Norwalk, Conn, Appleton & Lange, 1991.

Potential Complications You Should Keep in Mind

Alexander, TP: *Make Room for Twins: A Complete Guide to Pregnancy, Delivery and the Childhood Years.* New York, Bantam Books, 1987.

Bash, DM: Monitoring high–risk pregnancy. *FDA Consumer* 1992; 26(#2): 34–38.

Blatt, RJR: *Prenatal Tests: What They Are, Their Benefits and Risks, and How to Decide Whether to Have Them or Not.* New York, Vintage, 1988.

Diabetes in Pregnancy. (Technical bulletin) Washington, DC, American College of Obstetricians and Gynecologists, December 1986.

Elixhauser, A; Weschler, JM; Kitzmiller, JL; et al: Cost–benefit analysis of preconception care for women with established diabetes mellitus. *Diabetes Care* 1993; 16(#8): 1146–1157.

Feinbloom, RI; Forman, BY; *Pregnancy, Birth, and the Early Months: A Complete Guide.* Reading, Mass, Addison–Wesley, 1985.

Freeman, RK; Pescar, SC: *Safe Delivery: Protecting Your Baby During High Risk Pregnancy.* New York, Facts on File, 1982.

Hales, D; Creasy, RK: *New Hope for Problem Pregnancies: Helping Babies BEFORE They're Born.* New York, Harper & Row, 1982.

High Blood Pressure During Pregnancy. (Technical bulletin) Washington, DC, American College of Obstetricians and Gynecologists, November 1992.

Holohan, TV; Green, I: *Home Uterine Monitoring.* Rockville, Md, Agency for Health Care Policy and Research, 1992.

Katz, M; Gill, P; Turiel, J: *Preventing Preterm Birth: A Parent's Guide.* San Francisco, Health, 1988.

Kohn, I; Moffitt, P–L; Wilikins, IA: *A Silent Sorrow: Pregnancy Loss. Guidance and Support for You and Your Family.* New York, Dell, 1992.

Management of Diabetes Mellitus in Pregnancy. (Technical bulletin) Washington, DC, American College of Obstetricians and Gynecologists, May 1986.

Management of Preeclampsia. (Technical bulletin) Washington, DC, American College of Obstetricians and Gynecologists, February 1986.

Premature Rupture of Membranes. (Technical bulletin) Washington, DC, American College of Obstetricians and Gynecologists, April 1988.

Preterm Labor. (Technical bulletin) Washington, DC, American College of Obstetricians and Gynecologists, October 1989.

Preterm Labor. (Technical bulletin) Washington, DC, American College of Obstetricians and Gynecologists, March 1991.

The problem with problem pregnancies. *Psychology Today* 1993; 26(#5): 9.

Raab, D: *Getting Pregnant and Staying Pregnant: A Guide to Infertility and High–Risk Pregnancy.* Montreal, Sirdan, 1989.

Rich, LA: *When Pregnancy Isn't Perfect: A Layperson's Guide to Complications in Pregnancy.* New York, Dutton, 1991.

Robertson, PA; Berlin, PH: *The Premature Labor Handbook: Successfully Sustaining Your High–Risk Pregnancy.* New York, Doubleday, 1986.

Russell, KP: *Eastman's Expectant Motherhood*, ed 7. Boston, Little, Brown & Co, 1983. (Revised)

Scher, J; Dix, C: *Preventing Miscarriage: The Good News.* New York, Harper & Row, 1990.

Semchyshyn, S; Colman, C: *How to Prevent Miscarriage and Other Crises of Pregnancy: A Leading High–Risk Pregnancy Doctor's Prescription for Carrying Your Baby to Term.* New York, Macmillan, 1989.

Tapley, DF; Todd, WD; Subak–Sharpe, GJ; et al: *The Columbia University College of Physicians and Surgeons Complete Guide to Pregnancy.* New York, Crown Publishers Inc, 1988.

What to Expect During Labor and Delivery

Childbirth: A Guide to Labor, Delivery and Postpartum Care. Washington, DC, The American College of Obstetricians and Gynecologists, 1984.

Dunn, Leo J: Cesarean section and other obstetric operations, in: *Danforth's Obstetrics and Gynecology.* Philadelphia, JB Lippincott Co, 1990.

Fraser, W, et al: Effect of Early Amniotomy on the Risk of Dystocia in Nulliparous Women. *New England Journal of Medicine* 1993; 328: 1145–1149.

Gabbe, Steven G, et al (eds.): *Clinical Briefs in Obstetrics.* 1993; 1: 1–11.

Gimovsky, Martin L; Petrie, Roy A: Breech presentation: alternatives to routine C/S. *Contemporary OB/GYN* 1992; 37(#1): 35–48.

Hannah, Mary E, et al: Induction of labor as compared with serial antenatal monitoring in post–term pregnancy. *New England Journal of Medicine* 1992; 326: 1587–1592.

Jones, Monica M: Obstetric anesthesia and analgesia, in: *Danforth's Obstetrics and Gynecology.* Philadelphia, JB Lippincott Co, 1990.

Levine, Richard U: Labor and delivery, in: *The Columbia University College of Physicians and Surgeons Complete Guide to Pregnancy.* New York, Crown Publishers Inc, 1988.

Lopez–Zeno, Jose A, et al: A controlled trial of a program for the active management of labor. *New England Journal of Medicine.* 1992; 326: 450-454.

Pollycove, Ricki; Corrigan, Teresa; Coon, Gail; et al: *The Birth Book: Your Guide to Vaginal, Cesarean and VBAC Deliveries.* San Bruno, Calif, Krames Communications, 1991.

Quilligan, Edward J: Some safe alternatives to cesarean section. *Contemporary OB/GYN* 1991; 36(#12): 31–40.

Speroff, Leon (ed.): *OB/GYN Clinical Alert* 1993; (10, #2).

Speroff, Leon (ed.): *OB/GYN Clinical Alert* 1993; (10, #3).

Speroff, Leon (ed.): *OB/GYN Clinical Alert* 1993; (10, #4).

Wright, William C: Continuous epidural block for OB anesthesia. *Contemporary OB/GYN* 1991; 36(#11): 89–98.

Zlatnick, Frank J: Normal labor and delivery and its conduct, in: *Danforth's Obstetrics and Gynecology.* Philadelphia, JB Lippincott Co, 1990.

What To Do When Miscarriage Strikes

Cunningham, FG; MacDonald, PC; Gant, NF; et al (eds.): *Williams Obstetrics*, ed 19. East Norwalk, Conn, Appleton & Lange, 1993.

Danforth, DN (ed.): *Danforth's Obstetrics and Gynecology.* Philadelphia, JB Lippincott Co, 1990.

Friedman, EA; Acker, DB; Sachs, BP: *Obstetrical Decision–Making*, ed 2. Toronto, BC Decker, 1987.

Pernoll, ML (ed.): *Current Diagnosis & Treatment, Obstetrics & Gynecology*, ed 7. East Norwalk, Conn, Appleton & Lange, 1991.

Repeated Miscarriage. Washington, DC, American College of Obstetricians and Gynecologists, January 1993.

Todd, DW; Tapley, DF (eds): *The Columbia University College of Physicians and Surgeons Complete Guide to Pregnancy.* New York, Crown Publishers Inc, 1988.

Travel During Pregnancy. Washington, DC, American College of Obstetricians and Gynecologists, June 1993.

Section 5:
Coping With Menopause

Understanding the Change

Cone, Faye Kitchener: *Making Sense of Menopause.* New York, Simon & Schuster, 1993.

Cutler, Winnifred B; Garcia, Celso–Ramon: *Menopause: A Guide for Women and Those Who Love Them.* New York, WW Norton & Co, 1992. (Revised)

Doress, Paula Brown; Siegel, Diana Laskin: *Ourselves Growing Older.* New York, Simon & Schuster, 1987.

Utian, Wulf, H; Jacobowitz, Ruth S: *Managing Your Menopause.* New York, Prentice Hall, 1990.

Five Common Problems and Their Remedies

Cone, Faye Kitchener: *Making Sense of Menopause.* New York, Simon & Schuster, 1993.

Cutler, Winnifred B; Garcia, Celso–Ramon: *Menopause: A Guide for Women and Those Who Love Them.* New York, WW Norton & Co, 1992. (Revised)

Doress, Paula Brown; Siegel, Diana Laskin: *Ourselves Growing Older.* New York, Simon & Schuster, 1987.

Pernoll, Martin L, (ed.): *Current Obstetric & Gynecologic Diagnosis & Treatment*, ed 7. East Norwalk, Conn, Appleton & Lange, 1991.

University of California, Berkeley, Wellness Letter (ed.): *The Wellness Encyclopedia.* Boston, Houghton Mifflin Co, 1991.

Utian, Wulf, H; Jacobowitz, Ruth S: *Managing Your Menopause.* New York, Prentice Hall, 1990.

Holding Back Osteoporosis

Cone, Faye Kitchener: *Making Sense of Menopause.* New York, Simon & Schuster, 1993.

Cutler, Winnifred B; Garcia, Celso–Ramon: *Menopause: A Guide for Women and Those Who Love Them.* New York, WW Norton & Co, 1992. (Revised)

Doress, Paula Brown; Siegel, Diana Laskin: *Ourselves Growing Older.* New York, Simon & Schuster, 1987.

Henig, Robin Marantz, et al: *How a Woman Ages: Growing Older: What to Expect and What You Can Do About It.* New York, Ballantine Books, 1985.

Pernoll, Martin L, (ed): *Current Obstetric & Gynecologic Diagnosis & Treatment,* ed 7. East Norwalk, Conn, Appleton & Lange, 1991.

Utian, Wulf, H; Jacobowitz, Ruth S: *Managing Your Menopause.* New York, Prentice Hall, 1990.

Hormone Replacement Therapy: Weighing the Pros and Cons

Cutler, Winnifred B; Garcia, Celso–Ramon: *Menopause: A Guide for Women and Those Who Love Them.* New York, WW Norton & Co, 1992. (Revised)

Sandroff, Ronni: Menopause: Is it a medical problem? *The New York Times Magazine,* April 26, 1992.

Speroff, Leon: *Clinical Gynecological Endocrinology & Infertility,* ed 5. Baltimore, Williams & Wilkins, 1994.

Utian, Wulf, H; Jacobowitz, Ruth S: *Managing Your Menopause.* New York, Prentice Hall, 1990.

Section 6:
Conquering Emotional Problems

Coming to Grips With Stress

Bauman, Andrea: Second–hand stress. *American Health: Fitness of Body and Mind,* April 1991, 74.

Bloch, Gordon Bakoulis: Stress signals. *Working Woman Magazine,* February 1992, 80–82.

Drexler, Madeline: Why stress hurts your stomach. *Redbook,* November 1993, 44–46.

Gilbert, Evelyn: Stress common for working women. *National Underwriter Property & Casualty–Risk & Benefits Management,* September 23, 1991, 6–7.

Gutfield, Greg; Sangiorgio, Maureen; Rao, Linda: Hectic hearts. *Prevention,* July 1992, 11–12.

Houston, B Kent; Cates, David S; Kelly, Karen E: Job stress, psychosocial strain, and physical health problems in women employed full–time outside the home and homemakers. *Women & Health,* September/October 1992, 1–26.

Kabat–Zinn, Jon: *Full Catastrophe Living.* New York, Delacourt Press, 1990.

Klein, TW: Stress and infections. *Journal of Florida Medical Association,* 1993; 80(#6): 409–411.

Larson, David E (ed.): *Mayo Clinic Family Heath Book.* New York, William Morrow Co Inc, 1990.

Leatz, Christine A: *Career Success/Personal Stress.* New York, McGraw–Hill Inc, 1993.

McEwen, BS; Stellar, E: Stress and the individual. Mechanisms leading to disease. *Archives of Internal Medicine,* 1993; 153(#18): 2093–2101.

Miller, Benjamin F; Brackman Keane, Claire (eds.): *The Encyclopedia and Dictionary of Medicine, Nursing and Allied Health,* ed 5. San Diego, Calif, Harcourt Brace Jovanovich, 1992.

Perlmutter, Cathy; McCord, Holly; Sangiorgio, Maureen: Women's health confidential. *Prevention,* June 1993, 46–56.

Raymond, Chris Anne: Studies question how much role menopause plays in some women's emotional distress. *The Journal of the American Medical Association,* 1988; 259(#24): 3522–3524.

Reese, Alan M; Willey, Charlene D (eds.): *Personal Health Reporter.* Detroit, Gale Research, Inc. 1993.

Stress test (Women are more likely to eat under stress than men). *Tufts University Diet & Nutrition Letter,* June 1993, 1–2.

Thompson, Charlotte E: Stress and the single girl. *Executive Female,* March April 1991, 18 20.

Weiss, Robert J; Subak–Sharpe, Genell: *40+ Guide to Good Health.* New York, The Columbia University School of Public Health, Consumers Union of America, 1993.

Dealing With Anxiety, Depression, and Chronic Fatigue Syndrome

A Guide to CFIDS. Charlotte, NC, CFIDS Association, September 1993.

Anxiety. Rockville, Md, The Anxiety Disorder Association of America, 1993.

Anxiety. Winston-Salem, NC, Council on Anxiety Disorders, 1993.

Baer, Katie: Still puzzling after all these years. *Harvard Health Letter,* 1993; 18:1.

Bell, David: *CFIDS: The Disease of a Thousand Names.* Nauvoo, Ill, Pollard Publications, 1991.

Berne, Katrina: *Running on Empty.* Alameda, Calif, Hunter House Publishing, 1992.

Bower, B: Mood swings and creativity: new clues. *Science News,* October 24, 1987, 262.

Bower, B: Weighing the causes of severe depression. *Science News* 1993; 144: 102.

Chronic Fatigue Syndrome. Bethesda, Md, National Institute of Allergy and Infectious Diseases, 1993.

The Chronic Fatigue Syndrome. Atlanta, Ga, Centers for Disease Control, 1990.

Chronic Fatigue Syndrome, A Pamphlet for Physicians. Bethesda, Md, U.S. Department of Health and Human Services, 1992.

Chronic fatigue: all in the mind? *Consumer Reports,* October 1990.

Coleman, D: Critics challenge reliance on drugs in psychiatry. *The New York Times,* October 17, 1989.

Cowley, Geoffrey: Chronic fatigue syndrome: a modern medical mystery. *Newsweek,* November 12, 1990.

Depression. Chicago, National Depressive and Manic-Depressive Association, 1993.

Depression gets anxious. *Science News* 1991; 140:295.

Elson, John; Horowitz, Janice: Is Freud finished? *Time Magazine,* July 6, 1992.

Faulty circuits. *Time Magazine,* September 28, 1992.

Freedman, Daniel; Stahl, Stephen: Psychiatry. *Journal of the American Medical Association* 1992; 268: 403.

Freedman, Daniel; Stahl, Stephen: Psychiatry. *Journal of the American Medical Association* 1993; 270: 252.

Fuerst, ML: Worried to death. *American Health* 1991; 10:27.

Fuhr, Susan; Shean, Glenn: Subtypes of depression, efficacy and the depressive experiences questionnaire. *Journal of Psychology* 1992; 126: 495.

Goldberg, Ivan K: *Questions and Answers About Depression and Its Treatment.* Philadelphia, Charles Press, 1993.

Goode, EE; Linnon, N; et al: Beating depression. *U.S. News & World Report,* March 5, 1990.

Goodwin, FK; Gause, EN: From the alcohol, drug abuse and mental health administration. *Journal of the American Medical Association* 1991; 265: 1926.

Guze, BH; Freedman, DX: Psychiatry. *Journal of the American Medical Association* 1991; 265: 3164.

Hickie, Ian; Lloyd, AR; Wakefield, Dennis; et al: Psychiatric status of patients with chronic fatigue syndrome. *The British Journal of Psychiatry* 1990; 156: 534.

Holmes, Gary, et al: Chronic fatigue syndrome: a working class definition. *Annals of Internal Medicine* 1988; 108: 387.

If at first you do succeed. *The Lancet* 1991; 337:650.

Katzenstein, Larry: Sick and tired. *American Health,* May 1992, 51.

Klimas, Nancy, et al: Immunologic abnormalities in chronic fatigue syndrome. *Journal of Clinical Microbiology* 1990: 28: 1403.

Kramer, Peter: The transformation of personality. *Psychology Today* 1993; 26: 42.

Lane, Thomas; Manu, Peter; Matthews, Dale: Depression and somatizations in the chronic fatigue syndrome. *The American Journal of Medicine* 1991; 91: 335.

Levine, D: Heart drugs for head troubles. *American Health* 1992; 11: 40.

Michels, Robert; Marzuk, Peter: Progress in psychiatry. *New England Journal of Medicine* 1993; 329: 552–560, 628–638.

Palca, Joseph: On the track of an elusive disease. *Science* 1991; 254: 1726.

Powerless chemistry of depression. *Science News* 1992; 141: 396.

Price, Rumi; North, Carol; Wessely, Simon; et al: Estimating the prevalence of chronic fatigue syndrome. *Public Health Reports* 1992; 107: 515.

Recurrent brief depression and anxiety. *The Lancet* 1991; 337: 586.

Smith, JM: Prospective study of postpartum blues. *Journal of the American Medical Association* 1991; 266: 2817.

Squire, S: Shock therapy's return to respectability. *The New York Times Magazine,* November 22, 1987.

Van Amerigen, Michael; Smith, Jeanette; et al: Fluoxetine efficacy in social phobia. *Journal of the American Medical Association* 1993; 269: 2606.

When imagination turns ugly. *Science News* 1993; 143:08.

Winslow, Ron: Virus May Have Role in Causing Chronic Fatigue. *The Wall Street Journal,* September, 16, 1991.

Battling Anorexia, Bulimia...and Obesity

Abraham, S; Llewellyn–Jones, D: *Eating Disorders: The Facts,* ed 2. Oxford, Oxford University Press, 1987.

Bower, B: Tracing bulimia's roots. *Science News* 1993; 143: 366.

Diagnostic and Statistical Manual of Mental Disorders, Third Edition, Revised. Washington, DC, American Psychiatric Association, 1987.

Duker, M; Slade, R: *Anorexia Nervosa and Bulimia: How to Help.* Philadelphia, Open University Press, 1988.

Eating and Exercise Disorders. Eugene, Ore, Anorexia and Related Eating Disorders Inc, 1992.

Edelstein, EL: *Anorexia Nervosa and Other Dyscontrol Syndromes.* Berlin, Springer–Verlag, 1989.

Fairburn, CG; Agras, WS; Wilson, GT: The research on the treatment of bulimia nervosa: practical and theoretical implications, in: Anderson, GH; Kennedy, SH (eds.): *The Biology of Feast and Famine.* San Diego, Academic Press, 1992, 317–337.

Garfinkel, PE; Halmi, K; Shaw, B: Applications of current research findings: what we need for the future, in: Anderson, GH; Kennedy, SH (eds.): *The Biology of Feast and Famine.* San Diego, Academic Press, 1992, 369–383.

Kennedy, SH; Goldbloom, DS; Vaccarino, FJ: New drugs, new directions, in: Anderson, GH; Kennedy, SH (eds.): *The Biology of Feast and Famine.* San Diego, Academic Press, 1992, 341–353.

Matthews, JR: *Eating Disorders.* New York, Facts on File, 1991.

National Survey on Anorexia Nervosa and Bulimia. Highland Park, Ill, National Association of Anorexia Nervosa and Associated Disorders, (not dated).

Tierney, LM Jr; McPhee, SJ; Papadakis, MA (eds.): *Current Medical Diagnosis & Treatment.* East Norwalk, Conn, Appleton & Lange, 1994.

Coping After a Sexual Assault

Bartol, Curt R: *Criminal Behavior.* Englewood Cliffs, NJ, Prentice Hall, 1991, 248–289.

Carlson, Nancy; Quina, Katherine: *Rape, Incest, and Sexual Harassment.* New York, Praeger, 1989.

DeGroot, JM; Kennedy, S; Roden, C: Correlates of sexual abuse in women with anorexia nervosa and bulimia nervosa. *Canadian Journal of Psychiatry*, September 1992, 516–518.

Dinitz, Simon; Dynes, Russell; Clark Alfred: *Deviance.* New York, Oxford University Press, 1975, 53–58.

Jenny, Carole; Bowers, Thomas; et al: Sexually transmitted diseases in victims of rape. *New England Journal of Medicine* 1990; 322: 713–716.

Mauro-Cochrane, Jeanette: *Self-Respect and Sexual Assault.* Blue Ridge Summit, Pa, McGraw–Hill Inc, 1993.

Moscarello, R: Victims of Violence. *The Canadian Journal of Psychiatry*, September 1992, 497–500.

Shepard, SL; Hebert, CA: Long–term effects of unresolved sexual trauma. *American Family Physician* 1987; 36(#4): 169–175.

Snyder, Solomon H: *Biological Aspects of Mental Disorder.* New York, Oxford University Press, 1980, 18–29.

Stacey, William A; Shupe, Anson: *The Family Secret.* Boston, Beacon Press, 1983.

Viscott, David: *The Language of Feelings.* New York, Pocket Books, 1976, 128–139.

Walch, Anne; Broadhead, Eugene: Prevalence of lifetime sexual victimization among female patients. *Journal of Family Practice*, November 1992, 511–516.

Warshaw, Robin: *I Never Called it Rape.* New York, HarperCollins, 1988.

Winfred, Idee; George, Linda; Swart, Marvinn; et al: Sexual assault and psychological disorders among a community sample of women. *American Journal of Psychiatry* 1990; 147: 335–341.

Section 7: Dealing with Cancer

Breast Cancer: Great Odds of a Cure

Berkow, Robert (ed.): *The Merck Manual of Diagnosis and Therapy*, ed 16. Rahway, NJ, Merck & Co Inc, 1992.

Cancer Committee of the Medical Association of Georgia: *About Breast Cancer.* Atlanta, Ga, The Composite State Board of Medical Examiners.

Danforth, David N; Scott, James R (eds.): *Obstetrics and Gynecology*, ed 5. Philadelphia, JB Lippincott Co, 1986.

DiSaia, Philip J; Creasman, William T: *Clinical Gynecologic Oncology.* St. Louis, The CV Mosby Co, 1984.

Georgiade, Nicholas, G: Reconstructive and aesthetic breast surgery, in: Sabiston, David C Jr (ed.): *Textbook of Surgery: The Biological Basis of Modern Practice*, ed 13. Philadelphia, WB Saunders, 1986, 573–577.

Isselbacher, Kurt H; Adams, RD; Braunwald, Eugene; et al (eds.): *Harrison's Principles of Internal Medicine*, ed 9. New York, McGraw–Hill Inc, 1980.

Messner, Carolyn: Women in the Work Place: *The Challenge of Breast Cancer.* New York, Cancer Care Inc, 1991.

National Cancer Institute: *Adjuvant Therapy: Facts for Women with Breast Cancer.* Washington, DC, U.S. Department of Health and Human Services, 1987.

National Cancer Institute: *Advanced Cancer: Living Each Day.* Washington, DC, U.S. Department of Health and Human Services, 1987.

National Cancer Institute: *After Breast Cancer: A Guide to Follow–Up Care.* Washington, DC, U.S. Department of Health and Human Services, 1990.

National Cancer Institute: *Breast Cancer: Understanding Treatment Options.* Washington, DC, U.S. Department of Health and Human Services, 1990.

National Cancer Institute: *Chemotherapy and You: A Guide to Self–Help During Treatment.* Washington, DC, U.S. Department of Health and Human Services, 1990.

National Cancer Institute: *Diet, Nutrition, and Cancer Prevention: The Good News.* Washington, DC, U.S. Department of Health and Human Services, 1987.

National Cancer Institute: *Eating Hints: Tips and Recipes for Better Nutrition During Cancer Treatment.* Washington, DC, U.S. Department of Health and Human Services, 1990.

National Cancer Institute: *Taking Time: Support for People with Cancer and the People Who Care About Them.* Washington, DC, U.S. Department of Health and Human Services, 1990.

National Cancer Institute: *What Are Clinical Trials All About? A Booklet for Patients with Cancer.* Washington, DC, U.S. Department of Health and Human Services, 1989.

National Cancer Institute: *What You Need to Know About Breast Cancer.* Washington, DC, U.S. Department of Health and Human Services, 1990.

Your Best Insurance Against Breast Cancer

Breast implant special report. *National Women's Health Report*. 1992; 14(#2): 1–9.

Cancer–Related Check–Ups. Atlanta, Ga, American Cancer Society, 1993.

Coleman, Cathy; Rabinowitz, F Barbara; Jeffrey, Stefanie: *Breast Health*. Daly City, Calif, Krames Communications, 1990.

Gabbe, Steven G, et al (eds.): Mammography under age 50, in: *Clinical Briefs in Obstetrics and Gynecology*. Atlanta, Ga, American Health Consultants Inc, 1993.

Hanson, Kirsten A: Ask the expert: mammography Q & A. *National Women's Health Report* 1993; 15(#5): 8–9.

Hiott, Yvonne P (ed.): Mammography programs provide patient–focused care. *Women's Health Center Management* 1993; 1(#4): 66–69.

Hiott, Yvonne P (ed.): Women's centers brace for new mammography regulations. *Women's Health Center Management*. 1994; 2(#1): 6–9.

National Cancer Institute: *Breast exams: What you should know*. Washington, DC, U.S. Department of Health and Human Services, 1992.

National Cancer Institute: *Questions and Answers About Breast Lumps*. Washington, DC, U.S. Department of Health and Human Services, 1992.

National Cancer Institute: *Questions and Answers About Choosing a Mammography Facility*. Washington DC, U.S. Department of Health and Human Services, 1993.

The older you get, the more you need a mammogram. Atlanta, American Cancer Society, 1993.

Parker, Steve H; et al: Nonpalpable breast lesions: stereotactic automated large–core biopsies. *Radiology* 1991; 180: 403–407.

Stevenson, R; King, Carole: Common problems of the breasts, in: *Adult Nursing in Hospital and Community Settings*. East Norwalk, Conn, Appleton & Lange, 1992.

Trien, Susan Flamholtz: *The Menopause Handbook*. New York, Ballantine Books, 1986.

Cervical Cancer: The One That's Preventable

An Abnormal Pap. What Now? Philadelphia, Family Planning Council of Southeastern Pennsylvania.

Blakeslee, Sandra: In research on cervical cancer, a wart virus is the prime suspect. *The New York Times*, January 21, 1992, C3.

Ciotti, Mary C: Screening for gynecologic and colorectal cancer: is it adequate? *Women's Health Issues* 1992; 2(#2).

Gusbberg, SB; Cancer of the female reproductive tract, in: *The American Cancer Society Cancer Book*. New York, Doubleday & Co Inc, 1986; 479–508.

Haylock, Pamela J; McGinn, Kerry A: *Women's Cancers: How to Prevent Them, How to Treat Them, How to Beat Them*. Alameda, Calif, Hunter House Inc, 1993.

National Cancer Institute: *What You Need to Know About Cancer of the Cervix*. Washington, DC, U.S. Department of Health and Human Services, 1991.

What you should know about pap tests. *People's Medical Society Newsletter*, April 1991.

Making Sense of Your Pap Test

Cervical Cytology: evaluation and management of abnormalities. *American College of Obstetrics and Gynecology Technical Bulletin* 1993; (#183).

Herbst, AL, et al (eds.): *Comprehensive Gynecology*, ed 2. St. Louis, Mosby–Year Book, 1992.

Koss, Leopold: The papanicolaou test for cervical cancer detection: a triumph and a tragedy. *Journal of the American Medical Association* 1989; 261(#5): 737–743.

Lundberg, George: Quality assurance in cervical cytology; the papanicolaou smear. *Journal of the American Medical Association* 1989; 262(#12): 1672–1679.

Ovarian Cancer: Facing the Facts

Cancer and steroid hormone study: the reduction in risk of ovarian cancer associated with oral contraceptive use. *New England Journal of Medicine* 1987; 316: 650–655.

Herbst, AL, et al (eds.): *Comprehensive Gynecology*, ed 2. St. Louis, Mosby–Year Book, 1992.

Rubin, S: Monoclonal antibodies in the management of ovarian cancer. *Cancer* 1993; 71(#4, suppl): 1602–1612.

Short, RV: Why menstruate? *Healthright* 1985; 4(#4): 9.

Wilson, JD, et al: *Harrison's Principles of Internal Medicine*, ed 12. New York, McGraw–Hill, Inc, Health Professions Division, 1991.

Stopping Endometrial Cancer in Time

Fox, H; Buckley, CH; *Pathology for Gynecologists*. Baltimore, University Park Press, 1989.

Holleb, AI, et al: *Clinical Oncology*. Atlanta, American Cancer Society, 1990.

National Cancer Institute: *Cancer of the Uterus: Endometrial Cancer*. Washington, DC, U.S. Department of Health and Human Services, 1991.

National Cancer Institute: *What You Need to Know About Cancer of the Uterus*. Washington, DC, U.S. Department of Health and Human Services, 1988.

Clarke–Pearson, Daniel; Dawood, MYusoff (eds.): *Green's Gynecology: Essentials of Clinical Practice*, ed 4. Boston, Little, Brown & Co, 1990.

Peckham, BM; Shapiro, SH: *Signs and Symptoms in Gynecology*. New York, JB Lippincott Co, 1988.

Shingleton, HM, Hurt, WG: *Postreproductive Gynecology*. New York, Churchill Livingstone Inc, 1990.

Disease and Disorder Index

Use this index to find out which drugs are available for a specific medical problem. Both brand and generic names are listed; the generic ingredients are shown in italics. Only brands covered in the drug profiles are included.

Acne
Accutane, 497
Achromycin V Capsules, 499
A/T/S. *See* Erythromycin, Topical
Benzac W. *See* Desquam-E
Benzagel. *See* Desquam-E
Benzamycin, 526
BenzaShave. *See* Desquam-E
Benzoyl Peroxide.
　See Desquam-E
Cleocin T, 544
Clindamycin. See Cleocin T
Desquam-E, 565
Doryx, 574
Doxycycline. See Doryx
Dynacin. *See* Minocin
Erycette.
　See Erythromycin, Topical
Erythromycin with Benzoyl
　Peroxide. See Benzamycin
Erythromycin, Topical, 587
Isotretinoin. See Accutane
Minocin, 665
Minocycline. See Minocin
Retin-A, 735

Sumycin.
　See Achromycin V Capsules
Tetracycline. See Achromycin V
　Capsules
Theroxide. *See* Desquam-E
Tretinoin. See Retin-A
T-Stat.
　See Erythromycin, Topical
Vibramycin. *See* Doryx
Vibra-Tabs. *See* Doryx

Adrenal gland tumors
Inderal, 622
Propranolol. See Inderal

AIDS and AIDS-related infections
See Infections, HIV

Alcohol withdrawal
Chlordiazepoxide. See Librium
Diazepam. See Valium
Libritabs. *See* Librium
Librium, 634
Valium, 786

Alzheimer's Disease
Cognex, 552
Tacrine. See Cognex

Angina
Inderal, 622
Propranolol. See Inderal

Anxiety disorders
Alprazolam. See Xanax
Ativan, 517
BuSpar, 527
Buspirone Hydrochloride.
　See Buspar
Centrax, 538
Chlordiazepoxide. See Librium

Clorazepate. See Tranxene
Diazepam. See Valium
Librium, 634
Libritabs. *See* Librium
Lorazepam. See Ativan
Oxazepam. See Serax
Prazepam. See Centrax
Serax, 742
Tranxene, 769
Tranxene-SD. *See* Tranxene
Tranxene-SD Half Strength.
　See Tranxene
Valium, 786
Xanax, 795

Arthritis
Anaprox, 505
Ansaid, 510
Aspirin, 515
Cataflam. *See* Voltaren
Choline Magnesium Trisalicylate.
　See Trilisate
Clinoril, 548
Daypro, 560
Diclofenac. See Voltaren
Diflunisal. See Dolobid
Dolobid, 572
Ecotrin. *See* Aspirin
Empirin. *See* Aspirin
Etodolac. See Lodine
Feldene, 594
Fenoprofen. See Nalfon
Flurbiprofen. See Ansaid
Genuine Bayer. *See* Aspirin
Indocin, 625
Indomethacin. See Indocin
Ketoprofen. See Orudis

General Index

L isted in this index are the diseases, treatments, and other key subjects discussed in part 1, "A Woman's Special Health Concerns." Also shown, are the names of the drug profiles described in Part 2, "A Woman's Handbook of Medicines." Drugs and diseases mentioned within the text of the profiles are not included in the index.

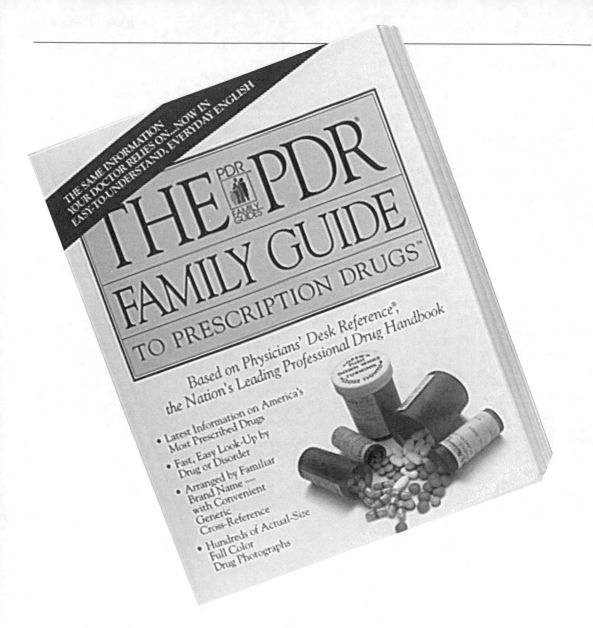

An Extra Measure of Safety for the Entire Family

Complete Your Set!

The PDR® Family Guide to Prescription Drugs®
Free Shipping and Handling

Yes! *Send me The PDR® Family Guide to Prescription Drugs® for only $24.95.*
I understand that shipping and handling are free.
NJ residents add 6% tax; in IA add 5%; in GA add 4%

Name _____

Address _____

City, State, Zip _____

Phone ( ) _____

Payment:

☐ My check for $24.95 plus tax is enclosed.

Charge:

☐ MasterCard   ☐ Visa   ☐ American Express   ☐ Discover

Number _____   Expiration _____

Only prepaid orders are accepted. Allow 2 weeks for delivery.
To order, insert in envelope and mail to:

The PDR Family Guide to Prescription Drugs
Medical Economics
Five Paragon Drive
Montvale, NJ 07645-1742

For Faster Service,

FE 50001-F110

CALL TOLL FREE: 1-800-331-0072

or fax your order to 1-201-573-4956

8092